INTRAVENOUS
MEDICATIONS

INTRAVENOUS MEDICATIONS

A Handbook for Nurses and Allied Health Professionals

BETTY L. GAHART, RN

Nurse Consultant in Education
Napa, California

Formerly Director, Education and Training
Queen of the Valley Hospital
Napa, California

ADRIENNE R. NAZARENO, PharmD

Clinical Coordinator, Department of Pharmacy
Queen of the Valley Hospital
Napa, California

FIFTEENTH EDITION

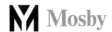 Mosby

St. Louis   Baltimore   Boston   Carlsbad
Chicago   Minneapolis   New York   Philadelphia   Portland
London   Milan   Sydney   Tokyo   Toronto

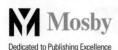

Mosby

Dedicated to Publishing Excellence

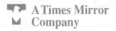

A Times Mirror
Company

Publisher: Nancy Coon
Editor: N. Darlene Como
Senior Developmental Editor: Dana L. Knighten
Project Manager: Deborah L. Vogel
Production Editor: Cindy Deichmann
Book Design Manager: Bill Drone
Manufacturing Manager: Dave Graybill
Cover Art: Dominic Doyle

Composition by Graphic World, Inc.
Printing/binding by R.R. Donnelley and Sons

Mosby, Inc.
11830 Westline Industrial Drive
St. Louis, Missouri 63146

International Standard Book Number: 0-8151-2988-2

98 99 00 01 02 / 9 8 7 6 5 4 3 2 1

Nursing and Pharmacology Consultants

ROBERT S. AUCKER, PharmD
Clinical Pharmacist, Saint Joseph's Hospital of Atlanta;
Adjunct Professor
Mercer Southern School of Pharmacy/Kennesaw State College of Nursing
Atlanta, Georgia

DANIAL E. BAKER, PharmD, FASHP, FASCP
Director, Drug Information Center
Director, Clinical Pharmacy Programs
Professor of Pharmacy Practice, Washington State University
Spokane, Washington

JACKSON COMO, PharmD
Director, Therapeutic Policy Management
University of Alabama Hospital
Birmingham, Alabama

CHARLOTTE DENEEN, BSN, MPA
Quality Improvement Consultant
Pleasant Hill, California

LINDA GRANT, RN, MSN
Clinical Coordinator for the Meditec Project
Queen of the Valley Hospital
Napa, California

PATRICIA HOWARD, PharmD, FCCP, BCPS
Clinical Associate Professor
School of Pharmacy, Department of Pharmacy Practice
University of Kansas Medical Center
Kansas City, Kansas

GREGORY D. NAZARENO, PharmD
Staff Pharmacist
Kaiser Permanente
Vallejo, California

MERRILEE NEWTON, RN, MSN
Director of Quality Clinical Resource Management
Alta Bates Medical Center
Berkeley, California

ROBERT T. REILLY, PharmD
Associate Director of Pharmacy, Thomason Hospital;
Clinical Instructor
University of Texas—El Paso
El Paso, Texas

Preface

This 1999 edition marks the twenty-sixth year of publication of *Intravenous Medications*.

The prolific approval of new IV drugs by the FDA continues. Twelve newly approved drugs are included in this fifteenth edition. In addition, at the request of users of *Intravenous Medications,* alfentanil (now being used for monitored anesthesia care) has been included to bring the total to twelve. The new drugs, and additions of the last several years, represent phenomenal changes and improvements in drug development and methods of delivery (e.g., liposomal and recombinant preparations). In addition, there are many important updates, such as changes in dose, new pediatric doses, additional disease-specific doses, refinements in dosing applications, new indications, new drug interactions, additional precautions, and new information in antidotes. Helpful charts for dilution and/or rate of administration are incorporated in selected monographs. A diluent compatibility chart is inside the back cover. Appendix E provides a generic dilution chart to simplify calculations. To maintain our commitment to provide the most current information available, any new drugs that are released after the composition of this edition is completed are made available in Appendix G. Front material provides a key to abbreviations and Important IV Therapy Facts.

Health care today is an intense environment. The speed of change is overwhelming, but the authors and publisher of *Intravenous Medications* have a commitment to provide all health professionals who have the responsibility to administer IV medications with annual editions incorporating complete, accurate, current information in a clear, concise, accessible, and reliable tool. Each specific drug must be able to be interpreted for a specific patient. All drugs currently approved for intravenous use (with the exception of opaque dyes used in radiology, some general anesthetics used only in OR, and a few rarely used drugs [see Appendix B]) are included. In addition, all information has been thoroughly revised to incorporate the most current documented knowledge available.

Intravenous Medications is designed for use in critical care areas, at the nursing station, in the office, in public health and home care settings, and by students and the armed services. Pertinent information can be found in a few seconds. Take advantage of its availability and quickly review every intravenous medication before administration.

The nurse is frequently placed in a variety of difficult situations. While the physician verbally requests or writes an order, the nurse must evaluate it for appropriateness, prepare it, administer it, and observe the effects. Intravenous drugs are instantly absorbed into the bloodstream, leading, it is hoped, to a prompt therapeutic action, but the risk of an inappropriate reaction is a constant threat that can easily become a frightening reality. It will be the nurse who must initiate emergency measures should adverse effects occur. This is an awesome responsibility.

If, after reviewing the information in *Intravenous Medications*, you have any questions about any order you are given, clarify it with the physician, consult with the pharmacist, or consult your supervisor. The circumstances will determine whom you approach first. If the physician thinks it is imperative to carry out an order even though you have unanswered questions or concerns, never hesitate to request that the physician administer the drug, drug combination, or dose himself or herself. In this era of constant change, the physician should be very willing to supply you, your supervisor, and/or the pharmacist with current studies documenting the validity and appropriateness of orders.

All information presented in this handbook is pertinent only to the intravenous use of the drug and not necessarily to intramuscular, subcutaneous, oral, or other means of administration.

Our sincere appreciation is extended to Gregory Nazareno, Charlotte Deneen, Linda Grant, and Merrilee Newton for their assistance. Thanks to each of you, the users of this reference, for your quest for information and your loyalty to the references that serve your needs and thus your patients' needs. We will continue to strive to earn your trust and confidence as we look forward together to an exciting future for health care.

Betty L. Gahart

Adrienne R. Nazareno

To my husband,

Bill,

for his patience, support, and many hours of much needed and appreciated assistance and to our children, their spouses, and our grandchildren for their encouragement and understanding.

BLG

To my husband,

Greg,

for his loving support and encouragement and to my children, Danielle, Bryan, Emily, and Mark, for allowing me the freedom to pursue my professional practice.

ARN

Contents

Format and Content of
Intravenous Medications

Designed to facilitate quick reference, each entry begins with the generic name of the drug in boldface type. Drug categories follow. The primary category may be followed by additional ones representing the multiple uses of a drug. Associated trade names are under the generic name. Boldface type and alphabetical order enable the reader to verify correct drug names easily. The use of a Canadian maple leaf symbol (♣) preceding a trade name indicates availability in Canada only. The pH is listed in the lower right-hand corner of the title section. While this information is not consistently available, it is provided whenever possible. It represents the pH of the undiluted drug, the drug after reconstitution, or the drug after dilution for administration.

Headings within drug monographs are as follows:

Usual dose: Doses recommended are the usual range for adults unless specifically stated otherwise. This information is presented first to enable the nurse to verify that the physician order is within acceptable parameters while checking the order and before preparation. If there are any questions, much time can be saved in clarifying them.

Pediatric dose: Pediatric doses are specifically stated if they vary from mg/kg of body weight or M^2 dose recommended for adults. Not all drugs are recommended for use in children.

Infant and/or neonatal dose: Included if available and distinct from Pediatric dose.

Dose adjustments: Any situation that requires increasing or decreasing a dose will be mentioned here. The range will cover adjustments needed for the elderly, debilitated, or patients with hepatic or renal impairment, to adjustments required in the presence of other medications or as physical conditions are monitored.

Dilution: Specific directions for dilution are given for all drugs if dilution is necessary or permissible. Appropriate diluents are listed. Additional solution compatibilities may be found in the chart on the back cover. This is the only reference that provides calculation examples to simplify dilution and accurate dose measurement. Charts are available in selected monographs. If recommendations for pediatric dilutions are available, they are listed. In some situations mcg or mg/ml dilutions partially account for this variation. If there are any doubts, consult with the pharmacist and/or pediatric specialist. Generic dilution charts for grams to milligrams and milligrams to micrograms are in Appendix E.

Storage: A subheading. Content here includes such items as stability, refrigeration versus room temperature, predilution versus postdilution.

Incompatible with: Incompatible drugs are alphabetized by generic name for ease in locating the drugs with which you are working. To make identification easier, common trade names accompany generic names, or examples are presented for drug categories. Again, no other reference consistently provides this helpful information. Not all incompatibilities are absolute. They are intended to alert the nurse to a problem requiring consultation with a pharmacist or the physician. It may be that a specific order of mixing is required or that particular drugs are compatible only in a specific solution. Knowledge is growing daily in this field. After receiving specific directions from the pharmacist on correctly mixing two drugs that have a compatibility problem, write the directions on the patient's medication record or nursing care plan so others will not have to retrace your research steps when the medication is to be given again. For some drugs, additive and/or Y-site compatibilities are listed.

Requests have been received to include compatibilities for all drugs. While there is no question that this is valuable information, the specifics involved make it difficult to include. All compatibility data are based on specific concentrations of both drugs, and these concentrations may or may not be related to usual dose and dilution. Detailing all concentrations is beyond the scope of this handbook. The pharmacist has access to extensive references dedicated to compatibilities and is the best reference source when questions arise.

Rate of administration: Accepted rates of administration are clearly stated. As a general rule, a slow rate is preferred. 25-gauge needles aid in giving a small amount of medication over time. Problems with rapid or slow injection rates are indicated here. Adjusted rates for infants, children, or the elderly are listed when available. Charts are available in selected monographs.

Actions: Clear, concise statements outline the origin of each drug, how it affects body systems, its length of action, and methods of excretion. If a drug crosses the placental barrier or is secreted in breast milk, it will be mentioned here.

Indications and uses: Uses recommended by the manufacturer are listed. Investigational or unlabeled uses are stated as such.

Contraindications: Contraindications are those specifically listed by the manufacturer. Consult with the physician if an ordered drug is contraindicated for the patient. The physician may have additional historical information that alters the situation or may decide that use of the drug is indicated in a critical situation.

Precautions: The section on precautions covers many areas of information needed before injecting any drug. The range covers all facets not covered under specific headings. There is no prioritizing; each listing is as important as the next. To make it easier for spot checks (after reading the entire monograph), additional subdivisions are now included.

Monitor: A subheading that includes information such as required prerequisites for drug administration, parameters for evaluation, and patient assessments.

Patient education: A subheading that addresses only specific, important issues required for short-term IV use. It is expected that the health professional will always review the major points in the drug profile with any conscious patient, side effects to expect, how to cope with them, when to report them, special requirements such as the intake of extra fluids, and an overall review of what the drug does, why it is needed, and how long the patient can anticipate receiving it.

Maternal/child: A subheading that addresses FDA pregnancy categories (see Appendix C for a complete explanation), any known specifics affecting patients capable of conception, safety for use during lactation, safety for use in children, and any special impact on infants and neonates.

Elderly: A subheading that is included whenever specific information impacting this patient group is available. Always consider age-related organ impairment (e.g., cardiac, hepatic, renal, insufficient bone marrow reserve) and route of excretion when determining dose and evaluating side effects.

Drug/lab interactions: Drug/drug or drug/lab interactions are listed here. If a conflict with the patient's drug profile is noted, consult a pharmacist immediately. Increasing or decreasing the effectiveness of a drug can be a potentially life-threatening situation. Check with the lab first on drug/lab interactions; acceptable alternatives are usually available. After this consultation, notify the physician if appropriate. To facilitate recognition, common trade names accompany generic names or examples are presented for drug categories. No other reference consistently provides this helpful information.

Side effects: Alphabetical order simplifies confirmation that a patient's symptom could be associated with specific drug use. Where there is a distinct line of tolerance for side effects, they are listed as minor or major and alphabetized after each of these subheadings. If a manufacturer provides percent of frequency, that information is listed.

Antidote: Specific antidotes are listed in this section. In addition, specific nursing actions to reverse undesirable side effects are clearly stated—an instant refresher course for critical situations.

Key to Abbreviations

<	less than
>	more than
1/2 NS	one-half normal saline (0.45%)
ACE	angiotensin converting enzyme
ACT	activated coagulation time
AIDS	acquired immune deficiency syndrome
ALT	(SGPT) alanine aminotransferase
aPTT	activated partial thromboplastin time
AST	(SGOT) aspartate aminotransferase
BP	blood pressure
BUN	blood urea nitrogen
C	Celsius; centigrade
Ca	calcium
CBC	complete blood count
CHF	congestive heart failure
Cl	chloride
CNS	central nervous system
CO_2	carbon dioxide
CPK	creatine-kinase
CrCl	creatinine clearance
CRT	controlled room temperature (20° to 25°C [68° to 77°F])
CSF	cerebrospinal fluid
C/S	culture and sensitivity
CVP	central venous pressure
D10/NS	10% dextrose in normal saline
D10W	10% dextrose in water
D5/0.2NS	5% dextrose in one-quarter NS (0.2%)
D5/0.45NS	5% dextrose in one-half normal saline (½NS)
D5/LR	5% dextrose in lactated Ringer's solution
D5/NS	5% dextrose in normal saline
D5/R	5% dextrose in Ringer's solution
D5W	5% dextrose in water
DC	discontinued
dL	deciliter(s) (100 ml)
DNA	deoxyribonucleic acid
ECG	electrocardiogram
EEG	electroencephalogram
F	Fahrenheit
GI	gastrointestinal
gm	gram(s)
gr	grain(s)
gtt	drop(s)
GU	genitourinary
Hb	hemoglobin
Hct	hematocrit
Hg	mercury
HIV	human immunodeficiency virus
hr	hour

HR	heart rate
IgA	immune globulin A
IM	intramuscular
IU	international unit(s)
IV	intravenously
K	potassium
KCL	potassium chloride
kg	kilogram(s)
L	liter(s)
lb	pound(s)
LDH	lactic dehydrogenase
LR	lactated Ringer's injection or solution
M	molar
M^2	meter squared
MAO	monoamine oxidase
mcg	microgram(s)
mCi	millicurie(s)
mEq	milliequivalent
Mg	magnesium
mg	milligram(s)
MI	myocardial infarction
min	minute
ml	milliliter
mmol	millimole(s)
Na	sodium
NaCl	sodium chloride
ng	nanogram (millimicrogram)
NS	normal saline (0.9%)
NSAID	nonsteroidal antiinflammatory drug
NSR	normal sinus rhythm
Pao_2	arterial oxygen pressure
PCA	patient controlled analgesia
pH	hydrogen ion concentration
PSVT	paroxysmal supraventricular tachycardia
PT	prothrombin time
PTT	partial thromboplastin time
R	Ringer's injection or solution
RBC	red blood cell or count
RNA	ribonucleic acid
SC	subcutaneous
SrCr	serum creatinine
S/S	signs and symptoms
SW	sterile water for injection
TT	thrombin time
VF	ventricular fibrillation
VT	ventricular tachycardia
WBC	white blood cell or count
WBCT	whole blood clotting time

Important IV Therapy Facts

- Read the Preface and Format and Contents sections at least once. They'll answer many of your questions and save time.

USUAL DOSE

- Doses calculated on body weight are usually based on pretreatment weight and not on edematous weight.
- Normal renal or hepatic function is usually required for drugs metabolized by these routes.
- Formula to calculate creatinine clearance (CrCl) from serum creatine value:

males: $\dfrac{\text{Weight in kg} \times (140 - \text{age in years})}{72 \times \text{serum creatinine (mg/dl)}} = \text{CrCl}$

females: $0.85 \times$ male CrCl value calculated from above formula.

DILUTION

- Check all labels (drugs, diluents, and solutions) to confirm appropriateness for IV use.
- Sterile technique is imperative in all phases of preparation.
- Use a filter needle when withdrawing IV meds from ampoules to eliminate possible pieces of glass.
- Pearls: 1 Gm in 1 Liter yields 1 mg/ml
  1 mg in 1 Liter yields 1 mcg/ml
  % of a solution equals the number of grams/100 ml
  (5% = 5 Gm/100 ml)
- Pediatric dilution: If you dilute 6.0 mg/kg in 100 ml, 1 ml/hr equals 1.0 mcg/kg/min
  If you dilute 0.6 mg/kg in 100 ml, 1 ml/hr equals 0.1 mcg/kg/min
- Do not use bacteriostatic diluents containing benzyl alcohol for neonates.
- Ensure adequate mixing of all drugs added to a solution.
- Examine solutions for clarity and any possible leakage.
- Syringe prepackaging for use in specific pumps is now available for many drugs. Concentrations are often the strongest permissible, but length of delivery is accurate.

INCOMPATIBILITIES

- Some manufacturers routinely suggest discontinuing the primary IV for intermittent infusion; usually done to avoid any possibility of incompatibility. Flushing the line before and after administration may be indicated and/or appropriate for some drugs.
- The brand of intravenous fluids or additives, concentrations, containers, rate and order of mixing, pH, and temperature all affect solubility and compatibility. Consult your pharmacist with any question, and document appropriate instructions on care plan.

TECHNIQUES

- Never hang plastic containers in a series connection; may cause air embolism.
- Confirm patency of peripheral and/or central sites. Avoid extravasation.

• Avoid accidental arterial injection; can cause gangrene.

RATE OF ADMINISTRATION

• Life-threatening reactions (time-related overdose or allergy) are frequently precipitated by a too-rapid rate of injection.

PATIENT EDUCATION

• A well-informed patient is a great asset; review all appropriate drug information with every conscious patient.

SIDE EFFECTS

• Reactions may be caused by a side effect of the drug itself, allergic response, overdose, or the underlying disease process.

FOR FURTHER READING

Additional and more detailed information on included drugs may be found in the following publications:

American Hospital Formulary Service Drug Information 98: Bethesda, MD, 1998, American Society of Hospital Pharmacists. (Updated quarterly.)

Facts and comparisons, St. Louis, 1998, Facts and Comparisons Division, JB Lippincot Company. (Updated monthly.)

Fisher, David S et al: The cancer chemotherapy handbook, ed 5, St. Louis, 1997, Mosby–Year Book.

The Johns Hopkins Hospital: The Harriet Lane handbook, ed 14, St Louis, 1996, Mosby–Year Book.

Journal of the American Medical Association: Guidelines for cardiopulmonary resuscitation and emergency cardiac care; recommendation of the 1992 National Conference, Oct 28, 1992, 268(16):2171-2302.

Manufacturer's literature.

Merck Manual of Diagnosis and Therapy, ed 16, 1992, Merck Research Laboratories, Rahway N.J.

Skidmore-Roth, Linda: Nursing drug reference, St Louis, 1998, Mosby–Year Book.

Tatro DS, Pharm D, eds: Drug Interaction Facts, St Louis, 1998, Facts and Comparisons Division, JB Lippincot Company. (Updated quarterly.)

Trissel LA: Handbook on injectable drugs, ed 9, 1996, and supplement, 1997. American Society of Hospital Pharmacists, Inc.

United States Pharmacopeia: Drug Information for the Health Care Professional, ed 18, Rockville, MD, 1997, United States Pharmacopeial Convention. (Updated monthly.)

Wingard LB, et al: Human pharmacology, St Louis, 1991, Mosby–Year Book.

ABCIXIMAB	Platelet aggregation inhibitor Antithrombotic Monoclonal antibody
ReoPro, c7E3, 7E3	pH 7.2

USUAL DOSE

Recommendations in this monograph are based on protocols from the clinical trials and communications with the manufacturer, as well as the package insert.

In all situations, premedication with histamine H_2 antagonists (e.g., famotidine [Pepcid], ranitidine [Zantac]) may be appropriate; prophylaxis should be considered when certain conditions are present (e.g., patients with HACA antibodies, readministration of abciximab).

Percutaneous coronary intervention: 0.25 mg/kg administered 10 to 60 minutes before percutaneous transluminal coronary angioplasty or atherectomy (PCTA). Follow with a continuous infusion of 0.125 mcg/kg/min (weight adjusted) to a maximum of 10 mcg/min (non-weight adjusted) for 12 hours. Used concurrently with heparin and aspirin. Establish a separate IV site for heparin. The initial bolus of heparin should be based on the results of the baseline ACT according to low-dose weight-adjusted guidelines in the following chart, but not exceeding a total bolus dose of 7000 units.

Low-Dose Weight-Adjusted Heparin *Target ACT* *≥200 seconds*			Standard-Dose Weight-Adjusted Heparin *Target ACT* *≥300 seconds*		
Initial Bolus	ACT (sec)	Heparin	Initial Bolus	ACT (sec)	Heparin
Not to exceed 7,000 units in patients >100 kg	<150	70 units/kg	Not to exceed 10,000 units in patients >100 kg	<150	100 units/kg
	150 to 199	50 units/kg		150 to 225	75 units/kg
	≥ 200	No heparin		226 to 229	50 units/kg
				≥300	No heparin
Additional bolus every 30 min or a 7-unit/kg/hr continuous infusion	<200	20 units/kg	Additional bolus every 30 min or a 10-unit/kg/hr continuous infusion	<275	50 units/kg
	≥200	No heparin		275 to 299	25 units/kg
				≥300	No heparin

Check the ACT (Hemochron instrument used to measure) a minimum of 2 minutes after the initial and each additional heparin bolus. Give additional bolus doses of 20 units/kg until the target ACT of 200 seconds is achieved before PTCA (a target ACT of up to 300 seconds using standard weight-adjusted doses of heparin has been used, but may increase the risk of severe bleeding [see preceding chart]). During the procedure administer additional bolus doses every 30 minutes to maintain the target ACT. Alternately, after the target ACT is reached, a 7-unit/kg/hr continuous infusion may be administered with no further measurement of ACT for the duration of the procedure. Unless contraindicated, administer aspirin, 325 mg, 2 hours before PTCA and once daily thereafter. At the completion of the procedure it is recommended that the heparin be discontinued and that the removal of the sheath be accomplished within 6 hours (see Monitor for specific criteria). If prolonged therapy or later sheath removal is clinically indicated, do not discontinue heparin, but continue the 7 unit/kg/hr heparin infusion. Check the aPTT in 6 hours and adjust rate of heparin based on a target aPTT of 60 to 85 seconds. (Note Precautions/Monitor.)

Unstable angina not responding to conventional medical therapy with planned PTCA intervention within 24 hours: Heparin is started before the abciximab; use a separate IV line. Maintain the APTT between 60 and 85 seconds during the Abciximab and heparin infusion period. Recent recommendations suggest that the low-dose weight adjusted doses of heparin and anticoagulation guidelines described under percutaneous coronary intervention are also appropriate for the planned PTCA intervention in unstable angina. The recommended dose of abciximab is 0.25 mg/kg as an IV bolus followed by a continuous infusion of 10 mcg/min for a minimum of 18 hours up to a maximum of 26 hours (PTCA usually accomplished between 18 and 24 hours). Discontinue abciximab 1 hour after the PTCA (i.e., removal of guidewire). Unless contraindicated, administer at least 250 mg of aspirin at the time heparin is begun and aspirin 50 to 500 mg daily through day 30. Oral or IV Nitroglycerin may also be indicated throughout the course of treatment. The process after the completion of the procedure is the same as in percutaneous coronary intervention.

DILUTION

Available in 5 ml vials (2 mg/ml). Solution must be clear. Must be filtered with a non-pyrogenic, low-protein binding 0.2 to 0.22 micron filter before administering the bolus and the infusion. Filtering of the infusion may be done during preparation or at administration, using the appropriate in-line filter. Do not shake.

Direct IV: Bolus injection may be given undiluted.

Infusion: Withdraw desired dose and further dilute with NS or D5W (5 ml [10 mg] diluted with 250 ml NS or D5W equals 40 mcg/ml).

Storage: Refrigerate prior to use. Do not freeze. Check expiration date on vial. Contains no preservative; discard any unused portion.

INCOMPATIBLE WITH

Manufacturer states that abciximab should be administered through a separate intravenous line; no other medication should be added to the infusion solution.

RATE OF ADMINISTRATION

Direct IV: An initial dose as a bolus injection, filter at this point if not done when withdrawing from vial.

Infusion: See Usual Dose. Must be administered through an in-line non-pyrogenic, low protein binding filter (0.2 or 0.22 microns), if not done during preparation, and controlled by a continuous infusion pump. A 40-mcg/ml solution (10 mg in 250 ml) at a rate of 10.5 ml/hr will deliver 7 mcg/min, and 15 ml/hr will deliver 10 mcg/min. Discard unused portion at the end of the infusion.

ACTIONS

The fab fragment of the chimeric human-murine monoclonal antibody, abciximab binds to the glycoprotein IIb/IIIa (GPIIb/IIIa) receptor of human platelets and produces rapid dose-dependent inhibition of platelet function. It inhibits platelet aggregation by preventing the binding of fibrinogen, von Willebrand factor, and other adhesive molecules to GPIIb/IIIa receptor sites on activated platelets. Inhibition of platelet function is temporary following a bolus dose, but can be sustained at > 80% by continuous IV infusion. Has prevented acute thrombosis and resulted in lower rates of thrombosis as compared to aspirin and/or heparin. Initial half-life is 10 minutes. Second phase half-life is 30 minutes. A bolus dose followed by an infusion produces approximately constant free plasma concentrations throughout the infusion. Median bleeding time increases to over 30 minutes as contrasted to a base line average of 5 minutes before administration. After the infusion is ended, free plasma concentration falls rapidly for 6 hours then more slowly. Platelet function generally recovers gradually over 48 hours. In most patients, bleeding time returns to < 12 minutes within 12 to 24 hours. Some abciximab remains in the circulation for 15 days or more.

INDICATIONS AND USES

An adjunct to percutaneous coronary intervention (PCI) (balloon angioplasty, atherectomy, or stent placement) for the prevention of cardiac ischemic complications in patients undergoing PCI and in patients with unstable angina not responding to conventional medical therapy when PCI is planned within 24 hours. Abciximab use in patients not undergoing PCI has not been studied. Used concurrently with aspirin and heparin.

CONTRAINDICATIONS

Active internal bleeding, administration of oral anticoagulants (e.g., warfarin [Coumadin]) within 7 days unless PT is ≤ 1.2 times control, aneurysm, arteriovenous malformation, bleeding diathesis, clinically significant GI or GU bleeding within 6 weeks, history of CVA within 2 years, history of CVA with significant residual neurologic deficit, history of vasculitis (presumed or documented), hypertension (severe and uncontrolled), intracranial neoplasm, known hypersensitivity to any component of abciximab or to murine proteins, major surgery or trauma within 6 weeks, thrombocytopenia (< 100,000/ mm³/dl), or the use of IV dextran before PTCA or intent to use it during PTCA.

PRECAUTIONS

Administered only in the hospital under the direction of a physician knowledgeable in its use and with appropriate diagnostic, laboratory, and surgical facilities available. ■ Frequently causes major bleeding complications (e.g., retroperitoneal bleeding, spontaneous GI and GU bleeding, bleeding at the arterial access site). ■ Incidence of major bleeding was reduced in clinical trials that used weight-adjusted dosing of abciximab and low-dose weight-adjusted doses of heparin, with adherence to stricter anticoagulation guidelines, and early sheath removal. This was true in patients weighing less than 75 kg (165 lb) that had increased incidences of bleeding with standard weight-adjusted heparin doses, as well as previously recommended heparin doses (up to 20,000 units all inclusive). ■ Incidence of major bleeding is increased in patients with a history of prior GI disease, those over 65 years of age, and those receiving thrombolytics (e.g., alteplase [tPA], anistreplase [Eminase], streptokinase, urokinase). Consider if benefits will outweigh risks, and proceed with extreme caution if use is considered necessary. ■ Incidence of major bleeding is also increased if PTCA occurs within 12 hours of the onset of symptoms of an acute MI, if the PTCA procedure is prolonged (lasting more than 70 minutes), or if PTCA procedure fails. ■ Extreme care must be taken in accessing the femoral artery for femoral sheath placement. Only the anterior wall of the femoral artery should be punctured (use of a single-walled needle versus double-walled [Seldinger through and through technique] is important). If both walls are punctured, massive bleeding could occur. ■ Avoid concurrent sheath placement in the femoral vein if possible (sometimes used to access right coronary artery or administer large amounts of medication). ■ Use of heparin concurrently also increases the risk of bleeding. ■ Anaphylaxis has not been reported, but can occur at any time. Emergency drugs and equipment must always be available. In addition, use may result in the formation of human anti-chimeric antibody (HACA). Can cause hypersensitivity reactions including anaphylaxis, thrombocytopenia, or diminished benefit if abciximab is readministered at another time or other monoclonal antibodies are administered. Consider premedication as outlined under Usual Dose. ■ Note Drug/lab interactions.

Monitor: Before initiating, obtain results of base line CBC, platelet count, prothrombin time (PT), ACT, and aPTT. Type and cross-match would also be appropriate. ■ Monitor heparin anticoagulation (ACT or aPTT) and PT closely. ■ While a femoral sheath is in place, the patient must be on strict bed rest, head of the bed should be < 30°, and the appropriate limb(s) restrained in a straight position. Monitor sheath insertion site(s) and distal pulses of affected leg(s) frequently while sheath is in place and for 6 hours after removal. Measure any hematoma and monitor for enlargement. ■ Monitor platelet count 2 to 4 hours following the bolus dose and at 24 hours or prior to discharge, whichever is first. More frequent monitoring may be indicated. ■ Monitor the patient carefully and frequently for signs of bleeding; take vital signs (avoiding automatic BP cuffs), observe any invaded sites at least every 15 minutes (e.g., sheaths, IV sites, cutdowns, punctures, foleys, NGs); watch for hematuria, hematemesis, bloody stool, petechiae, hematoma, flank pain, muscle weakness; and do neuro checks every hour. Continue until clotting functions move toward normal. ■ Use care in handling patient; avoid arterial puncture, venipuncture, and IM injection. Use extreme precautionary methods and only compressible sites if these procedures absolutely necessary. Apply pressure for 30 minutes to any invaded site and then apply pressure dressings. Saline or heparin locks suggested to facilitate blood draws. ■ Discontinue heparin at least 2 to 4 hours before femoral sheath(s) are to be removed. Sheath removal should not occur until aPTT ≤50 seconds or ACT ≤175 seconds (approaching normal limits). In the past, sheath removal usually occurred 16 hours after the initiating of abciximab (12 hours for abciximab and heparin infusions plus 4-hour waiting period, but in recent clinical trials heparin was discontinued after PTCA, and the sheath was removed no sooner than 2 hours and no later than 6 hours after heparin was discontinued and while the abciximab is still infusing (aPTT must be ≤50 seconds or ACT ≤175 seconds). After removal, apply pressure to the femoral artery for at least 30 minutes. when hemostasis is confirmed, apply a pressure dressing. Maintain strict bed rest for at least 6 to 8 hours after sheath removal and/or abciximab is discontinued, whichever is later. ▪ Throughout process medicate as needed for back or groin pain and nausea or vomiting. ▪ Remove pressure dressing before ambulation. ▪ If complications arise that indicate the need for surgery within 48 to 72 hours of treatment with abciximab, an Ivy bleeding time should be obtained. Platelet function may be partly restored with platelet transfusions. ▪ Note Precautions, Drug/lab interactions, and Antidote.

Patient education: Compliance with all measures to minimize bleeding (e.g., strict bed rest, positioning) is imperative. ▪ Avoid use of razors, toothbrushes, and other sharp items. ▪ Use caution while moving to avoid excessive bumping. ▪ Report all episodes of bleeding and apply local pressure if indicated. ▪ Expect oozing from IV sites.

Maternal/child: Pregnancy Category C. Use only if clearly needed and with extreme caution. ▪ Safety for use during lactation not established. Not known if it is secreted in breast milk; use extreme caution; probably best to postpone breast feeding until bleeding time approaches normal. ▪ Safety and effectiveness for use in children not established. Incidence of side effects may be increased with a weight under 75 kg.

Elderly: Increased risk of major bleeding complications if weight less than 75 kg or age over 65 years; note Precautions. ▪ Consider age-related organ impairment; may also increase risk of bleeding.

DRUG/LAB INTERACTIONS

Use with extreme caution with other drugs that affect hemostasis, (e.g., thrombolytics [e.g., alteplase (tPA), anistreplase (Eminase), streptokinase, urokinase], oral anticoagulants [e.g., warfarin (Coumadin), NSAIDs [e.g., ibuprofen (Motrin), dipyridamole [Persantine], ticlopidine [Ticlid], selected antibiotics [e.g., cefamandole, cefoperazone, cefotetan, ticarcillin]). ▪ Dextran solutions increased the risk of major bleeding events when used concurrently with abciximab. (Note Contraindications.) ▪ HACA titer may precipitate an acute hypersensitivity reaction with other diagnostic or therapeutic monoclonal antibodies (e.g., muromonab CD3).

SIDE EFFECTS

May cause major bleeding incidents (e.g., femoral artery or other access site, intracranial hemorrhage, spontaneous gross hematuria and other GU bleeds, spontaneous hematemesis and other GI bleeds, retroperitoneal bleeding). Decreases in hemoglobin greater than 5 g/dl or intracranial hemorrhage were defined as major during trials. Thrombocytopenia is common and may require platelet transfusion. Abdominal pain, back pain, bradycardia, chest pain, headache, hypotension, nausea, peripheral edema, positive HACA response, puncture site pain, and vomiting may occur. Other side effects that may occur are anemia, arrhythmias (e.g., atrial fibrillation/flutter, bradycardia, complete AV block, supraventricular tachycardia, ventricular PVCs, tachycardia, or fibrillation), confusion, hyperesthesia, intermittent claudication, leukocytosis, limb embolism, pericardial effusion, pleural effusion or pleurisy, pneumonia, pulmonary embolism, pulmonary edema, and visual disturbances. Anaphylaxis has not been reported but may occur.

ANTIDOTE

Stop the infusions of abciximab and heparin if any serious bleeding not controllable with pressure occurs. Stop infusion in patients with failed PTCAs. Stop infusion if a hypersensitivity reaction occurs and treat with epinephrine, dopamine (Intropin), theophylline, antihistamines (e.g., diphenhydramine [Benadryl]), and/or corticosteroids as indicated. Keep physician informed. If an acute platelet decrease occurs (< 100,000/mm^3 or a decrease of at least 25% from pretreatment value), obtain additional platelet counts in separate tubes containing ethylenediaminetetraacetic acid (EDTA), citrate, or heparin. This is to exclude pseudothrombocytopenia due to anticoagulant interaction. If true thrombocytopenia is verified, discontinue abciximab immediately. Platelet transfusions may be required. Heparin and aspirin should also be avoided if the platelet count drops below 60,000/mm^3.

ACETAZOLAMIDE SODIUM

Antiglaucoma
Anticonvulsant
Diuretic
Urinary alkalinizer

Diamox   pH 9.2

USUAL DOSE

Antiglaucoma agent: 250 mg to 1 Gm/24 hr. May be given as 250 mg doses at 4- to 6-hour intervals. To rapidly lower intraocular pressure, give an initial single dose of 500 mg followed by 125 to 250 mg at 4 hour intervals.

Edema of congestive heart failure or drug therapy: 250 to 375 mg or 5 mg/kg of body weight as a single dose daily; when loss of edematous fluid stops, reduce to every other day or give for 2 days followed by a day of rest.

Anticonvulsant: Adults and Children: Dose in epilepsy may range from 8 to 30 mg/kg/24 hr in divided doses every 6 to 12 hours. Reduce initial daily dose when given with other anticonvulsants.

Urinary alkalinization: Adults and Children: 5 mg/kg/dose every 8 to 12 hours.

PEDIATRIC DOSE

Acute antiglaucoma agent: 5 to 10 mg/kg every 6 hours.

Edema of congestive heart failure or drug therapy: 5 mg/kg as a single dose daily or every other day (note comment under adult Usual dose).

Slowly progressive hydrocephalus in infants 2 weeks to 10 months: 25 mg/kg/24 hr in equally divided doses every 8 hours. Up to 100 mg/kg/24 hr or a maximum dose of 2 Gm/24 hr has been used.

DOSE ADJUSTMENTS

Reduced dose required when introducing acetazolamide into a treatment regimen with other anticonvulsants.

DILUTION

Each 500 mg should be diluted in 5 ml sterile water for injection. May then be given directly IV or added to standard IV fluids.

Storage: Use within 24 hours of dilution.

INCOMPATIBLE WITH

Diltiazem (Cardizem), multivitamin infusion.

COMPATIBLE WITH

Cimetidine (Tagamet), ranitidine (Zantac).

RATE OF ADMINISTRATION

500 mg or fraction thereof over at least 1 minute or added to IV fluids to be given over 4 to 8 hours.

ACTIONS

A potent carbonic anhydrase inhibitor and nonbacteriostatic sulfonamide, acetazolamide depresses the tubular reabsorption of sodium, potassium, and bicarbonate. Excreted unchanged in the urine, producing diuresis, alkalinization of the urine, and a mild degree of metabolic acidosis.

INDICATIONS AND USES

Glaucoma. ▪ Epilepsy ▪ Urine alkalinization to treat toxicity of weakly acidic medications (e.g., phenobarbital, lithium, salicylates). Note Drug/lab interactions. ▪ No longer the drug of choice for congestive heart failure or drug-induced edema (e.g., steroids). ▪ Used orally for acute mountain sickness and hypo/hyperkalemia of familial periodic paralysis.

Investigational uses: Prevention or treatment of alkalosis following open heart surgery, treatment of acute pancreatitis and gastric ulcers (inhibits pancreatic and gastric secretions).

CONTRAINDICATIONS

Depressed sodium and potassium levels, hyperchloremic acidosis, marked kidney or liver disease, adrenocortical insufficiency, hypersensitivity to acetazolamide or any of its components. Long-term use contraindicated in some glaucomas.

PRECAUTIONS

Chemically related to sulfonamides; may cause serious reactions in sensitive patients. ▪ May be alternated with other diuretics to achieve maximum effect. ▪ Greater diuretic action is achieved by skipping a day of treatment rather than increasing dose; failure in therapy may be due to overdose or too frequent dosage. ▪ Direct IV administration is preferred. ▪ Use with caution in impaired respiratory function (e.g., pulmonary disease, edema, infection, obstruction); may cause severe respiratory acidosis. ▪ Potassium excretion is proportional to diuresis. Hypokalemia may result from diuresis or with severe cirrhosis. ▪ Introduce or withdraw gradually when used as an anticonvulsant.

Monitor: Obtain baseline CBC and platelet count prior to use and monitor during therapy.

Patient education: Consider birth control options.

Maternal/ child: Category D: avoid pregnancy; may cause premature delivery and congenital anomalies. ▪ Discontinue nursing or discontinue acetazolamide. ▪ Safety for use in children not established but no problems are documented.

Elderly: Use caution; no documented problems but age-related renal impairment may be a factor.

DRUG/LAB INTERACTIONS

May cause hypokalemia with concurrent use of steroids. ▪ Hypokalemia may cause toxicity and fatal cardiac arrhythmias with digitalis or interfere with insulin or oral antidiabetic agent response, thus causing hyperglycemia. ▪ Alkalinization of urine potentiates amphetamines, ephedrine, flecainide (Tambocor), methenamine, pseudoephedrine (Sudafed), procainamide, quinidine, and tricyclic antidepressants (e.g., amitriptyline [Elavil]) by decreasing rate of excretion. ▪ May decrease response to lithium, methotrexate, some antidepressants, phenobarbital, salicylates, and urinary antiinfectives by increasing rate of excretion. ▪ Metabolic acidosis induced by acetazolamide may potentiate salicylate toxicity (anorexia, tachypnea, lethargy, coma and death can occur with high-dose aspirin). ▪ Alkalinity may cause false-positive urinary protein and possibly urinary steroid tests. ▪ May depress iodine uptake by the thyroid.

SIDE EFFECTS

Minimal with short-term therapy. Respond to symptomatic treatment or withdrawal of drug: acidosis, anorexia, bone marrow depression, confusion, crystalluria, drowsiness, fever, hemolytic anemia, hypokalemia (ECG changes, fatigue, muscle weakness, vomiting), paresthesias, photosensitivity, polyuria, rash, renal calculus, thrombocytopenic purpura.

ANTIDOTE

Notify physician of any adverse effects and discontinue drug if necessary. Treat allergic reactions as indicated.

ACYCLOVIR   Antiviral
Acycloguanosine, Zovirax   pH 10.5 to 11.6

USUAL DOSE

Mucocutaneous HSV infections in immunocompromised patients: 5 to 10 mg/kg of body weight every 8 hours for 7 to 10 days.

Severe initial clinical episodes of herpes genitalis: 5 mg/kg every 8 hours for 5 days.

Varicella zoster infections (shingles) in immunocompromised patients and disseminated zoster in nonimmunocompromised patients: 10 mg/kg every 8 hours for 7 days. Calculate dose by ideal body weight in obese individuals. Do not exceed 500 mg/M^2 every 8 hours.

Herpes simplex encephalitis: 10 mg/kg every 8 hours for 10 days.

PEDIATRIC DOSE

Children under 12 years of age:

Mucocutaneous HSV infections in immunocompromised patients: 250 mg/M^2 every 8 hours for 7 days.

Severe initial clinical episodes of herpes genitalis: 250 mg/M^2 every 8 hours for 5 days.

Varicella zoster infections (shingles) in immunocompromised patients and disseminated zoster in nonimmunocompromised patients: 500 mg/M^2 every 8 hours for 7 days. Do not exceed this dose.

Varicella zoster (chickenpox): Children under 1 year: 10 mg/kg every 8 hours for 7 days. *Children over 1 year:* 500 mg/M^2 every 8 hours for 7 days.

Herpes simplex encephalitis: Children over 6 months of age: 500 mg/M^2 every 8 hours for 10 days.

Neonatal disseminated herpes simplex virus: 10 mg/kg every 8 hours for 10 to 14 days.

DOSE ADJUSTMENTS

Reduce dose in impaired renal function based on creatinine clearance. Specific calculation required (see literature).

DILUTION

Now available in liquid form (no reconstitution required) or each 500 mg vial of the dry product must be reconstituted with 10 ml sterile water for injection (50 mg/ml). Do not use bacteriostatic water containing parabens; will cause precipitation. Shake well to dissolve completely. Withdraw the desired dose from either preparation and further dilute in an amount of solution to provide a concentration less than 7 mg/ml (70 kg adult at 5 mg/kg equals 350 mg dissolved in a total of 100 ml of solution equals 3.5 mg/ml). Compatible with most infusion solutions. Use reconstituted solution within 12 hours.

Storage: Use solution fully diluted for administration within 24 hours.

INCOMPATIBLE WITH

Amifostine (Ethyol), blood products, diltiazem (Cardizem), dobutamine (Dobutrex), dopamine (Intropin), fludarabine (Fludara), foscarnet (Foscavir), idarubicin (Idamycin), meperidine (Demerol), morphine, ondansetron (Zofran), piperacillin-tazobactam (Zosyn), sagramostim (Leukine), vinorelbine (Navelbine).

RATE OF ADMINISTRATION

A single dose must be administered at a constant rate over 1 hour as an infusion. Renal tubular damage will occur with too rapid rate of injection. Acyclovir crystals will occlude renal tubules. Use of an infusion pump or microdrip (60 gtt/ml) recommended.

ACTIONS

An antiviral agent that inhibits DNA replication in viruses (e.g., herpes simplex virus, varicella zoster virus, Epstein-Barr virus, and cytomegalovirus). Onset of action is prompt and therapeutic levels maintained for 8 hours. Widely distributed in tissues and body fluids. Excreted in the urine. Crosses placental barrier. Secreted in breast milk.

INDICATIONS AND USES

Treatment of initial and recurrent mucosal and cutaneous herpes simplex infections in immunosuppressed patients. ■ Severe initial clinical episodes of herpes genitalis in patients who are not immunocompromised. ■ Varicella zoster infections (shingles) in immunocompromised patients. ■ Herpes simplex encephalitis in patients over 6 months of age.

Investigational uses: Cytomegalovirus and HSV infection after bone marrow or renal transplantation. ▪ Disseminated primary eczema herpeticum. ▪ Varicella pneumonia. ▪ Various herpes simplex infections (e.g., erythema multiforme, ocular, proctitis).

CONTRAINDICATIONS

Hypersensitivity to acyclovir or ganciclovir.

PRECAUTIONS

Confirm diagnosis of herpes simplex virus (HSV-1 or HSV-2) through laboratory culture. Initiate therapy as quickly as possible after symptoms identified. ▪ Use caution in patients with underlying neurologic abnormalities, in patients receiving interferon or intrathecal methotrexate, or with patients who have had previous neurologic reactions to cytotoxic drugs. ▪ Confirm patency of vein; will cause thrombophlebitis. Rotate site of infusion.

Monitor: Maintain adequate hydration and urine flow before and during infusion. Encourage fluid intake of 2 to 3 L/day.

Patient education: Virus remains dormant and can still spread to others. ▪ Avoid sexual intercourse when visible herpes lesions are present. Use condoms routinely.

Maternal/child: Category C: Use extreme caution in pregnancy and lactation. May cause chromosomal damage with high concentrations. CDC recommends use during pregnancy only for life-threatening disease. ▪ Breast milk concentrations can be higher than maternal serum concentrations. Discontinue nursing or evaluate very carefully.

DRUG/LAB INTERACTIONS

Note Precautions. May cause neurotoxicity (e.g., severe drowsiness and lethargy) with zidovudine. ▪ Side effects increased by other nephrotoxic drugs. ▪ Potentiated by probenecid. ▪ Synergistic effects with ketoconazole and interferon have been noted. Clinical importance not established. ▪ In one case report, a patient stabilized on phenytoin and valproic acid experienced seizures and a reduction in antiepileptic drug serum concentrations when acyclovir was added to the regimen.

SIDE EFFECTS

Acute renal failure, agitation, coma, confusion, diaphoresis, hallucinations, headache, hematuria, hives, hypotension, lethargy, nausea, obtundation, phlebitis, rash, seizures, transient increased serum creatinine levels, tremors, vomiting. Some patients (fewer than 1%) may have abdominal pain, anemia, anorexia, anuria, chest pain, edema, fever, hemoglobinemia, hypokalemia, ischemia of digits, leukocytosis, lightheadedness, neutropenia, neutrophilia, pulmonary edema with cardiac tamponade, rigors, thirst, thrombocytosis, thrombocytopenia.

ANTIDOTE

Notify physician of all side effects. Discontinue drug with onset of CNS side effects. Treatment will be symptomatic and supportive. Removed by hemodialysis. Treat anaphylaxis and resuscitate as necessary.

ADENOSINE

Antiarrhythmic
Diagnostic agent

Adenocard, Adenoscan, ATP

pH 4.5 to 7.5

USUAL DOSE

Conversion of acute paroxysmal supraventricular tachycardia (PSVT)
(Adenocard): 6 mg initially. If supraventricular tachycardia not eliminated in 1 to 2 minutes, give 12 mg. An additional 12 mg dose may be repeated once if required. Do not exceed 12 mg in any single dose. Patients with central lines may respond to lesser doses; peripheral lines usually require standard doses.

Do not administer a repeat dose to patients who develop a high-level block on one dose of adenosine.

Adenosine is not blocked by atropine. Digitalis; quinidine; beta-adrenergic blocking agents (e.g., atenolol, esmolol); calcium channel blocking agents (verapamil [Isoptin]); angiotensin-converting enzyme inhibitors (e.g., enalapril [Vasotec]); and other cardiac drugs can be administered without delay if indicated because of the short half-life of adenosine. Repeat episodes may be treated with adenosine or calcium channel blockers (e.g., diltiazem, verapamil).

Noninvasive diagnosis of coronary artery disease with thallium tomography
(Adenoscan): 140 mcg/kg/min as a 6-minute continuous infusion. Inject thallium at 3 minutes. Dose should be based on total body weight. ▪ Note Drug/lab interactions.

PEDIATRIC DOSE

Conversion of acute paroxysmal supraventricular tachycardia (PSVT)
(Adenocard): 0.1 mg/kg. May increase dose by 0.05 mg/kg increments every 2 min until PSVT terminated or maximum dose reached (0.25 mg/kg or 12 mg). ▪ Note comments in Usual dose.

DOSE ADJUSTMENTS

Metabolism of adenosine is independent of hepatic or renal function. No dose adjustment indicated. ▪ Note Drug/lab interactions; alternative therapy (e.g., calcium channel blockers) may be indicated.

DILUTION

Solution must be clear; do not use if discolored or particulate matter present.

Conversion of acute PSVT (Adenocard): Give undiluted directly into a vein. If given into an IV line, use the closest port to the insertion site and follow with a rapid NS flush (+/- 50 ml) to be certain the solution reaches the systemic circulation. Discard unused portion.

Pharmacological stress testing (Adenoscan): Dilute a single dose in sufficient NS to distribute over 6 minutes.

Storage: Store at room temperature; refrigeration will cause crystallization. If crystals do form, dissolve by warming to room temperature.

INCOMPATIBLE WITH

Any other drug in syringe or solution due to pharmacologic actions and specific use.

RATE OF ADMINISTRATION

Conversion of acute PSVT (Adenocard): Must be given as a rapid bolus IV injection over 1 to 2 seconds. Follow with NS flush if indicated (see Dilution).

Pharmacological stress testing (Adenoscan): (See Usual dose).

ACTIONS

A naturally occurring nucleoside present in all cells of the body. Has many functions. When given as a rapid IV bolus, adenosine has anti-arrhythmic properties, slowing cardiac conduction (particularly at the AV node) and it restores sinus rhythm in patients with PSVT. When used as a diagnostic aid and given as a continuous infusion, adenosine acts as a vasodilator. Adenocard and Adenoscan have the same molecular structure, same solvent, diluent, and concentration. The difference in their actions is in the rate of administration; however, the FDA has approved Adenocard for converting PSVT and Adenoscan for pharmacologic stress testing. Effective within 1 minute. Half-life is estimated to be less than 10 seconds. Adenosine is salvaged immediately by erythrocytes and blood vessel endothelial cells and metabolized for natural uses throughout the body (regulation of coronary and systemic vascular tone, platelet function, lipolysis in fat cells, intracardiac conduction).

INDICATIONS AND USES

To convert acute paroxysmal supraventricular tachycardia (PSVT) to normal sinus rhythm; a first-line agent according to JAMA. Includes PSVT associated with accessory bypass tracts (Wolff-Parkinson-White syndrome). Effective in up to 92% of patients. ▪ To convert wide-complex tachycardia (even if tachycardia may respond to lidocaine). ▪ Adjunct in diagnosis of atrial flutter or fibrillation. ▪ Noninvasive diagnosis of coronary artery disease with thallium tomography. (Results are similar to IV dipyridamole or exercise stress testing.)

Investigational uses: Studies of the use of adenosine with BCNU as an adjuvant to treatment of brain tumors and in the prevention of myocardial reperfusion damage are underway.

CONTRAINDICATIONS

Atrial flutter or fibrillation and ventricular tachycardia (not effective in converting these arrhythmias to normal sinus rhythm [NSR]). ▪ Known or suspected bronchospastic or bronchoconstrictive lung disease (e.g., asthma). ▪ Known hypersensitivity to adenosine. ▪ Symptomatic bradycardia, sick sinus syndrome, and second- or third-degree AV block unless a functioning artificial pacemaker is in place.

PRECAUTIONS

Absolutely confirm labeling for IV use. Do not use adenosine phosphate, which is for IM use in the symptomatic relief of varicose vein complications. ▪ Valsalva maneuver may be used before use of adenosine in PSVTs if clinically appropriate. ▪ Emergency resuscitation drugs and equipment must always be available. ▪ Could produce bronchoconstriction in patients with asthma. ▪ Considered the emerging drug of choice by many investigators, especially for terminating narrow-complex PSVT; others limit use to hemodynamically stable patients who do not require direct-current cardioversion but do require rapid conversion to a normal sinus rhythm. Also used in patients who have not responded to cumulative doses of verapamil 10 mg IV or those with congestive heart failure, concomitant beta blockade, hypotension, or left ventricular dysfunction when verapamil is relatively contraindicated. ■ Some slowing of ventricular response may occur if atrial flutter or fibrillation is also present. ■ Adenosine will not terminate arrhythmias not caused by reentry involving the AV node but may clarify the diagnosis by producing a transient AV or ventriculoatrial block. ■ Patients with unstable angina may be at greater risk for major side effects. ■ During pharmacologic stress testing, women, heavy to obese patients, and younger patients may be at greater risk for side effects.

Monitor: Conversion of acute PSVT: Must reach systemic circulation (See Dilution). ■ ECG monitoring during administration recommended. Monitor blood pressure. At the time of conversion to normal sinus rhythm, PVCs, PACs, sinus bradycardia, sinus tachycardia, skipped beats, and varying degrees of AV nodal block are seen on the ECG in many patients. Usually last only a few seconds and resolve without intervention. ■ Less likely to precipitate hypotension if arrhythmia does not terminate.

Pharmacologic stress testing: ECG monitoring during administration recommended. Monitor heart rate and blood pressure at regular intervals during infusion. ■ Obtain images when infusion complete and redistribution images 3 to 4 hours later.

Maternal/child: Category C: use in pregnancy only if clearly needed. Some references recommend avoiding early pregnancy. ■ Controlled studies have not been conducted in pediatric patients, but preliminary trials indicate similar response rate and side effects. Safety for use in pharmacologic stress testing in patients under 18 years not established.

Elderly: Patients over 70 years of age are at greater risk of AV block during an infusion of adenosine.

DRUG/LAB INTERACTIONS

Effects antagonized by methylxanthines (e.g., caffeine, theophylline); larger doses may be required or adenosine may not be effective. ■ Potentiated by dipyridamole (Persantine); smaller doses of adenosine may be indicated. ■ Cardiovascular effects increased by nicotine; lower doses of adenosine may be indicated. ■ May produce a higher degree of heart block with carbamazepine (Tegretol). ■ Before using Adenoscan for pharmacologic stress testing, avoid, or withhold for at least 5 half-lives, adenosine antagonists (e.g., methylxanthines) and/or potentiators (e.g., dipyridamole, papaverine). ■ Note Usual dose.

SIDE EFFECTS

Generally predictable, short lived, and easily tolerated. Most will appear immediately and last less than 1 minute. Chest pressure (7%), dizziness (1%), dyspnea and/or shortness of breath (12%), facial flushing (18%), headache (2%), lightheadedness (2%), nausea (3%), numbness (1%), PACs, PVCs, sinus bradycardia, sinus tachycardia, skipped beats, varying degrees of AV nodal block. Less than 1% of patients complain of apprehension, blurred vision, burning, chest pain, head pressure, heavy arms, hyperventilation, hypotension, metallic taste, neck and back pain, palpitations, pressure in groin, sweating, tight throat, and tingling in arms.

Major: Arrhythmias (persistent), bronchospasm (severe), myocardial infarction, pulmonary edema, third degree AV block.

ANTIDOTE

Notify physician of any side effect that lasts more than 1 minute. If a side effect persists, decrease rate of infusion (pharmacologic stress testing). With either use, for progression to a major side effect discontinue adenosine. Treat symptomatically if indicated. Bradycardia may be refractory to atropine. Short half-life generally precludes overdose problems, but aminophylline 50 to 125 mg as a slow infusion is a competitive antagonist. Resuscitate as necessary.

ALATROFLOXACIN MESYLATE

Antibacterial
Fluoroquinolone

Trovan   pH 3.5 to 4.3

USUAL DOSE

200 to 300 mg once every 24 hours. Dose and duration of treatment are based on degree of infection and specific diagnosis based on the chart below. Dose and serum levels similar by oral or IV route: no dose adjustment necessary. Transfer to oral dose as soon as practical.

INFECTION/LOCATION AND TYPE	DAILY UNIT DOSE AND ROUTE OF ADMINISTRATION	TOTAL DURATION
Nosocomial pneumonia*	300 mg. I.V. followed by 200 mg oral	10-14 days
Community-acquired pneumonia	200 mg oral or 200 mg I.V. followed by 200 mg oral	7-14 days
Complicated intra-abdominal infections, including postsurgical infections	300 mg I.V. followed by 200 mg oral	7-14 days
Gynecological and pelvic infections	300 mg I.V. followed by 200 mg oral	7-14 days
Surgical prophylaxis—elective colorectal surgery or elective abdominal and vaginal hysterectomy†	200 mg I.V. or oral	Single intravenous or oral dose within 30 min. to 4 hours before surgery
Skin and skin structure infections, complicated, including diabetic foot infections	200 mg oral or 200 mg I.V. followed by 200 mg oral	10-14 days

*If *Pseudomonas aeruginosa* is a documented or presumptive pathogen, combination therapy with either an aminoglycoside or aztreonam may be clinically indicated.
†If surgical prophylaxis with oral trovafloxacin is indicated, Bicitra® should not be given within 2 hours.

DOSE ADJUSTMENTS

No dose reduction required in impaired renal function, severe renal deficiency (Crcl < 20 ml/min), hemodialysis, or in the elderly.
■ Half-life is prolonged in impaired hepatic function and dose reduction is recommended in patients with mild to moderate cirrhosis based on the following chart. No data available for patients with severe cirrhosis.

INDICATED DOSE (Normal hepatic function)	CHRONIC HEPATIC DISEASE DOSE
300 mg I.V.	200 mg I.V.
200 mg I.V. or oral	100 mg I.V. or oral
100 mg oral	100 mg oral

DILUTION

Available in single-use vials. Withdraw desired dose (5 mg/ml) from vial. Each 100 mg must be further diluted with a minimum of 30 ml D5W, ½NS, D5/0.45NS, D5/0.2NS, D5/LR. Desired concentration is 1 to 2 mg/ml (see chart below). No preservatives; enter vial only once.

DOSAGE STRENGTH (mg)	VOLUME TO WITHDRAW (ml)	DILUENT VOLUME (ml)	TOTAL VOLUME (ml)	INFUSION CONCENTRATION (mg/ml)
100 mg	20	30	50	2
100 mg	20	80	100	1
200 mg	40	60	100	2
200 mg	40	160	200	1
300 mg	60	90	150	2
300 mg	60	240	300	1

Storage: Vials stable until expiration date stored at 15° to 30° C (59° to 86° F). Protect from light. Do not freeze. Concentrations of diluted solutions between 0.5 and 2 mg/ml are stable in glass or PVC plastic containers for up to 7 days if refrigerated and for up to 3 days at CRT. Discard any unused portion of vial or diluted solution.

INCOMPATIBLE WITH

Manufacturer recommends alatrofloxacin be administered separately. Never administer in the same IV or through the same tubing as any solution containing multivalent cations (e.g., magnesium, calcium). Always flush line with solution compatible to both drugs before and after administration of any other drug through the same IV line.

RATE OF ADMINISTRATION

A single dose must be equally distributed over 60 minutes as an infusion. Too-rapid administration may cause hypotension. May be given through a Y-tube or three-way stopcock of infusion set. Temporarily discontinue other solutions infusing at the same site and flush tubing with compatible solutions before and after alatrofloxacin.

ACTIONS

A fourth-generation fluoroquinolone antibacterial agent. Has a unique spectrum of activity to a wide range of organisms including grampositive, gram-negative, aerobic, anaerobic, and atypical microorganisms. Bactericidal through inhibition of DNA gyrase (an essential enzyme involved in synthesis, repair, recombination, and transposition of bacterial DNA) and topoisomerase IV (an enzyme key to the partitioning of DNA during bacterial cell division). Mechanism of fluoroquinolones differs from that of aminoglycosides, penicillins, cephalosporins, macrolides, and tetracyclines, and flororoquinolones may be active against pathogens resistant to these antibiotics. There is no cross-resistance between fluoroquinolones and these other antibiotics. Alatrofloxacin is rapidly converted to trovafloxacin. Widely distributed into body tissues in concentrations higher than in plasma within 5 to 10 minutes of completion of a 1-hour infusion. Half-life is approximately 11 hours. Steady-state concentrations are achieved by the third daily dose. Metabolized by conjugation in the liver (effect of cytochrome P_{450} oxidative metabolism is minimal). No significant age or gender differences. Some excretion occurs in urine and feces. Crosses the placental barrier. Secreted in breast milk.

INDICATIONS AND USES

Treatment of infection caused by susceptible strains of specific organisms (see literature for complete list). Used IV for repiratory tract infecions (e.g., nosocomial or community-acquired pneumonia); complicated intraabdominal infections including postsurgical infections, gynecologic and pelvic infections (e.g., endomyometritis, parametritis, septic abortion, postpartum); complicated skin and skin structure infections; sexually transmitted diseases; and surgical prophylaxis in elective colorectal surgery and abdominal or vaginal hysterectomy. Oral uses include all of the above, as well as acute bacterial exacerbation of chronic bronchitis, acute sinusitis, uncomplicated skin and skin structure infections, uncomplicated urinary tract infections (e.g., cystitis), chronic bacterial prostatitis, uncomplicated urethral gonorrhea in males, endocervical and rectal gonorrhea in females, cervicitis due to *Chlamydia trachomatis,* mild to moderate pelvic inflammatory disease.

CONTRAINDICATIONS

History of hypersensitivity to alatrofloxacin, traovafloxacin, any components of these products, or any other quinolone antimicrobial agents (e.g., ciprofloxacin [Cipro], levofloxacin [Levaquin], norfloxacin [Noroxin], ofloxacin [Floxin]).

PRECAUTIONS

For IV use only. ■ Culture and sensitivity studies indicated to determine susceptibility of the causative organism to alatrofloxacin. ■ Prolonged use may cause superinfection because of overgrowth of nonsusceptible organisms. ■ Use with caution in patients with known CNS disorders that predispose to seizures or alter seizure threshold (e.g., epilepsy, severe cerebral arteriosclerosis, concomitant drug therapy). Convulsions, toxic psychosis, increased intracranial pressure and CNS stimulation (confusion, depression, hallucinations, insomnia, lightheadedness, nightmares, paranoia, restlessness, tremor) have been reported with quinolones. ▪ Use caution in patients with impaired liver function (see Dose adjustments). ▪ May cause pseudomembranous colitis. ▪ Cross-resistance may occur with other fluoroquinolones, but some microorganisms resistant to other fluoroquinolones may be susceptible to alatrofloxacin. ▪ Rupture of shoulder, hand, and Achilles tendon has been reported in patients receiving quinolones. ▪ Not effective in the treatment of syphilis—antimicrobial treatment may mask symptoms; all patients with gonorrhea should have a serologic test for syphilis at the time of diagnosis. ▪ Safety and effectiveness for the treatment of osteomyelitis or for periods longer than 4 weeks have not been studied. ▪ Note Antidote.

Monitor: Hypersensitivity reactions, including anaphylaxis with the first or succeeding doses, have been reported in patients receiving quinolones, even in those without known hypersensitivity. Emergency equipment must always be available. ▪ Obtain baseline CBC with differential and platelets and liver function tests (e.g., ALT, AST, alkaline phosphatase). ▪ Monitor vital signs. ▪ Periodic monitoring of organ systems, including hematopoietic, hepatic, and renal, is recommended. ▪ Maintain adequate hydration to prevent concentrated urine throughout treatment. Other quinolones have formed crystals. ▪ Monitor infusion site for inflammation and/or extravasation. ▪ Note Precautions, Drug/Lab interactions, and Antidote.

Patient education: Report skin rash, difficult breathing or swallowing, swelling (e.g., lips, tongue, face), or any other hypersensitivity reaction promptly. ▪ Report diarrhea promptly; consult physician before taking any antidiarrhea medication (e.g., Imodium, Kaopectate, Pepto-Bismol). ▪ Dizziness or lightheadedness may interfere with ambulation and motor coordination; request assistance for ambulation. ▪ Drink fluids liberally. ▪ Has low potential for photosensitivity, but it may occur; best to avoid excessive sunlight or artificial ultraviolet light. ▪ Report tendon pain or inflammation promptly. ▪ Additional instruction required with transfer to oral trovalfoxacin. ▪ Note Precautions, Monitor, Drug/lab interactions, and Antidote.

Maternal/child: Category C: safety for use in pregnancy not established; benefits must outweigh risks. Has caused skeletal malformations in rat fetuses. ▪ Discontinue breast feeding. ▪ Safety for use in children and adolescents under 18 years of age not established. Quinolones have caused arthropathy and osteochondrosis in juvenile animals.

Elderly: No age-related differences noted.

DRUG/LAB INTERACTIONS

Concimitant administration with cimetidine may reduce alatrofloxacin renal clearance, but dose adjustment is not required. ▪ Interactions with theophylline that occur with other quinolones have not been noted, but monitoring of theophylline levels may be indicated with concomitant use. ▪ Interactions with warfarin that occur with other quinolones have not been noted, but monitoring of PT may be indicated with concomitant use. ▪ No dose adjustment required for either drug when alatrofloxacin is administered concomitantly with cyclosporine or digoxin. ▪ Note literature for additional drug/drug interactions on transfer to oral trovafloxacin.

SIDE EFFECTS

Abdominal pain, diarrhea, dizziness, headache, increased liver function tests (e.g., ALT, AST, alkaline phosphatase), lightheadedness, nausea, pain at injection site, pruritus, rash, vaginitis, and vomiting have occurred in more than 1% of patients. Capable of numerous other reactions (e.g., photosensitivity) in less than 1% of patients.

Major: Allergic reactions (e.g., anaphylaxis, cardiovascular collapse, death, dyspnea, edema [facial, laryngeal, or pharyngeal], hypotension, shock); CNS stimulation (e.g., anxiety, confusion, depression, hallucinations, insomnia, restlessness, nightmares, paranoia, tremor), increased intracranial pressure, and toxic psychoses; fever, rash, and severe dermatologic reactions (e.g., toxic epidermal necrolysis, Stevens-Johnson syndrome); pseudomembranous colitis; and pain, inflammation, and ruptures of the shoulder, hand, and Achilles tendon have all been reported in patients receiving quinolones.

ANTIDOTE

Keep physician informed of all side effects. Most minor side effects will be treated symptomatically or will resolve with continued dosing (e.g., dizziness, lightheadedness); monitor closely. Discontinue alatrofloxacin at the first sign of any major side effect (hypersensitivity, CNS symptoms, dermatologic reactions, pseudomembranous colitis, tendon rupture) or phototoxicity. Treat allergic reactions as indicated with epinephrine, airway management, oxygen, IV fluids, antihistamines (e.g., diphenhydramine [Benadryl]), corticosteroids (e.g., Solu-Cortef), and pressor amines (e.g., dopamine [Intropin]). Treat CNS symptoms as indicated, may require diazepam (Valium) for seizures. Oral vancomycin (Vancocin) or metronidazole (Flagyl) is the treatment of choice for antibiotic-related pseudomembranous colitis. Adequate hydration and supplementation of electrolytes and proteins usally indicated. Complete rest is indicated for an affected tendon until treatment is available. Maintain hydration in overdose. No specific antidote; not removed by hemodialysis. Maintain patient until drug is excreted and symptoms subside.

ALBUMIN (HUMAN)

Plasma volume expander
(Plasma protein fraction)

Albuminar-5 and -25, Albunex 5% , Albutein 5% & 25%,
Buminate 5% & 25%, Normal serum albumin,
Plasbumin-5 and -25

pH 6.4 to 7.4

USUAL DOSE

Variable, depending on patient condition (e.g., presence of hemorrhage, hypovolemia, or shock, pulse, blood pressure, hemoglobin and hematocrit, and amount of pulmonary or venous congestion present). Range is from 5 to 75 Gm/24 hr. Available as 5% solution (5 Gm/100 ml) in 50 ml, 250 ml, 500 ml, and 1,000 ml vials, or 25% solution (25 Gm/100 ml) in 20 ml, 50 ml, and 100 ml vials. Maximum dose is 2 Gm/kg/24 hr or 250 Gm in 48 hours (5 liters of 5% or 1 liter of

25%). Selection of 5% or 25% solution based on desired fluid volume and underlying condition.

Hypoproteinemia (hypoalbuminemia): 50 to 75 Gm as a 25% solution. Repeat doses may be required in patients who continue to lose albumin.

Hypovolemia: 25 Gm as a 5% or 25 % solution. May be repeated in 15 to 30 minutes if response inadequate. If 25% solution is used, additional fluids may be needed.

Burns: Electrolyte replacement and crystalloids (e.g., IV fluids) to maintain plasma volume are required in the first 24 hours. Then begin with 25 Gm and adjust as necessary to maintain albumin level from 2 to 3 Gm/dl.

Acute nephrosis or acute nephrotic syndrome: 25 Gm of a 25% solution with an appropriate diuretic daily for 7 to 10 days.

Hemodialysis: 25 Gm of a 25% solution.

Red blood cell resuspension: 20 to 25 Gm of a 25% solution/liter of red blood cells (RBC).

Cardiopulmonary bypass: Achieve a plasma albumin of 2.5 Gm/dl and hematocrit concentration of 20% with either a 5% or 25% solution. Use crystalloids (IV fluids) as a pump prime.

PEDIATRIC DOSE

0.6 to 1 Gm/kg/dose. 25% solution is usually used in infants and children, do not use in preterm infants. Maximum dose 6 Gm/kg/24 hr.

Hypoproteinemia (Hypoalbuminemia): 1 Gm/kg/dose. A second source recommends 25 Gm of a 25% solution.

Hypovolemia: 0.5 to 1 Gm/kg/dose. May be repeated in 15 to 30 minutes if response inadequate.

Hemolytic disease of the newborn: 1 Gm/kg of body weight 1 to 2 hours before blood transfusion or with transfusion (exchange 50 ml of albumin 25% for 50 ml plasma).

Burns: See Adult Dose.

DILUTION

May be given undiluted or further diluted with NS, D5W, or sodium lactate for infusion. The 5% product is isotonic and osmotically approximates human plasma. One volume of 25% to four volumes of diluent is isotonic. Use a filter needle to withdraw albumin into a syringe from the 20 ml vial. Use only clear solutions. Use within 4 hours after opening. Discard unused portions.

Storage: Store at contolled room temperature.

INCOMPATIBLE WITH

Alcohol-containing solutions, amino acid solutions, Ionosol D-CM, Ionosol G with dextrose 10%, midazolam (Versed), IV fat emulsion, protein hydrolysates, verapamil (Isoptin). Do not add directly to packed RBC (unless used as a resuspension vehicle), plasma, or whole blood. May be administered at Y-site.

RATE OF ADMINISTRATION

Variable, depending on indication, present blood volume, patient response, and concentration of solution. Any rate greater than 10 ml/min may cause circulatory overload and pulmonary edema.

Averages are: Normal blood volume: 5%, 5 to 10 ml/min, 25%, 2 to 3 ml/min.

Deficient blood volume (hypovolemia): A single dose as rapidly as tolerated. Repeat dose as rapidly as tolerated if indicated. As volume approaches normal, slow 5% to 2 to 4 ml/min and 25% to 1 ml/min to prevent circulatory overload and pulmonary edema.

Hypoproteinemia: 2 to 3 ml/min in adults, a single dose over 30 to 120 minutes in children.

Infants and children: For uses other than hypovolemia and hypoproteinemia, the rate of administration should be about one-fourth to one-half the adult rate.

ACTIONS

A sterile natural plasma protein substance prepared by a specific process, which makes it free from the danger of serum hepatitis. A blood volume expander that accounts for 70% to 80% of the colloid oncotic pressure of plasma. Expands blood volume proportionately to amount of circulating blood, improves cardiac output, prevents marked hemoconcentration, aids in reduction of edema, and raises serum protein levels. Low sodium content helps to maintain electrolyte balance and should promote diuresis in presence of edema (contains 130 to 160 mEq sodium/L). Also acts as a transport protein that binds both endogenous and exogenous substances, including bilirubin and certain drugs.

INDICATIONS AND USES

Hypovolemia (with or without shock [actual or impending], with or without hemorrhage); 5% if hypovolemic, 25% if adequate hydration or edema is present. ■ Hypoalbuminemia from inadequate production (e.g., burns, congenital analbuminemia, endocrine disorders, infection, liver disease, major injury, malignancy, malnutrition). ■ Hypoalbuminemia from excessive catabolism (e.g., burns, major injury, nephrosis, pancreatitis, pemphigus [chronic relapsing skin disease], thyrotoxicosis). ■ Hypoalbuminemia from loss from the body (e.g., hemorrhage, burn exudates, excessive renal excretion, exfoliative dermatoses, exudative enteropathy [e.g., inflammatory bowel disease]). ■ Hypoalbuminemia from redistribution within the body (e.g., cirrhosis with ascites, inflammatory conditions, major surgery). ■ Hypoalbuminemia secondary to pulmonary edema in adult respiratory distress syndrome (ARDS) (25%). ■ Raising plasma oncotic pressure to treat edema of nephrosis (25%). ■ Cardiopulmonary bypass surgery (25%). ■ Hemolytic disease of the newborn (bilirubin binding activity) as adjunct to exchange transfusion (25%). ■ Provide adequate volume and prevent hypoproteinemia as an adjunct to red blood cell resuspension.

CONTRAINDICATIONS

Anemia (severe), cardiac failure, history of allergic reaction to albumin, pulmonary edema.

PRECAUTIONS

Whole blood or packed cells probably indicated if more than 1,000 ml 5% albumin required in hemorrhage; are adjunctive to use of large amounts of serum albumin to prevent anemia. Is not a substitute for whole blood in situations where both the oxygen-carrying capacity and plasma volume expansion provided by whole blood are required. ■ May be given regardless of patient blood group. ■ Use caution in hypertension, low cardiac reserve, hepatic or renal failure, or lack of albumin deficiency. ■ Use caution in patients with normal or increased intravascular volume, however, patients with hypoproteine-mia may have normal blood volume. ■ 25 Gm of albumin is the osmotic equivalent of 2 units of fresh-frozen plasma. 25 Gm of albumin provides as much plasma protein as 500 ml of plasma or 2 units of whole blood. ■ Albumin is not a source of nutrition.

Monitor: Monitor blood pressure. ■ Hemoglobin, hematocrit, electro-lyte, and serum protein evaluations are mandatory during therapy. Alkaline phosphatase may be elevated. ■ Observe patient carefully for increased bleeding resulting from more normal blood pressure, cir-culatory embarrassment, pulmonary edema, or lack of diuresis. Central venous pressure readings are most helpful. ■ Maintain hydra-tion with additional fluids especially in dehydrated patients. ■ Normal plasma albumin is 3.5 to 6 Gm/100 ml.

Maternal/child: Category C: safety for use during pregnancy not estab-lished. ■ Do not use 25% solution in preterm infants.

Elderly: Monitor fluid intake carefully; more susceptible to circulatory overload and pulmonary edema. ■ Plasma albumin levels may be more volatile.

SIDE EFFECTS

Minor: Fever, nausea, salivation, vomiting.

Major: Circulatory failure, dyspnea, elevated central venous pressure, precipitous hypotension, pulmonary edema.

ANTIDOTE

Notify the physician of all side effects. Minor side effects are gener-ally tolerated and treated symptomatically. For major side effects, dis-continue albumin and treat symptomatically. Resuscitate as necessary.

ALDESLEUKIN

Antineoplastic
Immunomodulator
Biological response modifier
Recombinant interleukin-2

interleukin-2 recombinant, Proleukin, rIL-2   pH 7.2 to 7.8

> **Numerous changes for aldesleukin were recently approved by the FDA. Information was not available in time to update this monograph. Please turn to Appendix G, p. 908, for a revised monograph incorporating these recent changes.**

USUAL DOSE

Patient selection restricted. Prescreening and baseline studies required; note Precautions/Monitor.

Intermittent IV: Standard high-dose regimen: 600,000 IU/kg (0.037 mg/kg) every 8 hours for 14 doses. After 9 days of rest repeat for up to 14 more doses; this constitutes one course (two 5-day [14 or fewer doses] treatment cycles separated by a rest period of 9 days). Treat with 28 doses or until dose-limiting toxicity requiring ICU level support occurs.

Low-dose regimen (investigational): Intermittent: 72,000 IU/kg every 8 hours. Cycles same as standard regimen. Low-dose regimens are especially useful in patients at greater risk with a higher dose.

In all situations, evaluate for response 4 weeks after course completion and again before scheduling start of the next course. Additional courses are considered if there is some tumor shrinkage following the previous course, a CT scan rules out disease progression, and retreatment is not contraindicated. At least 7 weeks from hospital discharge should elapse before a second course is administered. Sometimes given in combination with other agents (see Indications).

Investigational protocols: Other investigational protocols have been used (see below). These various protocols expressed doses of aldesleukin in Cetus, Roche, or international units. Aldesleukin is available only in international units, 1 Cetus unit = 6IU, 1 Roche unit = 3 IU. Results from studies include stable disease or disease regression with some decreased toxicity, but efficacy not established.

Continuous IV (Investigational): 18,000,000 IU/M^2/day as a continuous infusion. Each daily dose is given over 24 hours (interrupted as indicated by patient symptoms) for two 5-day cycles with 5 to 8 days of rest before the second cycle. Another investigational study administers the daily dose for 4 days followed by 3 days off. This cycle is repeated for 4 weeks followed by 2 weeks off. Based on patient tolerance, the entire sequence is usually repeated until some response occurs. Another investigational low-dose regimen given on an outpatient basis uses 18,000,000 IU given as a clysis over 6 to 8 hours, Monday through Friday, 4 weeks on and 2 weeks off. Beginning with the second cycle, doses on day 1 and 2 are reduced to 9,000,000 IU. Other investigational studies are using SC injection.

DOSE ADJUSTMENTS

Doses are frequently withheld for toxicity. Doses are actually withheld, not reduced in amount. Median number of doses actually administered in a first course is 20. ▪ Hold doses and restart based on the following:

Hold dose for	May give next dose if
Cardiovascular:	
Atrial fibrillation, supraventricular tachycardia, bradycardia that requres treatment or is recurrent or persisent.	Patient is asymptomatic with full recovery to normal sinus rhythm.
Systolic BP < 90 mm Hg with increasing requirements for pressors.	Systolic BP > 90 mm Hg and stable or improving requirements for pressors.
Any ECG change consistent with MI or ischemia with or without chest pain; suspicion of cardiac ischemia.	Patient is asymptomatic, MI has been ruled out, clinical suspicion of angina is low.
Pulmonary:	
O_2 saturation < 94% on room air or < 90% with 2 L O_2 by nasal prongs.	O_2 saturation > 94% on room air or > 90% with 2 L O_2 by nasal prongs.
Central Nervous System:	
Mental status changes (e.g., agitation, confusion, lethargy, somnolence).	Mental status changes completely resolved.
Systemic:	
Sepsis syndrome; patient is clinically unstable.	Sepsis syndrome has resolved, patient is clinically stable, infection is under treatment.
Renal:	
Serum creatinine > 4.5 mg/dl or a serum creatinine of 4 mg/dl in presence of severe volume overload, acidosis, or hyperkalemia.	Serum creatinine < 4 mg/dl, and fluid and electrolyte status is stable.
Persistent oliguria, urine output of < 10 ml/hr for 16 to 24 hr with rising serum creatinine.	Urine output > 10 ml/hr with a decrease of serum creatinine > 1.5 mg/dl or normalization of serum creatinine.
Hepatic:	
Signs of hepatic failure including encephalopathy, increasing ascites, liver pain, hypoglycemia.	Discontinue for remainder of current course. May consider a new course of treatment in 7 weeks if all signs of hepatic failure have resolved.

Hold dose for	May give next dose if
Gastrointestinal:	
Stool guaiac repeatedly > 3 to 4$^+$.	Stool guaiac negative.
Skin:	
Bullous dermatitis or marked worsening of preexisting skin condition (avoid topical steroid therapy).	Resolution of all signs of bullous dermatitis.

- After withholding a dose, no dose should be given until patient is globally assessed and specific criteria for restarting aldesleukin are met.

DILUTION

Each 22,000,000 IU vial (1.3 mg) must be reconstituted with 1.2 ml of preservative-free sterile water for injection (18,000,000 IU/ml [1.1 mg/ml]). Sterile technique imperative. Direct diluent to side of vial and gently swirl to avoid excess foaming. Do not shake. Plastic infusion containers are preferred over glass. Do not use any filters for dilution or administration. Do not use any other diluent or infusion solution; may cause increased aggregation. Bring to room temperature before administration. Each single dose must be further diluted in 50 ml of D5W in water and given as an intermittent IV.

Continuous IV (Investigational): A single dose may be further diluted in D5W, but for each 50 ml of D5W, 1 ml of 5% human serum albumin (0.2 ml of 25%) must be added to the plastic infusion bag before adding reconstituted dose of aldesleukin. For 500 ml of diluent (D5W) 10 ml of 5% HSA or 2 ml of 25% HSA would be required. Final concentration of aldesleukin in D5W should be under 60 mcg/ml or over 100 mcg/ml. Solution unstable between 60 and 100 mcg/ml. Manufacturer provides a worksheet to guide dilution for continuous IV infusion with a programmed infusion pump.

Storage: Store in refrigerator before and after reconstitution and dilution. Do not freeze. No stability problems will occur at controlled room temperature for 48 hours after dilution but has no preservatives. Do not use beyond expiration date on vial. Stable for up to 6 days in a programmed infusion pump in a concentration of 100 to 500 mcg/ml.

INCOMPATIBLE WITH

Manufacturer states "do not mix with any other drug." Bacteriostatic water for injection or normal saline will increase aggregation.

Y-site: Ganciclovir (Cytovene), lorazepam (Ativan), pentamidine (Pentam 300), prochlorperazine (Compazine), promethazine (Phenergan).

RATE OF ADMINISTRATION

Intermittent IV: A single dose as an intermittent infusion over 15 minutes. Flush main line IV with D5W before and after each use. Manufacturer recommends that any keep-open IV in place for intermittent administration be D5W with no more than 10 mEq of potassium added.

Continuous IV (investigational): A single dose equally distributed over 24 hours. Only compatible with D5W. Must be administered through a programmed infusion pump. The Pharmacia Deltec CADD system has been used in clinical studies. Use of a central venous catheter is appropriate. All recommendations under Dilution (e.g., concentration and addition of albumin) are indicated.

ACTIONS

A genetically engineered recombinant protein that possesses the biologic activity of naturally occurring interleukin-2. It boosts immune system function by increasing production of immune system cells (e.g., T lymphocytes), inducing interferon-gamma activity, and enhancing the activity of other lymphokines. Lymphocytes exposed to interleukin-2 become capable of killing cancer cells and are called lymphokine activitated killer (LAK) cells. Clinically significant numbers of lymphokines become available as contrasted to a smaller quantity generated naturally. It can result in an immune response—related destruction of cancer cells and the reduction or elimination of tumor mass. 30% of a dose initally distributes to plasma and then to extravascular, extracellular spaces; 70% of a dose distributes rapidly into the liver, kidney, and lung. Half-life is from 13 to 85 minutes (distribution to elimination). Metabolized to amino acids in proximal convoluted tubules of the kidney. No active drug is found in urine. May cross blood-brain barrier. Not known if it crosses placental barrier or is secreted in breast milk.

INDICATIONS AND USES

Prescreening mandatory. Eligibility requirements for treatment are specific and directly impact response rate and toxicity (asymptomatic preferred; symptomatic and fully ambulatory may be considered). ▪ Treatment of metastatic renal cell carcinoma in adults over 18 years of age. May be used as a single agent, in combination with interferon-alfa, or in combination with interferon-alfa and 5-fluorouracil. Response rate is about 15% but may last an average of 2 years; may be complete or partial. ▪ Treatment of adults with metastatic melanoma. May be used as a single agent, in combination with interferon-alfa, in combination with chemotherapy, or in combination with interferon-alfa and chemotherapy. Several chemotherapy combinations have been used (Dartmouth regimen [carmustine, dacarbazine, cisplatin, and tamoxifen]; CVD regimen [cisplatin, vinblastine, and dacarbazine]).

Investigational uses: Kaposi's sarcoma in combination with zidovudine. ▪ Colorectal cancer. ▪ Non-Hodgkin's lymphoma. ▪ Lung cancer. ▪ Ovarian cancer.

CONTRAINDICATIONS

Abnormal thallium stress test or pulmonary function tests. ▪ Known hypersensitivity to interleukin-2 or any component of aldesleukin. ▪ Patients with organ allografts. ▪ Exclude from treatment any patient with significant cardiac, pulmonary, renal, hepatic or CNS impairment, any patient requiring treatment with steroidal agents, and any patient at higher risk for cardiovascular adverse events during periods of hypotension and fluid shifts.

Retreatment is permanently contraindicated in patients who experienced specific toxicities in a previous course of therapy, i.e.,

Organ system	Symptom
Cardiovascular	Sustained ventricular tachycardia ≥5 beats. Cardiac rhythm disturbances not controlled or unresponsive to management. Recurrent chest pain with ECG changes consistent with angina or myocardial infarction. Pericardial tamponade.
Pulmonary	Intubation required more than 72 hours.
Renal	Renal dysfunction requiring dialysis over 72 hours.
Central Nervous System	Coma or toxic psychosis lasting more than 48 hours. Repetitive or difficult to control seizures.
Gastrointestinal	Bowel ischemia or perforation. Bleeding requiring surgery.

PRECAUTIONS

Administered in the hospital under the supervision of a qualified physician (usually a medical oncologist and/or immunologist). Intensive care facilitites and specialists in cardiopulmonary and/or intensive care medicine must be available. ■ Capillary leak syndrome (CLS [extravasation of plasma proteins and fluid into the extravascular space and loss of vascular tone]) can begin immediately after aldesleukin treatment starts and results in hypotension and reduced organ perfusion that can be severe enough to result in death. ■ Therapy should be restricted to patients with normal cardiac, pulmonary, renal, hepatic, and CNS functions as defined by appropriate tests. Patients who have had a nephrectomy are eligible for treatment if serum creatinine is below 1.5 mg/dl (85% of patients in one study). ■ Use extreme caution in patients with normal thallium stress tests and pulmonary function tests who have a history of prior cardiac or pulmonary disease. ■ May exacerbate disease symptoms in clinically unrecognized or untreated CNS metastases. Thoroughly evaluate and treat CNS metastases prior to aldesleukin therapy. Should be neurologically stable and have a negative CT scan. ■ Use extreme caution in patients with a history of seizures (may cause seizures), patients with fixed requirements for large volumes of fluid (e.g., hypercalcemia), those with autoimmune disorders (e.g., Crohn's disease, ulcerative colitis, or psoriasis), previous cytotoxic drug therapy or radiation therapy, and patients sensitive to *Escherichia coli*-derived proteins. ■ Associated with impaired neutrophil function and an increased risk of disseminated infection, including sepsis and bacterial endocarditis. Preexisting bacterial infections should be adequately treated before beginning therapy. ■ Induces significant hypotension; discontinue antihypertensives during treatment. ■ May impair thyroid function; thyroid replacement therapy has been required in a few patients. ■ Note Drug/lab interactions.

Monitor: A central venous catheter (double or triple lumen) is frequently ordered on admission (required for continuous infusion). A minimum of two IV lines is usually required (one for the aldesleukin and its keep-open IV and one for other needed fluids and medications). One line could suffice if absolutely necessary since aldesleukin would be discontinued when colloids are administered. Flushing of line with D5W before and after aldesleukin is imperative. Ability to record CVP and draw blood samples should be available. ■ Admission chest x-ray, ECG, SMA-20, CBC with differential and platelet-count, T_3, T_4, PT, PTT, urinalysis and body weight should be obtained. Adequate pulmonary function, normal arterial blood gases, and normal ejection fraction and unimpaired wall motion (confirmed by thallium stress test and/or a stress echocardiogram) should be documented. ■ Continuous cardiac monitoring is indicated (required with blood pressure below 90 mm Hg or any cardiac irregularity). ■ Monitoring and flexibility in management of fluid and organ perfusion status is imperative. Requires constant management and balancing of effects of fluid shifts to prevent the consequences of hypovolemia (e.g., impaired organ function [such as breakdown of blood-brain barrier]) or fluid accumulation (e.g., edema, pulmonary edema, ascites, pulmonary effusion), which may exceed the patient's tolerance. ■ Assess hypovolemia by central venous catheterization and frequent central venous pressure monitoring. Administer colloids (albumin, plasmanate) or crystalloids (IV fluids) as indicated for a blood pressure drop of 20 mm Hg or greater or a CVP reading lower than 3 to 4 mm H_2O. ■ Neuro checks (note agitation, blurred vision, and persistent somnolence), vital signs, and strict I and O are required every 2 to 4 hours (much more frequently as side effects develop). ■ Weigh daily. ■ Blood is drawn twice daily (AM: CBC with differential and platelet count, SMA-20, PT, PTT; PM: SMA-6, electrolytes and creatinine [to check if evening dose can be given; significant changes in creatinine usually do not occur in less than 12 hr]). ■ Assess thyroid function periodically. ■ An ECG is indicated for any abnormal complex or rhythm. ■ Obtain a urinalysis as indicated, and draw a magnesium level for any respiratory problems, arrhythmias, or other electrolyte disturbances. ■ Assess pulmonary function through examination, vital signs, and pulse oximetry. Arterial blood gases are indicated for any dyspnea or respiratory impairment. ■ Some routine medications are indicated prophylactically to reduce incidence of side effects and to promote patient comfort. The morning of the first treatment begin acetaminophen 650 mg p.o. q 4 hr and indomethacin 25 mg q 6 hr (may increase nephrotoxicity) or naprosyn 500 mg q 12 hr p.o. for fever and arthralgia. Use ranitidine 150 mg p.o. q 12 hr or cimetidine 300 mg q 6 hr to prevent GI bleeding. Continue administration of these drugs until 12 hours after last dose of aldesleukin. Low-dose dopamine 1 to 5 mcg/kg can help maintain organ perfusion and urine output if given at initial onset of CLS before hypotension occurs. Give prophylactic ciprofloxacin 250 mg p.o. q 12 hr for patients with central venous lines (may be given IV [200 mg] or can substitute cefazolin, oxacillin, nafcillin, or vancomycin [must be active against *S. aureus*]; begin when line is placed and continue for 5 days after removal). Antiemetics, antidiarrheals, antichill/rigors (meperidine), antihistamines, and moisturizing skin lotions will also be used throughout treatment (note Antidote for specifics). ▪ If fever occurs several days into treatment or recurs after subsiding, assume infection first, then drug. Draw cultures; administer appropriate antibiotics. ▪ Patients who have had nephrectomies may be more at risk for increases in serum BUN or creatinine, electrolyte shifts, and reduced urine output. Evaluate fluid, electrolyte and acid base status promptly if any of the above occur. Gradual increases without other complications (marked fluid overload, hyperkalemia, acidosis) are frequently tolerated (serum creatinine must not exceed 4.5 mg/dl). ▪ Maintain pulmonary status as needed with O_2, diuretics (furosemide) and maintain serum bicarbonate above 15 mEq/L. Assess pulmonary status with chest x-rays. ▪ Monitor central and peripheral IV sites to reduce potential for infection. Change peripheral sites every 3 days. ▪ No restrictions on activity; use caution ambulating (orthostatic hypotension). ▪ No restrictions on diet. Encouragement may be required (anorexia and/or mouth sores). ▪ Specific preparation required for discharge; refer to literature. ▪ Manufacturer supplies excellent brochures with detailed guidelines in chart form on all aspects of monitoring, toxicity, and treatment for nurses and physicians. ▪ Complete review and adequate preparation of all aspects of this therapy with the patient and family are imperative. Can reduce psychological stress of toxicity. ▪ Tumor regression has continued for up to 12 months after one or more courses of therapy. ▪ Note Dose adjustments, Contraindications, and Antidote.

Patient education: Many side effects will occur; report any changes you perceive so they can be evaluated and treated if needed (e.g., changes in breathing, chest or other pain, temperature, mood, lightheadedness, fatigue). ▪ Request assistance for ambulation and always sit on the side of the bed first. ▪ Take only prescribed medications. ▪ Avoid alcohol. ▪ Use of effective contraceptive measures recommended for fertile men and women. ▪ Use 15 SPF sunscreen in sunlight to protect against photosensitivity. ▪ See Appendix D, p. 900, for additional information. ▪ Manufacturer supplies a patient education booklet; review thoroughly and discuss with your physicain and nurse.

Maternal/child: Pregnancy Category C: animal studies not conducted; effects unknown. Benefits must outweigh risks. Contraceptive measures required before initial administration and throughout treatment. ▪ Discontinue breast feeding. ▪ Safety for use in children under 18 years of age not established; studies show responsiveness and toxicity similar.

Elderly: May not tolerate toxicity; use caution, consider age-related organ impairment.

DRUG/LAB INTERACTIONS

May cause interactions with psychotropic drugs (e.g, analgesics, antiemetics, narcotics, sedatives, tranquilizers) because aldesleukin also affects central nervous function. ▪ Concomitant use with cardiotoxic agents (e.g., doxorubicin [Adriamycin]), hepatotoxic agents (e.g., methotrexate, asparaginase), myelotoxic agents (e.g., cytotoxic chemotherapy, radiation therapy), and nephrotoxic agents (e.g., aminoglycosides, indomethacin) may increase toxicity in these organ systems. ▪ Effects may be potentiated by drugs that also cause blood dyscrasias (e.g., penicillins, phenothiazines). ▪ May cause severe allergic reactions with iodinated contrast media. ▪ Glucocorticoids (e.g., dexamethasone [Decadron]) reduce aldesleukin-induced side effects but also reduce its antitumor effectiveness. ▪ Aldesleukin-induced hypotension may be potentiated by beta-blockers (e.g., metoprolol, atenolol) and antihypertensive agents (e.g., nitroglycerin IV, nitroprusside). ▪ Capable of altering numerous lab values, see literature.

SIDE EFFECTS

Frequent, predictable, often severe; are usually clinically manageable and frequently require intensive care management. Begin to occur shortly after therapy begins (chills, fatigue, fever, hypotension, nausea, vomiting). Frequency and severity are dose-related and schedule-dependent. Most are reversible within 2 or 3 days of discontinuation of therapy. Even with intensive management, side effects can progress to death.

Average dose: Initially anorexia, arthralgia, chills, fatigue, fever, nausea, and vomiting occur. Initial symptoms of capillary leak syndrome are edema, electrolyte abnormalities, hypotension, oliguria, respiratory distress, significant weight gain, tachycardia. Effects of CLS **successively** result in *hypovolemia* which in turn leads to→ hypotension→ hypoperfusion→ sinus tachycardia→ myocardial ischemia→ arrhythmias→ decreased renal perfusion→ prerenal azotemia→ oliguria→ anuria; *fluid retention/weight gain* which in turn leads to→ rales→ dyspnea→ cough→ tachypnea→ hypoxia→ pleural effusion→ diarrhea→ edema of the bowel→ refractory acidosis→ edema→ ascites; *and breakdown of blood-brain barrier* (neuropsychiatric toxicity [e.g., agitation, combativeness, confusion, hallucinations, lethargy, psychosis, somolence]). Abdominal pain and GI bleeding may be related to diarrhea, vomiting, stomatitis, duodenal ulcer formation, bowel ischemia or perforation. Cerebral edema and concomitant medications may impact many side effects. Lethargy and/or somnolence may lead to coma. Anemia and thrombocytopenia may occur; coagulation abnormalities (PT, PTT) reflect liver dysfunction. Hemodynamic effects similar to septic shock may be caused by tumor necrosis factor. Erythematous rash and pruritus (can progress to dry desquamation) can occur in almost all patients and are extremely uncomfortable.

ANTIDOTE

Temporarily discontinue aldesleukin and notify physician immediately of arrhythmias or rhythm changes, chest pain, marked changes in heart rate, positive neuropsychiatric check (agitation, blurred vision, persistent extreme somnolence), systolic blood pressure below 90 mm Hg, apical heart rate over 120, temperature over 38° C (100.4° F), respirations over 25/min, complaints of dyspnea, decreased breath sounds, or increased sputum production, urinary output less than 200 ml/4 hr, CVP reading below 3 to 4 mm H_2O, weight increase over 4 kg or 10% of baseline over 5 days, abnormal blood or urine tests (e.g., serum bicarbonate < 15 mEq/L, serum creatinine > 4 to 4.5 mg/dl [based on gradual or sudden rise and if accompanied by other complications]), severe diarrhea associated with refractory acidosis, vomiting refractory to treatment, acute changes in GI status. May be restarted based on patient response. Hold any subsequent dose for failure to maintain organic perfusion (see Dose adjustments). Fever is routinely treated with acetaminophen and indomethacin or naprosyn; increased doses may be needed; administer rectally if nausea and vomiting are present. Suggested treatments include slow IV meperidine (Demerol) 25 to 50 mg for chills and rigidity; kaopectate, diphenoxylate (Lomotil), or loperamide (Imodium) p.o. for diarrhea (these meds may not help and diarrhea may be dose limiting); diphenhydramine (Benadryl) 25 mg p.o. q 6 hr, a soothing skin cream (Eucerin), and oatmeal baths for urticaria and pruritus; temazepam (Restoril) for insomnia; ondansetron (Zofran) or prochlorperazine (Compazine) for nausea. Treat edema with furosemide (Lasix). IV fluids, albumin or plasmanate, and Trendelenburg positioning are used to maintain fluid balance and blood pressure. If organ perfusion and blood pressure are not sustained by dopamine 2 to 5 mcg/kg as a continuous infusion, increase to 6 to 10 mcg/kg or add phenylephrine (1 to 5 mcg/kg/min). Prolonged use of pressors at relatively high doses may cause cardiac arrhythmias. Treat arrhythmias as indicated (usually sinus or supraventricular tachycardia [adenosine, verapamil]). Use O_2 for decreased PaO_2. Use packed red blood cells for anemia and to ensure maximum oxygen carrying capacity. Platelet transfusions are indicated for thrombocytopenia or to reduce risk of GI bleeding. Special precautions may be required (e.g., avoid IM injections; test urine, emesis, stool, secretions for occult blood). All treatment is supportive; recovery should begin within a few hours of cessation of aldesleukin. With normalized blood pressure, diuretics (furosemide [Lasix]) can hasten recovery. Low-dose haloperidol (Haldol) may help severe mental status changes.

More rapid onset of dose-limiting toxicities will occur with overdose. **Dexamethasone (Decadron)** is indicated to counteract life-threatening toxicities. May result in loss of therapeutic effect.

ALFENTANIL HYDROCHLORIDE

General anesthetic
Narcotic analgesic agonist
Anesthesia adjunct

Alfenta　　　　　　　　　　　　　　　　　　　　　　pH 4 to 6

USUAL DOSE

Adults and children 12 years of age and older: Dose must be individualized and titrated to the desired effect in each patient according to body weight, physical status, underlying pathological condition, use of other drugs, and type and duration of surgical procedure and anesthesia. Usually used in conjunction with short-acting barbiturates (e.g., thiopental [Pentothal]), neuromuscular blocking agents (e.g, pancuronium [Pavulon], succinycholine [Anectine], and an inhalation anesthetic (e.g., nitrous oxide) to maintain balanced anesthesia. Use reduced doses of a neuromuscular blocking agent prophylactically to prevent muscle rigidity or to induce muscle relaxation after rigidity occurs. Full paralyzing doses may be used after loss of consciousness. Use of a benzodiazepine (e.g., diazepam [Valium], midazolam [Versed]) may reduce induction dose requirements, decrease time to loss of consciousness, and diminish patient recall (note Drug/lab interactions). Note Dose adjustments.

FOR USE DURING GENERAL ANESTHESIA	
SPONTANEOUSLY BREATHING/ ASSISTED VENTILATION Procedures lasting up to 30 minutes	Induction of Analgesia: 8-20 mcg/kg Maintenance of Analgesia: 3-5 mcg/kg q 5-20 min or 0.5 to 1 mcg/kg/min Total dose: 8-40 mcg/kg
ASSISTED OR CONTROLLED VENTILATION Incremental Injection in procedures lasting longer than 30 minutes (To attenuate response to laryngoscopy and intubation)	Induction of Analgesia: 20-50 mcg/kg Maintenance of Analgesia: 5-15 mcg/kg q 5-20 min Total dose: Up to 75 mcg/kg
Continuous Infusion in procedures lasting longer than 30 minutes (To provide attenuation of response to intubation and incision)	Infusion rates are variable and should be titrated to the desired clinical effect. SEE INFUSION DOSAGE GUIDELINES (NEXT PAGE) Induction of Analgesia: 50-75 mcg/kg Maintenace of Analgesia: 0.5 to 1.5 mcg/kg/min or general anethestic Total dose: Dependent on duration of procedure
Anesthetic Induction Procedures lasting 45 minutes or longer	Induction of Anesthesia: 130-245 mcg/kg Maintenance of Analgesia: 0.5 to 1.5 mcg/kg/min or general anesthetic Total dose: Dependent of duration of procedure At these doses, truncal rigidity should be expected and a muscle relaxant should be utilized Administer slowly (over 3 minutes) Concentration of inhalation agents reduced by 30%-50% for initial hour.
MONITORED ANESTHESIA CARE (MAC) (For sedated and responsive, spontaneously breathing patients)	Induction of MAC: 3-8 mcg/kg Maintenance of MAC: 3-5 mcg/kg q 5-20 min or 0.25 to 1 mcg/kg/min Total dose: 3-40 mcg/kg

FOR USE DURING GENERAL ANESTHESIA
INFUSION DOSAGE
Continuous infusion: 0.5-3 mcg/kg/min administered with nitrous oxide/ oxygen in patients undergoing general surgery. Following an anesthetic induction dose of alfentanil, infusion rate requirements are reduced by 30%-50% for the first hour of maintenance.
Changes in vital signs that indicate a response to surgical stress or lightening of anesthesia may be controlled by increasing the alfentanil to a maximum of 4 mcg/kg/min and/or administration of bolus doses of 7 mcg/kg. If changes are not controlled after three bolus doses given over a 5-minute period, a barbiturate, vasodilator, and/or inhalation agent should be used. Infusion rates should always be adjusted downward in the absence of these signs until there is some response to surgical stimulation.
Rather than an increase in infusion rate, 7 mcg/kg bolus doses of alfentanil or a potent inhalation agent should be administered in response to signs of lightening of anesthesia within the last 15 minutes of surgery. Alfentanil infusion should be discontinued at least 10 to 15 minutes before the end of surgery.
Discontinue 10 to 15 minutes before end of procedures in general anesthesia. Continue infusion to end of procedure during MAC, then discontinue.

PEDIATRIC DOSE

Half-life and duration of action is decreased in children; more frequent supplemental doses may be required. Not recommended for use in children under 12 years of age.

DOSE ADJUSTMENTS

Reduce dose of one or both agents when given in combination with other CNS depressants (e.g., barbiturates, inhalation anesthetics, narcotic analgesics, tranquilizers). ■ Calculate dose based on lean body weight in obese patients (more than 20% above ideal body weight). ■ Reduced initial dose required in elderly or debilitated patients (a 40% reduction was required in one study); reduced supplemental doses, a slower infusion rate, or longer intervals between doses may be required based on effects of initial dose. ■ Reduced dose may be required in hypothyroidism and in impaired hepatic function. ■ Note Drug/lab interations.

DILUTION

IV injection: Small volumes may be given undiluted (usually by the anesthesiologist). Use of tuberculin syringe recommended (1 ml equals 500 mcg). Further dilution with 5 ml of SW or NS to facilitate titration is appropriate.

Infusion: Dilute 20 ml alfentanil with 230 ml NS, D5/NS, D5W, or LR to achieve a conentration of 40 mcg/ml. Desired concentration range is 25 to 80 mcg/ml.

Storage: Store ampules at CRT; protect from light.

INCOMPATIBLE WITH

Diazepam (Valium), thiopental (Pentothal).

RATE OF ADMINISTRATION

IV injection: Administer over a minimum of 3 minutes. Rapid administration of lower doses or administration of full anesthetic doses will result in muscle rigidity, apnea, respiratory paralysis, loss of vascular tone, and hypotension. Titrate rate to desired patient response.

Infusion: See Usual dose.

ACTIONS

An opioid derivative, narcotic analgesic, and descending CNS depressant. Less potent than fentanyl milligram for milligram, but achieves higher plasma concentrations. Produces hypnosis and respiratory depressant actions that outlast its analgesic effect. Onset of action is immediate. Produces analgesic effects in 1 minute. Peak effect (respiratory depression and analgesia) occurs within 1½ to 2 minutes. With induction doses, loss of consciousness occurs within 1 to 2 minutes. Provides dose-related protection against hemodynamic responses to surgical stress. Histamine release rarely occurs. May cause rigidity of chest, pharynx, and abdominal muscles inhibiting ventilation (see Precautions/Monitor, Side effects, and Antidote). Duration of action is 5 to 10 minutes. Has a terminal half-life of 90 to 111 minutes. Cumulative effects are somewhat less than with fentanyl or sufentanil, but with repeat doses recovery may be prolonged. Recovery should occur within 10 to 15 minutes of end of procedure or 25 to 30 minutes after last incremental dose or discontinuing the infusion. Metabolized in the liver. Excreted as metabolites in urine. Crosses the placental barrier. Secreted in breast milk.

INDICATIONS AND USES

Analgesic adjunct given in incremental doses in the maintenance of anesthesia with barbiturate/nitrous oxide/oxygen. ■ Analgesic administered by continuous infusion with nitrous oxide/oxygen in the maintenance of general anesthesia. ■ Primary anesthetic agent for the induction of anesthesia in patients undergoing general surgery requiring endotracheal intubation and mechanical ventilation. ■ Analgesic component for monitored anesthesia care (MAC) during surgical or diagnostic procedures.

CONTRAINDICATIONS

Known hypersensitivity to alfentanil or known intolerance to other opioid agonists (e.g., fentanyl, sufentanil).

PRECAUTIONS

For IV use only. ■ Administered by or under the direct observations of the anesthesiologist. Must have responsibility only for anesthesia and continous observation of the patient during surgery and/or procedure. ■ Staff must be skilled in medical management of critically ill patients, cardiovascular resuscitation, and airway management. ■ Use caution; plasma clearance reduced and recovery time prolonged in the elderly and in patients with impaired liver function (half-life prolonged [up to 5.8 hours]); reduced dose may be indicated. ■ Use caution in patients with pulmonary disease, decreased respiratory reserve, or potentially compromised respiration. May cause rigidity of chest and abdominal muscles, decrease respiratory drive, and increase airway resistance; may require assisted or controlled ventilation. ■ Use caution in patients with head injury or increased intracranial pressure; risk of respiratory depression is increased. ■ Respiratory depression may cause an increased PCO_2 cerebral vasodilation, and increased intracranial pressure. Clinical course of head injury may be obscured. ■ Use caution in patients with bradyarrhythmias. ■ Use caution in patients with hypothyroidism; risk of respiratory depression and prolonged CNS depression is increased. Reduced doses may be indicated. ■ Note Drug/lab interactions.

Monitor: Oxygen, controlled ventilation equipment, opioid antagonists (e.g., naloxone [Narcan], nalmefene [Revex], and neuromuscular blocking agents (e.g., pancuronium [Pavulon], succinylcholine [Anectine]) and all emergency drugs and equipment must be immediately available. Can cause rigidity of respiratory muscles; concurrent use of a neuromuscular blocking agent can prevent or reverse muscle rigidity to permit controlled ventilation. ▪ Adequate preoperative hydration is recommended to reduce incidence of hypotension. ▪ Observe for hypotension, apnea, upper airway obstruction, and/or oxygen desaturation. Monitor vital signs and oxygen saturation continuously. If not unconscious, pateint will appear to be asleep and forget to breathe unless commanded to do so. ▪ Additional doses of alfentanil can be used to control tachycardia and hypertension during surgery. ▪ Prolonged postoperative monitoring may be indicated; respiratory depression, respiratory arrest, bradycardia, asystole, arrhythmias, and hypotension may occur after initial recovery ▪ Keep patient supine; orthostatic hypotension and fainting may occur. ▪ Has a short duration of action; pain medication may be required soon after initial recovery. ▪ Note Precautions and Drug/lab interactions.

Patient education: Avoid alcohol or other CNS depressants (e.g., antihistamines, benzodiazepines (e.g., diazepam [Valium]). ▪ Blurred vision, dizziness, drowsiness, or lightheadedness may occur; use caution. ▪ Review all medication for interactions.

Maternal/child: Pregnancy category C: safety for use in pregnancy not established. ▪ Not recommended for use during labor and delivery. ▪ Postpone breast feeding for at least 24 hours after use of alfentanil. ▪ Safety for use in children under 12 years of age not established.

Elderly: Note Dose adjustments and Precautions. ▪ May markedly decrease pulmonary ventilation. ▪ Decreased protein binding, decreased clearance, and possible increased brain sensitivity may make the elderly more sensitive to effects (e.g., respiratory depression, extended recovery time, urinary retention, constipation). ▪ Analgesia should be effective with lower doses. ▪ Consider age-related organ impairment; elimination half-life is extended, postoperative recovery may be delayed.

DRUG/LAB INTERACTIONS

Use of benzodiazepines (e.g., diazepam [Valium], midazolam [Versed]) may decrease dose of alfentanil required and decrease patient recall, but when given immediately before or in conjunction with high doses of alfentanil, benzodiazepines may produce vasodilation, severe hypotension, and result in delayed recovery. ▪ After an anesthetic induction dose of alfentanil, requirements for volatile inhalation anesthetics (e.g., nitrous oxide) and/or alfentanil infusion are reduced by 30% to 50% for the first hour of maintenance. ▪ Beta-adrenergic blocking agents (e.g., metoprolol, timolol) may be used preoperatively to decrease hypertensive episodes during surgical procedures, but chronic use (including ophthalmic preparations) may also increase the risk of initial bradycardia. ▪ Respiratory depression, CNS depression, hypotensive effects, and duration of action increased with concomitant administration of other CNS depressants (e.g., antidepressants, antihistamines, barbiturates, benzodiazepines, haloperidol, inhalation anesthetics, narcotic analgesics, phenothiazines). Reduced doses of one or both agents usually required. ▪ Clearance significantly decreased by erythromycin; risk of prolonged or delayed respiratory depression may be increased. ▪ Respiratory depressant effects are additive with neuromuscular blocking agents (e.g., pancuronium, succinylcholine). ▪ Clearance decreased by cimetidine (Tagamet); even if doses of alfentanil are reduced with prolonged administration, duration of action may be extended. ▪ Other opioids have caused severe hypertension with MAO inhibitors (e.g., selegiline [Eldepryl]). Use extreme caution; beta blockers (e.g., propranolol) and vasodilators (e.g., nitroglycerin) should be available. ▪ Duration of action may be prolonged with other agents that inhibit hepatic enzymes (e.g., beta blockers [e.g., metoprolol (Lopressor), propranolol (Inderal), timolol (Novo-Timol)], calcium channel blockers [e.g., diltiazem (Cardizem), verapamil (Isoptin)], fluoroquinolones [e.g., ciprofloxacin (Cipro), levofloxacin (Levaquin)], MAO inhibitors). ▪ Use of naltrexone (ReVia) would require increased doses of alfentanil; may cause prolonged respiratory depression and/or circulatory collapse. Discontinue naltrexone several days before elective surgery if use of an opioid is necessary. ▪ Cerebrospinal fluid pressure may be increased. ▪ May delay gastic emptying and invalidate diagnostic tests. ▪ May interfere with some hepatobiliary imaging. ▪ Delay plasma amylase and lipase measurements for at least 24 hours.

SIDE EFFECTS

Average dose: Bradycardia and hypotension may occur shortly after administration. Respiratory depression caused by alfentanil and/or muscle rigidity may progress to apnea. Agitation, allergic reactions (e.g., anaphylaxis, bronchospasm, itching, laryngospasm, urticaria), arrhythmias (e.g., bradycardia, tachycardia), blurred vision, bradypnea, chest wall rigidity, dizziness, euphoria, headache, hypercapnia (increased CO_2), hypertension, hypotension, muscle rigidity (skeletal muscles including abdomen, chest, pharynx, neck, and extremities), myoclonic movements, nausea, postoperative confusion, respiratory sedation, skeletal muscle movements, shivering, sleepiness, vomiting.

Overdose: Bradycardia; circulatory depression; cold, clammy skin; dizziness (severe); drowsiness (severe); hypotension; nervousness or restlessness (severe); pinpoint pupils of eyes; respiratory depression; weakness (severe).

ANTIDOTE

Many side effects are medical emergencies. Manage respiratory depression during surgery via endotracheal intubation and assisted or controlled ventilation; prolonged mechanical ventilation may be required. Treat postoperative respiratory depression with naloxone (Narcan) or nalmefene (Revex); titrate dose carefully to improve respirations without reversing analgesic effects or causing other adverse effects (hypertension and tachycardia may result in left ventricular failure and pulmonary edema, especially in cardiac patients). Treat bradycardia with atropine, or alfentanil-induced bradycardia can be antagonized with the use of a neuromuscular blocking agent with vagolytic activity (e.g., pancuronium). Treat hypotension by placing the patient in a Trendelenburg position, if possible; administer IV fluids and a vasopressor (e.g., norepinephrine [Levophed], dopamine [Intropin]) if indicated. Naloxone or nalmefene may reverse hypotension postoperatively. Muscle rigidity during anesthesia induction or surgery must be controlled with neuromuscular blocking agents and controlled ventilation with oxygen. Use a neuromuscular blocking agent prophylactically to prevent muscle rigidity or to induce muscle relaxation after rigidity occurs. Neuromuscular blocking agents with vagolytic activity (e.g., pancuronium) may decrease risk of alfentanil-induced bradycardia and hypotension, but may increase the risk of hypertension or tachcardia in some patients. In patients with compromised cardiac function and/or those receiving a beta-adrenergic blocking agent preoperatively, a nonvagolytic neuromuscular blocking agent (e.g., succinylcholine) may increase the incidence and severity of bradycardia and hypotension. Respiratory depressant effects of neuromuscular blocking agents are additive with alfentanil. Postoperatively, naloxone or nalmefene may be used in small incremental doses to reverse skeletal muscle rigidity. Resuscitate as necessary.

ALGLUCERASE

Enzyme Replenisher
(glucocerebrosidase)

Ceredase   pH 5.5 to 6.0

USUAL DOSE

Individuals now taking alglucerase will be transferred to imiglucerase (Cerezyme) as production levels of imiglucerase increase. This phase-in process began in 1997 and will continue until all patients are on imiglucerase. Once patients are transferred to imiglucerase, they should remain on imiglucerase. Dose is individualized to each patient based on the severity of illness and patient response. The recommended initial dose range is 15 to 60 Units/kg/infusion once every 2 weeks or up to 120 Units/kg per 4-week period. Recent studies indicate that lower range initial doses may be effective. Based on disease severity, patient response, or patient convenience, the frequency can be adjusted to as often as every other day or as infrequently as every 4 weeks. Alglucerase should be given at least every 4 weeks or symptoms and condition may relapse to pretreatment status. Patients beginning alglucerase therapy are usually given higher range initial doses for a limited time to stabilize their disease. Patients with very severe Gaucher's disease also may require higher range initial doses and/or increased frequency because they have accumulated more lipid throughout their bodies, requiring more enzyme to remove the excess stored lipid and bring their disease under control.

Investigational low-dose/high-frequency therapy for adults and children: 2.3 Units/kg three times a week. A study of this cost-saving regimen produced comparable results to high-dose, low-frequency doses recommended in Usual dose. All patients had implanted venous access devices to allow a home treatment program. Local anesthetic ointments were also used to reduce discomfort.

PEDIATRIC DOSE

9 to 30 Units/kg used in one study. Dose increased based on age of a child followed from 4 to 10 years.

DOSE ADJUSTMENTS

To utilize each bottle fully and reduce wasting, a single dose may be increased or decreased slightly as long as the total monthly dose (120 Units/kg) remains unaltered. ■ After patient response is well established (disease symptoms lessen and the accumulated lipid is reduced), the dose may be adjusted downward to achieve the optimum individualized maintenance dose. Usually progressively lowered at 3- to 6-month intervals while response parameters are closely monitored. Optimum goal is to establish the lowest dose that is effective in maintaining control of the disease and preventing recurrence of symptoms for each patient. Evidence suggests that this therapy works with doses as low as 1 Unit/kg.

DILUTION

A single dose must be diluted with NS to a total volume not to exceed 100 ml. Do not shake; may render the glycoprotein biologically inactive. Available as a single-use package containing 400 Units/5 ml (80 Units/ml) and in a vial containing 10 Units/ml.

Storage: Store unopened vials at 4° C (39° F). Do not use if discolored, particulate matter present, or after expiration date on bottle. Contains no preservative; do not store opened vials for future use.

INCOMPATIBLE WITH

Do not use as an additive with any other drug. Do not mix in any solution other than normal saline.

RATE OF ADMINISTRATION

A single dose equally distributed over 1 to 2 hours. Use an inline microfilter. Use of a microdrip (60 gtt/ml) or an infusion pump helpful.

ACTIONS

A modified form of the enzyme beta-glucocerebrosidase made from human placental tissue from selected donors and purified by specific processes. Gaucher's disease is characterized by a functional deficiency in beta-glucocerebrosidase enzymatic activity and the resultant accumulation of lipid glucocerebroside in tissue macrophages (Gaucher's cells). These cells are found in the liver, spleen, bone marrow and occasionally the lung, kidney, and intestine. Alglucerase acts like glucocerebrosidase to facilitate the release of the lipid glucocerebrosides. Effective in controlling and actually reversing disease symptoms. Increase in appetite and energy level and improvement in hemoglobin are often the first observable effects and may occur in 2 to 4 months. Cachexia and wasting in children are reduced. Within 6 months splenomegaly and hepatomegaly are significantly reduced, and hemoglobin, hematocrit, erythrocyte, and platelet counts improved. Replenishment of bone marrow and improving mineralization of bone may take several years.

INDICATIONS AND USES

Long-term enzyme replacement therapy for patients with confirmed diagnosis of Type I Gaucher's disease, with signs and symptoms severe enough to result in one or more of the following conditions: moderate-to-severe anemia, thrombocytopenia with bleeding tendency, bone disease, significant hepatomegaly or splenomegaly.

CONTRAINDICATIONS

None known. Discontinue if there is significant clinical evidence of hypersensitivity to alglucerase.

PRECAUTIONS

Effective only via IV route. ■ Should be used under the direction of a physician knowledgeable in the management of Gaucher's disease. ■ Special processing minimizes risk of HIV and hepatitis. Inactivation of all viruses cannot be guaranteed. Assess benefits and risks of treatment prior to use. ■ No obvious toxicity was detected after single doses up to 234 Units/kg; no experience with higher doses.

Monitor: Evaluation of hemoglobin, hematocrit, platelets, white blood cell count, acid phosphatase (AP), plasma glucocerebroside, liver and/or spleen size, and bone changes are required before and during therapy. Frequency determined by patient response; more frequent when determining response to initial dose and when dose is being adjusted (i.e., every 3 to 6 months). Blood tests will be done more frequently, since anemia is the first symptom to improve. ■ MRI provides the best evaluation of liver and spleen. ■ Standard x-rays provide adequate evaluation of bone changes. ■ Determine patency of vein; discomfort, burning and swelling may occur at the site. ■ Observe patient closely for signs of improvement (e.g., increased energy, reduced bleeding tendency, reduction in size of liver and/or spleen, reduced joint swelling, reduced bone pain).

Patient education: Treatment required for life. No longer than 1 month should elapse between treatments, or symptoms and condition may relapse to the pretreatment state.

Maternal/child: Category C: use in pregnancy only if clearly needed. No studies available on fetal harm or reproductive capacity. ■ Safety for use during lactation not established. Not known if alglucerase is secreted in breast milk.

DRUG/LAB INTERACTIONS

None indicated; limited information available.

SIDE EFFECTS

Burning, discomfort, and swelling at the injection site are most common. Abdominal discomfort, chills, fever, nausea and vomiting have occurred. A protein immune reaction may develop.

ANTIDOTE

Keep physician informed of side effects; may be treated symptomatically if indicated. Discontinue alglucerase for severe clinical evidence of hypersensitivity. Treat anaphylaxsis and resuscitate as necessary.

ALLOPURINOL SODIUM

Antigout
Antihyperuricemic

Zyloprim for injection

pH 10.8 to 11.8

USUAL DOSE

300 to 600 mg/day as a single infusion or in equally divided doses at 6-, 8-, or 12-hour intervals. Usually given at 8 hour intervals. An alternate dosing regimen is 40 to 150 mg/M^2 every 8 hours. Higher dose range possibly more effective in adults. Total dose should not exceed 800 mg/day. IV and oral doses are therapeutically equivalent. Oral dose can replace an IV dose at any time. (See Precautions/Monitor).

PEDIATRIC DOSE

Recommended starting dose is 200 mg/M^2/day. An alternate source suggests 10 mg/kg/day with a maximum total dose of 600 mg/day. Usually given in equally divided doses at 6- to 8-hour intervals. Studies found no significant difference in dose response in pediatric patients. Note comments in Usual dose.

DOSE ADJUSTMENTS

Reduced dose based on creatinine clearance (CrCl) required for renal insufficiency. Reduce to 200 mg/day with a CrCl between 10 and 20 ml/min, 100 mg/day with a CrCl between 3 and 10 ml/min, and 100 mg/day extending intervals between doses with a CrCl below 3 ml/min. ▪ Dose with normal renal function may be increased or decreased based on electrolytes and serum uric acid levels. Note Drug/lab interactions.

DILUTION

Available as a single dose vial containing 500 mg of allopurinol. Reconstitute with 25 ml of sterile water for injection (yields 20 mg/ml). Swirl until completely dissolved. Must be further diluted with normal saline or 5% dextrose for injection. Maximum concentration for administration is 6 mg/ml. 19 ml of additional diluent per 20 mg (1 ml) yields 1 mg/ml, 9 ml yields 2 mg/ml, and 2.3 ml yields 6 mg/ml.

Storage: Store unopened vials at controlled room temperature. Use reconstituted solution within 24 hours.

INCOMPATIBLE WITH

Manufacturer recommends administering sequentially and flushing before and after administration. Amikacin (Amikin), amphotericin B (Fungizone), carmustine (BiCNU), cefotaxime (Claforan), chlorpromazine (Thorazine), cimetidine (Tagamet), clindamycin (Cleocin), cytarabine (ARA-C), dacarbazine (DTIC), daunorubicin (Cerubidine), diphenhydramine (Benadryl), doxorubicin (Adriamycin), doxycycline (Vibramycin), droperidol (Inapsine), floxuridine (FUDR), gentamicin (Garamycin), haloperidol (Haldol), hydroxyzine (Atarax), idarubicin (Idamycin), imipenem-cilastatin (Primaxin), mechlorethamine (Mustargen), meperidine (Demerol), methylprednisolone (Solu-Medrol), metoclopramide (Reglan), minocycline (Minocin), nalbuphine (Nubain), netilmicin (Netromycin), ondansetron (Zofran), prochlorperazine

(Compazine), promethazine (Phenergan), sodium bicarbonate, strepto-zocin (Zanosar), tobramycin (Nebcin), vinorelbine (Navelbine).

RATE OF ADMINISTRATION

Manufacturer's recommendation not available. A maximum dose should take at least ½ to 1 hour or more based on volume with diluent and patient comfort and/or requirements. Include in hydration fluids. Note Incompatible with.

ACTIONS

A xanthine oxidase inhibitor. Metabolized to oxypurinol. Acts on purine catabolism without disrupting the biosynthesis of purines. It reduces the production of uric acid by inhibiting the biochemical reactions immediately preceding its formation. Onset of action is within 10 minutes. Peak concentrations are related to dose. Pharmacokinetic and plasma profiles of allopurinol and oxypurinol as well as half-lives and systemic clearance are similar with IV or oral administration. Systemic exposure to oxypurinol is also similar by both routes at each dose level. Cleared by glomerular filtration, some oxypurinol is reabsorbed in the kidney tubules. Secreted in breast milk.

INDICATIONS AND USES

Management of patients with leukemia, lymphoma, and solid tumor malignancies who are receiving cancer therapy that causes elevations of serum and urinary uric acid levels and who cannot tolerate oral therapy. Consider prophylactic use before initiation of and during chemotherapy in patients who are NPO, are nauseated and vomiting, or have malabsorption problems, dysphagia, or GI tract dysfunctions. Also helpful to attain rapid, significant blood levels, accurately dose pediatric patients, and dose patients with questionable compliance. Used prophylactically before the initiation of and during chemotherapy to prevent tumor lysis syndrome (TLS), and its sequela, acute uric acid nephropathy (AUAN).

Investigational uses: Preservation of cadaveric kidneys for transplantation.

CONTRAINDICATIONS

Any patient who has had a severe reaction to allopurinol (usually a hypersensitivity reaction).

PRECAUTIONS

Recently approved by the FDA. Is available commercially through Burroughs Wellcome Co. for patients receiving chemotherapy treatment for malignancies who cannot tolerate oral therapy. Has been available on a compassionate use basis since 1969.

Monitor: Assess serum uric acid levels and electrolytes before and during therapy. ■ Hydration with 3,000 ml/M^2/day (twice the level of maintenance fluid replacement) is recommended to promote a high volume of urine output with low urate concentration. ■ Increase alkalinity of urine with sodium bicarbonate to increase solubility of uric acid. ■ Monitor renal and hepatic systems before and during therapy. ■ Observe for symptoms of tumor lysis syndrome (e.g., hyperuricemia, hyperkalemia, hyperphosphatemia, and hypocalcemia). If untreated, may develop acute uric acid nephropathy leading to renal failure requiring hemodialysis.

Patient education: Report promptly blood in the urine, painful urination, irritation of the eyes, skin rash, or swelling of the lips or mouth. ■ Major acute toxicities may be allergic or renal.

Maternal/child: Category C. Potential benefits must justify potential risks to fetus. ■ Use caution if required during lactation.

Elderly: Consider age-related impaired organ function.

DRUG/LAB INTERACTIONS

Inhibits metabolism and increases effects and toxicity of thiopurines (e.g., azathioprine [Imuran], mercaptopurine [Purinethol]). Reduce dose of thiopurine by one third to one fourth. ■ Uricosuric agents (e.g., sulfinpyrazone [Anturane], probenicid [Benemid], colchicine) may increase elimination of active metabolites of allopurinol; could result in an additive effect. ■ Prolongs half-life of dicumarol; monitor PT or PTT, and adjust anticoagulant dose as indicated. ■ Frequency of skin rash increased with ampicillin/amoxicillin. ■ Bone marrow suppression may be increased concurrently with cytotoxic agents (e.g., cyclophosphamide [Cytoxan]); risk of bleeding or infection may be increased. ■ May prolong half-life of chlorpropamide (Diabinase). ■ Hypersensitivity reactions may be increased with ACE inhibitors (e.g., enalaprilat) or thiazide diuretics (e.g., chlorothiazide [Diuril]). ■ Larger doses (>600 mg/day) may decrease clearance and increase toxicity of theophyllines (e.g., Aminophyllin).

SIDE EFFECTS

Fewer than 1% of patients have had side effects directly attributable to allopurinol. All were allergic in nature (nausea and vomiting, rash, and renal failure/insufficiency) and of mild to moderate severity. Xanthine crystalluria has been rarely reported in long-term therapy with oral allopurinol.

ANTIDOTE

Discontinue allopurinol at the first sign of skin rash or any other allergic reaction. Do not restart. Keep physician informed of all side effects. Symptoms of tumor lysis syndrome require immediate intervention and correction of electrolyte abnormalities to avoid kidney damage. Treat allergic reactions as indicated; may require epinephrine (Adrenalin), diphenhydramine (Benadryl), corticosteroids (hydrocortisone), and/or oxygen.

ALPHA₁-PROTEINASE INHIBITOR (HUMAN)

Alpha antitrypsin replenisher

Alpha₁-PI, Prolastin

pH 6.6 to 7.4

USUAL DOSE

60 mg/kg once a week.

Every patient should be immunized against hepatitis B before administration. If immediate treatment is required, give a single dose of hepatitis B immune globulin (human) at the same time as the initial dose of hepatitis B vaccine.

DILUTION

Sterile water for injection supplied by manufacturer. Should yield approximately 20 mg/ml alpha₁-PI when reconstituted. Must be given within 3 hours of reconstitution.

Storage: Store in refrigerator before reconstitution and at room temperature after reconstitution.

INCOMPATIBLE WITH

Sufficient information not available. Do not mix with other drugs.

RATE OF ADMINISTRATION

0.08 ml/kg/min is recommended. May be given at a faster rate. A 50 kg (110 lb) woman would receive 3,000 mg (150 ml reconstituted solution) over no more than 37 minutes (4 ml/min).

ACTIONS

A sterile, stable, lyophilized preparation obtained from human plasma. Increases and maintains functional levels of alpha₁-PI in the epithelial lining of the lower respiratory tract. Provides adequate antineutrophil elastase activity in the lungs of individuals with alpha₁-antitrypsin deficiency.

INDICATIONS AND USES

Treatment of congenital alpha₁-antitrypsin deficiency, a potentially fatal disease; used for chronic replacement only in individuals with clinically demonstrated panacinar emphysema.

CONTRAINDICATIONS

None known when used for the specific indication listed.

PRECAUTIONS

Confirm diagnosis of congenital alpha₁-antitrypsin deficiency with clinically demonstrated panacinar emphysema. ▪ Each unit of plasma tested and found nonreactive to HIV antibody and hepatitis B surface antigen. Transmission of these viruses is still possible.

Monitor: Blood levels of alpha₁-PI have been maintained above the functional level of 80 mg/dl with this replacement therapy. Serum levels determined by commercial immunologic assays may not reflect actual functional alpha₁-PI levels. ▪ Assess lung sounds and rate and quality of respirations prior to each infusion.

Patient education: Inform of risks and of safety precautions taken during manufacturing process. ▪ Note changes in breathing pattern or sputum production; avoid smoking.

Maternal/child: Category C: use in pregnancy only when clearly needed. Potential hazard to fetus. ▪ Safety for use in children not yet established.

DRUG/LAB INTERACTIONS

No specific information available

SIDE EFFECTS

Mild transient leukocytosis several hours after transfusion. Dizziness, fever, or light-headedness may occur. Consider risk potential of contracting AIDS or hepatitis.

ANTIDOTE

All side effects except AIDS and hepatitis usually subside spontaneously. Keep the physician informed. Treat anaphylaxis (antihistamines, epinephrine, corticosteroids) and resuscitate as necessary.

ALPROSTADIL

Prostaglandin
(Ductus Arteriosus Patency Adjunct)

PGE₁, Prostaglandin E₁, Prostin VR Pediatric

USUAL DOSE

Begin with 0.05 to 0.1 mcg/kg of body weight/min. When therapeutic response is achieved, reduce infusion rate to lowest dose that maintains the response. (0.1 mcg to 0.05 to 0.025 to 0.01 mcg/min). If necessary dose may be increased gradually to a maximum of 0.4 mcg/kg/min. Generally these higher rates do not produce greater effects. May be given through infusion into a large vein or, if necessary, through an umbilical artery catheter placed at the ductal opening.

DILUTION

Each 500 mcg must be further diluted with NS or D5W. Various volumes may be used depending on infusion pump capabilities and desired infusion rate.

Diluent	Concentration	Desired dose	Rate of infusion
250 ml	2 mcg/ml	0.1 mcg/kg/min	0.05 ml/min/kg
25 ml	20 mcg/ml	0.1 mcg/kg/min	0.005 ml/min/kg

Storage: Refrigerate until dilution. Prepare fresh solution for administration every 24 hours.

INCOMPATIBLE WITH

Specific information not available.

RATE OF ADMINISTRATION

See Usual dose. Infusion pump capable of delivering 0.005, 0.01, 0.02, or 0.05 ml/min/kg required. Use for the shortest time possible at the lowest rate therapeutically effective. Decrease rate of infusion stat if a significant fall in arterial pressure occurs.

ACTIONS

A naturally occurring acidic lipid. Smooth muscle of the ductus arteriosus is susceptible to its relaxing effect, which reduces blood pressure and peripheral resistance and increases cardiac output and rate. In newborns it relaxes and may open the ductus. Metabolized by oxidation almost instantly (80% in one pass through the lungs). Remainder excreted as metabolites in the urine.

INDICATIONS AND USES

Temporarily maintain the patency of the ductus arteriosus until corrective or palliative surgery can be performed on infants with pulmonary atresia, pulmonary stenosis, tricuspid atresia, tetralogy of Fallot, interruption of the aortic arch, coarctation of the aorta, or transposition of the great vessels. ■ Used by intercavernosal injection to treat impotence.

CONTRAINDICATIONS

None known. Not indicated for respiratory distress syndrome (hyaline membrane disease).

PRECAUTIONS

Usually administered by trained personnel in pediatric intensive care facilities. ■ Establish a diagnosis of cyanotic heart disease (restricted pulmonary blood flow). ■ Response is poor in infants with Po$_2$ values of 40 mm Hg or those more than 4 days old. More effective with lower Po$_2$. ■ Use caution in neonates with bleeding tendencies; inhibits platelet aggregation.

Monitor: Monitor respiratory status continuously. Ventilatory assistance must be immediately available. May cause apnea (10% to 12% experience), especially in infants under 2 kg. ■ Monitor arterial pressure intermittently by umbilical artery catheter, auscultation, or Doppler transducer. Decrease rate of infusion stat if a significant fall in arterial pressure occurs. ■ Measure effectiveness with increase of Po$_2$ in infants with restricted pulmonary blood flow and increase of blood pressure and blood pH in infants with restricted systemic blood flow.

DRUG/LAB INTERACTIONS

Inhibits platelet aggregation.

SIDE EFFECTS

Cardiac arrest, cerebral bleeding, cortical proliferation of long bones, diarrhea, DIC, hyperextension of the neck, hyperirritability, hypothermia, seizures, sepsis, tachycardia. Many other side effects have occurred in 1% or less of infants receiving alprostadil.

Overdose: Apnea, bradycardia, flushing, hypotension, pyrexia.

ANTIDOTE

Notify physician of all side effects. Discontinue immediately if apnea or bradycardia occurs. Institute emergency measures. If infusion is restarted use extreme caution. Decrease rate if pyrexia, hypotension, or fall in arterial pressure occurs. Flushing is usually caused by incorrect intraarterial catheter placement. Reposition.

ALTEPLASE, RECOMBINANT

Thrombolytic Agent
(Recombinant)

Activase, Lysatec, rt-PA, Tissue Plasminogen Activator, tPA

pH 7.3

USUAL DOSE

Total dose is based on patient weight, and should not exceed 100 mg. In all situations follow total dose with at least 30 ml of NS or D5W through the IV tubing to ensure administration of total dose. Concurrent administration of heparin, aspirin, and/or dipyridamole (Persantine) has been consistently used in MI patients receiving alteplase therapy. MI patients in the *accelerated infusion* studies received a loading dose of heparin 5,000 units, followed by 1,000 units/hr by continuous infusion for 48 hours. Aspirin therapy was usually concurrent (e.g., 160 mg chewable aspirin on admission, followed by 160 to 325 mg/day) or followed with aspirin after 48 hours. 90% of MI patients receiving the 3-hour infusion also received heparin as a continuous infusion with or without a loading dose and either aspirin or dipyridamole. (Note Precautions and Monitor.)

Acute myocardial infarction: Accelerated Infusion > 67 kg: 100 mg titrated over 90 minutes as an IV infusion. Initially give a bolus of 15 mg over 2 minutes. Follow with 50 mg evenly distributed over 30 minutes. Infuse the remaining 35 mg dose evenly distributed over 60 minutes.

Accelerated Infusion < 67 kg: Initially give a bolus of 15 mg over 2 minutes. Follow with 0.75 mg/kg (not to exceed a 50 mg dose) evenly distributed over 30 minutes. Then infuse 0.5 mg/kg (not to exceed a 35 mg dose) evenly distributed over 60 minutes.

3-hour Infusion > 65 kg: 100 mg titrated over 3 hours as an IV infusion. Initially, give a bolus of 6 to 10 mg over 2 minutes. Follow with 50 to 54 mg (total 60 mg dose) evenly distributed over the first hour. Follow with 20 mg/hr for 2 hours.

3-hour Infusion < 65 kg: Calculate total dose using 1.25 mg/kg of body weight. Give three fifths of this total calculated dose divided as above into a bolus and first-hour dose. Give one fifth of this total calculated dose/hr for 2 hours.

The earlier intervention occurs, the better the results. Most effective administered within 4 to 6 hours of onset of symptoms of acute myocardial infarction.

Acute ischemic stroke: 0.9 mg/kg. Maximum dose is 90 mg. Give a bolus of 10% of the calcuted dose over 1 minute followed by balance of calculated dose (90%) as an infusion evenly distributed over 60 minutes. Treatment must start within 3 hours of onset of symptoms, but after bleeding in the brain has been ruled out (usually by a CT scan of the brain).

Pulmonary embolism: 100 mg titrated over 2 hours as an IV infusion. Diagnosis should be confirmed by objective means (e.g., lung scan, pulmonary angiography).

DILUTION

Must be diluted with SW without preservatives (provided by manufacturer). Available in 50- and 100-mg vials (1 mg/ml). **50-mg vials:** Use a large-bore (18-gauge) needle and direct the stream of diluent into the lyophilized cake. A vacuum must be present when the diluent is added to the powder for injection. Do not use if vacuum not present. Slight foaming is expected; let stand for several minutes to dissipate large bubbles. May be further diluted to 0.5 mg/ml immediately before administration with an equal volume of NS or D5W. Mix by swirling or slow inversion; avoid agitation during dilution. Use balance (at least 30 ml) of 250-ml bottle of NS or D5W to clear tubing after infusion and assure delivery of total dose. Connect NS or D5W to metriset and pump tubing. Clamp between solution and metriset. Add alteplase to metriset. Prime tubing with alteplase. Bolus dose can be given when indicated by direct IV through a med port or by IV pump. Administer balance of dose as outlined in Usual dose section, adjusting pump rate of delivery as required. Complete by flushing tubing with IV solution. **100-mg vial:** Diluent and transfer device provided (does not contain a vacuum). Insert one end of transfer device into upright vial of diluent (do not invert diluent vial yet). Hold alteplase vial upside down and push center of vial down onto piercing pin. Now invert vials and allow diluent to flow into alteplase. Small amount (0.5 ml) of diluent will not transfer. Swirl gently to dissolve. Do not shake. Process takes several minutes. An infusion set may be inserted into puncture site created by piercing pin. Hang by plastic capping on bottom of vial. Prime tubing with alteplase and administer as outlined above for 20 and 50 mg vials.

Storage: Refrigerate before dilution. Discard unused solution.

INCOMPATIBLE WITH

Manufacturer states "do not add other medications to infusion solution."

Y-site: Dobutamine (Dobutrex), dopamine (Intropin), heparin, nitroglycerin.

COMPATIBLE WITH

Lidocaine, metoprolol (Lopressor), and propranolol (Inderal) are compatible through Y-site of free-flowing alteplase infusion.

RATE OF ADMINISTRATION

Note specific rates for each diagnosis under Usual dose. In all situations use a metriset with microdrip (60 gtt/ml), or an infusion pump and IV tubing without a filter to facilitate accurate administration. Do not use any filters. Distribute final flush over 30 minutes.

ACTIONS

A tissue plasminogen activator and enzyme produced by recombinant DNA. It binds to fibrin in a thrombus and converts plasminogen to plasmin. Plasmin digests fibrin and dissolves the clot. With therapeutic doses, a decrease in circulating fibrinogen makes the patient susceptible to bleeding. Onset of action is prompt, effecting patency of the vessel within 1 to 2 hours in most patients. Prompt opening of arteries increases probability of improved function. Cleared from the plasma by the liver within 5 (50%) to 10 (80%) minutes after the infusion is discontinued. Some effects may linger for 45 minutes to several hours.

INDICATIONS AND USES

Management of acute myocardial infarction in adults for the lysis of thrombi obstructing coronary arteries, the reduction of infarct size, the improvement of ventricular function, and the reduction of the incidence of congestive heart failure. Recent studies suggest alteplase or reteplase are the drugs of choice. ■ Current AHA and JAMA recommendations identify thrombolytic agents as Class I therapy in patients younger than 70 years with recent onset of chest pain (within 6 hours) consistent with acute MI and at least 0.1 mV of ST segment elevation in at least two ECG leads. Use in all other patients based on age, accurate diagnosis, and time from onset of chest pain. ■ Management of acute ischemic stroke in adults to improve neurological recovery and reduce incidence of disability. ■ Management of acute massive pulmonary embolism in adults for the lysis of acute pulmonary emboli either obstructing blood flow to a lobe or multiple segments of the lung or accompanied by unstable hemodynamics (e.g., failure to maintain blood pressure).

Investigational uses: Treatment of unstable angina pectoris and deep vein thrombosis. Has been shown to restore blood flow to frostbitten limbs (0.075 mg/kg/hr for 6 hours). Has been used to clear thrombi in central venous catheters (2-mg bolus into the blocked catheter, in the occlusion of small blood vessels by microthrombi, and in management of peripheral thromboembolism (0.5 to 1 mg/hr intra-arterially).

CONTRAINDICATIONS

Acute myocardial infarction/pulmonary embolism: Active internal bleeding, arteriovenous malformation or aneurysm, bleeding diathesis, cerebral vascular accident, intracranial or intraspinal surgery or trauma within 2 months, intracranial neoplasm, severe uncontrolled hypertension.

Acute ischemic stroke: Active internal bleeding, evidence of intracranial hemorrhage on pretreatment evaluation, history of intracranial hemorrhage; intracranial neoplasm, arteriovenous malformation, or aneurysm; known bleeding diathesis (e.g., current use of oral anticoagulants [e.g., warfarin] with PT > 15 seconds, administration of heparin within 48 hours before onset of stroke with an elevated aPTT as presentation, platelet count <100,000/mm^3), recent intracranial surgery or serious head trauma or recent previous stroke, seizure at the onset of stroke, suspicion of subarachnoid hemorrhage, uncontrolled hypertension at time of treatment (e.g., systolic above 185 or diastolic above 110).

PRECAUTIONS

All indications: A 150-mg dose has caused increased intracranial bleeding; do not use. Administered under the direction of a physician knowledgeable in its use and with appropriate emergency drugs and diagnostic and laboratory facilities available. ▪ A greater alteration of hemostatic status than with heparin. Strict bed rest indicated to reduce risk of bleeding. Use extreme care with the patient; avoid any excessive or rough handling or pressure (including too frequent BPs); avoid invasive procedures (e.g., arterial puncture, venipuncture, IM injection). If these procedures are absolutely necessary, use extreme precautionary methods (use radial artery instead of femoral; small-gauge catheters and needles, and sites that are easily observed and compressible where bleeding can be controlled; avoid handling of catheter sites; and use extended pressure application of up to 30 minutes). Minor bleeding occurs often at catheter insertion sites. Avoid use of razors and toothbrushes. ▪ Use extreme caution in the following situations: major surgery, trauma, GI or GU bleeding, or puncture of noncompressible vessels (e.g., spinal puncture, thoracentesis) within the previous 10 days; cerebrovascular disease; hypertension (systolic above 180 or diastolic above 110); mitral stenosis with atrial fibrillation (likelihood of left heart thrombus); acute pericarditis; subacute bacterial endocarditis; coagulation disorders, including those secondary to severe hepatic or renal disease; severe liver dysfunction; pregnancy and first 10 days postpartum; hemorrhagic ophthalmic conditions (e.g., diabetic hemorrhagic retinopathy); septic thrombophlebitis; patients on anticoagulants; patients over 75 years of age; any situation where bleeding might be hazardous or difficult to manage because of location. ▪ *Myocardial infarction:* Reperfusion arrhythmias occur frequently (e.g., sinus bradycardia, accelerated idioventricular rhythm, PVCs, ventricular tachycardia); have antiarrhythmic meds available at bedside. ▪ Simultaneous therapy with continuous infusion of heparin (with or without a loading dose and aspirin or dipyridamole) is used to reduce the risk of rethrombosis.

Increases risk of bleeding (see Usual Dose). ▪ Standard treatment for myocardial infarction continues simultaneously with alteplase therapy except if temporarily contraindicated (e.g., arterial blood gases, unless absolutely necessary). ▪ **Acute ischemic stroke:** Treatment facility must be able to provide evaluation and management of intracranial hemorrhage. ▪ Use of heparin and aspirin during the first 24 hours has not been evaluated. ▪ Risks of alteplase therapy in the treatment of acute ischemic stroke may be increased in patients with severe neurological deficit at presentation (increased risk of intracranial hemorrhage), patients with major early infarct signs on CT scan (e.g., substantial edema, mass effect, or midline shift). ▪ Treatment may begin before coagulation study results are known in patients without recent use of oral anticoagulants or heparin. Discontinue infusion if pre-treatment PT > 15 seconds or an elevated aPTT is identified. ▪ Benefits of therapy have not been studied in patients treated with alteplase more than 3 hours after the onset of symptoms; use is not recommended; may cause cerebral edema with fatal brain herniation. ▪ Safety and efficacy in patients with minor neurological deficit or rapidly improving symptoms before treatment is begun has not been studied. ▪ **Pulmonary emboli:** Begin heparin at end of infusion or immediately after it is complete. Thrombin time (TT) or PTT should be twice normal or less.

Monitor: All indications: Best to establish a separate IV line for alteplase. ▪ Obtain appropriate clotting studies (e.g., PT, TT, PTT, aPTT, CBC, fibrinogen levels, platelets). ▪ Diagnosis specific baseline studies (e.g., ECG, CPK in myocardial infarction, CT brain scan and neurological assessment in acute ischemic stroke, and lung scan or pulmonary angiography in pulmonary embolism) are indicated. ▪ Baseline assessment (patient condition, pain, hematomas, petechiae, or recent wounds) should be completed before administration. ▪ Type and cross-match may also be ordered. ▪ Start IV if indicated (not previously established, other medications being administered through current IV, to have a line available for additional treatment). ▪ Maintain strict bed rest, monitor the patient carefully and frequently for pain and signs of bleeding; observe catheter sites at least every 15 minutes and apply pressure dressings to any recently invaded site; watch for hematuria, hematemesis, bloody stool, petechiae, hematoma, flank pain, muscle weakness; and do neuro checks every hour (or more frequently if indicated). Continue until normal clotting function returns. ▪ Watch for extravasation; may cause ecchymosis and/or inflammation. Restart IV at another site. Moist compresses may be helpful. ▪ Note Precautions and Drug/lab interactions. ▪ **Myocardial infarction:** Monitor ECG continuously, and record strips with greatest ST segment elevation initially and every 15 minutes for at least 4 hours. A 12-lead ECG is indicated when therapy is complete. ▪ **Acute ischemic stroke:** Hemorrhage in the brain occurs frequently during treatment with alteplase during the first 36 hours; monitor carefully. Studies did not show an increase in mortality and did confirm that more patients had minimal or no disability at 3 months.

Patient education: Compliance with all measures to minimize bleeding (e.g., strict bed rest) is very important. ▪ Avoid use of razors, toothbrushes, and other sharp items. Use caution while moving to avoid excessive bumping. ▪ Report all episodes of bleeding and apply local pressure if indicated. Expect oozing from IV sites.

Maternal/child: Pregnancy Category C. Safety for use in pregnancy, lactation, and children not established.

Elderly: Note Indications and Precautions. ▪ May have poorer prognosis following acute MI and pre-existing conditions that may increase risk of intracranial bleeding. Select patients carefully to maximize benefits.

DRUG/LAB INTERACTIONS

Use caution with drugs that may alter platelet function (e.g., aspirin, dipyridamole [Persantine], indomethacin, phenylbutazone). Risk of bleeding will be increased if used concomitantly. ▪ Risk of bleeding with concomitant use of heparin is markedly increased. ▪ Concurrent use with nitroglycerin decreases plasma concentrations of alteplase, impairing the thrombolytic effect. Coagulation tests will be unreliable; specific procedures can be used; notify the lab of alteplase use.

SIDE EFFECTS

Bleeding is most common: internal (GI tract, GU tract, retroperitoneal, or intracranial sites), epistaxis, gingival, and superficial or surface bleeding (venous cutdowns, arterial punctures, sites of recent surgical intervention). Mild allergic reactions (urticaria) have occurred. Fever, hypotension, nausea, and vomiting, reperfusion arrhythmias, and stroke have occurred. Cholesterol embolization syndrome (e.g., acute renal failure, bowel infarction, cerebral infarction, gangrenous digits, hypertension, livedo reticularis, myocardial infarction, pancreatitis, purple toe retinal artery occlusion, rhabdomyolysis, spinal cord infarction) can occur with thrombolytics but has been reported rarely.

ANTIDOTE

Notify physician of all side effects. Note even the minutest bleeding tendency. Oozing at IV sites is expected. Control minor bleeding by local pressure. For severe bleeding in a critical location discontinue alteplase and any heparin therapy immediately. Whole blood, packed red blood cells, cryoprecipitate, fresh-frozen plasma, platelets, desmopressin, tranexamic acid, and aminocaproic acid may all be indicated. Topical preparations of aminocaproic acid may stop minor bleeding. Consider protamine if heparin has been used. Treat bradycardia with atropine, reperfusion arrhythmias with lidocaine or procainamide; VT or VF may require cardioversion. If hypotension occurs, reduce rate promptly. If not resolved, vasopressors (e.g., dopamine [Intropin]), Trendelenburg position, and suitable plasma expanders (e.g., albumin, plasma protein fraction [plasmanate], or hetastarch) may be indicated. Treat minor allergic reactions symptomatically. Discontinue drug and treat anaphylaxis as indicated; resuscitate as necessary.

AMIFOSTINE

Ethyol

Antidote
Antineoplastic adjunct
Cytoprotective agent

USUAL DOSE

Must be administered in conjuction with cisplatin.

Premedication: Premedication to prevent severe nausea and vomiting is recommended prior to each dose. Usual regimen includes dexamethasone 20 mg IV and a serotonin $5HT_3$ receptor antagonist (e.g., ondansetron [Zofran], granisetron [Kytril]) given before and in conjunction with amifostine infusion.

Amifostine: 910 mg/M^2. Cisplatin dose must be given within 30 minutes of starting the amifostine infusion, but only after the full dose of amifostine is administered.

PEDIATRIC DOSE

Specific information not available. Experience is limited.

DOSE ADJUSTMENTS

Temporarily discontinue the infusion if the systolic BP decreases significantly from the baseline value. See chart below:

Infusion may be restarted to deliver the full dose if the BP returns to normal within 5 minutes and the patient is asymptomatic. If the BP does not return to baseline within 5 minutes and/or the patient is symptomatic (e.g., bradycardia, fainting, unconscious), the full dose cannot be delivered and subsequent doses should be reduced to 740 mg/M^2.

Guideline for Interrupting Amifostine Infusion Due to Decrease in Systolic Blood Pressure					
	Baseline Systolic Blood Pressure (mm Hg)				
	< 100	100-119	120-139	140-179	≥ 180
Decrease in systolic blood pressure during infusion of Amifostine (mm Hg)	20	25	30	40	50

DILUTION

Each 500 mg vial should be reconstituted with 9.5 ml of NS (50 mg/ml). May be further diluted with NS to concentrations from 5 to 40 mg/ml. An additional 2.5 ml of NS will yield 40 mg/ml, 90 ml NS will yield 5 mg/ml.

Storage: Store in refrigerator before reconstitution. Reconstituted or diluted solution is stable for 5 hours at room temperature or 24 hours if refrigerated.

INCOMPATIBLE WITH

Known to be compatible only with NS; use of any other additive, diluent or solution is not recommended.

Y-site: Acyclovir (Zovirax), amphotericin B, cefoperazone (Cefobid), cisplatin (Platinol), ganciclovir (Cytovene), hydroxyzine (Atarax), minocycline (Minocin), prochlorperazine (Compazine). May be compatible at Y-site with some drugs in specific concentrations, consult pharmacist.

RATE OF ADMINISTRATION

A single dose evenly distributed over 15 minutes. May be given by direct IV push or by infusion. Complete amifostine dose but begin cisplatin within 30 minutes after beginning amifostine. Amifostine must be given over 15 minutes; longer infusion times increase the risk of side effects, especially hypotension. Shorter infusion times have not been studied.

ACTIONS

A cytoprotective agent. Rapidly metabolized by alkaline phosphatase in tissues to an active metabolite that can reduce the nephrotoxic effects of cisplatin. This protective metabolite occurs in greater amounts in normal tissues versus tumor tissues and is available to bind to and detoxify reactive metabolites of cisplatin. It reduces the incidence of cisplatin nephrotoxicity but does not cause other toxic reactions. May adversely affect antitumor effects of cisplatin. Rapidly cleared from plasma with an elimination half-life of 8 minutes. Pretreatment with antiemetics does not alter its actions. Measurable levels of the metabolite have been found in bone marrow, minimal excretion in urine.

INDICATIONS AND USES

Reduce the cumulative renal toxicity associated with repeated administration of cisplatin in patients with advanced ovarian cancer or non-small cell lung cancer. May allow higher cumulative doses of cisplatin and cyclophosphamide, improved response rates and duration.

Investigational use: Reduce the damaging effects of paclitaxel on lung fibroblasts.

CONTRAINDICATIONS

Known sensitivity to aminothiol compounds or mannitol. ▪ Not recommended for patients receiving chemotherapy for malignancies that are potentially curable; may interfere with effectiveness of chemotherapy regimen and reduce incidence of cure. ▪ Not recommended for patients who are hypotensive, dehydrated, or for those receiving antihypertensive therapy that cannot be stopped for 24 hours before amifostine is administered.

PRECAUTIONS

Use caution in the elderly, patients with preexisting cardiovascular or cerebrovascular conditions (e.g., arrhythmias, congestive heart failure, history of stroke, history of ischemic heart disease). ▪ Hypotension and nausea and vomiting can be severe; use caution in any situation where these side effects may have serious consequences.

Monitor: Adequate hydration required prior to administration of amifostine. ▪ See Usual dose for premedication requirements. Additional antiemetics may be required to offset nausea and vomiting of chemotherapy drugs. ▪ Obtain baseline BP and monitor at least every 5 minutes during and immediately after the infusion. Hypotension can occur at any time but is more frequent toward the end of the infusion and recovery usually begins within 5 to 6 minutes after infusion is discontinued. ■ Keep patient in supine position during and immediately after the infusion. ■ Monitor fluid balance carefully, especially in conjunction with highly emetogenic chemotherapy (e.g., cisplatin). ■ Monitor serum calcium. Risk of hypocalcemia increased in some patients (e.g., nephrotic syndrome). Calcium supplements may be required. ■ Note Dose adjustments, Rate of administration, and Antidote.

Patient education: Void prior to administration. ■ May produce significant hypotension. Effects may be additive with medications currently being taken. Review all medications (prescription and nonprescription) with nurse and/or physician. ■ Must remain in supine position until BP stabilized, then request assistance for ambulation. ■ Report feelings of faintness or nausea promptly.

Maternal/child: Pregnancy Category C: use only if potential benefits justify risk to fetus; embryotoxic in rabbits at doses lower than required for humans. ■ Discontinue breast feeding. ■ Safety for use in children not established, experience is limited. In clinical trials, a few children received single doses up to 2700 mg/M^2 with no unexpected effects.

Elderly: Safety for use not established. Monitor fluid balance closely, avoid dehydration. ■ Hypotension may be sudden and severe, monitor closely. ■ Note Contraindications and Precautions.

DRUG/LAB INTERACTIONS

Antihypertensive therapy (e.g., ACE inhibitors [e.g., enalaprilat], calcium channel blocking agents [e.g., nicardipine, verapamil], diuretics [e.g., furosemide, torsemide], nitroglycerin, nitroprusside sodium) should be discontinued 24 hours before amifostine administration. (Note Contraindications.) ■ Use extreme caution in any patient receiving medications with hypotensive effects (antidepressants, benzodiazepines, beta-adrenergic blocking agents [e.g., atenolol, esmolol, metoprolol, propranolol], bretylium, lidocaine, magnesium, narcotics, nitrates, paclitaxel, procainamide); will cause additive hypotension.

SIDE EFFECTS

Hypotension (62%) and nausea and vomiting (severe) occur frequently. Chills, dizziness, feelings of warmth, flushing, hiccups, hypocalcemia, loss of consciousness, mild allergic reactions, sneezing, and somnolence may occur. Anaphylaxis has not been reported.

Overdose: Up to 3 doses have been given within 24 hours without unexpected side effects.

ANTIDOTE

Keep physician informed of side effects. Treatment of nausea and vomiting imperative to encourage patients to continue treatment with full doses of chemotherapeutic agents. Hypotension may be dose limiting. If the systolic BP decreases significantly (see Dose adjustments chart), temporarily discontinue the infusion, place the patient in Trendelenburg position, and administer an infusion of NS at a separate site. Vasopressors (e.g., dopamine [Intropin], norepinephrine [Levophed]) may be required. Restart infusion if BP returns to baseline within 5 minutes and patient is asymptomatic.

AMIKACIN SULFATE

Antibacterial
(Aminoglycoside)

Amikin

pH 3.5 to 5.5

USUAL DOSE

Up to 15 mg/kg of body weight/24 hr equally divided into 2 or 3 doses at equally divided intervals. Dosage based on ideal weight of lean body mass. Do not exceed a total adult dose of 15 mg/kg/24 hr in average weight patient or 1.5 Gm in heavier patients by all routes in 24 hours.

Recent studies suggest that a total daily dose administered as a single dose (instead of divided into 2 or 3 doses) may provide higher peak levels and enhance drug effectiveness while actually reducing or having no adverse effects on risk of toxicity. Monitor with trough levels.

Mycobacterium avium complex: 15 mg/kg/24 hr in equally divided doses every 8 to 12 hours (part of a 3 to 5 agent regimen).

PEDIATRIC DOSE

15 to 22.5 mg/kg/24 hr equally divided into 2 or 3 doses and given every 8 to 12 hours. Do not exceed 1.5 Gm/24 hr.

NEWBORN DOSE

10 mg/kg of body weight as a loading dose, then 7.5 mg/kg/dose. Give every 24 hours if *under 28 weeks gestation and less than 7 days of age.*

Give every 18 hours if *under 28 weeks gestation and over 7 days or 28 to 34 weeks gestation and under 7 days of age.*

Give every 12 hours if *28 to 34 weeks gestation and over 7 days of age or over 34 weeks gestation and under 7 days of age.*

Give every 8 hours if *over 34 weeks gestation and over 7 days of age.*

DOSE ADJUSTMENTS

Reduce daily dose commensurate with amount of renal impairment and/or increase intervals between injections. ■ Reduced dose or extended intervals may be required in the elderly. ■ Note Drug/lab interactions.

DILUTION

Each 500 mg or fraction thereof is diluted with 100 to 200 ml IV D5W, D5/NS, or NS. Amount of diluent may be decreased proportionately with dosage for children and infants. Available for pediatric injection as 50 mg/ml.

Storage: Diluted solution stable at room temperature for 24 hrs.

INCOMPATIBLE WITH

Administer separately as recommended by manufacturer. Note precautions. Allopurinol, aminophylline, amphotericin B, ampicillin, cefazolin (Kefzol), cephalothin (Keflin), cephapirin (Cefadyl), chlorothiazide (Diuril), dexamethasone (Decadron), erythromycin (Ilotycin), heparin, hetastarch (Hespan), phenytoin (Dilantin), potassium chloride, thiopental (Pentothal), warfarin. Inactivated by carbenicillin, warfarin (Coumadin), ticarcillin, and other penicillins.

RATE OF ADMINISTRATION

A single dose over at least 30 to 60 minutes. Infants should receive a 1 to 2 hour infusion.

ACTIONS

An aminoglycoside antibiotic with neuromuscular blocking action. Bactericidal against many gram-negative organisms resistant to other antibiotics including other aminoglycosides such as gentamicin (Garamycin), kanamycin (Kantrex), and tobramycin (Nebcin). Well distributed through all body fluids. Usual half-life is 2 to 3 hours. Half-life is prolonged in infants, postpartum females, fever, liver disease and ascites, spinal cord injury, cystic fibrosis, and the elderly; shorter in severe burns. Crosses the placental barrier. Excreted in the kidneys. Cross-allergenicity does occur between aminoglycosides.

INDICATIONS AND USES

Short-term treatment of serious infections caused by susceptible organisms (e.g., gram-negative bacteria) generally resistant to alternate drugs that have less potential toxicity. ▪ Effective in infections of the respiratory and urinary tracts, CNS (including meningitis), skin and soft tissue, intraabdominal (including peritonitis), bacterial septicemia (including neonatal sepsis), burns and postoperative infections. ▪ Considered initial therapy in suspected gram-negative infections after culture and sensitivity is drawn. ▪ Penicillins may be required concomitantly in neonatal sepsis to treat possible infections from gram-positive organisms.

Unlabeled uses: Treatment of *Mycobacterium avium* complex; a common infection in AIDS (part of a multiple [3 to 5] drug regimen).

CONTRAINDICATIONS

Known amikacin or aminoglycoside sensitivity. Sulfite sensitivity may be a contraindication.

PRECAUTIONS

Sensitivity studies indicated to determine susceptibility of causative organism to amikacin. ▪ Response should occur in 24 to 48 hours. Use extreme caution if therapy is required over 7 to 10 days. ▪ Superinfection may occur from overgrowth of nonsusceptible organisms. ▪ May contain sulfites; use caution in patients with asthma.

Monitor: Maintain good hydration. ▪ Narrow range between toxic and therapeutic levels. Periodically monitor peak and trough concentrations to avoid peak serum concentrations above 30 mcg/ml and trough concentrations above 5 to 10 mcg/ml. ▪ Monitor urine protein, presence of cells and casts, and decreased specific gravity. Watch for decrease in urine output, rising BUN and serum creatinine, and declining creatinine clearance levels. Dose adjustment may be necessary. ▪ Routine serum levels and evaluations of hearing are recommended. ▪ Monitor serum calcium, magnesium, and sodium; levels may decline. ▪ In extended treatment, monitor serum levels, electrolytes, renal, auditory, and vestibular functions frequently. ▪ Note Drug/lab interactions.

Patient education: Report promptly any changes in balance, hearing loss, weakness, or dizziness. ▪ Consider birth control options.

Maternal/child: Category D: avoid pregnancy. Potential hazard to fetus.

- Safety for use during lactation not established; use extreme caution.
- Peak concentrations are generally lower in infants and young children. ■ Use extreme caution in premature infants and neonates; immature kidney function will result in prolonged half-life.

Elderly: Consider less toxic alternatives. ■ Longer intervals between doses may be more important than smaller doses. ■ Monitor renal function and drug levels carefully. Measurement of creatinine clearance more useful than BUN or serum creatinine to assess renal function. ■ Half-life prolonged.

DRUG/LAB INTERACTIONS

Synergistic when used in combination with beta-lactam antibiotics (e.g., sulbactam sodium, clavulanate potassium, cephalosporins, penicillins), and vancomycin. Dose adjustment and appropriate spacing required due to physical incompatibilities and interactions. Synergism may be inconsistent; measure aminoglycoside levels. ■ Concurrent use topically or systemically with any other ototoxic or nephrotoxic agents should be avoided. May have dangerous additive effects with anesthetics (e.g., enflurane), other neuromuscular blocking antibiotics (e.g., kanamycin), diuretics (e.g., furosemide [Lasix]), beta-lactam antibiotics (e.g., cephalosporins), vancomycin, and many others. ■ Neuromuscular blocking muscle relaxants (e.g., doxacurium [Nuromax], succinylcholine [Anectine]) are potentiated by aminoglycosides. *Apnea can occur.* ■ Aminoglycosides are also potentiated by anticholinesterases (e.g., edrophonium), antineoplastics (e.g., nitrogen mustard, cisplatin). ■ May be antagonized by bacteriostatic antibiotics (e.g., chloramphemicol, erythromycin, and tetracyclines); bacterial action may be impacted.

SIDE EFFECTS

Occur more frequently with impaired renal function, higher doses, prolonged administration, in dehydrated or elderly patients, and in patients receiving other ototoxic or nephrotoxic drugs.

Minor: Fever, headache, hypotension, nausea, paresthesias, skin rash, tremor, vomiting.

Major: Albuminuria, anemia, arthralgia, azotemia, eosinophilia, loss of balance, neuromuscular blockade, oliguria, ototoxicity, red and white blood cells or casts in urine, respiratory depression or arrest, rising serum creatinine.

ANTIDOTE

Notify physician of all side effects. If minor side effects persist or any major symptom appears, discontinue drug and notify the physician. Treatment is symptomatic, or a reduction in dose may be required. In overdose hemodialysis may be indicated. Monitor fluid balance, creatinine clearance, and plasma levels carefully. Complexation with ticarcillin or carbenicillin (12 to 30 Gm/day) may be as effective as hemodialysis. Consider exchange transfusion in the newborn. Calcium salts or neostigmine may reverse neuromuscular blockade. Resuscitate as necessary.

AMINOCAPROIC ACID

Antifibrinolytic
Antihemorrhagic

Amicar pH 6.8

USUAL DOSE

5 Gm initially. Follow with 1 to 1.25 Gm/hr for 6 to 8 hours. Maximum dose is 30 Gm/24 hr.

Prevent recurrence of subarachnoid hemorrhage: 36 Gm/24 hr equally divided into 6 doses.

Reduce need for platelet transfusion in management of amegakaryocytic thrombocytopenia: 8 to 24 Gm/24 hr for 3 days to 13 months.

PEDIATRIC DOSE

100 mg/kg of body weight or 3 Gm/M^2 during the first hour. Follow with a continuous infusion of 33.3 mg/kg/hr or 1 Gm/M^2/hr. Do not exceed 18 Gm/M^2/24 hr. See Maternal/child.

DOSE ADJUSTMENTS

May be required with impaired renal or hepatic function.

DILUTION

1 Gm equals 4 ml of prepared solution. Further dilute with compatible infusion solutions (NS, D5/NS, D5W, DW [sterile water for injection], or Ringer's solution). Do not use DW in patients with subarachnoid hemorrhage.

Up to 50 ml of diluent may be used for each 1 Gm.

Storage: Prior to use store at controlled room temperature.

INCOMPATIBLE WITH

Sodium lactate.

RATE OF ADMINISTRATION

5 Gm or fraction thereof over first hour in 250 ml of solution; then administer each succeeding 1 Gm over 1 hour in 50 to 100 ml of solution. Use of an infusion pump for accurate dose recommended. Rapid administration or insufficient dilution may cause hypotension, bradycardia, and/or arrhythmia.

ACTIONS

A monaminocarboxylic acid with the specific action of inhibiting plasminogen activator substances; to a lesser degree inhibits plasmin activity. Increases fibrinogen activity in clot formation by inhibiting the enzyme required for destruction of formed fibrin. Onset of action is prompt, but will last less than 3 hours. Readily excreted in the urine. Easily penetrates red blood cells and tissue cells after prolonged administration.

INDICATIONS AND USES

Hemorrhage caused by overactivity of the fibrinolytic system. ■ Systemic hyperfibrinolysis (pathologic), which may result from heart surgery, portacaval shunt, prostatectomy, nephrectomy, aplastic anemia, abruptio placentae, hepatic cirrhosis, or carcinoma of the prostate, lung, stomach, and cervix. ■ Urinary fibrinolysis (normal physiologic phenomenon), which may result from severe trauma, anoxia, shock, surgery of the genitourinary system, or carcinoma of the genitourinary system. ■ Prophylaxis and treatment of postsurgical hemorrhage. ▪ Intra- and postoperative treatment of hemorrhage in patients with clotting defects other than hemophilia. ▪ Prophylaxis and treatment of hemophiliacs during surgery or dental surgery. ▪ Treat severe hemorrhage caused by thrombolytic agents (e.g., alteplase [tPA], streptokinase).

Investigational uses: Prevent recurrence of subarachnoid hemorrhage. ▪ Reduce need for platelet transfusions in management of amegakaryocytic thrombocytopenia.

CONTRAINDICATIONS

Disseminated intravascular coagulation, evidence of thrombosis, first and second trimester of pregnancy.

PRECAUTIONS

Use only in conjunction with general and specific tests to determine the amount of fibrinolysis present. ▪ Use extreme care in cardiac, hepatic, or renal diseases. Endocardial hemorrhage, myocardial fat degeneration, teratogenicity, and kidney stones have resulted in animals. ▪ Whole blood transfusions may be given if necessary.

Monitor: Vital signs, intake and output, any signs of bleeding, and neurologic assessment should be monitored based on patient condition. ▪ Observe for thromboembolic complications (e.g., chest pain, dyspnea, edema, hemoptysis, leg pain, or positive Homan's sign). ▪ Monitor lab evaluations as appropriate for diagnosis (e.g., platelet count, clotting factors, CPK, AST [SGOT]).

Patient education: Move slowly with help to avoid orthostatic hypotension.

Maternal/child: Category C: safety for use in pregnancy and lactation not established. Note Contraindications. ▪ Safety for use in children not established but is used.

Elderly: Consider age-related impaired organ function; reduced dose may be indicated.

DRUG/LAB INTERACTIONS

Potential for thrombus formation increased with concurrent use of estrogens. ▪ Frequently used with clotting factor complexes (e.g., factor IX complex, antiinhibitor coagulant complex) but risk of thrombus formation may be increased. Delay administration for 8 or more hours after clotting factor complexes. ▪ May elevate serum potassium, especially with impaired renal function; reduced dose may be indicated.

SIDE EFFECTS

Cramps, diarrhea, dizziness, grand mal seizure, headache, malaise, nausea, skin rash, stuffy nose, tearing, thrombophlebitis, tinnitus.

ANTIDOTE

Treat side effects symptomatically. Discontinue use of drug with any suspicion of thrombophlebitis, thromboembolic complications, or if CPK is elevated (myopathy). May be removed by hemodialysis or peritoneal dialysis.

AMINOPHYLLINE

Bronchodilator
Respiratory stimulant

(79% Theophylline), Theophylline ethylenediamine   pH 8.6 to 9.0

USUAL DOSE

Must be individualized based on serum theophylline concentration and patient response. Monitor frequently to avoid toxicity. Doses listed are milligrams of aminophylline to be administered.

Bronchodilation in acute asthma or bronchospasm: Loading dose: For patients not currently receiving a theophylline preparation, give an initial loading dose of 5 to 6 mg/kg of lean body weight (theophylline does not distribute into fatty tissue). Maintain by following with a continuous infusion. For patients who are currently receiving a theophylline preparation, the loading dose should be withheld if possible until a theophylline concentration can be obtained. Each 0.5 mg/ml of theophylline should result in a 1 mcg/ml increase in serum theophylline concentration. If a level cannot be obtained rapidly, a smaller loading dose may be administered, carefully evaluating the patient condition and risk versus benefit. For example, if significant respiratory distress is present, a smaller loading dose of 2.5 mg/kg should increase the level by approximately 5 mcg/ml. Such an increase is unlikely to cause significant side effects and may improve the clinical picture.

Maintenance dose: Most maintenance doses can be reduced within the first 12 hours based on serum theophylline levels and depending on patient condition and response. Usually given as a continuous infusion, but total daily dose can be calculated and given in equally divided doses every 4 to 6 hr. Current thinking is leaning toward lower serum theophylline levels than the present desired recommendation of 10 to 20 mcg/ml for adults.

Adult non-smokers: 0.5 to 0.7 mg/kg/hr.
Young adult smokers: 0.8 to 1 mg/kg/hr.
Older adults and patients with cor pulmonale: 0.3 to 0.6 mg/kg/hr.
Adults with CHF or liver failure: 0.1 to 0.5 mg/kg/hr.

PEDIATRIC DOSE

Bronchodilation in acute asthma or bronchospasm: Loading dose: For patients not currently receiving a theophylline preparation, 6 mg/kg of lean body weight is the maximum IV loading dose. Follow with a continuous infusion. For patients who are currently receiving a theophylline preparation, see comments under adult dose.

Maintenance dose: See all comments under adult maintenance dose. Present desired serum theophylline level recommendations for neonates are less than 10 mcg/ml and, for older infants, less than 20 mcg/ml.

Neonates: 0.2 mg/kg/hr.
Infants 6 weeks to 6 months: 0.5 mg/kg/hr.
Infants 6 months to 1 year: 0.6 to 0.7 mg/kg/hr.
Children 1 to 9 years: 0.8 to 1.2 mg/kg/hr.

Children 9 to 12 years and young adult smokers: 0.7 to 0.9 mg/kg/hr.
Children 12 to 16 years: 0.8 mg/kg/hr.

NEONATAL DOSE

Bronchodilation: See Pediatric dose. An alternate protocol calls for a loading dose of 1 mg/kg for each 2 mcg/ml serum theophylline concentration desired. Maintain with *(preterm [less than 40 weeks postconception])* 1 mg/kg lean body weight every 12 hours; *(term [40 weeks postconception] and up to 4 weeks postnatal)* 1 to 2 mg/kg every 12 hours; *(4 to 8 weeks)* 1 to 2 mg/kg every 8 hours; *(over 8 weeks)* 1 to 3 mg/kg every 6 hours.

Apnea and bradycardia of prematurity: Loading dose: 5 to 6 mg/kg given over 20 min.

Maintenance dose: One source recommends 1 to 2 mg/kg/dose every 6 to 8 hours. Other protocols use an intermittent infusion of 1 to 1.5 mg/kg given over 30 minutes every 12 hours. Other protocols are in use, for example: 3 to 8 mg/kg/day in 3 to 4 divided doses, 1 to 2 mg/kg every 6 or 8 hours, or a continuous infusion of 0.1 mg/kg/hr for *infants 0 to 24 days of age* and 0.15 mg/kg/hr for *infants over 24 days of age.* Maintain serum theophylline level between 6 and 13 mcg/ml for apnea.

DOSE ADJUSTMENTS

Dose adjustments should be based on patient response and measurement of serum theophylline concentration. ■ Reduced dose may be required in the elderly and in patients with cor pulmonale, congestive heart failure, or liver disease. ■ Smokers (especially those under 40 years) may require a higher dose. ■ Note Precautions.

DILUTION

Check vial carefully; must state for IV use. Warm to room temperature. Only the 25 mg/ml solution may be given by direct IV administration undiluted, but further dilution for infusion in at least 100 to 200 ml of D5W is preferred. Available prediluted. Crystals will form if solution pH falls below 8.0.

INCOMPATIBLE WITH

Acid solutions, amikacin (Amikin), ascorbic acid, atracurium (Tracrium), bleomycin (Blenoxane), cephalothin (Keflin), cephapirin (Cefadyl), chloramphenicol, chlorpromazine (Thorazine), cimetidine (Tagamet), ciprofloxacin (Cipro IV), clindamycin (Cleocin), codeine, corticotropin (Acthar), dimenhydrinate (Dramamine), dobutamine (Dobutrex), doxapram (Dopram), doxorubicin (Adriamycin), doxycycline (Vibramycin), epinephrine (Adrenalin), erythromycin (Ilotycin), fat emulsion 10%, fructose solution, heparin, hetastarch (Hespan), hydralazine, hydroxyzine (Vistaril), insulin, invert sugar solutions, isoproterenol (Isuprel), levorphanol (Levo-Dromoran), meperidine (Demerol), methadone, methicillin (Staphcillin), methylprednisolone (Solu-Medrol), morphine, nafcillin, norepineprine (Levophed), ondansetron (Zofran), papaverine, penicillin G sodium and potassium, pentazocine (Talwin), phenobarbital (Luminal), phenytoin (Dilantin), procaine, prochlorperazine (Compazine), promazine (Sparine), promethazine (Phenergan), succinylcholine (Anectine), vancomycin (Vancocin), verapamil (Isoptin).

RATE OF ADMINISTRATION

A single dose over a minimum of 20 to 30 minutes. Do not exceed an average rate of 1 ml or 20 mg/min when giving direct IV or as an infusion. Rapid administration may cause cardiac arrhythmias. Discontinue primary infusion if theophylline administered by piggyback or additive tubing and a possible incompatibility problem exists.

ACTIONS

An alkaloid xanthine derivative, it relaxes smooth muscle and the bronchial tubes. Cardiac output, urinary output, and sodium excretion are increased. Skeletal and cardiac muscles are stimulated, as is the CNS to a lesser degree. There is peripheral vasodilation. It decreases pulmonary artery pressure and lowers the threshold of the respiratory center to CO_2. Well distributed throughout the body and excreted in a changed form in the urine. Crosses the placental barrier. Secreted in breast milk.

INDICATIONS AND USES

Bronchial asthma. ■ Reversible bronchospasm of chronic bronchitis or emphysema.
Unlabeled uses: Apnea and bradycardia of prematurity. ■ Reduce bronchospasm in cystic fibrosis and acute descending respiratory infections. ■ Relieve periodic apnea and increase arterial blood pH in patients with Cheyne-Stokes respirations.

CONTRAINDICATIONS

Known sensitivity to theophylline or ethylenediamine, infants under 6 months of age except for apnea and bradycardia of prematurity.

PRECAUTIONS

Use with caution in cardiac disease, congestive heart failure, coronary occlusion, cor pulmonale, peptic ulcer disease, renal and hepatic disease, severe hypertension, severe hypoxemia, severe myocardial damage, hyperthyroidism, glaucoma, and in the elderly. Initiate oral therapy as soon as symptoms are adequately improved. Wait 4 to 6 hours after last IV dose or measure serum levels. ■ Note Maternal/child.
Monitor: Monitor serum levels to achieve maximum benefit with minimum risk. Each 0.5 mg/kg will increase serum theophylline by 1 mcg/ml. 10 to 20 mcg/ml is considered therapeutic. Peak serum level is best measured 20 to 30 minutes after initial loading dose or 12 to 14 hours into continuous infusion. ■ Monitor vital signs, including lung sounds. ■ Monitor for all signs of toxicity (see Side effects). Serious toxicity may not be preceded by less severe side effects. Maintain hydration. ■ Note Drug/lab interactions.
Maternal/child: Category C: use in pregnancy only if clearly indicated. ■ Neonates may have therapeutic blood levels and may develop apnea from theophylline withdrawal. ■ Elimination of drug is prolonged in premature infants, neonates, and children up to 1 year. Use with extreme caution in children. Has caused fatal reactions; note Contraindications. ■ Secreted in breast milk, some sources recommend discontinuing breast-feeding. If the decision is made to breast-feed, monitor infant for evidence of side effects.
Elderly: Note Dose adjustments. ■ Plasma clearance may be decreased and cause toxicity in patients over 55.

DRUG/LAB INTERACTIONS

Do not use one xanthine derivative concurrently with another xanthine derivative, ephedrine, or other sympathomimetic drugs. ▪ Xanthines antagonize or potentiate or are themselves antagonized or potentiated by many drug groups. Review of patient drug profile by pharmacist imperative. Examples are: inhibited (serum level decreased) by amino-glutenide, barbiturates, hydantoins (e.g., phenytoin [Dilantin]), keto-conazole (Nizoral), loop diuretics (e.g., furosemide [Lasix]), smoking; potentiated (serum level increased) by allopurinol, beta-adrenergic blockers (e.g., propranolol [Inderal]), caffeine (dietary), calcium channel blockers (e.g., diltiazem [Cardizem], verapamil [Isoptin]), cimetidine (Tagamet), erythromycin, interferon alfa-2b (recombinant [Intron A]), quinolone antibiotics (e.g., ciprofloxacin [Cipro]); potenti-ates erythromycin; inhibits nondepolarizing muscle relaxants (e.g., doxacurium [Nuromax], tubocurarine [Curare]). ▪ Carbamazipine (Tegretol) and loop diuretics (e.g., furosemide [Lasix]) may increase or decrease serum levels. ▪ May cause tachycardia with reserpine. ▪ Metabolism increases and plasma levels decrease in smokers. Higher dose ranges of aminophylline may be required. ▪ Reduces sedative effect of benzodiazepines (e.g., diazepam [Valium] and of propofol [Diprivan]). ▪ May decrease lithium levels. Dose adjustment and monitoring of lithium levels may be indicated. ▪ Concurrent use with halothane may induce cardiac arrhythmias. ▪ Concurrent use with ketamine may induce seizures.

SIDE EFFECTS

Toxicity resulting in death may occur suddenly, especially with serum levels above 20 mcg/ml. Anxiety, cardiac arrest, convulsions, delirium, dizziness, flushing, headache, hyperpyrexia, nausea, periph-eral vascular collapse, restlessness, temporary hypotension, ventricular fibrillation, vomiting.

ANTIDOTE

With onset of any side effect, discontinue the drug and notify the phy-sician. For mild symptoms the physician may choose to continue the drug at a decreased dose and rate of administration. All side effects will be treated symptomatically. Maintain adequate ventilation and adequate hydration. Grand mal seizures may not respond to anticon-vulsants. Diazepam (Valium) may be most effective. Treat atrial arrhythmias with verapamil, ventricular arrhythmias with lidocaine or procainamide. Use dopamine (Intropin) for hypotension. Do not use stimulants. Consider charcoal hemoperfusion dialysis for serum levels above 40 mcg/ml. Resuscitate as necessary.

AMIODARONE HYDROCHLORIDE

Antiarrhythmic

Cordarone

pH 4.08

USUAL DOSE

1,000 mg over the first 24 hours in 3 distinct segments; two loading infusions and a maintenance infusion. Use of a dedicated central venous catheter preferred.

Rapid loading infusion: 150 mg specifically diluted solution (1.5 mg/ml) over 10 minutes. Follow immediately with the slow loading infusion.

Slow loading infusion: 360 mg specifically diluted solution (1.8 mg/ml) at 1 mg/min over the next 6 hours.

Maintenance infusion: 540 mg of 1.8 mg/ml solution at 0.5 mg/min over 18 hours. Maintenance infusion is usually continued at 0.5 mg/min for 48 to 96 hours or until ventricular arrhythmias are stabilized. May be continued with caution for up to 2 to 3 weeks. Transfer to oral therapy as soon as feasible (guidelines are in package insert).

Treatment of breakthrough ventricular fibrillation (VF) or hemodynamically unstable ventricular tachycardia (VT): At any time that breakthrough VF or hemodynamically unstable VT occurs during administration, a supplemental rapid loading infusion (150 mg over 10 minutes) may be repeated. May be specifically diluted 1.5 mg/ml solution or rate of the maintenance infusion (1.8 mg/ml) may be temporarily increased to equal 150 mg (83.33 ml) over 10 minutes. During trials total doses above 1800 to 2100 mg (including added doses for breakthrough VF/VT) increased the risk of hypotension.

DOSE ADJUSTMENTS

Not required for the elderly or in renal or hepatic disease.

DILUTION

Do not use evacuated glass intravenous bottles. Use only commercially available D5W solutions in polyolefin or glass containers in any prepared solution that will be given over more than 2 hours. PVC containers are suitable only for dilution of the rapid loading dose.

Rapid loading infusion: Dilute 150 mg (3 ml) in 100 ml D5W (1.5 mg/ml).

Slow loading infusion and maintenance infusion: Dilute 900 mg (18 ml) in 500 ml D5W (1.8 mg/ml). Dilutions from 1 to 6 mg/ml have been used for maintenance solutions after the first 24 hours. Concentrations over 2 mg/ml for longer than 1 hour must be administered through a central venous catheter. Higher concentrations (3 to 6 mg/ml) have caused peripheral vein phlebitis.

Storage: Store ampuls in their carton at controlled room temperature. Use solutions diluted in PVC containers within 2 hours, diluted in glass or polyolefin containers within 24 hours.

INCOMPATIBLE WITH

Manufacturer recommends administration through a dedicated IV line (central venous catheter preferred). Y-site incompatibilities: aminophylline, cefamandole (Mandol), cefazolin (Kefzol), furosemide (Lasix), heparin, mezlocillin (Mezlin), sodium bicarbonate.

RATE OF ADMINISTRATION

A volumetric pump is required for administration. Surface properties of diluted solution reduce drop size; use of a drop counter infusion set causes underdosing. Use of a 0.2-micron in-line filter is also recommended. Filtering does not affect potency. Adhere to prescribed rates; risk of hypotension is increased in the first hours of treatment, with increased doses and increased rates; may cause secondary renal or hepatic failure.

Rapid loading infusion or breakthrough treatment of VF/VT: 150 mg over 10 minutes (15 mg/min). Do not exceed a rate of 30 mg/min.

Slow loading infusion: 1 mg/min or 33.3 ml/hr of 1.8 mg/ml solution for 6 hours.

Maintenance infusion: 0.5 mg/min or 16.6 ml/hr of 1.8 mg/ml solution for 18 hours. A continuing maintenance solution should deliver 720 mg/24 hr at 0.5 mg/min whether the concentration is 1.8 mg/ml or 6 mg/ml. May be continued at this rate for up to 2 to 3 weeks as described in Usual dose.

ACTIONS

An antiarrhythmic agent possessing several antiarrhythmic effects that result in a decreased number of VT/VF events. It prolongs the duration of action potentials in cardiac fibers, depresses conduction velocity, slows conduction at the AV node, and exhibits some alpha and beta blockade activity. Also has vasodilatory effects that decrease cardiac workload and myocardial oxygen consumption. Uptake by the myocardium is rapid; antiarrhythmic effect is prompt (clinically relevant within hours); however, full effect may take days. Has an exceptionally long half-life. Metabolized in the liver using cytochrome P-450 enzymes. Primarily excreted in bile. Crosses placental barrier. Secreted in breast milk.

INDICATIONS AND USES

Treatment of acute life-threatening VT/VF and prophylaxis of frequently recurring VF and hemodynamically unstable VT in patients refractory to other therapy (e.g., bretylium, lidocaine, procainamide). Used until ventricular arrhythmias are stabilized; usually 48 to 96 hours, but may be given for longer periods (i.e., up to 3 weeks). ■ Treatment of patients taking oral amiodarone who are unable to take oral medication.

CONTRAINDICATIONS

Cardiogenic shock, known hypersensitivity to amiodarone or any of its components, marked sinus bradycardia, second- or third-degree AV block unless a functioning pacemaker is available.

PRECAUTIONS

Usually administered by or under the direction of the physician specialist. ■ Adequate facilities and emergency resuscitation drugs and equipment must always be available. ■ Correct hypokalemia and hypomagnesemia before use; may exaggerate a prolonged QTc and cause arrhythmias (e.g., torsades de pointes). ■ Does absorb to PVC tubing but loss accounted for in specified dose; follow infusion regimen closely. ■ May cause transient increases in liver enzymes but abnormal baseline hepatic enzymes is not a contraindication to use. ■ May worsen existing arrhythmias or precipitate new ones, primarily torsades de pointes or new-onset VF. ■ May cause visual impairment (e.g., optic neuropathy or optic neuritis); has progressed to permanent blindness. ■ May cause pulmonary toxicity, especially with long-term use. ■ Note Drug/lab interactions.

Monitor: Continuous ECG and HR monitoring is mandatory to observe for arrhythmias. Watch for QTc prolongation; may cause proarrhythmia (torsades de pointes). ■ Monitor for bradycardia and AV block. A temporary pacemaker should be available. ■ Monitor blood pressure closely to minimize hypotension (occurs frequently with initial rates). ■ Confirm patency of vein. Reduce rate or concentration for pain or redness at injection site. Incidence of phlebitis markedly increased with concentrations above 2.5 mg/ml; central venous administration preferred. ■ Monitor serum electrolytes and acid-base balance, especially in patients with prolonged diarrhea and those receiving diuretics. ■ Monitor liver enzymes (AST, ALT, GGT) for elevations indicating progressive injury. ■ Regular ophthalmic exams, including fundoscopy and slit lamp exams, are recommended. Prompt ophthalmic exams recommended at first sign of visual impairment. May require discontinuation of amiodarone therapy. ■ Note Precautions and Drug/lab interactions.

Patient education: Report promptly any feelings of faintness, difficulty breathing, or pain or stinging along injection site. ■ Nonhormonal birth control recommended. ■ Avoid excessive sunlight. May cause sunburn for weeks (extended half-life). Protective clothing and dark glasses may be appropriate outdoors.

Maternal/child: Category D: avoid pregnancy or use only if benefit to mother justifies risk to fetus. Has caused infrequent neonatal congenital goiter/hypothyroidism and hyperthyroidism in addition to other adverse effects in animals. ■ Discontinue breast-feeding. ■ Safety for use during labor and delivery and in children not established.

Elderly: Clearance is slower and half-life may be doubled (up to 47 days).

DRUG/LAB INTERACTIONS

Amiodarone has a long half-life; drug interactions may persist long after it is discontinued.

Should not be given concurrently with ibutilide (Corvert). ■ Risk of cardiotoxicity increased with pimozide (Orap), ritonavir (Norvir), and sparfloxacin (Zagam), concurrent use not recommended. ■ Prothrombin time increased with warfarin (Coumadin). ■ May decrease metabolism and increase serum levels of cyclosporine (Sandimmune), digoxin, hydantoins (e.g. phenytoin [Dilantin]), lidocaine, procainamide (Pronestyl), quinidine, and theophyllines (Aminophylline). May cause toxicity; monitor serum levels. ■ Increases QT prolongation with disopyramide (Norpace); may cause arrhythmia. ■ May cause bradycardia, decreased cardiac output, and hypotension with fentanyl (Sublimaze). ■ Therapeutic plasma concentrations of flecainide (Tambocor) can be maintained with reduced doses because amiodarone interferes with flecainide metabolism. ■ Amiodarone metabolism increased and serum levels decreased with cholestyramine (Questran) and phenytoin (Dilantin). Cimetidine (Tagamet) decreases metabolism and increases serum amiodarone levels. ■ May increase risk of bradycardia and hypotension with beta-blockers (e.g., propranolol [Inderal]).

■ May increase risk of AV block and hypotension with calcium channel blockers (e.g., diltiazem [Cardizem], verapamil [Calan]).

■ Use for longer than 2 weeks may decrease metabolism and increase serum levels of dextromethorphan (Robitussin DM), methotrexate, and phenytoin.

SIDE EFFECTS

Hypotension or pain at the IV site are the most common side effects. Arrhythmias (e.g., AV block, bradycardia, new onset VT/VF, torsades de pointes), adult respiratory distress syndrome (ARDS), cardiac arrest, cardiogenic shock, congestive heart failure, dry eyes, hepato-toxicity (liver function test abnormalities), photosensitivity, and visual impairment/loss of vision may occur. In addition to these side effects, overdose or extended use may cause hepatic and/or renal failure secondary to hypotension.

ANTIDOTE

Keep physician informed of all side effects and treat promptly as appropriate; many are life-threatening. Reduce rate and/or concentration for pain at IV site. Monitor hepatic enzymes closely. Reduce rate or discontinue for progressive hepatic injury. Treat hypotension and cardiogenic shock by slowing the infusion rate. Vasopressors (e.g., dopamine [Intropin], norepinephrine [Levophed]), inotropic agents (e.g., digoxin), and volume expansion may be indicated. Slow infusion rate or discontinue if bradycardia and/or AV block occur; may require a temporary pacemaker. If torsades de pointes occurs, stop all cardioactive drugs (e.g., antiarrhythmics, digoxin, antidepressants, phenothiazines) and normalize electrolytes (e.g., potassium, magnesium). Atrial overdrive pacing may be required to stabilize cardiac rhythm. Amiodarone is not dialyzable. Resuscitate as necessary.

AMMONIUM CHLORIDE

Electrolyte Replenisher
Acidifying Agent

pH 4.5 to 6.0

USUAL DOSE

Dependent on patient condition and tolerance. Monitor serum bicarbonate or carbon dioxide combining power repeatedly to determine individualized dosage. Begin with contents of 1 or 2 vials (100 to 200 mEq). Use minimal effective dose initially. Usual adult dose is 1.5 Gm every 6 hours. Maximum effect of a single dose not fully apparent for several days. Each gram of ammonium chloride reduces the carbon dioxide combining power of 70 kg adult by 1.1 volume %.

26.75% solution contains 5 mEq NH_4 and 5 mEq Cl/ml. 1 Gm of ammonium chloride contains 18.7 mEq of NH_4 and 18.7 mEq of Cl.

PEDIATRIC DOSE

75 mg/kg/24 hr. Divide equally and give every 6 hours.

DILUTION

Each 100 mEq (20 ml) of 26.75% solution must be diluted with 500 ml NS to achieve the desired 1% to 2% solution. Potassium chloride,

20 to 40 mEq/L, may be added to the ammonium infusion (serum potassium usually low). For infants dilute each 1 ml of ammonium chloride in a minimum of 5 to 10 ml diluent. If crystals form, warm in a water bath to room temperature before administration.

Storage: Store at controlled room temperature.

INCOMPATIBLE WITH

Codeine, dimenhydrinate (Dramamine), levorphanol (Levo-Dromoran), methadone hydrochloride, warfarin (Coumadin). All alkalis

RATE OF ADMINISTRATION

Up to 5 ml diluted solution/min for adults. Reduce rate significantly for infants. Slow infusion rate for pain along venipuncture site.

ACTIONS

Acidifying agent. Ammonium chloride dissociates into an ammonium cation and a chloride anion. Ammonium ions are converted to urea by the liver, freeing hydrogen ions and chloride ions. Hydrogen ion reacts with bicarbonate to form water and carbon dioxide (excreted by the lungs). Chloride ion combines with fixed bases (mostly sodium) to produce diuresis. Combined process reduces the alkaline reserve of the body. A compensatory action occurs within the body to halt this process within 3 days.

INDICATIONS AND USES

Treatment of hypochloremic states and metabolic alkalosis, which may be due to chloride loss from vomiting (including vomiting due to pyloric stenosis in infants); gastric fistula drainage; gastric suction; or excessive alkalinizing medication to prevent tetany or renal damage due to persistent severe alkalemia.

CONTRAINDICATIONS

Impaired renal function, metabolic alkalosis with sodium loss resulting in excretion of sodium bicarbonate in the urine (usually due to vomiting of hydrochloric acid or gastric suction), severe hepatic impairment (can cause ammonia retention, intoxication and hepatic coma).

PRECAUTIONS

Use caution in cardiac edema, impaired renal or hepatic function, pulmonary insufficiency, or primary respiratory acidosis with a high total CO_2 and buffer base.

Monitor: Accurate blood chemistry data required before, during, and after therapy to avoid serious metabolic acidosis and deficiencies. Replacement of sodium or potassium ions may be required. ■ Observe respirations closely (increased ventilation at rest and exertional dyspnea indicate acidosis). ■ Monitor closely for metabolic acidosis (coma, confusion, disorientation) and ammonium toxicity (bradycardia, cardiac arrhythmias, coma, irregular breathing, local and general twitching, pallor, retching, sweating, tonic convulsions). ■ Record intake and output.

Maternal/child: Category C: safety for use during pregnancy or lactation not established; use only if clearly needed. ■ Safety for use in children not established.

DRUG/LAB INTERACTIONS

Inhibits or potentiates many drugs as an acidifying agent.

SIDE EFFECTS

Most side effects are caused by ammonia toxicity. Calcium-deficient tetany, cardiac arrhythmias including bradycardia, coma, convulsions (tonic), depression, disorientation, EEG abnormalities, excitability, glycosuria, headache, hyperglycemia, hypokalemia, increased rate and depth of breathing (Kussmaul), irregular respiration, metabolic acidosis, nausea, pain along injection site, pallor, retching, skin rash, stupor, sweating, twitching, vomiting, weakness. Note Precautions.

ANTIDOTE

For all side effects reduce rate of administration or discontinue drug and notify the physician. Treat hypokalemia with potassium and tetany with calcium. Sodium lactate or sodium bicarbonate IV may be used to treat acidosis. Resuscitate as necessary.

AMOBARBITAL SODIUM

Barbiturate
Sedative/Hypnotic
Anticonvulsant

Amytal sodium

pH 9.6 to 10.4

USUAL DOSE

Hypnotic: 65 to 200 mg/dose.

Sedative: 30 to 50 mg. May repeat 2 to 3 times daily.

Anticonvulsant: 65 to 500 mg (gr 1 to 71/2). 1 Gm (gr 15) is the maximum single adult dose.

PEDIATRIC DOSE

Children over 6 years: Same as adult doses.

Children under 6 years: Sedative: 3 to 5 mg/kg/dose.

Anticonvulsant: 3 to 5 mg/kg/dose or 125 mg/M^2.

DOSE ADJUSTMENTS

Reduce dose in impaired renal or hepatic function, usually required in the debilitated or elderly. ■ Note Drug/lab interactions.

DILUTION

Each 125 mg (gr 2) must be diluted with a minimum of 1.25 ml of sterile water for injection to make a 10% solution. Inject diluent slowly and rotate vial to dissolve powder. Do not shake. Hydrolyzes in dry or solution form when exposed to air. Solution should be absolutely clear after 5 minutes. Discard powder or solution that has been exposed to air for 30 minutes.

INCOMPATIBLE WITH

Cefazolin (Kefzol), cephalothin (Keflin), chlorpromazine (Thorazine), cimetidine (Tagamet), clindamycin (Cleocin), codeine, dimenhydrinate (Dramamine), diphenhydramine (Benadryl), droperidol (Inapsine), hydrocortisone sodium succinate (Solu-Cortef), hydroxyzine (Vistaril), insulin (aqueous), levorphanol (Levo-Dromoran), meperidine (Demerol), methadone, morphine, norepinephrine (Levophed), pancuronium (Pavulon), penicillin G potassium, pentazocine (Talwin), phytonadione (Aquamephyton), procaine, prochlorperazine (Compazine), streptomycin, thiamine (Betalin S), vancomycin (Vancocin).

RATE OF ADMINISTRATION

Each 50 to 100 mg or fraction thereof over 1 minute for adults and 60 mg/M^2 for children. Titrate slowly and use only enough medication to achieve desired effect. Do not exceed 1 ml of a 10% solution/min. Rapid injection may cause symptoms of overdose (e.g., serious respiratory depression).

ACTIONS

A sedative, hypnotic barbiturate of intermediate duration with anticonvulsant effects. Amobarbital is a CNS depressant. Onset of action is prompt by the IV route and lasts about 4 to 6 hours. Pain perception is unimpaired. Rapidly absorbed by all body tissues and excreted fairly quickly in changed form in the urine. Crosses the placental barrier. Secreted in breast milk.

INDICATIONS AND USES

Control of convulsive seizures due to eclampsia, meningitis, poisons, tetanus or chorea. ▪ Short term sedation. ▪ Narcoanalysis and narcotherapy. ▪ Control agitated behavior in acute psychosis.

CONTRAINDICATIONS

History of porphyria, severely impaired liver function especially with any signs of hepatic coma, known hypersensitivity to barbiturates, severe respiratory depression.

PRECAUTIONS

IV route usually reserved for critical situations. Use of large veins preferred to prevent thrombosis. Intraarterial injection causes gangrene. ▪ Treat the cause of a convulsion. ▪ Use caution in asthma, cardiovascular diseases, hypertension, hypotension, impaired hepatic or renal function, pulmonary diseases, depressive states after convulsions, shock, and in the elderly. ▪ Use caution in the presence of fever, diabetes, hyperthyroidism, or severe anemia; untoward reactions may occur. ▪ May be habit forming; use caution in acute or chronic pain. ▪ Status epilepticus can occur from too-rapid withdrawal. ▪ Benzodiazepines (diazepam [Valium]) generally preferred for sedation.

Monitor: Highly alkaline, determine absolute patency of vein; avoid extravasation. ▪ Record blood pressure, pulse, and respiration every 3 to 5 minutes. Keep patient under constant observation. ▪ Keep equipment for artificial ventilation available. Maintain a patent airway. ▪ Monitor hematopoietic, renal and hepatic systems in extended therapy. ▪ Note Drug/lab interactions.

Patient education: Avoid alcohol or other CNS depressants (e.g., antihistamines, diazepam [Valium]). ▪ May be habit forming. ▪ Consider birth control options.

Maternal/child: Category D: avoid pregnancy; will cause birth defects. ▪ Withdrawal symptoms have occurred in infants born to mothers receiving barbiturates. ▪ Drowsiness has been reported in nursing infants. ▪ May cause paradoxical excitement in children.

Elderly: Note Dose adjustments. ▪ Often have increased sensitivity to barbiturates, may cause marked excitement, depression, confusion and increased risk of barbiturate induced hypothermia.

DRUG/LAB INTERACTIONS

Use with extreme caution if any other CNS depressants have been given, such as alcohol, narcotic analgesics, anesthetics, antidepressants, antihistamines, hypnotics, MAO inhibitors, phenothiazines, sedatives, neuromuscular blocking antibiotics, and tranquilizers. Potentiation with respiratory depression may occur. ▪ Inhibits corticosteroids, doxycycline (Vibramycin), griseofulvin, oral anticoagulants, oral contraceptives, quinidine, theophylline, and beta adrenergic blockers (e.g., propranolol [Inderal]). Capable of innumerable interactions with many drugs. ■ May increase orthostatic hypotension with furosemide (Lasix). ■ Monitor phenytoin and barbiturate levels when both drugs are used concurrently. ■ May inhibit Vitamin D metabolism with extended use.

SIDE EFFECTS

Average dose: Depression, dermatitis, facial edema, fever, hypotension, neonatal apnea, respiratory depression (hypoventilation), thrombocytopenic purpura.

Overdose: Apnea, coma, cough reflex depression, flat EEG (reversible unless hypoxic damage has occurred), hypotension, hypothermia, laryngospasm, pulmonary edema, reflexes (sluggish or absent), renal shutdown, respiratory depression.

ANTIDOTE

Notify the physician of any side effect. Symptomatic and supportive treatment is most important in overdose. Maintain an adequate airway with artificial ventilation if indicated. Keep the patient warm. IV volume expanders (dextran) and other IV fluids will help maintain adequate circulation. Osmotic diuretics (mannitol) or hemodialysis will promote elimination of the drug. Vasopressors (e.g., dopamine [Intropin]) will maintain blood pressure.

AMPHOTERICIN B/AMPHOTERICIN B LIPOSOME INJECTION

Antifungal

Fungizone / Abelcet, AmBisome, Amphotec

pH 5.7 to 8.0 / 5.0 to 6.0

USUAL DOSE

Abelcet (amphotericin B lipid complex injection [liposomal]):
Adults and children: 5 mg/kg/24 hr as an infusion. Repeat daily until clinical response or mycological cure.

Amphotec (amphotericin B cholesteryl sulfate complex for injection [liposomal]):
Adults and children: 3 to 4 mg/kg/24 hr as an infusion. Pretreatment with antipyretics, antihistamines, or corticosteroids may be indicated, see Precautions and Antidote. On the first day of treatment, begin with a test dose of 10 ml of the final diluted preparation and infuse over 15 to 30 minutes. Observe the patient for the next 30 minutes. If there is no adverse reaction, continue with the calculated dose. May be increased to 6 mg/kg/24 hr if there is no improvement or if the fungal infection progresses. Note Indications.

AmBisome (amphotericin B liposome for injection):
Adults, children, and infants over 1 month of age: All doses are by infusion.

Empirical therapy: 3 mg/kg/24 hr.

Systemic fungal infections (e.g., Aspergillus, Candida, Cryptococcus): 3 to 5 mg/kg/24 hr.

Visceral Leishmaniasis in immunocompetent patients: 3 mg/kg/24 hr on days 1 through 5. Repeat 3 mg/kg on day 14 and on day 21. A repeat course of therapy may be useful if parasitic clearance is not achieved.

Visceral Leishmaniasis in immunocompromised patients: 4 mg/kg/24 hr on days 1 through 5. Repeat 4 mg/kg on days 10, 17, 21, 31, and 38. During clinical studies parasitic clearance was not achieved or relapse within 6 months occurred in 88.2% of patients. Usefulness of repeat courses not determined.

Fungizone/generic (traditional amphotericin B):
Adults and children: Begin with a test dose of 0.1 mg/kg up to 1 mg maximum dose in 20 to 50 ml D5W. Infuse over 10 to 30 minutes. Determine size of therapeutic dose by intensity of reaction over a 4-hour period. Usual is 0.25 mg/kg of body weight/24 hr gradually increased in 0.125- to 0.25-mg/kg increments to 1 mg/kg/24 hr or a maximum of 50 mg/day (average dose is 0.5 mg/kg) as tolerance permits. Maximum dose for children is 1 mg/kg/day or 30 mg/M^2/day. Up to 1.5 mg/kg/24 hr may be given on alternate-day therapy. Several months of therapy are usually required and recommended for cure. Dosage must be adjusted to each specific patient. In some instances higher doses can be used.

Mannitol 12.5 Gm immediately before and after each dose of Fungizone or generic amphotericin B may reduce nephrotoxic effects. See Precautions for additional suggestions.

DOSE ADJUSTMENTS

Abelcet: Full dose usually required; base on serum creatinine and overall patient condition.

Amphotec/AmBisome: No dose adjustments suggested.

Fungizone/generic: Full dose required even in impaired renal function, but reduce dose or discontinue drug if BUN above 40 mg/100 ml or serum creatinine above 3 mg/100 ml. ▪ Gradual dose increases are essential. Whenever medicine is not given for 7 days or longer, restart treatment at lowest dosage level.

DILUTION

Abelcet: Shake 20 ml (100 mg) vial until all yellow sediment is dissolved. Maintain aseptic technique. Withdraw an exact total daily dose from one or more vials using one or more 20-ml syringes and 18-gauge needles. Replace needle(s) on syringe(s) with the 5-micron filter(s) supplied with each vial. A new filter must be used for each 20 ml of Abelcet. Empty syringe contents through filter into an infusion of D5W. 4 ml of diluent (D5W) is required for each 1 ml (5 mg) of Abelcet to achieve a final concentration of 1 mg/ml. For *pediatric* and/or fluid restricted patients (e.g., cardiovascular disease) reduce diluent by half (approximate concentration of 2 mg/ml). Use only clear solutions and discard unused portion. pH 5.5 to 6.0.

Amphotec: Available in 50-mg or 100-mg vials. Reconstitute by rapidly adding 10 ml of SW for each 50 mg of Amphotec (5 mg/ml). Use of a 20-gauge needle is recommended. Shake gently, rotating the vial until all solids have dissolved. May be opalescent or clear. Must be further diluted for infusion with D5W (see chart). Final desired concentration is approximately 0.6 mg/ml (range with recommended amounts of diluent is 0.16 mg/ml to 0.83 mg/ml). Do not filter or use an in-line filter. Note Incompatible with and Rate of Administration.

Dose of AMPHOTEC	Volume of Reconstituted AMPHOTEC	Infusion Bag Size for D5W for Injection
10 - 35 mg	2 - 7 mL	50 mL
35 - 70 mg	7 - 14 mL	100 mL
70 - 175 mg	14 - 35 mL	250 mL
175 - 350 mg	35 - 70 mL	500 mL
350 - 1000 mg	70 - 200 mL	1000 mL

AmBisome: Reconstitute each 50-mg vial with 12 ml SW (without a bacteriostatic agent) to yield 4 mg/ml. Shake vial vigorously for 30 seconds; forms a yellow translucent suspension. Withdraw an exact total daily dose from one or more vials using one or more 20-ml syringes and needles. Replace needle(s) with the 5-micron filter(s) supplied with each vial. A new filter must be used for each 50-mg vial. Empty syringe contents through filter into an infusion of D5W. Use sufficient diluent to achieve a final concentration of 1 to 2 mg/ml, pH 5 to 6.

Pediatric dilution: May be further diluted to concentrations of 0.2 to 0.5 mg/ml for infants and small children to provide adequate volume for infusion.

Fungizone/generic: A 50-mg vial is initially diluted with 10 ml of sterile water for injection (without a bacteriostatic agent); 5 mg equals 1 ml. Shake well until solution is clear. Further dilute each 1 mg in at least 10 ml of D5W. Dextrose must have a pH above 4.2. Concentration of solution must not be greater than 0.1 mg/ml. Do not use any other diluent. Use a sterile 20-gauge or larger needle at each step of the dilution. Maintain aseptic technique. Larger-pore 1-micron filters may be used. Use only fresh solutions without evidence of precipitate or foreign matter. Light sensitive but protection from light not required unless solution exposed over 8 hours. pH 5.7 to 8.0.

Storage: Abelcet: Prior to reconstitution, refrigerate vials and protect from light. Do not freeze. Diluted solution is stable 15 hours if refrigerated and an additional 6 hours at room temperature.

Amphotec: Store unopened vials in carton at controlled room temperature. Refrigerate reconstituted or diluted solutions, must be used within 24 hours. Do not freeze. Discard unused drug.

AmBisome: Refrigerate unopened vials. Vials reconstituted with SW may be refrigerated for up to 24 hours. Do not freeze. Infusion of fully diluted solution must begin within 6 hours. Discard unused drug.

Fungizone/generic: Prior to reconstitution, refrigerate vials and protect from light. Do not freeze. Preserve concentrate in refrigerator up to 7 days or 24 hours at room temperature. Use diluted solution promptly.

INCOMPATIBLE WITH

Abelcet: Do not mix with any other diluent, drug, or solution. Use only D5W. Manufacturer states compatibility with any other diluent has not been established.

Amphotec/AmBisome: Do not mix with any other diluent, drug, or solution. Use only SW for reconstitution and D5W for dilution for infusion. Use of any other solution or the presence of a bacteriostatic agent (e.g., benzyl alcohol) may cause precipitation.

Fungizone/generic: Do not mix with any drug unless absolutely necessary. Allopurinol (Zyloprim), amifostine (Ethyol), amikacin (Amikin), calcium chloride, calcium gluconate, calcium disodium edetate, carbenicillin (Geopen), chlorpromazine (Thorazine), chlortetracycline (Aureomycin), cimetidine (Tagamet), diphenhydramine (Benadryl), dopamine (Intropin), electrolyte solutions, enalaprilat (Vasotec IV), fat emulsion 20%, filgrastim (Neupogen), fluconazole (Diflucan), fludarabine (Fludara), foscarnet (Foscavir), gentamicin (Garamycin), heparin, kanamycin (Kantrex), magnesium sulfate, melphalan (Alkeran), metaraminol (Aramine), methyldopa (Aldomet), multivitamin infusions, normal saline, ondansetron (Zofran), paclitaxel (Taxol), penicillin G, potassium, or sodium, piperacillin-tazobactam (Zosyn), polymyxin B (Aerosporin), potassium chloride, preservatives such as benzyl alcohol, prochlorperazine (Compazine), ranitidine; saline solutions (Zantac), sargramostim (Leukine), streptomycin, verapamil (Isoptin), vinorelbine (Navelbine). Not compatible in any solution with a pH below 4.2.

RATE OF ADMINISTRATION

All amphotericins: Rapid infusion may cause hypotension, hypokalemia, arrhythmia, and shock. Infusion reactions can occur with all amphotericin B formulations. Note Precautions, Side Effects and Antidote. With all formulations, flush existing line with D5W before and after administration or use a separate IV line.

Abelcet: Total daily dose as an infusion at 2.5 mg/kg/hr. Contents of diluted solution must be mixed by shaking at least every 2 hours. Do not use any in-line filter less than 5 microns.

Amphotec: Note rate for test dose in usual dose. Give total daily dose as an infusion at 1 mg/kg/hr. Infusion time may be shortened to a minimum of 2 hours for patients who show no evidence of intolerance or infusion-related reactions. May be extended for acute reactions or if infusion volume is not tolerated. Do not use filters.

AmBisome: Total daily dose as an infusion over 2 hours. Use of a controlled infusion device is recommended. Infusion time may be shortened to a minimum of 1 hour for patients who show no evidence of intolerance or infusion related reactions. Infusion time may be extended for patient discomfort or acute reactions or if infusion volume is not tolerated. Do not use any in-line filter less than 1 micron.

Fungizone/generic: Daily dose over 2 to 6 hours by slow IV infusion. Expected reactions usually less severe with slower rate. A minimum 1-micron filter may be used.

ACTIONS

Antifungal antibiotic agents that bind to fungal cell membranes resulting in leakage of cellular contents. May be fungistatic or fungicidal according to body fluid concentration and susceptibility of the fungus. Abelcet is amphotericin B complexed with two phospholipids in a 1:1 drug-to-lipid ratio. Amphotec is amphotericin B complexed with cholesteryl sulfate in a 1:1 drug-to-lipid ratio. AmBisome is amphotericin B intercalated into a liposomal membrane with several components. While assay tests cannot distinguish lipid complexed amphotericin (Abelcet and Amphotec) from uncomplexed (Fungizone/generic), the lipid complex can affect properties of a drug (e.g., incidence of renal toxicity and other side effects somewhat reduced). Lipid complexed agents are not uncomplexed until in the presence of lipase release (usually areas where fungi are) so it does less harm to the rest of the body. Not effective against bacteria, rickettsiae, or viruses. Remains in the body at a therapeutic level up to 20 hours after each infusion (Abelcet has the longest elimination half-life [up to 173 hours]). Route of metabolism not known. Excreted very slowly in the urine.

INDICATIONS AND USES

Abelcet: Treatment of invasive fungal infections in patients who are refractory to or intolerant of traditional amphotericin B therapy (e.g., aspergillosis, candidiasis, cryptococcosis, cryptococcal meningitis, fusariosis, zygomycosis). Has orphan drug approval for invasive coccidioidomycosis, invasive prototheccosis, and invasive sporotrichosis.

Amphotec: Treatment of invasive aspergillosis in patients refractory to or intolerant of traditional amphotericin B or in patients where traditional amphotericin treatment has failed.

AmBisome: Empirical therapy for presumed fungal infection in febrile, neutropenic patients. ■ Treatment of patients with aspergillosis, candida, and/or cryptococcus infections refractory to traditional amphotericin B or in patients in whom renal impairment or unacceptable toxicity precludes the use of traditional amphotericin B. ■ Treatment of visceral Leishmaniasis. ▪ Has orphan drug approval for treatment of cryptococcal meningitis. Specific information not yet available.

Fungizone/generic: Treatment of fungal infections that are progressive and potentially fatal, such as aspergillosis, cryptococcosis, blastomycosis, and disseminated forms of candidiasis, coccidioidomycosis, and histoplasmosis, mucormycosis, and sporotrichosis. These infections must be caused by specific organisms.

Investigational use: Abelcet is used to prevent fungal infections in bone marrow transplant patients (0.1 mg/kg/day).

CONTRAINDICATIONS

All amphotericin formulations: Known sensitivity to amphotericin B or any components of its formulations unless a life-threatening situation is present.

PRECAUTIONS

All amphotericin formulations: Diagnosis should be positively established by culture or histologic study. ▪ Close clinical observation is imperative. Anaphylaxis has occurred; emergency equipment and supplies must be available. ▪ Infusion reactions are common, pretreatment with antipyretics, antihistamines (e.g., diphenhydramine [Benadryl]), and/or selective use of corticosteroids may be indicated. ▪ Use caution in patients receiving leukocyte transfusions, may cause acute pulmonary toxicity. Separate times of administration as much as possible. ▪ Diabetics must be well controlled before treatment with amphotericin is begun.

Abelcet: Renal toxicity is dose dependent but has been consistently less nephrotoxic than uncomplexed amphotericin B.

Amphotec/AmBisome: Incidence of renal toxicity significantly lower than with uncomplexed amphotericin B.

Fungizone/generic: Hospitalization preferred to initiate therapy. ▪ A small amount of heparin added to the infusion may reduce the incidence of thrombophlebitis. ▪ Meperidine (Demerol) or nonsteroidal antiinflammatory agents (e.g., ibuprofen) prior to administration or hydrocortisone 0.7 mg/kg of body weight added to the infusion may prevent febrile reactions including chills; corticosteroids not recommended for concomitant use in other situations; they exaggerate hypokalemia. ▪ Prophylactic antiemetics and antihistamines are also appropriate.

Monitor: All amphotericin formulations: Obtain baseline CBC, serum electrolytes, renal (e.g., serum creatinine, BUN) and liver function (e.g., ALT, AST) tests. Repeat frequently during therapy, recommended weekly. Discontinue or reduce dose until renal function improves if BUN > 40 mg/dl or serum creatinine > 3 mg/dl. Side effects (e.g., hypokalemia, hypomagnesemia, impaired renal function) may be life threatening. ▪ Monitor vital signs and intake output. Record every 30 minutes for up to 4 hours after infusion is complete. ▪ Encourage fluids to maintain hydration.

Patient education: All amphotericin formulations: Discomfort associated with infusion. ▪ Report difficulty breathing promptly. ▪ Long-term therapy required to effect a cure. ▪ Report diarrhea, fever, increased or decreased urination, loss of appetite, stomach pain, sore throat, and any unusual bleeding or bruising, tiredness, or weakness.

Maternal/child: All amphotericin formulations: Pregnancy category B: Has been used successfully during pregnancy but adequate studies not available. Use only if clearly needed. ▪ Safety for use in lactation and children not established. Discontinue nursing. ▪ Fungizone/generic has been used in children. Liposomal preparations have been used in children without any unexpected side effects. Safety of use of AmBisome in infants under 1 month of age not established.

Elderly: Consider age-related impaired body functions. Liposomal preparations have been used without unexpected side effects.

DRUG/LAB INTERACTIONS

Drug interaction studies have not been done for liposomal preparations, but interactions similar to Fungizone/generic are expected.

Corticosteroids and corticotropin (ACTH) will increase hypokalemia and may cause arrhythmias. Use with caution only if indicated to control drug reactions or, if necessary, monitor serum electrolytes and cardiac function closely. ▪ Hypokalemic effect may be increased with thiazides, may potentiate digitalis toxicity, and/or enhance the curariform effect of neuromuscular blocking agents (e.g., doxacurium [Nuromax], rocuronium [Zemuron], succinylcholine [Anectine]); monitor serum potassium levels. ▪ Avoid use or use extreme caution with other nephrotoxic drugs; aminoglycosides (e.g., gentamicin [Garamycin], tobramycin [Nebcin]), selected antibiotics (e.g., polymyxin B, vancomycin), antineoplastics (e.g., cisplatin, nitrogen mustard), anesthetics (e.g., methoxyflurane [Penthrane]), antituberculars (e.g., capreomycin [Capestat]), cyclosporine (Sandimmune), diuretics (e.g., furosemide [Lasix], torsemide [Demadex]), pentamidine (Pentam). Nephrotoxic effects are additive. Frequent monitoring of renal function indicated if any other nephrotoxic drug must be used. ▪ Nephrotoxicity and myelotoxicity are both increased when given concurrently with zidovudine (AZT). ▪ Potentiates nephrotoxicity of cyclosporine; alternate immunosuppressive therapy recommended. ▪ Concurrent use with antineoplastic agents (e.g., methotrexate) or radiation therapy may increase renal toxicity and incidence of bronchospasm and hypotension. ▪ Enhances antifungal effects of flucytosine (Ancobon) and other antibiotics. May increase toxicity. ▪ May antagonize effect of imidazoles (e.g., ketoconazole, miconazole, fluconazole). ▪ Acute pulmonary toxicity occurred in patients receiving leukocyte transfusion; separate administration times as much as possible.

SIDE EFFECTS

Liposomal preparations: Most side effect similar to Fungizone but occur with less frequency and intensity. Acute reactions including fever and chills may occur within 1 to 2 hours of starting the infusion. More common with initial doses and subside with subsequent doses. Arrhythmia, bronchospasm, hypotension, and shock can occur. Anaphylaxis and cardiac arrest from overdose have been reported.

Fungizone/generic: Common even at doses below therapeutic; may begin to occur within 15 to 20 minutes: anorexia, chills, convulsions, diarrhea, fever, headache, phlebitis, vomiting. Anaphylactoid reactions, anemia, cardiac disturbances (including fibrillation and arrest), coagulation defects, hypertension, hypokalemia, hypotension, and numerous other side effects occur fairly frequently. Renal function impaired in 80% of patients. May reverse after treatment ends but some permanent damage likely.

ANTIDOTE

All amphotericin formulations: Notify the physician of all side effects. Many are reversible if the drug is discontinued. Some will respond to symptomatic treatment. Acute reactions (e.g., fever, chills, hypotension, nausea, and vomiting) usually lessen with subsequent doses. These acute infusion-related reactions can be managed by pretreatment with antipyretics, antihistamines, and/or corticosteroids or reduction of the rate of infusion and prompt treatment with antihistamines and/or corticosteroids and meperidine (Demerol) for chills. If anaphylaxis or serious respiratory distress occurs, discontinue amphotericin and treat as necessary. Give no further infusions. Hemodialysis not effective in overdose. Discontinue if BUN and alkaline phosphatase are abnormal. Dantrolene has been used to prevent (50 mg PO) or treat (50 mg IV) severe, shaking chills.

Fungizone/generic: Administration of Fungizone/generic on alternate days may decrease the incidence of some side effects. Urinary alkalinizers may minimize renal tubular acidosis.

Abelcet, Amphotec: Overdose has caused cardiac arrest. Discontinue drug and treat symptomatically.

AMPICILLIN SODIUM   Antibacterial
                                                 (penicillin)

❈Ampicin, ❈Ampilean, Omnipen-N,
❈Penbritin, Polycillin N, Totacillin-N   pH 8.0 to 10

USUAL DOSE

Weight over 20 kg: Range is from 1 to 12 Gm/24 hr. Larger doses may be indicated based on the seriousness of the infection. Some clinicians suggest a weight of 40 kg to receive adult dose range.

Respiratory tract or skin and skin structure infections: 250 to 500 mg every 6 hours.

GI or GU infections: 500 mg every 6 hours.

Septicemia or bacterial meningitis: 8 to 14 Gm or 150 to 200 mg/kg/24 hr in equally divided doses every 3 to 4 hours. Administer IV a minimum of 3 days; then may be given IV or IM.

Treatment of gonorrhea: 500 mg. Repeat in 8 to 12 hours. May repeat 2-dose regimen IV or IM if indicated. Ceftriaxone (Rocephin) IV or IM is most commonly used.

Prevention of bacterial endocarditis in dental, respiratory tract, GI or GU tract surgery or instrumentation: 2 Gm 30 minutes before procedure. For dental and respiratory tract prophylaxis, repeat ampicillin or give oral amoxicillin 1.5 Gm in 6 hours. For GI or GU prophylaxis, give gentamicin 1.5 mg/kg (up to 80 mg) concurrently 30 minutes before procedure. Give 1.5 Gm of oral amoxicillin in 6 hours or repeat ampicillin dose in 8 hours.

Prophylaxis in high-risk cesarean section patients: 1 to 2 Gm immediately after clamping cord.

PEDIATRIC DOSE

Weight under 20 kg: Range is from 25 to 400 mg/kg of body weight/24 hours. Some clinicians suggest a weight up to 40 kg is appropriate for pediatric use. Do not exceed adult dose or 12 Gm.

Respiratory tract or skin and skin structure infections: 25 to 50 mg/kg/24 hr in equally divided doses every 6 hours.

GI or GU infections: 50 to 100 mg/kg/24 hr in equally divided doses every 6 hours.

Septicemia or bacterial meningitis: 100 to 200 mg/kg/24 hr in equally divided doses every 3 to 4 hours. Some clinicians recommend 200 to 400 mg/kg/24 hr in equally divided doses every 4 to 6 hours in children 1 month to 12 years of age in conjunction with chloramphenicol. Satisfactory response should occur within 48 hours or initiate alternate therapy. Administer any regimen IV a minimum of 3 days, then may be given IV or IM.

NEONATAL DOSE

Age up to 7 days: under 2,000 Gm: 25 mg/kg every 12 hours. **Over 2,000 Gm:** 25 mg/kg every 8 hours.

Over 7 days of age: under 2,000 Gm: 25 mg/kg every 8 hours. **Over 2,000 Gm:** 25 mg/kg every 6 hours.

Bacterial meningitis in neonates and infants under 1 month of age: 100 to 300 mg/kg/24 hr in equally divided doses in conjunction with IM gentamicin. Administer any regimen IV a minimum of 3 days, then may be given IV or IM. An alternate dose schedule is:

Age up to 7 days: under 2,000 Gm: 50 to 75 mg/kg every 12 hours. **Over 2,000 Gm:** 50 to 75 mg/kg every 8 hours.

Over 7 days of age: under 2,000 Gm: 50 mg/kg every 8 hours. **Over 2,000 Gm:** 50 mg/kg every 6 hours.

DOSE ADJUSTMENTS

Reduce dose by increasing interval to 12 hours in severe renal impairment.

DILUTION

Each 500 mg or fraction thereof must be reconstituted with at least 5 ml of sterile water for injection. May be further diluted in 50 ml or more of NS, D5W, D5/0.45 NS, 10% invert sugar in water, or ⅙ sodium lactate solution and given as an infusion over not more than 4 hours. Final concentration should not exceed 30 mg/ml. In NS, potency is maintained over 8 hours. After initial dilution, may also be added to the last 100 ml of a compatible IV solution. Also available in ADD-Vantage vials for use with Abbott ADD-Vantage diluent containers. Use within 1 hour of reconstitution unless diluted in aforementioned solutions.

INCOMPATIBLE WITH

Do not use as an additive with any other drug. Do not mix in any solutions other than those specifically recommended. **Y-site:** Midazolam (Versed). Some drugs may be administered through the Y-tubing in small amounts. Consult with the pharmacist.

RATE OF ADMINISTRATION

A single dose over 10 to 15 minutes when given direct IV. In 100 ml or more of solution, administer at prescribed infusion rate but never exceed direct IV rate. Too-rapid injection may cause seizures.

ACTIONS

A semisynthetic penicillin. Bactericidal against many gram-positive and some gram-negative organisms. Appears in all body fluids. Appears in cerebrospinal fluid only if inflammation is present. Crosses the placental barrier. Excreted in urine. Secreted in breast milk.

INDICATIONS AND USES

Highly effective against severe infections caused by gram-positive and some gram-negative organisms (e.g., respiratory tract, skin and skin structure, bacterial meningitis, septicemia). Not effective with penicillinase-producing staphylococci. ■ Prevention of bacterial endocarditis in dental, respiratory tract, GI or GU surgery or instrumentation. Used concurrently with gentamicin. ■ Drug of choice during labor for prevention of neonatal group B streptococcal infections.

Unlabeled use: Prophylaxis in high-risk cesarean section patients.

CONTRAINDICATIONS

Known penicillin or cephalosporin sensitivity (not absolute). Infectious mononucleosis because of increased incidence of rash.

PRECAUTIONS

Sensitivity studies indicated to determine susceptibility of the causative organism to ampicillin. ■ Avoid prolonged use of this drug; superinfection caused by overgrowth of nonsusceptible organisms may result. ■ Side effects increased in some patients; note Side effects.

Monitor: Watch for early symptoms of allergic reaction, especially in individuals with a history of allergic problems. ■ AST (SGOT) may be increased. Renal, hepatic, and hematopoietic function should be checked during prolonged therapy. ■ Electrolyte imbalance and cardiac irregularities from sodium content are possible. Contains 2.9 mEq sodium/Gm. May aggravate CHF. Observe for hypokalemia.

Patient education: May require alternate birth control.

Maternal/child: Pregnancy category B: Use only if clearly needed. ■ May cause diarrhea, candidiasis, or allergic response in nursing infants. ■ Elimination rate markedly reduced in neonates.

Elderly: Consider degree of age-related impaired renal function.

DRUG/LAB INTERACTIONS

Streptomycin potentiates bactericidal activity against enterococci. ■ May be used concurrently with aminoglycosides (e.g., gentamicin [Garamycin]) but must be administered in separate infusions; inactivates aminoglycosides. ■ May be antagonized by bacteriostatic antibiotics (e.g., chloramphenicol, erythromycin, and tetracyclines), bactericidal action may be negated. ■ Concomitant use with beta adrenergic blockers (e.g., propranolol [Inderal]) may increase risk of anaphylaxis and inhibit treatment. ■ Potentiated by probenecid (Benemid); toxicity may result. ■ Increased risk of bleeding with heparin. ■ May decrease clearance and increase toxicity of methotrexate. ■ Decreases effectiveness of oral contraceptives; breakthrough bleeding or pregnancy could result. ■ Ampicillin-induced skin rash potentiated by allopurinol (Zyloprim). ■ False-positive glucose reaction with Clinitest and Benedict's or Fehling's solution. ■ May cause false values in other lab tests; see literature.

SIDE EFFECTS

Primarily hypersensitivity reactions such as anaphylaxis, exfoliative dermatitis, rashes, and urticaria. May cause pseudomembranous colitis. Hypersensitivity myocarditis can occur (fever, eosinophilia, rash, sinus tachycardia, ST-T changes, and cardiomegaly). Anemia, leukopenia, and thrombocytopenia have been reported. Thrombophlebitis will occur with long-term use. Higher than normal doses may cause neurologic adverse reactions including convulsions; especially with impaired renal function. Incidence of side effects increased in patients with viral infections, or those taking allopurinol (Zyloprim).

ANTIDOTE

Notify the physician of any side effect. For severe symptoms, discontinue the drug, treat allergic reaction (antihistamines, epinephrine, corticosteroids), and resuscitate as necessary. Hemodialysis is effective in overdose.

AMPICILLIN SODIUM AND SULBACTAM SODIUM

Antibacterial
(penicillin and beta-lactamase inhibitor)

Unasyn   pH 8.0 to 10.0

USUAL DOSE

1.5 to 3 Gm every 6 hours. All commercial preparations in the U.S. have a 2:1 ratio of ampicillin to sulbactam (e.g., 1.5 Gm = 1 Gm ampicillin plus 0.5 Gm sulbactam. Do not exceed 4 Gm sulbactam/24 hr.

PEDIATRIC DOSE

Skin and skin structure infections in pediatric patients over 1 year of age and under 40 kg: 300 mg/kg/24 hr in equally divided doses as an intermittent infusion every 6 hours.

NEONATAL DOSE

Under 7 days of age: 150 mg/kg/24 hr in equally divided doses. Give at 12-hour intervals.

Over 7 days of age: 150 mg/kg/24 hr in equally divided doses. Give at 6-to 8-hour intervals. Another source suggests doses of 300 to 600 mg/24 hr in equally divided doses have been used for children up to 12 years.

DOSE ADJUSTMENTS

May be required in impaired renal function. Average doses usually given less frequently based on creatinine clearance; see literature. May be given to patients on dialysis; see literature. ■ May be indicated in the elderly.

DILUTION

Each 1.5 Gm or fraction thereof must be initially reconstituted with at least 3.2 ml of sterile water for injection (375 mg/ml). Allow to stand to dissipate foaming. Solution should be clear. Must be further diluted to a final concentration of 3 to 45 mg/ml in one of the following solutions and given by slow IV injection or as an intermittent IV infusion: D5W, D5/0.45 NS, 10% invert sugar in water, LR, 1/6 sodium lactate solution, or NS. 3 Gm/L equals 3 mg/ml, 3 Gm/125 ml equals 24 mg/ml. Also available in piggyback vials and Add-Vantage vials (see manufacturer's directions).

Storage: Store at controlled room temperature before dilution. Stable in all specifically listed solutions in any dilution for at least 2 hours. Stability in each solution varies (see literature).

INCOMPATIBLE WITH

Do not use as an additive with any other drug. Do not mix in any solutions other than those specifically recommended. **Y-site:** Ciprofloxacin (Cipro IV). Some drugs may be administered through the Y-tubing in small amounts. Consult with the pharmacist.

RATE OF ADMINISTRATION

Direct IV: A single dose over a minimum of 15 minutes.

Intermittent IV: A single dose over 15 to 30 minutes or longer, depending on amount of solution. Too-rapid injection may cause seizures.

ACTIONS

A semisynthetic penicillin. The addition of sulbactam improves ampicillin's bactericidal activity against beta-lactamase-producing strains resistant to penicillins and cephalosporins. A broad-spectrum antibiotic and beta-lactamase inhibitor effective against selected gram-positive, gram-negative, and anaerobic organisms (see literature). Peak serum levels achieved by end of infusion. Appears in all body fluids. Crosses the placental barrier. Excreted in the urine. Secreted in breast milk.

INDICATIONS AND USES

Treatment of skin and skin structure and intraabdominal and gynecologic urinary tract infections due to susceptible strains of specific organisms.

CONTRAINDICATIONS

Known penicillin, cephalosporin, or beta-lactamase inhibitor sensitivity (not absolute); infectious mononucleosis because of increased incidence of rash.

PRECAUTIONS

Studies indicated to determine the causative organism and susceptibility to ampicillin/sulbactam. ■ Avoid prolonged use of this drug; superinfection caused by overgrowth of nonsusceptible organisms may result. ■ Elimination of sulbactam increased in cystic fibrosis patients. ■ Use caution in patients with CHF, a history of bleeding disorders, or GI disease (e.g., colitis).

Monitor: Watch for early symptoms of allergic reaction, especially in individuals with a history of allergic problems. ■ AST (SGOT) may be increased. Renal, hepatic, and hematopoietic function should be checked during prolonged therapy. ■ May cause thrombophlebitis. Observe carefully and rotate infusion sites. ■ Electrolyte imbalance and cardiac irregularities from sodium content are possible. Contains 5 mEq sodium/1.5 Gm. May aggravate CHF. Observe for hypokalemia.

Patient education: Report promptly; fever, rash, sore throat, unusual bleeding or bruising, severe stomach cramps, and/or diarrhea, seizures. ■ May require alternate birth control.

Maternal/child: Pregnancy category B: Studies in rabbits have not shown adverse effects on fertility or in the fetus. Use only if clearly needed. ■ May cause diarrhea, candidiasis, or allergic response in nursing infants. ■ Safety for use in infants and children under 12 years of age not established but is in use. Elimination rate markedly reduced in neonates.

Elderly: Consider degree of age-related impaired renal function. ▪ Note dose adjustments.

DRUG/LAB INTERACTIONS

Streptomycin potentiates bactericidal activity against enterococci. ▪ May be used concurrently with aminoglycosides (e.g., gentamicin [Garamycin]) but must be administered in separate infusions (at least 1 hour apart); inactivates aminoglycosides. ▪ May be antagonized by bacteriostatic antibiotics (e.g., chloramphenicol, erythromycin, tetracyclines); bactericidal action may be negated. ▪ Concomitant use with beta-adrenergic blockers (e.g., propranolol [Inderal]) may increase risk of anaphylaxis and inhibit treatment. ▪ Potentiated by probenecid (Benemid); higher blood levels may be a positive interaction. ▪ Increased risk of bleeding with heparin. ▪ May decrease clearance and increase toxicity of methotrexate. ▪ Decreases effectiveness of oral contraceptives; breakthrough bleeding or pregnancy could result. ▪ Ampicillin-induced skin rash potentiated by allopurinol (Zyloprim). ▪ False-positive glucose reaction with Clinitest and Benedict's or, Fehling's solution. ▪ May cause false values in other lab tests, see literature.

SIDE EFFECTS

Full scope of allergic reactions including anaphylaxis are possible. Burning, discomfort, and pain at injection site; diarrhea, rash, and thrombophlebitis occur most frequently. Abdominal distention; candidiasis; chest pain; chills; decreased hemoglobin, hematocrit, RBC, WBC, lymphocytes, neutrophils, and platelets; decreased serum albumin and total protein; dysuria; edema; epistaxis; erythema; facial swelling; fatigue; flatulence; glossitis; headache; hypersensitivity myocarditis (fever, eosinophilia, rash, sinus tachycardia, ST-T changes and cardiomegaly); increased alkaline phosphatase, BUN, creatinine, LDH, AST (SGOT), ALT (SGPT); increased basophils, eosinophils, lymphocytes, monocytes and platelets; itching; malaise; mucosal bleeding; nausea and vomiting; RBCs and hyaline casts in urine; substernal pain; tightness in throat; and urine retention can occur. May cause pseudomembranous colitis. Higher than normal doses may cause neurologic adverse reactions, including convulsions; especially with impaired renal function.

ANTIDOTE

Notify the physician of any side effect. For severe symptoms, discontinue the drug, treat allergic reaction (antihistamines, epinephrine, corticosteroids), and resuscitate as necessary. Hemodialysis may be effective in overdose.

AMRINONE LACTATE

Inocor

Inotropic agent

pH 3.2 to 4.0

USUAL DOSE

Adults and children: 0.75 mg/kg of body weight as the initial loading dose (52.5 mg [10.5 ml] for a 70 kg person).

Loading dose determination 0.75 mg/kg (undiluted)										
Patient weight in kg	30	40	50	60	70	80	90	100	110	120
ml of undiluted Inocor Inj	4.5	6	7.5	9	10.5	12	13.5	15	16.5	18

Follow with a maintenance infusion of 5 to 10 mcg/kg/min. The initial dose (0.75 mg/kg) may be repeated once in 30 minutes if indicated. Do not exceed a total dose of 10 mg/kg/24 hr including loading doses.

INFANT AND NEONATAL DOSE

0.75 mg/kg as the initial loading dose. May be repeated in 30 minutes if necessary. Another source suggests up to 3 to 4.5 mg/kg as a loading dose. Give in divided doses to desired effect. Maintain *infants* with an infusion of 5 to 10 mcg (0.005 to 0.01 mg)/kg/min and *neonates* with an infusion of 3 mcg (0.003 mg) to 5 mcg (0.005 mg)/kg/min.

DOSE ADJUSTMENTS

May be required in impaired renal or hepatic function or if thrombocytopenia occurs.

DILUTION

May be given undiluted, or each 5 mg (1 ml) may be diluted in 1 ml NS or 0.45 NS. For infusion dilute 300 mg (60 ml) in 60 ml NS or 0.45 NS. 1 ml will deliver 2.5 mg (2,500 mcg). May be given through Y-tube or three-way stopcock of IV infusion set. Use diluted solution within 24 hours.

INCOMPATIBLE WITH

Dextrose solutions (direct dilution only), furosemide (Lasix), procainamide (Pronestyl), sodium bicarbonate.

RATE OF ADMINISTRATION

Loading dose: A single dose over 2 to 3 minutes.

Infusion: Using a microdrip (60 gtt/ml) or an infusion pump deliver amrinone in recommended doses. See dosage chart defining selected dose in mcg/min/body weight in ml/hr.

Incor I.V. (amrinone) Infusion rate (ml/hr) (2.5 mg/ml infusion concentration)*										
Patient weight (kg)	30	40	50	60	70	80	90	100	110	120
Dosage 5 mcg/kg/min	4	5	6	7	8	10	11	12	13	14
7.5 mcg/kg/min	5	7	9	11	13	14	16	18	20	22
10 mcg/kg/min	7	10	12	14	17	19	22	24	26	29

*A 70-kg patient receiving 7.5 mcg/kg/min would have a flow rate of 13 ml/hr with a 2.5 mg/ml concentration.

Adjust as indicated by physician's orders and progress in patient's condition. Reduce rate or stop infusion for excessive drop in blood pressure.

ACTIONS

A new class of cardiac inotropic agent that differs in chemical structure and mode of action from digitalis glycosides and catecholamines. With a bolus dose, peak effect occurs within 10 minutes. Continuous administration is required to maintain serum levels. It has positive inotropic action with vasodilator activity. Reduces afterload and preload by direct relaxant effect on vascular smooth muscle. Cardiac output is increased without measurable increase in myocardial oxygen consumption or changes in arteriovenous oxygen difference. Pulmonary capillary wedge pressure, total peripheral resistance, diastolic blood pressure, and mean arterial pressure are decreased. Heart rate generally remains the same. Metabolized by conjugated pathways, it is primarily excreted in the urine.

INDICATIONS AND USES

Short-term management of congestive heart failure in patients who have not responded adequately to digitalis, diuretics, or vasodilators. ▪ Short-term management of congestive heart failure, pulmonary hypertension, and postop low cardiac output in neonates and infants up to 2 years.

CONTRAINDICATIONS

Hypersensitivity to amrinone or bisulfites, severe aortic or pulmonic valvular disease where surgical relief of the obstruction is required.

PRECAUTIONS

May increase ventricular response in atrial flutter/fibrillation. Pretreat with digitalis (recommended). ▪ May be given to digitalized patients without causing signs of digitalis toxicity. ▪ Use caution in impaired renal or liver function; serum levels may increase considerably. ▪ Not recommended for use in the acute phase of myocardial infarction due to lack of clinical trials to date. ▪ May aggravate outflow tract obstruction in hypertrophic subaortic stenosis.

Monitor: Observe patient continuously; monitoring of ECG, cardiac index, pulmonary capillary wedge pressure, central venous pressure, and plasma concentration are recommended (steady state plasma concentrations of ≈ 3 mcg/ml suggested). ■ Monitor blood pressure, urine output, and body weight. Observe for orthopnea, dyspnea, and fatigue. ■ Obtain platelet count before and during therapy to monitor onset of thrombocytopenia. ■ Additional fluids and electrolytes may be required to facilitate appropriate response in patients who have been vigorously diuresed and may have insufficient cardiac filling pressure. Use caution. ■ Monitor electrolytes; hypokalemia secondary to improved cardiac output with improved diuresis may cause arrhythmias. ■ Monitor IV site, avoid extravasation.

Maternal/child: Pregnancy category C: Use during pregnancy only if benefits outweigh risks. ■ Safety during lactation not established. ■ Safety for use in children not established but has been used effectively.

Elderly: No problems documented; consider possible renal impairment; see Dose adjustment.

DRUG/LAB INTERACTIONS
May cause excessive hypotension with disopyramide (Norpace).

SIDE EFFECTS
Abdominal pain, anorexia, burning at site of injection, chest pain, dysrhythmias, fever, hepatotoxicity, hypotension, nausea and vomiting, thrombocytopenia. Hypersensitivity reactions manifested by ascites, myositis with interstitial shadowing on chest x-ray and elevated sedimentation rate, pericarditis, pleuritis, vasculitis with nodular pulmonary densities, hypoxemia, and jaundice have been reported.

ANTIDOTE
Notify the physician of any side effect. Based on degree of severity and condition of the patient, may be treated symptomatically, and dose may remain the same, be decreased, or the amrinone may be discontinued. Reduce rate or discontinue the drug at the first sign of marked hypotension and notify the physician. May be resolved by these measures alone or vasopressors (e.g., dopamine [Intropin]) may be required. Treat arrhythmias with the appropriate drug. Resuscitate as necessary.

ANISTREPLASE   Thrombolytic agent
APSAC, Eminase   pH 7.3

USUAL DOSE
30 units direct IV as soon as possible after onset of symptoms of acute myocardial infarction. Most effective when given within 4 to 6 hours. Note Monitor section under Precautions.

DOSE ADJUSTMENTS
May be required in the elderly.

DILUTION
Each single-dose vial must be diluted with 5 ml SW for injection. Add diluent slowly, direct to sides of vial, and roll and tilt gently to mix. Do not shake. No further dilution recommended. Should be clear

to pale yellow with no particulate matter. May be given through Y-tube or three-way stopcock of infusion set. Discard if not administered within 30 minutes of dilution.

Storage: Refrigerate before dilution.

INCOMPATIBLE WITH

Manufacturer states "do not add to any infusion fluid. Do not add any other medication to vial or syringe."

RATE OF ADMINISTRATION

A single dose evenly distributed over 2 to 5 minutes (4 to 5 minutes is usual).

ACTIONS

A thrombolytic agent. An inactive derivative of a fibrinolytic enzyme (panisoylated lys-plasminogen streptokinase activator complex). Made from streptokinase and human plasminogen. Activation begins with dilution; on injection activation continues in a progressive and controlled manner. The process converts plasminogen to plasmin, which degrades fibrin clots, fibrinogen, and other plasma proteins. This activation takes place within a thrombus as well as on the surface. Onset of action is prompt. It has a slow rate of degradation and an active half-life up to 2 hours. Anistreplase is 10 times more potent than streptokinase as a thrombolytic. Fibrin binding compares favorably to alteplase.

INDICATIONS AND USES

Management of acute myocardial infarction in adults for the lysis of thrombi obstructing coronary arteries, the reduction of infarct size, the improvement of ventricular function, and the reduction of mortality. ■ Current AHA and JAMA recommendations identify thrombolytic agents as Class I therapy in patients younger than 70 years of age with recent onset of chest pain (within 6 hours) consistent with acute MI and at least 0.1 mV of ST segment elevation in at least two ECG leads. Use in all other patients based on age, accurate diagnosis, and time from onset of chest pain.

CONTRAINDICATIONS

Known hypersensitivity to anistreplase or streptokinase. Active internal bleeding, arteriovenous malformation or aneurysm, bleeding diathesis, cerebrovascular accident, intracranial or intraspinal surgery or trauma within 2 months, intracranial neoplasm, severe uncontrolled hypertension.

PRECAUTIONS

Administered under the direction of a physician knowledgeable in its use and with appropriate diagnostic and laboratory facilities available. ■ Reperfusion arrhythmias occur frequently (e.g., sinus bradycardia, accelerated idioventricular rhythm, PVCs, ventricular tachycardia); have antiarrhythmic medications available at bedside. ■ Establish a separate IV line for anistreplase. ■ Maintain strict bed rest and apply pressure dressings to any recently invaded site. ■ A greater alteration of hemostatic status than with heparin; use extreme care with the patient, avoid any excessive or rough handling or pressure (including too-frequent BPs), avoid invasive procedures (e.g., arterial puncture, venipuncture, IM injection). If these procedures absolutely necessary, use extreme precautionary methods (use radial artery instead of femoral, small-gauge catheters and needles, and sites that are easily observed and compressible where bleeding can be controlled; avoid handling of catheter sites; use extended pressure application of up to 30 minutes). Minor bleeding occurs often at catheter insertion sites. Avoid use of razors and toothbrushes. ■ Follow-up therapy with continuous infusion of heparin (without a loading dose) is frequently used to reduce the risk of rethrombosis. Increases risk of bleeding. ■ Use extreme caution in the following situations: major surgery, trauma, GI or GU bleeding, or puncture of noncompressible vessels (e.g., spinal puncture, thoracentesis) within the previous 10 days; cerebrovascular disease; hypertension (systolic above 180 or diastolic above 110); mitral stenosis with atrial fibrillation (likelihood of left heart thrombus); acute pericarditis; subacute bacterial endocarditis; coagulation disorders, including those secondary to severe hepatic or renal disease; severe liver dysfunction; pregnancy and first 10 days postpartum; hemorrhagic ophthalmic conditions (e.g., diabetic hemorrhagic retinopathy); septic thrombophlebitis; patients taking anticoagulants; patients over 75 years of age; any situation where bleeding might be hazardous or difficult to manage because of location. ■ Standard treatment for MI continues simultaneously with anistreplase therapy except if temporarily contraindicated (arterial blood gases, etc., unless absolutely necessary). ■ Repeat injections of anistreplase or streptokinase 5 days to 6 months after first injection or after streptococcal infection may not be effective (increased antistreptokinase antibodies) or may increase incidence of allergic reactions.

Monitor: Baseline ECG, CPK, and clotting studies (PT, PTT, CBC, fibrinogen level, platelets) and baseline assessment (patient condition, blood pressure, pain, hematomas, petechiae, or recent wounds) should be completed before administration. Type and cross-match may also be ordered. ■ Monitor ECG continuously, and record strips with greatest ST segment elevation initially and every 15 minutes for at least 4 hours. May cause severe hypotension; monitor blood pressure with caution to prevent bruising or bleeding. A 12-lead ECG is indicated when therapy is complete. ■ Start IV if indicated (not previously established, other medications being administered through current IV, or to have a line available for additional treatment). ■ Monitor the patient carefully and frequently for anginal pain and any signs of bleeding; observe catheter sites at least every 15 minutes; watch for hematuria, hematemesis, bloody stool, petechiae, hematoma, flank pain, muscle weakness; and do neuro checks every hour. Continue until normal clotting function returns. ■ Strict bed rest indicated to reduce risk of bleeding.

Patient education: Compliance with all measures to minimize bleeding (e.g., strict bed rest) is very important. ■ Avoid use of razors, toothbrushes, and other sharp items. Use caution while moving to avoid excessive bumping. ■ Report all episodes of bleeding and apply local pressure if indicated. Expect oozing from IV sites.

Maternal/child: Pregnancy category C: Use during pregnancy only if clearly needed. ■ Discontinue breast feeding temporarily. ■ Safety for use in children not established.

Elderly: May have poorer prognosis following MI and pre-existing conditions that may increase risk of intercranial bleeding. Select patients carefully to maximize benefits. ■ Safety for use in patients over 75 years of age not established. ▪ Note Dose adjustments, Indications and Precautions.

DRUG/LAB INTERACTIONS

Use caution with drugs that may alter platelet function (e.g., aspirin, dipyridamole [Persantin], indomethacin, phenylbutazone). Risk of bleeding will be increased if used concomitantly. ▪ Risk of bleeding with concomitant use of heparin is markedly increased. ▪ Coagulation tests will be unreliable; specific procedures can be used; notify the lab of anistreplase use.

SIDE EFFECTS

Bleeding is most common: internal (GI tract, GU tract, intracranial, ocular, or retroperitoneal sites), epistaxis, gingival, and superficial or surface bleeding (venous cutdowns, arterial punctures, sites of recent surgical intervention). Delayed purpuric rash, eosinophilia, fever, flushing, hypotension (severe and not secondary to bleeding or anaphylaxis), itching, nausea and vomiting, rashes. Anaphylactic reactions such as angioedema and bronchospasm are rare but have occurred. No cases of hepatitis or AIDS have been reported. Manufacturing process includes a vapor heat treatment to inactivate viruses. Other side effects have occurred but may be due to the MI itself.

ANTIDOTE

Notify physician of all side effects. Note even the most minute bleeding tendency. Oozing at IV sites is expected. Control minor bleeding by local pressure. For severe bleeding in a critical location, discontinue anistreplase and any heparin therapy immediately. Whole blood, packed red blood cells, cryoprecipitate, fresh-frozen plasma, platelets, desmopressin, tranexamic acid, and aminocaproic acid may all be indicated. Topical preparations of aminocaproic acid may stop minor bleeding. Consider protamine if heparin has been used. Treat bradycardia with atropine, reperfusion, arrhythmias with lidocaine or procainamide. VT or VF may require cardioversion. If hypotension occurs, reduce rate promptly. If not resolved, vasopressors (e.g., dopamine [Intropin]), Trendelenburg position, and suitable plasma expanders (e.g., albumin, plasma protein fraction [Plasmanate], or hetastarch) may be indicated. Treat minor allergic reactions symptomatically. Discontinue drug and treat anaphylaxis with epinephrine, diphenhydramine (Benadryl), and corticosteroids. Resuscitate as necessary.

ANTIHEMOPHILIC FACTOR (HUMAN OR RECOMBINANT)

Antihemorrhagic

AHF, Alphanate, Antihemophilic Factor (Porcine) Hydate:C, Bioclate™ (Recombinant), Factor VIII, Helixate™ (Recombinant), Hemofil M, Humate-P, Koate HP, Kogenate [recombinant], Monoclate P, Profilate OSD, Profilate SD, Recombinate™

USUAL DOSE

Adults and children: Completely individualized. Based on degree of deficiency, desired antihemophilic factor level, body weight, severity of bleeding, and presence of factor VIII inhibitors. Identify factor VIII deficiency and level assays before administration. 1 International unit (IU) is approximately equal to the level of factor VIII activity in 1 ml of fresh pooled human plasma. Recombinant products may be substituted for plasma-derived products without disrupting treatment regimen. A plasma antihemophilic factor level of about 30% of normal is needed for effective hemostasis when hemorrhage is present; greater percentages are required for surgical procedures, and only 5% to 10% of normal may be needed to control hemarthrosis. Each preparation suggests a different formula; end results are similar. An example is:

$$\text{AHF/IU required} =$$
$$\text{body weight (kg)} \times \text{desired factor VIII increase (\% of normal)} \times 0.5$$

$$\text{Expected factor VIII increase (\% of normal)} =$$
$$\text{AHF/IU/kg dose administered} \times 2$$

Examples of doses are as follows:
Prophylactic management: (e.g., severe factor VIII deficiency with frequent hemorrhages). Raise factor VIII level to 15% of normal. Repeat every 1 to 2 days. Usually requires 250 units daily in patients weighing less than 50 kg, 500 units daily in patients weighing more than 50 kg. Increase dose until bleeding episodes are adequately controlled.
Early hemarthrosis (blood into a joint or its synovial cavity), muscle bleed, or oral bleed: Raise factor VIII level to 20% to 40%. Usually requires 5 to 10 units/kg initially. Repeat infusion every 12 to 24 hours for 1 to 3 days until the bleeding episode as indicated by pain is resolved or healing is achieved. If early hemarthrosis is treated promptly, lowest doses may be adequate.
More extensive hemarthrosis, muscle bleed, or hematoma: Raise factor VIII level to 30% to 60%. Usually requires 10 to 25 units/kg initially. Adjust dose based on circulating AHF levels and repeat infusion every 8 to 24 hours for 3 days or more until pain and disability are resolved.

Life-threatening bleeds (e.g., head injury, throat bleed, severe abdominal pain): Raise factor VIII level to 60% to 100%. Usually requires 40 to 50 units/kg initially. Adjust dose based on circulating AHF levels and repeat infusion every 8 to 24 hours until threat is resolved.

Minor surgery, including tooth extraction: Raise factor VIII level to 60% to 80%. Usually requires 25 to 40 units/kg. A single infusion plus oral antifibrinolytic therapy within 1 hour is sufficient in 70% of patients.

Major surgery: Raise factor VIII level to 80% to 100%. Usually requires 45 to 50 units/kg initially. Repeat infusion every 8 to 24 hours depending on state of healing. Reduce dose as indicated by state of healing. Increase dose if level falls below 30%.

Maintenance doses vary slightly with specific products; see literature.

DOSE ADJUSTMENTS

If AHF does not significantly improve the partial thromboplastin time, factor VIII antibodies are probable; may respond to an increased dose, especially if titer is less than 10 Bethesda Units/ml. Frequent determinations of circulating AHF levels indicated.

DILUTION

All preparations provide diluent. Actual number of AHF units shown on each vial. Use only the diluent provided, and maintain strict aseptic technique. Use a plastic syringe to prevent binding to glass surfaces. Warm to room temperature (25° C) before dilution and maintain throughout administration to avoid precipitation of active ingredients.

Plasma-based AHF: Usually provide administration equipment. Always use a new sterile needle and syringe or administration set for each vial. Gently agitate to mix; do not shake. Complete dissolution may take up to 10 minutes. Must be completely dissolved or active components may be removed by filter. Should be administered through a filter. Best if administered within 1 hour of dilution; must be used within 3 hours.

Recombinant products: Double-ended needle and 18-gauge needle provided. Initially insert double-ended needle into diluent. Invert diluent bottle over the upright recombinate bottle and rapidly insert other end of needle. Vacuum will draw in diluent. Remove diluent bottle; then remove needle. Swirl gently to dissolve completely. Attach 18-gauge needle to a disposable syringe and draw air into it. Inject air into bottle and withdraw solution. Multiple bottles may be drawn into the same syringe. Must be administered within 3 hours.

Kogenate (recombinant): Process similar. Direct diluent against wall to avoid excessive foaming. Swirl continuously to dissolve. Withdraw into a syringe using a filter needle (provided). Replace filter needle with administration set. Multiple bottles may be drawn into same syringe. Use a separate filter needle for each bottle. Must be administered within 3 hours.

Storage: Maintain at room temperature after dilution. Do not use beyond expiration dates on bottles.

Plasma-based AHF: Must be refrigerated before dilution. (Alphanate can be kept at controlled room temperature for up to 2 months.)

Recombinant products: May be refrigerated or stored at room temperature not to exceed (30° C [86° F]) for up to 3 months before dilution.

INCOMPATIBLE WITH

Sufficient information not available. Do not mix with other drugs.

RATE OF ADMINISTRATION

Reduce rate of infusion or temporarily discontinue if a significant increase in pulse rate occurs.

Plasma-based AHF: Preparations with less than 34 AHF IU/ml: infuse each 10 to 20 ml over 3 minutes. Preparations with more than 34 AHF IU/ml should infuse at a maximum rate of 2 ml/min. *Recombinate™ AHF, Bioclate:* Up to 10 ml/min. **Kogenate AHF, Helixate:** A single dose over 5 to 10 minutes is usually well tolerated.

ACTIONS

AHF is one of nine major factors in the blood that must act in sequence to produce coagulation, or clotting. It is the specific clotting factor deficient in patients with hemophilia A (classic hemophilia) and can temporarily correct the coagulation defect in these patients. Has a half-life of 10 to 18 hours. *Plasma-based AHF:* A lyophilized concentrate of coagulation factor VIII (antihemophilic factor) prepared by various processes (e.g., heat treatment, chemical inactivation, solvent detergent treatment, immunoaffinity chromatography). Obtained from fresh (less than 3 hours old) human plasma cryoprecipitate. Tested and determined free from hepatitis and HIV viruses and containing acceptable ALT (SGPT) concentrations. *Recombinant AHF:* Produced through genetic engineering technology. Purified using monoclonal antibody purification techniques, ion exchange chromatography and immunoaffinity chromatography. Risk of viral transmission eliminated because it is not derived from human blood. *Porcine AHF:* No evidence of viral transmission; pigs do not harbor hepatitis or HIV.

INDICATIONS AND USES

Temporary replacement of factor VIII in patients with a congenital deficiency (classic hemophilia A or acquired deficiency [Alphanate only]); used to correct or prevent bleeding episodes or to perform emergency or elective surgery.

CONTRAINDICATIONS

Hypersensitivity to mouse, hamster, or bovine protein (monoclonal-anti-body-derived factor VIII). Not effective for bleeding in patients with von Willebrand's disease.

PRECAUTIONS

Treatment of choice when volume or red blood cell replacement is not needed; avoids hypervolemia and hyperproteinemia. ▪ Desmopressin is preferred treatment in mild to moderate hemophilia A. ▪ Hepatitis B vaccination indicated in all patients with hemophilia; usually done at birth or time of diagnosis. ▪ Risk of transmitting hepatitis or HIV is markedly reduced with newer plasma-based products. There are no reported instances of new seroconversions to HIV with currently marketed products. ▪ No risk of any viral transmission (hepatitis or HIV) with recombinant products. ▪ Intravascular hemolysis can occur when large volumes are given to individuals with blood groups A, B, or AB. Monitor for progressive anemia. ▪ Type-specific cryoprecipitate has been used to maintain adequate factor VIII levels and is appropriate in selected cases; carries risk of possible delayed seroconversion after viral infection (HIV, hepatitis A, B, or C). ▪ Inhibitor titers above 10 Bethesda Units/ml may make hemostatic control with AHF impossible or impractical because of the large dose required. Inhibitor titer may rise after AHF infusion due to an anamnestic (immunologic memory) response to the AHF antigen.

Monitor: Identification of factor VIII deficiency with determination of circulating AHF levels should be obtained previous to administration and during treatment. Adjust dose as indicated. ▪ Monitor pulse before and during treatment. ▪ Note Precautions.

Patient education: Prophylactic hepatitis B vaccine recommended. ▪ Instruction for self-administration and proper preparation may be appropriate. ▪ Report skin rash or any other hypersensitivity reaction promptly. ▪ HIV screening every 2 to 3 months; not required with recombinant products.

Maternal/child: Pregnancy category C: Use only if clearly needed. ▪ Safe for use in children of all ages, including the newborn.

SIDE EFFECTS

Usually respond to reduced rate of administration. Massive doses may cause acute hemolytic anemia, hyperfibrinogenemia, increased bleeding tendency, or jaundice (rare).

Plasma-based AHF: Allergic reactions (anaphylaxis, backache, chills, erythema, fever, hives, hypotension, nausea, stinging at infusion site, tightness of chest, urticaria, wheezing); clouding or loss of consciousness, flushing, headache, lethargy, paresthesias, somnolence, tachycardia, or vomiting may occur. Consider risk potential of contracting AIDS or hepatitis; risk of withholding treatment outweighs any risk associated with use.

Recombinant products: No serious side effects have occurred and side effects have been self-limiting. Burning, erythema, and pruritus at injection site; chest discomfort, cold feet, diarrhea, dizziness, fever, flushing, hypotension (slight), nausea, rash, sore throat, or an unusual taste in the mouth occur occasionally.

ANTIDOTE

Most side effects usually subside spontaneously in 15 to 20 minutes and are generally related to the rate of infusion. Keep the physician informed. Discontinue immediately and treat allergic reactions (antihistamines, epinephrine, corticosteroids) and resuscitate as necessary.

ANTI-INHIBITOR COAGULANT COMPLEX

Antihemorrhagic

Autoplex-T, Feiba VH Immuno

USUAL DOSE

Range is 25 to 100 factor VIII correctional units/kg. May be repeated in 6 to 12 hours. Do not exceed 200 units/kg/24 hr. Completely individualized; subsequent doses should be adjusted according to patient response. Identification of factor VIII inhibitor levels and prothrombin time (PT) mandatory prior to administration.

DILUTION

All preparations provide diluent for IV infusion. Actual number of factor VIII inhibitor bypassing activity units shown on each vial. Use only the diluent provided and maintain strict aseptic technique. May be given through Y-tube or three-way stopcock of infusion set. To avoid hypotension from prekallikrein activator (PKA), give Autoplex-T within 1 hour of dilution and Feiba VH Immuno within 3 hours.

Storage: Refrigerate before reconstitution; do not refrigerate after.

INCOMPATIBLE WITH

Specific information not available. Do not mix directly with other drugs.

RATE OF ADMINISTRATION

10 ml or less per minute. If symptoms of too-rapid infusion (headache, flushing, changes in blood pressure or pulse rate) occur, discontinue until symptoms subside. Restart at 2 ml/min.

ACTIONS

A 1-unit volume of factor VIII correctional activity (quantity of activated prothrombin complex) will correct clotting time to normal (35 seconds) when added to an equal volume of factor VIII deficient or inhibitor plasma. A dried or freeze-dried concentrate prepared from human plasma by a specific process.

INDICATIONS AND USES

To control hemorrhagic episodes in hemophiliacs (hemophilia A) with factor VIII inhibitors who are bleeding or will undergo elective or emergency surgery. Most frequently indicated if factor VIII inhibitor levels are above 2 to 10 Bethesda Units or rise to that level following treatment with AHF.

CONTRAINDICATIONS

Disseminated intravascular coagulation (DIC), symptoms (signs) of fibrinolysis, known hypersensitivity.

PRECAUTIONS

Could transmit HIV and hepatitis. ▪ Use extreme caution in newborns and patients with liver disease. ▪ Note Drug/lab interactions.

Monitor: Monitor prothrombin time (PT) before and after treatment. Only accurate means of treatment evaluation. Must be two thirds of preinfusion value after treatment if patient is to receive any additional doses.

Maternal/child: Pregnancy category C: Use only if clearly needed.

DRUG/LAB INTERACTIONS

Not recommended for use with antifibrinolytic products (aminocaproic acid, tranexamic acid). ▪ aPTT, WBCT, and other clotting factor tests do not correlate with actual results and may lead to overdose and DIC.

SIDE EFFECTS

Anaphylaxis, bradycardia, chest pain, chills, cough, decreased fibrinogen concentration, decreased platelet count, fever, flushing, headache, hypertension, hypotension, prolonged partial thromboplastin time (PTT), prolonged thrombin time, prolonged PT, respiratory distress, tachycardia, urticaria. Consider risk potential of contracting AIDS or hepatitis.

ANTIDOTE

If side effects occur, discontinue the infusion and notify the physician. May be resumed at a slower rate or an alternate product may be used.

Symptoms of DIC (blood pressure and pulse rate changes, respiratory discomfort, chest pain, cough, prolonged clotting tests) require immediate treatment. Treat anaphylaxis (antihistamines, epinephrine, corticosteroids) and resuscitate as necessary.

ANTITHROMBIN III

Anticoagulant
Antithrombotic

AT-III, ATnativ, Thrombate III

pH 6.5 to 7.5

USUAL DOSE

Loading dose, maintenance dose, and dosing intervals are completely individualized based on confirmed diagnosis (See Precautions) , specific product, patient weight, clinical condition, degree of deficiency, type of surgery or procedure involved, physician judgment, desired level of antithrombin III (AT-III), and actual plasma levels achieved as verified by appropriate lab tests. 1 Unit/kg should raise the level of AT-III by 1% to 2.1%. The desired AT-III level after the first dose should be about 120% of normal (normal is 0.1 to 0.2 Gm/L). AT-III levels must be maintained at normal or at least above 80% of normal for 2 to 8 days depending on individual patient factors. Usually achieved by administration of a maintenance dose once daily. Concomitant administration of heparin usually indicated. (See Drug/lab interactions).

Calculate the initial loading dose using the following formula (assumes a plasma volume of 40 ml/kg):

$$\text{Dosage units} = \frac{(\text{desired AT-III level [\%]} - \text{baseline AT-III [\%]}) \times \text{body weight (kg)}}{\div 1\% \text{ (1 International Unit/kg) with ATnativ or } 1.4\% \text{ with Thrombate III}}$$

For a 70-kg patient with a baseline AT-III level of 57% the initial dose of ATnativ would be $(120\% - 57\%) \times 70 \div 1 = 4410$ IU and Thrombate III would be $[120\% - 57\%] \times 70 \div 1.4 = 3150$ IU. Plasma AT-III levels should be measured preceding the initial dose and 30 minutes later to calculate the in vivo recovery. For Thrombate III, measurement of plasma levels is suggested preinfusion, 10 minutes postinfusion (peak), 12 hours postinfusion, and preceding next infusion (trough). If recovery differs from the anticipated rise of 1% to 1.4% for each IU/kg, modify the formula accordingly. If the above patient receiving ATnativ has a 30-minute AT-III level of 147%, the increase in AT-III measured for each 1 IU/kg administered is $(147\% - 57\%) \times 70$ kg $\div 4410$ Units = 1.43% rise for each IU/kg administered. This in vivo recovery would be used to calculate future doses. A maintenance dose of approximately 60% of the loading dose every 24 hours is the average required to maintain plasma levels between 80% and 120%. Dose and interval based on plasma levels.

DOSE ADJUSTMENTS

Note Drug/lab interactions.

DILUTION

ATnativ: Each 500 IU must be reconstituted with 10 ml of sterile water for injection (preferred), NS or D5W. Swirl to dissolve. Do not shake. Bring solution to room temperature. May be further diluted with additional amounts of the same infusion solutions if desired.

Thrombate III: Diluent, double-ended needles for dilution and filter needle for aspiration into a syringe are provided. Warm unopened diluent and concentrate to room temperature. Enter diluent bottle first. Enter vacuum concentrate bottle with needle at an angle. Direct diluent from above to sides of vial to gently moisten all contents. Remove diluent bottle and transfer needle, swirl continuously until completely dissolved. Draw into a syringe through the filter needle. Remove filter needle; replace with an administration set (not provided). For larger doses, several bottles may be drawn into one syringe. Use a separate filter needle for each bottle.

Storage: Store in refrigerator before dilution; avoid freezing. Use within 3 hours of reconstitution.

INCOMPATIBLE WITH

ATnativ: Specific information not available.

Thrombate III: Manufacturer states, "give alone; do not mix with other agents or dilution solutions."

RATE OF ADMINISTRATION

Too-rapid injection may cause dyspnea.

ATnativ: Each 50 IU or fraction thereof should be given over 1 minute. Do not exceed a rate of 100 IU/min.

Thrombate III: A single dose over 10 to 20 minutes.

ACTIONS

Manufactured from human plasma, purified and heat treated through specific processes, AT-III is a plasma-based protein produced by the body to inactivate specific clotting proteins and control clot formation. Identical to heparin cofactor I, a factor in plasma necessary for heparin to exert its anticoagulant effect. It inactivates thrombin and the activated forms of factors IX, X, XI, and XII (all coagulation enzymes except factors VIIa and Factor XIIIa). Increases AT-III levels within 30 minutes and has a half-life of up to 3 days.

INDICATIONS AND USES

Treatment of patients with hereditary AT-III deficiency to prevent thrombosis during surgical or obstetric procedures (replacement therapy) or during acute thrombotic episodes.

CONTRAINDICATIONS

None when used as indicated.

PRECAUTIONS

For IV use only. ■ Confirm diagnosis of hereditary AT-III deficiency based on a clear family history of venous thrombosis as well as decreased plasma AT-III levels and the exclusion of acquired deficiency. Present laboratory tests may not be able to identify all cases of congenital AT-III deficiency. ■ Every unit of plasma used to manufacture AT-III is tested and found nonreactive for HBsAg and negative for antibody to HIV by FDA-approved tests, then heat-treated by a special process. Even with these precautions, individuals who receive multiple infusions may develop viral infection, particularly non-A, non-B hepatitis. HIV infection remains a remote possibility. ■ May reverse heparin resistance.

Monitor: Note varying methods for measuring AT-III levels under Usual dose. Should be measured at least twice daily until the patient is stabilized and peak and trough levels established, then measured daily. All blood work should be drawn immediately before the next infusion of AT-III.

Patient education: Inform of risks of thrombosis in connection with pregnancy and surgery and the fact that AT-III deficiency is hereditary.

Maternal/child: Neonatal AT-III levels should be measured immediately after birth if parents are known to have AT-III deficiency (fatal neonatal thromboembolism [e.g., aortic thrombi] has occurred). Treatment of the neonate should be under the direction of a physician knowledgeable about coagulation disorders. Normal full-term and premature infants have lower than adult averages of AT-III plasma levels. ■ Pregnancy category C: use only if clearly indicated. Fetal abnormalities not noted when administered in the third trimester. ■ Safety for use in children not established.

DRUG/LAB INTERACTIONS

Half-life of AT-III decreases with concurrent heparin treatment. The anticoagulant effect of heparin is enhanced and a reduced dose of heparin is indicated to avoid bleeding.

SIDE EFFECTS

None noted with ATnativ in patients with hereditary AT-III deficiency. Bowel fullness, chest pain, chest tightness, chills, cramps, dizziness, fever, film over eye, foul taste in mouth, hives, light-headedness, oozing and hematoma formation, and shortness of breath have occurred with Thrombate III. Some patients with acquired AT-III deficiency diagnosed with disseminated intravascular coagulation (DIC) have had diuretic and vasodilatory effects. Rapid infusion may cause dyspnea.

ANTIDOTE

Levels of 150% to 210% found in a few patients have not caused any apparent complications. Observe for bleeding. Reduce rate of infusion immediately for dyspnea. Decrease rate or interrupt infusion as indicated until side effects subside. Keep physician informed of patient's lab values and condition.

ANTIVENIN (CROTALIDAE) POLYVALENT

Antivenin

USUAL DOSE

Testing for sensitivity to horse serum required before use. (See Precautions and Monitor for additional pretreatment requirements.) Dosage based on severity of envenomation when patient is initially assessed.

No envenomation: None.

Minimal envenomation: 2 to 4 vials (20 to 40 ml).

Moderate envenomation: 5 to 9 vials (50 to 90 ml).

Severe envenomation: 10 to 15 vials (100 to 150 ml).

Additional antivenin need based on clinical response and progression of symptoms. If condition deteriorates, 1 to 5 additional vials (10 to 50 ml) may be given. Most effective within 4 hours of the bite, less effective after 8 hours, but in the presence of envenomation is to be given even after 24 hours have elapsed.

PEDIATRIC DOSE

Not based on weight. Small children bitten by large snakes may require larger doses of antivenin.

DILUTION

Each single vial must be diluted with 10 ml sterile water for injection (supplied). Must be further diluted with NS or D5W to a 1:1 to 1:10 solution (1 ml antivenin to 10 ml infusion solution preferred unless patient's condition limits fluid intake). Avoid foaming by gently swirling to mix thoroughly.

Storage: Store vials at controlled room temperature; do not freeze. Use reconstituted solution within 48 hours and diluted solutions within 12 hours.

INCOMPATIBLE WITH

Specific information not available. Do not mix with any other drug in syringe or solution because of specific use.

RATE OF ADMINISTRATION

Infuse 5 to 10 ml over a minimum of 3 to 5 minutes. If no adverse reaction occurs, give remaining initial dose at maximum rate of administration based on severity of envenomation and fluid tolerance appropriate for this patient's body weight and condition.

ACTIONS

Prepared from the blood serum of horses immunized against the venom of crotalids (pit vipers) found in North, Central, and South America. Will neutralize the venom of rattlesnakes, copperheads, and cottonmouth moccasins. (See literature for specific species.)

INDICATIONS AND USES

Treatment of patients with symptoms of envenomation sustained from the bite of a rattlesnake, copperhead, cottonmouth moccasin, or other specific pit viper species of snake.

CONTRAINDICATIONS

Hypersensitivity to horse serum unless only treatment available for life-threatening situation. Several techniques, including preload of antihistamines and/or desensitization, may be considered (see literature).

PRECAUTIONS

Read drug literature supplied with antivenin completely before use. Essential to evaluate symptoms and individual status of each patient. ■ Determine patient response to any previous injections of serum of any type and history of any allergic type reactions. ■ Hospitalize patient. ■ Test every patient without exception for sensitivity to horse serum (1 ml vial of 1:10 dilution horse serum supplied). Conjunctival test and skin test recommended for maximum safety. Always begin with the conjunctival test.

Conjunctival test: Instill 1 drop 1:10 horse serum into conjunctival sac for adults (1 drop 1:100 dilution for children). Itching, redness, burning, and/or lacrimation within 30 minutes is a positive reaction. A drop of normal saline in the opposite eye is used as a control and should be asymptomatic. Reverse adverse effects of positive reaction with 1 drop epinephrine ophthalmic solution.

Scratch test: Make a ¼-inch skin scratch through a drop of 1:100 dilution in normal saline. Make a similar scratch through a drop of normal saline on a comparable skin site as a control. Compare sites in 20 minutes. An urticarial wheal surrounded by a zone of erythema is a positive reaction.

Skin test: Inject 0.02 to 0.1 ml of 1:100 horse serum intradermally. In patients with a history of allergies use a 1:1,000 solution. A similar injection of normal saline can be used as a control. Compare in 20 minutes. An urticarial wheal surrounded by a zone of erythema is a positive reaction.

Other testing methods may be used. Use at least two. ■ A systemic reaction may occur even when both sensitivity tests are negative. ■ Tetanus prophylaxis is indicated. ■ Corticosteroids are the drugs of choice if antivenin is not available until 24 hours after the snake bite but are not recommended for concomitant administration. ■ Consider use of broad-spectrum antibiotic. ■ Check with poison control center; many authorities do not recommend packing the bitten extremity in ice.

Monitor: Before antivenin is administered draw adequate blood for baseline studies (type and cross-match, CBC, hematocrit, platelet count, prothrombin time [PT], clot retraction, bleeding and coagulation times, BUN, electrolytes, and bilirubin). ■ Monitor all vital signs at frequent intervals. ■ Have urine specimens tested frequently for microscopic erythrocytes. ■ In most cases, the sooner a sensitivity reaction occurs, the greater the sensitivity. Observe patient continuously. ■ Initiate two IV lines as soon as possible; one to be used for supportive therapy, the other for antivenin and electrolytes. ■ Keep emergency equipment available at all times, including oxygen, epinephrine, antihistamines (e.g., diphenhydramine [Benadryl]), vasopressors (e.g., dopamine [Intropin]), corticosteroids, and ventilation equipment.

Maternal/child: Pregnancy category C: Use during pregnancy only if clearly needed. ■ Safety for use during lactation not established; no documented problems.

DRUG/LAB INTERACTIONS

Concomitant use of antihistamines may interfere with sensitivity tests.

SIDE EFFECTS

Acute anaphylaxis with urticaria, respiratory distress, and vascular collapse. Serum sickness may occur. Usually appears in 7 to 12 days. Local pain, local erythema, and urticaria without systemic reaction can occur.

ANTIDOTE

Discontinue the drug and notify the physician of all side effects. Treat anaphylaxis immediately. Epinephrine (Adrenalin) and diphenhydramine (Benadryl), oxygen, vasopressors (dopamine), corticosteroids, H_2 antagonists (Cimetidine), and ventilation equipment must always be available. Resuscitate as necessary.

ANTIVENIN *(LATRODECTUS MACTANS)*

Antivenin

Black Widow Spider Species Antivenin

USUAL DOSE

Testing for sensitivity to horse serum required before use. (See Precautions) for additional pretreatment requirements.)

Entire contents of 1 vial of antivenin (2.5 ml) is recommended for adults and children. One vial is usually enough but a second dose may be necessary in rare instances. Best results obtained if administered within 4 hours of envenomation.

PEDIATRIC DOSE

Same as adult dose.

DILUTION

Each single dose (6,000 antivenin units) must be initially diluted with 2.5 ml SW for injection (supplied). Keep needle in rubber stopper of antivenin and shake vial to dissolve contents completely. Must be further diluted in 10 to 50 ml NS for IV injection.

Storage: Refrigerate unopened vials; do not freeze. Refrigerate reconstituted and/or diluted solution; discard in 6 hours.

INCOMPATIBLE WITH

Specific information not available. Do not mix with any other drug in syringe or solution because of specific use.

RATE OF ADMINISTRATION

A single dose over a minimum of 15 minutes.

ACTIONS

Prepared from the blood serum of horses immunized against the venom of the black widow spider. One unit will neutralize one average mouse-lethal dose of black widow spider venom when both are injected simultaneously under lab conditions.

INDICATIONS AND USES

Treatment of patients with symptoms resulting from black widow spider bites *(Latrodectus mactans).*

CONTRAINDICATIONS

Hypersensitivity to horse serum unless only treatment available for a life-threatening situation. Several techniques including preload of antihistamine and/or desensitization may be considered (see literature).

PRECAUTIONS

Read drug literature supplied with antivenin completely before use. Essential to evaluate symptoms and individual status of each patient. ■ Determine patient response to any previous injections of serum of any type and history of any allergic-type reactions. ■ Hospitalize patient if possible. ■ Muscle relaxants may be the initial treatment of choice in healthy individuals between 16 and 60. Antivenin use may be deferred while patient is observed. ■ Test every patient without exception for sensitivity to horse serum (1-ml vial of 1:10 dilution horse serum supplied). Conjunctival test and skin test recommended for maximum safety. Always begin with the conjunctival test.

Conjunctival test: Instill 1 drop 1:10 horse serum into conjunctival sac for adults (1 drop 1:100 dilution for children). Itching, redness, burning, and/or lacrimation within 30 minutes is a positive reaction. A drop of normal saline in the opposite eye is used as a control and should be asymptomatic. Reverse adverse effects of positive reaction with 1 drop epinephrine ophthalmic solution.

Scratch test: Make a ¼-inch skin scratch through a drop of 1:100 dilution in normal saline. Make a similar scratch through a drop of normal saline on a comparable skin site as a control. Compare sites in 20 minutes. An urticarial wheal surrounded by a zone of erythema is a positive reaction.

Skin test: Inject 0.02 to 0.1 ml of 1:100 horse serum intradermally. In patients with a history of allergies use a 1:1,000 solution. A similar injection of normal saline can be used as a control. Compare in 20 minutes. An urticarial wheal surrounded by a zone of erythema is a positive reaction.

Other testing methods may be used. Use at least two. ■ A systemic reaction may occur even when both sensitivity tests are negative. ■ May be given IM. IV preferred in severe cases, if patient is in shock, or in children under 12 years of age.

Monitor: Supportive therapy is indicated. 10 ml of 10% calcium gluconate IV may control muscle pain. Morphine may be needed. Barbiturates or diazepam may be used for restlessness. Prolonged warm baths are helpful; corticosteroids have been used. ■ Observe patient constantly for respiratory paralysis. Can occur from toxin alone, and narcotics and sedatives may precipitate respiratory depression. ■ Observe for serum sickness for 8 to 12 days.

Maternal/child: Pregnancy category C: Use only if clearly needed. ■ Safety for use in lactation not established. ■ Safety for use in children not established, but there have been no adverse effects when used.

DRUG/LAB INTERACTIONS

Concomitant use of antihistamines may interfere with sensitivity tests. ■ Narcotics and sedatives may precipitate respiratory depression.

SIDE EFFECTS

Acute anaphylaxis with urticaria, respiratory distress, and vascular collapse. Serum sickness may occur. Usually appears in 7 to 12 days.

Local pain, local erythema, and urticaria without systemic reaction can occur.

ANTIDOTE

Discontinue the drug and notify the physician of all side effects. Treat anaphylaxis immediately. Epinephrine (Adrenalin), diphenhydramine (Benadryl), oxygen, vasopressors (dopamine), corticosteroids, H_2 antagonists (Cimetidine), and ventilation equipment must always be available. Resuscitate as necessary.

ANTIVENIN *(MICRURUS FULVIUS)*
Antivenin

North American Coral Snake Antivenin
pH 6.5 to 7.5

USUAL DOSE

Testing for sensitivity to horse serum required before use. (See Precautions) for additional pretreatment requirements.)

Entire contents of 3 to 5 vials (30 to 50 ml) is recommended depending on the nature and severity of envenomation. Up to 10 vials may be required if the snake's entire venom load was delivered by the bite. Best results obtained if administered within 4 hours of envenomation.

PEDIATRIC DOSE

Same as adult dose, not adjusted by weight of patient.

DILUTION

Each single vial must be diluted with 10 ml sterile water for injection (supplied). Start an IV infusion of 250 to 500 ml NS. May be administered through the tubing of the free-flowing IV or added to the infusion solution after initial 2 ml given without adverse reaction.

Storage: Store vials at controlled room temperature; do not freeze. Use reconstituted solution within 48 hours and diluted solution within 12 hours.

INCOMPATIBLE WITH

Specific information not available. Do not mix with any other drug in syringe or solution because of specific use.

RATE OF ADMINISTRATION

Inject the first 1 to 2 ml over a minimum of 3 to 5 minutes. If no adverse reaction, give remaining initial dose at maximum rate of administration based on severity of envenomation and fluid tolerance appropriate for patient's body weight and condition.

ACTIONS

Prepared from the blood serum of horses immunized against the venom of specific coral snakes. Will neutralize the venom of *M. fulvius fulvius* (eastern coral snake) and *M. fulvius tenere* (Texas coral snake). Response should be rapid and dramatic.

INDICATIONS AND USES

Treatment of patients with symptoms resulting from the venom of *M. fulvius fulvius* (eastern coral snake) and *M. fulvius tenere* (Texas coral snake). ▪ Not effective for *M. euryxanthus* (Arizona or Sonoran coral snake).

CONTRAINDICATIONS

Hypersensitivity to horse serum unless only treatment available for a life-threatening situation. Several techniques including preload of antihistamines and/or desensitization may be considered (see literature).

PRECAUTIONS

Read drug literature supplied with antivenin completely before use. Essential to evaluate symptoms and individual status of each patient. ▪ Determine patient response to any previous injections of serum of any type and history of any allergic type reactions. ▪ Immobilize victim. At a minimum, splint bitten extremity. Hospitalize patient if possible. ▪ Test every patient without exception for sensitivity to horse serum (1 ml vial of 1:10 dilution horse serum supplied). Conjunctival test and scratch test recommended for maximum safety. Always begin with the conjunctival test.

Conjunctival test: Instill 1 drop 1:10 horse serum into conjunctival sac for adults (1 drop 1:100 dilution for children). Itching, redness, burning, and/or lacrimation within 30 minutes is a positive reaction. A drop of normal saline in the opposite eye is used as a control and should be asymptomatic. Reverse adverse effects of positive reaction with 1 drop epinephrine ophthalmic solution.

Scratch test: Place 1 drop of 1:100 solution on the skin. Make a ¼-inch scratch through this drop. Establish a normal saline control in the same manner on a similar skin surface. Compare in 20 minutes. An urticarial wheal surrounded by a zone of erythema is a positive reaction.

Skin test: Inject 0.02 to 0.03 ml of a 1:100 dilution of horse serum in NS. In patients with a history of allergies use a 1:100 dilution. A similar injection of NS can be used as a control. Compare sites in 5 to 30 minutes. An urticarial wheel surrounded by a zone of erythema is a positive reaction.

Other testing methods may be used. Use at least two. ▪ A systemic reaction may occur even when both sensitivity tests are negative. ▪ Tetanus prophylaxis indicated.

Monitor: Observe patient constantly. Additional antivenin may be needed. Paralysis can occur within 2 to 2½ hours. Local tissue reaction does not reflect the amount of envenomation. Observe signs and symptoms to assess amount of toxin injected. Symptoms may begin in 1 hour or be delayed up to 18 hours. ▪ Supportive therapy is indicated. Respiratory depressants (e.g., narcotics, sedatives) are contraindicated or used with extreme caution. Keep equipment for artificial ventilation immediately available.

Maternal/child: Pregnancy category C: Use only if clearly needed. ▪ Safety for use during lactation not established; problems not documented.

DRUG/LAB INTERACTIONS

Concomitant use of antihistamines may interfere with sensitivity tests. ▪ Narcotics and sedatives may precipitate respiratory depression.

SIDE EFFECTS

Acute anaphylaxis with urticaria, respiratory distress, and vascular collapse. Serum sickness may occur. Usually appears in 7 to 12 days.

Local pain, local erythema, and urticaria without systemic reaction can occur.

ANTIDOTE

Discontinue the drug and notify the physician of all side effects. Treat anaphylaxis immediately. Epinephrine (Adrenalin) and diphenhydramine (Benadryl), oxygen, vasopressors (dopamine), H_2 antagonists (Cimetidine), and ventilation equipment must always be available. Resuscitate as necessary.

APROTININ INJECTION

Antifibrinolytic
Antihemorrhagic

Trasylol

pH 4.5 to 6.5

USUAL DOSE

Regimen A consists of a test dose, a loading dose, a constant infusion dose, and a dose to be added to the priming fluid of the cardiopulmonary bypass circuit ("pump prime" dose). IV doses must be given through a central venous line with the patient in a supine position. Do not administer any other drug using the same line. Total cumulative doses of more than 7 million KIU (Kallikrein inhibitor units) have not been studied in controlled trials. Requires concurrent use of heparin (heparin dose-response required prior to administration of aprotinin, see below). Note Precautions/Monitor.

Test dose: 1 ml (1.4 mg or 10,000 KIU). Must be given IV at least 10 minutes before the loading dose.

Loading dose: 200 ml (280 mg or 2.0 million KIU). Given slowly IV over 20 to 30 minutes, after induction of anesthesia but prior to sternotomy. When complete, follow with a *constant infusion* of 50 ml/hr (70 mg/hr or 500,000 KIU/hr). Continue until the surgery is complete and the patient leaves the operating room.

"Pump prime dose": 200 ml (280 mg or 2.0 million KIU). Add to the priming fluid of the cardiopulmonary bypass circuit, by replacing an aliquot of priming fluid before instituting cardiopulmonary bypass.

Heparin: May be administered by a titration regimen or a fixed regimen.

Heparin titration regimen: Prior to administration of aprotinin, obtain a heparin dose response assessed by protamine titration to determine the heparin loading dose. Obtain heparin levels by protamine titration during bypass. Heparin levels during bypass should not be allowed to drop below 2.7 units/ml (2 mg/kg) or below the level indicated by heparin dose-response testing performed prior to aprotinin administration.

Fixed heparin regimen: A standard loading dose of heparin, administered prior to cannulation of the heart, and the quantity of heparin added to the prime volume of the cardiopulmonary bypass (CPB) circuit should total at least 350 units/kg. Additional heparin should be administered in a fixed-dose regimen based on patient weight and duration of CPB.

DOSE ADJUSTMENTS

Not required with age or impaired renal function; changes in pharmacokinetics of aprotinin are not great enough. ■ No information available for patients with preexisting hepatic disease, note side effects. ■ Regimen B doses are exactly one-half of Regimen A. Experience with this lower-dose regimen is limited. Donor blood use is reduced but Regimen A is considered most effective at this time.

DILUTION

Supplied as a solution. Each 1 ml contains 1.4 mg or 10,000 KIU. May be used without further dilution.

Storage: Store at controlled room temperature. Protect from freezing.

INCOMPATIBLE WITH

Corticosteroids, heparin, nutrient solutions (e.g., amino acids or fat emulsion), tetracyclines. All drugs given concomitantly should be administered separately through different venous lines or catheters.

RATE OF ADMINISTRATION

Test dose: A single dose over 1 minute.

Loading dose: A single dose over 20 to 30 minutes. Follow with an infusion at 50 ml/hr. Too-rapid administration can cause a transient fall in blood pressure.

ACTIONS

A natural proteinase inhibitor obtained from bovine lung. Has a variety of effects on the coagulation system. The net effect is inhibition of both fibrinolysis and turnover of coagulation factors (common results of CPB) and decrease in bleeding. Precise mechanism of this effect is unclear. Significantly reduces the donor blood transfusion requirement. Rapidly distributed into the total extracellular space with a rapid initial decrease in plasma concentration. Plasma half-life is 150 minutes. Terminal elimination half-life is about 10 hours. Accumulated in the kidney, and slowly degraded by lysosomal enzymes. Some excretion in urine.

INDICATIONS AND USES

Prophylactic use to reduce perioperative blood loss and the need for blood transfusion in patients undergoing repeat coronary artery bypass graft surgery (CABG). May be used in selected primary CABG patients where the risk of bleeding is especially high (impaired hemostasis [e.g., presence of aspirin or other coagulopathy]) or where transfusion is unavailable or unacceptable. Use in primary CABG patients is also based on the risk of renal dysfunction and the risk of anaphylaxis if a second procedure is needed.

CONTRAINDICATIONS

Hypersensitivity to aprotinin.

PRECAUTIONS

Should be used under the direction of a physician specialist and an anesthesiologist. ■ Do not administer to a patient who experiences any allergic reaction to aprotinin. ■ Risk of anaphylaxis (even with test dose) is increased in patients who have received aprotinin in the past (especially within the previous 6 months). Emergency equipment and drugs must be immediately available. Do not administer the test dose or loading dose until the conditions for rapid cannulation (if necessary) are present. Delay addition of aprotinin into the pump prime solution until after the loading dose has been safely administered.

Consider prophylactic administration of H_1 and H_2 blockers before the test dose (note Monitor). ■ Use caution in patients with a history of allergic reactions. ■ May cause increased renal failure and mortality in patients undergoing deep hypothermic circulatory arrest during surgery of the aortic arch. ■ Use caution in patients with impaired liver function.

Monitor: Primary patient monitoring under the direction of the anesthesiologist. ■ Premedication with diphenhydramine (Benadryl) and H_2 blockers (e.g., ranitidine [Zantac]) is recommended 15 minutes before the loading dose in any patient who has received aprotinin previously.
■ In prolonged extracorporeal circulation, patients may require additional heparin, even in the presence of activated clotting time (ACT) levels that appear to represent adequate anticoagulation. Maintain a minimal celite-ACT of >750 seconds or a kaolin-ACT of >480 seconds, independent of the effects of hemodilution and hypothermia. Administer heparin either in a fixed-dose regimen based on patient weight and duration of CPB or on the basis of heparin levels measured by a method not affected by aprotinin (e.g., protamine titration); see Usual dose. ■ Note Precautions, Antidote.

Patient education: Explain risk of allergic reaction.

Maternal/child: Pregnancy category B: Use only if clearly needed.
■ Safety and effectiveness in children not established.

Elderly: Dose adjustment not required.

DRUG/LAB INTERACTIONS

Had antifibrinolytic activity, may inhibit the effects of fibrinolytic agents (e.g., heparin, alteplase [tPA], anistreplase [Eminase]). ■ May block the acute hypotensive effect of captopril (Capoten). ■ Prolongs the ACT in the presence of heparin but is not a heparin-sparing agent (note Monitor).

SIDE EFFECTS

Hypersensitivity reactions including anaphylaxis can occur at any time even if the test dose is negative; risk increased with repeated administration. Elevated PTT and ACT are expected for several hours after surgery. Elevated ALT (SGOT) is more frequent with repeated administration. Increased serum creatinine (reversible renal dysfunction), serum creatinine kinase, and serum glucose may occur. There may be an increased incidence of myocardial infarction and of saphenous vein graft closure. Many reported side effects are not attributable to aprotinin but are common in open-heart surgery (e.g., apnea, arrhythmias, asthma, cardiac arrest, confusion, congestive heart failure, dyspnea, fever, hypotension, kidney failure, myocardial infarction, pneumonia, sepsis, shock).

ANTIDOTE

Discontinue aprotinin and treat anaphylaxis immediately (epinephrine [Adrenalin], corticosteroids, diphenhydramine [Benadryl], ranitidine [Zantac], airway management, oxygen). Keep physician informed. To reverse heparin activity, the amount of protamine administered should be based on the actual amount of heparin given and not on the ACT values. Give protamine by very slow IV injection over a 10-minute period in doses not to exceed 50 mg; too-rapid injection of protamine can cause bradycardia, severe hypotension, and anaphylaxis. Treat all side effects (e.g., arrhythmias) appropriately and resuscitate as necessary.

ARBUTAMINE HYDROCHLORIDE
GenESA

Diagnostic agent

pH 3.8

USUAL DOSE
The GenESA system is a combination product. The diagnostic agent (arbutamine) in its special prefilled syringe is intended for direct IV infusion only with an automated delivery device called the GenESA Device. Complete directions for operating the GenESA Device must be read before use. Arbutamine must not be diluted or transferred to another syringe. The GenESA Device is a minicomputer containing a single-channel ECG (R wave) detector, a noninvasive BP monitor, computer software (closed-loop algorithm) that controls drug delivery, an IV syringe pump, display functions, and an operator key pad. The GenESA Device individualizes the dosing regimen of arbutamine according to the heart rate response of the patient using the closed loop algorithm. The physician selects the desired rate of heart rate rise (HR slope) and the maximum heart rate to be achieved (HR target).

DILUTION
Arbutamine must not be diluted or transferred to another syringe. To prepare the syringe: Remove the prefilled glass syringe and plunger rod from the package. Inspect the grey tip cap and stopper for proper engagement. Evidence of leakage or a loose tip cap may indicate a violation of sterility. Thread the plunger rod into the stopper clockwise until fully seated (approximately one full revolution). Hold the syringe vertically (tip UP), remove the tip cap, and manually express any air from the syringe. Attach the IV administration set to the syringe luer lock. Use a push and twist (clockwise) action until fully engaged. Load the assembled syringe/IV set into the GenESA Device as instructed in The GenESA System Directions For Use.

Storage: Store the prepackaged syringes at 2° to 8° C. Protect from light.

INCOMPATIBLE WITH
Any other drug in syringe or solution due to specific use.

RATE OF ADMINISTRATION
Upon starting the test, the GenESA Device delivers a small dose (0.1 mcg/kg/min for 1 minute) and measures the patient's HR response. It then calculates the difference between the desired and actual HR responses and adjusts the infusion rate appropriately. The maximum infusion rate delivered is 0.8 mcg/kg/min. Specific alerts warn of conditions that may require attention. Specific alarms stop drug delivery due to potential safety hazards. The physician may interrupt delivery manually at any time it is clinically appropriate. The device includes a "hold HR" feature that, when activated, allows HR to be maintained at approximately that level for 5 minutes. Drug delivery will stop

automatically when the target HR has been reached or a total of 10 mcg/kg of arbutamine has been delivered.

ACTIONS

A synthetic catecholamine with chronotropic and inotropic properties. Specifically designed to simulate the cardiac effects of exercise for use in stress testing. Its beta-adrenergic activity produces parallel increases in heart rate and cardiac contractility while also increasing systolic blood pressure. The adjunctive use of atropine is not required and not recommended. It mimics exercise and provokes myocardial ischemia in patients with compromised coronary arteries. Probably limits tissue oxygenation by its increase in heart rate. Acts principally on the myocardium. Onset of action is within 1 minute. Half-life is approximately 8 minutes. Within 16 minutes after the infusion is stopped, heart rate is decreased by 50% from maximum achieved or target rate. Primarily metabolized in the liver and excreted in urine and feces.

INDICATIONS AND USES

The GenESA system with arbutamine is an aid in diagnosing the presence or absence of cardiovascular disease (CAD) in patients with suspected CAD who cannot exercise adequately. It is used in conjunction with echocardiography and radionuclide myocardial perfusion imaging.

CONTRAINDICATIONS

Patients with idiopathic hypertrophic subaortic stenosis, history of recurrent sustained ventricular tachycardia, congestive heart failure (NYHA Class III or IV), hypersensitivity to arbutamine or its components (contains sulfites). *Do not use in the presence of an implanted cardiac pacemaker or automated cardioverter/defibrillator.* ▪ Note Precautions.

PRECAUTIONS

Administered by or under the direct supervision of the physician specialist. ▪ May precipitate or exacerbate supraventricular and ventricular arrhythmias. Not recommended for use in patients with a history of sustained arrhythmias or in patients receiving Class I antiarrhythmic agents (e.g., quinidine, lidocaine, flecainide). ▪ Not recommended for use in patients with unstable angina, mechanical left ventricular outflow obstruction (e.g., severe valvular aortic stenosis), uncontrolled systemic hypertension, heart transplant, a history of CVA, or peripheral vascular disorder resulting in cerebral or aortic aneurysm. ▪ Not recommended for use in patients with narrow-angle glaucoma or uncontrolled hyperthyroidism. ▪ Not recommended for use in patients receiving anticholinergic agents (e.g., atropine), digoxin, or tricyclic antidepressants (e.g., amitriptyline [Elavil]). ▪ The GenESA Device is not designed to detect arrhythmias and may record an inaccurate HR in the presence of an arrhythmia. Must be used in conjunction with a diagnostic-quality ECG machine. ▪ Safety for use within 30 days of a myocardial infarction has not been established. ▪ Use caution in patients with allergies; contains sulfites. ▪ Note Drug/lab interactions. ***Monitor:*** Complete cardiac and pulmonary emergency resuscitation equipment and supplies must always be available (e.g., defibrillator, oxygen, controlled ventilation, drugs). Beta-adrenergic antagonists (e.g., esmolol [Brevibloc], metoprolol [Lopressor], propranolol [Inderal]) must be immediately available. ▪ Monitor ECG continuously for inaccurate heart rates and/or arrhythmias. Immediate treatment or discontinuation of the arbutamine may be indicated. ▪ Monitor BP continuously. ▪ May cause rapid increases or paradoxical decreases in HR and sytolic BP that will reverse if the infusion is discontinued. May be restarted if clinically appropriate. ▪ GenESA will stop drug delivery when the target HR is achieved or after a total dose of 10 mcg/kg has been delivered. ▪ Continue monitoring the patient until HR and BP have returned to acceptable levels. ▪ Note Precautions, Drug/lab interactions, Side effects, and Antidote.

Patient education: Report any difficulty in breathing promptly.

Maternal/child: Category B. Use during pregnancy only if clearly needed. ▪ Specific information not available regarding use during lactation or in children.

Elderly: Specific information not available.

DRUG/LAB INTERACTIONS

Beta-adrenergic antagonists (e.g., atenolol [Tenormin], esmolol [Brevibloc], metoprolol [Lopressor], propranolol [Inderal]) may negate the desired pharmacologic effects of arbutamine. Discontinue at least 48 hours before conducting a GenESA System Test. ▪ Use of atropine to enchance the chronotropic response to arbutamine is not recommended. ▪ Not recommended for use in patients receiving anticholinergic agents (e.g., atropine), digoxin, or tricyclic antidepressants (e.g., amitriptyline [Elavil]) ▪ Because of their proarrhythmic effects, arbutamine is not recommended for concurrent use with Class I antiarrhythmic agents (e.g., quinidine, lidocaine, flecainide). ▪ No evidence to date of interactions with platelet aggregation inhibitors (e.g., abciximab [ReoPro], dipyridamole [Persantine]), nitroprusside sodium, nitroglycerin, or calcium channel blockers (e.g., diltiazem [Cardizem], verapamil [Isoptin]).

SIDE EFFECTS

Superventricular or ventricular arrhythmias (isolate PVCs and PACs are most frequent); but although most arrhythmias have been self-limiting, multiple arrhythmias may occur in any one patient. Some have been life-threatening (e.g., VF, VT, heart blocks), but to this date no deaths have occurred. May cause rapid increases or paradoxical decreases in HR and BP. Some side effects result from symptoms of catecholamine excess (e.g., angina, anxiety, diaphoresis, dizziness, dry mouth, headache, hot flashes, flushing, hypotension, nausea, paresthesia, tremor). Others result from positive chronotropic and inotropic effects on the myocardium (e.g., hypertension, myocardial infarction [occurred in one patient], tachyarrhythmias, and ventricular fibrillation). Chest pain, dyspnea, fatigue, hypoesthesia (abnormal decrease to sensory stimulation), nonspecific pain, palpitation, taste perversion, and vasodilation have also been reported. May also cause a transient decrease in serum potassium (rarely hypokalemia) and transient increases in QT interval (not associated with arrhythmias).

ANTIDOTE

Discontinue infusion when a diagnostic endpoint (e.g., ST segment deviation on ECG) has been reached, if clinically significant symptoms or arrhythmias occur, or if clinically appropriate for any reason (e.g., catecholamine excess is not tolerable, rapid increases or paradoxical decreases in HR and systolic BP). Establish an adequate airway and ensure adequate oxygenation and ventilation. Treat severe symptoms (e.g., angina, hypotension, ST segment abnormalities, tachyarrhythmias) that have not been quickly resolved by discontinuing the infusion with IV beta-blocking antagonists (e.g., esmolol 10 to 80 mg, metoprolol 7.5 to 50 mg, propranolol 0.5 to 2 mg). Sublingual nitroglycerin may be indicated. Short half-life generally precludes prolonged side effects or overdose problems. Treat unresolved side effects symptomatically (e.g., arrhythmias, hypotension, hypertension, myocardial infarction). Resuscitate as necessary.

ARGININE HYDROCHLORIDE   Diagnostic Agent
R-Gene 10   pH 5.0 to 6.5

USUAL DOSE
300 ml as a single test dose under specific clinical conditions and procedures. Confirm serum electrolyte balance before administration.

PEDIATRIC DOSE
5 ml/kg of body weight.

DILUTION
Available as 10% solution in 500-ml bottles ready for use as an IV infusion. Inspect each bottle; discard if not clear or vacuum is not present.

INCOMPATIBLE WITH
Specific information not available. Should be considered incompatible with any other drug or solution because of specific use.

RATE OF ADMINISTRATION
A single dose evenly distributed over 30 minutes. Recommended dose must be infused in 30 minutes to ensure accurate test results.

ACTIONS
A diagnostic aid, it is an IV stimulant to the pituitary that often induces a pronounced rise in plasma level of human growth hormone (HGH) in normal individuals. This rise does not occur if pituitary function is diminished or absent.

INDICATIONS AND USES
IV stimulant to pituitary as a diagnostic aid. May be useful in panhypopituitarism, pituitary dwarfism, chromophobe adenoma, postsurgical craniopharyngioma, hypophysectomy, pituitary trauma, acromegaly, gigantism, and problems of growth or stature.

CONTRAINDICATIONS
Individuals with known severe allergic tendencies.

PRECAUTIONS
Confirm absolute patency of vein; hypertonic and acidic, infiltration may cause necrosis of tissue. ■ False-positive or false-negative results 30% of time. Cross-check or confirm result with insulin hypoglycemia test and a second arginine test. Allow 1 day between each test.
  ■ High chloride content; may cause bicarbonate deficit and/or potas-

sium excess. ▪ Use caution in renal impairment; high nitrogen content.

Monitor: Specific test procedure must be observed. Schedule in morning; patient must be fasting overnight and have had a normal night's rest. Maintain bed rest and calming atmosphere from 30 minutes before infusion to completion of test process. Draw blood samples from opposite arm of infusion 30 minutes before, at time infusion is begun, and every 30 minutes times 5. Technician should promptly centrifuge and store all samples at −20° C until processed.

Maternal/child: Pregnancy category B: Pregnancy will cause a false-positive result. Do not use. ▪ Safety for use during lactation not established.

DRUG/LAB INTERACTIONS
Oral contraceptives will cause false-positive results.

SIDE EFFECTS
Usually result from rate or hypertonicity of solution. Flushing, headache, local venous irritation, nausea, numbness, rash, tissue necrosis at site of infiltration, vomiting.

Overdose: May cause transient metabolic acidosis with hyperventilation.

ANTIDOTE
Slow infusion to reduce side effects, but must be infused in 30 minutes for accurate results. Notify physician of all side effects. Discontinue drug and treat allergic reaction with diphenhydramine (Benadryl) or epinephrine. If metabolic acidosis persists, calculation of deficit and use of an alkalizing agent (e.g., sodium bicarbonate) may be required. Resuscitate as necessary.

ASCORBIC ACID
Nutritional supplement (Vitamin)

Cenolate, Cevalin, ✚Redoxon, sodium ascorbate, vitamin C

pH 5.5 to 7.0

USUAL DOSE
Up to 6 Gm/24 hr has been given without toxicity.

Nutritional protection: 70 to 150 mg daily. 100 to 200 mg daily may be required during chronic dialysis.

Prevention or treatment of scurvy: 100 to 250 mg 1 to 3 times daily. Give for a minimum of several days; up to 2 to 3 weeks may be indicated.

Enhance wound healing: 300 to 500 mg daily for 7 to 10 days.

Burns: 1 to 2 Gm daily.

PEDIATRIC DOSE
Nutritional protection: 30 mg daily. *Premature infants* may require 75 to 100 mg daily.

Prevention or treatment of scurvy: 100 to 300 mg/24 hr. Give in divided doses. Give for a minimum of several days, up to 2 to 3 weeks may be indicated.

DILUTION

May be given undiluted or may be administered diluted in IV infusion solutions. Soluble in the more commonly used solutions, such as D5W, D5/NS, NS, LR, Ringer's injection, or sodium lactate injection. Slight coloration does not affect the medication.

Storage: Protect from freezing and from light.

INCOMPATIBLE WITH

Aminophylline, bleomycin (Blenoxane), cefazolin (Kefzol), cephapirin (Cefadyl), chloramphenicol (Chloromycetin), chlordiazepoxide (Librium), chlorothiazide (Diuril), conjugated estrogens (Premarin), dextran, doxapram (Dopram), erythromycin (Erythrocin), fat emulsion 10%, hydrocortisone, nafcillin (Unipen), phytonadione (Aquamephyton), sodium bicarbonate, sulfisoxazole, triflupromazine (Vesprin), vitamin B_{12} (e.g., Redisol), warfarin (Coumadin).

RATE OF ADMINISTRATION

Direct IV: 100 mg or fraction thereof over 1 minute.

Infusion: Administer at ordered rate for standard infusion (e.g., over 4 to 8 hr).

ACTIONS

This water-soluble vitamin is necessary for the formation of collagen in all fibrous tissue, carbohydrate metabolism, connective tissue repair, maintenance of intracellular stability of blood vessels, and many other body functions. Not stored in the body. Daily requirements must be met. Completely utilized; excess is excreted unchanged in the urine. Crosses placental barrier. Secreted in breast milk.

INDICATIONS AND USES

Prevention and treatment of Vitamin C, deficiency which may lead to scurvy. ■ Give pre- and post-op to enhance wound healing. ■ Prolonged IV therapy. ■ Increased vitamin requirements or replacement therapy in severe burns, extensive injuries, and severe infections. ■ Prematurity. ■ Deficient intestinal absorption of water-soluble vitamins. ■ Prolonged or wasting diseases. ■ Hemovascular disorders and delayed fracture and wound healing require increased intake.

CONTRAINDICATIONS

There are no absolute contraindications.

PRECAUTIONS

Vitamin C is better absorbed and utilized by IM injection. ■ Use caution in cardiac patients. Sodium or calcium content may antagonize other drugs or overall condition. ■ Use caution in diabetics and patients prone to recurrent renal calculi or undergoing stool occult blood tests. May contain sulfites; use caution in allergic individuals.

Monitor: Increased urinary excretion is diagnostic for vitamin C saturation. ■ Continue curative doses until clinical symptoms subside or urinary saturation occurs.

Maternal/child: Use caution in pregnancy; high dose may adversely affect fetus.

DRUG/LAB INTERACTIONS

Potentiates oral contraceptives, ferrous iron absorption, salicylates, and sulfonamides. ■ May antagonize anticoagulants. ■ 2 Gm/day will lower urine pH and will cause reabsorption of acidic drugs and crystallization with sulfonamides. ■ May inhibit phenothiazines. ■ Plasma levels decreased by smoking cigarettes; increased doses of ascorbic acid may be required. ■ May cause false-negative occult blood in stool. ■ May cause false-positive or false-negative in urine glucose tests. ■ Can alter numerous test results, must be individually evaluated.

SIDE EFFECTS

Occur only with too-rapid injection: temporary dizziness or faintness. Diarrhea or renal calculi may occur with large doses.

ANTIDOTE

Discontinue administration temporarily. Resume administration at a decreased rate. If side effects persist, discontinue drug and notify the physician.

ASPARAGINASE

Antineoplastic
(Enzyme)

Elspar, ✚Kidrolase

pH 7.4

USUAL DOSE

Skin test: Required before initial dose and whenever 7 days or more elapse between doses. See Dilution for preparation. Give 2 IU intradermally and observe for 1 hour for the appearance of a wheal or erythema.

Intermittent IV: Very specific amount to be given on a specific day or days in a specific regimen of other chemotherapeutic agents, i.e., 1,000 IU/kg of body weight/day for 10 successive days beginning on day 22 of regimen with specific prednisone and vincristine doses. When used as a single agent (rare), the usual dose for adults and children is 200 IU/kg/day for 28 days.

Desensitization process for administration: Extensive process. See drug literature.

DILUTION

Specific techniques required; (See Precautions). Initially reconstitute each 10-ml vial (10,000 IU) with 4 ml of SW for Kidrolase and 5 ml of SW or NS for Elspar. Both result in 2,000 IU/ml.

Skin test: Withdraw 0.1 ml from the above solution and further dilute with 9.9 ml NS (20 IU/ml). 0.1 ml of this solution equals 2 IU.

Intermittent IV: Use 2,000 IU/ml solution. Should be further diluted with 50 to 100 ml of D5W or NS and administered as an infusion through Y-tube or three-way stopcock of a free-flowing infusion of D5W or NS. Use only clear solutions. May contain fiberlike particles; use of 5.0 micron filter recommended.

Storage: Refrigerate before and after dilution. Discard Elspar after 8 hours. Reconstituted Kidrolase may be refrigerated up to 14 days. Discard any solution that is cloudy.

INCOMPATIBLE WITH

Specific information not available. Consider incompatible in syringe or solution because of toxicity and specific use.

RATE OF ADMINISTRATION

Intermittent IV: Each dose evenly distributed over at least 30 minutes.

ACTIONS

An enzyme derived from *Escherichia coli* that rapidly depletes asparagine from cells. Some malignant cells have a metabolic defect that makes them dependent on exogenous asparagine for survival, but they are unable to synthesize asparagine as normal cells do. Undergoes metabolic degradation. Range of plasma half-life is 8 to 30 hours. Trace amounts excreted in urine.

INDICATIONS AND USES

Induces remissions in acute lymphocytic leukemia. Primarily used in specific combinations with other chemotherapeutic agents. ▪ May be useful in other leukemias and non-Hodgkin's lymphoma.

CONTRAINDICATIONS

Hypersensitivity to asparaginase, pancreatitis, or past history of pancreatitis.

PRECAUTIONS

▪ Follow guidelines for handling cytotoxic agents. See Appendix A, p. 893. ▪ A lethal drug; administered by or under the direction of the physician specialist. ▪ Rarely used as a single agent; not recommended for maintenance therapy. ▪ Impairs liver function; may increase toxicity of other drugs.

Monitor: Toxicity and short-term effectiveness limit use. More toxic in adults than in children. ▪ Avoid giving at night. ▪ Observe patient carefully during and after infusion. Monitor blood pressure every 15 minutes for at least 1 hour. ▪ Appropriate treatment for anaphylaxis must always be available. Risk increased if patient has received asparaginase before. ▪ Allopurinol, increased fluid intake and alkalinization of the urine may be required to reduce uric acid levels. ▪ Frequent blood counts, bone marrow evaluation, serum amylase, blood sugar, and evaluation of liver and kidney function are necessary. ▪ Nausea and vomiting can be severe. Prophylactic administration of antiemetics recommended to increase patient comfort. ▪ Predisposition to infection probable. Prophylactic antibiotics may be indicated pending results of C/S in a febrile neutropenic patient.

Patient education: Report all symptoms promptly; verbalize all questions. ▪ Assess birth control requirements. Nonhormonal contraception advised. ▪ See Appendix D, p. 900.

Maternal/child: Pregnancy category C: Will produce teratogenic effects on the fetus. Evaluation of benefit versus risk for anyone who is pregnant or may become pregnant. ▪ Discontinue breast feeding.

Elderly: Toxicity may be more severe. ▪ Consider age-related organ impairment.

DRUG/LAB INTERACTIONS

Toxicity of all agents may be increased if asparaginase is given before or concurrently with vincristine and prednisone. May be less pronounced if asparaginase is given 12 to 24 hours after vincristine and prednisone. ▪ Blocks the effects of methotrexate for as long as asparagine concentrations are suppressed. Some references suggest administering asparaginase 24 hours after methotrexate; others suggest these agents should not be used together while asparagine concentrations are suppressed. ▪ May interfere with thyroid function test interpretation. ▪ Do not administer any live vaccine to patients receiving antineoplastic drugs. ▪ Note Precautions.

SIDE EFFECTS

Occur frequently (usually within 30 minutes), even with the initial dose, and may cause death. Allergic reactions including anaphylaxis (even if skin test negative and/or allergic symptoms have not occurred with previous doses), agitation, azotemia, bleeding, bone marrow depression, coma, confusion, depression, fatigue, hallucinations, hyperglycemia, hyperthermia (fatal), pulmonary embolism or thrombosis from hypofibrinogenemia and depression of other clotting factors, nausea and vomiting, fulminating pancreatitis (fatal).

ANTIDOTE

Notify physician of all side effects. Asparaginase may have to be discontinued until recovery or permanently discontinued. Symptomatic and supportive treatment is indicated. Treat anaphylaxis with epinephrine, corticosteroids, oxygen, and antihistamines. There is no specific antidote.

ATENOLOL

Tenormin

Beta-Adrenergic blocking agent

pH 5.5 to 6.5

USUAL DOSE

5 mg. Initiate as soon as the patient's hemodynamic condition has stabilized and eligibility has been established. If initial dose well tolerated, repeat in 10 minutes. If full IV dose is well tolerated, give 50 mg orally 10 minutes after last bolus. Repeat in 12 hours. Follow with an oral maintenance dose of 100 mg daily or 50 mg twice a day for 6 to 9 days or until discharged from hospital. Discontinue if bradycardia or hypotension requiring treatment occurs. Best results achieved if administered within 2 to 4 hours of symptom onset or thrombolytic therapy.

Used concurrently with digitalis, alpha-adrenergic blockers (e.g., phentolamine [Regitine]), vasodilators (e.g., nitroglycerin), and clot-dissolving drugs (e.g., alteplase recombinant [tPA], anistreplase [Eminase]), as indicated.

DOSE ADJUSTMENTS

Use with caution and reduce dose by one half in patients with asthma or other bronchospastic disease. Isoproterenol (Isuprel) should be available. ■ Reduced dose may be indicated in patients already taking a beta blocker (e.g., propranolol [Inderal]). Titrate by clinical observations. ■ Reduce dose by one half in renal impairment with a creatinine clearance less than 35 ml/min (see literature).

DILUTION

May be given undiluted by direct IV or diluted in 10 to 50 ml D2½W, D5W, D10W, D5/0.45NS, D5/NS, or NS and given as an infusion.

Storage: Stable for 48 hours after dilution.

INCOMPATIBLE WITH

Any other drug in syringe or solution because of specific use.

COMPATIBLE WITH

May be compatible with meperidine (Demerol) or morphine at Y-site.

RATE OF ADMINISTRATION

Distribute a single dose evenly over 5 minutes. Monitor ECG, heart rate, and blood pressure and discontinue atenolol if adverse symptoms occur (bradycardia less than 45 beats/min, heart block greater than first degree, systolic blood pressure less than 90 mm Hg, or moderate to severe cardiac failure).

ACTIONS

Atenolol is a cardioselective (beta$_1$-) adrenergic blocking agent. Its mechanism of action in patients with suspected or definite myocardial infarction is not known. Reduces heart rate, cardiac output, blood pressure, and myocardial oxygen consumption. Promotes redistribution of blood flow from adequately supplied areas of the heart to ischemic areas. May also reduce chest pain. It reduces the incidence of recurrent myocardial infarctions (MI) and reduces the size of the infarct and the incidence of fatal arrhythmias. Inhibits isoproterenol-induced tachycardia and reduces reflex orthostatic tachycardia. Well distributed throughout the body, it acts within 1 to 2 minutes and lasts about 3 to 4 hours. Undergoes little or no metabolism by the liver. Excreted in urine. Secreted in breast milk.

INDICATIONS AND USES

Reduces cardiac mortality, recurrent MI, and incidence of ventricular fibrillation in hemodynamically stable individuals with suspected or definite MI. ▪ Reduces incidence of ventricular fibrillation in post MI patients who do not receive thrombolytic agents. ▪ Used within 2 to 4 hours of thrombolytic agents, may reduce rate of nonfatal reinfarction and recurrent ischemia; used within 2 hours of symptom onset, may reduce mortality and recurrent MI. ▪ Oral form also used to treat hypertension and angina pectoris.

CONTRAINDICATIONS

Sinus bradycardia, heart block greater than first degree, cardiogenic shock, overt cardiac failure.

PRECAUTIONS

Use caution in the presence of heart failure. ▪ Use caution in heart failure controlled by digitalis; both drugs slow AV conduction. ▪ Use caution in any patient with lung disease and/or bronchospasm. ▪ May mask tachycardia occurring with hypoglycemia in diabetes and tachycardia of hyperthyroidism. Abrupt withdrawal in patients with thyroid disease may precipitate a thyroid storm. ▪ Discontinuation of beta blockers prior to OR is controversial (beta blockade interferes with cardiac response to reflex stimuli and can cause severe hypotension and difficulty starting or maintaining a heartbeat during surgery); however, some authorities recommend administering throughout the perioperative period. May cause arrhythmia, angina, MI, or death if stopped abruptly. ▪ Reduce oral dose gradually to avoid rebound angina, MI, or ventricular dysrhythmias.

Monitor: Continuous ECG, heart rate, and blood pressure monitoring are mandatory during administration of IV atenolol. ▪ Note Drug/lab interactions.

Patient education: Report any breathing difficulty promptly.

Maternal/child: Use with caution and only when specifically indicated in pregnancy and lactation. ▪ May have to postpone breast feeding. ▪ Safety for use in children not established.

DRUG/LAB INTERACTIONS

Synergistic with digitalis; both drugs slow AV conduction. (See Precautions). ■ Beta-adrenergic blocking agents may be inhibited by nonsteroidal antiinflammatory agents, sympathomimetics (e.g., epinephrine, norepinephrine, isoproterenol [Isuprel], dopamine [Intropin], dobutamine [Dobutrex]), and ritodrine. ■ May potentiate catecholamine-depleting drugs (e.g., reserpine), lidocaine, prazosin (Minipress), disopyramide (Norpace), and verapamil (Isoptin). ■ Use with calcium channel blockers (e.g., diltiazem [Cardizem], verapamil [Isoptin]), may potentiate both drugs and result in severe depression of myocardium and AV conduction. ■ May cause severe hypotension and/or bradycardia with catecholamine-depleting drugs (e.g., reserpine); observe patient closely. ■ Use with clonidine may precipitate acute hypertension. May aggravate rebound hypertension if clonidine stopped abruptly; discontinue atenolol several days before gradual withdrawal of clonidine. ■ Some authorities recommend that beta-adrenergic blockers be discontinued 48 hours before major surgery (beta blockage interferes with cardiac response to reflex stimuli). If continued, use caution administering general anesthetics that depress the myocardium (e.g., cyclopropane, trichloroethylene). ■ May be potentiated by atropine.

SIDE EFFECTS

AV conduction delays, bradyarrhythmias, bronchospasm, cardiac arrest, cardiac failure, cold extremities, depression, diarrhea, dizziness, dreaming, drowsiness, dyspnea, fatigue, heart block, hypotension, lightheadedness, nausea, postural hypotension, pulmonary emboli, supraventricular tachycardia, ventricular tachycardia, vertigo, wheezing.

ANTIDOTE

For any side effect, discontinue the drug and notify the physician immediately. Physician may elect to continue atenolol at a reduced dose. Patients with MI may be more hemodynamically unstable; treat with caution. Bradycardia and hypotension may respond spontaneously after atenolol discontinued. If indicated, use atropine for bradycardia; use isoproterenol with caution if atropine is not effective. Glucagon, 5 to 10 mg IV, may be effective if atropine and isoproterenol are not (investigation use). Transvenous cardiac pacing may be needed. Treat hypotension with IV fluids if indicated or vasopressors (epinephrine rather than norepinephrine [levarterenol] or isoproterenol [Isuprel]; treat cause of hypotension (e.g., bradycardia). Use all vasopressors with extreme caution; severe hypotension can result. Use digitalis and diuretics at first signs of cardiac failure; dobutamine, isoproterenol, or glucagon may be required. Use aminophylline or isoproterenol with extreme care for bronchospasm. Use IV glucose for hypoglycemia. Treat other side effects symptomatically and resuscitate as necessary. Hemodialysis is effective in overdose.

ATRACURIUM BESYLATE

Neuromuscular
blocking agent
(Nondepolarizing)
Anesthesia Adjunct

Tracrium

pH 3.25 to 3.65

USUAL DOSE

Adjunct to general anesthesia for adults and children over 2 years of age:
Must be individualized, depending on previous drugs administered
and degree and length of muscle relaxation required. 0.4 to 0.5 mg/kg
of body weight initially as an IV bolus. Patient should be unconscious
before administration. Determine need for maintenance dose based on
beginning symptoms of neuromuscular blockade reversal determined
by a peripheral nerve stimulator. To maintain muscle relaxation a
maintenance dose may be given as a bolus injection of 0.08 to 0.10
mg/kg and is required in approximately 25 to 40 minutes and every
15 to 25 minutes. May alternately be given as a continuous IV infusion of 2 to 15 mcg/kg/min. Repeated doses have no cumulative
effect if recovery is allowed to begin prior to administration.

Adjunct to general anesthesia for infants and children 1 month to 2 years of age:
0.3 to 0.4 mg/kg for infants and children under halothane anesthesia.
See Usual dose for maintenance dose, may be required on a more frequent basis.

Support of intubated, mechanically ventilated or respiratory controlled adult ICU
patients (Investigational): An initial infusion rate of 11 to 13 mcg/kg/
min (range 4.5 to 29.5), provides adequate neuromuscular blockade.
Published reports describe a wide interpatient variability in dosing
requirements for maintenance ranging from 2.3 to 23 mcg/kg/min
(0.14 to 1.38 mg/kg/hr) in adult ICU patients. Occasional adult
patients have needed very high infusion rates (>60mcg/kg/min). In
Pediatric ICU patients maintenance doses ranged from 10 to 30 mcg/
kg/min (0.6 to 1.8 mg/kg/hr). A specific initial dose for pediatric
patients has not yet been defined.

In adults or children, adjust infusion rate according to clinical assessment of the patient's response. Use of a peripheral nerve stimulator is
recommended.

DOSE ADJUSTMENTS

Reduce dose by one third (0.25 to 0.35 mg/kg) if isoflurane or enflurane are used as general anesthetics. ■ Reduce dose to 0.3 to 0.4
mg/kg if using halothane anesthetic, in patients with a history of cardiovascular disease, or a history suggesting greater risk of histamine
release (allergies), or following succinylcholine administration. Succinylcholine must show signs of wearing off before atracurium is given.
Use caution. ■ Reduce maintenance dose by one-half where hypothermia is induced (e.g., cardiac bypass). ■ Note Drug/lab interactions.

DILUTION

Initial IV bolus may be given undiluted. Maintenance dose for anesthesia and mechanical ventilation support must be further diluted in
NS, D5W, or D5/NS and given as a continuous infusion titrated to

symptoms of neuromuscular blockade reversal. 20 mg (2 ml) diluted in 98 ml yields 200 mcg/ml (0.2 mg/ml). 50 mg (5 ml) diluted in 95 ml yields 500 mcg/ml (0.5 mg/ml).

Storage: Refrigerate. Diluted solution stable for 24 hours refrigerated or at room temperature.

INCOMPATIBLE WITH

Alkaline solutions, aminophylline, barbiturates, cefazolin (Kefzol), diazepam (Valium), heparin, procainamide (Pronestyl), quinidine, ranitidine (Zantac), Ringer's lactate, sodium nitroprusside (Nitropress). Do not mix in the same syringe or simultaneously through the same needle. A precipitate will form.

RATE OF ADMINISTRATION

Adjunct to general anesthesia: Initial IV bolus over 30 to 60 seconds.

Maintenance dose: In the 200 mcg/ml dilution, 5 mcg/kg/min will be delivered by a rate of 0.025 ml/kg/min or 1.75 ml/min for a 70-kg patient. Adjust rate to specific dose desired. Drug literature has additional rate calculations.

Mechanical ventilation support in ICU: See Usual dose for specific rates and criteria.

ACTIONS

A nondepolarizing skeletal muscle relaxant with duration of blockade one-third to one-half that of tubocurarine chloride (curare). A less potent histamine releaser than tubocurarine or metocurine. Causes paralysis by interfering with neural transmission at the myoneural junction. Onset of action is dose dependent. Produces maximum neuromuscular blockade within 3 to 5 minutes and lasts about 25 minutes. When infusion is discontinued, some recovery occurs within 30 minutes. Recovery to 75% averages 60 minutes (range 32 to 108 minutes). It may be several hours before complete recovery occurs. Excreted as metabolites in bile and urine. Crosses the placental barrier.

INDICATIONS AND USES

Adjunctive to general anesthesia to facilitate endotracheal intubation and to relax skeletal muscles during surgery or mechanical ventilation.

Investigational use: Support of intubated, mechanically ventilated or respiratory controlled patients in ICU.

CONTRAINDICATIONS

Known hypersensitivity to atracurium.

PRECAUTIONS

For IV use only. ▪ Administered by or under the observation of the anesthesiologist. ▪ Use extreme caution in patients with significant cardiovascular disease or a history of allergies or allergic reaction. ▪ Myasthenia gravis and other neuromuscular diseases increase sensitivity to drug. Can cause critical reactions. ▪ Respiratory depression with propofol (Diprivan) or morphine may be preferred in some patients requiring mechanical ventilation. ▪ Bradycardia fairly common since atracurium will not counteract the bradycardia produced by many anesthetic agents or vagal stimulation.

Monitor: This drug produces apnea. Controlled artificial ventilation with oxygen must be continuous and under direct observation at all times. Maintain a patent airway. ▪ Use a peripheral nerve stimulator to monitor response to atracurium and avoid overdose. ▪ Patient may be conscious and completely unable to communicate by any means. Has no analgesic properties. ■ Action potentiated by hypokalemia and some carcinomas. ■ Action is altered by dehydration, electrolyte imbalance, body temperature, and acid-base imbalance.

Maternal/child: Pregnancy category C: Use in pregnancy only if use justifies potential risk to fetus. has been used during cesarean section; monitor infant carefully. ■ Use caution during lactation. ■ Safety for use in infants under 1 month of age not established. ■ Contains benzyl alcohol; may cause "gasping syndrome" in premature infants.

Elderly: No adjustments identified.

DRUG/LAB INTERACTIONS

Potentiated by general anesthetics (e.g., enflurane, isoflurane, halothane), many antibiotics (e.g., lincosamides [clindamycin (Cleocin)], aminoglycosides [kanamycin (Kantrex), gentamicin (Garamycin)], polypeptides [bacitracin, colistimethate]), corticosteroids, diuretics, diazepam (Valium) and other muscle relaxants, magnesium sulfate, morphine, meperidine, procainamide (Pronestyl), quinidine, succinylcholine, verapamil, and others. May need to reduce dose of atracurium; use with caution. ■ Antagonized by acetylcholine, anticholinesterases, azathioprine, carbamazepine, phenytoin, and theophylline. ■ Succinylcholine must show signs of wearing off before atracurium is given. Use caution.

SIDE EFFECTS

Prolonged action resulting in respiratory insufficiency or apnea. Airway closure caused by relaxation of epiglottis, pharynx, and tongue muscles. Hypersensitivity reactions including anaphylaxis are possible. Bradycardia, bronchospasm, dyspnea, flushing, histamine release, hypotension, laryngospasm, reaction at injection site, shock, and tachycardia may occur. Rare reports of seizures with use of atracurium in ICU could be caused by other conditions or medications. Malignant hyperthermia is rare but may occur.

ANTIDOTE

All side effects are medical emergencies. Treat symptomatically. Controlled artificial ventilation must be continuous. Pyridostigmine (Mestinon) or neostigmine (Prostigmin) given with atropine will probably reverse the muscle relaxation. Not effective in all situations; may aggravate severe overdosage. Resuscitate as necessary.

ATROPINE SULFATE

Anticholinergic
Antiarrhythmic
Antidote

pH 3.5 to 6.5

USUAL DOSE

Bradyarrhythmias: 0.5- to 1-mg bolus repeated every 3 to 5 minutes up to a total dose of 2 mg can be used to achieve a desired pulse rate above 60. Subsequent doses of 0.5 to 1 mg may be given at 4- to 6-hour intervals. Doses under 0.5 mg may cause paradoxical slowing of heart rate.

Smooth muscle relaxation and suppression of secretions: 0.4 to 0.6 mg every 4 to 6 hours.

During surgery: Above doses appropriate except during cyclopropane anesthesia. Start with 0.4 mg or less. Administer very slowly to avoid ventricular arrhythmias.

Cardiac asystole: 1 mg bolus recommended in asystole with specific protocol. May be repeated in 3 to 5 minutes if asystole persists. Usual total dose does not exceed 2 to 2.5 mg within 2½ hours, but 0.4 mg/kg may be given only in cardiac asystole. Use caution; a total dose of 3 mg causes full vagal blockade.

Antidote to reverse muscarinic effects of anticholinesterase agents: 0.6 to 1.2 mg for each 0.5 to 2.5 mg of neostigmine or 10 to 20 mg of pyridostigmine administered. Administer in a separate syringe, concurrently or a few minutes before the anticholinesterase agent. If bradycardia present bring pulse up to 80 by giving IV atropine first. See neostigmine, pyridostigmine, or physostigmine monographs.

Antidote for acute poisoning from exposure to anticholinesterase compounds (e.g., organophosphate pesticides, nerve gases, and mushroom poisoning): 1 to 2 mg may be given in a single dose and repeated every 5 to 60 minutes. In severe poisoning 2 to 6 mg may be given and repeated at 5- to 60-minute intervals until muscarinic signs and symptoms subside and repeated if they appear. Up to 50 mg may be required in the first 24 hours. Use oral atropine for maintenance, withdraw gradually to avoid recurrence of symptoms (e.g., pulmonary edema). A cholinase reactivator (e.g., pralidoxime) is administered concomitantly except in carbamate exposure.

PEDIATRIC DOSE

Bradyarrhythmias: 0.01 to 0.03 mg/kg of body weight can be used to achieve a pulse rate above 80 in a distressed infant under 6 months or above 60 in a child. Minimum dose is 0.1 mg. Maximum single dose is 0.5 mg in a child, 1 mg for an adolescent. May be repeated in 5-minute intervals times 2. Maximum total dose for a child is 1 mg, for an adolescent 2 mg. When used for bradycardia or asystole in infants and small children, vagolytic doses are required. Smaller doses may cause paradoxical bradycardia.

Smooth muscle relaxation and suppression of secretions: 0.01 mg/kg. Minimum dose is 0.1 mg in the newborn; up to 0.4 mg for a 12-year-old. Usually given SC. May repeat every 4 to 6 hours.

Bronchospasm: 0.05 mg/kg in 2.5 ml NS every 6 to 8 hours. Minimum dose 0.25 mg; maximum dose is 1 mg.

Antidote to reverse muscarinic effects of anticholinesterase agents: 0.02 mg/kg of atropine concomitantly with 0.04 mg/kg of neostigmine. See adult dose for additional information.

Antidote for acute poisoning from exposure to anticholinesterase compounds (e.g., organophosphate compounds, nerve gases, mushroom poisoning): 0.05 mg/kg, repeated every 10 to 30 minutes until muscarinic signs and symptoms subside and repeated if they appear. See adult dose for additional information.

DOSE ADJUSTMENTS

May be indicated in the elderly. ■ Note Drug/lab interactions and Pediatric dose.

DILUTION

May be given undiluted, but may prefer to dilute desired dose in at least 10 ml or sterile water for injection. Do not add to IV solutions. Inject through Y-tube or three-way stopcock of infusion set. Also available in combination with edrophonium (Enlon-Plus) to reverse cholinesterase toxicity caused by reversal of nondepolarizing muscle relaxants.

INCOMPATIBLE WITH

Amobarbital (Amytal), ampicillin (Omnipen), chloramphenicol (chloromycetin), chlortetracycline (Aureomycin), cimetidine (Tagamet), epinephrine (Adrenalin), heparin, isoproterenol (Isuprel), metaraminol (Aramine), methicillin (Staphcillin), methohexital (Brevital), norepinephrine (Levophed), pentobarbital (Nembutal), promazine (sparine), sodium bicarbonate, sodium iodide, thiopental (Pentothal), warfarin (Coumadin).

RATE OF ADMINISTRATION

1 mg or fraction thereof over 1 minute.

ACTIONS

Atropine is an anticholinergic drug and a potent belladonna alkaloid. It produces local, central, and peripheral effects on the body. The main therapeutic uses of atropine are peripheral, affecting smooth muscle, cardiac muscle, and gland cells. Reverses cholinergic mediated decreases in heart rate, systemic vascular resistance, and blood pressure. This drug can interfere with vagal stimuli. It is widely distributed in all body fluids. Metabolized by the liver and excreted in urine and bile. Crosses placental barrier. Secreted in breast milk.

INDICATIONS AND USES

Treatment of symptomatic sinus bradycardia, syncope from Stokes-Adams syndrome, and high-degree atrioventricular block with profound bradycardia. ■ Cardiac asystole. ■ Suppression of salivary, gastric, pancreatic, and respiratory secretions. ■ To relieve pylorospasm, hypertonicity of the small intestine, and hypermotility of the colon. ■ To relieve biliary and ureteral colic. ■ Antidote to reverse cholinesterase toxicity (muscarinic effects) caused by reversal of nondepolarizing muscle relaxants by neostigmine, physostigmine, and pyridostigmine. ■ Antidote for specific poisons such as organophosphorus insecticides, nerve gases and mushroom poisoning (*Amanita muscaria*). ■ Used in combination with many other drugs to produce a desired effect (e.g., edrophonium [Enlon, Enlon-Plus]).

CONTRAINDICATIONS

Hypersensitivity to atropine, acute glaucoma, acute hemorrhage with unstable cardiovascular status, asthma, hepatic disease, intestinal atony of the elderly or debilitated, myasthenia gravis, myocardial ischemia, obstructive disease of the GI or GU tracts, paralytic ileus, pyloric stenosis, renal disease, severe ulcerative colitis, tachycardia, toxic megacolon.

PRECAUTIONS

Use caution in prostatic hypertrophy, chronic lung disease, infants and small children, the elderly and debilitated, in urinary retention, during cyclopropane anesthesia, and in myocardial ischemia or infarction. ■ Increases myocardial oxygen demand and can trigger tachyarrhythmias. ■ Doses less than 0.5 mg may further slow heart rate. ■ May be given endotracheally. ▪ Considered possibly harmful in AV block at the His-Purkinje level or with newly appearing wide QRS complexes.

Monitor: Vital signs and/or ECG based on specific situation.

Patient education: Use caution if task requires alertness; may cause blurred vision, dizziness, or drowsiness. ▪ Report eye pain, flushing, or skin rash promptly. ▪ Report dry mouth, difficulty urinating, constipation, or increased light sensitivity.

Maternal/child: Pregnancy category C: Safety for use in pregnancy, lactation, and children not established. ▪ Toxicity to nursing infants probable.

Elderly: May produce excitement, agitation, confusion or drowsiness. ▪ May precipitate undiagnosed glaucoma. ▪ Potential for constipation and urinary retention increased. ▪ Has potential to increase memory impairment. ▪ Note Dose adjustments and Precautions.

DRUG/LAB INTERACTIONS

Potentiated by amantadine, tricyclic antidepressants (e.g., amitriptyline [Elavil]). Reduce dose of atropine. ▪ Effects of atropine and phenothiazines (e.g., prochlorperazine [Compazine]) will both be potentiated if given concomitantly. Reduce dose of both. ▪ Potentiates effects of many oral drugs by delaying gastric emptying and increasing rate of absorption (e.g., atenolol, digoxin, nitrofurantoin, thiazide diuretics). ▪ Antagonistic to many drugs (e.g., edrophonium [Tensilon], pyridostigmine [Mestinon]).

SIDE EFFECTS

Average dose: Anhidrosis, anticholinergic psychosis, blurred vision, bradycardia (temporary), constipation, dilation of the pupils, dryness of the mouth, flushing, gastroesophageal reflux, heat prostration from decreased sweating, nausea, paralytic ileus, postural hypotension, tachyarrhythmias, urinary hesitancy and retention (especially in males), and vomiting may occur.

Overdose: Coma, death, delirium, elevated blood pressure, fever, paralytic ileus, rash, respiratory failure, stupor, tachycardia.

ANTIDOTE

Discontinue if side effects increase or are severe. Notify physician. Use standard treatments to manage cardiac arrhythmias. Physostigmine salicylate (Antilirium) reverses most cardiovascular and CNS effects; however, it may cause profound bradycardia, seizures, or asystole. Administer pilocarpine, 10 mg (SC), until the mouth is moist. Sustain physiologic functions at a normal level. Use diazepam (Valium), short-acting barbiturates (amobarbital), or chloral hydrate to relieve excitement. Neostigmine methylsulfate (Prostigmin) is an alternate antidote.

AZATHIOPRINE SODIUM

Immunosuppressant

Imuran

pH 9.6

USUAL DOSE

3 to 5 mg/kg of body weight/24 hr. Begin treatment within 24 hours of renal homotransplantation. Some authorities recommend doses of 1 to 5 mg/kg for several days previous to transplant. Maintenance dose is 1 to 2 mg/kg/24 hr. Individualized adjustment is imperative and may be required on a daily basis.

DOSE ADJUSTMENTS

Reduce dose in impaired kidney function (especially immediately after transplant or with cadaveric kidneys) and in persistent negative nitrogen balance. ■ Note Drug/lab interactions and Precautions/Monitor.

DILUTION

Specific techniques suggested; see Precautions. Each 100 mg should be initially reconstituted with 10 ml of SW. Swirl the vial gently until completely in solution. May be further diluted in a minimum of 50 ml of NS, D5W, or D5/NS and given as an infusion. Note Incompatible with. Use within 24 hours.

INCOMPATIBLE WITH

Preservatives (e.g., methyl and propyl parabens, phenol). Administer separately. Converts to 6-mercaptopurine in alkaline solutions and sulfhydryl compounds (e.g., cysteine).

RATE OF ADMINISTRATION

A single dose properly diluted over 30 to 60 minutes. Actual range may be 5 minutes to 8 hours.

ACTIONS

An immunosuppressive drug. It is a derivative of the antineoplastic preparation mercaptopurine. Maximum response occurs if administered when antibody response begins. Has a selective action but achieves good response in many situations. Metabolized readily with small amounts excreted in the urine.

INDICATIONS AND USES

Adjunct to prevent rejection in renal homotransplantation.

CONTRAINDICATIONS

Anuria, known hypersensitivity, severe rejection.

PRECAUTIONS

■ Follow guidelines for handling cytotoxic agents. See Appendix A, p. 893. Oral route preferred; begin as soon as feasible. ■ May increase possibility of malignant tumor growth. ■ Use caution with other myelosuppressive drugs or radiation therapy. ■ Toxic hepatitis or biliary status may necessitate discontinuing drug.

Monitor: Monitor platelet count, RBC, WBC, and BUN frequently. Drug should be withdrawn or dose reduced at first sign of abnormally large fall in the leukocyte count or other evidence of persistent bone marrow depression. ■ Observe constantly for signs of infection. Prophylactic antibiotics may be indicated pending results of C/S in a febrile neutropenic patient.

Patient education: Avoid pregnancy ■ See Appendix D, p. 900.

Maternal/child: Pregnancy category D: Avoid pregnancy. Can cause fetal harm. ▪ Discontinue breast feeding.

DRUG/LAB INTERACTIONS

Potentiated by allopurinol (Zyloprim). Reduce dose to one third or one fourth of usual. ▪ Inhibits nondepolarizing muscle relaxants (e.g., tubocurarine), cyclosporine (Sandimmune), and anticoagulants (e.g., heparin). ▪ Concurrent use with ACE inhibitors (e.g., captopril [Capoten]) may induce leukemia. ▪ Plasma levels of the metabolite 6-MP may be increased by methotrexate. ▪ Avoid vaccinations and do not use live vaccines in patients receiving azathioprine.

SIDE EFFECTS

Alopecia, anemia, anorexia, arthralgia, bleeding, diarrhea, fever, jaundice, leukopenia, nausea, oral lesions, pancreatitis, skin rash, thrombocytopenia, vomiting.

ANTIDOTE

Notify the physician of all side effects. Most can be treated symptomatically. Drug may be decreased or discontinued or other immunosuppressive agents utilized. Hematopoietic depression may require temporary or permanent withholding of treatment.

AZITHROMYCIN

Antibacterial
(Azalide/macrolide)

Zithromax

USUAL DOSE

Community acquired pneumonia: 500 mg as a single daily dose for a minimum of 2 days. Follow with 500 mg of oral azithromycin as a single daily dose. Total course of therapy (IV + oral) should be 7 to 10 days.

Pelvic inflammatory disease: 500 mg as a single daily dose for 1 to 2 days. Follow with 250 mg of oral azithromycin as a single daily dose. Total course of therapy (IV + oral) should be 7 days. If anaerobic microorganisms are also suspected, concurrent administration of an antibacterial agent with anaerobic activity is recommended (e.g., metronidazole [Flagyl]).

PEDIATRIC DOSE

Safety and effectiveness for children under 16 years of age not established; (See Maternal/child).

DOSE ADJUSTMENTS

Reduced dose may be required in impaired liver or renal function (note Precautions). ▪ Note Drug/lab interactions.

DILUTION

Each 500-mg vial must be reconstituted with 4.8 ml SW. Shake well to ensure dilution (100 mg/ml). Further dilute each 500 mg of reconstituted solution with 250 to 500 ml of one of the following solutions: D5, NS, 0.45%NS, D5/0.3%NS, D5/0.45%NS, D5/0.45%NS with 20 mEq KCL, LR, D5/LR, D5/Normosol M, D5/Normosol R. 500 ml diluent yields 1 mg/ml, 250 ml yields 2 mg/ml. Concentrations greater than 2 mg/ml have caused local IV site reactions and should be avoided.

Storage: Reconstituted or diluted solution stable at controlled room temperature for 24 hours. Diluted solution stable for up to 7 days if refrigerated.

INCOMPATIBLE WITH

Specific information not available.

RATE OF ADMINISTRATION

1 mg/ml dilution: A single dose equally distributed over a minimum of 1 hour; over 3 hours is preferred.

2 mg/ml dilution: A single dose equally distributed over at least 1 hour.

ACTIONS

An azalide (subclass of macrolide) antibiotic. Bactericidal and bacteriostatic to selected organisms, including aerobic gram-positive and gram-negative organisms, *Chlamydia*, and *Mycoplasma pneumoniae*. It is derived from erythromycin but is chemically different. Interferes with microbial protein synthesis by binding to a ribosomal subunit of a susceptible microorganism. Concentration in phagocytes and fibroblasts may contribute to distribution in inflamed tissues. Activity not affected by beta-lactamase production. Compared to oral dosing, IV route plasma concentrations are consistently higher throughout a 24-hour interval. Trough levels increase with successive doses. Has a long tissue half-life permitting once-a-day dosing. Metabolized in the liver. Primarily excreted as unchanged drug in bile. Up to 14% excreted in urine within 24 hours.

INDICATIONS AND USES

Treatment of community acquired pneumonia and pelvic inflammatory disease caused by specific organisms (e.g., *Staphylococcus aureus, Streptococcus pneumoniae, Haemophilus influenzae, Neisseria gonorrhoeae, Chlamydia trachomatis.* See product insert for complete list). Many other indications for oral use.

CONTRAINDICATIONS

Known hypersensitivity to azithromycin, erythromycin, or any macrolide antibiotic.

PRECAUTIONS

Specific sensitivity studies are indicated to determine susceptibility of the causative organism to azithromycin. ▪ Has demonstrated cross-resistance with erythromycin-resistant gram-positive organisms. Most strains of *Enterococcus faecalis* and methicillin-resistant staphylococci are resistant to azithromycin. ▪ Use extreme caution; allergic symptoms have recurred even after azithromycin was discontinued and allergic symptoms treated. Anaphylaxis resulting in fatalities has been reported rarely. ▪ Principally eliminated in the liver; use caution in patients with impaired hepatic function. ▪ Use caution in patients with impaired renal function; no data available on effects of IV azithromycin. ▪ Use caution in patients with prolonged QT intervals; other macrolide antibiotics have caused ventricular arrhythmias, including ventricular tachycardia and torsades de pointes. One patient suffered an MI. ▪ Timing of transfer to oral therapy should be based on clinical response. ▪ Avoid prolonged use; superinfection caused by overgrowth of nonsusceptible organisms may result. ▪ Pseudomembranous colitis has been reported. ▪ May cause photosensitivity.

Monitor: Monitor vital signs. ▪ Observe closely for signs of allergic reaction. ▪ Monitoring of liver function may be indicated. ▪ Monitor infusion site for inflammation and/or extravasation. ▪ Note Drug/lab interactions and Antidote.

Patient education: Discontinue azithromycin and report any signs of an allergic reaction immediately (difficulty breathing, itching, rash, swelling). ▪ Oral azithromycin should be taken 1 hour before or 2 hours after a meal, should not be taken with food. ▪ Do not take antacids containing aluminum or magnesium simultaneously with oral azithromycin.

Maternal/child: Pregnancy category B: Safety for use during pregnancy and lactation not established; use with caution and only if clearly needed. ▪ Has been administered to pediatric patients age 6 months to 16 years by the oral route.

Elderly: Specific information not available. Consider age-related organ impairment.

DRUG/LAB INTERACTIONS

Other macrolide antibiotics cause interactions when given concomitantly with the following drugs; azithromycin has not been studied. May increase serum concentrations of theophylline; monitoring of theophylline levels indicated. ▪ May increase anticoagulant effects of warfarin (Coumadin); monitoring of PT indicated. ▪ May increase digoxin levels; monitoring of digoxin levels indicated. ▪ May cause acute ergot toxicity (severe peripheral vasospasm and dysesthesia) with ergotamine or dihydroergotamine. ▪ May inhibit metabolism and increase serum levels and effects of triazolam (Halcion) and drugs metabolized by the cytochrome P_{450} system (e.g., carbamazepine (Tegretol), cimetidine (Tagamet), cyclosporine (Sandimmune), phenytoin (Dilantin), terfenadine (Seldane); reduced doses of these drugs may be indicated.

SIDE EFFECTS

Usually mild to moderate in severity and reversible after azithromycin discontinued. Abdominal pain, anorexia, diarrhea; dizziness, dyspnea; increase in AST (SGOT), ALT (SGPT), and/or alkaline phosphatase levels; injection site pain or local inflammation, nausea, rashes, stomatitis, vaginitis, vomiting. Acute interstitial nephritis (fever, joint pain, skin rash) is rare but may cause acute renal failure. Allergic reactions (e.g., angioedema, anaphylaxis, and dermatologic reactions including Stevens-Johnson syndrome and toxic epidermal necrolysis) have been reported rarely and may be fatal; note Precautions. Pseudomembranous colitis has been reported.

ANTIDOTE

Notify physician of any side effects. Discontinue azithromycin for allergic reaction. Treat allergic reaction as indicated and resuscitate as necessary. Additional allergic symptoms have recurred after azithromycin has been discontinued and initial allergic treatment completed. Prolonged observation is required. Mild cases of colitis may respond to discontinuation of azithromycin. Fluids, electrolytes, and protein supplements may be indicated. Oral vancomycin (Vancocin) or metronidazole (Flagyl) is the treatment of choice for antibiotic-related pseudomembranous colitis.

AZTREONAM

Antibacterial
(monobactam)

Azactam

pH 4.5 to 7.5

USUAL DOSE

Range is from 500 mg to 2 Gm every 6, 8, or 12 hours. Dosage based on severity of infection. Use the full suggested dose. Do not exceed 8 Gm/24 hr. Normal renal function required. Continue for at least 2 days after all symptoms of infection subside. Can produce therapeutic serum levels given intraperitoneally in dialysis fluid.

PEDIATRIC DOSE

90 to 120 mg/kg/24 hr. Give in equally divided doses every 6 to 8 hours. Maximum dose 8 Gm/24 hr.

Cystic fibrosis: 50 mg/kg every 6 to 8 hours. Maximum dose 8 Gm/24 hr.

Neonatal dose: 30 mg/kg/dose. Give every 12 hours if *less than 1,200 Gm and 0 to 4 weeks of age* or *less than 2,000 Gm and 0 to 7 days of age.* Give every 8 hours if *1,200 to 2,000 Gm and over 7 days of age* or *over 2,000 Gm and 0 to 7 days of age.* Give every 6 hours if *over 2,000 Gm and 7 days of age.*

DOSE ADJUSTMENTS

Reduce total daily dose in the elderly and if renal function impaired. Calculated according to degree of impairment (see literature).

DILUTION

Usually light yellow, may become slightly pink on standing; does not affect potency.

Direct IV: Reconstitute a single dose with 6 to 10 ml of sterile water for injection. Shake immediately and vigorously. Use immediately and discard any unused solution.

Intermittent IV: Initially reconstitute each single dose with a minimum of 3 ml of sterile water for injection. Shake immediately and vigorously. Must be further diluted in at least 50 ml of D5W, NS, or other compatible infusion solutions for each 1 Gm of aztreonam (see chart on back cover or literature). Concentration should not exceed 20 mg/ml. Available in 15-ml vials and 100-ml infusion bottles.

Storage: Stable for 48 hours at room temperature or up to 7 days if refrigerated. When specific diluents are used, may be frozen for up to 3 months. Thaw at room temperature (see literature); do not refreeze.

INCOMPATIBLE WITH

Ampicillin, cefoxitin (Mefoxin), cephradine (Velosef), metronidazole (Flagyl IV), nafcillin, vancomycin (Vancocin).

COMPATIBLE WITH

Compatible and stable for 48 hours with Ampicillin, cefoxitin (Mefoxin), cephradine (Velosef), metronidazole (Flagyl IV), nafcillin, vancomycin (Vancocin), clindamycin, gentamicin, tobramycin, or cefazolin in normal saline or 5% dextrose in water. Compatible and stable for 24 hours with ampicillin in normal saline or for 2 hours in 5%

dextrose in water. Mixing of these drugs is not suggested by manufacturers of the other drugs at this time.

RATE OF ADMINISTRATION

Direct IV: A single dose equally distributed over 3 to 5 minutes.

Intermittent IV: A single dose over 20 to 60 minutes. May be given through Y-tube or three-way stopcock of infusion set. Do not infuse simultaneously with other drugs or solutions except in proven compatibility. Flush common IV tubing before and after administration.

ACTIONS

A synthetic monobactam antibiotic. Bactericidal through inhibition of bacterial cell wall synthesis to a wide spectrum of specific gram-negative aerobic organisms including *Pseudomonas aeruginosa*. Effective against many otherwise resistant organisms. Therapeutic levels widely distributed into many body fluids and tissues. Primarily excreted in the urine with some excretion through feces. Crosses placental barrier. Secreted in breast milk.

INDICATIONS AND USES

Treatment of serious lower respiratory tract, urinary tract, skin and skin structure, gynecologic, and intraabdominal infections and bacterial septicemia. Most effective against specific organisms (see literature). ▪ Adjunctive therapy to surgery for the management of infections.

CONTRAINDICATIONS

Known hypersensitivity to aztreonam.

PRECAUTIONS

Specific studies are indicated to identify the causative organism and susceptibility to aztreonam. ▪ Avoid prolonged use of drug; superinfection caused by overgrowth of nonsusceptible organisms may result.

Monitor: Watch for early symptoms of allergic reaction. Use extreme caution in the penicillin-sensitive patient. ▪ Monitor renal and hepatic function, especially in the elderly. ▪ May cause thrombophlebitis. Use small needles, large veins, and rotate infusion sites.

Maternal/child: Pregnancy category B: Use only if clearly needed in pregnancy and lactation. ▪ Consider discontinuation of breast feeding. ▪ Safety for use in infants and children not established.

DRUG/LAB INTERACTIONS

Adverse interaction may occur with beta-lactamase-inducing antibiotics (e.g., cefoxitin, imipenem); do not use concurrently. ▪ May be used concomitantly with aminoglycosides in severe infections. Nephrotoxicity and ototoxicity can be markedly increased when both drugs utilized. ▪ Probenecid and furosemide do increase blood levels; not clinically significant. ▪ Note Side effects.

SIDE EFFECTS

Full scope of allergic reactions including anaphylaxis. Burning, discomfort, and pain at injection site; diarrhea; nausea and vomiting; pseudomembranous colitis; and rash occur most frequently. Abdominal cramps, altered taste, confusion, diaphoresis, diplopia, dizziness, dyspnea, elevated alkaline phosphatase, AST (SGOT), ALT (SGPT), and serum creatinine, eosinophilia, erythema multiforme, exfoliative dermatitis, fever, halitosis, headache, hematologic changes, hepatitis, hypotension, insomnia, jaundice, mouth ulcer, nasal congestion, numb tongue, paresthesia, petechiae, positive Coombs' test, prolonged pro-thrombin time (PT) and PTT, pruritus, purpura, transient ECG changes (ventricular bigeminy and PVCs), seizures, sneezing, tinnitus, urticaria, vaginitis, vertigo can occur.

ANTIDOTE

Notify physician of any side effects. Discontinue the drug if indicated. Treat allergic reaction as indicated and resuscitate as necessary. Mild causes of colitis may respond to discontinuation of drug. Oral vanco-mycin is the treatment of choice for antibiotic-related pseudomembra-nous colitis. Hemodialysis or peritoneal dialysis may be useful in overdose.

BENZTROPINE MESYLATE

Cogentin

Antidyskinetic
Antiparkinson
Anticholinergic

pH 5.0 to 8.0

USUAL DOSE

1 to 2 mg. May be increased gradually to 4 to 6 mg/24 hr if required.

DOSE ADJUSTMENTS

Required if an inability to move particular muscle groups persists.
■ Use lower dose range in the elderly or debilitated.

DILUTION

1 ml of prepared solution equals 1 mg. May be given undiluted.

INCOMPATIBLE WITH

No specific incompatibilities are known.

RATE OF ADMINISTRATION

1 mg or fraction thereof over 1 minute.

ACTIONS

Anticholinergic and antihistaminic agent. Effectively relieves tremor, rigidity, drooling, dysphagia, gait disturbances, pain caused by muscle spasm, and other annoying symptoms of parkinsonism. Provides excellent relief in combination with levodopa. Onset of action is prompt by IV or IM route. Primarily excreted in the urine.

INDICATIONS AND USES

Parkinsonism: drug-induced (especially phenothiazines and reserpine), postencephalitic, idiopathic, or arteriosclerotic.

CONTRAINDICATIONS

Known hypersensitivity in children under 3 years. Ineffective in tardive dyskinesia.

PRECAUTIONS

IV route seldom used except in acute drug reactions or psychotic patients; IM and oral routes are satisfactory. ■ Treatment of drug-induced parkinsonism can precipitate toxic psychosis. ■ Do not dis-continue other antiparkinsonian drugs abruptly; reduce gradually.

Monitor: Has a potent cumulative action; the patient must be under close observation. ■ Observe carefully in patients with hypotension, narrow-angle glaucoma, myasthenia gravis, tachycardia, prostatic hypertrophy, urinary retention, intestinal obstruction, and in the elderly.

Maternal/child: Pregnancy category C: Safety for use in pregnancy, and lactation not established. ■ Has been used in children over 3 years of age with caution. ■ May inhibit lactation.

Elderly: Note Dose adjustments and Precautions. ■ May produce agitation, confusion, disorientation, hallucinations, or psychotic-like symptoms. ■ Has potential to increase memory impairment. ■ Chronic use may precipitate glaucoma.

DRUG/LAB INTERACTIONS

Side effects may be potentiated by alcohol, antihistamines, barbiturates, narcotic analgesics, phenothiazines, quinidine, and tricyclic antidepressants. ■ May reduce amount of levodopa absorbed in the GI tract. ■ Inhibits haloperidol and phenothiazines. ■ May potentiate oral digoxin.

SIDE EFFECTS

Average dose: Allergic reactions including skin rash, blurred vision, constipation, depression, dizziness, dry mouth, listlessness, nausea, nervousness, numbness of the fingers, vomiting.

Overdose: Anhidrosis, circulatory collapse, coma, dilation of the pupils, dry mucous membranes, flushed skin, hyperpyrexia, incipient glaucoma, paralytic ileus, respiratory depression, tachycardia, urinary retention.

ANTIDOTE

Notify the physician of all side effects. Symptoms of an average dose may be relieved by reducing the dose or discontinuing for a day or so and then resuming at a lesser dose. Treat overdose symptomatically, including respiratory support. Physostigmine salicylate (Antilirium) will reverse symptoms of anticholinergic intoxication. Observe for relapses up to 12 hours. Diazepam (Valium) reduces CNS excitation. Resuscitate as necessary.

BLEOMYCIN SULFATE

Antineoplastic (Antibiotic)

Blenoxane

pH 4.5 to 6.0

USUAL DOSE

0.25 to 0.5 unit/kg of body weight/24 hr (10 to 20 units/M^2), once or twice weekly. The first 2 doses in lymphoma patients should not exceed 2 units in order to rule out hypersensitivity.

Hodgkin's disease: Dosage as above. After a 50% response, a maintenance dose of 1 unit/daily or 5 units weekly is recommended.

DOSE ADJUSTMENTS

Unit/kg dose based on average weight in presence of edema or ascites. ■ Reduce dose in impaired renal function. Based on creatinine clearance, see literature.

DILUTION

Specific techniques required; see Precautions. Each 15 units or fraction thereof must be reconstituted with 5 ml or more of sterile water for injection, 5% dextrose, or sodium chloride for injection. Further dilution with 50 to 100 ml of same solution is recommended. May be given through Y-tube or three-way stopcock of a free-flowing IV.

Storage: Refrigerate powder. Diluted solution stable at room temperature for 24 hours.

INCOMPATIBLE WITH

Amino acids, aminophylline, ascorbic acid, cefazolin (Kefzol), cephalothin (Keflin), diazepam (Valium), furosemide (Lasix), hydrocortisone sodium succinate (Solu-Cortef), methotrexate (Folex), mitomycin (MTC), nafcillin (Unipen), penicillin G sodium, riboflavin, and sulfhydryl groups (e.g., cysteine), terbutaline (Brethine). Consider toxicity and specific use.

RATE OF ADMINISTRATION

Each 15 units or fraction thereof over 10 minutes.

ACTIONS

An antibiotic antineoplastic agent, cell cycle phase specific, that seems to act by splitting and fragmentation of double-stranded DNA, leading to chromosomal damage. It localizes in tumors. Improvement usually noted within 2 weeks. Well distributed in skin, lungs, kidneys, peritoneum, and lymphatics. About 60% to 70% excreted in urine.

INDICATIONS AND USES

Testicular carcinoma; may induce complete remission with vinblastine and cisplatin. ■ Palliative treatment, adjunct to surgery or radiation, in patients not responsive to other chemotherapeutic agents or those with squamous cell carcinoma of the skin, head, esophagus, neck, or GU tract, including the cervix, vulva, scrotum, and penis; in Hodgkin's disease and other lymphomas. ■ Injected into pleural cavity to treat malignant pleural effusion.

CONTRAINDICATIONS

Known hypersensitivity to bleomycin, elderly patients with pulmonary disease.

PRECAUTIONS

■ Follow guidelines for handling cytotoxic agents. See Appendix A, p. 893. ■ Administered by or under the direction of the physician specialist. ■ May be used with other antineoplastic drugs to achieve tumor remission. ■ May cause severe anaphylaxis with lymphomas; use a test dose.

Monitor: Obtain a baseline chest x-ray, and recheck every 1 to 2 weeks to detect pulmonary changes. ■ Monitor renal, hepatic, and central nervous systems and skin for symptoms of toxicity. ■ Determine patency of vein; avoid extravasation. ■ Pulmonary toxicity increases markedly with advancing age, larger doses, or in smokers; may occur at lower doses when bleomycin is used in combination with other antineoplastic agents. To identify subclinical pulmonary toxicity, monitor pulmonary diffusion capacity for carbon monoxide monthly. Should remain 30% to 35% above pretreatment value. Most toxic when total cumulative dose exceeds 350 to 450 units. ■ Maintain adequate hydration. ■ Prophylactic antiemetics may reduce nausea and vomiting and increase patient comfort. ■ Observe closely for all

signs of infection. Prophylactic antibiotics may be indicated pending results of C/S in a febrile neutropenic patient. ▪ Acetaminophen, diphenhydramine (Benadryl) and steroids (e.g., hydrocortisone) may be used prophylactically to reduce incidence of fever and anaphylaxis. *Patient education:* Use nonhormonal contraception. ▪ Report any possible side effects promptly. ▪ Report stinging or burning at IV site promptly. ▪ See Appendix D, p. 900. ▪ Pulmonary toxicity more likely in smokers.
Maternal/child: Avoid pregnancy. ▪ Not recommended during lactation.
Elderly: Increased risk of pulmonary toxicity. ▪ Consider age-related renal impairment.

DRUG/LAB INTERACTIONS

Note Precautions. ▪ Vascular toxicities (e.g., myocardial infarction, CVA, thrombotic microangiopathy, cerebral arteritis) or Raynaud's phenomenon have occurred rarely when bleomycin is used in combination with other antineoplastic agents. ▪ May decrease GI absorption of digoxin and hydantoins (e.g., phenytoin). ▪ Do not administer live vaccines to patients receiving antineoplastic drugs. ▪ Causes sensitization of lung tissue to O_2; increases risk of pulmonary toxicity with O_2 and general anesthetics. ▪ Cisplatin may inhibit renal elimination and increase toxicity.

SIDE EFFECTS

Minor: Alopecia, anorexia, chills, dyspnea, fever, hypotension, nausea, phlebitis (infrequent), rales, tenderness of the skin, tumor site pain, vomiting, weight loss.
Major: Anaphylaxis (up to 6 hours after test dose), chest pain (acute with sudden onset suggestive of pleuropericarditis), pneumonitis, pulmonary fibrosis, skin toxicity (including nodules on hands, desquamation of skin, hyperpigmentation, and gangrene).

ANTIDOTE

Notify the physician of all side effects. Minor side effects will be treated symptomatically. Discontinue the drug immediately and notify the physician of any symptom of major side effects. Provide immediate treatment (epinephrine [Adrenalin] and diphenhydramine [Benadryl] for anaphylaxis, antibiotics and steroids for pneumonitis) or supportive therapy as indicated.

BRETYLIUM TOSYLATE

Antiarrhythmic

♣Bretylate, Bretylium tosylate PF

pH 4.5 to 7.0

USUAL DOSE

Life-threatening ventricular arrhythmias: 5 mg/kg of body weight. Defibrillate. If ventricular arrhythmia persists, increase to 10 mg/kg and repeat every 5 to 30 minutes as necessary. Maximum total dose is 35 mg/kg.

Other ventricular arrhythmias: 5 to 10 mg/kg by IV infusion. Repeat in 1 to 2 hours if arrhythmia persists.

Maintenance dose: 5 to 10 mg/kg by intermittent infusion every 6 hours or a continuous infusion at 1 to 2 mg/min. Replace with oral antiarrhythmic therapy as soon as practical, usually within 24 hours. Reduce dose under ECG monitoring.

PEDIATRIC DOSE

Same as adult doses except total dose should not exceed 30 mg/kg.

DOSE ADJUSTMENTS

May be required in impaired renal function.

DILUTION

May be given undiluted in ventricular fibrillation. For other ventricular arrhythmias each dose must be diluted with 50 ml or more of D5W or NS to be given as an intermittent infusion. Larger amounts may be further diluted in any amount of the above solutions and given as a continuous infusion (1 Gm in 1,000 ml equals 1 mg/ml). 1 Gm in 250 ml (4 mg/ml) may be used to deliver bolus doses. Available premixed as 500 or 1,000 mg in 250 ml D5W.

INCOMPATIBLE WITH

Dobutamine (Dobutrex), phenytoin (Dilantin).

COMPATIBLE WITH

Is physically compatible with Dobutamine (Dobutrex), phenytoin (Dilantin), calcium chloride, dopamine, lidocaine, nitroglycerin, potassium chloride, procainamide, and verapamil; however, therapeutic rates of administration may differ.

RATE OF ADMINISTRATION

Life-threatening ventricular arrhythmias: A single dose over 1 minute.

Intermittent infusion: A single dose over a minimum of 8 to 10 minutes. More rapid infusion may cause nausea and vomiting.

Continuous infusion: 1 to 2 mg diluted solution/min. Use an infusion pump or microdrip (60 gtt/ml). Adjust as indicated by progress in patient's condition.

ACTIONS

A quaternary ammonium compound with antiarrhythmic effects. It increases the ventricular fibrillation threshold, suppresses ventricular arrhythmias and aberrant impulses, and increases the refractory period without increasing heart rate. Probably effective through its adrenergic blocking action. Antifibrillatory effects occur within minutes; suppression of ventricular tachycardia and other ventricular arrhythmias develop over 15 to 20 minutes. Suppression of premature beats requires constant plasma levels. Half-life ranges from 4 to 17 hours. Excreted in the urine.

INDICATIONS AND USES

Prophylaxis and treatment of ventricular fibrillation and treatment of life-threatening ventricular arrhythmias. Not a first-line antiarrhythmic agent. Recommended when defibrillation, epinephrine, and lidocaine have failed to convert VF, when VF has recurred despite epinephrine and lidocaine, when lidocaine and procainamide have not controlled VT associated with a pulse, or when lidocaine and adenosine have not controlled wide-complex tachycardias.

CONTRAINDICATIONS

None when used as indicated.

PRECAUTIONS

May cause severe hypotension if fixed cardiac output present (aortic stenosis, pulmonary hypertension). ■ May cause transient hypertension and increased frequency of arrhythmias. ■ Use caution if renal function impaired.

Monitor: Monitor the patient's ECG and BP continuously. ■ Keep patient in supine position; postural hypotension is almost always present. Tolerance to hypotensive effect may develop after several days. ■ Correct dehydration or hypovolemia. ■ Observe for increased anginal pain in susceptible patients.

Maternal/child: Used during pregnancy or in children only in life-threatening situations.

DRUG/LAB INTERACTIONS

May aggravate digitalis toxicity; use with caution if patient receiving digitalis; avoid simultaneous initiation of therapy. ■ Will potentiate catecholamines (e.g., dopamine [Intropin]); use diluted solution and monitor BP closely. ■ Risk of cardiotoxicity increased with pimozide (Orap) and sparfloxacin (Zagam); concurrent use not recommended.

SIDE EFFECTS

Anginal attacks, bradycardia, dizziness, hypotension and postural hypotension, increased frequency of PVCs, initial increase in arrhythmias, light-headedness, nausea and vomiting, substernal pressure, syncope, transitory hypertension, vertigo.

ANTIDOTE

Notify the physician of all side effects. Nausea and vomiting may subside with reduction in rate of administration. Use dopamine or norepinephrine (Levophed) and IV fluids to correct hypotension. Treat hypertension with a short-acting antihypertensive agent (e.g., nitroprusside [Nipride]). Resuscitate as necessary.

BUMETANIDE
Bumex

USUAL DOSE

0.5 to 1.0 mg. May be repeated at 2- to 3- hour intervals. Do not exceed 10 mg/24 hr. Can be used for patients allergic to furosemide. 1:40 mg ratio (bumetanide to furosemide) is used to determine dose.

DOSE ADJUSTMENTS

Reduced dose or extended intervals may be appropriate in the elderly.

DILUTION

May be given undiluted. Not usually added to IV solutions but compatible with D5W, NS, and LR infusion solutions. Usually given through Y-tube or three-way stopcock of infusion set. Use only freshly prepared solutions for infusion. Discard after 24 hours.

INCOMPATIBLE WITH

Dobutamine (Dobutrex), midazolam (Versed), milrinone (Primacor). Note Precautions.

RATE OF ADMINISTRATION

A single dose direct IV over 1 to 2 minutes. Give infusion at prescribed rate.

ACTIONS

A sulfonamide diuretic, antihypertensive, and antihypercalcemic agent related to the thiazides. A loop diuretic agent. Extremely potent. Onset of action is within minutes and duration of action may last 4 to 6 hours. Apparently acts on the proximal and distal ends of the tubule and the ascending limb of the loop of Henle to excrete water, sodium, chloride, and potassium. Will produce diuresis in alkalosis or acidosis. Rapidly distributed, it is excreted primarily in the urine.

INDICATIONS AND USES

Edema associated with congestive heart failure, cirrhosis of the liver with ascites, renal diseases including nephrotic syndrome. ▪ Acute pulmonary edema. ▪ Edema unresponsive to other diuretic agents. ▪ Diuresis in patients allergic to furosemide.

CONTRAINDICATIONS

Anuria, known hypersensitivity to bumetanide. Use caution in patients with hepatic coma or in states of severe electrolyte depletion. Do not use until condition is improved or corrected.

PRECAUTIONS

May be used concurrently with aldosterone antagonists (e.g., spironolactone [Aldactone]) for more effective diuresis and to prevent excessive potassium loss. ▪ May increase blood glucose; has precipitated diabetes mellitus. ▪ May lower serum calcium level, causing tetany. ▪ In rare instances may precipitate an acute attack of gout. ▪ Risk of ototoxicity increased with higher doses, rapid injection, decreased renal function, or concurrent use with other ototoxic drugs (See Drug/lab interactions) ▪ Patients allergic to sulfonamides may have an allergic reaction to bumetamide.

Monitor: May precipitate excessive diuresis with water and electrolyte depletion. Routine checks on electrolyte panel, CO_2, serum glucose, uric acid, and BUN are necessary during therapy. Potassium chloride replacement may be required.

Patient education: Hypotension may cause dizziness; move slowly, and request assistance to sit on edge of bed or ambulate. ■ May decrease potassium levels and require a supplement.

Maternal/child: Category C: use in pregnancy only if clearly needed. ■ Consider discontinuing breast feeding. ■ Safety for use in children not established.

Elderly: Consider increased sensitivity to hypotensive and electrolyte effects and increased risk of circulatory collapse or thromboembolic episodes. ■ Consider possibility of decreased renal function.

DRUG/LAB INTERACTIONS

May cause transient or permanent deafness with doses exceeding the usual or when given in conjunction with other ototoxic drugs (e.g., cisplatin, aminoglycosides [e.g., gentamicin]). ■ May increase activity of anticoagulants; monitor PT. ■ May increase serum levels of beta-blockers (e.g., propranolol [Inderal]) and lithium (may cause toxicity). ■ May cause cardiac arrhythmias with digitalis. ■ May enhance or inhibit actions of non-depolarizing muscle relaxants (e.g., mivacurium [Mivacron]) or theophyllines. ■ May cause hyperglycemia with sulfo-nylureas (e.g., tolbutamide) by decreasing glucose tolerance. ■ Effects may be inhibited by NSAIDS (e.g., ibuprofen [Motrin]), probenecid, or in patients with cirrhosis and ascites on salicylates. ■ May cause profound diuresis and serious electrolyte abnormalities with thiazide diuretics (e.g., chlorothiazide [Diuril]) because of synergistic effects. ■ Note Precautions.

SIDE EFFECTS

Usually occur in prolonged therapy, seriously ill patients, or following large doses.

Minor: Abdominal pain, arthritic pain, azotemia, dizziness, ECG changes, elevated serum creatinine, encephalopathy, headache, hyper-glycemia, hyperuricemia, hypochloremia, hyponatremia, hypotension, impaired hearing, muscle cramps, nausea, pruritus, rash.

Major: Anaphylactic shock, blood volume reduction, circulatory col-lapse, dehydration, excessive diuresis, hypokalemia, metabolic acido-sis, thrombocytopenia, vascular thrombosis and embolism.

ANTIDOTE

If minor side effects are noted, discontinue the drug and notify the physician, who may treat the side effects symptomatically and con-tinue the drug. If side effects are progressive or any major side effect occurs, discontinue the drug immediately and notify the physician. Treatment of major side effects is symptomatic and aggressive and includes fluid and electrolyte replacement. Resuscitate as necessary.

BUPRENORPHINE HYDROCHLORIDE

Narcotic analgesic
(Agonist-antagonist)
Anesthesia adjunct

Buprenex

pH 3.5 to 5.5

USUAL DOSE

Pain control: 0.3 mg (1ml). Repeat every 6 hours as necessary. May be repeated in 30 to 60 minutes, if indicated. These dose recommendations have been lowered because of excessive respiratory depression with doses up to 0.6 mg. 25 to 250 mcg/hr has been given as a continuous infusion to manage post operative pain.

Reverse fentanyl-induced anesthesia (unlabeled): 0.3 to 0.8 mg 1 to 4 hours after induction of anesthesia and 30 minutes prior to end of surgery.

PEDIATRIC DOSE

2 to 12 years of age: Pain control: 2 to 6 mcg/kg of body weight every 4 to 8 hours. A repeat dose in 30 to 60 minutes is not recommended. Longer intervals (6 to 8 hours) are suggested and should provide sufficient pain relief. Determine appropriate interval through clinical assessment.

DOSE ADJUSTMENTS

Reduce dose by one half in high-risk patients (e.g., elderly or debilitated, respiratory disease), when other CNS depressants have been given, and in the immediate postoperative period (Note Drug/lab interactions). ▪ Reduced dose may be required in impaired liver function.

DILUTION

Direct IV: May be given undiluted.

Infusion: May be further diluted with NS, D5W, D5/NS, or lactated Ringer's injection and given as an infusion. 1 mg in 250 ml = 4 mcg/ml, 3 mg in 250 ml = 12 mcg/ml.

Storage: Prior to use, store at controlled room temperature. Avoid freezing and/or prolonged exposure to light.

INCOMPATIBLE WITH

Alcohol solutions, diazepam (Valium), furosemide (Lasix), lorazepam (Ativan).

COMPATIBLE WITH

Atropine, diphenhydramine (Benedryl), droperidol (Inapsine), glycopyrrolate (Robinul), haloperidol (Haldoll), hydroxyzine (Atarax), promethazine (Phenergan), scopalamine.

RATE OF ADMINISTRATION

Titrate slowly according to symptom relief and respiratory rate.

Direct IV: A single dose over 3 to 5 minutes.

Infusion: See Usual dose, use of a metriset (60 gtt/min) or a controlled infusion device recommended.

ACTIONS

A synthetic narcotic agonist-antagonist analgesic. Thirty times as potent as morphine in analgesic effect (0.3 mg equivalent to 10 mg morphine) and has the antagonist effect of naloxone in larger doses. Does produce respiratory depression. Pain relief is effected in 2 to 3 minutes and lasts up to 6 hours. Metabolized in the liver. Primarily excreted through feces. Crosses the placental barrier. Secreted in breast milk.

INDICATIONS AND USES

Relief of moderate to severe pain.

Unlabeled use: Reverse fentanyl induced anesthesia.

CONTRAINDICATIONS

Children 2 years of age and younger, hypersensitivity to buprenorphine.

PRECAUTIONS

Usually given IM. ■ May precipitate withdrawal symptoms if stopped too quickly after prolonged use or if patient has been on opiates. ■ Use caution in asthma, respiratory depression or difficulty from any source, impaired renal or hepatic function, the elderly or debilitated, myxedema or hypothyroidism, adrenocortical insufficiency, CNS depression or coma, toxic psychoses, prostatic hypertrophy or urethral stricture, acute alcoholism, delirium tremens, or kyphoscoliosis. ■ May elevate cerebrospinal fluid pressure; use caution in head injury, intracranial lesions, and other situations with increased intracranial pressure.

Monitor: Naloxone (Narcan), oxygen, and controlled respiratory equipment must be available. Naloxone is only partially effective in reversing respiratory depression. ■ Observe patient frequently and monitor vital signs. ■ Keep patient supine to minimize side effects; orthostatic hypotension and fainting may occur. Observe closely during ambulation. ■ Pain control usually more effective with routinely administered doses. Determine appropriate interval through clinical assessment.

Patient education: Avoid use of alcohol or other CNS depressants (e.g., antihistamines, diazepam [Valium]). ■ Use caution performing any task requiring alertness; may cause dizziness, euphoria, and sedation. ■ Request assistance for ambulation. ■ May be habit forming.

Maternal/child: Safety for use during pregnancy, labor and delivery, or lactation not established. Use only when clearly needed. ■ Not recommended in children under 2 years of age but has been used in children as young as 9 months of age.

Elderly: Note Dose adjustments. ■ May be more sensitive to effects (e.g., respiratory depression, urinary retention, constipation, dizziness). ■ Analgesia should be effective with lower doses. ■ Consider possibility of decreased organ function.

DRUG/LAB INTERACTIONS

Potentiated by cimetidine (Tagamet), phenothiazines (e.g., chlorpromazine [Thorazine]), and CNS depressants such as narcotic analgesics, general anesthetics, alcohol, anticholinergics, antihistamines, barbiturates, benzodiazepines (e.g., diazepam [Valium]), hypnotics, MAO inhibitors, neuromuscular blocking agents (e.g., mivacurium [Mivacron]), psychotropic agents, and sedatives. Reduced doses of both drugs may be indicated. ■ May decrease analgesic effects of other narcotics; avoid concurrent use.

SIDE EFFECTS

Excessive sedation is a major side effect. Has caused death from respiratory depression. Anaphylaxis, bradycardia, clammy skin, constipation, cyanosis, dizziness, dyspnea, headache, hypertension, hypotension, nausea, pruritus, tachycardia, vertigo, visual disturbances, vomiting.

ANTIDOTE

With increasing severity of any side effect or onset of symptoms of overdose, discontinue the drug and notify the physician. Naloxone hydrochloride (Narcan) will help to reverse respiratory depression, but is not as effective as with other narcotics. A patent airway, artificial ventilation, oxygen therapy, and other symptomatic treatment must be instituted promptly. Treat anaphylaxis and resuscitate as necessary.

BUTORPHANOL TARTRATE

Narcotic analgesic
(Agonist-antagonist)
Anesthesia Adjunct

Stadol   pH 3.0 to 5.5

USUAL DOSE

Pain control: 1 mg. Repeat every 3 to 4 hours as necessary. Range is 0.5 to 2 mg.

Preoperative or preanesthetic: 2 mg 30 to 60 minutes before surgery. Individualize dose. Usually given IM

Labor: 1 to 2 mg at full term in early labor; may be repeated after 4 hours.

Adjunct to balanced anesthesia: 2 mg just before induction or 0.5 to 1 mg in increments during anesthesia. Increments may be up to 0.06 mg/kg. Total dose ranges from 4 to 12.5 mg. Administered only under the direction of the anesthesiologist.

DOSE ADJUSTMENTS

Reduce dose by one-half and double the intervals between doses in high-risk patients (e.g., elderly or debilitated, respiratory disease); adjust as indicated by patient response. ■ Reduce dose when other CNS depressants have been given and in the immediate postoperative period. ■ Extend intervals to 6 or 8 hours in impaired liver or renal function; adjust as indicated by patient response. ■ Note Drug/lab interactions.

DILUTION

May be given undiluted.

Storage: Prior to use, store at controlled room termperature. Avoid freezing and/or prolonged exposure to light.

INCOMPATIBLE WITH

Barbiturates (e.g., pentobarbital [Nembutal]), dimenhydrinate (Dramanate).

RATE OF ADMINISTRATION

Each 2 mg or fraction thereof over 3 to 5 minutes. Frequently titrated according to symptom relief and respiratory rate.

ACTIONS

A potent narcotic analgesic with some narcotic agonist-antagonist effects. Exact mechanism of action is unknown. Analgesia similar to morphine is produced. Does produce respiratory depression, but this does not increase markedly with larger doses. Pain relief is effected almost immediately, peaks at 30 minutes, and lasts about 3 hours. Causes some hemodynamic changes that increase the workload of the heart. Metabolized in the liver. Excreted in urine. Crosses the placental barrier. Secreted in breast milk.

INDICATIONS AND USES

Relief of moderate to severe pain. ▪ Preoperative medication. ▪ Obstetric analgesia during labor.

CONTRAINDICATIONS

Hypersensitivity to butorphanol.

PRECAUTIONS

Not used for narcotic-dependent patients because of antagonist activity. ▪ Use in myocardial infarction, ventricular dysfunction, and coronary insufficiency only if the patient is hypersensitive to morphine or meperidine. ▪ Use caution in respiratory depression or difficulty from any source, obstructive respiratory conditions, head injury, biliary surgery, and impaired liver or kidney function.

Monitor: Naloxone (Narcan), oxygen, and controlled respiratory equipment must be available. ▪ Observe patient frequently and monitor vital signs. ▪ Keep patient supine to minimize side effects; orthostatic hypotension and fainting may occur. Observe closely during ambulation. ▪ Pain control usually more effective with routinely administered doses. Determine appropriate interval through clinical assessment.

Patient education: Avoid use of alcohol or other CNS depressants (e.g., antihistamines, diazepam [Valium]). ▪ Use caution performing any task requiring alertness, may cause dizziness, euphoria, and sedation. ▪ Request assistance for ambulation. ▪ May be habit forming.

Maternal/child: Pregnancy Category C: safety for use in pregnancy not established; could result in neonatal withdrawal. ▪ Has been used safely during labor and delivery of term infants, but use caution during labor and delivery of premature infants. ▪ Discontinue breast-feeding. ▪ Not recommended for children under 18 years.

Elderly: May be more sensitive to effects (e.g., respiratory depression, urinary retention, constipation, dizziness). ▪ Analgesia should be effective with lower doses. ▪ Consider possibility of decreased organ function.

DRUG/LAB INTERACTIONS

Potentiated by cimetidine (Tagamet), phenothiazines (e.g., chlorpromazine [Thorazine]), droperidol (Inapsine), and CNS depressants such as narcotic analgesics, general anesthetics, alcohol, anticholinergics, antihistamines, barbiturates, benzodiazepines (e.g., diazepam [Valium]), hypnotics, MAO inhibitors, neuromuscular blocking agents (e.g., mivacurium [Mivacron]), psychotropic agents, and sedatives. Reduced doses of both drugs may be indicated. ▪ May decrease analgesic effects of other narcotics; avoid concurrent use. ▪ Will cause an increase in conjunctival changes with pancuronium (Pavulon).

SIDE EFFECTS

Anaphylaxis, clammy skin, confusion, diplopia, dizziness, dry mouth, floating feeling, flushing, hallucinations, headache, lethargy, light-headedness, nausea, respiratory depression, sedation, sensitivity to cold, sweating, unusual dreams, vertigo, vomiting, warmth. May cause increased pulmonary artery pressure, pulmonary wedge pressure, left ventricular end-diastolic pressure, systemic arterial pressure, pulmonary vascular resistance and cardiac workload.

ANTIDOTE

With increasing severity of any side effect or onset of symptoms of overdose, discontinue the drug and notify the physician. Treat side effects symptomatically. Naloxone hydrochloride (Narcan) will reverse respiratory depression. A patent airway, artificial ventilation, oxygen therapy, and other symptomatic treatment must be instituted promptly.

CAFFEINE AND SODIUM BENZOATE

CNS stimulant
Respiratory stimulant adjunct

pH 6.5 to 8.5

USUAL DOSE

500 mg to 1 Gm. Maximum dose is 2.5 Gm/24 hr.

PEDIATRIC DOSE

8 mg/kg of body weight up to 500 mg every 4 hours.

Neonatal apnea: Do not use in neonates; sodium benzoate can displace bilirubin from its protein-binding sites. Caffeine citrate or caffeine without sodium benzoate is preferred for IV dosage in neonates. These alternate IV formulations must be prepared and sterilized by the pharmacy. Caffeine citrate should be available as a prepared solution by late fall 1998. An initial dose of up to 10 mg/kg of body weight (20 mg/kg if caffeine citrate is used). Follow with a maintenance dose of 2.5 mg/kg/day (5 mg/kg caffeine citrate). Plasma concentrations of 5 to 20 mcg/ml have controlled apnea. Oral therapy with caffeine only is preferred.

DOSE ADJUSTMENTS

Note Drug/lab interactions.

DILUTION

May be given undiluted.

INCOMPATIBLE WITH

Chlorpromazine (Thorazine).

RATE OF ADMINISTRATION

250 mg or fraction thereof over 1 minute. Extend rate of administration in neonate.

ACTIONS

A xanthine derivative and descending analeptic CNS stimulant. Small doses cause wakefulness and mental alertness. Larger doses stimulate the respiratory center and increase heart action. It is believed to constrict the intracranial blood vessels and lower intracranial pressure. Widely distributed throughout the body and excreted in the urine. Crosses the placental barrier. Secreted in breast milk.

INDICATIONS AND USES

Rarely used. Alleviate headaches after spinal cord puncture. ▪ Alcoholic stupor/excitement. ▪ Barbiturate poisoning antidote. ▪ Narcotic poisoning antidote if naloxone (Narcan) or nalmefene (Revex) is not available.

Unlabeled use: Treatment of neonatal apnea in citrate form.

CONTRAINDICATIONS

Acute myocardial infarction, hypersensitivity to drug or its components.

PRECAUTIONS

Usually given IM; IV route is for emergencies only. ▪ Most people have developed a tolerance level for caffeine because of daily ingestion of coffee or tea. ▪ Death has occurred with IV administration. ▪ Use as an analeptic considered ineffective by most clinicians. ▪ May reactivate duodenal ulcers. ▪ Doses over 1 Gm may increase depression in depressed individuals.

Monitor: Observe frequently and monitor vital signs. ▪ Monitor blood glucose; may cause hyperglycemia.

Maternal/child: Category C: safety not established in pregnancy or lactation. Excessive intake causes fetal loss, low birth weight, and premature delivery.

DRUG/LAB INTERACTIONS

MAO inhibitors (e.g., selegiline [Eldepryl]) potentiate caffeine and can cause an acute hypertensive crisis. ▪ May produce convulsions with overdose of propoxyphene (Darvon). ▪ Metabolism inhibited by oral contraceptives, cimetidine (Tagamet), disulfiram (Antabuse), and fluoroquinolones (e.g., ciprofloxacin [Cipro]); a lower dose of caffeine may be indicated. ▪ Smoking promotes elimination of caffeine; may inhibit effectiveness. ▪ Serum levels increased by phenylpropanolamine (Phenoxine, Dexatrim). ▪ May increase urine levels of VMA, cate-cholamines, 5-HIAA, and false-positive serum urate elevations. May cause false diagnosis of pheochromocytoma or neuroblastoma; avoid caffeine when testing for these disorders.

SIDE EFFECTS

Cardiac irregularities, diarrhea, diuresis, excessive irritability, excitement, flushing, headache, hypertension (transient), insomnia, lightheadedness, muscle twitching, nausea and vomiting, nervousness, palpitations, restlessness, scintillating scotoma (lightning flashes in the eyes), tachycardia, tinnitus, and death.

Neonatal: Bradycardia, coarse tremors, hypertonicity alternating with hypotonicity, hypotension, intracranial hemorrhage, opisthotonic posturing, and severe acidosis.

ANTIDOTE

For major symptoms, discontinue drug and notify the physician. Diazepam (Valium), phenytoin (Dilantin), or phenobarbital (Luminal) will quiet CNS stimulation or seizures. Resuscitate as necessary.

CALCIUM CHLORIDE

Electrolyte replenisher
Antihypocalcemic
Cardiotonic
Antihyperkalemic
Antihypermagnesemic

pH 5.5 to 7.5

USUAL DOSE

Hypocalcemia/maintenance: 5 to 10 ml (500 mg to 1 Gm) at intervals of 1 to 3 days. Repeat doses may be required and are based on patient response or serum calcium levels. *In a 10% solution 10 ml (1 Gm) contains 13.6 mEq (272 mg) of calcium; 1 ml (100 mg) 1.36 mEq (27.2 mg).*

Magnesium intoxication: 5 ml (500 mg). Observe for signs of recovery before giving any additional calcium.

Hyperkalemia ECG disturbances of cardiac function: 1 to 10 ml (100 mg to 1 Gm); titrate dose by monitoring ECG changes.

Cardiac resuscitation: (see Indications). 2 to 4 mg/kg; repeat at 10-minute intervals as indicated or as measured by serum deficits of calcium. Consider need for calcium (usually gluconate or gluceptate) for every 500 ml of whole blood if arrest occurs in a situation requiring copious blood replacement.

PEDIATRIC DOSE

Hypocalcemic disorders: 0.2 ml of a 10% solution/kg of body weight (20 mg/kg). Up to 10 ml (1 Gm)/day may be required.

Cardiac resuscitation: 0.2 ml of a 10% solution/kg (20 mg/kg) (See Indications). Repeat at 10-minute intervals.

DILUTION

May be given undiluted, but preferably diluted with an equal amount of distilled water or normal saline for injection to make a 5% solution. Solution should be warmed to body temperature.

INCOMPATIBLE WITH

Amphotericin B (Fungizone), cefamandole (Mandol), cephalothin (Keflin), chlorpheniramine (Chlortrimeton), chlortetracycline (Aureomycin), digitalis (e.g., digitoxin), dobutamine (Dobutrex), epinephrine (Adrenalin), fat emulsion 10% IV (Intralipid 10%), sodium bicarbonate, warfarin. Calcium salts not generally mixed with carbonates (Coumadin), phosphates, sulfates, or tartrates.

RATE OF ADMINISTRATION

0.5 to 1 ml of solution over 1 minute. Stop or slow infusion rate if patient complains of discomfort. Rapid administration may cause bradycardia; heat waves; local burning sensation; metallic, calcium or chalky taste; moderate drop in blood pressure; peripheral vasodilation; or a sense of oppression.

ACTIONS

Calcium is a basic element prevalent in the human body. It affects bones, nerves, muscles, glands, cardiac and vascular tone, and normal coagulation of the blood. It is excreted in the urine and feces.

INDICATIONS AND USES

Calcium preparations other than calcium chloride are often preferred except in cardiac resuscitation or verapamil toxicity. ■ Increase plasma calcium levels in hypocalcemic disorders (e.g., tetany [neonatal, parathyroid deficiency], vitamin D deficiency, alkalosis, conditions associated with intestinal malabsorption). ■ Treat ECG disturbances caused by hyper-kalemia or verapamil-induced hypotension. ■ Adjunctive therapy in sensitivity reactions (especially with urticaria), insect bites or stings (relieve muscle cramping), acute symptoms of lead colic, rickets, or osteomalacia. ■ Cardiac resuscitation only to treat hypocalcemia, hyperkalemia, or calcium-channel blocker toxicity (verapamil, diltiazem), or after open heart surgery if epinephrine does not produce effective myocardial contractions. ■ Antidote for cardiac and respiratory depression of magnesium sulfate toxicity.

Investigational uses: Treatment of verapamil overdose, acute hypotension from verapamil; and prevention of initial hypotension when it could be detrimental to a specific patient and verapamil is required.

CONTRAINDICATIONS

Digitalized patients, hypercalcemia, ventricular fibrillation.

PRECAUTIONS

Three times more potent than calcium gluconate. ■ For IV use only. ■ Note Drug/lab interactions.

Monitor: Confirm patency of vein, select a large vein, and use a small needle to reduce vein irritation. Necrosis and sloughing will occur with IM or SC injection or extravasation. ■ Keep patient recumbent after injection to prevent postural hypotension. ■ Monitor vital signs carefully.

Maternal/child: Category C: safety for use in pregnancy and lactation not established. Use only when clearly needed.

DRUG/LAB INTERACTIONS

Will increase digitalis toxicity and may cause arrhythmias. If necessary, give small amounts very slowly. ■ Potentiated by thiazide diuretics (e.g., chlorothiazide [Diuril]); may cause hypercalcemia or calcium toxicity. ■ May reduce plasma levels of atenolol (Tenormin). ■ Can reduce neuromuscular paralysis and respiratory depression produced by antibiotics such as kanamycin (Kantrex). ■ Antagonizes verapamil; can reverse clinical effects. ■ May cause metabolic alkalosis and inhibit binding of potassium with sodium polystyrene sulfonate.

SIDE EFFECTS

Usual doses will produce a local burning sensation, moderate drop in blood pressure, and peripheral vasodilation. May cause bradycardia, cardiac arrest, heat waves; metallic, calcium or chalky taste; prolonged state of cardiac contraction, sense of oppression, or tingling sensation, especially with a too rapid rate of administration.

Overdose: Coma, intractable nausea and vomiting, lethargy, markedly elevated plasma calcium level, weakness, and sudden death.

ANTIDOTE

If side effects occur, further dilution and decrease in the rate of administration may be necessary. If side effects persist, discontinue the drug and notify the physician. IV infusion of sodium chloride (to maintain normovolemia) and furosemide (Lasix) 80 to 100 mg IV every 2 to 4 hours (with caution) is recommended in overdose. Sodium chloride competes with calcium for reabsorption in the renal tubules; furosemide enhances the activity. Together they will reduce hypercalcemia by causing a marked increase in calcium excretion. Monitoring of fluid, electrolytes, cardiac and respiratory status is imperative. Disodium edetate may be used with extreme caution as a calcium chelating agent if overdose is critical. For extravasation inject affected area with 1% procaine hydrochloride and hyaluronidase to reduce venospasm and dilute calcium. Use a 27- or 25-gauge needle. Warm moist compresses may be helpful. Resuscitate as necessary.

CALCIUM GLUCEPTATE

Electrolyte replenisher
Antihypocalcemic
Antihypermagnesemic

pH 5.6 to 7.0

USUAL DOSE

Hypocalcemia/maintenance: 5 to 20 ml. May be repeated if indicated. 5 ml (1.1 Gm) contains 4.5 mEq (90 mg) of calcium.

Cardiac resuscitation: (See Indications). 5 to 7 ml; repeat at 10-minute intervals as indicated by clinical condition or serum calcium level.

Newborn exchange transfusion: 0.5 ml (0.11 Gm) after each 100 ml of blood exchanged.

DILUTION

May be given undiluted. Solution should be warmed to body temperature. Solution must be clear and free of crystals. Discard unused portion.

INCOMPATIBLE WITH

Cefamandole (Mandol), cefazolin (Kefzol), cephalothin (Keflin), magnesium sulfate, prednisolone sodium phosphate (Hydeltrasol), prochlorperazine (Compazine), tetracyclines. Calcium salts are not generally mixed with carbonates, phosphates, sulfates, or tartrates.

RATE OF ADMINISTRATION

1 ml or fraction thereof over 1 minute. Do not exceed 2 ml/min. Stop or slow infusion rate if patient complains of discomfort. Rapid administration may cause bradycardia; heat waves; local burning sensation; metallic, calcium, or chalky taste; or a sense of oppression.

ACTIONS

Calcium is a basic element prevalent in the human body. It affects bones, nerves, muscles, glands, cardiac and vascular tone, and normal coagulation of the blood. It is excreted in the urine and feces.

INDICATIONS AND USES

Increase plasma calcium levels in hyopcalcemic disorders (e.g., tetany [neonatal, parathyroid deficiency], vitamin D deficiency, alkalosis, conditions associated with intestinal malabsorption). ■ Prevention of hypocalcemia during exchange transfusions. ■ Cardiac resuscitation only to treat hypocalcemia, hyperkalemia, or calcium channel-blocker toxicity (verapamil, diltiazem). ▪ Antidote for cardiac and respiratory depression of magnesium sulfate toxicity.

Investigational uses: Treatment of verapamil overdose, acute hypotension from verapamil, and prevention of initial hypotension when it could be detrimental to a specific patient and verapamil is required.

CONTRAINDICATIONS
Digitalized patients, hypercalcemia, ventricular fibrillation.

PRECAUTIONS
IV use is preferred in adults, infants, and young children. ▪ Mild to serious local reactions may occur with IM or subcutaneous injection or extravasation.

Monitor: Confirm patency of vein. ▪ Keep patient lying down after injection to prevent postural hypotension. ▪ Monitor vital signs carefully.

Maternal/child: Category C: safety for use in pregnancy not established. Use only when clearly needed. ▪ According to some authorities IM use is contraindicated in infants and small children. If IM route necessary, use lateral thigh site for injection.

DRUG/LAB INTERACTIONS
Will increase digitalis toxicity and may cause arrhythmias. If necessary, give small amounts very slowly. ▪ Potentiated by thiazide diuretics (e.g., chlorothiazide [Diuril]); may cause hypercalcemia or calcium toxicity. ▪ May reduce plasma levels of atenolol (Tenormin). ▪ Antagonizes verapamil; can reverse clinical effects. ▪ May cause metabolic alkalosis and inhibit binding of potassium with sodium polystyrene sulfonate.

SIDE EFFECTS
Usually occur only with rapid administration and may include bradycardia; heat waves; local burning sensation; metallic, calcium or chalky taste; a sense of oppression; and tingling sensations.

Overdose: Coma, intractable nausea and vomiting, lethargy, markedly elevated plasma calcium level, weakness, and sudden death.

ANTIDOTE
If side effects occur, further dilution and decrease in the rate of administration may be necessary. If side effects persist, discontinue the drug and notify the physician. Further dilution and decrease in the rate of administration may be necessary. IV infusion of sodium chloride (to maintain normovolemia) and furosemide (Lasix) 80 to 100 mg IV every 2 to 4 hours (with caution) are recommended in overdose. Sodium chloride competes with calcium for reabsorption in the renal tubules; furosemide enhances the activity. Together they will reduce hypercalcemia by causing a marked increase in calcium excretion. Monitoring of fluid, electrolytes, and cardiac and respiratory status is imperative. Disodium edetate may be used with extreme caution as a calcium chelating agent if overdosage is critical. For extravasation inject affected area with 1% procaine hydrochloride and hyaluronidase to reduce venospasm and dilute calcium. Use a 27- or 25-gauge needle. Warm moist compresses may be helpful. Resuscitate as necessary.

CALCIUM GLUCONATE

Electrolyte replenisher
Antihypocalcemic
Cardiotonic
Antihyperkalemic
Antihypermagnesemic

pH 6.0 to 8.2

USUAL DOSE

Hypocalcemia/Maintenance: 5 to 20 ml (2.3 to 9.3 mEq). Repeat as required. Daily dose ranges from 4.65 to 70 mEq. Larger amounts may be given as an intermittent or continuous IV infusion. 10 ml (1 Gm in a 10% solution) contains 4.65 mEq (93 mg) of calcium.

Emergency elevation of serum calcium: 15 to 30.1 ml (7 to 14 mEq). Repeat every 1 to 3 days based on patient response.

Cardiac resuscitation: (See Indications). 5 to 8 ml (2.3 to 3.6 mEq). Repeat at 10-minute intervals as indicated by clinical condition or serum calcium level.

Hyperkalemia with secondary cardiac toxicity: 4.8 to 30.1 ml (2.25 to 14 mEq). ECG monitoring required; observe results and repeat in 1 to 2 minutes if indicated.

Hypocalcemic tetany: 9.7 to 34.4 ml (4.5 to 16 mEq). Repeat as indicated to control tetany.

Magnesium intoxication: 9.7 to 19.4 ml (4.5 to 9 mEq). Repeat as indicated by patient response; observe for signs of recovery before giving additional calcium.

Exchange transfusion: Approximately 2.9 ml (1.35 mEq) with each 100 ml of citrated blood.

PEDIATRIC DOSE

Hypocalcemia/Maintenance: 5 ml/kg/day (2.3 mEq/kg/day) or 120 ml/M^2/day (56 mEq/M^2/day) in divided doses.

Emergency elevation of serum calcium: 2.2 to 15 ml (1 to 7 mEq). Repeat every 1 to 3 days based on patient response.

Hypocalcemic tetany: 1.1 to 1.5 ml/kg (0.5 to 0.7 mEq/kg) 3 or 4 times daily until tetany is controlled.

NEONATAL DOSE

Hypocalcemia/Maintenance: Not more than 2 ml (0.93 mEq).

Emergency elevation of serum calcium: Up to 2.2 ml (1 mEq). Repeat every 1 to 3 days based on patient response.

Hypocalcemic tetany: 5.2 ml/kg/24 hr (2.4 mEq/kg/24 hr) in divided doses.

Exchange transfusion: 1 ml (0.45 mEq) with each 100 ml of citrated blood.

DILUTION

May be given undiluted or may be further diluted in up to 1,000 ml of normal saline solution for infusion. Solution should be warmed to body temperature. Solution must be clear and free of crystals. Crystals can be dissolved by heating to 80° C (146° F) in a dry heat oven for at least 1 hour. Shake vigorously; cool to room temperature. Discard if crystals persist.

Pediatric and neonatal dilution: Must be further diluted with NS.

INCOMPATIBLE WITH

Amphotericin B (Fungizone), ampicillin (Polycillin-N), cefamandole (Mandol), cefazolin (Ancef), cephalothin (Keflin), chlortetracycline (Aureomycin), digitalis (e.g., Digitoxin), dobutamine (Dobutrex), epinephrine (Adrenalin), fat emulsion 10% IV (Intralipid 10%), fluconazole (Diflucan), hydrocortisone phosphate, indomethacin (Indocin), kanamycin (Kantrex), magnesium sulfate, metoclopramide (Reglan), methylprednisolone (Solucortef), potassium phosphate, prochlorperazine (Compazine), promethazine (Phenergan), sodium bicarbonate, streptomycin, tetracycline. Calcium salts are not generally mixed with carbonates, phosphates, sulfates, or tartrates.

RATE OF ADMINISTRATION

In all situations stop or slow infusion rate if patient complains of discomfort. Rapid administration may cause vasdodilation, decreased blood pressure, cardiac arrhythmias, syncope, and cardiac arrest.

Direct IV: Undiluted, each 0.5 ml or fraction thereof over 1 minute. Do not exceed 2 ml/min (200 mg).

Intermittent IV: Do not exceed a rate of 200 mg/min (direct IV rate).

Infusion: Diluted in 1,000 ml of normal saline, it may be given over 12 to 24 hours. Do not exceed 200 mg/min.

Pediatric and neonatal rate of administration: Slow rate of administration considerably. Observe continuously.

ACTIONS

Calcium is a basic element prevalent in the human body. It affects bones, nerves, glands, cardiac and vascular tone, and normal coagulation of the blood. Crosses the placental barrier and is secreted in breast milk. It is excreted in the urine and feces.

INDICATIONS AND USES

■ Increase plasma calcium levels in hypocalcemic disorders (e.g., tetany [neonatal, parathyroid deficiency], vitamin D deficiency, alkalosis, conditions associated with intestinal malabsorption). ■ Adjunctive therapy in sensitivity reactions (especially with urticaria), insect bites or stings (relieve muscle cramping), acute symptoms of lead colic, rickets, or osteomalacia. ■ Cardiac resuscitation only to treat hypocalcemia or hyperkalemia or calcium-channel blocker toxicity (verapamil, diltiazem). ■ Antidote for cardiac and respiratory depression of magnesium sulfate toxicity. ■ Prevention of hypocalcemia during exchange transfusions. ■ Decrease capillary permeability in allergic conditions, nonthrombocytopenic purpura and exudative dermatoses (e.g., dermatitis herpetiformis). ■ Treat pruritus of eruptions caused by drugs. ■ Treat ECG disturbances caused by hyperkalemia or verapamil-induced hypotension.

Investigational uses: Treatment of verapamil overdose, acute hypotension from verapamil, and prevention of initial hypotension when it could be detrimental to a specific patient and verapamil is required.

CONTRAINDICATIONS

IM use in infants and small children. Digitalized patients, hypercalcemia, ventricular fibrillation.

PRECAUTIONS

Has only one third the potency of calcium chloride. ■ For IV use only; IM use permitted in adults only if IV administration cannot be accomplished (note Monitor).

Monitor: Confirm patency of vein; select a large vein, and use a small needle to reduce vein irritation. Local necrosis and abscess formation can occur with IM or SC injection or extravasation. ▪ Keep patient recumbent after injection to prevent postural hypotension. ▪ Monitor vital signs carefully.

Maternal/ child: Category C: safety for use in pregnancy not established; benefits must outweigh risk. ▪ Note Contraindications.

DRUG/LAB INTERACTIONS

Will increase digitalis toxicity and may cause arrhythmias. If necessary, give small amounts very slowly. ▪ Potentiated by thiazide diuretics (e.g., chlorothiazide [Diuril]); may cause hypercalcemia or calcium toxicity. ▪ May reduce plasma levels of atenolol (Tenormin). ▪ Antagonizes verapamil; can reverse clinical effects. ▪ May cause metabolic alkalosis and inhibit binding of potassium with sodium polystyrene sulfonate.

SIDE EFFECTS

Rare when given as recommended: bradycardia, cardiac arrhythmias, cardiac arrest, heat waves, hypotension; metallic, calcium, or chalky taste; sense of oppression, syncope, tingling, and vasodilation can occur with too rapid rate of administration. Depression of neuromuscular function, flushing, prolonged state of cardiac contraction can occur.

Overdose: Coma, intractable nausea and vomiting, lethargy, markedly elevated plasma calcium level, weakness, and sudden death.

ANTIDOTE

If side effects occur, further dilution and decrease in the rate of administration may be necessary. If side effects persist, discontinue the drug and notify the physician. IV infusion of sodium chloride (to maintain normovolemia) and furosemide (Lasix) 80 to 100 mg IV every 2 to 4 hours (with caution) are recommended in overdose. Sodium chloride competes with calcium for reabsorption in the renal tubules; furosemide enhances the activity. Together, they will reduce hypercalcemia by causing a marked increase in calcium excretion. Monitoring of fluid, electrolytes, cardiac and respiratory status is imperative. Disodium edetate may be used with extreme caution as a calcium chelating agent if overdosage is critical. For extravasation inject affected area with 1% procaine hydrochloride and hyaluronidase to reduce venospasm and dilute calcium. Use a 27- or 25-gauge needle. Warm moist compresses may be helpful. Resuscitate as necessary.

CARBOPLATIN

Antineoplastic
(Alkylating agent)

Paraplatin

pH 5.0 to 7.0

USUAL DOSE

Before giving any dose, platelets must be above $100,000/mm^3$ and neutrophils above $2,000/mm^3$.

As a single agent: With normal renal function (creatinine clearance > 60 ml/min), give 360 mg/M^2 on day 1 every 4 weeks.

Recently a new dosing formula based on preexisting renal function and/or desired platelet nadir has been suggested (see package insert).

In combination with cyclophosphamide: Carboplatin 300 mg/M^2 plus cyclophosphamide 600 mg/M^2 on day 1 every 4 weeks for 6 cycles.

DOSE ADJUSTMENTS

Single agent or combination therapy

Platelets/mm^3	Neutrophils/mm^3	Adjusted dose (from prior course)
> 100,000	> 2,000	↑ to 125%
50,000–100,000	500–2,000	No adjustment
< 50,000	< 500	↓ to 75%

Once the dose has been increased to 125% of the starting dose, no further dose increases are indicated. ■ With impaired renal function (creatinine clearance 16 to 40 ml/min), give 200 mg/M^2, (40 to 59 ml/min) give 250 mg/M^2. Adjust dose by percentages and criteria as indicated for normal renal function. ■ Bone marrow suppression is more severe in patients who have had prior therapy, especially with cisplatin, and when carboplatin is used with other bone marrow-suppressing therapies or radiation and may be more severe in the elderly. Reduced dose may be indicated. Monitor carefully and manage dose and timing to reduce additive effects.

DILUTION

Specific techniques required; see Precautions. Immediately before use dilute each 10 mg of carboplatin with 1 ml of sterile water for injection, 5% dextrose in water, or normal saline (50 mg with 5 ml, 150 mg with 15 ml, 450 mg with 45 ml). All yield 10 mg/ml. Should be further diluted with normal saline or 5% dextrose in water to 1 to 4 mg/ml (add 10 ml additional diluent to each 10 mg to obtain 1mg/ml and 2.5 ml to each 10 mg to obtain 4 mg/ml). Do not use needles or IV tubing with aluminum parts to mix or administer; a precipitate will form and decrease potency. Best to mix immediately before use. Discard solution 8 hours after dilution at room temperature, 24 hours if refrigerated.

Storage: Store unopened vials at 15° to 30° C (59° to 86° F). Protect from light.

INCOMPATIBLE WITH

Aluminum, fluorouracil (5FU), mesna, sodium bicarbonate. Should be considered incompatible in syringe or solution with any other drug because of toxicity and specific use.

COMPATIBLE WITH

0.3 mg/ml carboplatin is compatible with etoposide, 0.4 mg/ml in NS or D5W.

RATE OF ADMINISTRATION

A single dose as an infusion over a minimum of 15 minutes. Extend administration time based on amount of diluent and patient condition.

ACTIONS

An alkylating agent. An improved platinum-based compound similar to cisplatin but with improved therapeutic effects. Better tolerated by patients, carboplatin causes less nausea and vomiting, less neurotoxicity, and less nephrotoxicity than cisplatin. Myelosuppression is generally reversible and manageable with antibiotics and transfusions. Produces interstrand DNA cross-links and is cell cycle nonspecific. Not as heavily protein bound as cisplatin. Majority of carboplatin is excreted in the urine within 24 hours.

INDICATIONS AND USES

Initial treatment of advanced ovarian cancer in combination with other approved chemotherapeutic agents (e.g., cyclophosphamide). ■ Palliative treatment of recurrent ovarian cancer after prior chemotherapy, including patients treated with cisplatin.

Investigational uses: To replace cisplatin in treatment of cervical, endometrial, head and neck, lung and testicular cancers and relapsed and refractory acute leukemia. Used as a single agent but most effective in protocols.

CONTRAINDICATIONS

Hypersensitivity to cisplatin or other platinum-containing compounds or mannitol; severe bone marrow depression; significant bleeding.

PRECAUTIONS

■ Follow guidelines for handling cytotoxic agents. See Appendix A, p. 893. ■ Usually administered by or under the direction of the physician specialist. ■ Peripheral neurotoxicity is infrequent but may increase in patients over 65 years of age and in patients previously treated with cisplatin.

Monitor: BUN and serum creatinine should be done before each dose. CrCl, WBC, platelet count, and hemoglobin are recommended before each dose and weekly thereafter. Platelet count must be 100,000/mm^3 and neutrophils 2,000/mm^3 before a dose can be repeated. Anemia is frequent and cumulative. Transfusion is often indicated. ■ Excessive hydration or forced diuresis not required, but maintain adequate hydration and urinary output. ■ Nausea and vomiting are frequently severe but less than with cisplatin; generally last 24 hours. Prophylactic administration of antiemetics is indicated. Various protocols, including metoclopramide (Reglan), ondansetron (Zofran); dexamethasone (Decadron), and lorazepam (Ativan); droperidol (Inapsine) or haloperidol (Haldol) and dexamethasone; or prochlorperazine (Compazine) are used. ■ Observe for symptoms of allergic reaction during administration; epinephrine, corticosteroids, and antihistamines should be available. ■ Observe closely for symptoms of infection. Prophylactic antibiotics may be indicated pending results of C/S in a febrile neutropenic patient.

Patient education: Nonhormonal birth control recommended. ■ See Appendix D, p. 900.

Maternal/ child: Category D: avoid pregnancy. ■ Discontinue breast feeding.

Elderly: Neurotoxicity and myelotoxicity may be more severe. ■ Consider possibility of decreased renal function. ■ Note Dose adjustments and Precautions.

DRUG/LAB INTERACTIONS

Nephrotoxicity and ototoxicity potentiated by aminoglycosides (e.g., gentamicin [Garamycin]). Use caution if patient receiving both drugs. ■ Do not administer live virus vaccines to patients receiving antineoplastic drugs. ■ Note Dose adjustments.

SIDE EFFECTS

Allergic reactions including anaphylaxis can occur during administration. Alopecia (rare), anemia, anorexia, bleeding, bone marrow suppression (usually reversible), bronchospasm, bruising, changes in taste, constipation, death, decreased urine output, decreased serum electrolytes, dehydration, diarrhea, erythema, fatigue, fever, hemolytic uremic syndrome (rare, cancer associated), hypotension, infection, laboratory test abnormalities (alkaline phosphatase, aspartate aminotransferase [AST], BUN, serum creatinine, total bilirubin), nausea and vomiting (severe), neutropenia, ototoxicity, peripheral neuropathies, pruritus, rash, thrombocytopenia, urticaria, visual disturbances, weakness.

ANTIDOTE

Notify physician of all side effects. Symptomatic and supportive treatment is indicated. Withhold carboplatin until myelosuppression is reversed. Transfusions or epoetin alfa (Epogen, Procril) may be indicated for anemia. Filgrastin or sargramostin may be indicated for neutropenia. Oprelvekin (Numega) may be indicated for thrombocytopenia. Treat anaphylaxis with epinephrine, corticosteroids, oxygen, and antihistamines. There is no specific antidote.

CARMUSTINE (BCNU)

Antineoplastic
(Alkylating agent/Nitrosourea)

BiCNU

pH 5.6 to 6.0

USUAL DOSE

Initial dose is 150 to 200 mg/M^2. May be given as a single dose or one half of the calculated dose may be given initially and repeated the next day. Repeat every 6 weeks if bone marrow sufficiently recovered. Repeat doses adjusted according to hematologic response of previous dose; (See Dose Adjustments).

DOSE ADJUSTMENTS

Nadir after prior dose		Percentage of prior dose to be given
Leukocytes/mm^3	Platelets/mm^3	%
> 4000	> 100,000	100
3000–3999	75,000–99,999	100
2000–2999	25,000–74,999	70
< 2000	< 25,000	50

DILUTION
Specific techniques required; see Precautions. Initially dilute 100-mg vial with supplied sterile diluent (3 ml of absolute ethanol). Further dilute with 27 ml of sterile water for injection. Each ml will contain 3.3 mg carmustine. Withdraw desired dose and further dilute in 100 to 500 ml D5W or NS and give as an infusion. Use of glass containers preferred; loss of potency occurs in PVC containers and IV tubing.

Storage: Protect from light. Store in refrigerator (2° to 8° C [35° to 46° F]) in all forms. Stable 24 hours after reconstitution and up to 48 hours after dilution. Temperatures above 27° C (80° F) will cause liquefaction of the drug powder; discard immediately.

INCOMPATIBLE WITH
Consider incompatible with any other drug in syringe or solution because of toxicity and specific use. Allopurinol (Zyloprim), sodium bicarbonate.

RATE OF ADMINISTRATION
Each single dose must be given as an infusion over a minimum of 1 hour. Reduce rate for pain or burning at injection site, flushing of the skin, or suffusion of the conjunctiva. Usually given over 1 to 2 hours.

ACTIONS
An alkylating agent of the nitrosourea group with antitumor activity, cell cycle phase nonspecific. Degraded to metabolites within 15 minutes of administration. Effectively crosses the blood-brain barrier; concentration higher in cerebrospinal fluid than in plasma. Excreted in changed form in urine. Small amounts excreted as respiratory CO_2.

INDICATIONS AND USES
Suppress or retard neoplastic growth of brain tumors; multiple myeloma; GI, breast, bronchogenic, and renal carcinomas; meningeal leukemia; Hodgkin's disease; and some non-Hodgkin's lymphomas.

CONTRAINDICATIONS
Hypersensitivity to carmustine, previous chemotherapy, or other causes that result in insufficient circulating platelets, leukocytes, or erythrocytes.

PRECAUTIONS
■ Follow guidelines for handling cytotoxic agents. See Appendix A, p. 893. ■ Administered by or under the direction of the physician specialist. ■ Often used with other antineoplastic drugs in reduced doses to achieve tumor remission. ■ Pulmonary toxicity associated with cumulative dose > 1400 mg/M^2. Delayed onset pulmonary fibrosis has occurred up to 15 years after treatment with injectable carmustine in patients who received it in childhood or early adolescence.

Monitor: Determine absolute patency and quality of vein and adequate circulation of extremity. Severe cellulitis may result from extravasation. ■ Delayed toxicity probable in 4 to 6 weeks; wait at least 6 weeks between doses; frequent CBCs including leukocyte and platelet counts indicated. ■ Nausea and vomiting can be severe. Prophylactic administration of antiemetics recommended. ■ Avoid contact of carmustine solution with the skin. ■ Observe for any signs of infection. Prophylactic antibiotics may be indicated pending results of C/S in a febrile neutropenic patient. ■ Maintain hydration.

Patient education: Nonhormonal birth control recommended. ■ Report stinging or burning at IV site promptly. ■ See Appendix D, p. 900.

Maternal/child: Category D: avoid pregnancy; will produce teratogenic effects in rats; has mutagenic potential. ▪ Discontinue breast
feeding.

Elderly: Consider age-related renal impairment, toxicity may be
increased.

DRUG/LAB INTERACTIONS

Potentiates or is potentiated by hepatotoxic or nephrotoxic medications and radiation therapy. ▪ Potentiated by cimetidine (Tagamet);
may cause increased myelosuppression. ▪ Inhibits digoxin and phenytoin (Dilantin); may reduce serum levels. ▪ May cause corneal and
conjunctival epithelial damage with mitomycin. ▪ Do not administer
vaccine or chloroquine to patients receiving antineoplastic drugs.
▪ Note Dose adjustments.

SIDE EFFECTS

Most are dose related and can be reversed. Bone marrow toxicity
(especially leukopenia and thrombocytopenia) most pronounced at 4
to 6 weeks; can be severe and cumulative with repeated dosage.
Anemia, elevated liver function test results, flushing of skin and suffusion of conjunctiva from too-rapid infusion rate, hyperpigmentation
and burning of skin (from actual contact with solution), nausea and
vomiting, pulmonary infiltrates or fibrosis with long-term therapy,
renal abnormalities, retinal hemorrage.

ANTIDOTE

Notify physician of all side effects. Most will decrease in severity
with reduced dosage, increased time span between doses, or symptomatic treatment. May reduce therapeutic effectiveness. Hematopoietic
depression may require withholding carmustine until recovery occurs.
There is no specific antidote. Supportive therapy as indicated will help
sustain the patient in toxicity. For extravasation, elevate extremity,
consider injection of long-acting dexamethasone (Decadron LA) or
hyaluronidase (Wydase) throughout extravasated tissue. Use a 27- or
25-gauge needle. Apply warm moist compresses.

CEFAMANDOLE NAFATE

Mandol

Antibacterial
Cephalosporin

pH 6.0 to 8.5

USUAL DOSE

Range is from 500 mg to 2 Gm every 4 to 8 hours. Severe infections may require 1 Gm every 4 to 6 hours. Life-threatening infections may require 2 Gm every 4 hours. Larger doses may also be required with less susceptible organisms. Do not exceed 12 Gm/24 hr.

Uncomplicated pneumonia, skin and soft tissue infections: 500 mg every 6 hours.

GU infections: 500 mg every 8 hours. Increase to 1 Gm every 8 hours in serious GU infections.

Perioperative prophylaxis: 1 or 2 Gm 30 minutes to 1 hour before incision. Follow with 1 to 2 Gm every 6 hours for 24 to 48 hours. Extend to 72 hours in patients undergoing prosthetic arthroplasty. During **cesarean section**, initial dose is given immediately prior to surgery or just after the cord is clamped.

PEDIATRIC DOSE

50 to 100 mg/kg of body weight/24 hr in equally divided doses every 4 to 8 hours. May be increased to 150 mg/kg/24 hr in serious infections. Do not exceed 150 mg/kg/24 hr or maximum adult dose.

Perioperative prophylaxis; infants over 3 months of age: 50 to 100 mg/kg/24 hr in equally divided doses. Give first dose 30 minutes to 1 hour before incision and then every 6 hours for up to 24 to 48 hours.

DOSE ADJUSTMENTS

Reduce total daily dose if renal function impaired. Calculated according to degree of impairment (see literature). ■ Note Drug/lab interactions.

DILUTION

Forms carbon dioxide after initial dilution; use caution when drawing from vial; do not store in syringe.

Direct IV: Each 1 Gm or fraction thereof must be reconstituted with at least 10 ml SW, D5W, or NS. (1 Gm in 22 ml sterile water is isotonic).

Intermittent infusion: Further dilute in 50 to 100 ml D5W or NS for infusion and give through Y-tube, three-way stopcock, or additive infusion set. Also available in Add-Vantage vials for use with Abbott ADD-Vantage diluent containers.

Continuous infusion: May be further diluted in up to 1,000 ml compatible infusion solutions (e.g., D5W, D10W, 2%, 0.45%, or 0.9% NS with or without dextrose, 1/6 molar lactate).

Storage: Administer within 24 hours of preparation if unrefrigerated or within 96 hours if refrigerated.

INCOMPATIBLE WITH

Manufacturer recommends temporarily discontinuing other solutions infusing at the same site to avoid compatibility problems. Acetated Ringer's injection, all aminoglycosides (e.g., amikacin [Amikin], gentamicin [Garamycin], tobramycin [Nebcin]), amiodarone (Cordarone), calcium, carbenicillin (Geopen), cimetidine (Tagamet), D5/Isolyte M, diltiazem (Cardizem), hetastarch (Hespan), lidocaine (Xylocaine), magnesium, metronidazole (Flagyl IV), Plasma-Lyte, ranitidine (Zantac), Ringer's and lactacted Ringer's injection.

RATE OF ADMINISTRATION

Note Incompatible with. Each 1 Gm or fraction thereof over 3 to 5 minutes or longer as indicated by amount of solution and condition of the patient. Rate of continuous infusion should be by physician order.

ACTIONS

A semisynthetic second-generation broad-spectrum cephalosporin antibiotic that is bactericidal to specific gram-positive, gram-negative, and anaerobic organisms. Peak serum levels achieved by end of infusion. Widely distributed in most tissues, body fluids (CSF minimal), bone, gallbladder, myocardium, and skin and soft tissue. Crosses the placental barrier. Excreted rapidly in the urine. Secreted in breast milk.

INDICATIONS AND USES

Treatment of serious respiratory tract, GU tract, bone, joint, soft tissue, and skin infections; septicemia, and peritonitis. Effective only if the causative organism is susceptible. ▪ Perioperative prophylaxis.

CONTRAINDICATIONS

Previous allergic reaction to cephalosporins or related antibiotics (penicillins). Absolute only if reaction was serious.

PRECAUTIONS

Sensitivity studies indicated to determine susceptibility of the causative organism to cefamandole. ▪ Continue for at least 2 to 3 days after all symptoms of infection subside. ▪ Avoid prolonged use of drug; superinfection caused by overgrowth of nonsusceptible organisms may result. ▪ Use caution in patients with impaired renal function; a history of GI disease (especially colitis), bleeding disorders, or allergies; and those receiving an extended course of cephalosporins.

Monitor: Watch for early symptoms of allergic reaction. ▪ Use extreme caution in the penicillin-sensitive patient; incidence of cross-sensitivity may range from 3% to 16%. ▪ Observe for electrolyte imbalance and cardiac irregularities. Each gram contains 3.3 mEq of sodium. ▪ May cause hypoprothrombinemia (deficiency of prothrombin [Factor II]); 10 mg/week of prophylactic vitamin K may be indicated in elderly, debilitated, or other patients with vitamin K deficiency. Monitor prothrombin times. ▪ Note Drug/lab interactions; additional monitoring may be indicated (e.g., renal function, drug serum levels, prothrombin times).

Patient education: Avoid alcohol or alcohol-containing preparations; may cause abdominal cramps, headache, flushing, nausea and vomiting, shortness of breath, sweating and tachycardia. ▪ Report promptly any bleeding or bruising, diarrhea, symptons of allergy (e.g., difficulty breathing, hives, itching, rash).

Maternal/child: Category B: safety for use during pregnancy and lactation not established. No problems documented. ▪ Safety for use in infants under 1 month of age not established; immature renal function will increase blood levels.

Elderly: No specific problems documented. Consider age-related impaired organ function and nutritional status; reduced dose or extended intervals may be indicated.

DRUG/LAB INTERACTIONS

May produce symptoms of acute alcohol intolerance with alcohol (a disulfiramlike reaction [abdominal cramps, headache, flushing, nausea and vomiting, shortness of breath, sweating, tachycardia]). Patient must abstain from alcohol during treatment until at least 72 hours after discontinued. ■ Frequently used concomitantly with aminoglycosides in severe infections, but these drugs must never be mixed in the same infusion or given concurrently. ■ Risk of nephrotoxicity may be increased with aminoglycosides and other nephrotoxic agents (e.g., loop diuretics [such as furosemide [Lasix]). ■ Probenecid inhibits excretion and may require reduction in dosage. ■ May be antagonized by bacteriostatic antibiotics (e.g., chloramphenicol, erythromycin, tetracyclines); bactericidal action may be negated. ■ Bleeding tendency may be increased with any medicine that affects blood clotting (e.g., heparin and oral anticoagulants [warfarin (Coumadin)], thrombolytic agents [e.g., alteplase (tPA)], salicylates, NSAIDs [e.g., ibuprofen (Motrin), sulfinpyrazone [Anturane]) ■ Large amounts of cephalosporins and/or salicylates may induce hypoprothrombinemia. ■ False-positive reaction for urine glucose except with Tes-Tape or Chemstik. ■ May produce false-positive test for proteinuria. ■ Note Side effects.

SIDE EFFECTS

Allergic reactions including anaphylaxis; anorexia; bleeding episodes; diarrhea; jaundice; leukopenia; local site pain; nausea and vomiting; neutropenia; oral thrush; phlebitis; positive direct Coombs' test; prolonged prothrombin time, pseudomembranous colitis; transient elevation of AST (SGOT), ALT (SGPT), BUN, and alkaline phosphatase; proteinuria; seizures (large doses); thrombophlebitis; vaginal itching or discharge. Hypoprothrombinemia may occur (rare).

ANTIDOTE

Notify physician of any side effects. Discontinue the drug if indicated. Treat allergic reaction as indicated and resuscitate as necessary. Hemodialysis or peritoneal dialysis may be useful in overdose. Vitamin K, fresh-frozen plasma, packed red cells, or platelet concentrates may be indicated in abnormal bleeding tendencies confirmed by lab evaluations. If bleeding due to platelet dysfunction, discontinue and use an alternate antibiotic. Treat antibiotic-related pseudomembranous colitis with oral metronidazole (Flagyl) or vancomycin.

CEFAZOLIN SODIUM

Antibacterial
(Cephalosporin)

Ancef, Kefzol, Zolicef

pH 4.5 to 7.0

USUAL DOSE

250 mg to 1.5 Gm every 6 to 8 hours. Up to 6 Gm is usual but 12 Gm in 24 hours has been used, depending on severity of infection.

Mild infections: 250 to 500 mg every 8 hours.

Moderate to severe infections: 500 mg to 1 Gm every 6 to 8 hours.

Life-threatening infections (e.g., endocarditis, septicemia): 1 to 1.5 Gm every 6 hours.

Pneumococcal pneumonia: 500 mg every 12 hours.

Uncomplicated GU infections: 1 Gm every 12 hours.

Perioperative prophylaxis: 1 Gm 30 minutes to 1 hour before incision. 0.5 to 1 Gm may be repeated in 2 hours in the OR and every 6 to 8 hours for 24 hours or for up to 5 days in specific situations.

PEDIATRIC DOSE

Over 1 month of age: 25 to 50 mg/kg of body weight/24 hr in 3 or 4 equally divided doses. May be increased to 100 mg/kg/24 hr in severe infections. Do not exceed adult dose.

NEONATAL DOSE

Note Maternal/Child.

Less than 7 days of age or over 7 days but under 2,000 Gm: 20 mg/kg every 12 hours.

7 days to 1 month of age and over 2,000 Gm: 20 mg/kg every 8 hours.

DOSE ADJUSTMENTS

Reduce total daily dose if renal function impaired. Calculated according to degree of impairment (see literature).

DILUTION

Each 1 Gm or fraction thereof must be reconstituted with at least 10 ml of sterile water for injection. To reduce the incidence of thrombophlebitis, may be further diluted in 50 to 100 ml of D5W, NS, or other compatible infusion solutions (see chart on back cover or literature) and given as an intermittent infusion. Available premixed and in ADD-Vantage vials for use with Abbott ADD-Vantage diluent containers. May be administered through Y-tube, three-way stopcock, or additive infusion set.

Storage: Give within 24 hours of preparation, or within 96 hours if under refrigeration.

INCOMPATIBLE WITH

Aminoglycosides (e.g., amikacin [Amikin], gentamicin [Garamycin], tobramycin [Nebcin]), amiodarone (Cordarone), amobarbital (Amytal), ascorbic acid, atracurium (Tracrium), bleomycin (Blenoxane), calcium gluceptate, calcium gluconate, cimetidine (Tagamet), colistimethate (Coly-Mycin M), erythromycin, hetastarch (Hespan), hydromorphone (Dilaudid), idarubicin (Idamycin), lidocaine (Xylocaine), pentamidine (Pentam 300), pentobarbital (Nembutal), polymyxin B, vinorelbine (Navelbine).

RATE OF ADMINISTRATION

Each 1 Gm or fraction thereof over 5 minutes or longer as indicated by amount of solution and condition of patient.

ACTIONS

A semisynthetic first-generation broad-spectrum cephalosporin antibiotic that is bactericidal through inhibition of cell wall synthesis to some gram-positive and gram-negative organisms, including staphylococci and streptococci. A number of organisms are resistant to this cephalosporin. Peak serum levels achieved by end of infusion. Widely distributed in most tissues, body fluids (CSF minimal), bone, gallbladder, myocardium, and skin and soft tissue. Crosses the placental barrier. Excreted rapidly in the urine. Secreted in breast milk.

INDICATIONS AND USES

Treatment of serious infections of the bone, joints, skin, soft tissue, respiratory tract, biliary tract, and GU tract; septicemia and endocarditis. Effective only if the causative organism is susceptible. ▪ Perioperative prophylaxis.

CONTRAINDICATIONS

Previous allergic reaction to cephalosporins or related antibiotics (penicillins). Absolute only if reaction was serious.

PRECAUTIONS

Sensitivity studies indicated to determine susceptibility of the causative organisms to cefazolin. ▪ Continue for at least 2 to 3 days after all symptoms of infection subside. ▪ Avoid prolonged use of drug; superinfection caused by overgrowth of nonsusceptible organisms may result. ▪ Use caution in patients with impaired renal function, allergies, or a history of GI disease (especially colitis). ▪ Continuous IV infusion not recommended; markedly increases incidence of phlebitis. *Monitor:* Watch for early symptoms of allergic reaction. ▪ Use extreme caution in the penicillin-sensitive patient; incidence of cross-sensitivity may range from 3% to 16%. ▪ Observe for electrolyte imbalance and cardiac irregularities. Contains 2.1 mEq sodium per Gm. ▪ Note Drug/lab interactions; additional monitoring may be indicated (e.g., renal function, drug serum levels, prothrombin times).

Patient education: Report promptly any bleeding or bruising, diarrhea or symptons of allergy (e.g., difficulty breathing, hives, itching, rash).

Maternal/child: Category B: safety for use during pregnancy and lactation not established. No problems documented. ▪ Safety for use in infants under 1 month of age not established; immature renal function will increase blood levels.

Elderly: No specific problems documented. Consider age-related impaired organ function and nutritional status; reduced dose or extended intervals may be indicated.

DRUG/LAB INTERACTIONS

Frequently used concomitantly with aminoglycosides in severe infections, but these drugs must never be mixed in the same infusion or given concurrently. Risk of nephrotoxicity may be increased with aminoglycosides and other nephrotoxic agents (e.g., loop diuretics [e.g., furosemide (Lasix)]). ▪ Probenecid inhibits excretion and may require reduced dose. ▪ May be antagonized by bacteriostatic antibiotics (e.g., chloramphenicol, erythromycin, tetracyclines); bactericidal action may be negated. ▪ Large amounts of cephalosporins and/or salicylates may induce hypoprothrombinemia (deficiency of prothrombin [Factor II]). The addition of agents which may affect platelet aggregation and/or may have GI ulcerative potential (e.g., NSAIDs [ibuprofen (Motrin)] or sulfinpyrazone [Anturane]) may increase risk of hemorrhage. ▪ False-positive reaction for urine glucose except with Tes-Tape or Chemstik. ▪ Note Side effects.

SIDE EFFECTS

Allergic reactions including anaphylaxis; anorexia, diarrhea, leukopenia, local site pain, nausea and vomiting, neutropenia, oral thrush, phlebitis, positive direct and indirect Coombs' test, prolonged prothrombin time, pseudomembranous colitis, transient elevation of AST (SGOT), ALT (SGPT), BUN, and alkaline phosphatase, seizures (large doses), thrombophlebitis, vaginal itching or discharge. Hypoprothrombinemia may occur (rare).

ANTIDOTE

Notify the physician of any side effects. Discontinue the drug if indicated. Treat antibiotic-related pseudomembranous colitis with oral metronidazole (Flagyl) or vancomycin. Treat allergic reaction as indicated, and resuscitate as necessary. Hemodialysis may be useful in overdose.

CEFEPIME HYDROCHLORIDE

Maxipime

Antibacterial
(Cephalosporin)

pH 4.0 to 6.0

USUAL DOSE

Adults and children over 12 years of age: Range is from 0.5 Gm to 2 Gm. Usually given every 12 hours. Dose based on severity of disease and/or specific organism according to the following chart.

Site and type of infection	Dose	Frequency	Duration (days)
Mild to Moderate Uncomplicated or Complicated Urinary Tract Infections	0.5-1g IV/IM	q12h	7-10
Severe Uncomplicated or Complicated Urinary Tract Infections	2 g IV	q12h	10
Moderate to Severe Pneumonia	1-2 g IV	q12h	10
Moderate to Severe Uncomplicated Skin and Skin Structure Infections	2 g IV	q12h	10
Empiric Therapy for febrile neutropenic patients.	2 g IV	q8h	7 or until neutropenia resolves.
Complicated Intraabdominal Infections	Cefepime 2 g IV + metronidazole 500 mg or 7.5 mg/kg not to exceed 4g/24 hr	q12h q6h	7 to 10 7 to 10

DOSE ADJUSTMENTS

In impaired renal function, the initial dose should be as above, but all remaining doses should be reduced based on creatinine clearance according to chart below (e.g., if the normal dose is 1 Gm every 12 hr with a CrCl >60 the maintenance dose would be reduced to 1 Gm every 24 hr with a CrCl between 30 and 60 ml/min).

Creatinine Clearance (ml/min)	Recommended Maintenance Schedule (relative to normal dosing schedule)		
Normal recommended dosing schedule (>60)	**500 mg q12h**	**1 g q12h**	**2 g q12h**
30-60	500 mg q24h	1 g q24h	2 g q24h
11-29	500 mg q24h	500 mg q24h	1 g q24h
≤10	250 mg q24h	250 mg q24h	500 mg q24h

Consult literature for conversion formula if dose is to be based on serum creatinine. ■ Give a repeat dose equal to the initial dose at the end of a hemodialysis session. ■ Give the Usual dose to patients on continuous ambulatory peritoneal dialysis, but increase intervals between each dose to 48 hours. ■ Reduced dose may be required in the elderly based on renal function. ■ Dose adjustment not required in impaired hepatic function.

DILUTION

Available in vials (IM/IV), piggyback, and ADD-Vantage preparations.

Vials may be reconstituted (see table below) and then further diluted with NS, D5W, D10W, D5/NS, D5/LR, M/6 sodium lactate, Normosol-R, or D5/Normosol M. Concentrations between 1 mg/ml and 40 mg/ml are acceptable. (500 mg reconstituted with 5 ml = 100 mg/ml, further diluted with 95 ml = 5 mg/ml, with 45 ml = 10 mg/ml.)

Piggyback preparations must be diluted with 50 to 100 ml of any of the above compatible solutions.

ADD-Vantage vials must only be diluted with 50 to 100 ml of NS or D5W in Abbott ADD-Vantage diluent containers.

Single-Dose Vials for Intravenous/ Intramuscular Administration	Amount of Diluent to Be Added (ml)	Approximate Available Volume (ml)	Approximate Cefepime Concentration (mg/ml)
Cefepime vial content			
500 mg (iv)	5	5.6	100
500 mg (im)	1.3	1.8	280
1 g (iv)	10	11.3	100
1 g (im)	2.4	3.6	280
2 g (iv)	10	12.5	160
Piggyback (100 ml)			
1 g bottle	50	50	20
1 g bottle	100	100	10
2 g bottle	50	50	40
2 g bottle	100	100	20
ADD-Vantage			
1 g vial	50	50	20
1 g vial	100	100	10

Storage: Store cefepime in the dry state between 2° to 25°C (36° to 77° F), protect from light. Reconstituted or diluted solutions are stable for 24 hours at controlled room temperature and 7 days if refrigerated.

INCOMPATIBLE WITH

Manufacturer recommends temporarily discontinuing other solutions infusing at the same site. Acyclovir (Zovirax), aminophylline, amphotericin B (Fungizone, Abelcet), ampicillin, chlordiazepoxide (Librium), chlorpromazine (Thorazine), cimetidine (Tagemet), ciprofloxacin (Cipro IV), cisplatin (Platinol), dacarbazine (DTIC), daunorubicin (Cerubidine, Daunoxome), diazepam (Valium), diphenhydramine (Benadryl), dobutamine (Dobutrex), dopamine (Intropin), doxorubicin (Adriamycin, Doxil), droperidol (Inapsine), enalaprilat (Vasotec IV), etoposide (VePesid), famotidine (Pepcid IV), filgrastim (Neupogen), floxuridine, gallium nitrate (Ganite), ganciclovir (Cytovene), gentamicin (Garamycin), haloperidol (Haldol), hydroxyzine (Atarax), idarubicin (Idamycin), ifosfamide (Ifex), magnesium sulfate, mannitol (Osmitrol), mechlorethamine (Nitrogen mustard), meperidine (Demerol), metoclopramide (Reglan), metronidazole (Flagyl IV), miconazole (Monistat IV), mitomycin (Mutamycin), mitoxantrone (Novantrone), morphine, nalbuphine (Nubain), netilimicin (Netromycin), ofloxacin (Floxin IV), ondansetron (Zofran), plicamycin (Mithramycin), prochlorperazine (Compazine), promethazine (Phenergan), streptozocin (Zanosar), tobramycin (Nebcin), vancomycin (Lyphocin), vinblastine (Velban), vincristine (Oncovin).

COMPATIBLE WITH

Physically compatible with many drugs in specific concentrations. See package insert for selected admixtures or consult pharmacist. Manufacturer provides extensive references.

RATE OF ADMINISTRATION

May be given through Y-tube or three-way stopcock of infusion set; note Incompatible with.

Intermittent infusion: A single dose equally distributed over 30 minutes.

ACTIONS

A semisynthetic extended-spectrum fourth-generation cephalosporin antibiotic. Bactericidal to both gram-positive and gram-negative organisms, including many strains resistant to third-generation cephalosporins and aminoglycosides. Acts by inhibition of bacterial wall synthesis. Has a well-balanced spectrum with good antistaphylococcal activity, enhanced activity against gram-negative organisms, and good antipseudomonal activity. Peak serum levels achieved by end of infusion; half-live is 2.2 hours. Therapeutic levels last for 12 hours, allowing for twice-daily dosing. Well distributed into many body fluids and tissues. Crosses inflamed meninges to enter CSF. Partially metabolized; 85% excreted unchanged in urine. May cross placental barrier. Secreted in breast milk.

INDICATIONS AND USES

Treatment of moderate to severe pneumonia caused by susceptible nosocomial pathogens, as well as severe pneumonias complicated by pneumococcal bacteremia. ■ Treatment of uncomplicated and complicated urinary tract infections caused by susceptible organisms, including pyelonephritis and cases associated with concurrent bacteremia. ■ Treatment of uncomplicated skin and skin structure infections caused by susceptible organisms. ■ Empiric monotherapy in the treatment of febrile neutropenic patients. ■ See literature for list of susceptible organisms.

CONTRAINDICATIONS

Patients who have shown immediate hypersensitivity reactions to cefepime, any cephalosporin, cephamycins, penicillamine, penicillins, or other beta-lactam antibiotics.

PRECAUTIONS

Specific sensitivity studies are indicated to determine susceptibility of the causative organism to cefepime. ■ Use extreme caution in the penicillin-sensitive patient; incidence of cross-sensitivity among beta-lactam antibiotics may be up to 10%. ■ IM injection is used only for mild to moderate urinary tract infections. ■ Avoid prolonged use of drug; superinfection caused by overgrowth of nonsusceptible organisms may result. ■ Continue for at least 2 days after all symptoms of infection subside. ■ May decrease prothrombin activity, especially in patients with impaired renal or hepatic function, those in a poor nutritional state, and those receiving extended courses of antimicrobial therapy. ■ Use caution in patients with a history of GI disease (especially colitis). ■ Contains arginine, which may alter glucose metabolism and elevate serum potassium. ■ Higher end doses may increase incidence and severity of rash and require cefepime to be discontinued. ■ Insufficient data exist for treatment of febrile neutropenia in patients at high risk for severe infection (e.g., history of recent bone marrow transplant, hypotension on presentation, underlying hematologic malignancy, severe or prolonged neutropenia). No data are available for patients with septic shock.

Monitor: Watch for early symptoms of allergic reaction. ■ Obtain baseline CBC with differential and platelets and serum creatinine. ■ Record vital signs at least 3 times daily. ■ Obtain baseline prothrombin time and monitor, especially in at-risk patients (See Precautions) ; vitamin K may be indicated. ■ Monitoring of serum glucose and electrolytes (e.g., potassium, calcium) may be indicated. ■ May cause thrombophlebitis. ■ Monitor and re-evaluate frequently the need for continued antimicrobial treatment in patients whose fever resolves but who remain neutropenic for more than 7 days. ■ Note Drug/lab interactions.

Patient education: Promptly report any bleeding or bruising, diarrhea, or symptons of allergy (e.g., difficulty breathing, hives, itching, rash).

Maternal/child: Category B: safety for use during pregnancy and lactation not established; use only if clearly needed. ■ A nursing infant consuming 1 quart of breast milk in a day would receive about 0.5 mg of cefepime. ■ Safety and effectiveness not established for children under 12 years of age. ■ Immature renal function of infants and small children will increase blood levels of all cephalosporins.

Elderly: No specific problems documented. Consider age-related impaired organ function and nutritional status; reduced dose or extended intervals may be indicated. Monitor for hypocalcemia.

DRUG/LAB INTERACTIONS

May be used concomitantly with aminophylline, aminoglycosides (gentamicin, netilimicin, tobramycin), ampicillin at concentrations < 40 mg/ml, clindamycin (Cleocin), metronidazole (Flagyl), and vancomycin, but these drugs must never be mixed in the same infusion or given concurrently (the exception is amikacin in specific concentrations and solutions). Monitor renal function carefully, especially with high doses of aminoglycosides. ■ Risk of nephrotoxicity may be increased with aminoglycosides and other nephrotoxic agents (e.g., loop diuretics [e.g., furosemide (Lasix)]); monitor renal function closely. ■ May cause a false-positive direct Coombs's test. ■ May have a false-positive reaction for urine glucose except with Tes-Tape or Clinistix. ■ Note Side effects. ■ While it has not been specifically studied with cefepime, other cephalosporins have the following drug interactions. May be antagonized by bacteriostatic antibiotics (e.g., chloramphenicol, erythromycin, tetracyclines); bactericidal action may be negated. ■ Large amounts of cephalosporins and/or salicylates may induce hypoprothrombinemia (deficiency of prothrombin [Factor II]). The addition of agents that affect platelet aggregation and/or may have GI ulcerative potential (e.g., NSAIDs [ibuprofen (Motrin)] or sulfinpyrazone [Anturane]) may increase risk of hemorrhage.

SIDE EFFECTS

Full scope of allergic reactions (e.g., anaphylaxis, itching, rash, urticaria). Burning, discomfort, pain, or phlebitis at injection site; diarrhea; elevated alkaline phosphotase, AST (SGOT), ALT (SGPT), BUN; fever; headache; nausea and vomiting; oral moniliasis; prolonged prothrombin time; pseudomenbranous colitis; seizures (large doses or standard doses in renally impaired); vaginitis.

Overdose: Encephalopathy, neuromuscular excitability, seizures.

ANTIDOTE

Notify physician of any side effects. Discontinue cefepime and treat allergic reaction as indicated (airway, oxygen, IV fluids, epinephrine, corticorsteroids, pressor amines [e.g., dopamine], antihistamines [e.g., diphenhydramine]). Resuscitate as necessary. Discontinue cefepime if seizures occur and treat with anticonvulsants (e.g., diazepam [Valium]). Mild cases of colitis may respond to discontinuation of cefepime. Oral vancomycin (Vancocin) or metronidazole (Flagyl) is the treatment of choice for antibiotic-related pseudomembranous colitis. Hemodialysis may be useful in overdose.

CEFMETAZOLE SODIUM   Antibacterial
                                          (Cephalosporin)
Zefazone   pH 4.2 to 6.2

USUAL DOSE

2 Gm every 6, 8, or 12 hours. Dose based on severity of disease and patient's condition.

Perioperative prophylaxis: Dose requirements and time frames vary with specific surgery (see specific doses below). In all situations repeat the preoperative dose if the surgery lasts more than 4 hours. Preoperative bowel preparation recommended.

Vaginal hysterectomy: 2 Gm 30 to 90 minutes before surgery as a single dose or 1 Gm 30 to 90 minutes before surgery repeated in 8 hours and again in 16 hours.

Abdominal hysterectomy or high-risk cholecystectomy: 1 Gm 30 to 90 minutes before surgery. Repeat in 8 hours and again in 16 hours.

Colorectal surgery: 2 Gm 30 to 90 minutes before surgery. May be given as a single dose or repeated in 8 hours and again in 16 hours.

Cesarean Section: 2 Gm after clamping the cord as a single dose or 1 Gm after clamping the cord, repeated in 8 hours and again in 16 hours.

DOSE ADJUSTMENTS

Reduce total daily dose if renal function impaired. Calculated according to degree of impairment (see literature).

DILUTION

Initially reconstitute with SW, bacteriostatic water for injection, or NS. For 1 Gm use 3.7 ml (250 mg/ml) or 10 ml (100 mg/ml). For 2 Gm use 7 ml (250 mg/ml) or 15 ml (125 mg/ml). Shake to dissolve and let stand until clear. May be further diluted with NS, D5W or LR to solutions containing 1 to 20 mg/ml. Usually given as an intermittent infusion but may be given direct IV in otherwise healthy patients when used for surgical prophylaxis.

Storage: Stable after dilution for 24 hours at room temperature, 7 days if refrigerated. May be frozen for up to 6 weeks after initial dilution; thaw at room temperature (see literature); do not refreeze.

INCOMPATIBLE WITH

Manufacturer recommends temporarily discontinuing other solutions infusing at the same site to avoid compatibility problems. Inactivates heparin; administer heparin at another site. Should be considered incompatible in syringe or solution with any other bacteriostatic agents and all aminoglycosides (e.g., gentamicin [Garamycin]).

COMPATIBLE WITH

May have additive compatibility with clindamycin (Cleocin) and KCL; consult pharmacist.

RATE OF ADMINISTRATION

Note Incompatible with. Either route may be given through a Y-tube or three-way stopcock of infusion set.

Direct IV for surgical prophylaxis: A single dose equally distributed over 3 to 5 minutes.

Intermittent IV: A single dose over 10 to 60 minutes.

ACTIONS

A semisynthetic, second-generation broad-spectrum cephalosporin antibiotic. Bactericidal through inhibition of cell wall synthesis to a wide range of selected aerobic and anaerobic gram-negative and gram-positive organisms. Onset of action is prompt, and serum levels are dose related. Half-life averages 1.2 hours. Peak serum levels achieved at end of infusion. Widely distributed in most tissues, body fluids (CSF minimal), bone, gallbladder, myocardium, and skin and soft tissue (e.g., vaginal, uterine, adnexal). 85% excreted unchanged in the urine within 12 hours. Crosses placental barrier. Secreted in breast milk.

INDICATIONS AND USES

Treatment of serious urinary tract, lower respiratory tract, skin and skin structure, and intraabdominal infections. Most effective against specific organisms (see literature). ■ Perioperative prophylaxis. ■ Not indicated for infections caused by methicillin-resistant staphylococci.

CONTRAINDICATIONS

Previous allergic reaction to cephalosporins or related antibiotics (penicillins). Absolute only if reaction was serious.

PRECAUTIONS

Specific sensitivity studies are indicated to determine susceptibility of the causative organism to cefmetazole. ■ Continue for 5 to 14 days (at least 2 to 3 days after all symptons of infection subside). ■ Avoid prolonged use of drug; superinfection caused by overgrowth of non-susceptible organisms may result. ■ Use caution in patients with impaired renal function; a history of GI disease (especially colitis), bleeding disorders, or allergies; and those receiving an extended course of cephalosporins.

Monitor: Watch for early symptoms of allergic reaction. Use caution in patients with histories of asthma or other allergies. ■ Use extreme caution in the penicillin-sensitive patient; incidence of cross-sensitivity may range from 3% to 16%. ■ May cause hypoprothrombinemia (deficiency of prothrombin [Factor II]); 10 mg/week of prophylactic vitamin K may be indicated in elderly, debilitated or other patients with vitamin K deficiency. Monitor prothrombin times. ■ May cause thrombophlebitis. Use small needles and large veins, and rotate infusion sites. ■ Observe for electrolyte imbalance and cardiac irregularities; contains 2 mEq of sodium/Gm. ■ Note Drug/lab interactions; additional monitoring may be indicated (e.g., renal function, drug serum levels, prothrombin times).

Patient education: Avoid alcohol or alcohol-containing preparations; may cause abdominal cramps, headache, flushing, nausea and vomiting, shortness of breath, sweating, and tachycardia. ■ Report promptly any bleeding or bruising, diarrhea, symptons of allergy (e.g., difficulty breathing, hives, itching, rash).

Maternal/child: Category B: Safety for use in pregnancy not established. ■ Discontinue breast feeding until course of therapy complete. (One reference says no problems documented in nursing infants.) ■ Safety for use in children not established. Some testicular atrophy occurred in young rats given high doses.

Elderly: No specific problems documented. Consider age-related impaired organ function and nutritional status; reduced dose or extended intervals may be indicated.

DRUG/LAB INTERACTIONS

Frequently used concomitantly with aminoglycosides (e.g., gentamicin [Garamycin]) in severe infection, but these drugs must never be mixed in the same infusion or given concurrently. ■ Risk of nephrotoxicity may be increased with aminoglycosides and other neprotoxic agents (e.g., loop diuretics such as furosemide [Lasix]). ■ May be antagonized by bacteriostatic antibiotics (e.g., chloramphenicol, erythromycin, tetracyclines); bactericidal action may be negated. ■ May produce symptons of acute alcohol intolerance with alcohol (a disulfiramlike reaction [abdominal cramps, headache, flushing, nausea and vomiting, shortness of breath, sweating, tachycardia]). Patient must abstain from alcohol during treatment and until at least 48 to 72 hours after discontinuing. ■ Probenecid inhibits excretion and may require reduced dosage. ▪ Bleeding tendency may be increased with any medicine that affects blood clotting (e.g., heparin and oral anticoagulants [warfarin (Coumadin)], thrombolytic agents [e.g., alteplase (tPA)], salicylates, NSAIDs [e.g., ibuprofen (Motrin)], sulfinpyrazone [Anturane]). ▪ Large amounts of cephalosporins and/or salicylates may induce hypoprothrombinemia. ▪ Note Monitor and Side effects.

SIDE EFFECTS

Generally well tolerated. Full scope of allergic reactions including anaphylaxis. Bleeding; burning, discomfort, and pain at injection site; candidiasis; changes in color perception; decreased serum albumin and total serum protein; diarrhea; dyspnea; elevated alkaline phosphatase, AST (SGOT), ALT (SGPT), bilirubin, and LDH; elevated prothrombin time (PT), PTT, and other differential blood cell abnormalities (e.g., lymphocytopenia); elevated serum glucose; epigastric pain; headache; hot flashes; hypotension; nausea and vomiting; pleural effusion; pseudomembranous colitis; seizures; shock. Many additional side effects are possible. Hypoprothrombinemia may occur (rare).

ANTIDOTE

Notify physician of any side effects. Discontinue the drug if indicated. Treat allergic reaction as indicated and resuscitate as necessary. Mild cases of colitis may respond to discontinuation of cefmetazole. Oral vancomycin (Vancocin) or metronidazole (Flagyl) is the treatment of choice for antibiotic-related pseudomembranous colitis. Vitamin K, fresh-frozen plasma, packed red cells, or platelet concentrates may be indicated in abnormal bleeding tendencies confirmed by lab evaluations. If bleeding due to platelet dysfunction, discontinue and use an alternate antibiotic. Overdose may precipitate seizures, especially in patients with renal impairment; may require anticonvulsants (e.g., diazepam [Valium]). Hemodialysis may be useful.

CEFONICID SODIUM

Antibacterial (Cephalosporin)

Monocid

pH 3.5 to 6.5

USUAL DOSE

1 Gm/24 hr. Range is 0.5 to 2 Gm/ 24 hr.

Perioperative prophylaxis: 1 Gm IV 1 hour before incision except during cesarean birth. Given only after clamping the umbilical cord in **cesarean birth.** Daily dose may be repeated for 2 days in prosthetic arthroplasty or open heart surgery.

DOSE ADJUSTMENTS

Reduce total daily dose if renal function impaired. Calculated according to degree of impairment (see literature).

DILUTION

Direct IV: reconstitute 0.5 Gm with 2 ml of sterile water for injection and each 1 Gm with 2.5 ml.

Intermittent IV: A single dose may be further diluted or piggyback vials initially diluted with 50 to 100 ml of D5W, NS, or other compatible infusion solution (see chart on back cover or literature). Shake well. (1 Gm in 18 ml sterile water is isotonic).

Storage: Administer within 24 hours of preparation, or within 72 hours if refrigerated. Slight yellowing does not affect potency.

INCOMPATIBLE WITH

Aminoglycosides (e.g., gentamicin [Garamycin]), filgrastim (Neupogen), hetastarch (Hespan), sagramostim (Leukine). Should be considered incompatible in syringe or solution with any other bacteriostatic agent.

RATE OF ADMINISTRATION

May be given through Y-tube or three-way stop-cock of infusion set.

Direct IV: A single dose equally distributed over 3 to 5 minutes.

Intermittent IV: A single dose over 30 minutes.

ACTIONS

A broad-spectrum second-generation cephalosporin antibiotic. Bactericidal to selected gram-negative, gram-positive, and anaerobic organisms. Effective against many otherwise resistant organisms. Peak serum levels achieved by end of infusion. Widely distributed in most tissues, body fluids (CSF minimal), bone, gallbladder, myocardium, and skin and soft tissue. 99% excreted in the urine. Crosses placental barrier. Secreted in breast milk.

INDICATIONS AND USES

Treatment of serious lower respiratory tract, urinary tract, bone and joint, skin and skin structure infections, and septicemia. Most effective against specific organisms (see literature). ■ Perioperative prophylaxis.

CONTRAINDICATIONS

Previous allergic reaction to cephalosporins, or related antibiotics (penicillins). Absolute only if reaction was serious.

PRECAUTIONS

Specific sensitivity studies are indicated to determine susceptibility of the causative organism to cefonicid. ■ Continue for at least 2 to 3 days after all symptoms of infection subside. ■ Use caution in patients with impaired renal function, allergies, or a history of GI disease (especially colitis). ■ Avoid prolonged use of drug; superinfection caused by overgrowth of nonsusceptible organisms may result.

Monitor: Watch for early symptoms of allergic reaction. ■ Use extreme caution in the penicillin-sensitive patient; incidence of cross-sensitivity may range from 3% to 16%. ■ Single daily dose reduces incidence of thrombophlebitis. Use of small needles and large veins and rotation of infusion sites is still preferred. ■ Observe for electrolyte imbalance and cardiac irregularities. Contains 3.7 mEq sodium per Gm. ■ Note Drug/lab interactions; additional monitoring may be indicated (e.g., renal function, drug serum levels, prothrombin times).

Patient education: Report promptly any bleeding or bruising, diarrhea, or symptons of allergy (e.g., difficulty breathing, hives, itching, rash).

Maternal/child: Category B: safety for use during pregnancy and lactation not established. No problems documented. ■ Has been used in children over 1 year of age but safety not established. Immature renal function of infants and small children will increase blood levels of all cephalosporins.

Elderly: No specific problems documented. Consider age-related impaired organ function and nutritional status; reduced dose or extended intervals may be indicated.

DRUG/LAB INTERACTIONS

Frequently used concomitantly with aminoglycosides in severe infections, but these drugs must never be mixed in the same fusion or given concurrently. ■ Risk of nephrotoxicity may be increased with aminoglycosides and other nephrotoxic agents (e.g., loop diuretics such as furosemide [Lasix]). ■ Probenicid inhibits excretion and may require reduced dose. ■ May be antagonized by bacteriostatic antibiotics (e.g., chloramphenicol, erythromycin, tetracyclines); bactericidal action may be negated. ■ Large amounts of cephalosporins and/or salicylates may induce hypoprothombinemia (deficiency of prothrombin [Factor II]). The addition of agents which affect platelet aggregation and/or may have GI ulcerative potential (e.g., NSAIDs [ibuprofen (Motrin)], or sulfinpyrazone [Anturane]) may increase risk of hemorrhage. ■ Note Side effects.

SIDE EFFECTS

Full scope of allergic reactions including anaphylaxis. Burning, discomfort, and pain at injection site; diarrhea; increase in platelets and eosinophils; elevated alkaline phosphatase, AST (SGOT), ALT (SGPT), GGTP, and LDH; positive direct Coombs' test; prolonged prothrombin time; pseudomembranous colitis; and seizures (large doses). Hypoprothrombinemia may occur (rare).

ANTIDOTE

Notify physician of any side effects. Discontinue the drug if indicated. Treat allergic reaction as indicated and resuscitate as necessary. Mild cases of colitis may respond to discontinuation of cefonicid. Oral vancomycin (Vancocin) or metronidazole (Flagyl) is the treatment of choice for antibiotic-related pseudomembranous colitis. Only small amounts are removed by hemodialysis.

CEFOPERAZONE SODIUM

Antibacterial
(Cephalosporin)

Cefobid

pH 4.5 to 6.5

USUAL DOSE

Moderate infections: 1 to 2 Gm every 12 hours.

Severe infections: 2 to 4 Gm every 8 hours. Up to 12 to 16 Gm has been given in 24 hours.

PEDIATRIC DOSE

50 to 100 mg/kg of body weight every 12 hours. (See Maternal/child).

DOSE ADJUSTMENTS

Reduce total daily dose to 1 to 2 Gm/24 hr if both renal and hepatic function are impaired. ■ Reduce total daily dose to 2 to 4 Gm/24 in impaired hepatic function or biliary obstruction. ■ Note Drug/lab interactions.

DILUTION

Each 1 Gm must be reconstituted with 5 ml sterile water. Difficult to put into solution. Shake vigorously to ensure solution; then allow to sit and examine for clarity. Should be further diluted with 20 to 40 ml D5W, NS, or other compatible solutions (see chart on back cover or literature) to a maximum dilution of 50 mg/ml and given as an intermittent infusion. Available pre-mixed in 50 ml diluent. May be further diluted to 2 to 25 mg/ml and given as a continuous infusion.

Storage: Administer within 24 hours of preparation. Selected solutions may be preserved 5 days with refrigeration.

INCOMPATIBLE WITH

Manufacturer recommends temporarily discontinuing other solutions infusing at the same site to avoid compatibility problems. Amifostine (Ethyol), diltiazem (Cardizem), doxapram (Dopram), filgrastim (Neupogen), hetastarch (Hespan), labetalol (Trandate), meperidine (Demerol), ondansetron (Zofran), pentamidine (Pentam 300), perphenazine (Trilafon), promethazine (Phenergan), sargramostim (Leukine), vinorelbine. Should be considered imcompatible in syringe or solution with all aminoglycosides (e.g., gentamicin [Garamycin] (Navelbine), and any other bacteriostatic agents.

RATE OF ADMINISTRATION

Note Incompatible with.

Intermittent IV: A single dose over 15 to 30 minutes.

Continuous infusion: 500 to 1,000 ml over 6 to 24 hours, depending on total dose and concentration.

ACTIONS

A broad-spectrum third-generation cephalosporin antibiotic. Bactericidal to many gram-negative, gram-positive, and anaerobic organisms. Effective against organisms resistant to other second- and third-generation cephalosporins. Peak serum levels achieved by end of infusion. Widely distributed in most tissues, body fluids (including inflamed meninges), bone, gallbladder (high biliary concentrations), myocardium, and skin and soft tissue. Excreted in bile. Crosses placental barrier. Secreted in breast milk.

INDICATIONS AND USES

Treatment of serious respiratory tract, intraabdominal, skin and skin structure, gynecologic infections, and bacterial septicemia. Most effective against specific organisms (see literature).

CONTRAINDICATIONS

Previous allergic reaction to cephalosporins or related antibiotics (penicillins). Absolute only if reaction was serious.

PRECAUTIONS

Sensitivity studies indicated to determine susceptibility of the causative organism to cefoperazone. ▪ Continue for at least 2 to 3 days after all symptoms of infection subside. ▪ Avoid prolonged use of drug; superinfection caused by overgrowth of nonsusceptible organisms may result. ▪ Use caution in patients with impaired liver function or biliary obstruction, impaire renal function; a history of GI disease (especially colitis), bleeding disorders, or allergies; and those receiving an extended course of cephalosporins.

Monitor: Watch for early symptoms of allergic reaction. ▪ Use extreme caution in the penicillin-sensitive patient; incidence of cross-sensitivity may range from 3% to 16%. ▪ May cause thrombophlebitis. Use small needles and large veins, and rotate infusion sites. ▪ Observe for electrolyte imbalance and cardiac irregularities. Contains 1.5 mEq sodium per Gm. ▪ May cause hypoprothrombinemia (deficiency of prothrombin [Factor II]); 10 mg/week of prophylactic vitamin K may be indicated in elderly, debilitated, or other patients with vitamin K deficiency. Monitor prothrombin times. ▪ Note Drug/lab interactions; additional monitoring may be indicated (e.g., renal function, drug serum levels, prothrombin times).

Patient education: Avoid alcohol or alcohol-containing preparations; may cause abdominal cramping, flushing, headache, nausea and vomiting, shortness of breath, sweating, and tachycardia. ▪ Report promptly any bleeding or bruising, diarrhea, symptoms of allergy (e.g., difficulty breathing, hives, itching, rash).

Maternal/child: Category B: safety for use during pregnancy and lactation not established. No problems documented. ▪ Safety and effectiveness for use in children under 12 years not established.

Elderly: No specific problems documented. Consider age-related impaired organ function and nutritional status, reduced dose or extended intervals may be indicated.

DRUG/LAB INTERACTIONS

May produce symptons of acute alcohol intolerance with alcohol (a disulfiramlike reaction with abdominal cramps, headache, flushing, nausea and vomiting, shortness of breath, sweating, tachycardia). Patient must abstain from alcohol during treatment and until at least 72 hours after discontinued. ▪ Frequently used concomitantly with aminoglycosides in severe infections, but these drugs must never be mixed in the same infusion or given concurrently. Use individual secondary tubings and irrigate primary tubing between doses. ▪ Risk of nephrotoxicity may be increased with aminoglycoside and other nephrotoxic agents (e.g., loop diuretics such as furosemide [Lasix]). ▪ Is not inhibited by probencid as other cephalosporins are because of biliary excretion. ▪ May be antagonized by bacteriostatic antibiotics (e.g., chloramphenicol, erythromycin, tetracyclines); bactericidal action may be negated. ▪ Bleeding tendency may be increased with any medicine that affects blood clotting (e.g., heparin and oral anticoagulants [warfarin (Coumadin)], thrombolytic agents [e.g., alteplase (tPA)], salicylates, NSAIDs [e.g., ibuprofen (Motrin)], sulfinpyrazone [Anturane]). ▪ Large amounts of cephalosporins and/or salicylates may induce hypoprothrombinemia. ▪ Positive Coombs' test. ▪ False-positive reaction for urine glucose except with TesTape or Chemstix. ▪ Note Side effects.

SIDE EFFECTS

Full scope of allergic reactions including anaphylaxis. Abnormal bleeding; decreased hemoglobin or decreased hematocrit; decreased platelet functions; diarrhea, eosinophilia; elevation of AST (SGOT), ALT (SGPT), total bilirubin, alkaline phosphatase, LDH, and BUN (transient); fever; leukopenia; local site pain; positive Coombs' test; prolonged prothrombin time; pseudomembranous colitis; seizures (large doses); thrombocytopenia; thrombophlebitis; transient neutropenia; vaginitis; vomiting. Hypoprothrombinemia may occur (rare).

ANTIDOTE

Notify the physician of any side effects. Discontinue the drug if indicated. Treat allergic reaction as indicated and resuscitate as necessary. Mild cases of colitis may respond to discontinuation of cefoperazone. Oral vancomycin (Vancocin) or metronidazole (Flagyl) is the treatment of choice for antibiotic-related pseudomembranous colitis. Hemodialysis only slightly useful in overdose. Vitamin K, fresh-frozen plasma, packed red cells, or platelet concentrates may be indicated in abnormal bleeding tendencies confirmed by lab evaluations. If bleeding due to platelet dysfunction, discontinue and use an alternate antibiotic.

CEFOTAXIME SODIUM

Antibacterial
(Cephalosporin)

Claforan

pH 4.5 to 7.5

USUAL DOSE

Range is 2 to 12 Gm/24 hr. Depends on seriousness of infection. Maximum daily dose is 12 Gm.

Uncomplicated infections: 1 Gm every 12 hours.

Moderate to severe infections: 1 to 2 Gm every 8 hours.

Serious infections: 2 Gm every 6 to 8 hours.

Life-threatening infections: 2 Gm every 4 hours.

Higher doses often reduced with positive clinical response.

Perioperative prophylaxis: 1 Gm 30 to 90 minutes before incision. May be repeated in a lengthy procedure. In *cesarean section* give initial dose after cord is clamped; then 1 Gm at 6 and 12 hours postoperatively.

PEDIATRIC DOSE

Newborn to 1 week: 50 mg/kg of body weight every 12 hours. Same dose used for *newborn to 4 weeks if weight under 1,200 Gm.*

1 to 4 weeks, over 1,200 Gm: 50 mg/kg every 8 hours.

1 month to 12 years: Weight less than 50 kg, 100 to 200 mg/kg/24 hr in 3 to 4 divided doses.

Meningitis: 50 mg/kg every 6 hours.

DOSE ADJUSTMENTS

In impaired renal function with a creatinine clearance <20 ml/min, reduce dose by one/half. ■ Note Usual dose and Drug/lab interactions.

DILUTION

Each single dose must be reconstituted with 10 ml sterile water, D5W, NS, or other compatible infusion solution (see chart on back cover or literature). Available premixed and in ADD-Vantage vials for use with Abbott ADD-Vantage diluent containers. May be further diluted with compatible solutions and given as an intermittent infusion or added to larger volumes and given as a continuous infusion. (1 Gm in 14 ml of sterile water is isotonic.)

Storage: Administer within 24 hours or within 5 days if refrigerated.

INCOMPATIBLE WITH

Manufacturer recommends temporarily discontinuing other solutions infusing at the same time to avoid compatibility problems. Should be considered incompatible in syringe or solution with any other bacteriostatic agent; all aminoglycosides; all diluents with a pH of 7.5 or more (e.g., aminophylline and sodium bicarbonate) (e.g., gentamicin [Garamycin]), allopurinol (Zyloprim), doxapram (Dopram), filgrastim (Neupogen), fluconazole (Diflucan), hetastarch (Hespan), pentamidine (Pentam 300).

RATE OF ADMINISTRATION

Note Incompatible with. Injection and intermittent infusion may be given through Y-tube or three-way stopcock of infusion set.

Direct IV: A single dose equally distributed over 3 to 5 minutes.

Intermittent IV: A single dose over 30 minutes.

Continuous infusion: 500 to 1,000 ml over 6 to 24 hours, depending on total dose and concentration.

ACTIONS

A broad-spectrum third-generation cephalosporin antibiotic. Bactericidal to many gram-negative, gram-positive, and anaerobic organisms. Effective against many otherwise resistant organisms. Peak serum levels achieved within 30 minutes. Distributed into most body tissues and fluids including inflamed meninges. Some metabolites formed. Excreted in the urine. Crosses placental barrier. Secreted in breast milk.

INDICATIONS AND USES

Treatment of serious lower respiratory tract, urinary tract, skin and skin structure, intraabdominal, bone and joint, CNS, and gynecologic infections; bacteremia/septicemia, disseminated gonococcal infection, and gonococcal ophthalmia. Most effective against specific organisms (see literature). ■ Perioperative prophylaxis.

CONTRAINDICATIONS

Previous allergic reation to cephalosporins or related antibiotics (penicillins). Absolute only if reaction was serious.

PRECAUTIONS

Sensitivity studies indicated to determine susceptibility of the causative organism to cefotaxime. ■ Continue for 2 to 3 days after all symptoms of infection subside. ■ Avoid prolonged use of drug; superinfection caused by overgrowth of nonsusceptible organisms may result. ■ Use caution in patients with impaired renal function, allergies, or a history of GI disease (especially colitis).

Monitor: Watch for early symptoms of allergic reaction. ■ Use extreme caution in the penicillin-sensitive patient; incidence of cross-sensitivity may range from 3% to 16%. ■ May cause thrombophlebitis. Use small needles and large veins, and rotate infusion sites. ■ Observe for electrolyte imbalance or cardiac irregularities. Contains 2.2 mEq sodium per Gm. ■ Note Drug/lab interactions; additional monitoring may be indicated (e.g., renal function, drug serum levels, prothrombin times).

Patient education: Report promptly any bleeding or bruising, diarrhea, or symptons of allergy (e.g., difficulty breathing, hives, itching, rash).

Maternal/child: Category B: safety for use during pregnancy and lactation not established. No problems documented. ■ Immature renal function of infants and small children will increase blood levels of all cephalosporins.

Elderly: No specific problems documented. Consider age-related impaired organ function and nutritional status; reduced dose or extended intervals may be indicated.

DRUG/LAB INTERACTIONS

Frequently used concomitantly with aminoglycosides in severe infections, but these drugs must never be mixed in the same infusion or given concurrently. ■ Risk of nephrotoxicity may be increased with aminoglycosides (not reported with cefotaxime) and other nephrotoxic agents (e.g., loop diuretics [such as furosemide (Lasix)]). ■ Probenecid inhibits excretion and may require reduced dosage. ■ May be antagonized by bacteriostatic antibiotics (e.g., chloramphenicol, erythromycin, tetracyclines); bactericidal action may be negated. ■ Large amounts of cephalosporins and/or salicylates may induce hypoprothrombinemia (deficiency of prothrombin [Factor II]). The addition of agents which affect platelet aggregation and/or may have GI ulcerative potential (e.g., NSAIDs [ibuprofen (Motrin)], or sulfinpyrazone [Anturane]) may increase risk of hemorrhage. ■ Note Side effects.

SIDE EFFECTS

Full scope of allergic reactions including anaphylaxis. Decreased hemoglobin or decreased hematocrit; decreased platelet functions; diarrhea; dyspnea; elevation of AST (SGOT), ALT (SGPT), total bilirubin, alkaline phosphatase, LDH, and BUN (transient); eosinophilia; fever; leukopenia; local site pain; nausea; oral thrush; positive direct Coombs' test; prolonged prothrombin time, pseudomembranous colitis; seizures (large doses); thrombocytopenia; thrombophlebitis; transient neutropenia; vaginitis; vomiting. Hypoprothrombinemia may occur (rare).

ANTIDOTE

Notify the physician of any side effects. Discontinue the drug if indicated. mild cases of colitis may respond to discontinuation of cefotaxime. Oral vancomycin (Vancocin) or metronidazole (Flagyl) is the treatment of choice for antibiotic-related pseudomembranous colitis. Treat allergic reaction as indicated and resuscitate as necessary. Hemodialysis may be useful in overdose.

CEFOTETAN DISODIUM

Antibacterial
(Cephalosporin)

Cefotan

pH 4.0 to 6.5

USUAL DOSE

Range is 1 to 6 Gm/24 hours for 5 to 10 days. Do not exceed 6 Gm/24 hr.

Urinary tract infections: 500 mg to 2 Gm every 12 hours or 1 to 2 Gm every 24 hours.

Moderate infections: 1 or 2 Gm every 12 hours.

Serious infections: 2 Gm every 12 hours.

Life-threatening infections: 3 Gm every 12 hours.

Perioperative prophylaxis: 1 to 2 Gm IV 30 to 60 minutes before incision except during *cesarean section.* Given only after clamping the umbilical cord in cesarean section.

PEDIATRIC DOSE

20 to 40 mg/kg of body weight every 12 hours; note Maternal/Child.

DOSE ADJUSTMENTS

Reduce total daily dose if renal function impaired. Calculated according to degree of impairment (see literature).

DILUTION

Available in vials, piggyback, and ADD-Vantage preparations. With all preparations, after dilution shake well and let stand until clear.

Direct IV: Reconstitute each 1 Gm with 10 ml of sterile water for injection (2 Gm with 20 ml).

Intermittent IV: Vials: A single dose may be further diluted or initially diluted with 50 to 100 ml of D5W or NS.

Piggyback preparations may be diluted with 50 to 100 ml D5W or NS.

ADD-Vantage preparations must be diluted with 50, 100, or 250 ml of NS or D5W provided in flexible diluent containers for administration. Follow manufacturer's instructions.

Storage: Administer within 24 hours of preparation, or within 96 hours if refrigerated. Stable after dilution for 1 week if frozen; thaw at room temperature before use, discard remaining solution, do not refreeze. Slight yellowing does not affect potency.

INCOMPATIBLE WITH

Manufacturer recommends temporarily discontinuing other solutions infusing at the same site to avoid compatibility problems. Should be considered incompatible in syringe or solution with any other bacteriostatic agent; all aminoglycosides (e.g., gentamicin [Garamycin]), doxapram (Dopram), heparin, vinorelbine (Navelbine).

RATE OF ADMINISTRATION

Note Incompatible with. May be given through Y-tube or three-way stopcock of infusion set.

Direct IV: A single dose equally distributed over 3 to 5 minutes.

Intermittent IV: A single dose over 30 minutes.

ACTIONS

A broad-spectrum second-generation cephalosporin antibiotic. Bactericidal to selected gram-negative, gram-positive, and anaerobic organisms. Effective against many otherwise resistant organisms. Peak serum levels achieved at end of infusion. Widely distributed in most tissues, body fluids (CSF minimal), bone, gallbladder, myocardium, and skin and soft tissue. Primarily excreted in the urine. Crosses placental barrier. Secreted in breast milk.

INDICATIONS AND USES

Treatment of serious lower respiratory tract, urinary tract, skin and skin structure, gynecologic, intraabdominal, and bone and joint infections. Most effective against specific organisms (see literature).
 ▪ Perioperative prophylaxis.

CONTRAINDICATIONS

Previous allergic reaction to cephalosporins, or related antibiotics (penicillins). Absolute only if reaction was serious.

PRECAUTIONS

Specific sensitivity studies are indicated to determine susceptibility of the causative organism to cefotetan. ▪ Continue for at least 2 or 3 days after all symptoms of infection subside. ▪ Avoid prolonged use of drug; superinfection caused by overgrowth of nonsusceptible organisms may result. ▪ Use caution in patients with impaired renal function; a history of GI disease (especially colitis); bleeding disoreders, or allergies; and those receiving an extended course of cephalosporins. *Monitor:* Watch for early symptoms of allergic reaction. ▪ Use extreme caution in the penicillin-sensitive patient; incidence of cross-sensitivity may range from 3% to 16%. ▪ May cause hypoprothrombinemia (deficiency of prothrombin [Factor II]); 10 mg/week of prophylactic vitamin K may be indicated in elderly, debilitated, or other patients with vitamin K deficiency. Monitor prothrombin times. ▪ May cause thrombophlebitis. Use small needles and large veins, and rotate infusion sites. ▪ Observe for electrolyte imbalance and cardiac irregularities. Contains 3.5 mEq sodium per Gm. ▪ Note Drug/lab interactions; additional monitoring may be indicated (e.g., renal function, drug serum levels, prothrombin times).

Patient education: Avoid alcohol or alcohol-containing preparations; may cause abdominal cramps, flushing, headache, nausea and vomiting, shortness of breath, sweating and tachycardia. ▪ Report promptly any bleeding or bruising, diarrhea, symptoms of allergy (e.g., difficulty breathing, hives, itching, rash).

Maternal/child: Category B: safety for use during pregnancy and lactation not established. No problems documented. ▪ Safety for use in children not established. Immature renal function of infants and small children will increase blood levels of all cephalosporins.

Elderly: No specific problems documented. Consider age-related impaired organ function and nutritional status, reduced dose or extended intervals may be indicated.

DRUG/LAB INTERACTIONS

May produce symptons of acute intolerance with alcohol (a disulfiramlike reaction with abdominal cramps, headache, flushing, nausea and vomiting, shortness of breath, sweating, tachycardia). Patient must abstain from alcohol during treatment and until at least 72 hours after discontinued. Frequently used concomitantly with aminoglycosides in severe infections, but these drugs must never be mixed in the same infusion or given concurrently. ▪ Risk of nephrotoxicity may be increased with aminoglycosides and other nephrotoxic agents (e.g., loop diuretics [furosemide (Lasix)]). ▪ Sources differ on inhibition of excretion by probenecid. ▪ May be antagonized by bacteriostatic antibiotics (e.g., chloramphenicol, erythomycin, tetracyclines); bactericidal action may be negated. ▪ Bleeding tendency increased with any medicine that affects blood clotting (e.g., heparin and oral anticoagulants [warfarin (Coumadin)], thrombolytic agents [e.g., alteplase (tPA)], salicylates, NSAIDs [e.g., ibuprofen (Motrin)], sulfinpyrazone [anturane]). ▪ Large amounts of cephalosporins and/or salicylates may induce hypoprothrombinemia. ▪ False increases in creatinine levels with Jaffe method. ▪ False-positive for urine glucose except with Tes-Tape or Chemstix. ▪ Positive direct Coombs' test. ▪ Note Side effects.

SIDE EFFECTS

Full scope of allergic reactions, including anaphylaxis. Bleeding episodes; burning, discomfort, and pain at injection site; diarrhea; eosinophilia; elevated alkaline phosphatase, AST (SGOT), ALT (SGPT), and LDH; nausea; prolonged prothrombin time; pseudomembranous colitis; seizures (large doses); thrombocytosis. Hypoprothrom-binemia may occur (rare).

ANTIDOTE

Notify physician of any side effects. Discontinue the drug if indicated. Treat allergic reaction as indicated and resuscitate as necessary. Mild cases of colitis may respond to discontinuation of cefotetan. Oral vancomycin (Vancocin) or metronidazole (Flagyl) is the treatment of choice for antibiotic-related pseudomembranous colitis. Bleeding episodes may respond to Vitamin K or require discontinuation of drug. Fresh-frozen plasma, packed red cells, or platelet concentrates may be indicated in abnormal bleeding tendencies confirmed by lab evaluations. If bleeding due to platelet dysfunction, discontinue and use an alternate antibiotic. Hemodialysis only slightly useful in overdose.

CEFOXITIN SODIUM

Antibacterial
(Cephalosporin)

Mefoxin

pH 4.2 to 8.0

USUAL DOSE

1 to 2 Gm every 6 to 8 hours depending on severity of the infection up to 12 Gm/24 hr.

Uncomplicated infections: 1 Gm every 6 to 8 hours.

Moderately severe to severe infections: 1 Gm every 4 hours or 2 Gm every 6 to 8 hours.

Life-threatening infections: 2 Gm every 4 hours or 3 Gm every 6 hours.

Oral bacterial eikenella corrudens: 1 to 2 Gm every 6 hours.

Perioperative prophylaxis: 2 Gm 30 minutes to 1 hour before incision. Follow with 2 Gm every 6 hours for 24 hours (72 hours after prosthetic arthroplasty).

Prophylaxis during cesarean section: 2 Gm after clamping the umbilical cord. Repeat in 4 hours and again in 8 hours.

Prophylaxis during transurethral prostatectomy: 1 Gm before surgery. May be repeated every 8 hours for up to 5 days.

PEDIATRIC DOSE

Infants and children over 3 months of age: 80 to 160 mg/kg of body weight/24 hours in equally divided doses every 4 to 6 hours. Do not exceed adult dose.

Perioperative prophylaxis in infants and children over 3 months of age: 30 to 40 mg/kg 30 minutes to 1 hour before incision and every 6 hours for 24 hours.

NEONATAL DOSE

Use sterile cefoxitin sodium USP only. Components of other formulations may be harmful.

Prematures over 1,500 Gm and neonates to 1 week of age: 20 to 40 mg/kg every 12 hours.

Neonates 1 to 4 weeks of age: 20 to 40 mg/kg every 8 hours.

Infants 1 to 3 months of age: 20 to 40 mg/kg every 6 to 8 hours.

DOSE ADJUSTMENTS

Reduce total daily dose if renal function impaired; calculated according to degree of impairment (see literature). ■ Note Drug/lab interactions.

DILUTION

Each 1 Gm or fraction thereof must be reconstituted with at least 10 ml of sterile water, D5W, or NS. A single dose may be further diluted in 50 to 1,000 ml of most common infusion solutions (see chart on back cover and literature). Available pre-mixed, in piggyback vials, and in ADD-Vantage vials for use with ADD-Vantage diluent containers. May be given through a Y tube, three-way stopcock, additive infusion set, or as a continuous infusion.

Storage: Administer within 24 hours of preparation. Stable 2 to 7 days, if refrigerated, depending on diluent and concentration; consult pharmacist.

INCOMPATIBLE WITH

Manufacturer recommends temporarily discontinuing other solutions at the same site to avoid compatibility problems. All aminoglycosides (e.g., amikacin [Amikin], gentamicin [Garamycin], tobramycin [Nebcin]), aztreonam (Azactam), filgrastim (Neupogen), hetastarch (Hespan), pentamidine (Pentam 300), ranitidine (Zantac).

RATE OF ADMINISTRATION

Note Incompatible with. Each 1 Gm or fraction thereof over 3 to 5 minutes or longer as indicated by amount of solution and condition of the patient. Rate of continuous infusion should be by physician order.

ACTIONS

A semisynthetic second-generation cephalosporin antibiotic that is bactericidal to many gram-positive, gram-negative, and anaerobic organisms. Peak serum levels achieved by end of infusion. Widely distributed into most body tissues and fluids (CSF minimal), bone, gallbladder, myocardium, and skin and soft tissues. Crosses the placental barrier. Excreted rapidly in the urine. Secreted in breast milk.

INDICATIONS AND USES

Treatment of serious respiratory, GU, intraabdominal, gynecologic, bone and joint, skin and skin structure infections, and septicemia. Effective only if the causative organism is susceptible. ■ Treatment of oral bacterial eikenella corrudens. ■ Perioperative prophylaxis.

CONTRAINDICATIONS

Previous allergic reaction to cephalosporins or related antibiotics (penicillins). Absolute only if reaction was serious.

PRECAUTIONS

Sensitivity studies indicated to determine susceptibility of the causative organism to cefoxitin. ■ Continue for at least 2 to 3 days after all symptoms of infection subside. ■ Avoid prolonged use of drug; superinfection caused by overgrowth of nonsusceptible organisms may result. ■ Use caution in patients with impaired renal function, allergies, or a history of GI disease (especially colitis).

Monitor: Watch for early symptoms of allergic reaction. ■ Use extreme caution in the penicillin-sensitive patient; incidence of cross-sensitivity may range from 3% to 16%. ■ Use of scalp-vein needles may reduce incidence of phlebitis. ■ Observe for electrolyte imbalance or cardiac irregularities. Contains 2.3 mEq sodium/Gm. ■ Note Drug/lab interactions; additional monitoring may be indicated (e.g., renal function, drug serum levels, prothrombin times).

Patient education: Report promptly any bleeding or bruising, diarrhea, or symptoms of allergy (e.g., difficulty breathing, hives, itching, rash).

Maternal/child: Category B: safety for use during pregnancy and lactation not established. No problems documented. ■ A specific formulation is used in infants and children under 3 months but safety not established; immature renal function will increase blood levels. ■ Eosinophilia and elevated AST (SGOT) associated with higher doses in infants and children.

Elderly: No specific problems documented. Consider age-related impaired organ function and nutritional status; reduced dose or extended intervals may be indicated.

DRUG/LAB INTERACTIONS

Frequently used concomitantly with aminoglycosides in severe infections, but these drugs must never be mixed in the same infusion or given concurrently. Risk of nephrotoxicity may be increased with aminoglycosides and other nephrotoxic agents (e.g., loop diuretics such as furosemide [Lasix]). ■ Probenecid inhibits excretion and may require reduction in dosage. ■ May be antagonized by bacteriostatic antibiotics (e.g., chloramphenicol, erythromycin, tetracyclines); bactericidal action may be negated. ■ Large doses of cephalosporins and/or salicylates may induce hypoprothrombinemia (deficiency of prothrombin [Factor II]). The addition of agents which affect platelet aggregation and/or may have GI ulcerative potential (e.g., NSAIDs [ibuprofen (Motrin)], or sulfinpyrazone [Anturane]) may increase risk of hemorrhage. ■ False-positive reaction for urine glucose except with Tes-Tape or Chemstix. ■ Positive Coombs's test. ■ False increases in creatinine levels with Jaffe method. ■ Note Side effects.

SIDE EFFECTS

Allergic reactions including anaphylaxis; anorexia; leukopenia; local site pain; increased prothrombin time, nausea and vomiting; neutropenia; oral thrush; phlebitis; transient elevation of AST (SGOT), ALT (SGPT), BUN, and alkaline phosphatase; prolonged prothrombin time; proteinuria; pseudomembranous colitis; seizures (large doses); and thrombophlebitis. Hypoprothrombinemia may occur (rare).

ANTIDOTE

Notify physician of any side effects. Discontinue the drug if indicated. Oral vancomycin (Vancocin) or metronidazole (Flagyl) is the treatment of choice for antibiotic-related pseudomembranous colitis. Treat allergic reaction as indicated and resuscitate as necessary. Hemodialysis may be useful in overdose.

CEFTAZIDIME

Ceptaz, Fortaz, Tazicef, Tazidime

Antibacterial
(Cephalosporin)

pH 5.5 to 8.0

USUAL DOSE

Range is from 250 mg to 2 Gm every 8 to 12 hours. Dosage based on severity of disease and condition of the patient.

Uncomplicated GU infections: 250 mg every 12 hours.

Complicated GU infections: 500 mg every 8 to 12 hours.

Uncomplicated pneumonia and skin and skin structure infections: 500 mg to 1 Gm every 8 hours.

Bone and joint infections: 2 Gm every 12 hours.

Severe or life-threatening infections: 2 Gm every 8 hours.

Pseudomonal lung infections in cystic fibrosis patients: 30 to 50 mg/kg of body weight every 8 hours. Do not exceed 6 Gm/24 hr.

PEDIATRIC DOSE

Use sodium product only for children under 12 years. Components of other formulations may be harmful.

1 month to 12 years: 30 to 50 mg/kg of body weight every 8 hours. Do not exceed 6 Gm/24 hr.

Cystic fibrosis: 50 mg/kg every 8 hours.

NEONATAL DOSE

Use sodium product only. Components of other formulations may be harmful.

Up to 4 weeks and under 1,200 Gm or 0 to 7 days of age over 1,200 Gm: 30 to 50 mg/kg every 12 hours.

Over 7 days of age and over 1,200 Gm: 30 to 50 mg/kg every 8 hours.

DOSE ADJUSTMENTS

Reduce total daily dose if renal function impaired. Calculated according to degree of impairment (see literature).

DILUTION

Direct IV: Reconstitute 0.5 Gm with 5 ml of sterile water; 1 Gm or more with 10 ml of sterile water for injection. Shake well. Dilution generates CO_2. Invert vial and completely depress plunger of syringe. Insert needle through stopper and keep it within the solution. Expel bubbles from solution in syringe before injection.

Intermittent IV: A single dose may be further diluted in 50 to 100 ml of D5W, NS, or other compatible infusion solutions for injection (see literature or chart on back cover). Also available pre-mixed, in infusion packs, in piggyback vials, and in ADD-Vantage vials for use with ADD-Vantage diluent containers.

Storage: Administer within 24 hours of preparation, or refrigerate for up to 7 days. May be frozen for up to 3 months after initial dilution; thaw at room temperature (see instructions); do not refreeze. Will be light yellow to amber in color depending on concentration and diluent.

INCOMPATIBLE WITH

Manufacturer recommends temporarily discontinuing other solutions infusing at the same site to avoid compatibility problems. Should be considered incompatible in syringe or solution with any other bacteriostatic agent; all aminoglycosides (e.g., gentamicin [Garamycin]), fluconazole [Diflucan], idarubicin (Idamycin), midazolam (Versed), pentamidine (Pentam 300), ranitidine (Zantac), sargramostim (Leukine), vancomycin (will form a precipitate; flush thoroughly before and after if administered through same IV tubing).

RATE OF ADMINISTRATION

Note Incompatible with. May be given through Y-tube or three-way stopcock of infusion set.

Direct IV: A single dose equally distributed over 3 to 5 minutes.

Intermittent IV: A single dose over 30 minutes.

ACTIONS

A broad-spectrum third-generation cephalosporin antibiotic. Bactericidal to selected gram-negative, gram-positive, and anaerobic organisms. Effective against many otherwise resistant organisms including Pseudomonas aeroginosa. Peak serum levels achieved by end of infusion. Therapeutic levels distributed into many body fluids and tissues including CSF. Excreted unchanged in the urine. Crosses placental barrier. Secreted in breast milk.

INDICATIONS AND USES

Treatment of serious lower respiratory tract, urinary tract, skin and skin structure, bone and joint, gynecologic, intraabdominal, CNS infections (including meningitis), and bacterial septicemia. Most effective against specific organisms (see literature).

CONTRAINDICATIONS

Previous allergic reaction to cephalosporins or related antibiotics (penicillins). Absolute only if reaction was serious.

PRECAUTIONS

Specific sensitivity studies are indicated to determine susceptibility of the causative organism to ceftazidime. ■ Continue for at least 2 days after all symptons of infection subside. ■ Avoid prolonged use of drug; superinfection caused by overgrowth of nonsusceptible organisms may result. ■ Use caution in patients with impaired renal function, allergies, or a history of GI disease (especially colitis).

Monitor: Watch for early symptoms of allergic reaction. ■ Use extreme caution in the penicillin-sensitive patient; incidence of cross-sensitivity may range from 3% to 16%. ■ May cause thrombophlebitis. Use small needles and large veins, and rotate infusion sites. ■ Observe for electrolyte imbalance and cardiac irregularities. Contains 2.3 mEq of sodium/Gm. Ceptaz and Pentacef do not contain sodium. ■ Note Drug interactions; additional monitoring may be indicated (e.g., renal function, drug serum levels, prothrombin times).

Patient education: Report promptly any bleeding or bruising, diarrhea, or symptoms of allergy (e.g., difficulty breathing, hives, itching, rash).

Maternal/child: Category B: safety for use during pregnancy and lactation not established. No problems documented. ■ Immature renal function of infants and small children will increase blood levels of all cephalosporins. ■ Only specific solutions can be used in children.

Elderly: No specific problems documented. Consider age-related impaired organ function and nutritional status; reduced dose or extended intervals may be indicated.

DRUG/LAB INTERACTIONS

Frequently used concomitantly with aminoglycosides, vancomycin, and clindamycin in severe infections, but these drugs must never be mixed in the same infusion or given concurrently. ■ Risk of nephrotoxicity may be increased with aminoglycosides and other nephrotoxic agents (e.g., loop diuretics such as furosemide [Lasix]). ■ Probenecid does not increase blood levels as it does with other cephalosporins. ■ May be antagonized by bacteriostatic antibiotics (e.g., chloramphenicol, erythromycin, tetracyclines); bactericidal action may be negated. ■ Large amounts of cephalosporins and/or salicylates may induce hypoprothrombinemia (deficiency of prothrombin [Factor II]). The addition of agents which affect platelet aggregation and/or may have GI ulcerative potential (e.g., NSAIDs [ibuprofen (Motrin)], or sulfinpyrazone [Anturane]) may increase risk of hemorrhage. ■ False-positive Coombs's test. ■ May have a false-positive reaction for urine glucose except with Tes-Tape or Chemstix. ■ Note Side effects.

SIDE EFFECTS

Full scope of allergic reactions, including anaphylaxis. Burning, discomfort, and pain at injection site; diarrhea; elevated alkaline phosphotase, AST (SGOT), ALT (SGPT), GGT, and BUN; nausea and vomiting; prolonged prothrombin time; pseudomembranous colitis; seizures (large doses). Hypoprothrombinemia may occur (rare).

ANTIDOTE

Notify physician of any side effects. Discontinue the drug if indicated. Treat allergic reaction as indicated and resuscitate as necessary. Mild cases of colitis may respond to discontinuation of ceftazidime. Oral vancomycin (Vancocin) or metronidazole (Flagyl) is the treatment of choice for antibiotic-related pseudomembranous colitis. Hemodialysis may be useful in overdose.

CEFTIZOXIME SODIUM

Antibacterial (Cephalosporin)

Cefizox

pH 5.5 to 8.0

USUAL DOSE

Dependent on seriousness of infection. Range is 500 mg to 4 Gm every 8 to 12 hours.

Uncomplicated urinary tract infection: 500 mg every 12 hours.

Pelvic inflammatory disease: 2 Gm every 8 hours.

Other uncomplicated infections: 1 Gm every 8 to 12 hours.

Severe or refractory infections: 1 Gm every 8 hours or 2 Gm every 8 to 12 hours.

Life-threatening infections: 3 to 4 Gm every 8 hours.

PEDIATRIC DOSE

Children over 6 months of age: 50 mg/kg of body weight every 6 to 8 hours. Up to 200 mg/kg/24 hr has been used, but do not exceed adult dose.

DOSE ADJUSTMENTS

Higher doses often reduced with positive clinical response. ■ Reduce total daily dose if renal function impaired. Calculated according to degree of impairment (see literature). ■ Note Drug/lab interactions.

DILUTION

Each 1 Gm must be reconstituted with 10 ml sterile water. Shake well. May be further diluted in 50 to 100 ml of NS or other compatible solutions (see chart on back cover and literature) and given as an intermittent infusion. Available premixed, in piggyback vials, and in ADD-Vantage vials for use with ADD-Vantage diluent containers. Not given as a continuous infusion.

Storage: Administer within 24 hours of preparation, or within 96 hours if refrigerated.

INCOMPATIBLE WITH

Should be considered incompatible in syringe or solution with any other bacteriostatic agent; all aminoglycosides (e.g., gentamicin [Garamycin]), filgrastim [Neupogen].

RATE OF ADMINISTRATION

May be given through Y-tube or three-way stopcock of infusion set.

Direct IV: A single dose equally distributed over 3 to 5 minutes.

Intermittent IV: A single dose over 30 minutes.

ACTIONS

A broad-spectrum third-generation cephalosporin antibiotic. Bactericidal to many gram-negative, gram-positive, and anaerobic organisms.

Effective against many otherwise resistant organisms. Peak serum levels achieved by end of infusion. Widely distributed into most body tissues and fluids, including inflamed meninges and bone. Excreted in the urine. Crosses placental barrier. Secreted in breast milk.

INDICATIONS AND USES

Treatment of serious infections of the lower respiratory tract, urinary tract; intraabdominal, skin and skin structure, and bone and joint infections; gonorrhea; pelvic inflammatory disease; septicemia and meningitis. Most effective against specific organisms (see literature).

CONTRAINDICATIONS

Previous allergic reaction of cephalosporins or related antibiotics (penicillins). Absolute only if reaction was serious.

PRECAUTIONS

Specific sensitivity studies indicated to determine susceptibility of the causative organism to ceftizoxime. ■ Continue for at least 2 to 3 days after all symptons of infection subside. ■ Avoid prolonged use of drug; superinfection caused by overgrowth of nonsusceptible organisms may result. ■ Use caution in patients with impaired renal function, allergies, or a history of GI disease (especially colitis).

Monitor: Watch for early symptoms of allergic reaction. ■ Use extreme caution in the penicillin-sensitive patient; incidence of cross-sensitivity may range from 3% to 16%. ■ May cause thrombophlebitis. Use small needles and large veins, and rotate infusion sites. ■ Observe for electrolyte imbalance or cardiac irregularities. Contains 2.6 mEq of sodium/Gm. ■ Note Drug/lab interactions; additional monitoring may be indicated (e.g., renal function, drug serum levels, prothrombin times).

Patient education: Report promptly any bleeding or bruising, diarrhea, or sypmtons of allergy (e.g., difficulty breathing, hives, itching, rash).

Maternal/child: Category B: safety for use during pregnancy and lactation not established. No problems documented. ■ Not recommended for use in children under 6 months of age. ■ Transient elevation of eosinophils, ALT (SGOT), AST (SGPT), and CK have occurred in infants under 6 months of age; use not recommended.

Elderly: No specific problems documented. Consider age-related impaired organ function and nutritional status; reduced dose or extended intervals may be indicated.

DRUG/LAB INTERACTIONS

Frequently used concomitantly with aminoglycosides in severe infections, but these drugs must never be mixed in the same infusion or given concurrently. ■ Risk of nephrotoxicity may be increased with aminoglycosides and other nephrotoxic agents (e.g., loop diuretics such as furosemide [Lasix]). ■ Probenecid inhibits excretion and may require reduction in dosage. ■ May be antagonized by bacteriostatic antibiotics (e.g., chloramphenicol, erythromycin, tetracyclines); bactericidal action may be negated. ■ Large amounts of cephalosporins and/or salicylates may induce hypoprothrombinemia (deficiency of prothrombin [Factor II]). The addition of agents which affect platelet aggregation and/or may have GI ulcerative potential (e.g., NSAIDs [ibuprofen (Motrin)], or sulfinpyrazone [Anturane]) may increase risk of hemorrhage. ■ Positive Coombs's test.

SIDE EFFECTS

Full scope of allergic reactions including anaphylaxis. Decreased hemoglobin or decreased hematocrit; decreased platelet functions; diarrhea; dyspnea; elevation of AST (SGOT), ALT (SGPT), total bilirubin, alkaline phosphatase, LDH, and BUN (transient); eosinophilia; fever; leukopenia; local site pain; nausea; oral thrush; prolonged prothrombin time; pseudomembranous colitis; seizures (large doses), thrombocytopenia; thrombophlebitis; vaginitis; vomiting. Hypoprothrombinemia may occur (rare).

ANTIDOTE

Notify the physician of any side effects. Discontinue the drug if indicated. Oral vancomycin (Vancocin) or metronidazole (Flagyl) is the treatment of choice for antibiotic-related pseudomembranous colitis. Treat allergic reaction as indicated and resuscitate as necessary. Hemodialysis may be somewhat useful in overdose.

CEFTRIAXONE SODIUM

Antibacterial
(Cephalosporin)

Rocephin

pH 6.6 to 6.7

USUAL DOSE

Adults and children over 12 years: 1 to 2 Gm/24 hr. May be given as a single dose every 24 hours or equally divided into 2 doses and given every 12 hours. Do not exceed a total dose of 4 Gm/24 hr.

Disseminated gonococcal infections: 1 Gm once daily for 7 days.

Gonococcal meningitis/endocarditis: 1 to 2 Gm every 12 hours.

Lyme disease: 2 Gm daily for 10 to 21 days.

Perioperative prophylaxis: 1 Gm IV 30 minutes to 2 hours before incision. Used primarily in patients undergoing coronary artery bypass surgery and in contaminated or potentially contaminated surgeries.

PEDIATRIC DOSE

Children 1 month to 12 years: 50 to 75 mg/kg of body weight/24 hr as a single dose or in equally divided doses every 12 hours. Do not exceed a total dose of 2 Gm/24 hr.

Lyme disease: 50 to 100 mg/kg daily for 10 to 21 days.

Acute PID in prepubertal children: 100 mg/kg/24 hr in combination with erythromycin or sulfisoxazole.

Bacterial meningitis: Begin with a loading dose of 100 mg/kg (Do not exceed a total dose of 4 Gm), follow with 100 mg/kg/day (not ot exceed 4 Gm) as a single dose or in equally divided doses every 12 hours. An alternate regimen (American Academy of Pediatrics) begins with an 80 to 100 mg/kg loading dose (not over 4 Gm); follow with 80 mg/kg at 12-hour intervals for 2 doses, then 80 to 100 mg/kg every 24 hours.

NEONATAL DOSE

25 to 50 mg/kg/day as a single daily dose. Up to 75 mg/kg may be indicated in infants over 7 days old weighing over 2,000 Gm. Up to 100 mg/kg may be indicated in bacterial meningitis. Neonatal doses may also be given IM.

Infants born to mothers with gonococcal infections: 50 mg/kg one time only (do not exceed 125 mg).

DOSE ADJUSTMENTS

In adults with both hepatic and renal impairment, dose should not exceed 2 Gm daily unless serum concentrations of ceftriaxone are monitored. ■ Note Drug/lab interactions.

DILUTION

Initially reconstitute each 250 mg with 2.4 ml (500 mg with 4.8 ml, etc.) of sterile water, NS, D5W, D10W, D5/NS, or D10/NS for injection. Each ml will contain 100 mg. A single dose must be further diluted with 50 to 100 ml of the same solution and be given as an intermittent infusion. Shake well. Concentrations of 10 mg/ml to 40 mg/ml are recommended for intermittent infusion. Available premixed, in piggyback vials, and in ADD-Vantage vials for use with ADD-Vantage diluent containers.

Storage: Stable at room temperature for at least 24 hours in stated solutions or up to 10 days if refrigerated. Stability and color (clear to yellow) depend on concentration and diluent. Thaw frozen solutions at room temperature before use. Discard unused portions; do not refreeze.

INCOMPATIBLE WITH

Should be considered incompatible in syringe, solution, or IV tubing with any other bacteriostatic agent; all aminoglycosides (e.g., gentamicin [Garamycin]), clindamycin, filgrastim (Neupogen), fluconazole (Diflucan), pentamidine (Pentam 300), vancomycin (Lyphocin), vinorelbine (Navelbine).

RATE OF ADMINISTRATION

Intermittent IV: A single dose over 15 to 30 minutes.

ACTIONS

A broad-spectrum third-generation cephalosporin antibiotic. Bactericidal to selected gram-negative, gram-positive, and anaerobic organisms. Effective against many otherwise resistant organisms. Therapeutic concentrations achieved in many body fluids and tissues including CSF. Has a long half-life (range is 5.8 to 8.7 hours), once a day dosing sufficient. Peak serum levels achieved by end of infusion. Excreted through bile and urine. Crosses placental barrier. Secreted in breast milk.

INDICATIONS AND USES

Treatment of serious lower respiratory tract, urinary tract, skin and skin structure, bone and joint, and intraabdominal infections. ▪ Pelvic inflammatory disease. ▪ Bacterial septicemia. ▪ Meningitis. ▪ Most effective against specific organisms (see literature). ▪ Perioperative prophylaxis. ▪ Given IM for additional indications.

Investigational use: Treatment of Lyme disease.

CONTRAINDICATIONS

Previous allergic reaction to cephalosporins or related antibiotics (penicillins). Absolute only if reaction was serious.

PRECAUTIONS

Sensitivity studies are indicated to determine susceptibility of the causative organism to ceftriaxone. ▪ Continue for at least 2 to 3 days after all symptoms of infection subside. Usual course of therapy 4 to 14 days; S. pyogenes requires treatment for 10 days. In serious invasive infection, continue for 5 to 7 days after cultures are negative. ▪ Avoid prolonged use of drug; superinfection caused by overgrowth of nonsusceptible organisms may result. ▪ Use caution in patients with both impaired renal and hepatic function, allergies, or a history of GI disease (especially colitis). ▪ Prolonged use may lead to gallbladder disease.

Monitor: Watch for early symptoms of allergic reaction. ▪ Use extreme caution in the penicillin-sensitive patient; incidence of cross-sensitivity may range from 3% to 16%. ▪ Single daily dose reduces incidence of thrombophlebitis. Use of small needles, large veins, and rotation of infusion sites is preferred. ▪ Observe for electrolyte imbalance and cardiac irregularities. Contains 3.6 mEq sodium per Gm. ▪ Note Dose adjustments and Drug/lab interactions; additional monitoring may be indicated (e.g., renal function, drug serum levels, prothrombin times).

Patient education: Report promptly any bleeding or bruising, diarrhea, or symptoms of allergy (e.g., difficulty breathing, hives, itching, rash).

Maternal/child: Category B: Safety for use during pregnancy and lactation not established. No problems documented. ■ Immature renal function of infants and small children will increase blood levels of all cephalosporins. ■ Use with caution in hyperbilirubinemic neonates (especially premature infants), highly protein bound and may displace bilirubin from albumin.

Elderly: No specific problems documented. Consider age-related impaired organ function and nutritional status; reduced dose may be indicated.

DRUG/LAB INTERACTIONS

Frequently used concomitantly with aminoglycosides in severe infections, but these drugs must never be mixed in the same infusion or given concurrently. ■ Risk of nephrotocicity may be increased with aminoglycosides and other nephrotoxic agents (e.g., loop diuretics such as furosemide [Lasix]). ■ Probenecid does not increase blood levels as it does with other cephalosporins. ■ May be antagonized by bacteriostatic antibiotics (e.g., chloramphenicol, erythromycin, tetracyclines); bactericidal action may be negated. ■ Large amounts of cephalosporins and/or salicylates may induce hypoprothrombinemia (deficiency of prothrombin [Factor II]). The addition of agents which affect platelet aggregation and/or may have GI ulcerative potential (e.g., NSAIDs [ibuprofen (Motrin)], or sulfinpyrazone [Anturane]) may increase risk of hemorrhage. ■ False-positive Coombs' test. ■ May produce false-positive reaction for urine glucose except with Tes-Tape or Chemstix. ■ Note Side effects.

SIDE EFFECTS

Full scope of allergic reactions including anaphylaxis are possible. "Biliary sludge" or pseudolithiasis, bleeding episodes; burning, discomfort, and pain at injection site; casts in urine; diarrhea; dizziness; eosinophilia; elevated alkaline phosphatase, bilirubin, BUN, creatinine, AST (SGOT), and ALT (SGPT); headache; leukopenia; prolonged prothrombin time; pseudomembranous colitis; seizures (large doses); thrombophlebitis. Hypoprothrom-binemia may occur (rare).

ANTIDOTE

Notify physician of any side effects. Discontinue the drug if indicated. Treat allergic reaction as indicated and resuscitate as necessary. Mild cases of colitis may respond to discontinuation of ceftriaxone. Oral vancomycin (Vancocin) or metronidazole (Flagyl) is the treatment of choice for antibiotic-related pseudomembranous colitis. Vitamin K may be useful in bleeding episodes, or drug may have to be discontinued. Not removed by hemodialysis.

CEFUROXIME SODIUM

Antibacterial
(Cephalosporin)

Kefurox, Zinacef

pH 5.0 to 8.5

USUAL DOSE

Dependent on seriousness of infection. Range is from 750 mg to 3 Gm every 8 hours for 5 to 10 days.

Uncomplicated infections: 750 mg every 8 hours.

Severe or complicated infections and bone and joint infections: 1.5 Gm every 8 hours.

Life-threatening or infections due to less susceptible organisms: 1.5 Gm every 6 hours.

Bacterial meningitis: 3 Gm every 8 hours.

Acute pelvic inflammatory disease: 150 mg/kg of body weight/24 hr equally divided into 4 doses. May be given in combination with erythromycin, sulfisoxazole, or tetracycline. Continue IV until 2 days after symptoms subside. Continue other agents orally for 14 days.

Perioperative prophylaxis: 1.5 Gm IV 30 minutes to 1 hour before incision; then 750 mg every 8 hours for 24 hours or 1.5 Gm every 12 hours to total dose of 6 Gm in open heart surgery.

PEDIATRIC DOSE

Do not exceed adult dose.

Infants and children over 3 months of age: 50 to 100 mg/kg/24 hr in equal divided doses every 6 to 8 hours. Higher-end dosing used for more serious infections.

Bone and joint infections: 150 mg/kg/24 hr in equally divided doses every 8 hours.

Bacterial meningitis: 200 to 240 mg/kg/24 hr in equally divided doses every 6 to 8 hours.

Acute pelvic inflammatory disease in children over 7 years of age: 30 mg/kg/24 hr equally divided into 3 doses. See adult regimen for rest of protocol.

NEONATAL DOSE

Infants under 3 months of age: 10 to 25 mg/kg every 12 hours. Another source recommends 15 to 50 mg/kg every 12 hours.

Bacterial meningitis: 100 mg/kg/24 hr in equally divided doses every 8 to 12 hours.

DOSE ADJUSTMENTS

Reduce total daily dose if renal function impaired. Calculated according to degree of impairment (see literature). ■ Note Drug/Lab interactions.

DILUTION

Each 750 mg must be reconstituted with 8 ml sterile water, D5W, NS, or other compatible infusion solution for injection (see chart on back cover and literature). Shake well. May be further diluted with compatible solutions to 50 or 100 ml and given as an intermittent infusion, or added to 500 to 1,000 ml and given as a continuous infusion. Available pre-mixed, in piggyback vials, infusion packs, and in ADD-Vantage vials for use with ADD-Vantage diluent containers.

Storage: Administer within 24 hours of preparation or within 48 hours if refrigerated.

INCOMPATIBLE WITH

Manufacturer recommends temporarily discontinuing other solutions infusing at the same site to avoid compatibility problems. Should be considered incompatible in syringe or solution with any other bacteriostatic agent; all aminoglycosides (e.g., gentamicin [Garamycin]), doxapram (Dopram), filgrastim (Neupogen), Fluconazole (Diflucan), midazolam (Versed), ranitidine (Zantac), vinorelbine (Navelbine).

RATE OF ADMINISTRATION

Note Incompatible with. Injection or intermittent infusion may be given through Y-tube or three-way stopcock of infusion set.
Direct IV: A single dose equally distributed over 3 to 5 minutes.
Intermittent IV: A single dose over 30 minutes.
Continuous infusion: 500 to 1,000 ml over 6 to 24 hours, depending on total dose and concentration.

ACTIONS

A broad-spectrum, second-generation cephalosporin antibiotic. Bactericidal to selected gram-negative, gram-positive, and anaerobic organisms. Effective against many otherwise resistant organisms. Widely distributed in most tissues, body fluids (including inflamed meninges), bone, skin and soft tissue. Peak serum levels acheived by end of infusion. The only second-generation cephalosporin to achieve therapeutic levels in CSF. Excreted in the urine. Crosses placental barrier. Secreted in breast milk.

INDICATIONS AND USES

Treatment of serious lower respiratory tract, urinary tract, skin and skin structure infections, septicemia, meningitis, and gonorrhea. Most effective against specific organisms and when mixed organisms are present (see literature). ■ Perioperative prophylaxis.

CONTRAINDICATIONS

Previous allergic reaction to cephalosporins or related antibiotics (penicillins). Absolute only if reaction was serious.

PRECAUTIONS

Sensitivity studies indicated to determine susceptibility of the causative organism to cefuroxime. ■ Continue for at least 2 to 3 days after all symptoms of infection subside. ■ Avoid prolonged use of drug; superinfection caused by overgrowth of nonsusceptible organisms may result. ■ Use caution in patients with impaired renal function, allergies, or a history of GI disease (especially colitis).
Monitor: Watch for early symptoms of allergic reaction. ■ Use extreme caution in the penicillin-sensitive patient; incidence of cross-sensitivity may range from 3% to 16%. ■ May cause thrombophlebitis. Use small needles and large veins, and rotate infusion sites. ■ Observe for electrolyte imbalance and cardiac irregularities. Contains 2.4 mEq sodium/Gm. ■ Note Drug/lab interactions; additional monitoring may be indicated (e.g., renal function, drug serum levels, prothrombin times).
Patient education: Report promptly any bleeding or bruising, diarrhea, or symptons of allergy (e.g., difficulty breathing, hives, itching, rash).
Maternal/child: Category B: safety for use during pregnancy and lactation not established. No problems documented. ■ Is used in infants

under 3 months of age, but safety not established; immature renal function will increase blood levels.

Elderly: No specific problems documented. Consider age-related impaired organ function and nutritional status; reduced dose or extended intervals may be indicated.

DRUG/LAB INTERACTIONS

Frequently used concomitantly with aminoglycosides in severe infections, but these drugs must never be mixed in the same infusion or given concurrently. ■ Risk of nephrotoxicity may be increased with aminoglycosides and other nephrotoxic agents (e.g., loop diuretics such as furosemide [Lasix]). ■ Probenecid inhibits excretion and may require reduction in dosage. ■ May be antagonized by bacteriostatic antibiotics (e.g., chloramphenicol, erythromycin, tetracyclines); bactericidal action may be negated. ■ Large amounts of cephalosporins and/or salicylates may induce hypoprothrombinemia (deficiency of prothrombin [Factor II]). The addition of agents which affect platelet aggregation and/or may have GI ulcerative potential (e.g., NSAIDs [ibuprofen (Motrin)] or sulfinpyrazone [Anturane]) may increase risk of hemorrhage. ■ May cause a false-negative reaction in specific blood glucose tests (ferricyanide). ■ False-positive reaction for urine glucose except with Tes-Tape or Chemstix. ■ False-positive Coombs' test. ■ Note Side effects.

SIDE EFFECTS

Full scope of allergic reactions including anaphylaxis. Decreased hemoglobin, hematocrit, or platelet functions; diarrhea; dyspnea; elevation of AST (SGOT), ALT (SGPT), total bilirubin, alkaline phosphatase, LDH, and BUN (transient); eosinophilia; fever; leukopenia; local site pain; nausea; oral thrush; prolonged prothrombin time, pseudomembranous colitis; seizures (large doses); transient neutropenia; thrombocytopenia; thrombophlebitis; vaginitis; vomiting. Hypoprothrombinemia may occur (rare).

ANTIDOTE

Notify physician of any side effects. Discontinue the drug if indicated. Treat antibiotic-related pseudomembranous colitis with oral vancomycin (Vancocin) or metronidazole (Flagyl). Treat allergic reaction and resuscitate as necessary. Hemodialysis may be somewhat useful in overdose.

CEPHAPIRIN SODIUM

Antibacterial (Cephalosporin)

Cefadyl

pH 6.5 to 8.5

USUAL DOSE

500 mg to 1 Gm every 4 to 6 hours. 8 to 12 Gm/24 hr has been given in severe infections.

Perioperative prophylaxis: 1 to 2 Gm 30 minutes to 1 hour before incision. May be repeated in OR and every 6 hours for 24 hours or up to 5 days in specific situations.

PEDIATRIC DOSE

Infants and children over 3 months of age: 10 to 20 mg/kg of body weight every 6 hours. *Do not exceed adult dose.*

DOSE ADJUSTMENTS

Reduce total daily dose if renal function impaired. Calculated according to degree of impairment (see literature). ■ For perioperative prophylaxis, reduce dose to 7.5 to 15 mg/kg every 12 hours in patients who are moderately oliguric or those with a serum creatinine >5 mg/dl. ■ Note Drug/lab interactions.

DILUTION

Each 1 Gm or fraction thereof must be reconstituted with at least 10 ml of SW. To reduce incidence of thrombophlebitis, may be further diluted in 50 to 100 ml of D5W, NS, or other compatible infusion solutions (see chart on back cover and literature). Available in piggyback vials. May be administered through Y-tube, three-way stopcock, or additive infusion set.

Storage: Administer within 24 hours of preparation.

INCOMPATIBLE WITH

Manufacturer recommends temporarily discontinuing other solutions infusing at the same site to avoid compatibility problems. All aminoglycosides (e.g., amikacin [Amikin], gentamicin [Garamycin]), aminophylline, ascorbic acid (Cenolate), epinephrine (Adrenalin), mannitol, norepinephrine (Levophed), phenytoin (Dilantin), thiopental (Pentothal).

RATE OF ADMINISTRATION

Note Incompatible with. Each 1 Gm or fraction thereof over 5 minutes or longer as indicated by amount of solution and condition of patient.

ACTIONS

A semisynthetic first-generation cephalosporin antibiotic that is bactericidal through inhibition of cell wall synthesis to some gram-positive and gram-negative organisms, including staphylococci and streptococci. A number of organisms are resistant to this cephalosporin. Peak serum levels achieved by end of infusion. Widely distributed into most body fluids (CSF minimal) and excreted in the urine. Crosses the placental barrier. Secreted in breast milk.

INDICATIONS AND USES

Effective only if the causative organism is susceptible. Treatment of moderate to severe infections of the skin, soft tissue, respiratory tract, and GU tract. ▪ Septicemia. ▪ Endocarditis. ▪ Osteomyelitis. ▪ Perioperative prophylaxis.

CONTRAINDICATIONS
Previous allergic reaction to cephalosporins or related antibiotics (penicillins). Absolute only if reaction was serious.

PRECAUTIONS
Sensitivity studies necessary to determine susceptibility of the causative organism to cephapirin. ▪ Continue for at least 2 to 3 days after all symptoms of infection subside. ▪ Avoid prolonged use of drug; superinfection caused by overgrowth of nonsusceptible organisms may result. ▪ Use caution in patients with impaired renal function, allergies, or a history of GI disease (especially colitis).

Monitor: Watch for early symptoms of allergic reaction. ▪ Use extreme caution in the penicillin-sensitive patient; incidence of cross-sensitivity may range from 3% to 16%. ▪ May cause thrombophlebitis. Use small needles and large veins, and rotate infusion sites. ▪ Observe for electrolyte imbalance and cardiac irregularities. Contains 2.4 mEq sodium/Gm. ▪ Note Drug/lab interactions; additional monitoring may be indicated (e.g., renal function, drug serum levels, prothrombin times).

Patient education: Report promptly any bleeding or bruising, diarrhea or symptoms of allergy (e.g., difficulty breathing, hives, itching, rash).

Maternal/child: Category B: safety for use during pregnancy and lactation not established. No problems documented. ▪ Safety for use in infants under 3 months of age not established. Immature renal function will increase blood levels.

Elderly: No specific problems documented. Consider age-related impaired organ function and nutritional status; reduced dose or extended intervals may be indicated.

DRUG/LAB INTERACTIONS
Frequently used concomitantly with aminoglycosides in severe infections, but these drugs must never be mixed in the same infusion or given concurrently. ▪ Risk of nephrotoxicity may be increased with aminoglycosides and other nephrotoxic agents (e.g., loop diuretics such as furosemide [Lasix]). ▪ Probenecid inhibits excretion and may require reduction in dosage. ▪ May be antagonized by bacteriostatic antibiotics (e.g., chloramphenicol, erythromycin, tetracyclines); bactericidal action may be negated. ▪ Large amounts of cephalosporins and/or salicylates may induce hypoprothrombinemia (deficiency of prothrombin [Factor II]). The addition of agents which affect platelet aggregation and/or may have GI ulcerative potential (e.g., NSAIDs [ibuprofen (Motrin)], or sulfinpyrazone [Anturane]) may increase risk of hemorrhage. ▪ False-positive reaction for urine glucose except with Tes-Tape or Chemstix. ▪ False-positive Coombs' test. ▪ Note Side effects.

SIDE EFFECTS
Allergic reactions including anaphylaxis; anemia, diarrhea, jaundice, leukopenia, local site pain, neutropenia, phlebitis, prolonged prothrombin time, pseudomembranous colitis, seizures (large doses); and transient elevation of AST (SGOT), ALT (SGPT), BUN, and alkaline phosphatase. Hypoprothrombinemia may occur (rare).

ANTIDOTE

Notify the physician of any side effects. Discontinue the drug if indicated, treat allergic reaction as indicated, and resuscitate as necessary. Treat antibiotic-related pseudomembranous colitis with oral vancomycin (Vancocin) or metronidazole (Flagyl). Small amounts may be removed by hemodialysis.

CHLORAMPHENICOL SODIUM SUCCINATE

Chloromycetin

Antibacterial

pH 6.4 to 7.0

USUAL DOSE

For all age levels, determine baseline blood studies before administration. Avoid repeated courses of this drug.

Adults, children and infants over 2 weeks of age: 50 mg/kg/24 hr in equally divided doses every 6 hours. In severe infections an increase to 75 mg/kg/24 hr may be indicated. Up to 100 mg/kg/24 hr may be required in meningitis. These increased doses must be reduced as soon as possible. Maximum dose is 4 Gm/24 hr.

NEONATAL DOSE

Under 2,000 Gm: 25 mg/kg of body weight once daily.

Over 2,000 Gm, birth to 7 days of age: 25 mg/kg once daily.

Over 2,000 Gm and over 7 days of age: 25 mg/kg every 12 hours.

DOSE ADJUSTMENTS

Reduce dose and/or initiate oral therapy as soon as feasible. ■ Reduce dose to 25 mg/kg/24 hr in infants and children with immature metabolic processes. ■ In patients with immature or impaired hepatic or renal function, dose reduction may be required.

DILUTION

Each 1 Gm should be reconstituted with 10 ml of sterile water for injection or D5W to prepare a 10% solution (100 mg/ml). May be further diluted in 50 to 100 ml of D5W for intermittent infusion. Give through Y-tube, three-way stopcock, or additive infusion set. May also be further diluted and given as a continuous infusion.

Storage: Administer within 24 hours of preparation

INCOMPATIBLE WITH

Amobarbital (Amytal), ampicillin (Polycillin), carbenicillin (Geopen), chlorpromazine (Thorazine), digitoxin (Crystodigin), erythromycins (Ilotycin, Erythrocin), fluconazole (Diflucan), glycopyrrolate, hydrocortisone phosphate, hydroxyzine (Vistaril), metoclopramide (Reglan), oxacillin (Prostaphlin), pentobarbital (Nembutal), phenytoin (Dilantin), polymyxin B (Aerosporin), procaine (Novocain), prochlorperazine (Compazine), promazine (Sparine), promethazine (Phenergan), solutions with a pH below 5.5 or above 7.0, thiopental (Pentothal), tripelennamine hydrochloride (Pyribenzamine), vancomycin (Vancocin), warfarin (Coumadin).

RATE OF ADMINISTRATION
Direct IV: 1 Gm or fraction thereof over at least 3 to 5 minutes.
Intermittent infustion: A single dose over 30 to 60 minutes.
Continuous infusion: A single dose evenly distributed over 6 hours.

ACTIONS
Effective against many life-threatening organisms. Primarily bacteriostatic. May be bactericidal at high concentrations or against highly susceptible organisms. Acts by inhibiting protein synthesis. Well distributed in therapeutic doses throughout the body, especially in the liver and kidneys. Lowest concentrations are found in the brain and spinal fluid. Excreted in urine, bile, and feces. Crosses the placental barrier. Secreted in breast milk.

INDICATIONS AND USES
Only in serious infections in which potentially less dangerous drugs are ineffective or contraindicated; acute *Salmonella typhi* infections, meningeal infections, bacteremia, Rocky Mountain spotted fever, lymphogranuloma psittacosis, and others. ■ Cystic fibrosis regimens.

CONTRAINDICATIONS
Known chloramphenicol sensitivity; pregnancy, labor, delivery, and lactation.

PRECAUTIONS
This is a lethal drug. Sensitivity studies mandatory to determine susceptibility of the causative organism not only to chloramphenicol but to other less dangerous drugs. ■ Super-infection caused by overgrowth of nonsusceptible organisms, including fungi, is possible. ■ For IV use only; not effective IM. ■ Use caution in patients with acute intermittent porphyria or glucose 6-phosphate dehydrogenase deficiency.
Monitor: Obtain blood studies (CBC) prior to initiating therapy and at least every 2 to 3 days during therapy and discontinue drug if indicated. ■ Monitor serum levels at least weekly, and more often if indicated. Maintain trough levels between 5 to 10 mcg/ml and peak levels between 10 to 20 mcg/ml. ■ Monitor hepatic and renal function as indicated. ■ Note Drug/lab interactions.
Patient education: Report fever, sore throat, tiredness, unusual bleeding or bruising promptly.
Maternal/child: No studies documented. Use during pregnancy or lactation with extreme caution, may cause gray syndrome in fetus. Use caution in premature infants and newborns (causes gray syndrome); monitor serum levels (see Precautions/Monitor). ■ Note Contraindications.

DRUG/LAB INTERACTIONS
Decreases plasma clearance and prolongs duration of alfentanil (Alfenta). ■ May cause irreversible bone marrow depression. Avoid concurrent therapy with drugs that cause blood dyscrasias (e.g., penicillins, hydantoins [phenytoin (Dilantin)]), other bone marrow depressants (e.g., cytotoxic drugs, radiation therapy). ■ Increases serum levels of oral antidiabetics (e.g., chlorpropamide [Diabinase]) and increases hypoglycemic effects; dose reduction may be required. ■ May antagonize effects of erythromycin, clindamycin, lincomycin, and penicillins. (Is used with ampicillin in pediatric patients.) ■ Chloramphenicol can inhibit the P_{450} enzyme system; reduced metabolism and increased serum levels may occur in agents also metabolized by that route (e.g., phenobarbitol, phe-

nytoin, warfarin). ▪ May increase response to iron preparations. ▪ Phenobarbital may also increase metabolism and decrease effects of chloramphenicol. ▪ Rifampin increases chloramphenicol metabolism and decreases its effects. ▪ Inhibits effects of Vitamin B_{12}. ▪ May decrease effectiveness of oral contraceptives; breakthrough bleeding and pregnancy may result.

SIDE EFFECTS

Anaphylaxis, aplastic anemia, bone marrow depression (irreversible), confusion, depression, diarrhea, fever, granulocytopenia, gray syndrome of newborns and infants, headache, hypoplastic anemia, leukemia, nausea, optic and peripheral neuritis, paroxysmal nocturnal hemoglobinuria, rashes, stomatitis, thrombocytopenia, vomiting, and many others. *May be fatal.*

ANTIDOTE

Notify the physician immediately of any adverse symptoms. Discontinue the drug if indicated, treat allergic reaction as indicated, and resuscitate as necessary.

CHLORDIAZEPOXIDE HYDROCHLORIDE

Benzodiazepine
Antianxiety agent
Sedative/hypnotic

Librium   pH 2.5 to 3.5

USUAL DOSE

Maximum dose is 300 mg in a 6- to 24-hour period.

Acute alcohol withdrawal: 50 to 100 mg initially. Repeat in 2 to 4 hours if indicated.

Acute or severe anxiety: 50 to 100 mg initially, then 25 to 50 mg 3 or 4 times daily if necessary.

Pre-op apprehension or anxiety: 50 to 100 mg 1 hour before surgery. Usually given IM.

PEDIATRIC DOSE

Children over 12 years of age: 25 to 50 mg/dose or 0.5 mg/kg/24 hr in equally divided doses every 6 to 8 hours.

DOSE ADJUSTMENTS

Reduce dose by one-half (25 to 50 mg) for the elderly or debilitated, in impaired liver or renal function, in patients with limited pulmonary reserves, and in the presence of other CNS depressants. ▪ Note Drug/lab interactions.

DILUTION

Each 100 mg ampoule of sterile powder should be diluted with 5 ml of NS or sterile water for injection. Agitate gently to dissolve completely. *(Do not use diluent provided; for IM use only).* May not be mixed with infusion fluids. Give through Y-tube or three-way stopcock of infusion set. Observe closely for occurrence of fine white precipitate. Use only freshly prepared solutions; discard unused portion.

INCOMPATIBLE WITH

Ascorbic acid, heparin, pentobarbital (Nembutal), phenytoin (Dilantin), promethazine (Phenergan), Ringer's injection, secobarbital (Seconal).

RATE OF ADMINISTRATION

100 mg or fraction thereof over a minimum of 1 minute. Titrate to effect desired. Too-rapid injection may cause symptoms of overdose.

ACTIONS

A benzodiazepine that produces CNS depression, inducing sedation and reducing anxiety. Wide margin of safety between therapeutic and toxic doses. Response is extremely rapid by IV route. Slowly metabolized by the liver and excreted very slowly in the urine. Crosses the placental barrier. Secreted in breast milk.

INDICATIONS AND USES

Management of anxiety disorders ■ Short term relief of symptoms of anxiety. ■ Withdrawal symptoms of acute alcoholism. ■ Preoperative apprehension and anxiety.

CONTRAINDICATIONS

Known hypersensitivity to chlordiazepoxide.

PRECAUTIONS

Not recommended for use in depressed patients (may develop suicidal tendencies) or those with known psychoses. ■ Use extreme caution if indicated in shock or comatose states or in untreated narrow-angle glaucoma. ■ Use extreme caution in the elderly or very ill and in patients with limited pulmonary reserve (may cause cardiac and/or respiratory depression). ■ Withdrawal symptoms possible after long-term use or high doses. ■ Hypoalbuminemia may increase incidence of side effects.

Monitor: Bed rest required for a minimum of 3 hours after IV injection. ■ Monitor vital signs. ■ Keep resuscitation equipment and flumazenil (Romazicon) available.

Patient education: May produce drowsiness or dizziness. Request assistance with ambulation and use caution performing tasks that require alertness. ■ Avoid use of alcohol or other CNS depressants (e.g., antihistamines, barbiturates). ■ May be habit forming with long-term use or high-dose therapy. ■ Consider birth control options.

Maternal/child: Pregnancy category D. Increased risk of congenital malformation has occurred. ■ Not recommended during pregnancy, labor and delivery, lactation, or in children under 12 years of age.

Elderly: Note Dose adjustments. Start with a small dose and increase gradually based on response. ■ More sensitive to therapeutic and adverse effects (e.g., oversedation, ataxia, and dizziness.) ■ IV injection may be more likely to cause apnea, bradycardia, hypotension, and cardiac arrest. ■ Note Precautions and Drug/lab interactions.

DRUG/LAB INTERACTIONS

Concurrent use with other CNS depressants (e.g., alcohol, antihistamines, barbiturates, MAO inhibitors [e.g., selegiline (Eldepryl)], narcotics [e.g., morphine, meperidine (Demerol), fentanyl], phenothiazines [e.g., prochlorperazine (Compazine)], and tricyclic antidepressants [e.g., imipramine (Tofranil-PM)]) may result in additive effects. Reduced dose may be indicated. ■ May increase serum concentrations of digoxin and phenytoin (Dilantin); monitor digoxin and phenytoin serum levels. ▪ Concurrent use with beta-blockers (e.g., metoprolol [Lopressor], propranolol [Inderal]), cimetidine (Tagamet), estrogen containing oral contraceptives, disulfiram (Antabuse), fluoxetine (Prozac), isoniazid (Nydrazid), ketoconazole (Nizoral), probenecid, and valproic acid (Depakene), may inhibit hepatic metabolism, resulting in increased plasma concentrations of chlordiazepoxide. ▪ Decreases clearance and increase toxicity of zidovudine (AZT). ▪ May increase clearance and decrease effectiveness of levodopa. ▪ Hypotensive effects of benzodiazepines may be increased by any agent that induces hypotension (e.g., antihypertensives, bretylium, CNS depressants, diuretics, lidocaine, paclitaxel). ▪ Use with carbamazepine (Tegretol) or rifampin (Rifadin) increases clearance and reduces effects of chlordiazepoxide. ▪ Theophyllines (e.g., Aminophylline) antagonize sedative effects of benzodiazepines. ▪ Clozapine (Leponix) has caused respiratory distress or cardiac arrest in a few patients, use concurrently with extreme caution. ▪ Smoking increases metabolism and clearance of chlordiazepoxide, decreasing plasma levels and sedative effects.

SIDE EFFECTS

Average dose: Blood dyscrasias, constipation, EEG changes, hiccups, hypotension, menstrual irregularities, nausea, skin eruptions, syncope, tachycardia, urinary retention, urticaria.

Overdose: May be caused by too-rapid injection. Apnea, ataxia, bradycardia, cardiovascular collapse, confusion, coma, diminished reflexes, drowsiness, edema, hypotension (severe), paradoxical reactions, somnolence.

ANTIDOTE

Notify the physician of all side effects. Reduction of dosage may be required. Discontinue the drug for paradoxical reactions including hyperexcitability, hallucinations, and acute rage. Do not treat with barbiturates or CNS stimulants. Treat hypotension with dopamine (Intropin) or norepinephrine (Levophed). For overdose, flumazenil (Romazicon) will reverse all sedative effects of benzodiazepines. A patent airway, artificial ventilation, oxygen therapy, and other symptomatic and supportive treatment must be instituted promptly. Hemodialysis may be of limited value. Resuscitate as necessary.

CHLORPROMAZINE HYDROCHLORIDE

Phenothiazine
Antipsychotic
Antiemetic

❧Ormazine, Thorazine

pH 3.0 to 5.0

USUAL DOSE

Acute nausea and vomiting in surgery: 2 mg. May repeat at 2-minute intervals as indicated. Do not exceed 25 mg. Usually given as an infusion.

Intractable hiccups: 25 to 50 mg as an infusion in 500 to 1,000 ml of NS.

Tetanus: 25 to 50 mg as an infusion of at least 1 mg/ml. Individualize dose to patient response and tolerance. Repeat every 6 to 8 hr.

PEDIATRIC DOSE

Children over 6 months of age:

Acute nausea and vomiting in surgery: 1 mg. May repeat at 2-minute intervals as indicated. Maximum is usually 0.275 mg/kg. IV route rarely used for children.

Tetanus: 0.55 mg/kg of body weight every 6 to 8 hours. Do not exceed 40 mg/24 hours for up to 23 kg and 75 mg/24 hours for up to 50 kg.

DOSE ADJUSTMENTS

Reduce dose of any medication potentiated by phenothiazines by one fourth to one half. Note Drug/lab interactions. ■ Reduce dose by one fourth to one half in the elderly and increase very gradually by response.

DILUTION

Each 25 mg (1 ml) must be diluted with 24 ml of NS for injection. 1 ml will equal 1 mg. May be further diluted in 500 to 1,000 ml of NS and given as an infusion. Handle carefully; may cause contact dermatitis. Sensitive to light. Slightly yellow color does not alter potency. Discard if markedly discolored.

INCOMPATIBLE WITH

Allopurinol (Zyloprim), amifostine (Ethyol), ampicillin, aminophylline, amphotericin B (Fungizone), atropine, caffeine and sodium benzoate, cephalothin (Keflin), chloramphenicol (Chloromycetin), chlorothiazide (Diuril), cimetidine (Tagamet), dimenhydrinate (Dramanate), epinephrine (Adrenalin), folic acid, fludarabine (Fludara), furosemide (Lasix), heparin, hydrocortisone (Solu-Cortef), kanamycin (Kantrex), magnesium sulfate, melphalan (Alkeran), methicillin (Staphcillin), methohexital (Brevital), methotrexate (Folex), methylprednisolone (Solu-Medrol), paclitaxel (Taxol), paraldehyde, penicillin G potassium, pentobarbital (Nembutal), phenobarbital (Luminal), piperacillin tazobactam (Zosyn), ranitidine (Zantac), sargramostim (Leukine), secobarbital (Seconal), sodium bicarbonate, thiopental (Pentothal).

RATE OF ADMINISTRATION

Titrate to symptoms and vital signs. (See Precautions).

Direct IV: each 1 mg or fraction thereof over 1 minute.

Infusion: Given very slowly. Do not exceed 1 mg/min.

Pediatric rate: Do not exceed 1 mg or fraction thereof over 2 minutes.

ACTIONS

A phenothiazine derivative with effects on the central, autonomic, and peripheral nervous systems. Decreases anxiety and tension, relaxes muscles, produces sedation, and tranquilizes. Has an antiemetic effect, some antihistamine action, and potentiates CNS depressants. Onset of action is prompt and of short duration in small IV doses. Extensively metabolized in liver and kidney and excreted primarily in urine. Crosses the placental barrier. Secreted in breast milk.

INDICATIONS AND USES

Treatment of acute nausea and vomiting in surgery, severe hiccups, and as an adjunct in the treatment of tetanus. ■ Also indicated for management of psychotic disorders, control of nausea and vomiting, relief of restlessness and apprehension before surgery, management of acute intermittent porphyria, control of manic episodes in manic depressive illness, and treatment of severe behavioral problems in children; usually given by IM or oral routes.

Unlabeled uses: Treatment of Phencyclidine (PCP) psychosis. ▪ Treatment of migraine headaches (IV or IM).

CONTRAINDICATIONS

Bone marrow depression, cerebral arteriosclerosis, children under 6 months, circulatory collapse, coronary disease, comatose or severely depressed states, hypersensitivity to phenothiazines, lactation, Parkinson's disease, pregnancy, severe hypotension or hypertension, subcortical brain damage (even if only suspected).

PRECAUTIONS

▪ IV use is limited to above specific indications. IM injection preferred. ▪ Use caution in cardiovascular, liver, and chronic respiratory diseases, and acute respiratory diseases of children. ▪ Use with caution in patients with a history of glaucoma or seizure disorders. ▪ May mask diagnosis of brain tumor, drug intoxication, and intestinal obstruction. ▪ May cause paradoxical excitation in children and the elderly. ▪ Use phenothiazines with extreme caution in children with a history of sleep apnea, a family history of SIDS, or in the presence of Reye's syndrome.

Monitor: Keep patient in supine position. ▪ Monitor blood pressure and pulse before administration and between doses. ▪ Cough reflex is often depressed. ▪ Anticholinergic and cardiac effects may be troublesome during anesthesia. For patients receiving phenothiazines, taper and discontinue preoperatively if they will not be continued after surgery. ▪ May discolor urine pink to reddish brown. ▪ Photosensitivity of skin is possible. ▪ Note Drug/lab interactions.

Patient education: Request assistance for ambulation; may cause dizziness or fainting. ▪ Observe caution performing tasks that require alertness. ▪ Avoid use of alcohol and other CNS depressants (e.g., diazepam [Valium], narcotics). ▪ Possible eye and skin photosensitivity. Avoid unprotected exposure to sun. ▪ Urine may discolor to pink or reddish brown.

Maternal/child: Note Precautions and Contraindications. ▪ Not recommended during pregnancy. May depress spermatogenesis. ▪ May cause embryo toxicity, increase neonatal mortality, or cause permanent neurological damage. ▪ Not recommended during lactation. Increases risk of dystonia and tardive dyskinesia. ▪ Children are at increased risk to develop extrapyramidal actions, especially during acute illness (e.g., chickenpox, CNS infections, dehydration, gastroenteritis, measles); monitor closely.

Elderly: Note Dose adjustments and Precautions. ▪ May have increased sensitivity to postural hypotension, anticholinergic and sedative effects. ▪ Increased risk of extrapyramidal side effects (e.g., tardive dyskinesia, parkinsonism).

DRUG/LAB INTERACTIONS

Increased CNS, respiratory depression and hypotensive effects with CNS depressants, (e.g., narcotics, alcohol, anesthetics, and barbiturates), reduced doses of these agents usually indicated. ▪ Additive effects with MAO inhibitors (e.g., selegiline [Eldepryl]), anticholinergics, antihistamines, antihypertensives, hypnotics, muscle relaxants, rauwolfia alkaloids, and thiazide diuretics; dose adjustment may be necessary. ■ Barbiturates may also increase metabolism of chlorpromazine and reduce its effects. ■ Risk of cardiotoxicity increased with pimozide (Orap) and sparfloxacin (Zagam); concurrent use not recommended. ■ Use with epinephrine not recommended; may cause precipitous hypotension. ■ Chlorpromazine may lower the seizure threshold. It may also interfere with phenytoin and valproic acid clearance, increasing potential for toxicity. Dose adjustment of anticonvulsants may be necessary. ■ Concurrent use with tricyclic antidepressants (e.g., amitriptyline [Elavil]) or MAO inhibitors (e.g., selegiline [Eldepryl]) may increase effects of both drugs; risk of neuroleptic malignant syndrome may be increased. ■ Use with thyroid agents may increase risk of agranulocytosis. ■ Use with agents that produce hypotension (e.g., antihypertensives, benzodiazepines, diuretics, lidocaine, paclitaxel) may produce severe hypotension. ■ May inhibit antiparkinson effects of levodopa. ■ May decrease pressor response to ephedrine. ■ May increase cardiac depressant effects of quinidine. ■ May increase anticholinergic effect of orphenadrine. ■ May decrease effects of oral anticoagulants. ■ Concurrent use with haldol, droperidol, or metoclopramide may cause increased extrapyramidal effects. ■ Use with metrizamide (Amipaque) may lower seizure threshold; discontinue chlorpromazine 48 hours before myelography and do not resume for 24 hours after test completed. ■ Metabolism and clearance of chlorpromazine is increased in cigarette smokers; decreased plasma levels and effectiveness may occur; dose adjustment of chlorpromazine may be indicated. ■ Decreased drowsiness may occur in cigarette smokers. May be offset by increased doses of chlorpromazine. ■ Use caution during anesthesia with barbiturates (e.g., methohexital, triopental); may increase frequency and severity of hypotension and neuromuscular excitation. ■ Capable of innumerable other interactions. ■ May cause false-positive pregnancy test, and false-positive amylase, PKU, and other urine tests.

SIDE EFFECTS

Usually transient if drug discontinued, but may require treatment if severe. Anaphylaxis, cardiac arrest, distorted Q and T waves, excitement, extrapyramidal symptoms (e.g., abnormal positioning, extreme restlessness, pseudoparkinsonism, weakness of extremities), fever, hypersensitivity reactions, hypertension, hypotension (occurs less frequently in smokers), tachycardia, and many others. Overdose can cause convulsions, hallucinations, and death.

ANTIDOTE

Discontinue the drug at onset of any side effect and notify the physician. Counteract hypotension with dopamine (Intropin) or phenylephrine (Neo-Synephrine) and IV fluids. Counteract extrapyramidal symptoms with benztropine (Cogentin) or diphenhydramine (Benadryl). Use diazepam (Valium) or phenobarbital for convulsions or hyperactivity. Epinephrine is contraindicated for hypotension; further hypotension will occur. Phenytoin may be helpful in ventricular arrhythmias. Avoid analeptics such as caffeine and sodium benzoate in treating respiratory depression and unconsciousness; they may cause convulsions. Resuscitate as necessary.

CIDOFOVIR INJECTION

Antiviral
(nucleotide analog)

Vistide

pH 7.4

USUAL DOSE

A specific protocol is required; see chart, *Overview of treatment regimen for cidofovir*. A 4 Gm course of oral probenecid is required on the day of each infusion of cidofovir to reduce the risk of renal impairment. Hydration with 1 to 2 liters of normal saline is required to help reduce proteinuria and prevent increases in serum creatinine. Infrequent dosing schedule may eliminate need for an indwelling IV catheter, reducing discomfort and potential for infection.

Induction: 5 mg/kg in 100 ml NS once weekly for 2 weeks.

Maintenance: 5 mg/kg in 100 ml NS once every other week.

Overview of the Treatment Regimen for cidofovir		
Before cidofovir infusion	**During cidofovir infusion**	**After cidofovir infusion**
1. Patient takes 2 g of probenecid* (4 × 500 mg tablets) 3 hours prior to cidofovir infusion	1. Begin IV infusion of cidofovir (5 mg/kg body weight in 100 ml normal saline) at a constant rate over 1 hour‡	1. Patient takes 1 g of probenecid (2 × 500 mg tablets) 2 hours after the *end* of cidofovir infusion
2. Infuse first liter of normal saline over 1 to 2 hours immediately before starting cidofovir infusion	2. For patients who can tolerate the extra fluid load, infuse a second liter of normal saline. If administered, initiate either at the start of the cidofovir infusion or immediately afterward, and infuse over a 1- to 3-hour period	2. Patient takes 1 g of probenecid (2 × 500 mg tablets) 8 hours after the *end* of cidofovir infusion

*Patients receiving concomitant probenecid and zidovudine should temporarily discontinue zidovudine or decrease the zidovudine dose by 50% on days of combined zidovudine and probenecid administration.
‡The recommended dosage, frequency, or infusion rate must not be exceeded.

DOSE ADJUSTMENTS

Reduce dose to 3 mg/kg for the remainder of therapy, if serum creatinine increases by 0.3 to 0.4 mg/dl above baseline. ■ 5 mg/kg may be given to patients who develop a 2⁺ proteinuria but have a stable serum creatinine. Encourage oral hydration; additional IV hydration may be appropriate. ■ Discontinue cidofovir if the serum creatinine increases by ≥ 0.5 mg/dl above baseline or if proteinuria ≥ 3⁺ develops. ▪ Restarting cidofovir in patients whose renal function has returned to baseline after a serum creatinine elevation > 0.5 mg/dl is not recommended. ▪ Discontinue cidofovir in any patient who requires therapy with a nephrotoxic agent (note Contraindications). Cidofovir may be restarted after other nephrotoxic therapy is complete, an adequate washout period of at least 7 days has passed, and adequate renal function (serum creatinine <1.5 mg/dl) is confirmed (no adequate clinical experience with this regimen to date).

DILUTION

Specific techniques required; see Precautions. A calculated dose must be diluted in 100 ml of NS.

Storage: Store unopened vials at controlled room temperature. May be refrigerated but must be used within 24 hours of dilution with NS. Allow to return to room temperature before administration. Discard partially used vials.

INCOMPATIBLE WITH

Specific information not available.

RATE OF ADMINISTRATION

A single dose as an infusion at a constant rate over 1 hr. Use of an infusion pump is recommended.

ACTIONS

A nucleotide analog antiviral. Its active intracellular metabolite selectively inhibits CMV DNA synthesis. It is incorporated into the growing viral DNA chain resulting in reductions in the rate of viral DNA synthesis. This action is independent of virus infection (acyclovir or ganciclovir require activation by a virally encoded enzyme). Elimination half-life is short (2.6 hours) but it has a long intracellular half-life, which permits infrequent dosing. Primarily excreted in urine (70% to 85% in 24 hours with concomitant doses of probenecid).

INDICATIONS AND USES

Treatment of newly diagnosed or relapsing CMV retinitis in patients with AIDS. ▪ Safety and effectiveness have not been established for treatment of other CMV infections (e.g., pneumonitis, gastroenteritis, congenital or neonatal CMV disease) or for CMV disease in non–HIV-infected individuals.

CONTRAINDICATIONS

Preexisting renal dysfunction (e.g., baseline serum creatinine ≥ 1.5 mg/dl, calculated creatinine clearance < 55 ml/min, or a urine protein > 100 mg/dl [equivalent to a 2^+ proteinuria]). ▪ Patients receiving agents with nephrotoxic potential (e.g., aminoglycosides, amphotericin B, foscarnet, NSAIDs, IV pentamidine, vancomycin). No other nephrotoxic agent should be administered within 7 days of starting cidofovir or concomitantly during cidofovir therapy. ▪ Hypersensitivity to cidofovir and/or a history of clinically severe hypersensitivity (e.g., hypotension, respiratory distress) to probenecid or other sulfa-containing medications (e.g., sulfamethoxazole-trimethoprim [Bactrim]).

PRECAUTIONS

▪ Follow guidelines for handling cytotoxic agents. See Appendix A, p. 893. ▪ Administered by or under the direction of the physician specialist, preferably in an environment where emergency treatment is available. ▪ This formulation is for IV use only; DO NOT use for intraocular injection. ▪ Calculated creatinine clearance may not accurately estimate renal function in emaciated (e.g., patients with AIDS) or extremely muscular patients; a 24-hour urine collection may be required. ▪ CMV resistant to ganciclovir may also be resistant to cidofovir, but may be sensitive to foscarnet (Foscavir). ▪ CMV resistant to foscarnet may be sensitive to cidofovir. ▪ Do not exceed recommended doses, frequency, or rate of administration; may cause increased risk of renal toxicity. ▪ Renal function may not return to baseline after treatment with cidofovir. ▪ Proteinuria is an indicator of nephrotoxicity, which may lead to additional proximal tubular cell injury resulting in glycosuria, decreased serum phosphate, uric acid, and bicarbonate; increased serum creatinine; and/or acute renal failure, which may necessitate dialysis. ▪ Although some reference sources have published doses for patients with impaired renal function, this drug is contraindicated in such patients and should be given only to those who meet specific dosing criteria (see Contraindications).

Monitor: 24 to 48 hours before each cidofovir infusion, obtain a serum creatinine, urine protein (via dipstick or quantitative urinalysis), and a CBC with differential (absolute neutrophil count [ANC]). ▪ Administration of probenecid as ordered and adequate hydration (oral and IV) are imperative. ▪ Antiretroviral therapy may be continued with the exception of zidovudine; (See Drug/lab interactions). ▪ Probenecid frequently causes fever, flushing, headache, nausea with or without emesis, and rash. Use acetaminophen for prophylaxis or treatment of fever or headache. Encourage ingestion of food prior to each dose of probenecid to reduce nausea; prophylactic antiemetics (e.g., ondansetron [Zofran]) are appropriate. Consider use of antihistamines (e.g., diphenhydramine [Benadryl]) for prophylaxis or treatment in patients who develop mild hypersensitivity reactions (e.g., rash). Severe hypersensitivity reactions (e.g., laryngospasm, hypotension) have occasionally been reported with probenecid. Usually occur within several hours after patients have received probenecid even though they have received it before with no adverse reactions. Observe patient carefully for allergic reactions. Treatment for anaphylaxis (e.g., epinephrine, corticosteroids, and antihistamines) must be readily available. ▪ May increase intraocular pressure; monitor with a baseline ophthalmologic exam and periodically during therapy; risk may be increased in patients with preexisting diabetes mellitus.

Patient education: Not a cure for CMV retinitis. Retinitis may recur during maintenance or after treatment; regular ophthalmologic exams imperative. ▪ Full compliance with regimen imperative (e.g., probenecid with food, increased IV and oral hydration, regular lab testing). ▪ Report fever, rash, nausea, and vomiting promptly. ▪ Report concomitant medication changes or additions. ▪ Notify all health care personnel of treatment with probenecid to avoid interactions. ▪ Consider birth control options; note Maternal/child.

Maternal/child: Category C: should not be used during pregnancy; embryotoxic in animals. A potential carcinogen; knowledge of effects on women unknown. ▪ Women of childbearing age should use effective contraception during cidofovir therapy and for 1 month after completion. ▪ Men should use barrier contraception during cidofovir therapy and for 3 months after completion. ▪ Has caused reduced testical weight and hypospermia in animals. ▪ Do not administer to nursing mothers. HIV-infected mothers are advised not to breast feed to avoid transmission to an uninfected child. ▪ Safety and effectiveness for use in children not established. Use in children with extreme caution and only if the benefits of treatment outweigh the risks of long-term carcinogenicity and reproductive toxicity. Consult physician specialist for adjustments in probenecid and hydration.

Elderly: Effects have not been studied; monitor renal function carefully.

DRUG/LAB INTERACTIONS

Limited information available. Drug profile review by pharmacist imperative. ▪ Nephrotoxicity increased by other nephrotoxic agents (e.g., aminoglycosides [e.g., amikacin, gentamicin], amphotericin B [Fungizone, Abelcet], foscarnet [Foscovir], IV pentamidine [Pentam 300], NSAIDs [e.g., ibuprofen (Motrin), vancomycin [Vancocin]); (See Contraindications). ▪ Prior treatment with foscavir may also increase the risk of nephrotoxicity; monitor renal function carefully. ▪ Probenecid decreases clearance of zidovudine; temporarily discontinue or reduce dose of zidovudine by 50% on days of combined zidovudine and probenecid administration. ▪ Probenecid may have interactions with numerous other drugs (e.g., acetaminophen, acyclovir [Zovirax], ACE inhibitors [e.g., enalaprilat (Vasotec)], aminosalicylic acid, barbiturates, benzodiazepines [e.g., diazepam, lorazepam (Ativan), midazolam], bumetamide, clofibrate, ddC, famotidine, furosemide, chlorpropamide [Diabinese], methotrexate, NSAIDs [e.g., ketoprofen (Orudis)], theophyllines), usually decreasing their rate of excretion and increasing toxicity. Consider witholding any drug that may interact with probenecid on the day of cidofovir administration.

SIDE EFFECTS

Nephrotoxicity is dose limiting. Metabolic acidosis (Fanconi's syndrome), neutropenia, and ocular hypotony may be dose limiting and require prompt treatment. Asthenia, decreased serum bicarbonate, diarrhea, dyspnea, fever, headache, increased creatinine, infection, nausea and vomiting, pneumonia, and proteinuria may occur.

ANTIDOTE

There is no specific antidote. Keep physician informed. Adequate hydration, use of probenecid, and careful monitoring will help to reduce potential for renal impairment and may minimize other side effects. Filgrastim (Neupogen) may be used to treat neutropenia. (See Monitor) for management of probenecid side effects. Discontinue cidofovir based on criteria in Dose adjustments. Treat overdose for 3 to 5 days with probenecid 1 Gm three times daily and vigorous IV hydration to tolerance. Treat anaphylaxis and resuscitate as indicated. Hemodialysis may be helpful in overdose.

CIMETIDINE

Antiulcer
(H$_2$ antagonist)
Gastric acid inhibitor
Adjunct urticaria therapy

Tagamet   pH 3.8 to 6.0

USUAL DOSE

Direct or intermittent IV: 300 mg every 6 hours. Increase frequency of dose, not amount, if necessary for pain relief. Do not exceed 2,400 mg/24 hr.

Continuous IV: 900 mg evenly distributed over 24 hours (37.5 mg/hr). May be preceded by a loading dose of 150 to 300 mg if indicated (total dose from 1,050 to 1,200 mg/24 hr). To maintain intragastric acid secretory rates at 10 mEq/hr or less, dose range may be higher in patients with pathologic hypersecretory states. Product insert mentions a study that used a range of 40 to 600 mg/hr averaging 160 mg/hr; well beyond usual doses. Any dose beyond the normal should be administered with extreme caution.

Additive for total parenteral nutrition (TPN): 70% to 100% of an average 24-hour dose has been used equally distributed over 24 hours as a continuous infusion. May be supplemented with intermittent doses as needed.

Prevention of upper GI bleeding: A continuous infusion of 37.5 to 50 mg/hr for up to 7 days. Maintain gastric pH at 3.5 to 4. May be preceded by a loading dose of up to 300 mg.

Prevention of aspiration pneumonitis: 300 mg 60 to 90 minutes before anesthesia.

Erosive gastroesophageal reflux disease (GERD): 1,600 mg/day (IV or PO) in divided doses every 6 hours (400 mg) or 12 hours (800 mg) for 12 weeks.

PEDIATRIC DOSE

5 to 10 mg/kg of body weight every 6 hours.

INFANT DOSE

2.5 to 5 mg/kg every 6 hours.

DOSE ADJUSTMENTS

Increase intervals between injections to achieve pain relief with least frequent dosage in impaired renal function. ▪ Reduce dose by half in prevention of GI bleeding if creatinine clearance below 30 ml/min.

DILUTION

Direct IV: Each 300 mg must be diluted with 18 ml (total volume of 20 ml) of NS or other compatible solution for injection (see chart on back cover).

Intermittent infusion: Each 300 mg may be diluted in at least 50 ml of D5W or other compatible infusion solution and given piggyback. Available premixed. Do not use premixed plastic containers in series connections; may cause air embolism.

Continuous infusion: Total daily dose may be diluted in 100 to 1,000 ml of infusion solution. Compatible with most dextrose and saline solutions, lactated Ringer's solution, 5% sodium bicarbonate, and many others. Compatible in selected TPN solutions for 24 hours (consult pharmacist).

Storage: Stable at controlled room temperature for 48 hours after dilution.

INCOMPATIBLE WITH

Allopurinol (Zyloprim), aminophylline, amphotericin B (Fungizone), atropine, barbiturates, cefamandole (Mandol), cephalosporins (e.g., cetazolin [Ancef], cephalothin [Keflin]), chlorpromazine (Throazine), indomethacin (Indocin). Do not add any other drugs to premixed cimetidine in plastic containers.

RATE OF ADMINISTRATION

Direct IV: Each 300 mg or fraction thereof over a minimum of 5 minutes.

Intermittent infusion: Each 300 mg dose over 15 to 20 minutes.

Continuous infusion: Give loading dose at intermittent infusion rate and distribute balance of daily dose equally over 24 hours. Use of infusion pump preferred, especially with volumes of 250 ml or less, to avoid complications of overdose or too-rapid administration (note Side effects).

ACTIONS

A histamine H_2 antagonist, it inhibits both daytime and nocturnal basal gastric acid secretion. It also inhibits gastric acid secretion stimulated by food, histamine, pentagastrin, caffeine, and insulin. Onset of action is prompt and effective for 4 to 5 hours. Excreted in the urine. Crosses placental barrier. Secreted in breast milk.

INDICATIONS AND USES

Short-term treatment of active duodenal ulcers and active benign gastric ulcers. ▪ Pathologic hypersecretory conditions. ▪ Erosive gastroesophageal reflux disease (GERD) diagnosed by endoscopy. ▪ Prevention of GI bleeding in critically ill patients especially those with potential for stress-related mucosal damage (e.g., erosive gastritis, stress ulcers). ▪ Additive to TPN to simplify fluid and electrolyte management (decreases the volume and chloride content of gastric secretions).

Investigational uses: Preoperatively to prevent aspiration pneumonia. ▪ Treatment of itching and flushing of anaphylaxis, pruritus, urticaria, and contact dermatitis. ▪ Treatment of acetaminophen overdose (helps to reduce hepatotoxicity).

CONTRAINDICATIONS

Known hypersensitivity to cimetidine.

PRECAUTIONS

IV bolus administration has precipitated rare instances of cardiac arrhythmias, hypotension, and death. ▪ Gastric malignancy may be present even though patient is asymptomatic. ▪ Gastric pain and ulceration may recur after medication stopped.

Monitor: Use antacids concomitantly to relieve pain. ▪ Monitor prothrombin times. ▪ Note Drug/lab interactions. ▪ Change to oral doses when appropriate; usually discontinued after 4 to 8 weeks.

Patient education: Interacts with many medications. Check with pharmacist or physician before taking any other drugs. ▪ Abstain from smoking; at least avoid smoking after the last dose of the day.

Maternal/child: Pregnancy category B: no adequate studies available; benefits must outweigh risks. ▪ Discontinue breast feeding. ▪ Not recommended for children under 16, but 20 to 40 mg/kg/day has been used.

Elderly: Safety and effectiveness consistent with younger ages; renal clearance of cimetidine likely to be decreased.

DRUG/LAB INTERACTIONS

May potentiate warfarin-type anticoagulants; monitor prothrombin times. ■ Potentiates effects of alcohol, antimalarials (e.g., chloroquine), some benzodiazepines (e.g., diazepam [Valium]), beta blockers (e.g., propranolol [Inderal]), caffeine, calcium channel blockers (e.g., verapamil), carbamazepine, fluoroquinolones (e.g., ciprofloxacin [Cipro]), hydantoins (e.g., phenytoin [Dilantin]), lidocaine, metronidazole (e.g., Flagyl), pentoxifylline (Trental), procainamide (Pronestyl), quinidine, sulfonylureas, tricyclic antidepressants (e.g., imipramine [Tofranil]), theophyllines (e.g., aminophylline), and triamterene (Dyrenium). ■ May inhibit digoxin absorption. ■ Clinical effect (inhibition of nocturnal gastric secretion) reversed by cigarette smoking. ■ May precipitate apnea, confusion, and muscle twitching with morphine. ■ May cause increased myelosuppression with alkylating agents (e.g., carmustine). ■ Concurrent use with paroxetine (Paxil) may cause increased serum levels of paroxetine and an increase in BP. ■ May inhibit gastric absorption of ketoconazole (Nizoral). ■ Many unconfirmed reports of inhibiting pharmacologic action of other drugs.

SIDE EFFECTS

Average dose: Bradycardia, confusion, diarrhea, delirium, dizziness, elevated AST (SGOT), fever, galactorrhea, gynecomastia, hallucinations, impotence, interstitial nephritis, muscular pain, rash.

Overdose: Cardiac arrhythmias, death, hypotension, respiratory failure, tachycardia.

ANTIDOTE

Notify physician of all side effects. May be treated symptomatically or may respond to decrease in frequency of dose. Physostigmine may be useful to reverse CNS toxicity. In overdose, assisted ventilation is indicated and beta blockers (e.g., metoprolol [Lopressor], propranolol [Inderal]) may control tachycardia.

CIPROFLOXACIN

Antibacterial
(Fluoroquinolone)

Cipro I.V.

pH 3.3 to 4.6

USUAL DOSE

Dose based on severity and nature of the infection, susceptibility of the causative organism, integrity of host-defense mechanisms, and renal and hepatic status. Range is from 200 to 400 mg according to the following chart on p. 209. Continue for 7 to 14 days (at least 2 days after all symptoms of infection subside). Bone and joint infections may require treatment for 4 to 6 weeks or more. May be transferred to oral dosing when appropriate.

Infection	Type of Severity	Unit Dose	Frequency	Total 24-hr Dose
Urinary tract	Mild/moderate	200 mg	q12h	400 mg
	Severe/ complicated	400 mg	q12h	800 mg
Lower respiratory tract	Mild/moderate	400 mg	q12h	800 mg
	Severe/ complicated	400 mg	q8h	1200 mg
Nosocomial pneumonia	Mild/moderate/ severe	400 mg	q8h	1200 mg
Skin and skin structure	Mild/moderate	400 mg	q12h	800 mg
	Severe/ complicated	400 mg	q8h	1200 mg
Bone and joint	Mild/moderate	400 mg	q12h	800 mg
	Severe/ complicated	400 mg	q8h	1200 mg
Septicemia (Canada)		400 mg	q12h	800 mg
Intra-abdominal, Complicated	Ciprofloxacin + metronidazole	400 mg 500 mg	q12h q6h	800 mg 2000 mg
Empirical therapy in febrile neutropenic patients, Severe	Ciprofloxacin + piperacillin	400 mg 50 mg	q8h q4h	1200 mg Not to exceed 24 g/day

PEDIATRIC DOSE

Used only when alternate therapy cannot be used; see Maternal/ child. 10 to 15 mg/kg of body weight every 12 hours.

DOSE ADJUSTMENTS

Reduce time between doses (200 to 400 mg every 18 to 24 hours) if creatinine clearance is less than 30 ml/min (see literature for additional information). ■ Note Drug/lab interactions.

DILUTION

Available prediluted in NS or D5W in plastic infusion containers ready for use. A clear, colorless to slightly yellow solution. Do not hang plastic containers in a series; may cause air embolism. Also available in 20 and 40 ml vials containing 10 mg/ml (1% solution), which must be diluted with NS, D5W, SW, D10W, D5/0.2 NS, D5/0.45 NS, or LR to a final concentration of 0.5 to 2 mg/ml.

Storage: Store at room temperature before dilution; protect from light, excessive heat, and freezing. Stable for up to 14 days refrigerated or at room temperature in the final diluted concentration.

INCOMPATIBLE WITH

Manufacturer recommends ciprofloxacin be administered separately. Aminophylline, ampicillin (Polycillin-N), ampicillin sulbactam (Unasyn), clindamycin (Cleocin), ceftazidime (Tazicef), dexamethasone (Decadron), furosemide (Lasix), heparin, hydrocortison succinate (Solu-Cortef), magnesium sulfate, methylprednisolone (Solu-Medrol), mezlocillin (Mezlin), phenytoin (Dilantin), sodium bicarbonate.

RATE OF ADMINISTRATION

A single dose must be equally distributed over 60 minutes as an infusion. Too-rapid administration and/or the use of a small vein may increase incidence of anaphylaxis, local site inflammation, and other side effects. May be given through a Y-tube or three-way stopcock of infusion set. Temporarily discontinue other solutions infusing at the same site.

ACTIONS

A synthetic broad-spectrum antimicrobial agent, a fluoroquinolone. Bactericidal to a wide range of aerobic gram-negative and gram-positive organisms through interference with the enzyme needed for synthesis of bacterial DNA. Onset of action is prompt, and serum levels are dose related. Half-life averages 5 to 6 hours. Readily distributed to body fluids (saliva, nasal and bronchial secretions, sputum, skin blister fluid, lymph, peritoneal fluid, bile and prostatic secretions). Found in lung, skin, fat, muscle, cartilage, and bone. Distribution to cerebrospinal fluid and eye fluids is lower than plasma levels. Excreted as unchanged drug in the urine, usually within 24 hours. Crosses placental barrier. Secreted in breast milk.

INDICATIONS AND USES

Treatment of mild, moderate, severe, and complicated urinary tract infections; and mild to moderate lower respiratory, skin and skin structure, and bone and joint infections. Most effective against specific organisms (see literature). ■ Additional appropriate therapy required if anaerobic organisms are suspected of contributing to the infection. ■ Oral route of administration indicated for treatment of other infections (e.g., cystitis, prostatitis, acute sinusitis).
Investigational uses: Treatment of tuberculosis in combination with other antituberculosis agents (e.g., rifampin). ■ Treatment of *Mycobacterium avium* complex infection in AIDS patients.

CONTRAINDICATIONS

Known hypersensitivity to ciprofloxacin or any other quinolone antimicrobial agent (e.g., norfloxacin [Noroxin]).

PRECAUTIONS

Specific culture and sensitivity studies indicated to determine susceptibility of the causative organism to ciprofloxacin. ■ Pseudomonas aeruginosa may develop resistance during treatment. Ongoing culture and sensitivity studies indicated. ■ Prolonged use may cause superinfection because of overgrowth of nonsusceptible organisms. Monitor carefully. ■ Use caution in patients with impaired hepatic function and known CNS disorders (e.g., epilepsy, severe cerebral arteriosclerosis, or any other factors that predispose to seizures). ■ May cause ophthalmologic abnormalities (e.g., cataracts). Incidence increases with length of treatment.
Monitor: May cause anaphylaxis with the first or succeeding doses,

even in patients without known hypersensitivity. Emergency equipment must always be available. ▪ Maintain adequate hydration and acidity of urine throughout treatment. Will form crystals in alkaline urine. ▪ Monitor hematopoietic, hepatic, and renal systems during prolonged treatment. ▪ Use of large veins recommended to dilute toxicity, reduce incidence of allergic reactions, and reduce incidence of local irritation. Symptoms of local irritation do not preclude further administration of ciprofloxacin unless they recur or worsen. Generally resolve when infusion complete. ▪ Monitor serum levels with theophylline; observe with caffeine. ▪ Note Drug/lab interactions.

Patient education: Consider birth control options. ▪ Avoid exposure to sunlight or artificial ultraviolet light; may cause severe sunburn. Wear dark glasses outdoors. ▪ Request assistance for ambulation; may cause dizziness and lightheadedness. ▪ Effects of caffeine- or theophylline-containing preparations may be increased. Limit or eliminate concurrent use. Monitor if concurrent use necessary. ▪ Report skin rash or any other hypersensitivity reaction promptly.

Maternal/child: Category C: not recommended for use in pregnancy; is toxic to the fetus; benefits must outweigh risk. ▪ Discontinue breast feeding. ▪ Safety for use in children under 18 years of age not established. May erode cartilage of weight-bearing joints or cause other signs of arthropathy in infants and children.

DRUG/LAB INTERACTIONS

May cause serious or fatal reactions with theophylline (e.g., cardiac arrhythmias or arrest, respiratory failure, or seizures). If must be used concomitantly, monitor serum levels of theophylline and decrease dose as appropriate. Observe closely with caffeine intake; has caused similar problems. ▪ Use with cyclosporine may cause an increase in serum creatinine and nephrotoxic effects. ▪ May potentiate oral anticoagulants (e.g., warfarin [Coumadin]); monitor prothrombin times. ▪ Potentiated by probenicid; may require dose adjustment based on ciprofloxacin serum levels. ▪ Serum levels may be decreased with antineoplastic agents (e.g., cisplatin, doxorubicin [Adriamycin]). ▪ Serum levels may be increased with cimetidine (Tagamet). ▪ 2 case reports suggest concurrent administration with foscarnet (Foscavir) may cause seizures; monitor patient carefully. ▪ Note Side effects.

SIDE EFFECTS

Allergic reactions (anaphylaxis, cardiovascular collapse, death, dyspnea, edema [facial or pharyngeal], eosinophilia, fever, hepatic necrosis, itching, jaundice, loss of consciousness, rash, urticaria); cardiac arrest; CNS stimulation (confusion, hallucinations, lightheadedness, restlessness, seizures, tingling, toxic psychosis, tremors); decreased hemoglobin, hematocrit, and platelet count; diarrhea; elevation of eosinophil and platelet counts, blood glucose, BUN, serum creatine, serum creatine phosphokinase, uric acid, and triglycerides; headache; hepatic enzyme abnormalities (elevation of alkaline phosphatase, AST [SGOT], ALT [SGPT], LDH, serum bilirubin); increased intracranial pressure; local site reactions; nausea; phototoxicity and vision changes; pseudomembranous colitis; respiratory failure; status epilepticus. Capable of numerous other reactions in less than 1% of patients.

ANTIDOTE

Death may result from some of these side effects. Discontinue ciprofloxacin at the first appearance of a skin rash or any other sign of hypersensitivity, at the onset of any CNS symptom, or the onset of pseudomembranous colitis. Treat allergic reaction with epinephrine (Adrenalin), airway management, oxygen, IV fluids, antihistamines (diphenhydramine [Benadryl]), corticosteroids (Solu-cortef), and pressor amines (dopamine [Intropin]) as indicated. Treat CNS symptoms as indicated. May require diazepam (Valium) for seizures. Mild cases of colitis may respond to discontinuation of ciprofloxacin. Oral vancomycin (Vancocin) or metronidazole (Flagyl) is the treatment of choice for antibiotic-related pseudomembranous colitis. Keep physician informed of all side effects. Many will require symptomatic treatment; monitor closely. Maintain hydration in overdose. No specific antidote; up to 10% may be excreted by hemodialysis or peritoneal dialysis. Maintain patient until drug excreted.

CISATRACURIUM BESYLATE

Neuromuscular
blocking agent
(nondepolarizing)
Anesthesia adjunct

Nimbex   pH 3.25 to 3.65

USUAL DOSE

Must be individualized based on previous drugs administered (e.g., fentanyl [Sublimaze], midazolam [Versed]), desired time to intubation, and anticipated length of surgery. Patient should be unconscious before administration. Use of a peripheral nerve stimulator is indicated in all situations.

Adjunct to propofol/N_2O/O_2 anesthesia for adults (IV bolus): Initial dose: 0.15 to 0.2 mg/kg. 0.15 mg/kg should provide good to excellent conditions for intubation within 2 minutes and adequate muscle relaxation for 55 minutes (range 44 to 74 min). 0.2 mg/kg (7 ml [of a 2 mg/ml conc] for a 70-kg patient) should be effective within 1.5 minutes and last for 61 minutes (range 41 to 81 min). Up to 0.4 mg/kg has been used; has a dose-related length of effectiveness.

Maintenance dose: May be given by IV bolus or as a continuous infusion. Determine need for maintenance dose based on beginning symptoms of neuromuscular blockade reversal determined by a peripheral nerve stimulator. Usually required 40 to 60 minutes after a bolus dose. Do not administer before recovery begins. Repeated doses have no cumulative effect if recovery is allowed to begin prior to administration. Note Dose adjustments. *IV bolus:* 0.03 mg/kg (1 ml [of a 2 mg/ml conc] for a 70-kg patient) should provide an additional 20 minutes of muscle relaxation. Smaller or larger doses may be given based on expected duration of procedure. *Continuous infusion:* Begin infusion with 3 mcg/kg/min to rapidly counteract the spontaneous recovery, then decrease to 1 to 2 mcg/kg/min. Monitor maintenance infusion with a peripheral nerve stimulator.

Support of intubated, mechanically ventilated, or respiratory controlled adult ICU patients: After intubation is accomplished (usually with succinylcholine), an initial bolus dose of 0.1 mg/kg provides adequate neuromuscular blockade. Maintain with 3 mcg/kg/min (range 0.5 to 10.2 mcg/kg/min). Published reports describe a wide interpatient variability in dosing requirements that may change from day to day. Adjust infusion rate according to clinical assessment of the patient's response. Use of a peripheral nerve stimulator is recommended. Do not increase dose until there is a definite response to nerve stimulation. If recovery from neuromuscular block has progressed, readministration of a bolus dose may be necessary. Long-term use (beyond 6 days) has not been studied.

PEDIATRIC DOSE

Adjunct to halothane or opioid anesthesia for children 2 to 12 years of age: (IV bolus) initial dose: 0.1 mg/kg. Should provide good to excellent conditions for intubation within 2.8 minutes and adequate muscle relaxation for 28 minutes (range 21 to 38 min). Note all comments under adult dose and Maternal/child.

Maintenance dose: Same as adult dosing; note all comments.

DOSE ADJUSTMENTS

Reduce initial dose to 0.02 mg/kg in any condition that may result in a prolonged neuromuscular blockade (e.g., myasthenia gravis, myasthenic syndrome, carcinomatosis, debilitation, other drugs). Use a peripheral nerve stimulator to assess the level of neuromuscular block and to monitor dose requirements. Note Drug/lab interactions.
■ Increased initial and maintenance doses may be required in burn patients. Duration of action may be shortened. ■ Half-life is extended but no dose adjustment is required in patients with renal or hepatic disease or in the elderly. Time of onset may be slightly faster in patients with liver disease and slower in the elderly and patients with renal disease. Slower onset may require a delay of an additional minute before intubation. ■ Reduce maintenance dose by 30% to 40% in the presence of isoflurane or enflurane anesthesia. Larger reductions may be indicated in prolonged anesthesia. ■ May need to reduce maintenance dose by 50% in patients undergoing coronary artery bypass surgery with induced hypothermia.

DILUTION

IV bolus: May be given undiluted.

Infusion: Further dilute in NS, D5W, D5/NS, or D5/LR to a 0.1 mg/ml or 0.4 mg/ml solution. Using the 2 mg/ml solution, 10 mg diluted in 95 ml yields 0.1 mg/ml; 40 mg diluted in 80 ml yields 0.4 mg/ml.

ICU infusion: A 20 ml vial (10 mg/ml concentration) is available for use in ICU (200 mg/vial). 200 mg in 1,000 ml yields 0.2 mg/ml, in 500 ml yields 0.4 mg/ml.

Storage: Refrigerate in carton before use; protect from light; do not freeze. Use within 21 days if at room temperature even if it was rerefrigerated. Most diluted solutions are stable refrigerated or at room temperature for 24 hours. Solutions diluted in D5/LR can be refrigerated for up to 24 hours.

INCOMPATIBLE WITH

Solution: Alkaline solutions (e.g., aminophyline, barbiturates), LR.

Y-site: Propofol (Diprivan), ketorolac (Toradol).

COMPATIBLE WITH

Y-site: Alfentanil (Alfenta), droperidol (Inapsine), fentanyl (Subli-maze), midazolam (Versed), and sulfentanil (Sufenta), if drugs are diluted as directed.

RATE OF ADMINISTRATION

IV bolus: A single dose over 5 to 10 seconds.

Infusion for anesthesia adjunct or ICU: Use of a microdrip (60 gtt/ml) or volume infusion pump required. Adjust rate to desired dose based on charts below for 0.1 mg/ml and 0.4 mg/ml. For 0.2 mg/ml solution in ICU, multiply rates (ml/hr) of 0.1 mg/ml solution by 2 or divide rates (ml/hr) of 0.4 mg/ml solution in half.

Cisatracurium Infusion Rates for a Concentration of 0.1 mg/mL

Patient Weight (kg)	DRUG DELIVERY RATE (mcg/kg/min)				
	1	1.5	2	3	5
	Infusion Delivery Rate (mL/hr)				
10	6	9	12	18	30
45	27	41	54	81	135
70	42	63	84	126	210
100	60	90	120	180	300

Cisatracurium Infusion Rates for a Concentration of 0.4 mg/mL

Patient Weight (kg)	DRUG DELIVERY RATE (mcg/kg/min)				
	1	1.5	2	3	5
	Infusion Delivery Rate (mL/hr)				
10	1.5	2.3	3	4.5	7.5
45	6.8	10.1	13.5	20.3	33.8
70	10.5	15.8	21	31.5	52.5
100	15	22.5	30	45	75

ACTIONS

A nondepolarizing skeletal muscle relaxant with intermediate onset and duration of action. An isomer of atracurium (Tracrium) with three times its potency at a mg for mg dose. In contrast to most of the other neuromuscular blocking agents, cisatracurium has no clinically significant effect on heart rate or blood pressure with usual doses even in patients with serious cardiovascular disease and it also does not produce a dose related histamine release. Causes paralysis by interfering with neural transmission at the myoneural junction. Produces maximum neuromuscular blockade within 1.5 to 3 minutes and lasts about 50 minutes in adults. Recovery to 75% usually occurs within 30 minutes. Metabolized by a process that mostly bypasses both the kidney and the liver. Forms specific metabolites (e.g., alcohol, laudanosine) that do not have neuromuscular blocking activity.

Because of reduced dose requirements, laudanosine accumulation is lower than with atracurium, lowering the potential of seizures. Eliminated renally, primarily as metabolites.

INDICATIONS AND USES

Adjunctive to general anesthesia for inpatients and outpatients to facilitate endotracheal intubation and to relax skeletal muscles during surgery. ■ Relax skeletal muscles during mechanical ventilation in ICU.

CONTRAINDICATIONS

Known hypersensitivity to cisatracurium, other bis-benzylisoquinolinium compounds (e.g., atracurium), and benzyl alcohol (some preparations contain benzyl alcohol).

PRECAUTIONS

For IV use only. ■ Administered by or under the observation of the anesthesiologist. Adequate facilities, emergency resuscitation drugs and equipment, neuromuscular blocking antagonists (e.g., anticholinesterase agents [e.g., neostigmine, edrophonium]) and atropine must always be available. ■ Not recommended for rapid sequence intubation; succinylcholine is usually the drug of choice. ■ Myasthenia gravis and other neuromuscular diseases increase sensitivity to cisatracurium. Can cause critical reactions. ■ Sensitivity may be decreased in patients with burns or paralysis. Note Dose adjustments and Monitor. ■ In patients with renal or hepatic disease, half-life of metabolites is longer, and concentrations may be higher with long-term administration. ■ Did not trigger Malignant Hypertension (MH) in susceptible pigs at doses above those required for humans, but has not been studied in MH-susceptible humans. ■ Respiratory depression with propofol (Diprivan) or morphine may be preferred in some patients requiring mechanical ventilation. ■ Will not counteract the bradycardia produced by many anesthetic agents or vagal stimulation.

Monitor: This drug produces apnea. Controlled artificial ventilation with oxygen must be continuous and under direct observation at all times. Maintain a patent airway. ■ Use a peripheral nerve stimulator to monitor drug effect, determine the need for additional doses, confirm recovery from neuromuscular block, and avoid overdose. Place on a non-paralyzed limb in patients with paralysis. ■ Monitor vital signs and ECG continuously. ■ Has no analgesic properties or effect on consciousness. Use in conjunction with anesthesia, sedation, or analgesia as indicated. ■ Action potentiated by hypokalemia and some carcinomas. ■ Action may be potentiated or antagonized by dehydration, electrolyte imbalance, body temperature, or acid-base imbalance.

Maternal/child: Category B: use in pregnancy only if clearly needed. Safety for use during labor and delivery not established. ■ Use caution during lactation; probably best to defer breast feeding until after full recovery. ■ Safety for use in infants under 2 years of age not established. ■ 10 ml (2 mg/ml) multiple dose vials contain benzyl alcohol, do not use in newborns. ■ In children 2 to 12 years of age, onset is faster, duration shorter, and recovery faster than in adults.

Elderly: Safely administered even in patients with significant cardiac disease. ■ Onset to complete neuromuscular block slightly slower; delay intubation until fully effective. Recovery may be slower.

DRUG/LAB INTERACTIONS

Potentiated by general anesthetics (e.g., enflurane, isoflurane), many antibiotics (e.g., aminoglycosides [kanamycin (Kantrex), gentamicin (Garamycin)], lincosamides [clindamycin (Cleocin)], polypeptides [bacitracin, colistimethate], tetracyclines), muscle relaxants, diuretics, lithium, local anesthetics, magnesium sulfate, procainamide (Pronestyl), quinidine, succinylcholine, and others. May need to reduce initial or maintenance dose of cisatracurium, use with caution. ▪ Antagonized by acetylcholine and anticholinesterases. ▪ Duration of neuromuscular block may be shorter and dose requirements may be higher during maintenance infusion in patients stabilized on carbamazepine (Tegretol) or phenytoin (Dilantin). ▪ Time to onset of maximum block is faster when succinycholine is given before cisatracurium. Succinylcholine must show signs of wearing off before cisatracurium is given. Use caution.

SIDE EFFECTS

Bradycardia, bronchospasm, flushing, hypotension, and rash occurred in fewer than 1% of patients. Rare reports of seizures with similar agents in ICU could be caused by accumulated laudanosine, other conditions or medications. Excessive dosing or prolonged action may result in respiratory insufficiency or apnea. Airway closure may be caused by relaxation of epiglottis, pharynx, and tongue muscles. Hypersensitivity reactions including anaphylaxis are possible.

ANTIDOTE

Side effects can be medical emergencies. Treat symptomatically. Maintain a patent airway, and continuous controlled artificial ventilation and oxygenation until full recovery is ensured. The more profound the neuromuscular block, the longer it will take until recovery begins. Recovery from neuromuscular block must be confirmed by a peripheral nerve stimulator before anticholinesterase agents (e.g., neostigmine [Prostigmin], or edrophonium [Enlon]) can be given with an anticholinergic agent (e.g., atropine) to reverse the muscle relaxation. Neostigmine 0.04 to 0.07 mg/kg at 10% recovery in conjunction with atropine should be effective in 9 to 10 minutes. Edrophonium 1 mg/kg at 25% recovery in conjunction with atropine (Enlon + is edrophonium and atropine combined) should be effective in 3 to 5 minutes. Confirm recovery by 5 second head lift and grip strength. Recovery may be inhibited by cachexia, carcinomatosis, debilitation, or the concomitant use of certain drugs, note Drug/lab interactions. Resuscitate as necessary.

CISPLATIN

Antineoplastic
(Alkylating agent)

CDDP, Platinol, Platinol-AQ

pH 3.5 to 6.0

USUAL DOSE

Metastatic testicular tumors: 20 mg/M^2 daily for 5 days every 3 weeks for 3 courses. Bleomycin and vinblastine also indicated.

Metastatic ovarian tumors: 50 mg/M^2 once every 3 weeks with doxorubicin. 100 mg/M^2 every 4 weeks as a single agent.

Advanced bladder cancer: 50 to 70 mg/M^2 once every 3 to 4 weeks. Initial or repeat doses may not be given unless serum creatinine is below 1.5 mg/100 ml and/or the BUN is below 25 mg/100 ml; platelets should be 100,000/mm^3 and leukocytes 4,000/mm^3; verify auditory acuity as within normal limits. Numerous other doses and combinations are used.

DOSE ADJUSTMENTS

All doses adjusted based on prior radiation therapy or chemotherapy.
- Reduced dose indicated if creatinine clearance less than 50 ml/min; see literature.

DILUTION

Specific techniques required; see Precautions. Initially dilute each 10 (50) mg vial with 10 (50) ml of sterile water for injection (1 mg/ml). Platinol-AQ is prediluted to 1 mg/ml. Withdraw desired dose. Immediately before use each one half of a single dose should be diluted in 1 liter of 5% dextrose in 0.2%, 0.45% saline or NS containing 12.5 to 25 Gm of mannitol (optional). Will decompose if adequate chloride ion not available. Is also diluted in smaller amounts of NS (100 to 500 ml). Do not use needles or IV tubing with aluminum parts to administer; a precipitate will form and potency will decrease. (See Monitor) for additional optional additives.

Storage: Stable at room temperature for at least 24 hours. Use immediately if contains mannitol.

INCOMPATIBLE WITH

Amifostine (Ethyol), fluorouracil (5 FU), gallium nitrate (Ganite), mesna, metoclopramide. piperacillin tazobactam (Zosyn) (Reglan), thiotepa. Inactivated by alkaline solutions (e.g., sodium bicarbonate), sodium bisulfite, sodium thiosulfate.

COMPATIBLE WITH

Carmustine, cyclophosphamide, etoposide, mannitol, magnesium sulfate, and potassium chloride. Consultation with pharmacist required.

RATE OF ADMINISTRATION

Each 1 liter of infusion solution over 3 to 4 hours. Give total dose (2 liters) over 6 to 8 hours. Rate must be sufficient to maintain hydration and diuresis. Solutions from 100 to 500 ml are sometimes given over 30 min. Infusion time has also been extended to 24 hours/dose. Too-rapid administration (5 min) increases nephrotoxicity and ototoxicity.

ACTIONS

A heavy metal complex (platinum and chloride atoms). Has properties similar to alkylating agents and is cell cycle nonspecific. Concentrates in liver, kidneys, large and small intestines. Little distributes into normal cerebrospinal fluid but can be detected in intracerebral tumors. Heavily protein bound. Only one fourth to one half of the drug is excreted in the urine by the end of 5 days. Secreted in breast milk.

INDICATIONS AND USES

Treatment of metastatic tumors of the testes and ovaries, advanced bladder cancer, and osteogenic sarcoma. Most commonly used in specific combinations with other chemotherapeutic drugs.

Investigational uses: Treatment of cancers of the brain, adrenal cortex, breast, cervix, uterus, endometrium, head and neck, esophagus, lung, skin, prostate, and stomach; non-Hodgkins lymphoma; and trophoblastic neoplasms.

CONTRAINDICATIONS

Hypersensitivity to cisplatin or other platinum-containing compounds, myelosuppressed patients, preexisting impaired renal function or hearing deficit.

PRECAUTIONS

■ Follow guidelines for handling cytotoxic agents. See Appendix A, p. 893. ■ Administered by or under the direction of the physician specialist. ■ Neuropathies may occur with higher doses, greater frequency of average doses, or prolonged therapy. ■ Do not administer live virus vaccines to patients receiving antineoplastic agents.

Monitor: Hydrate patient with 1 to 2 liters of infusion fluid for 8 to 12 hours before injection. Urinary output should exceed 100 to 150 ml/hr. ■ Maintain adequate hydration and urinary output of at least 100 to 200 ml/hr for 24 hours after each dose. ■ The greater the dose, the more hydration is required (e.g., 20 mg/M^2, 1 liter; 40 mg/M^2, 2 liters). Potassium chloride (20 mEq) and magnesium sulfate (8 mEq) are frequently added to predosing fluids and/or cisplatin. ■ In addition to mannitol, furosemide (Lasix) may be added to cisplatin if fluid overload is a concern. ■ Frequent kidney function tests, blood counts, and electrolytes are indicated. Repeat doses based on these studies (note Usual dose). ■ Nausea and vomiting are frequently severe and prolonged (up to a week). Prophylactic administration of antiemetics recommended. Ondansetron (Zofran), metoclopramide (Reglan), dexamethasone or droperidol are effective in most patients. ■ Ototoxicity is cumulative; test hearing before administration and regularly during treatment. Ototoxicity increased in children. ■ Allopurinol may be indicated to reduce uric acid levels. ■ Observe closely for signs of infection. Prophylactic antibiotics may be indicated pending results of C/S in a febrile neutropenic patient.

Patient education: Nonhormonal birth control recommended. ■ See Appendix D, p. 900.

Maternal/child: Avoid pregnancy, will produce teratogenic effects on the fetus. Has a mutagenic potential. ■ Discontinue breast feeding. ■ Ototoxicity increased in children.

Elderly: No specific problems documented. ■ Consider age-related renal impairment.

DRUG/LAB INTERACTIONS

Ototoxicity and nephrotoxicity are potentiated with aminoglycosides (e.g., gentamicin) and loop diuretics (e.g., furosemide [Lasix], ethacrynic acid [Edecrin]). ■ May inhibit phenytoin (Dilantin). ■ Bone marrow toxicity increased with other antineoplastic agents and/or radiation therapy. ■ Synergistic with etoposide (VePesid); may be beneficial. ■ Potentiated by probenicid; may cause toxicity. ■ May affect renal excretion and increase toxicity of many drugs (e.g., bleomycin, doxorubicin, fluorouracil, methotrexate). ■ Concurrent use with high-dose cytarbine may increase ototoxicity. ■ Myclotoxicity may be increased if administered before paclitaxel rather than after.

SIDE EFFECTS

Are frequent; can occur with the initial dose and will become more severe with succeeding doses. Anaphylaxis (facial edema, hypotension, tachycardia, and wheezing within minutes of administration), hyperuricemia, myelosuppression, nausea and vomiting, nephrotoxicity (often noted in the second week after a dose), ototoxicity including tinnitus and hearing loss in the high-frequency range, and peripheral neuropathy (may be irreversible).

ANTIDOTE

Notify physician of all side effects. Cisplatin may have to be discontinued permanently or until recovery. Symptomatic and supportive treatment is indicated. Oprelvebin (Numega) may be indicated for treatment of thrombocytopenia. Treat anaphylaxis with epinephrine, corticosteroids, oxygen, and antihistamines. There is no specific antidote. Hemodialysis may be somewhat helpful in the first 1 to 1 1/2 hours after administration.

CLADRIBINE

Antineoplastic
(Antimetabolite)

2-CdA, 2-chlorodeoxyadenosine, Leustatin   pH 5.7 to 6.9

USUAL DOSE

In all situations, may be administered on an outpatient basis with an appropriate pump and a central venous line in place. Administer any subsequent course with extreme caution. Hematologic recovery must be considered.

Hairy cell leukemia: 0.1 mg/kg/24 hr equally distributed as a continuous infusion over 24 hours. Repeat daily for 7 consecutive days. Usually only one course of treatment is given.

Chronic multiple sclerosis (orphan designation): Dose and process is the same as for hairy cell leukemia except the regimen is repeated once each month for 4 months.

Non-Hodgkin's lymphoma (investigational): Dose and process is the same as for hairy cell leukemia except regimen is repeated every 28 days.

DOSE ADJUSTMENTS

May be required in subsequent courses, severe bone marrow impairment, with prior radiation or myelosuppressive agents. ■ May be required in severe renal insufficiency; effects of renal or hepatic impairment on excretion of cladribine not yet clarified for humans. ■ Note Drug/lab interactions.

DILUTION

Specific techniques required; see Precautions. Available in single-use 10 ml vials containing 10 mg (1 mg/ml). Contains no preservatives; aseptic technique imperative. May develop a precipitate at low temperatures. Warm naturally to room temperature and shake vigorously. Do not heat or microwave.

Inpatient continuous infusion: A single daily calculated dose must be added to 500 ml of NS.

Outpatient continuous infusion: A total 7-day dose is added to a calculated amount of bacteriostatic NS to make a total volume of 100 ml. Specific equipment (i.e., a sterile medication reservoir and pump capable of delivering accurate minute amounts into a central venous line [presently using Pharmacia Deltec medication cassette with Pharmacia Deltec pump]) and a specific process including the use of a 0.22 micron syringe filter are required. Preparation of cassette usually done by pharmacist. Line of cassette remains clamped until attached to central venous line and pump is functional. See literature for details and follow all specific instructions for medication pump.

Storage: Protect from light. Refrigerate or freeze before reconstitution. Never refreeze. Discard any unused concentrate. *500 ml dilution* may be refrigerated for up to 8 hours after dilution. Immediate use preferred. *100 ml dilution* is stable in reservoir of medication cassette for 7 days if correctly diluted.

INCOMPATIBLE WITH

D5W will cause degradation of cladribine. Manufacturer states "should not be mixed with other IV drugs or additives or infused simultaneously via a common IV line. Compatibility testing has not been performed."

RATE OF ADMINISTRATION

Inpatient continuous infusion: A single dose properly diluted evenly distributed as an infusion over 24 hours.

Outpatient continuous infusion: Administered through a central venous line (very concentrated solution). Medication reservoir and pump required (presently using Pharmacia Deltec medication cassette and pump worn as a fanny pak). Set rate for equal distribution of 100 ml over 7 days. Follow all specific instructions for pump.

ACTIONS

A synthetic antineoplastic agent. Mechanism of action is not known, but it is believed to be cytotoxic by inhibition of DNA synthesis and the accumulation of DNA strand breaks. Affects both dividing and resting cells. The 7-day course for hairy cell leukemia has resulted in complete remissions in a majority of patients with no evidence of persistent bone marrow disease. May potentially be a cure. Improvements in neurologic symptons are occurring in patients with multiple sclerosis. In all situations time to response is about 4 months. Has immunosuppressant activity. Lymphocyte subsets (e.g., CD4, CD8 T cells) are affected; may take 6 to 12 months for full recovery. Crosses the blood-brain barrier. Average half-life is 5.4 hours. Metabolized in all cells. Specific methods of metabolism and routes of excretion are not known. Some drug does appear in urine.

INDICATIONS AND USES

Treatment of hairy cell leukemia (HCL). ■ Management of chronic multiple sclerosis (*orphan designation*).

Investigational uses: Treatment of non-Hodgkin's lymphoma.

CONTRAINDICATIONS

Hypersensitivity to cladribine or any of its components; neonates (7 day dilution contains benzyl alcohol).

PRECAUTIONS

- Follow guidelines for handling cytotoxic agents. See Appendix A, p. 893. ■ Administered by or under the direction of the physician specialist. ■ Anticipate severe suppression of bone marrow function, including neutropenia, anemia, and thrombocytopenia. ■ Because of the possibility of increased toxicity, use caution in known or suspected renal insufficiency, or any severe bone marrow impairment, or prior cytoxic or radiation therapy. ■ Appears to be no relationship between serum concentrations and ultimate clinical outcome. ■ Additional courses did not improve overall response. ■ Current studies suggest that overall response rate may be decreased in patients previously treated with splenectomy, deoxycoformycin (Pentostatin), and in patients refractory to alpha-interferon. ■ May cause prolonged bone marrow hypocellularity; clinical significance not known.

Monitor: Obtain baseline CBC with differential (including CD4 and CD8 T cell counts) and platelets before therapy. May be repeated as indicated, but usually not required again until 7 or 8 days after treatment begins; then monitor as indicated for at least 4 to 8 weeks (anemia, neutropenia, thrombocytopenia, infection [bacterial, fungal, or viral], and bleeding are common and must be treated promptly). Monitoring schedule facilitates outpatient treatment; keep in close contact with patient. ■ Consider possibility of infection if fever occurs; appropriate lab tests, x-rays and broad-spectrum antibiotics may be indicated in suspected infection. ■ Monitor uric acid levels before and during treatment, maintain hydration; allopurinol may be indicated (preferred agent). Alkalinization of urine may also be indicated. ■ Monitor renal and hepatic function periodically. ■ Take precautions and limit invasive procedures in any patient with thrombocytopenia. Avoid constipation, and avoid alcohol and aspirin (risk of GI bleeding). ■ Platelet count usually returns to normal in 12 days (may be delayed if severe baseline thrombocytopenia was present), neutorphil count usually returns to normal in 5 weeks, and hemoglobin in 8 weeks. All should be normal by 9 weeks. ■ Complete response is indicated by an absence of hairy cells in bone marrow and peripheral blood and normalization of peripheral blood parameters. Confirm response with bone marrow aspiration and biopsy between 9 weeks and 4 months. ■ Prophylactic antiemetics may improve patient comfort.

Patient education: Avoid pregnancy; consider birth control options and future fertility. ■ Report fever, bleeding, cough, edema, injection site reactions, malaise, mouth sores, rashes, shortness of breath, stomach pain, and tachycardia promptly. Maintain hydration. ■ Manufacturer supplies a patient education booklet; review thoroughly and discuss with physician and nurse. ■ Review all literature provided with pump to deliver outpatient dosing. ■ See Appendix D, p. 900.

Maternal/child: Category D: avoid pregnancy; has potential to cause fetal harm. Has caused suppression of testicular cells in monkeys; effect on human fertility unknown. ■ Discontinue breast feeding. ■ Safety for use in children not established. Investigationally used in higher doses to treat relapsed acute leukemia. Dose-limiting toxicity occurred.

Elderly: Geriatric specific problems not encountered in studies to date. Consider age-related organ impairment.

DRUG/LAB INTERACTIONS

Increased toxicity with other myelosuppressive agents (e.g., methotrexate). ■ May raise concentration of blood uric acid, increased doses of antigout agents (e.g., allopurinol [Zyloprim]) may be indicated; avoid uricosurics (e.g., probenicid, sulfinpyrazone [Anturane]). ■ Do not administer live vaccines to patients receiving antineoplastic agents.

SIDE EFFECTS

Fever (69%) occurs first. Onset of thrombocytopenia (12%) begins in 7 to 10 days followed by anemia (severe [37%]) and neutropenia (severe [70%]). Fatigue (45%), headache (22%), injection site reactions (19%), infection (28%), nausea (28%), and rash (27%) are common. Many other side effects may or may not be related to cladribine; abdominal pain (6%), abnormal breath sounds (11%), abnormal chest sounds (9%), anorexia (17%), arthralgia (5%), chills (9%), constipation (9%), cough (10%), diaphoresis (9%), diarrhea (10%), dizziness (9%), edema (6%), epistaxis (5%), erythema (6%), insomnia (7%), malaise (7%), myalgia (7%), pain (6%), petechiae (8%), pruritus (6%), purpura (10%), shortness of breath (7%), tachycardia (6%), trunk pain (6%), weakness (9%), vomiting (13%).

Overdose: Acute nephrotoxicity, irreversible neurologic toxicity (paraparesis/quadriparesis), severe bone marrow depression (anemia, neutropenia, and thrombocytopenia).

ANTIDOTE

Keep physician informed of all side effects; many will be treated symptomatically as indicated. Platelet or red blood cell transfusions are frequently required to treat anemia or thrombocytopenia, especially during the first month. Filgrastim (Neupogen) may be used to increase neutrophil count, although recovery is usually spontaneous. Use specific antibiotics to combat infection. Discontinue cladribine if renal toxicity, neurotoxicity, or overdose occurs. No specific antidote for overdose. Supportive therapy as indicated will help sustain the patient in toxicity. Resuscitate if indicated.

CLINDAMYCIN PHOSPHATE

Antibacterial
Antiprotozoal
(Lincosamide)

Cleocin Phosphate   pH 5.5 to 7.0

USUAL DOSE

900 to 2,700 mg/24 hr in 2, 3, or 4 equally divided doses. Up to 4.8 Gm has been given in life-threatening infections.

Acute pelvic inflammatory disease (investigational): 900 mg every 8 hours for at least 4 days. Concurrent administration of 2 mg/kg of gentamicin as an initial dose and 1.5 mg/kg every 8 hours thereafter is recommended. Continue both drugs for at least 48 hours after patient improves. Complete 10-to 14-day treatment program with oral doxy-cycline or clindamycin.

CNS toxoplasmosis in AIDS (investigational): 1,200 to 2,400 mg/24 hr in divided doses. Up to 4.8 Gm has been required. Used in combination with pyrimethamine (Daraprim).

Pneumocystis carinii pneumonia (investigational): 600 mg every 6 hours or 900 mg every 8 hours. Used in combination with primaquine.

Babesiosis (investigational): 1,200 to 2,400 mg/24 hr in 4 equally divided doses. Continue for 7 to 10 days. Used in combination with quinine.

Prophylaxis of bacterial endocarditis: 300 mg IV or orally 30 minutes before procedure and 150 mg IV or orally in 6 hours.

PEDIATRIC DOSE

Minimum recommended dose regardless of weight is 300 mg/24 hours for severe infections.

Children over 1 month of age: 15 to 40 mg/kg of body weight/24 hr in 3 or 4 equally divided doses for serious infections. Alternately 350 mg/M^2/24 hr may be used. 450 mg/M^2/24 hr may be used for more serious infections if necessary.

Bone infections: 7.5 mg/kg every 6 hours.

Babesiosis (investigational): A suggested dose is 20 mg/kg/24 hr. Continue for 7 to 10 days. Used in combination with 25 mg/kg/24 hr of oral quinine.

Prophylaxis of bacterial endocarditis: 10 mg/kg IV or p.o. 30 minutes before procedure. Give 5 mg/kg IV or p.o. in 6 hours.

NEONATAL DOSE

Under 1 month of age, full term: 3.75 to 5 mg/kg every 6 hours or 5 to 6.7 mg/kg every 8 hours. Another source suggests:

Infants under 7 days of age weighing less than 2 kg: 5 mg/kg every 12 hours.

Infants under 7 days of age weighing over 2 kg: 5 mg/kg every 8 hours.

Infants over 7 days of age weighing less than 1.2 kg: 5 mg/kg every 12 hours.

Infants over 7 days of age weighing 1.2 to 2 kg: 5 mg/kg every 8 hours.

Infants over 7 days of age weighing over 2 kg: 5 mg/kg every 6 hours.

DOSE ADJUSTMENTS

May be required in severely impaired liver or renal function.

DILUTION

Available prediluted in 300, 600, and 900 mg ready-to-use Galaxy bags or ADD-Vantage vials for use with ADD-Vantage diluent containers, or each 18 mg must be reconstituted with a minimum of 1 ml of D5W, NS, or other compatible infusion solution (300 mg with 17 ml diluent, 600 mg with 34 ml, and 900 mg with 50 ml). Additional diluent may be used to lessen concentration, but never exceed a concentration of 18 mg/ml.

Acute pelvic inflammatory disease: May be further diluted in larger amounts of compatible infusion solutions and given as a continuous infusion after the initial dose.

INCOMPATIBLE WITH

Allopurinol (Zyloprim), aminophylline, ampicillin, barbiturates, calcium gluconate, ceftriaxone (Rocephin), ciprofloxacin (Cipro IV), filgrastim (Neupogen), fluconazole (Diflucan), gentamicin (Garamycin), idarubicin (Idamycin), magnesium sulfate, phenytoin (Dilantin), ranitidine (Zantac), Ringer's solution, tobramycin (Nebcin).

RATE OF ADMINISTRATION

Severe hypotension and cardiac arrest can occur with too-rapid injection. To maintain serum levels at 4 (5 or 6) mcg/ml, give initial dose at 10 (15 or 20) mg/min over 30 minutes. Do not exceed 30 mg or fraction thereof over at least 1 minute (each 300 mg over a minimum of 10 minutes). Do not give more than 1,200 mg in single 1-hour infusion.

Acute pelvic inflammatory disease: To maintain serum levels at 4 (5 or 6) mcg/ml give initial dose at 10 (15 or 20) mg/min over 30 minutes. Follow with maintenance infusion at 0.75 (1.00 or 1.25) mg/min.

ACTIONS

A semisynthetic antibiotic that quickly converts to active clindamycin. It inhibits protein synthesis in the bacterial cell, producing irreversible changes in the protein-synthesizing ribosomes. Widely distributed in most body fluids, tissues, and bones. There is no clinically effective distribution to cerebrospinal fluid. Excreted in urine and feces in small amounts. Most excreted in inactive form in the urine. Crosses placental barrier. Secreted in breast milk.

INDICATIONS AND USES

Treatment of serious infections caused by susceptible anaerobic bacteria; or susceptible aerobic bacterial infections in penicillin-allergic patients; or infections that do not respond or are resistant to other less toxic antibiotics, such as penicillins or cephalosporins. ■ Treatment of acute pelvic inflammatory disease.

Investigational uses: Alternative to sulfonamides with pyrimethamine to treat CNS toxoplasmosis in AIDS patients. ■ Treat Pneumocystis carinii pneumonia in combination with primaquine.

CONTRAINDICATIONS

Known hypersensitivity to clindamycin or lincomycin. Treatment of minor bacterial or viral infections.

PRECAUTIONS

A highly toxic drug, to be used only when absolutely necessary and when an alternate drug (e.g., erythromycin) is not acceptable. ■ Sensitivity studies indicated to determine susceptibility of the causative organism to clindamycin. ■ Avoid prolonged use; superinfection caused by overgrowth of nonsusceptible organisms may result. ■ Use caution with a history of GI, severe renal, or liver disease, and in patients with a history of asthma or significant allergies. ■ Not appropriate to treat meningitis.

Monitor: Capable of causing severe, even fatal, colitis; observe for symptoms of diarrhea. ■ Periodic blood cell counts and liver and kidney studies are indicated in prolonged therapy. ■ Each ml contains 9.45 mg benzyl alcohol. Monitor organ system functions if used in infants.

Patient education: Do not treat diarrhea without notifying physician.

Maternal/child: Safety for use in pregnancy not established. ■ Best to discontinue nursing, even though considered acceptable by pediatricians. ■ Note Monitor before using in infants.

Elderly: Monitor carefully for changes in bowel frequency; may not tolerate diarrhea well.

DRUG/LAB INTERACTIONS
May potentiate other neuromuscular blocking agents (e.g., kanamycin, streptomycin, tubocurarine, mivacurium) and cause profound respiratory depression. ■ Antagonized by erythromycin.

SIDE EFFECTS
Abdominal pain, agranulocytosis, allergic reactions, anaphylaxis, anorexia, azotemia, cardiac arrest, colitis, diarrhea, elevated ALT (SGOT), eosinophilia (transient), erythema multiforme, esophagitis, hypotension, jaundice, leukopenia, metallic taste, nausea, neutropenia (transient), oliguria, polyarthritis (rare), skin rashes, tenesmus (straining at stool), thrombocytopenic purpura, thrombophlebitis, urticaria, vomiting.

ANTIDOTE
Notify the physician of any side effects. Discontinue the drug if indicated (colitis, diarrhea, allergic reactions, etc.), treat allergic reaction as indicated, and resuscitate as necessary. Do not treat diarrhea with opiates or diphenoxylate with atropine (Lomitil). Condition will worsen. Treat colitis with fluid, electrolyte, and protein supplements, systemic corticosteroids, and corticoid retention enemas. Treatment with oral vancomycin (Vancocin), cholestyramine, and colestipol has been effective. Stagger administration times to prevent inappropriate binding of vancomycin. Hemodialysis or CAPD will not decrease blood levels in toxicity.

CONJUGATED ESTROGENS

Hormone (estrogen) Antihemorrhagic

Premarin intravenous

pH 7.2 to 7.4

USUAL DOSE
25 mg in 1 injection. May be repeated in 6 to 12 hours if indicated.

DILUTION
Withdraw all air from the vial of powder. Carefully withdraw contents from ampoule of sterile diluent provided. Direct flow of diluent gently against the side of the vial of powder. Mix solution by rotating the vial between the palms of the hands. Do not shake. Do not use if discolored or precipitate present.

Storage: Must be refrigerated before and after reconstitution. Most frequently used promptly, but it is stable for up to 60 days if protected from light.

INCOMPATIBLE WITH
Ascorbic acid, lactated Ringer's injection, protein hydrolysate, Ringer's injection, sodium lactate injection (⅙ molar lactate), any solution with an acid pH.

RATE OF ADMINISTRATION
5 mg or fraction thereof over 1 minute. Must be given direct IV or through IV tubing close to needle site. Infusion solution must be compatible (normal saline, dextrose, and invert sugar solutions). Perineal or vaginal burning may be caused by too-rapid injection.

ACTIONS

Produces a prompt increase in circulating prothrombin and accelerator globulin and decrease in antithrombin activities of the blood. The coagulability of the blood, especially in capillary beds, is enhanced. Promptly corrects bleeding due to estrogen deficiency. Metabolized primarily in the liver and excreted in the urine. Secreted in breast milk.

INDICATIONS AND USES

Dysfunctional uterine bleeding caused by hormonal imbalance in the absence of organic pathology.

Unlabeled use: Postcoital contraception.

CONTRAINDICATIONS

Breast cancer (except selected metastatic disease), estrogen-dependent neoplasia, pregnancy, thrombophlebitis or thromboembolic disorders, undiagnosed abnormal genital bleeding. Other specific contraindications for estrogens must be considered.

PRECAUTIONS

Dilution in an IV infusion is not recommended. ▪ Even though bleeding is controlled, the etiology of the bleeding must be determined and definitive therapy instituted. ▪ Follow immediately with oral estrogens as recommended for dysfunctional uterine bleeding. ▪ Use with caution in epilepsy, hypercalcemia, migraine, asthma, or cardiac, hepatic, or renal disease; induces salt and water retention. ▪ Estrogens may be carcinogenic; use only for specific indications.

Monitor: Monitor VS; may cause a temporary BP elevation.

Maternal/child: Category X: avoid pregnancy. Safety for use in children not established. Has adverse effects on epiphyseal closure of bone.

DRUG/LAB INTERACTIONS

May decrease effects of oral antidiabetics. ▪ Barbiturates (e.g., phenobarbital), phenytoin (Dilantin), and rifampin (Rifadin) increase metabolism and decrease serum levels and effects. ▪ May decrease metabolism and increase serum levels of cyclosporine. May increase risk of cyclosporine toxicity. ▪ Increased risk of hepatotoxicity with other hepatotoxic agents (e.g., dantrolene [Dantrium]). ▪ May increase blood glucose levels and serum lipids.

SIDE EFFECTS

Rare when used as directed; flushing, nausea, vomiting.

ANTIDOTE

No toxicity has been reported throughout years of clinical use. Discontinue if jaundice occurs.

CORTICORELIN OVINE TRIFLUTATE

Diagnostic agent
Hormone
(Adrenocorticotropic)

Acthrel

USUAL DOSE

1 mcg/kg as a single test dose. Produces maximal cortisol responses and significant ACTH responses. Doses above 1 mcg/kg are not recommended.

PEDIATRIC DOSE

Same as adult dose. Experience limited. No differences in response to the test have been reported.

DILUTION

Immediately before use reconstitute each 100 mcg vial with 2 ml NS. Roll the vial gently to dissolve; avoid bubbles; do not shake. Contains 50 mcg/ml.

Storage: Store unopened vials in refrigerator (2° to 8° C [36° to 46° F]) protected from light. Use reconstituted solution immediately and discard unused solution.

INCOMPATIBLE WITH

Specific information not available. Consider specific use.

RATE OF ADMINISTRATION

To reduce incidence of side effects, a single dose over 30 to 60 seconds is preferred to a bolus injection.

ACTIONS

A synthetic peptide that is an analog of the naturally occurring human corticotropin releasing hormone. A potent stimulator of adrenocorticotropic hormone (ACTH) release from the anterior pituitary. ACTH stimulates cortisol production from the adrenal cortex. IV injection results in a rapid and sustained increase of plasma ACTH levels and a near-parallel increase of plasma cortisol. With usual dosage (1 mcg/kg) ACTH levels increase within minutes and peak in 15 to 60 minutes, and cortisol levels increase within approximately 10 minutes and peak in 30 to 120 minutes. Levels remain elevated for up to 2 hours.

INDICATIONS AND USES

To differentiate pituitary and ectopic production of ACTH in patients with ACTH-dependent Cushing's syndrome.

CONTRAINDICATIONS

None noted; consider hypersensitivity to ovine products.

PRECAUTIONS

Administered by or under the direction of the physician specialist. ■ Prior to testing, a diagnosis of hypercortisolism consistent with Cushing's disease not caused by autonomous adrenal hyperfunction is usually established. Testing with corticorelin establishes the source of excessive ACTH secretions. ■ Corticorelin does not affect insulin, plasma renin activity, prolactin, or growth hormone release. ■ ACTH and cortisol levels will differ between AM and PM; any subsequent tests required should be done at the same time of day as the original. ■ False negative response may occur in 5% to 10% of patients with Cushing's disease.

Monitor: Obtain baseline vital signs. ■ Obtain instructions from the lab for handling of blood samples; determination of ACTH and cortisol content can be directly impacted. ■ Five samples are drawn; ACTH and cortisol testing will be done from each sample. ■ Draw venous blood samples 15 minutes before and just before administration of corticorelin (these are averaged to obtain ACTH baseline). Administer corticorelin and draw venous blood samples 15, 30, and 60 minutes after administration. ■ Monitor the patient closely until all side effects have subsided.

Patient education: Report dizziness, feeling faint, or shortness of breath immediately.

Maternal/child: Pregnancy Category C: use only if clearly needed. ■ Safety not established; use caution if necessary during lactation (breast feeding could be temporarily discontinued). ■ Limited experience in children; no difference in response has been reported.

Elderly: Specific information not available.

DRUG/LAB INTERACTIONS

Pretreatment with dexamethasone will inhibit plasma ACTH response. ■ Use of heparin to maintain IV cannula patency during blood draws is not recommended. While the interaction is unknown, it may cause severe hypotension.

SIDE EFFECTS

Flushing of the face, neck, and upper chest begins almost immediately and last 3 to 5 minutes. May cause an urge to take a deep breath.

Overdose: Doses over 1 mcg/kg may cause dyspnea, hypotension, prolonged flushing, tachycardia, and a feeling of compression or tightness in the chest. Asystole and loss of consciousness have occurred.

ANTIDOTE

Notify the physician of any symptoms of overdose. Treat symptomatically. Emergency drugs (e.g., oxygen, epinephrine, diphenhydramine, atropine, and vasopressors [e.g., dopamine]) should be available. Resuscitate as necessary.

CORTICOTROPIN INJECTION

Hormone
(Adrenocorticotropic)
Diagnostic agent

ACTH, Acthar   pH 2.5 to 6.0

USUAL DOSE

10 to 25 units. Up to 80 units as a single injection has been used. Other tests using different doses (e.g., 40 units by infusion every 12 hours for 48 hours) or multiple IM injections have been used. Skin test for allergy if a known sensitivity exists to polypeptides or to hogs. Cosyntropin is the preferred diagnostic agent.

PEDIATRIC DOSE
Cosyntropin recommended for diagnosis of adrenocortical function in children.

DOSE ADJUSTMENTS
May be required in the elderly.

DILUTION
Dilute lyophilized powder initially with 2 ml water or NS for injection. Withdraw desired dose of corticotropin and further dilute in 500 ml of D5W. NS may be used unless salt is restricted.

Storage: Refrigerate before and after reconstitution. Use reconstituted solution within 24 hours.

INCOMPATIBLE WITH
Aminophylline, sodium bicarbonate.

RATE OF ADMINISTRATION
Given as a continuous IV infusion over an 8-hour period.

ACTIONS
An anterior pituitary hormone that stimulates the adrenal gland to produce and secrete adrenocortical hormone. A polypeptide, not absorbed through the GI tract. Given IV, it rapidly disappears from the bloodstream and little effect remains 6 hours after termination of the infusion. Effective only when the adrenal glands are normal and can respond to its stimulation. A normal increase in plasma cortisol rules out primary adrenocortical failure. Excreted in the urine.

INDICATIONS AND USES
Diagnosis of adrenocortical function. ■ Has been used for treatment of idiopathic thrombocytopenia purpura in adults. ■ IM or SC injections used to treat selected disease processes.

CONTRAINDICATIONS
Do not use in ocular herpes simplex, acute psychoses, scleroderma, osteoporosis, systemic fungal infections or after recent surgery.

Relative contraindications: ■ Active or latent peptic ulcer, congestive heart failure, diabetes mellitus, diverticulitis, hypertension, lactation, pregnancy (especially during the first trimester), protein sensitivity, psychotic tendencies, renal insufficiency, thromboembolic tendencies, active or healed tuberculosis.

PRECAUTIONS
Vial must state "for IV use." ■ 30 minute cosyntropin test preferred for screening of primary adrenocortical insufficiency (Addison's disease); causes fewer alleric reactions. Use with caution in hypothyroidism and cirrhosis. ■ Use extreme caution in patients allergic to corticotropin, cosyntropin, or porcine derivatives.

Monitor: Continuous observation for at least the first 30 minutes is mandatory. Observe frequently throughout administration. ■ Check blood pressure frequently; may cause elevated blood pressure and salt and water retention. ■ Diabetes may require increased insulin or oral hypoglycemics ■ Note Drug/lab interactions.

Patient education: Report abdominal pain, headache, marked fluid retention, muscle weakness, or seizures promptly. ■ May mask signs of infection and/or decrease resistance. ■ Avoid immunization with live vaccines.

Maternal/child: Pregnancy Category C: will cause fetal abnormalities; benefits must outweigh risks. ■ Temporarily discontinue breast feeding.

Elderly: Note Dose adjustments and Monitor. ■ Increased risk of hypertension.

DRUG/LAB INTERACTIONS

Plasma cortisol may be falsely elevated for patients taking spironolactone when fluorometric procedure used; in patients receiving corticosteroids; and in individuals with increased plasma bilirubin levels or free hemoglobin in the plasma. ■ Response to corticotropin may be decreased by glucocorticoid corticosteroids (e.g., prednisolone). ■ Many drug reactions are possible with corticosteroids, but usually not a concern with specific IV diagnostic use. ■ Effects of anticoagulants may be decreased when used with corticotropin. ■ May block effects of nondepolarizing neuromuscular blockers (e.g., pancuronium, tubocurarine). ■ Potassium-depleting diuretics (e.g., acetazolamide [Diamox]) and amphotericin B may cause hypokalemia. Monitor serum potassium. ■ Amphotericin B may also decrease adrenocortical responsiveness. ■ Barbiturates may increase metabolism and decrease effects. ■ Avoid immunization with live vaccines. ■ Regular use of oral verapamil may cause a false-negative test result.

SIDE EFFECTS

Allergic reactions including anaphylaxis are most common with short term use for diagnostic testing. Side effects do occur, but are usually reversible; alteration of glucose metabolism including hyperglycemia, Cushing's syndrome (moon face, fat pads), electrolyte imbalance, increased blood pressure, increased intracranial pressure with papilledema, masking of infection, pancreatitis, perforation and hemorrhage from aggravation of peptic ulcer, protein catabolism with negative nitrogen balance, psychic disturbances (especially euphoria); suppression of growth, thromboembolism, and many others.

ANTIDOTE

Notify the physician of any side effect so that it can be treated if necessary. Keep epinephrine and diphenhydramine available to treat anaphylaxis. Resuscitate as necessary.

COSYNTROPIN

Cortrosyn

Diagnostic agent
(Adrenocorticotropic)

pH 5.5 to 7.5

USUAL DOSE

250 mcg (0.25 mg). Up to 750 mcg (0.75 mg) has been used.

PEDIATRIC DOSE

Children over 2 years of age: May use adult dose but 125 mcg (0.125 mg) is usually adequate.

Children under 2 years of age: 125 mcg (0.125 mg). Usually given IM.

DILUTION

Diluent provided (1.1 ml vial of NS). May be given direct IV after this initial dilution or further diluted in D5W or NS and given as an infusion (250 mcg in 250 ml equals 1 mcg/ml).

Storage: Stable after reconstitution for 24 hours at room temperature and 21 days if refrigerated. Infusion stable 12 hours at room temperature.

INCOMPATIBLE WITH

Blood and blood products. Should be considered incompatible with any other drug because of specific use.

RATE OF ADMINISTRATION

Direct IV: A single dose over 2 minutes.

Infusion: A single dose evenly distributed over 4 to 8 hours.

ACTIONS

A synthetic form of adrenocorticotropic hormone (ACTH). Stimulates the adrenal cortex to secrete adrenocortical hormone. Does not increase cortisol secretion in patients with primary adrenocortical insufficiency. Peak plasma cortisol levels occur in 1 hour after cosyntropin dose in patients with normal renal function.

INDICATIONS AND USES

Diagnostic aid for adrenocortical insufficiency.

CONTRAINDICATIONS

Hypersensitivity to cosyntropin.

PRECAUTIONS

Preferable to ACTH because it is less likely to cause allergic reactions. ■ May be used in patients who have had an allergic reaction to ACTH. ■ Infusion method used if greater stimulus needed to effect results.

Monitor: Continuous observation for at least the first 30 minutes is mandatory. Observe frequently thereafter. ■ Check blood pressure frequently; may cause elevated blood pressure and salt water retention. ■ Diabetes may require increased insulin or oral hypoglycemics. ■ Monitor correct collection of specimens. ■ Note Drug/lab interactions.

Patient education: May mask signs of infection. ■ May decrease resistance. ■ Avoid immunization with live vaccines.

Maternal/child: Use caution in pregnancy and lactation.

DRUG/LAB INTERACTIONS

Plasma cortisol may be falsely elevated for patients taking spironolactone when fluorometric procedure used; patients receiving corticosteroids; and individuals with increased plasma bilirubin levels or free hemoglobin in the plasma. ■ Many drug reactions are possible with corticosteroids, but usually not a concern with specific diagnostic use.

SIDE EFFECTS

Bradycardia, dizziness, dyspnea, fainting, fever, flushing, irritability, rash, seizures, urticaria.

ANTIDOTE

Notify the physician of any side effect. Keep epinephrine and diphenhydramine available to treat anaphylaxis. Resuscitate as necessary.

CYCLOPHOSPHAMIDE

Antineoplastic
(Alkylating agent/
nitrogen mustard)

Cytoxan, Cytoxan Lyophilized,
Neosar, ✷Procytox

pH 3.0 to 7.5

USUAL DOSE

Malignant diseases (adults and children): As a single agent the initial dose may be up to a maximum of 40 to 50 mg/kg of body weight, usually given in divided doses (10 to 20 mg/kg/24 hr) over 2 to 5 days. Maintenance doses vary from 3 to 5 mg/kg twice weekly to 10 to 15 mg/kg every 7 to 10 days. Numerous dosing regimens in use. Note Monitor section.

Polymyositis (investigational): 500 mg every 1 to 3 weeks as an IV infusion over 1 hour.

Polyarteritis nodosa (investigational): Begin with 4 mg/kg/24 hr. Adjust dose based on patient response.

DOSE ADJUSTMENTS

Dose based on average weight in presence of edema or ascites. ▪ Dose is reduced by one third to one half if hematologic disease is present or there has been extensive radiation therapy. ▪ Reduced dose may be required in the adrenalectomized patient and in impaired hepatic function. ▪ Often used with other antineoplastic drugs in reduced doses to achieve tumor remission.

DILUTION

Specific techniques required; see Precautions. Each 100 mg must be diluted with 5 ml of sterile water or bacteriostatic water for injection (paraben preserved only) yields 20 mg/ml. Shake solution gently and allow to stand until clear. Further dilution with up to 250 ml D5W, NS, or other compatible solution is recommended to reduce side effects. Do not use heat to facilitate dilution.

Storage: Diluted solution without preservative must be used within 6 hours, with preservative use within 24 hours. Stable up to 6 days if refrigerated. Do not store cyclophosphamide in temperatures over 37° C (90° F).

COMPATIBLE WITH

Physically compatible with many drugs (e.g., bleomycin, cisplatin, dacarbazine [DTIC], doxorubicin [Adriamycin], mesna and others). Consult pharmacist.

RATE OF ADMINISTRATION

Each 100 mg or fraction thereof over 15 minutes or longer. May be given by IV push, as an intermittent IV infusion or through the lumen of the rubber tubing or three-way stopcock if the IV solution is dextrose or saline.

ACTIONS

An alkylating agent of the nitrogen mustard group with antitumor activity, cell cycle phase nonspecific, but most effective in S phase. It is an inert compound but is activated by hepatic microsomal enzymes to produce regression in the size of malignant tumors. Elimination half-life is 3 to 10 hours. Metabolized in the liver, it or its metabolites are excreted in the urine. Secreted in breast milk.

INDICATIONS AND USES

To suppress or retard neoplastic growth. Good response has been experienced in lymphomas such as Hodgkin's disease, leukemia, and multiple myeloma, and in solid malignancies of the breast and ovary. Used to treat many other malignancies. ■ Treatment of biopsyproven nephrotic syndrome in children when disease fails to respond to primary therapy or primary therapy causes intolerable side effects.

Investigational uses: Severe rheumatologic conditions. ■ Polyarteritis nodosa. ■ Alone or in combination with corticosteroids to treat polymyositis.

CONTRAINDICATIONS

Previous hypersensitivity, severely depressed bone marrow function.

PRECAUTIONS

■ Follow guidelines for handling cytotoxic agents. See Appendix A, p. 893. ■ Administered by or under the direction of the physician specialist. ■ Use caution in cases of leukopenia, thrombocytopenia, bone marrow infiltrated with malignant cells, previous radiation therapy, previous cytotoxic therapy, and severe hepatic or renal disease. ■ Wait 5 to 7 days after a major surgical procedure before beginning treatment. May interfere with normal wound healing. ■ Do not administer any live vaccine to patients receiving antineoplastic drugs. ■ May cause syndrome of inappropriate antidiuretic hormone (SIADH) with normal doses because of fluid loading. ■ May result in reversible hemorrhagic ureteritis or renal tubular necrosis.

Monitor: Prehydration with 500 to 1,000 ml NS recommended especially with higher doses. ■ Marked leukopenia will occur after the initial dose. Recovery should begin in 7 to 10 days. ■ Monitor neutrophils and platelets and examine urine for red blood cells on a regular basis. ■ Maintenance doses are regulated by an acceptable leukocyte count (2,500 to 4,000 cells/mm^3) and the absence of serious side effects. The maximum effective maintenance dose should be used. ■ Observe continuously for infection. Prophylactic antibiotics may be indicated pending results of C/S in a febrile neutropenic patient. ■ Use antiemetics for patient comfort. ■ Acute hemorrhagic cystitis occurs in 7% to 12% of patients; administer before 4 PM to decrease amount of drug remaining in bladder overnight. Encourage fluid intake and frequent voiding to prevent cystitis.

Patient education: Nonhormonal birth control recommended. ■ Increase fluid intake and void frequently. ■ See Appendix D, p. 900.

Maternal/child: Pregnancy Category D: may produce teratogenic effects on the fetus. Has a mutagenic potential. ■ Discontinue breast feeding.

Elderly: Consider age-related organ impairment; toxicity may be increased.

DRUG/LAB INTERACTIONS

Half-life increased and metabolic concentrations decreased with chloramphenicol. ■ Thiazide diuretics (e.g., chlorothiazide [Diuril]) may prolong leukopenia. ■ Increased risk of bleeding with anticoagulants (e.g., warfarin [Coumadin]); dose reduction of anticoagulant may be indicated. ■ May reduce serum digoxin levels. ■ Can potentiate doxorubicin-induced cardiotoxicity. ■ May prolong neuromuscular blockade and prolonged respiratory depression caused by succinylcholine (Anectine). These effects are dose dependent and may occur up to several days after cyclophosphamide is discontinued. ▪ May decrease effectiveness of quinolone antibiotics (e.g., ciprofloxacin [Cipro]). ▪ Risk of bleeding or infection may be increased with allopurinol (Zyloprim). ▪ Chronic administration of high doses of phenobarbital may increase metabolism of cyclophosphamide and decrease its effectiveness. ▪ Capable of many other interactions.

SIDE EFFECTS
Minor: Alopecia (regrowth may be slightly darker), amenorrhea, gonadal suppression, leukopenia (See Precautions), mucosal ulcerations, nausea and vomiting, skin and fingernails become darker, susceptibility to infection.

Major: Bone marrow depression, hemorrhagic ureteritis (reversible), pulmonary fibrosis, renal tubular necrosis (reversible), secondary neoplasia, SIADH, sterile hemorrhagic cystitis, which can be fatal.

ANTIDOTE
Minor side effects will be treated symptomatically if necessary. Discontinue the drug and notify the physician of hematuria immediately. Formalin bladder instillation may control cystitis. Mesna has decreased incidence of cystitis. Oprelvekin (Numega) may be indicated for treatment of thrombocytopenia. There is no specific antidote. Supportive therapy as indicated will help sustain the patient in toxicity. Approximately 36% can be removed by hemodialysis.

CYCLOSPORINE   Immunosuppressant
Sandimmune

USUAL DOSE
5 to 6 mg/kg of body weight as a single dose 4 to 12 hours before transplantation. Repeat once each day until oral solution can be tolerated. Individualized adjustment is imperative and may be required on a daily basis.

PEDIATRIC DOSE
Same as adult dose. Note Maternal/child.

DOSE ADJUSTMENTS
Reduced dose may be required in impaired renal function. ▪ Higher doses may be required in children. ▪ Note Monitor and Drug/lab interactions.

DILUTION
Each 50 mg should be diluted immediately before use with 20 to 100 ml of NS or D5W and given as an infusion. May leach phthalate from polyvinylchloride containers; use diluents in glass infusion bottles. Dilute immediately before use and discard unused portion.

Storage: Discard diluted solution after 24 hours.

INCOMPATIBLE WITH

Limited information available. Administer separately. Magnesium sulfate.

RATE OF ADMINISTRATION

A single dose properly diluted over 2 to 6 hours.

ACTIONS

A potent immunosuppressive agent. Prolongs survival of kidney, liver, and heart allogeneic transplants in the human. Measured by specific or non-specific assays. Extensively metabolized by the cytochrome P_{450} hepatic enzyme system to metabolites and excreted in bile and urine. Crosses the placental barrier. Secreted in breast milk.

INDICATIONS AND USES

Prophylaxis of organ rejection in kidney, liver, and heart allogeneic transplants in conjunction with adrenocortical steroids. ■ Treatment of chronic rejection in patients previously treated with other immunosuppressive agents if oral administration not feasible.

Investigational uses: Prophylaxis of organ rejection in pancreas, bone marrow, and heart/lung transplantation. ■ Severe ulcerative colitis.

CONTRAINDICATIONS

Hypersensitivity to cyclosporine or polyoxyethylated castor oil.

PRECAUTIONS

Oral dosage preferred; begin as soon as feasible. ■ Usually administered in the hospital by or under the direction of a physician experienced in immunosuppressive therapy and management of organ transplant patients. ■ Adequate laboratory and supportive medical resources must be available. ■ Given concomitantly with adrenocortical steroids only. Do not administer any other immunosuppressive agent. ■ In impaired renal function, if rejection is severe, try other immunosuppressive therapy or allow rejection and removal of the kidney rather than increase dose of cyclosporine. ■ May cause lymphomas. ■ Note Drug/lab interactions.

Monitor: Monitor BUN, serum creatinine, serum bilirubin, and liver enzymes frequently. Timing and amount of rise in BUN and creatinine and degree of nephrotoxicity or hepatotoxicity distinguish between need for dose reduction or symptoms of organ rejection. ■ Monitor cyclosporine blood levels. Measured by specific or non-specific assay. 24-hour specific trough values of 100 to 200 ng/ml of whole blood or 24-hour non-specific trough values of 250 to 800 ng/ml of whole blood minimize side effects and rejection events. Non-specific assays trough values are higher because they include metabolites. Confirm assay method to evaluate appropriately. ■ Observe constantly for signs of infection (fever, sore throat, tiredness) or unusual bleeding or bruising. ■ Prophylactic antibiotics may be indicated pending results of C/S in a febrile neutropenic patient. ■ Monitor blood pressure. ■ Note Drug/lab interactions.

Patient education: Use nonhormonal birth control. Do not use oral contraceptives. See Appendix D, p. 900. ■ Do not make any changes in formulation (e.g., IV, capsules, oral solution) without physician direction. May require dose adjustment.

Maternal/child: Category C: safety for use in pregnancy and in men and women capable of conception not established. Embryotoxic and fetotoxic in rats. ▪ Discontinue breast feeding. ▪ Safety for use in children not established but has been used in patients as young as 6 months. Hypertension occurs more frequently in children.

DRUG/LAB INTERACTIONS

Nephrotoxicity may be increased because of additive nephrotoxic effects with amphotericin B, aminoglycosides (e.g., gentamicin), diclofenac (Cataflam), foscarnet (Foscavir), H_2 antagonists (e.g., cimetidine, ranitidine), ketoconazole (Nizoral), melphalan (Alkeran), NSAIDs, quinolones (e.g., ciprofloxacin [Cipro]), TMP SMZ (Bactrim); use extreme caution, monitor renal function closely. Concurrent use with melphalan may cause acute renal failure. May occur after the first dose of each drug. ▪ Metabolism decreased and serum levels increased by bromocriptine (Parlodel), calcium channel blockers (e.g., diltiazem [Ca rdizem], verapamil [Isoptin]), danozole (Danocrine), erythromycin, fluconazole (Diflucan), ketoconazole (Nizoral), metoclopramide (Reglan), methylprednisolone (Solu-Cortef). Monitor blood levels with concurrent use to avoid cyclosporine toxicity. ▪ Cyclosporine blood levels and effectiveness are decreased by barbiturates (e.g. phenobarbital), carbamazepine (Tegretol), hydantoins (e.g., phenytoin [Dilantin]) rifampin (Rifadin), TMP SMZ (Bactrim); transplant rejection may occur. ▪ Cyclosporine blood levels and effectiveness may be reduced when administered concurrently with famotidine (Pepcid) and ketoconazole (Nizoral). ▪ Cyclosporine reduces clearance and may increase blood levels of digoxin, lovastatin, and prednisolone; in addition it may increase the volume distribution of digoxin and cause toxicity rather quickly. Monitor digoxin levels. ▪ Impenimen-cilastin (Primaxin), may increase cyclosporine blood levels resulting in CNS toxicity. ▪ Potentiates nondepolarizing muscle relaxants (e.g., tubocurarine, doxacurium [Neuromax]); will prolong neuromuscular blockade. ▪ Do not use potassium-sparing diuretics (e.g., spironolactone [Aldactone]); may increase risk of hyperkalemia. ▪ May cause convulsions with methylprednisolone. Has additive effects with other immunosuppressive agents (except steroids), may increase risk of lymphoma. ▪ Serum levels may increase with chloroquine (Aralen). ▪ Avoid vaccinations and do not use live vaccines in patients receiving cyclosporine. ▪ Concurrent administration with colchicine may cause cyclosporine toxicity (e.g., GI, hepatic, renal, and neuromuscular toxicity).

SIDE EFFECTS

Acne, convulsions, cramps, diarrhea, gum hyperplasia, headache, hepatotoxicity, hirsutism, hyperkalemia, hypertension (more severe in children), hyperuricemia, infection, leukopenia, lymphoma, nausea and vomiting, paresthesia, renal dysfunction, and tremor. Mild allergic reactions have occurred.

ANTIDOTE

Notify the physician of all side effects. Most can be treated symptomatically. Drug may be decreased or discontinued or other immunosuppressive agents utilized. Nephrotoxicity, hepatotoxicity, or hematopoietic depression may require temporary reduction of dosage or permanent withholding of treatment. Dialysis is not effective in overdose.

CYSTEINE HYDROCHLORIDE

Protein substrate/nutritional (Amino acid)

pH 1.0 to 2.5

USUAL DOSE

Individually ordered by neonatologist; a component of total parenteral nutrition.

DILUTION

Each 0.5 Gm dose must be initially diluted with 12.5 Gm of crystalline amino acids (e.g., Aminosyn 5%), then must be further diluted with 250 ml or less of 50% dextrose. Equal volumes of Aminosyn and dextrose in the above example equal a final solution of 2.5% Aminosyn (preferred in infants and children) and 25% dextrose/ml. Sometimes diluted with lower percentages of dextrose to achieve a dilution of 2.5% Aminosyn and dextrose suitable for peripheral infusion. Give within 1 hour of mixing, or may be refrigerated and must be used within 24 hours. Cysteine is unstable over time and will precipitate.

INCOMPATIBLE WITH

Any other drug in syringe. Note incompatibilities under protein (amino acid) products.

RATE OF ADMINISTRATION

Should be specifically ordered by the neonatologist. See Protein amino acid monograph. *Total daily dose should be evenly distributed over the 24-hour period. Maintain a constant drip rate.* Use of infusion pump and microfilter is recommended.

ACTIONS

A sulfur-containing amino acid naturally synthesized in the adult. The enzyme necessary to accomplish this conversion is missing in newborn infants. An essential amino acid in infants. Provided as an additive to Aminosyn 5% to be mixed immediately before administration.

INDICATIONS AND USES

To meet the IV amino acid nutritional requirements of infants receiving total parenteral nutrition.

CONTRAINDICATIONS

Known hypersensitivity to any component, acidosis, anuria, azotemia, severe liver disease, metabolic disorders with impaired nitrogen utilization.

PRECAUTIONS

For use only after dilution with crystalline amino acids (e.g., Aminosyn 5%) and dextrose ■ If 50% dextrose is used, the resulting solution is suitable for administration by central venous infusion only. A 10% solution or less of dextrose may be administered peripherally. ■ Use caution in impaired hepatic function; may cause serum amino acid imbalances, metabolic alkalosis, prerenal azotemia, hyperammonemia, stupor and coma. ■ Use caution in impaired renal function;

may further increase BUN. ■ See all precautions listed under protein (amino acid) products.

Maternal/child: Hyperammonemia is of special significance in infants. Can cause mental retardation. Measure blood ammonia frequently.

SIDE EFFECTS

All side effects under protein (amino acid) products are possible; i.e., abdominal pains, anaphylaxis, convulsions, edema at the site of injection, electrolyte imbalances, glycosuria, hyperammonemia, hyperglycemia, hyperpyrexia, hyperchloremia, metabolic acidosis and/or alkalosis, neuromuscular paresthesias, osmotic dehydration, phlebitis and thrombosis, rebound hypoglycemia, septicemia, vasodilation, vomiting, and weakness.

ANTIDOTE

Notify the physician of all side effects. Amounts of cysteine, glucose, or other additives may be adjusted to correct the problem. Many of the side effects possible will respond to a reduced rate. Some will require catheter insertion at a new site. Treat symptomatically and resuscitate as necessary.

CYTARABINE

Antineoplastic
(Antimetabolite)

ARA-C, ✤Cytosar, Cytosar-U,
Cytosine arabinoside, Tarabine PFS   pH 5.0

USUAL DOSE

Acute lymphocytic leukemia in adults and children: In combination chemotherapy, variable depending on specific regime or protocol. 2 to 6 mg/kg/24 hr or 100 to 200 mg/M^2/24 hr as a continuous infusion or IV injection in divided doses every 12 hours. Repeat daily for 5 to 10 days depending on regimen. Maintain treatment until therapeutic effect or toxicity occurs. Modify on a day-to-day basis for maximum individualized effectiveness.

Acute myelocytic leukemia remission induction in adults and children: As a single agent, 100 to 200 mg/M^2/24 hr for 5 to 10 days as a continuous infusion or IV injection. Total dose is 1,000 mg/M^2. Repeat every 2 weeks.

Refractory acute leukemia remission induction: As a single agent, 3 Gm/M^2 as an IV infusion over 2 to 3 hours every 12 hours for 4 to 12 doses. Repeat at 2- to 3-week intervals.

DOSE ADJUSTMENTS

Dose (mg/kg) based on average weight in presence of edema or ascites. ■ Dose reduction may be indicated in impaired hepatic function. ■ Note Precautions/Monitor. ■ Usually used with other antineoplastic drugs in specific doses to achieve tumor remission.

DILUTION

Specific techniques required; see Precautions. Each 100 mg must be initially diluted with 5 ml (500 mg with 10 ml) of sterile water for injection with benzyl alcohol 0.9%. Solution pH about 5.0. May be given

by direct IV administration as is or further diluted in 50 to 100 ml or more of NS or D5W and given as an infusion. Direct IV administration should be through a free-flowing IV tubing. Use only clear solutions.
Storage: Stable at room temperature for 48 hours.

INCOMPATIBLE WITH

Allopurinol (Zyloprim), cephalothin (Keflin), fluorouracil, gallium nitrate (Ganite), ganciclovir (Cytovene), gentamicin (Garamycin), heparin, insulin, methylprednisolone sodium succinate (Solu-Medrol), oxacillin, penicillin G sodium, Nafcillin.

COMPATIBLE WITH

May be compatible with calcium, hydrocortisone, magnesium sulfate, methotrexate, daunorubicin, etoposide, and vincristine. Consult pharmacist. Consider toxicity and specific use.

RATE OF ADMINISTRATION

IV injection: Each 100 mg or fraction thereof over 1 to 3 minutes.
IV infusion: Single daily dose properly diluted over 30 minutes to 24 hours, depending on amount of infusion solution and dosage regime.

ACTIONS

An antimetabolite and pyrimidine antagonist that interferes with the synthesis of DNA. Cell cycle specific for S phase. Through various chemical processes this deprivation acts more quickly on rapidly growing cells and causes their death. Cytotoxic and cytostatic. A potent bone marrow depressant. Crosses the blood-brain barrier. Metabolized in the liver and excreted in the urine.

INDICATIONS AND USES

Induction and maintenance of remission in acute myelocytic leukemia of adults and children and other acute leukemias in adults and children.

CONTRAINDICATIONS

Hypersensitivity to cytarabine, preexisting drug-induced bone marrow depression.

PRECAUTIONS

Follow guidelines for handling cytotoxic agents. See Appendix A, p. 893. ■ Administered by or under the direction of the physician specialist. ■ Remissions induced by cytarabine are brief unless followed by maintenance therapy. ■ Use caution with impaired liver function.
Monitor: Leukocyte and platelet counts should be monitored daily. Discontinue therapy for platelet count under 50,000 or polymorphonuclear granulocytes under 1,000 cells/mm^3. ■ Monitor bone marrow, liver, and renal function at regular intervals during therapy. ■ Higher doses tolerated by IV injection compared with IV infusion, but the incidence and intensity of nausea and vomiting are increased. ■ Prophylactic administration of antiemetics recommended. ■ Be alert for signs of bone marrow depression, bleeding, or infection. These side effects are dose- and schedule-dependent. ■ Prophylactic antibiotics may be indicated pending results of C/S in a febrile neutropenic patient. ■ Monitor uric acid levels; maintain hydration; allopurinol may be indicated.
Patient education: Nonhormonal birth control recommended. ■ See Appendix D, p. 900.
Maternal/child: Category D: avoid pregnancy. May produce teratogenic

effects on the fetus especially during the first trimester. ■ Discontinue breast feeding. ■ Note Drug/lab interactions.

Elderly: Consider age-related organ impairment; toxicity may be increased.

DRUG/LAB INTERACTIONS

May inhibit digoxin absorption. ■ Do not administer any live vaccines to patients receiving antineoplastic drugs. ■ May cause acute pancreatitis in patients who previously received L-asparaginase. ■ May antagonize action of gentamicin against *Klebsiella.* ■ May antagonize antifungal actions of flucytosine (Ancobon). ■ Benzyl alcohol may cause a fatal "gasping syndrome" in premature infants. ■ Clearance decreased and toxicity increased with nephrotoxic agents (e.g., aminoglycosides [gentamicin]), may cause neurotoxic symptoms (e.g., ataxia, confusion, lethargy). ■ Concurrent use of high doses of cytarabine with cisplatin may increase ototoxicity.

SIDE EFFECTS

Abdominal pain, anemia, bone marrow depression, bone pain, cardiomyopathy, chest pain, conjunctivitis, diarrhea, esophagitis, fever, hepatic dysfunction, hyperuricemia, leukopenia, malaise, megaloblastosis, mucosal bleeding, myalgia, nausea, oral ulceration, rash, stomatitis, thrombocytopenia, thrombophlebitis, vomiting. Higher than usual dose regimens may cause severe coma, GI ulcerations and peritonitis, personality changes, pulmonary toxicity, somnolence, or death.

ANTIDOTE

Notify the physician of all side effects. Most will be treated symptomatically. Some toxicity is necessary to produce remission. Discontinue the drug for serious hematologic depression. Oprelvekin (Numega) has been used to treat thrombocytopenia. Drug must be restarted as soon as signs of bone marrow recovery occur, or its effectiveness will be lost. Use corticosteroids for cytarabine syndrome (fever, myalgia, bone pain, occasional chest pain, maculopapular rash, conjunctivitis, malaise). Usually occurs in 6 to 12 hours after administration. Continue cytarabine if patient responds to corticosteriods. There is no specific antidote; supportive therapy as indicated will help to sustain the patient in toxicity.

CYTOMEGALOVIRUS IMMUNE GLOBULIN INTRAVENOUS (HUMAN)

Passive immunizing agent
Antibacterial
Antiviral

CMV-IGIV, CytoGam

USUAL DOSE

150 mg/kg of body weight as a single dose IV infusion. This initial dose must be given within 72 hours of transplant. Do not exceed this dose. Follow with an infusion containing 100 mg/kg at 2, 4, 6, and 8 weeks post transplant.

DOSE ADJUSTMENTS

Reduce dose to 50 mg/kg per infusion at weeks 12 and 16 post transplant.

DILUTION

Absolute sterile technique required; contains no preservatives. Available in 20 and 50 ml vials (10 mg/ml); multiple vials may be required. Use only if clear and colorless. Enter vial only once and initiate infusion within 6 hours. Must be completely infused within 12 hours of dilution. Filters are not required, but an in-line filter may be used.

Storage: Store dry powder in refrigerator between 2° to 8° C (35° to 46° F).

INCOMPATIBLE WITH

Administration through a separate infusion line recommended. If absolutely necessary, may be piggy-backed into a preexisting line containing NS, 0.45 NS, dextrose 2.5%, 5%, 10%, or 20% in water or saline. Do not dilute CMV-IGIV, more than one part to two parts of any of these solutions.

RATE OF ADMINISTRATION

Use of a constant infusion pump (e.g., IVAC) is required. Begin with a rate of 15 mg/kg/hr. May be increased to 30 mg/kg/hr in 30 minutes if no discomfort or adverse effects. May be increased in another 30 minutes to 60 mg/kg/hr if no discomfort or adverse effects. Do not exceed the 60 mg/kg/hr rate or allow the volume infused to exceed 75 ml/hr regardless of mg/kg/hr dose. Slow rate of infusion at onset of patient discomfort or any adverse reactions. Infusion must be complete within 12 hours of dilution. Subsequent doses may be increased at 15-minute intervals using the same mg/kg/hr rates and adhering to the volume maximum of 75 ml/hr.

ACTIONS

A sterile solution of immunoglobulin G (IgG). Derived from pooled adult human plasma selected for high titers of antibody for cytomegalovirus (CMV). Purified by a specific process. Can raise the relevant antibody levels sufficiently to attenuate or reduce the incidence of serious CMV disease. Antibody levels will last 2 to 3 weeks.

INDICATIONS AND USES

Attenuation of primary (1°) CMV disease associated with kidney transplantation. Intended for use in all kidney transplant recipients who are seronegative for CMV and who receive a kidney from a CMV seropositive donor.

CONTRAINDICATIONS

History of a prior severe reaction associated with any human immuno-globulin preparations. Individuals with selective immunoglobulin A deficiency may develop antibodies to IgA and are at risk for anaphylaxis.

PRECAUTIONS

75% of untreated recipients would be expected to develop CMV disease. Use of CMV-IGIV has effected a 50% reduction in this disease rate. Effective results have been obtained with a variety of immunosuppressive regimens (e.g., combinations of azathioprine, cyclosporine, prednisone). ■ A fatal CMV infection occurred even with ganciclovir treatment in one patient, who inadvertently missed a single injection.

Monitor: Continuous monitoring of vital signs is preferred. Must be monitored before infusion, at every rate change, the midpoint, at the conclusion, and several times after completion. ■ All supplies for emergency treatment of acute anaphylatic reaction must be available (See Antidote)

Patient education: Adherence to the prescribed regimen is imperative.

Maternal/child: Pregnancy Category C: safety for use during pregnancy or lactation not established. Use only if clearly needed.

DRUG/LAB INTERACTIONS

Defer vaccination with any live virus vaccine (e.g., measles, mumps, rubella) until 3 months after CMV-IGIV administration.

SIDE EFFECTS

Incidence related to rate of administration; back pain, chills, fever, flushing, hypotension, muscle cramps, nausea, vomiting, wheezing. Allergic reactions including anaphylaxis are possible.

ANTIDOTE

With onset of any minor side effect reduce rate of infusion immediately or discontinue temporarily. Discontinue CMV-IGIV if symptoms persist and notify the physician. May be treated symptomatically, and infusion resumed at a slower rate if symptoms subside. Discontinue CMV-IGIV if hypotension or anaphylaxis occur and treat immediately. Epinephrine (Adrenalin), diphenhydramine (Benadryl), oxygen, vasopressors (e.g., dopamine [Intropin]), corticosteroids, and ventilation equipment must always be available. Resuscitate as necessary.

DACARBAZINE

Antineoplastic (Miscellaneous)

DTIC, DTIC-Dome, Imidazole carboxamide

pH 3.0 to 4.0

USUAL DOSE

Malignant melanoma: 2 to 4.5 mg/kg of body weight/24 hr for 10 days. May be repeated at 4-week intervals. May administer 250 mg/M^2 daily for 5 days. Repeat in 3 weeks. Has proved as effective in lesser doses as in larger doses. Individualized response determines dosage of subsequent treatments.

Hodgkin's disease: 150 mg/M^2/24 hr for 5 days. Repeat every 4 weeks. Used in combination with other drugs in a specific regimen. An alternate regimen is 375 mg/M^2 on day one in combination with a specific protocol. Repeat every 15 days.

DOSE ADJUSTMENTS

Dose (mg/kg) based on average weight in presence of edema or ascites. ■ Used with other antineoplastic drugs and radiation therapy in reduced doses to achieve tumor remission. ■ Dose reduction may be required in impaired liver and renal function.

DILUTION

Specific techniques required; see Precautions. Each 100-mg vial is diluted with 9.9 ml (200 mg with 19.7 ml) of sterile water for injection (10 mg/ml). Further dilution in 50 to 250 ml of D5W or NS for infusion is preferred. May be given through Y-tube or three-way stopcock of infusion set through a free-flowing IV.

Storage: Discard in 6 to 8 hours if kept at room temperature. Reconstituted solution stable for 72 hours, diluted solution for 24 hours if refrigerated at 4° C (39° F).

INCOMPATIBLE WITH

Limited information available; allopurinol (Zyloprim), heparin, hydrocortisone sodium succinate, hydrocortisone sodium phosphate, lidocaine.

COMPATIBLE WITH

Cyclophosphamide (Cytoxan), dactinomycin (Cosmogen), doxorubicin (Adriamycin), methotrexate, piperacillin sodium and tazobactam (Zosyn), vinblastine (Velban). Consult pharmacist.

RATE OF ADMINISTRATION

Total dose over 30 to 60 minutes. More rapid rate may cause severe venous irritation.

ACTIONS

An antineoplastic agent. Exact mechanism of action is not known; may inhibit DNA and RNA synthesis. It is an alkylating agent, cell cycle phase nonspecific. Probably localizes in the liver and is excreted in the urine.

INDICATIONS AND USES

Metastatic malignant melanoma. ■ Hodgkin's disease. ■ Soft-tissue sarcomas.

Investigational uses: Treatment of malignant pheochromocytoma with cyclophosphamide and vincristine. ■ Treatment of metastatic malignant melanoma with tamoxifen.

CONTRAINDICATIONS

Known hypersensitivity to dacarbazine.

PRECAUTIONS

■ Follow guidelines for handling cytotoxic agents. See Appendix A, p. 893. ■ Administered by or under the direction of the physician specialist. ■ Use caution in impaired liver and renal function.

Monitor: Determine absolute patency of vein; a stinging or burning sensation indicates extravasation; severe cellulitis and tissue necrosis will result. Discontinue injection; use another vein. ▪ Monitor bone marrow function, white and red blood cell and platelet count frequently. ▪ Nausea and vomiting may be reduced by restricting oral intake of fluid and foods for 4 to 6 hours before administration. Use prophylactic antiemetics. ▪ Be alert for signs of bone marrow depression, bleeding, or infection. ▪ Prophylactic antibiotics may be indicated pending results of C/S in a febrile neutropenic patient.

Patient education: Protect skin surfaces, may cause photosensitive skin reactions. ▪ Nonhormonal birth control recommended. ▪ Report burning or stinging at IV site promptly. ▪ See Appendix D, p. 900.

Maternal/child: Pregnancy Category C: safety for use in pregnancy or lactation and in men and women capable of conception not established. ▪ Discontinue breast feeding.

Elderly: Consider age-related organ impairment; toxicity may be increased.

DRUG/LAB INTERACTIONS

Do not administer any live vaccines to patients receiving antineoplastic drugs. ▪ Inhibited by phenobarbital and phenytoin (Dilantin). ▪ Potentiates allopurinol.

SIDE EFFECTS

Leukopenia and thrombocytopenia may be serious enough to cause death. Alopecia, anaphylaxis, anorexia, facial flushing, facial paresthesias, fever, hepatotoxicity, malaise, myalgia, nausea, skin necrosis, vomiting.

ANTIDOTE

Notify physician of all side effects. Most will be treated symptomatically. Hematopoietic depression may require temporary or permanent withholding of treatment. Oprelvekin (Numega) has been used to treat thrombocytopenia. Filgrastin (Neupogen) may be indicated to treat severe leukopenia. There is no specific antidote. Supportive therapy as indicated will help sustain the patient in toxicity. For extravasation, elevate extremity; consider injection of long-acting dexamethasone (Decadron LA) or hyaluronidase (Wydase) throughout extravasated tissue. Use a 27- or 25-gauge needle. Apply moist warm compresses.

DACLIZUMAB

Recombinant monoclonal antibody
Immunosuppressant

Zenapax   pH 6.9

USUAL DOSE

Used concurrently with cyclosporine (Sandimmune) and corticosteroids.

Organ rejection prophylaxis in renal transplant: 1 mg/kg as an infusion for a total of 5 doses. Administer the first dose no more than 24 hours before transplantation. Give the 4 remaining doses at intervals of 14 days.

PEDIATRIC DOSE

Safety for use in children not established; studies not complete. Note Maternal/child.

DOSE ADJUSTMENTS

No dose adjustments indicated in severe renal impairment or based on age, gender, race, or degree of proteinuria. ■ No data available in patients with severe impaired liver function.

DILUTION

Each single dose must be diluted with 50 ml of NS. Do not shake; gently invert to avoid foaming. Sterile technique is imperative. Discard any unused portion.

Storage: Store unopened vials in the refrigerator (2° to 8° C [36° to 45° F]). Do not shake or freeze. Protect from light. Should be used within 4 hours of dilution. If necessary, may be refrigerated for up to 24 hours. Discard prepared solution after 24 hours.

INCOMPATIBLE WITH

Manufacturer states, "Other drug substances should not be added or infused simultaneously through the same IV line."

RATE OF ADMINISTRATION

A single dose, properly diluted, as an infusion over 15 minutes. May be given through a peripheral or central vein.

ACTIONS

An immunosuppressive agent. A humanized IgG$_1$ monoclonal antibody produced by recombinant DNA technology. Acts as an IL-2 receptor antagonist that binds to the Tac subunit of the high-affinity IL-2 receptor complex and inhibits IL-2 mediated activation of lymphocytes, a critical pathway in the cellular immune response involved in allograft rejection. Blocks only those immune cells (T-cells) that are activated by a foreign substance, impairing the response of the immune system to antigenic challenges. During studies, trough levels of 5 to 10 mcg/ml were considered necessary for saturation of the Tac subunit to block the responses of activated T lymphocytes. Does not suppress the entire immune system, which would increase the risk of infection. Has reduced the incidence of kidney rejection episodes without increasing most side effects and may improve survival rates. Estimated terminal half-life is 20 days (range 11 to 38 days). May cross the placental barrier. May be secreted in breast milk.

INDICATIONS AND USES

Prophylaxis of acute organ rejection in patients receiving renal transplants. Used as part of an immunosuppressive regimen that includes cyclosporine and corticosteroids.

CONTRAINDICATIONS

Known hypersensitivity to daclizumab or any of its components (composite of human [90%] and murine [10%] antibodies).

PRECAUTIONS

Usually administered by or under the direction of a physician experienced in immunosuppressive therapy and management of organ transplant patients. Adequate laboratory and supportive medical resources must be available. ■ Use caution; allergic reactions have not been observed, but this is a protein substance—emergency equipment and drugs for treatment of severe hypersensitivity reactions must be immediately available. ■ Readministration after an initial course of therapy has not been studied in humans, but other monoclonal antibodies have precipitated anaphylactoid reactions. ■ It is not known whether daclizumab use will have a long-term effect on the ability of the immune system to respond to antigens first encountered during induced immunosuppression. ■ Low titers of antiidiotype antibodies to daclizumab have been detected in some patients during treatment; no adverse effects have been noted.

Monitor: Obtain baseline CBC with differential and platelets and baseline renal and liver tests if not already completed for other immunosuppressant agents. ■ Monitor vital signs. ■ Observe closely for signs of infection (e.g., fever, sore throat, tiredness) or unusual bleeding or bruising. ■ Prophylactic antibiotics may be indicated pending results of C/S in a febrile neutropenic patient. ■ Symptoms of cytokine release syndrome (e.g., chills, fever, dyspnea, and malaise) have not been reported but may occur; observe carefully. ■ Note Precautions and Drug/Lab interactions.

Patient education: Report difficulty in breathing, swallowing, rapid heart beat, rash, or itching immediately. ■ Avoid pregnancy; nonhormonal birth control preferred. Women with childbearing potential should use effective contraception before beginning daclizumab therapy, during therapy, and for 4 months after completion ■ See Appendix D, p. 900.

Maternal/child: Category C: use during pregnancy only if benefits justify the potential risk to the fetus. Avoid pregnancy; effective contraception required, see Patient education. ■ Discontinue breast feeding. ■ Has been used in children from 11 months to 17 years of age (average age 12 years), but safety not established; studies still in progress. Somewhat higher rates of hypertension and dehydration occurred in pediatric patients.

Elderly: Specific information not available. Use caution and observe closely.

DRUG/LAB INTERACTIONS

Has been administered concurrently with acyclovir (Zovirax), azathioprine (Imuran), corticosteroids, cyclosporine, ganciclovir (Cytovene), and mycophenolate mofetil (CellCept); no additional adverse reactions noted. ■ Limited experience with concurrent use of antithymocyte globulin, antilymphocyte globulin, muromonab-CD3 (Orthoclone), and tacrolimus (Prograf). ■ May increase fasting blood glucose.

SIDE EFFECTS

Daclizumab did not appear to alter the pattern, frequency, or severity of known side effects associated with the use of immunosuppressive drugs. Whereas 95% of a placebo-treated group reported side effects from concurrent immunosuppressants, 96% of the daclizumab group (also being treated with concurrent immunosuppressants) reported similar side effects. Side effects seen in patients receiving immunosuppressive therapy may include: abdominal distention, abdominal pain, back pain, bleeding, cellulitis, chest pain, constipation, coughing, dehydration, diarrhea, dizziness, dyspepsia, dyspnea, dysuria, edema, epigastric pain (not food related), fatigue, fever, headache, heartburn, hypertension, hypotension, impaired wound healing without infection, insomnia, lymphocele, musculoskeletal pain, nausea, oliguria, postoperative pain, pulmonary edema, renal tubular necrosis, tachycardia, thrombosis, tremor, vomiting, and wound infections. Daclizumab did not increase the number of posttransplant lymphomas.

ANTIDOTE

Notify physician of all side effects. Most will be treated symptomatically. Daclizumab may be discontinued or alternate immunosuppressive agents substituted. Discontinue immediately if anaphylaxis occurs and treat with oxygen, epinephrine, corticosteroids, and/or antihistamines (e.g., diphenhydramine [Benadryl]). Resuscitate as necessary.

DACTINOMYCIN

**Antineoplastic
(Antibiotic)**

ACT, Actinomycin D, Cosmegen

pH 5.5 to 7.0

USUAL DOSE

0.01 mg (10 mcg) to 0.015 mg (15 mcg)/kg/24 hr or 0.5 mg/M^2/24 hr for up to 5 days. May be repeated after 3 weeks if all signs of toxicity have disappeared. Daily dose may range from 0.25 to 0.6 mg/M^2 for up to 5 days. Do not exceed 15 mcg/kg of body weight or 400 to 600 mcg/M^2/day.

PEDIATRIC DOSE

0.01 mg (10 mcg) to 0.015 mg (15 mcg)/kg of body weight/24 hr for 5 days or a total dose of 2.5 mg/M^2 in equally divided doses over 7 days. May be repeated after 3 weeks if all signs of toxicity have disappeared. Maximum dose is 15 mcg/kg or 500 mcg/24 hr.

DOSE ADJUSTMENTS

Calculate dose based on body surface area in presence of edema or ascites. ■ Used with other antineoplastic drugs in reduced doses to achieve tumor remission. ■ Reduce dose of dactinomycin and radiation therapy when used concurrently, if either has been used previously, or if previous chemotherapy has been employed.

DILUTION

Specific techniques required; see Precautions. Dilute each 0.5 mg vial with 1.1 ml of preservative free sterile water for injection (0.5 mg/ml). Sterile water with preservative (benzyl alcohol or paraben) will cause precipitation. Use 2.2 ml to yield 0.25 mg/ml (vent vial to relieve pressure). Use sterile two-needle technique: one needle to dilute and withdraw and one needle to inject into the vein (rinse with blood or IV solution before removing). May be given direct IV, through the Y-tube or three-way stopcock of a free-flowing infusion of D5W or NS, or further diluted in 50 ml of the above solutions for infusion. Do not use a filter smaller than 5 microns. Loss of potency will occur. Discard any unused portion.
Storage: Light sensitive in dry form.

INCOMPATIBLE WITH

Diluents containing preservatives, filgrastim (Neupogen). Should be considered incompatible in syringe or solution with most drugs. May be compatible with dacarbazine (DTIC); consult pharmacist.

RATE OF ADMINISTRATION

Direct IV: A single dose over 2 to 3 minutes.
IV infusion: A single dose over 20 to 30 minutes.

ACTIONS

A highly toxic antibiotic antineoplastic agent, cell cycle phase nonspecific. Cytotoxic, it interferes with cell division by binding DNA to slow production of RNA. Found in high concentrations in the kidney, liver, and spleen. Metabolized in the liver. Elimination half-life is 30 to 40 hours. Excreted as unchanged drug in bile and urine.

INDICATIONS AND USES

Wilms' tumor. ▪ Rhabdomyosarcoma. ▪ Carcinoma of the testis and uterus. ▪ Choriocarcinoma. ▪ Ewing's sarcoma. ▪ Botryoid sarcoma. *Investigational uses:* Nonlymphocytic leukemia, Kaposi's sarcoma, melanoma, osteosarcoma, trophoblaxtic neoplasms, and cancers of the endometrium and ovary.

CONTRAINDICATIONS

Exposure to chicken pox, known sensitivity to dactinomycin, infants under 6 to 12 months of age.

PRECAUTIONS

▪ Follow guidelines for handling cytotoxic agents. See Appendix A, p. 893. ▪ Administered by or under the direction of the physician specialist.

Monitor: Determine absolute patency of vein; a stinging or burning sensation indicates extravasation; severe cellulitis and tissue necrosis will result. Discontinue injection; use another vein. ▪ Monitor renal, hepatic, and bone marrow function frequently. ▪ Except for immediate nausea and vomiting, side effects may not appear for 2 to 4 days. Always observe closely. Use prophylactic antiemetics. ▪ Allopurinol, increased fluid intake, and alkalinization of the urine may be required to reduce uric acid levels. ▪ Observe closely for signs of infection. Prophylactic antibiotics may be indicated pending results of C/S in a febrile neutropenic patient.

Patient education: Nonhormonal birth control recommended. ▪ Report burning or stinging at IV site promptly. ▪ See Appendix D, p. 900.

Maternal/child: Pregnancy Category C: safety for use in pregnancy not established. May produce teratogenic effects on the fetus; use caution in men and women capable of conception. ▪ Discontinue breast feeding. ▪ Note Contraindications.

Elderly: Consider age-related organ impairment; toxicity may be increased.

DRUG/LAB INTERACTIONS

Radiation therapy potentiates dactinomycin. ▪ Dactinomycin alone may reactivate erythema from previous radiation therapy. ▪ Do not administer live vaccines to patients receiving antineoplastic drugs. ▪ Inhibits action of penicillin. ▪ Note Dose adjustments. ▪ May interfere with bioassay procedures used in determining antibacterial drug levels.

SIDE EFFECTS

Abdominal pain, acne, alopecia, anaphylaxis, anemia, anorexia, ascites, cheilitis, diarrhea, dysphagia, erythema flare-up, esophagitis, fatigue, fever, GI ulceration, hepatitis, hepatomegaly, hypocalcemia, lethargy, leukopenia, liver function test abnormalities, malaise, myalgia, nausea, pharyngitis, proctitis, skin eruptions, thrombocytopenia, ulcerative stomatitis, vomiting.

ANTIDOTE

Any side effect can result in death. Notify the physician of all side effects. Most will be treated symptomatically. Hematopoietic depression may require withholding dactinomycin until recovery occurs. There is no specific antidote. Supportive therapy as indicated will help sustain the patient in toxicity. For extravasation, elevate extremity, apply cold compresses, flush area with normal saline, and inject long-acting dexamethasone (Decadron LA) or hyaluronidase (Wydase) throughout extravasated tissue. Use a 27- or 25-gauge needle.

DANTROLENE SODIUM

Skeletal muscle relaxant (Direct acting)

Dantrium Intravenous

pH 9.5

USUAL DOSE

In patients known to be susceptible to malignant hyperthermia, oral dantrolene is indicated prophylactically preoperatively and postoperatively for 1 to 3 days following therapeutic IV treatment. Postoperative dosing is indicated after emergency treatment.

Prophylactic dose: 2.5 mg/kg as an infusion administered over 1 hour prior to anesthesia. Oral dantrolene may be used.

Therapeutic or emergency dose: 1 mg/kg of body weight as an initial dose. Repeat as necessary until symptoms subside or a cumulative dose of 10 mg/kg is reached. Entire regimen may be repeated if symptoms reappear. Dose required depends on degree of susceptibility to malignant hyperthermia, length of time of exposure to triggering agent, and time lapse between onset of crisis and beginning of treatment.

Post crisis follow up: An oral dose of 4 to 8 mg/kg/day for 1 to 3 days to prevent recurrences. If oral dosing not feasible, begin IV dose at 1 mg/kg and individualize by increasing based on patient response.

PEDIATRIC DOSE

Prophylactic, therapeutic, and post crisis follow up doses are the same as for adults.

DILUTION

Each 20 mg must be diluted with 60 ml sterile water for injection without a bacteriostatic agent. Shake until solution is clear. May be administered through a Y-tube or three-way stopcock of infusion tubing. Protect diluted solution from direct light and discard after 6 hours.

Storage: Store undiluted vials between 15° and 30° C (59° and 86° F).

INCOMPATIBLE WITH

Specific information not available.

RATE OF ADMINISTRATION

Prophylactic dose: A single dose as an infusion distributed over 1 hour.

Therapeutic or emergency dose: Each single dose should be given rapid continuous IV push. Follow immediately with subsequent doses as indicated.

Follow up dose: Each single dose over 2 to 3 minutes.

ACTIONS

A direct-acting skeletal muscle relaxant. Inhibits excitation-contraction coupling by interfering with the release of the calcium ion from the sarcoplasmic reticulum to reverse the physiologic cause of malignant hyperthermia. Has no appreciable effect on cardiovascular or respiratory function. Onset of action is prompt and lasts about 5 hours. Metabolized in the liver and excreted in urine.

INDICATIONS AND USES

Perioperatively to prevent, treat, or minimize the severity of clinical and laboratory signs of malignant hyperthermia in individuals who may be or are known to be susceptible.

CONTRAINDICATIONS

None when used as indicated.

PRECAUTIONS

Use caution in patients with impaired pulmonary or cardiac function or history of liver disease. ▪ Discontinue all anesthetic agents immediately when onset of malignant hyperthermia is recognized. S/S of the fulminant hypermetabolism of skeletal muscle characteristic of malignant hyperthermia crisis are tachycardia, tachypnea, central venous desaturation, hypercapnia, metabolic acidosis, skeletal muscle rigidity, cyanosis, mottling of skin, fever, increased use of anesthesia circuit CO_2 absorber.

Monitor: Monitor ECG, vital signs, electrolytes, and urine output continuously. ▪ Oxygen needs are increased. ▪ Manage metabolic acidosis. ▪ Institute cooling measures. ▪ Confirm absolute patency of vein; avoid extravasation.

Patient education: May experience decreased grip strength, weakness in leg muscles and lightheadedness post op. May persist for 48 hours. ▪ Request assistance for ambulation. ▪ Use caution when eating; choking and difficulty swallowing has been reported on day of administration. ▪ Avoid alcohol and other CNS depressants (e.g., diazepam [Valium]). ▪ Avoid tasks that require alertness. ▪ Photosensitivity may occur; sunscreens or protective clothing may be required. ▪ May cause diarrhea, fatigue, nausea, and weakness. Notify physician if they persist. ▪ Promptly report bloody or tarry stools, itching, jaundice (yellow color) of eyes and skin, or skin rash.

Maternal/ child: Pregnancy Category C: embryocidal with larger doses in rats. Benefits must outweigh risks. ▪ Discontinue breast feeding. ▪ Use caution in children under 5 years; safety not established.

DRUG/LAB INTERACTIONS

Ability to bind to plasma proteins inhibited by warfarin and clofibrate; increased by tolbutamide. ▪ Avoid concurrent use of calcium channel blockers (e.g., diltiazem [Cardizem]) and dantrolene. Myocardial depression, arrhythmias, and hyperkalemia have been reported. ▪ May cause hepatotoxicity with estrogens, especially in women over 35.

SIDE EFFECTS

Erythema, pulmonary edema, urticaria, thrombophlebitis.

ANTIDOTE

No specific antidote is available or needed when used correctly. Notify physician and initiate supportive measures (adequate airway and ventilation, monitor ECG) in overdosage. Large amounts of IV fluids may be needed to prevent crystalluria. Treat anaphylaxis and resuscitate as necessary.

DAUNORUBICIN HYDROCHLORIDE/ DAUNORUBICIN CITRATE LIPOSOME INJECTION

Antineoplastic (Antibiotic)

Cerubidine, DNR/DaunoXome

pH 4.5 to 6.5 / 4.9 to 6.0

USUAL DOSE

Conventional daunorubicin

Acute myelogenous leukemia: Up to 60 mg/M^2/day for 3 days. Repeat every 3 to 4 weeks.

Adult acute nonlymphocytic leukemia: 45 mg/M^2/day in adults under age 60 (adults over age 60 may require reduction to 30 mg/M^2/day) for 3 days. Used in specific protocol combination therapy (e.g., cytarabine 100 mg/M^2/day for 7 days). Repeat daunorubicin, 30 to 45 mg/M^2/day depending on age for only 2 days in subsequent courses every 3 to 4 weeks.

Adult acute lymphocytic leukemia: 45 mg/M^2/day on days 1, 2, and 3. Used in combination therapy (e.g., vincristine, prednisone, and L-asparaginase).

In all situations, when remission is complete, an individual maintenance program should be established.

DaunoXome (liposomal daunorubicin)

Advanced, HIV-associated Kaposi's sarcoma: 40 mg/M^2 as an IV infusion. Repeat every 2 weeks. Continue treatment until there is evidence of disease progression (specifics outlined in package insert).

PEDIATRIC DOSE

Conventional daunorubicin:

Pediatric acute lymphocytic leukemia: 25 mg/M^2/day on day 1 each week, vincristine 1.5 mg/M^2 on day 1 each week, and prednisone 40 mg/M^2 orally daily. Remission should be obtained in 4 to 6 weeks.

DaunoXome: Safety for use in children not established.

DOSE ADJUSTMENTS

All daunorubicins: Note Precautions/Monitor.

Conventional daunorubicin: Reduce dose up to one half if liver or renal function impaired. Note Usual dose for adults over 60 years of age.

DaunoXome: Reduce dose to 75% of normal (30 mg/M^2) if serum bilirubin is 1.2 to 3 mg/dl. Reduce dose to 50% of normal (20 mg/M^2) if serum bilirubin or creatinine is > 3 mg/dl. ■ Withhold dose if absolute granulocyte count is < 750 cells/mm^3.

DILUTION

Specific techniques required; see precautions.

Conventional daunorubicin: Each 20 mg must be diluted with 4 ml of sterile water for injection (5 mg/ml). Agitate gently to dissolve completely. Further dilute each dose with 10 to 15 ml of NS. Usually given through Y-tube or three-way stopcock of a free-flowing infusion of D5W or NS. May be added to 100 ml NS and given as an infusion. Use extreme caution.

DaunoXome: A single dose must be diluted with an equal amount of D5W. Available as a 2 mg/ml preservative-free solution. Withdraw the calculated volume (dose of DaunoXome) from the vial and transfer to a sterile infusion bag that contains an equal volume of D5W. Desired concentration is 1 mg/ml. Do not use any other diluent. A translucent red liposomal dispersion; do not use if opaque. Do not use in-line filters for infusion. Note Incompatible with.

Storage: Conventional daunorubicin: Protect from sunlight. Diluted solution stable 24 hours at room temperature, 48 hours if refrigerated; then discard. *DaunoXome:* Refrigerate unopened vials; avoid freezing. Protect from light. Discard unused drug. Reconstituted solutions may be refrigerated for a maximum of 6 hours.

INCOMPATIBLE WITH

Conventional daunorubicin: Allopurinol (Zyloprim), dexamethasone (Decadron), fludarabine (Fludara), heparin, piperacillin sodium, and tazobactam (Zosyn). Should be considered incompatible with any other drug because of toxicity and specific use.

DaunoXome: Manufacturer states, "DaunoXome must not be mixed with saline, bacteriostatic agents such as benzyl alcohol, or any other solution."

COMPATIBLE WITH

Conventional daunorubicin: May be compatible with cytarabine (ARA-C), and etoposide (VePesid) ; consult pharmacist.

RATE OF ADMINISTRATION

Conventional daunorubicin: IV Injection: A single dose of properly diluted medication over 3 to 5 minutes.

IV infusion: A single dose evenly distributed over 30 to 45 minutes.

DaunoXome: A single dose as an infusion evenly distributed over 60 minutes. Do not use an in-line filter. Back pain, flushing, and chest tightness may occur. Usually subsides if infusion is stopped, and usually does not recur if infusion is restarted at a slower rate after symptoms subside.

ACTIONS

Conventional daunorubicin: A highly toxic antibiotic antineoplastic agent. Rapidly cleared from plasma, it inhibits synthesis of DNA. Cell cycle specific for S phase; exact method of action is unknown; antimitotic, cytotoxic, and immunosuppressive. Does not cross blood-brain barrier. Metabolized in the liver. Elimination half-life is 18 to 30 hours. Slowly excreted in bile and urine.

DaunoXome: A liposomal preparation of daunorubicin formulated to maximize selectivity for solid tumors. In the circulation, the liposomal preparation protects the entrapped daunorubicin from chemical and enzymatic degradation, minimizes protein binding, and generally decreases uptake by normal (non-reticuloendothelial system) tissues. The mechanism of delivery is not known, but may be through the often altered and/or compromised vasculature of tumors. In animals, it has been shown to accumulate in tumors to a greater extent than conventional daunorubicin. Released over time within the cells of the solid tumor. Persists at high levels within tumor tissue for several days. It differs from conventional daunorubicin because it mostly confines itself to vascular fluid volume. Plasma clearance is slower and the AUC (area under the curve) is larger.

INDICATIONS AND USES

Conventional daunorubicin: Treatment of acute myelogenous leukemia. Treatment of acute nonlymphocytic leukemia in adults. ■ Combination therapy for acute lymphocytic leukemia in adults and children.

DaunoXome: Currently approved only for first-line cytotoxic therapy for advanced HIV-associated Kaposi's sarcoma.

CONTRAINDICATIONS

Conventional daunorubicin: Not absolute; preexisting bone marrow suppression, impaired cardiac function, preexisting infection (See Precautions)

DaunoXome: History of hypersensitivity reaction to previous treatment with DaunoXome or any of its components (includes conventional daunorubicin). Not recommended in patients with less than advanced HIV-related Kaposi's sarcoma.

PRECAUTIONS

All daunorubicins: Follow guidelines for handling cytotoxic agents. See Appendix A, p. 893. ■ Administered by or under the direction of the physician specialist. ■ Urine may be reddish color (from dye not hematuria). ■ Use extreme caution in preexisting drug-induced bone marrow suppression, existing heart disease, previous treatment with other anthracyclines (e.g., doxorubicin [Adriamycin]), or radiation therapy encompassing the heart.

Monitor: All daunorubicins: Monitor CBC including differential and platelet count before each dose. ■ Monitoring of liver function, kidney function, ECG, chest x-ray, echocardiography, and systolic ejection fraction indicated before and during therapy; recommended before each course. ■ Evaluation of cardiac function by medical history and physical exam is recommended before each dose. ■ Determine absolute patency of vein; a stinging or burning sensation indicates extravasation; discontinue injection, use another vein. Severe cellulitis and tissue necrosis will result from extravasation with conventional daunorubicins; has not been observed with DaunoXome. ■ Prophylactic antiemetics may reduce nausea and vomiting and increase patient comfort. ■ Monitor uric acid levels; maintain hydration; allopurinol may be indicated. ■ Observe closely for all signs of infection. Prophylactic antibiotics may be indicated pending results of C/S in a febrile neutropenic patient.

Conventional daunorubicin: May cause acute congestive heart failure with total cumulative doses over 550 mg/M^2 in adults (400 mg/M^2 if previous treatment with doxorubicin or radiation therapy in area of heart), 300 mg/M^2 in children over 2 years, and 10 mg/kg in children under 2 years.

DaunoXome: May also cause cardiomyopathy. Monitoring of LVEF recommended at total cumulative doses of 320 mg/M^2, 480 mg/M^2, and every 240 mg/M^2 thereafter.

Patient education: Nonhormonal birth control recommended. ■ Report IV site burning or stinging promptly. ■ See Appendix D, p. 900.

Maternal/child: All daunorubicins: Pregnancy Category D: can cause fetal harm. Avoid pregnancy. ▪ Safety for use in lactation not established; discontinue breast feeding. ▪ Note Monitor. *DaunoXome:* Safety for use in children not established.

Elderly: Cardiotoxicity and myelotoxicity may be more severe. Consider age-related renal impairment. Safety of DaunoXome for use in the elderly has not been established.

DRUG/LAB INTERACTIONS

Do not administer vaccines or chloroquine to patients receiving antineoplastic drugs. ▪ Note Precautions.

SIDE EFFECTS

All daunorubicins: Bone marrow suppression and cardiomyopathy are dose related and dose limiting.

Conventional daunorubicin: Acute congestive heart failure, alopecia (reversible), bone marrow suppression (marked with average doses), chills, decrease in systolic ejection fraction, depressed QRS voltage, diarrhea, fever, gonadal suppression, mucositis, myocarditis, nausea, pericarditis, skin rash, vomiting.

DaunoXome: Granulocytopenia is most common. Symptoms common to conventional daunorubicin may also occur. Infusion related back pain, chest tightness, and flushing may be related to liposomal formulation.

Overdose: Will cause increased severity of myelosuppression, fatigue, nausea, and vomiting.

ANTIDOTE

Most side effects will be tolerated or treated symptomatically. Keep physician informed. Close monitoring of cumulative dosage, bone marrow, ECG, chest x-ray, echocardiography, and systolic ejection fraction may prevent most serious and potentially fatal side effects. There is no specific antidote. Supportive therapy as indicated will help sustain the patient in toxicity. For extravasation, aspirate as much infiltrated drug as possible, flood site with normal saline, and inject hydrocortisone sodium succinate (Solu-Cortef) or hyaluronidase (Wydase) throughout extravasated tissue. Use a 27- or 25-gauge needle. Cold moist compresses may be helpful; elevate extremity. Site should be observed promptly by a reconstructive surgeon.

DEFEROXAMINE MESYLATE

Antidote
Chelating agent

Desferal

pH 4.0 to 6.0

USUAL DOSE

Available on an allocation basis from the manufacturer. Hospitals and selected health facilities are allowed to keep 4 boxes on hand. See Precautions for ordering process.

Acute iron intoxication: 15 mg/kg/hr may be given up to a total dose of 90 mg/kg every 8 hours. *Do not exceed 6 Gm in 24 hours by way of any or all routes—IV, IM, clysis, or oral.*

Chronic iron overload: In addition to IM dose given with each unit of blood, give 2 Gm IV at a rate not to exceed 15 mg/kg/hr. Use a separate vein.

Aluminum toxicity: Dose must be individualized. 100 mg can bind 4.1 mg of aluminum.

Diagnosis of aluminum toxicity: 1 Gm infused at a rate not to exceed 15 mg/kg/hr. Usually given post dialysis, but may be given during the last two hours of dialysis.

PEDIATRIC DOSE

Acute iron intoxication in children over 3 years of age: A continuous infusion of 50 mg/kg of body weight up to 2 Gm every 6 hours or 90 mg/kg every 8 hours. *Do not exceed 6 Gm in 24 hours.*

Acute iron intoxication in children under 3 years of age: 15 mg/kg/hr as a continuous infusion.

Chronic iron overload: 50 mg/kg/dose every 6 hr at a rate not to exceed 15 mg/kg/hr. Maximum 2 Gm/dose or 6 Gm in 24 hours.

Diagnosis of aluminum toxicity: 15 to 20 mg/kg at a rate not to exceed 15 mg/kg/hr. See comment under adult dose.

DILUTION

Each 500 mg must be diluted in 2 ml of sterile water for injection. When completely dissolved, deferoxamine must be further diluted in an IV solution; NS, D5W, D10W, and Ringer's lactate solution are compatible.

Storage: Under sterile conditions, deferoxamine diluted with sterile water may be stored at room temperature for 1 week. Protect from light.

INCOMPATIBLE WITH

Must be diluted in specific IV solutions. *Do not mix with any other IV medication.*

RATE OF ADMINISTRATION

In all situations the fully diluted solution must not exceed a rate of 15 mg/kg of body weight/hr.

ACTIONS

An iron-chelating agent, deferoxamine complexes with iron to form ferrioxamine, a stable chelate that prevents the iron from entering into further chemical reactions. Readily soluble in water, it passes easily through the kidney, giving the urine a characteristic reddish color. It will remove iron from free serum iron, ferritin, and transferrin, but not from hemoglobin or cytochromes. Metabolized by plasma enzymes.

INDICATIONS AND USES

To facilitate the removal of iron in the treatment of acute iron intoxication or chronic iron overload from multiple transfusions.

Investigational use: Diagnosis and management of aluminum accumulation in bone of renal failure patients and in aluminum-induced dialysis encephalopathy.

CONTRAINDICATIONS

Severe renal disease or anuria.

PRECAUTIONS

IM administration is preferred. May be given SC by hypodermoclysis. IV administration should be used only in a state of cardiovascular shock or chronic iron overload. ▪ For long-term therapy, check for cataract development. ▪ Note Maternal/child. ▪ To order from manufacturer (Novartis), fax request to 1-973-503-5695 (24 hr line). Include a copy of the prescription or doctor's order, a written request for a 2 week supply, and the name and address of a wholesaler for billing purposes. Questions? Telephone 1-888-669-6682.

Monitor: Deferoxamine is adjunctive therapy. Standard measures for treating acute iron intoxication are also indicated: induction of emesis and/or gastric lavage; suction and maintenance of a clear airway; control of shock with IV fluids, blood, oxygen, and vasopressors; correction of acidosis. Monitor serum ferritin or iron concentration. ▪ In acute iron intoxication, larger than normal amounts of IV fluids are required to maintain intravascular volume and prevent kidney damage. Monitor blood gases, central venous pressure (CVP), and cardiac output frequently to assess effects of absorbed iron. Monitor renal function.

Patient education: Report any hearing or vision changes. ▪ Do not take vitamin C unless prescribed by physician.

Maternal/child: Category C: use only if clearly needed during early pregnancy or during child-bearing years. ▪ Use in children under 3 years only if there is iron mobilization greater than 1 mg/24 hours.

Elderly: Note Drug/lab interactions. ▪ Risk of cardiac decompensation increased.

DRUG/LAB INTERACTIONS

Risk of cardiac decompensation from increased tissue iron toxicity increased when given concurrently with ascorbic acid.

SIDE EFFECTS

Occur more frequently with too-rapid administration; abdominal discomfort, allergic type of reactions including anaphylaxis, blurring of vision, diarrhea, flushing of the skin, fever, hypotension, leg cramps, shock, tachycardia, urticaria.

ANTIDOTE

At first sign of side effects, decrease rate of administration. If side effects persist, discontinue drug and notify physician. Further dilution and decrease in rate of administration may be necessary. Readily dialyzable. Resuscitate as indicated.

DESMOPRESSIN ACETATE

DDAVP, 1-Deamino-8-D-Arginine Vasopressin

USUAL DOSE

Diabetes insipidus: 2 to 4 mcg daily in 2 divided doses. Adjust each dose individually for an adequate diurnal rhythm of water turnover. IV dose has 10 times the antidiuretic effect of intranasal desmopressin. Available as a tablet to manage cranial central diabetes insipidus.

Hemophilia A and von Willebrand's disease (Type 1): 0.3 mcg/kg of body weight. Administer 30 minutes preoperatively.

DOSE ADJUSTMENTS

Many specific requirements depending on diagnosis. (See Precautions/Monitor). ■ Reduce dose accordingly when transferring from intranasal to IV administration.

DILUTION

Diabetes insipidus: May be given undiluted.

Hemophilia A and von Willebrand's disease (Type 1): Dilute a single dose in 10 ml of NS for children under 10 kg; and 50 ml for adults and children over 10 kg. Must be given as an IV infusion.

INCOMPATIBLE WITH

Specific information not available.

RATE OF ADMINISTRATION

Diabetes insipidus: A single dose direct IV over 1 minute.

Hemophilia A and von Willebrand's disease (Type 1): A single dose as an IV infusion over 15 to 30 minutes.

ACTIONS

A synthetic analog of the natural hormone arginine vasopressin (human antidiuretic hormone—ADH). It is more potent than arginine vasopressin in increasing plasma levels of factor VIII activity in patients with hemophilia A and von Willebrand's disease (Type I). Produces dose-related increase in factor VIII levels within 30 minutes and peaks in 90 to 120 minutes. Onset of action as an antidiuretic is prompt and lasts from 8 to 20 hours. Increases water resorption in the kidney, increases urine osmolality, and decreases urine output. Clinically effective antidiuretic doses are usually below the levels needed to affect vascular or visceral smooth muscle.

INDICATIONS AND USES

Antidiuretic replacement therapy in the management of central (cranial) diabetes insipidus. ■ Management of the temporary polyuria and polydipsia following head trauma or surgery in the pituitary region. ■ Maintenance of hemostasis in patients with hemophilia A or von Willebrand's disease during surgical procedures and postoperatively. ■ To stop bleeding in patients with hemophilia A or von Willebrand's disease with episodes of spontaneous or trauma-induced injuries.

CONTRAINDICATIONS

Infants under 3 months in hemophilia A or von Willebrand's disease, known hypersensitivity to desmopressin.

PRECAUTIONS

Use caution in patients with coronary artery insufficiency or hypertension. ■ Excessive fluid intake may result in an extreme decrease in plasma osmolality. May lead to seizures and coma. ■ Use with caution in patients predisposed to thrombus formation. ■ Use with caution in patients with conditions associated with fluid and electrolyte imbalance (e.g., cystic fibrosis).

Monitor: Diabetes insipidus: Not effective for the treatment of nephrogenic diabetes insipidus. ■ Confirm diagnosis of diabetes insipidus by the water deprivation test, the hypertonic saline infusion test, and the response to ADH. Monitor continued response by measuring urine volume and osmolality. Plasma osmolality may be needed. Monitor serum electrolytes in therapy lasting longer than seven days. Accuracy and effectiveness of dose measured by duration of sleep and adequate, not excessive, water turnover.

Hemophilia A: May be considered for use in patients with factor VIII activity levels from 2% to 5% with careful monitoring. Generally used only when the factor VIII activity level is above 5%. ■ Not indicated in patients with hemophilia B or those with factor VIII antibodies. ■ Monitor factor VIII coagulant, factor VIII antigen, factor VIII ristocetin cofactor, and APTT.

Von Willebrand's disease (Type I): Most effective when factor VIII activity level above 5%. ■ Monitor bleeding time, factor VIII activity levels, ristocetin cofactor activity, and von Willebrand factor antigen during therapy to ensure adequate levels. ■ Not indicated for treatment of severe classic von Willebrand's disease (Type I), Type IIB von Willebrand's disease (will induce platelet aggregation), or if there is evidence of an abnormal molecular form of factor VIII antigen.

Hemophilia and von Willebrand's: Sometimes used with aminocaproic acid. ■ Monitor blood pressure and pulse during infusion.

Patient education: When antidiuretic effect is not needed, caution patients (especially the young and the elderly) to limit fluid intake to satisfy thirst needs only; this decreases potential occurrence of water intoxication and hyponatremia.

Maternal/child: Use only when clearly indicated in pregnancy and lactation. ■ Risk of hyponatremia and water intoxication increased in children. Restrict fluid intake. ■ Safety for use in children under 12 years with diabetes insipidus not established. ■ Note Contraindications.

Elderly: Risk of hyponatremia and water intoxication increased. Use caution and careful fluid intake restriction.

DRUG/LAB INTERACTIONS

May produce hypertension with other vasopressors (e.g., dopamine [Intropin]). ■ May be potentiated by chlorpropamide, clofibrate, or carbamazepine.

SIDE EFFECTS

Are infrequent. High doses may produce facial flushing, headache, hypertension (slight), mild abdominal cramps, nausea, and vulval pain. May cause burning, local erythema, and swelling at site of injection; hyponatremia; and water intoxication. Anaphylaxis has been reported.

ANTIDOTE

Notify physician of all side effects. Most will respond to reduction of dose or rate of administration, or symptomatic treatment. May need to discontinue drug. Resuscitate as necessary.

DEXAMETHASONE SODIUM PHOSPHATE

Hormone
(Adrenocorticoid/glucocorticoid)
Antiinflammatory, Antiemetic
Immunosuppressant, Diagnostic agent

Ak-Dek, Dalalone, Decadrol, Decadron,
Decadron phosphate, Decaject, Dexasone,
Dexone, Hexadrol phosphate, Solurex

pH 7.0 to 8.5

USUAL DOSE

Average dose range is 0.5 to 24 mg daily. May be divided into 2 to 4 doses. IV dexamethasone is usually given in an emergency situation or when oral dosing is not feasible. Larger doses may be justified by patient condition. Repeat until adequate response, then decrease dose as indicated. Total dose usually does not exceed 80 mg/24 hr. Dosage must be individualized. High dose treatment is utilized until patient condition stabilizes, usually no longer than 48 to 72 hours. IV replacement for oral therapy is usually one-half to one-third of the oral dose but may be increased.

Antiinflammatory: See average dose range above.

Shock: Several regimens have been suggested:

1 to 6 mg/kg as a single injection; or

40 mg. Repeat every 2 to 6 hours as needed; or

20 mg as a *loading dose,* followed by a continuous infusion of 3 mg/kg equally distributed over 24 hours.

Cerebral edema: Loading dose: 10 mg. *Maintenance dose:* 4 mg every 6 hours (usually given IM). Reduce dose after 2 to 4 days. Discontinue gradually over 5 to 7 days. A brain tumor requiring treatment before dexamethasone can be discontinued is the exception.

Cerebral edema (ICP) in recurrent or inoperable brain tumors: 2 mg every 8 to 12 hours (usually given IM). Adjust based on patient response.

Antiemetic in management of emesis-inducing chemotherapy: Several regimens have been used:

10 to 20 mg before chemotherapy. Lower doses may be given over the next 24 to 72 hours if necessary; or

give a loading dose of 4 to 8 mg/M^2. May repeat 2 to 4 mg/M^2 every 6 hours; or

20 mg 40 minutes before administration of chemotherapeutic agent. Given concurrently with metoclopramide and lorazepam or diphenhydramine; or

10 mg 30 minutes before administration of chemotherapeutic agent. Given concurrently with oral dexamethasone 8 mg beginning prior evening, 4 mg every 4 to 6 hr continuing through treatment day, with droperidol or haloperidol.

Airway edema: Adults and children: 0.25 to 0.5 mg/kg every 6 hours for croup or beginning 24 hours before elective extubation. Repeat for 4 to 6 doses. Up to 1 mg/kg/24 hr may be given in divided doses before and after extubation.

Allergic conditions: (Usually given IM or PO) 4 to 8 mg on the first day, then orally in decreasing doses (1.5 mg every 12 hours on day 2 and 3; 0.75 mg every 12 hours on day 4; and 0.75 mg on day 5 and 6).

Meningitis: Adults and children: 0.15 mg/kg/dose every 6 hours for 4 days.

Primary or secondary adrenocortical insufficiency (physiologic replacement): 0.03 to 0.15 mg/kg/24 hr or 0.6 to 0.75 mg/M^2/24 hours given in divided doses every 6 to 12 hours (usually given IM). Dexamethasone has minimal mineralocorticoid properties; may require a concomitant mineralocorticoid (e.g., hydrocortisone IV or fludrocortisone [Florinef] PO). Hydrocortisone is the drug of choice for this indication.

PEDIATRIC DOSE

Cerebral edema: Loading dose: 0.5 to 1.5 mg/kg of body weight. *Maintenance dose:* 0.2 to 0.5 mg/kg/24 hours in equally divided doses every 6 hours for 5 days, then gradually decrease.

Airway edema: See adult dose.

Antiemetic: Loading dose: 4 to 8 mg/M^2. May repeat 2 to 4 mg/M^2 every 6 hours.

Antiinflammatory: 0.03 to 0.15 mg/kg/24 hours in equally divided doses every 6 to 12 hours.

Meningitis: See adult dose.

DOSE ADJUSTMENTS

Reduced dose may be required in the elderly and with cyclophosphamide. ▪ Note Drug/lab interactions.

DILUTION

May be given undiluted or added to IV glucose or saline solutions and given as an infusion.

Storage: Use diluted solutions within 24 hours. Sensitive to heat. Protect from freezing.

INCOMPATIBLE WITH

Amikacin (Amikin), ciprofloxacin (Cipro IV), daunorubicin (Cerubidine), diphenhydramine (Benadryl), doxorubicin (Adriamycin), glycopyrrolate (Robinul), hydromorphone (Dilaudid), idarubicin (Idamycin), metaraminol (Aramine), midazolam (Versed), prochlorperazine (Compazine), vancomycin (Vancocin). Limited information available. Give other drugs concurrently through a three-way stopcock.

RATE OF ADMINISTRATION

A single dose over 1 minute or less if necessary. As an IV infusion, give at prescribed rate.

ACTIONS

An antiinflammatory glucocorticoid. A synthetic adrenocortical steroid with little sodium retention. Very soluble in water. Seven times as potent as prednisolone and 20 to 30 times as potent as hydrocortisone. Has minimal mineralocorticoid activity. Primarily used for antiinflammatory and immunosuppressive effects. May be used in conjunction with other forms of therapy, such as epinephrine for acute allergic reactions or antibiotics for acute infections. Metabolized primarily in the liver and excreted as inactive metabolites in urine. Crosses the placental barrier. Excreted in urine and breast milk.

INDICATIONS AND USES

Supplementary therapy for severe allergic reactions. ▪ Reduction of acute edematous states (cerebral edema, airway edema). ▪ Shock unresponsive to conventional therapy. ▪ Acute exacerbations of disease for patients receiving steroid therapy. ▪ Adrenocortical insufficiency; total, relative, and operative. ■ Antiemetic for chemotherapy induced vomiting (e.g., cisplatin). Has numerous other uses by other routes of administration (e.g., IM, intraarticular, intralesional, intrasynovial, soft-tissue injection, oral inhalant).

Unlabeled use: Adjunct to treatment of meningitis with antibiotics (to reduce incidence of ototoxicity). ■ Dexamethasone or betamethasone are given IM to the mother to accelerate the production of lung surfactant in utero in the prevention of respiratory distress syndrome of premature infants.

CONTRAINDICATIONS

Hypersensitivity to any product component including sulfites, systemic fungal infections.

Relative contraindications: active or latent peptic ulcer, acute or healed tuberculosis, acute or chronic infections (especially chickenpox), acute psychoses, diabetes mellitus, diverticulitis, fresh intestinal anastomoses, myasthenia gravis, ocular herpes simplex, osteoporosis, pregnancy, psychotic tendencies, renal insufficiency, thromboembolic tendencies.

PRECAUTIONS

Withdrawal from therapy should be gradual to avoid precipitation of symptoms of adrenal insufficiency. The patient is observed, especially under stress, for up to 2 years. ■ Prophylactic antacids may prevent peptic ulcer complications. ■ Use with caution in hypothyroidism and cirrhosis.

Monitor: May increase insulin needs in diabetes. ■ Monitor electrolytes periodically. May cause sodium retention and potassium and calcium excretion. May cause hypertension secondary to fluid and electrolyte disturbances. ■ May mask signs of infection. ■ Administer a single dose before 9 AM to reduce suppression of individual's adrenocortical activity. ■ Periodic ophthalmic exams may be necessary with prolonged treatment. ■ Note Drug/lab interactions.

Patient education: Report edema, tarry stools, or weight gain promptly. Anorexia, diarrhea, dizziness, fatigue, low blood sugar, nausea, weakness, weight loss, and vomiting promptly. May indicate adrenal insufficiency after dose reduction or discontinuing therapy; report any of these symptoms. ■ May mask signs of infection and/or decrease resistance. ■ Diabetics may have an increased requirement for insulin or oral hypoglycemics. ■ Avoid immunization with live vaccines. ■ Carry ID stating steroid dependent if receiving prolonged therapy.

Maternal/child: Pregnancy Category C: has caused birth defects; benefits must outweigh risks. ■ Observe newborn for hypoadrenalism if mother has received large doses. ■ Monitor growth and development of children receiving prolonged treatment.

Elderly: Reduced muscle mass and plasma volume may necessitate a reduced dose. Monitor blood pressure, blood glucose, and electrolytes carefully. ■ Increased risk of hypertension. ■ Higher risk of glucocorticoid-induced osteoporosis. ■ Avoid aluminum-based antacids (risk of Alzheimer's disease).

DRUG/LAB INTERACTIONS

Aminoglutethimide (Cytadren) and mitotane (Lysodren) suppress adrenal function and increase metabolism of dexamethasone two-fold. Not recommended for concurrent use, or dexamethasone dose may require doubling to be effective. Use of hydrocortisone suggested. ■ Metabolism increased and effects reduced by hepatic enzyme inducing agents (e.g., alcohol, barbiturates [e.g., phenobarbital], hydantoins [e.g., phenytoin (Dilantin)], rifampin [Rifadin]); dose adjustments may be required when adding or deleting from drug profile. ■ Risk of hypokalemia increased with amphotericin B or potassium-depleting diuretics (e.g., thiazides, furosemide, ethacrynic acid). Monitor potassium levels and cardiac function. ■ Increased risk of digitalis (e.g., digoxin) toxicity secondary to hypokalemia. ■ May also decrease effectiveness of potassium supplements; monitor serum potassium. ■ Diuretics decrease sodium and fluid retention effects of corticosteroids; corticosteroids decrease sodium excretion and diuretic effects of diuretics. ■ Clearance increased and effects decreased with ephedrine. ■ May antagonize effects of anticholinesterases (e.g., neostigmine), isoniazid, salicylates, and somatrem; dose adjustments may be required. ■ Clearance decreased and effects increased with estrogens, oral contraceptives, and ketoconazole (Nizoral). ■ May interact with anticoagulants, nondepolarizing muscle relaxants (e.g., doxacurium [Nuromax]) or theophyllines; may inhibit or potentiate action; monitor carefully. ■ Monitor patients receiving insulin or thyroid hormones carefully; dose adjustments of either or both agents may be required. ■ Use with ritodrine (Yutopar) has caused pulmonary edema in the mother; discontinue both agents with onset of S/S of pulmonary edema. ■ Do not vaccinate with attenuated-virus vaccines (smallpox, etc.) during therapy. ■ Altered protein binding capacity will impact effectiveness of this drug. ■ Smoking may antagonize therapeutic effects. ■ Note Precautions. ■ Decreases uptake of radioactive material in cerebral edema; will alter brain scan.

SIDE EFFECTS

Do occur but are usually reversible: burning, Cushing's syndrome, electrolyte imbalance, embolism, euphoria, glycosuria, headache, hyperglycemia, hypersensitivity reactions including anaphylaxis; hypertension, menstrual irregularities, peptic ulcer, perforation and hemorrhage, protein catabolism, sweating, thromboembolism, tingling, weakness, and many others.

ANTIDOTE

Notify the physician of any side effect. Will probably treat the side effect. Resuscitate as necessary for anaphylaxis and notify physician. Keep epinephrine immediately available.

DEXRAZOXANE

Antidote
Antineoplastic adjunct
Chelating agent

Zinecard

pH 3.5 to 5.5

USUAL DOSE

Administered in conjunction with doxorubicin. Dose ratio of dexrazoxane to doxorubicin (Adriamycin) is 10:1 (500 mg/M^2 dexrazoxane to 50 mg/M^2 doxorubicin). Doxorubicin dose must be given within 30 minutes of starting the dexrazoxane injection, but only after the full dose of dexrazoxane is administered.

PEDIATRIC DOSE

Safety for use in children not established. One source indicates that 3500 mg/M^2/24 hr for 3 days is the maximum tolerated dose based on coagulation parameters.

DOSE ADJUSTMENTS

No specific adjustments recommended; note Antidote.

DILUTION

Specific techniques required; see Precautions. Initially reconstitute each 250 mg (500 mg) with 25 ml (50 ml) of 1/6 molar sodium lactate diluent provided by manufacturer (10 mg/ml). May be further diluted with D5W or NS. Concentration should range from 1.3 to 5 mg/ml. An additional 25 ml (50 ml) of diluent would yield 5 mg/ml; 75 ml (150 ml) would yield 2.5 mg/ml.

Storage: Store unopened vials at controlled room temperature. Reconstituted or diluted solution stable for 6 hours at controlled room temperature or refrigerated. Discard unused solutions.

INCOMPATIBLE WITH

Manufacturer states "should not be mixed with other drugs"; degrades rapidly at a pH above 7.0.

RATE OF ADMINISTRATION

A single dose may be given by slow IV push or rapid infusion (given over 10 to 15 minutes in one study). Complete dexrazoxane dose but begin doxorubicin within 30 minutes of beginning dexrazoxane.

ACTIONS

A cardioprotective agent. A potent intracellular chelating agent that readily penetrates cell membranes and interferes with iron-mediated free radical generation thought to be, in part, responsible for anthracycline-induced cardiomyopathy. Reduces the incidence of doxorubicin cardiomyopathy. Rapidly distributed, at least partly metabolized. Elimination half-life is 2.5 hours. Primarily excreted in urine. (See Drug/lab interactions).

INDICATIONS AND USES

Reduce the incidence and severity of cardiomyopathy associated with cumulative doses of doxorubicin exceeding 300 mg/M^2. May allow higher doses of doxorubicin and improved response rates and duration. Currently approved only for use in women with metastatic breast cancer who would benefit from continuing doxorubicin therapy above this cumulative dose.

CONTRAINDICATIONS

Do not use with chemotherapy regimens that do not contain an anthracycline or in the initiation of doxorubicin therapy.

PRECAUTIONS

■ Follow guidelines for handling cytotoxic agents. See Appendix A, p. 893. Usually administered by or under the direction of the physician specialist. ■ May cause coagulation abnormalities (e.g., increased PT, PTT, and decreased levels of fibrinogen and clotting factors).

Monitor: Obtain baseline ECG, serum levels of iron and zinc, and liver and renal function tests. Monitor at intervals. Baseline left ventricular ejection fraction (LVEF) helpful. ■ Obtain baseline CBC, PT, and PTT and monitor frequently for increased bone marrow depression and coagulation abnormalities. ■ Reduces but does not eliminate the risk of doxorubicin-induced cardiotoxicity. Monitor for signs of congestive heart failure (e.g., basilar rales, S_3 gallop, paroxysmal nocturnal dyspnea, significant dyspnea on exertion, cardiomegaly by x-ray, or progressive decline from baseline of LVEF). A decline in QRS voltage on a 6 lead ECG of >30% may indicate cardiomyopathy. ■ Use of prophylactic antiemetics may be indicated.

Patient education: Non-hormonal birth control recommended. ■ Report pain at injection site promptly.

Maternal/child: Category C: safety for use in pregnancy, lactation and children not established. ■ Embryotoxic and teratogenic in rats at doses lower than required for humans. May cause testicular atrophy. ■ Discontinue breast feeding.

Elderly: No specific recommendations. Consider age-related impaired organ function.

DRUG/LAB INTERACTIONS

Not indicated for use in initiation of doxorubicin therapy; may interfere with antitumor effects of combination regimens. ■ May have additive bone marrow depressant effects with other bone marrow depressants (e.g., fluorouracil [5FU], cyclophosphamide [Cytoxan]).

SIDE EFFECTS

Increased myelosuppression (e.g., granulocytopenia, leukopenia, and thrombocytopenia); may be dose limiting. Coagulation abnormalities, decreased serum zinc, increased serum iron, increased AST and ALT, increased serum triglycerides, pain at injection site do occur. Alopecia, anorexia, diarrhea, and nausea and vomiting as well as other side effects do occur but are most likely caused by chemotherapeutic regimen.

ANTIDOTE

Keep physician informed of side effects; most will be treated symptomatically. Recovery from myelosuppression similar with or without dexrazoxane. A reduced dose may be indicated if coagulation abnormalities develop. Hemodialysis or peritoneal dialysis may be useful in overdose.

DEXTRAN HIGH MOLECULAR WEIGHT

Plasma volume expander

Dextran 70, Dextran 75,
Gentran 75, Macrodex

pH 3.0 to 7.0

USUAL DOSE

Variable, depending on amount of fluid loss and resultant hemoconcentration. Initially 30 Gm (500 ml). Total dose should not exceed 1.2 Gm/kg (20 ml/kg) of body weight in the first 24 hr for adults and children. May give 0.6 Gm/kg (10 ml/kg) every 24 hr thereafter if indicated. *Use of Dextran 1 is indicated for prophylaxis of serious anaphylactic reactions.*

DILUTION

Available as a 6% solution in 500 ml bottles properly diluted in NS or D5W and ready for use. Dextran 70 (Cutter) is available in a 250 ml bottle. Use only clear solution. Crystallization of dextran can occur at low temperatures. Submerge in warm water and dissolve all crystals before administration.

Storage: Store at constant temperature not above 25° C (76° F). Discard partially used solution; no preservative added.

INCOMPATIBLE WITH

Do not add any drug to a bottle of dextran solution. Ascorbic acid, phytonadione (Aquamephyton), promethazine (Phenergan).

RATE OF ADMINISTRATION

Variable, depending on indication, present blood volume, and patient response. Initial 500 ml may be given at 20 to 40 ml/minute if hypovolemic If additional high-molecular-weight dextran is required, reduce flow to lowest rate possible to maintain hemodynamic status desired. In normovolemic patients, rate should not exceed 4 ml/min.

ACTIONS

A glucose polymer that approximates colloidal properties of human albumin. Provides hemodynamically significant plasma volume expansion in excess of the amount infused for about 24 hours. Dilutes total serum proteins and hematocrit values. Smaller dextran molecules are eliminated in urine; larger molecules are degraded to glucose.

INDICATIONS AND USES

Adjunct in treatment of shock or impending shock caused by burns, hemorrhage, surgery, or trauma.

Unlabeled uses: Treatment of nephrosis, toxemia of late pregnancy, and prevention of postoperative deep vein thrombosis.

CONTRAINDICATIONS

Severe bleeding disorders, marked hemostatic defects (e.g., thrombocytopenia, hypofibrinogenemia), even if drug-induced (e.g., heparin, warfarin), known hypersensitivity to dextran, lactation and pregnancy unless a lifesaving measure, severe congestive cardiac failure, renal failure.

PRECAUTIONS

For IV use only. ▪ Used when whole blood or blood products are not available. Not a substitute for whole blood or plasma proteins. ▪ Use extreme caution in heart disease, impaired hepatic or renal function, congestive heart failure, pulmonary edema, in patients with edema and sodium retention of pathological abdominal conditions, and in patients receiving anticoagulants or corticosteroids.

Monitor: Monitor pulse, blood pressure, central venous pressure, and urine output every 5 to 15 minutes for the first hour and hourly thereafter while indicated. ▪ Maintain hydration of patient with additional IV fluids; dextran promotes tissue dehydration. Avoid overhydration with dilution of electrolyte balance. ▪ Change IV tubing or flush well with normal saline before infusing blood. Dextran will promote coagulation of blood in the tubing (glucose content). ▪ May reduce coagulability of the circulating blood. Observe patient for increased bleeding; maintain hematocrit above 30%. ▪ Hemoglobin, hematocrit, electrolyte, and serum protein evaluations are necessary during therapy. ▪ 500 ml contains 77 mEq of sodium and chloride. ▪ Note Drug/lab interactions.

Maternal/child: Pregnancy Category C: safety for use in pregnancy and lactation not established.

DRUG/LAB INTERACTIONS

Draw blood for laboratory tests and type and cross-match before giving dextran, or notify laboratory of its use. May alter type and cross-match, blood sugar, total protein, and total bilirubin evaluation. ▪ May produce elevated urine specific gravity (also symptom of dehydration) and increase AST (SGOT) and ALT (SGPT). ▪ Note Monitor for interaction with blood.

SIDE EFFECTS

Bleeding, dehydration, fever, hypotension, joint pain, nausea, overhydration, tightness of the chest, urticaria, vomiting, wheezing. Severe anaphylaxis and death have occurred. Excessive doses have caused wound hematoma, seroma, and bleeding; distant bleeding (hematuria, melena); and pulmonary edema.

ANTIDOTE

Notify the physician of any side effect. Discontinue the drug immediately at the first sign of an allergic reaction, provided other means of sustaining the circulation are available. Use epinephrine (Adrenalin) and/or antihistamines (diphenhydramine [Benadryl]) as indicated. Factor VIII infusion may reverse excessive bleeding. Resuscitate as necessary.

DEXTRAN LOW MOLECULAR WEIGHT

Plasma volume expander

Dextran 40, Gentran 40,
L.M.D. 10%, Rheomacrodex

pH 3.0 to 7.0

USUAL DOSE

Adjunct in shock: Variable, depending on amount of fluid loss and resultant hemoconcentration. Do not exceed 2 Gm/kg (20 ml) of body weight total over first 24 hours and 1 Gm/kg (10 ml) total over each succeeding 24 hours. Discontinue infusion after 5 days of therapy. *Dextran 1 is indicated for prophylaxis of serious anaphylactic reactions.*

Prophylaxis of venous thrombosis and/or pulmonary embolism: 10 mg/kg of body weight on day of surgery. 500 ml daily for 2 to 3 days, then 500 ml every 2 to 3 days up to 2 weeks. Length of treatment based on risk of thromboemboli complication. *Note comment on dextran 1 above.*

As priming fluid: 10 to 20 ml/kg of body weight. Do not exceed this dose. May be used in conjunction with other priming fluids.

DILUTION

Available as a 10% solution in 500 ml bottles properly diluted in NS or D5W and ready for use. Use only clear solution. Crystallization of dextran can occur at low temperatures. Submerge in warm water and dissolve all crystals before administration.

Storage: Store at constant temperature not above 25° C (76° F). Discard partially used solution; no preservative added.

INCOMPATIBLE WITH

Do not add any drug to a bottle of dextran solution. Ascorbic acid, phytonadione (Aquamephyton), promethazine (Phenergan).

RATE OF ADMINISTRATION

Initial 500 ml may be given rapidly. Remainder of any desired daily dose should be evenly distributed over 8 to 24 hours depending on use. Slow rate, or discontinue dextran for rapid increase of central venous pressure.

ACTIONS

A low-molecular-weight, rapid, but short-acting plasma volume expander. A colloid hypertonic solution, it increases plasma volume by once or twice its own volume. Helps to restore normal circulatory dynamics, increasing arterial and pulse pressure, central venous pressure, and cardiac output. Improves microcirculatory flow and prevents sludging in venous channels. Mobilizes water from body tissues and increases urine output.

INDICATIONS AND USES

Adjunctive therapy in the treatment of shock caused by hemorrhage, burns, trauma, or surgery. ■ Prophylaxis during surgical procedures with a high incidence of venous thrombosis and pulmonary embolism. ■ Pump priming during extracorporeal circulation.

CONTRAINDICATIONS

Severe bleeding disorders, marked hemostatic defects (e.g., thrombocytopenia, hypofibrinogenemia) even if drug induced (e.g., heparin, warfarin), known hypersensitivity to dextran, lactation and pregnancy unless a lifesaving measure, severe congestive cardiac failure, renal failure.

PRECAUTIONS

For IV use only. ▪ Use caution in heart disease, renal shutdown, congestive heart failure, pulmonary edema, patients with edema and sodium retention, and patients taking corticosteroids.

Monitor: Monitor pulse, blood pressure, central venous pressure (if possible), and urine output every 5 to 15 minutes for the first hour and hourly thereafter while indicated. ▪ Slow rate or discontinue dextran for rapid increase of central venous pressure (normal 7 to 14 mm H_2O pressure). ▪ If anuric or oliguric after 500 ml of dextran, discontinue the dextran. Mannitol may help increase urine flow. ▪ Maintain hydration of patient with additional IV fluids; dextran promotes tissue dehydration. Avoid overhydration and dilution of serum electrolytes. ▪ Change IV tubing or flush well with normal saline before superimposing blood. Dextran will promote coagulation of blood in the tubing (glucose content). ▪ May reduce coagulability of the circulating blood slightly. Observe for bleeding complications, particularly following surgery or if patient is being anticoagulated. Maintain hematocrit above 30%. ▪ 500 ml contains 77 mEq of sodium and cloride. ▪ Note Drug/lab interactions.

Maternal/child: Pregnancy Category C: safety for use in pregnancy and lactation not established.

DRUG/LAB INTERACTIONS

Draw blood for laboratory tests and type and cross-match before giving dextran, or notify laboratory of its use. May alter type and cross-match, blood sugar, total protein, and total bilirubin evaluation. ▪ May produce elevated urine specific gravity (also a symptom of dehydration) and increase AST (SGOT) and ALT (SGPT). ▪ Note Monitor for interaction with blood.

SIDE EFFECTS

Bleeding, dehydration, fever, hypotension, joint pain, nausea, overhydration, tightness of chest, urticaria, vomiting, wheezing. Severe anaphylaxis and death can occur. Excessive doses have caused wound hematoma, wound seroma, wound bleeding, distant bleeding (hematuria, melena), and pulmonary edema.

ANTIDOTE

Notify the physician of any side effect. Discontinue the drug immediately at the first sign of an allergic reaction, provided other means of sustaining the circulation are available. Use epinephrine (Adrenalin) and/or antihistamines (diphenhydramine [Benadryl]) as indicated. Factor VIII infusion may reverse excessive bleeding. Resuscitate as necessary.

DEXTRAN 1

Dextran adjunct
Antidote

Promit

USUAL DOSE

20 ml (150 mg/ml) 1 to 2 minutes before every IV clinical dextran infusion. If 15 minutes or more elapses before the clinical dextran infusion is started, a full dose of dextran 1 must be repeated before the infusion.

PEDIATRIC DOSE

0.3 ml/kg of body weight. To be given in same manner as adult dose.

DILUTION

May be given undiluted. May be given through Y-tube or three-way stopcock of an infusion set if there is minimum dilution with the primary IV. May not be diluted with or administered through an IV tubing containing clinical dextran infusion.

INCOMPATIBLE WITH

Dextran, low molecular weight; dextran, high molecular weight.

RATE OF ADMINISTRATION

A single dose over 1 minute.

ACTIONS

A monovalent hapten, it binds to one of two available sites on dextran-reacting antibodies. An adequate dose (molar excess) given just before the IV administration of clinical dextran solution prevents the formation of immune complexes with the polyvalent clinical dextrans and helps to prevent severe anaphylaxis. Incidence of anaphylaxis is 15 to 20 times less. Rapidly excreted in urine.

INDICATIONS AND USES

Prophylaxis of serious anaphylactic reactions associated with IV infusion of clinical dextran solutions.

CONTRAINDICATIONS

Do not give if clinical dextran is contraindicated (severe bleeding disorders, marked hemostatic defects [e.g., thrombocytopenia, hypofibrinogenemia], even if drug induced [e.g., heparin, warfarin], lactation and pregnancy unless a lifesaving measure, severe congestive cardiac failure, renal failure).

PRECAUTIONS

For IV use only. ■ Will not prevent mild allergic reactions induced by clinical dextran solutions. ■ If any reaction occurs to dextran 1, *do not administer clinical dextran infusion.*

Monitor: May cause severe hypotension and bradycardia.

Maternal/child: Pregnancy Category B: note Contraindications.

DRUG/LAB INTERACTIONS

Note Precautions and Dilution.

SIDE EFFECTS

Bradycardia, cutaneous reactions, hypotension (moderate to severe), nausea, pallor, shivering.

ANTIDOTE

Discontinue drug immediately and notify physician at the first sign of allergic reaction or side effect. Do not administer clinical dextran solution. Use epinephrine (Adrenalin) and/or antihistamines (diphenhydramine [Benadryl]) as indicated. Resuscitate as necessary.

DEXTROSE

Nutritional
(Carbohydrate)

Glucose

pH 3.5 to 6.5

USUAL DOSE

Depends on use and age, weight, and clinical condition of the patient. 50 to 1,000 ml 2 1/2% (25 Gm/L) or 5% (50 Gm/L) dextrose. May be repeated as indicated. Consider total amount of fluid.

5 ml of 10% dextrose. May repeat as necessary.

500 to 1,000 ml of 10% dextrose (100 Gm/L) once or twice every 24 hours as indicated.

500 ml of 20% dextrose (200 Gm/L) once or twice every 24 hours as indicated.

20 to 50 ml of 50% dextrose (25 Gm). 10 to 25 Gm for *insulin-induced hypoglycemia*. May repeat if indicated.

500 to 1,500 ml/24 hr of 30% (300 Gm/L), 38.5% (385 Gm/L), 40% (400 Gm/L), 50% (500 Gm/L), 60% (600 Gm/L), 70% (700 Gm/L) as dextrose for nutrition.

NEONATAL DOSE

Acute symptomatic hypoglycemia: 250 to 500 mg/kg of body weight of 10 to 25% dextrose.

DILUTION

May be given undiluted in prepared solutions or further diluted to achieve desired final concentration. Dextrose solutions are excellent media for bacterial growth. Do not use unless the solution is entirely clear and the vial is sterile. Do not store after adding additives.

INCOMPATIBLE WITH

Cyanocobalamin (vitamin B_{12}), kanamycin (Kantrex), sodium bicarbonate, warfarin (Coumadin), whole blood.

RATE OF ADMINISTRATION

2 1/2% and 5% solution, rate dependent on amount.

10% solution, 5 ml over 10 to 15 seconds.

10% solution, 1,000 ml over at least 3 hours.

20% solution, 500 ml over 30 to 60 minutes.

50% solution, 3 ml over 1 minute.

500 ml of 30% to 70% solution over 4 to 12 hours, depending on body weight. A rate of 0.5 Gm/kg/hr will not cause glycosuria. At 0.8 Gm/kg/hr 95% is retained and will cause glycosuria. May cause hyperosmolar syndrome.

ACTIONS

A monosaccharide, it provides glucose calories for metabolic needs. Metabolized to CO_2 and water. Its oxidation provides water to sustain volume and may help lower excess ketone production and prevent protein loss. Hypertonic solutions (20% to 50%) act as a diuretic and reduce CNS edema. Readily excreted by the kidneys, producing diuresis.

INDICATIONS AND USES

To provide calories and fluid by peripheral infusion when calories and fluid are required (2 1/2%, 5%, 10%). ▪ To provide calories by central IV infusion in conditions requiring a minimum volume of fluid (20%). ▪ To provide calories by central IV infusion in combination with other amino acid solutions as total parenteral nutrition (10% to 70%). ▪ Treatment of insulin hypoglycemia (50%). ▪ Treatment of acute symptomatic episodes of hypoglycemia in the neonate and infant (25%). ▪ Shock (sustain blood volume). ▪ Diuresis (20% to 50% solution). ▪ Hyperkalemia (20% solution). ▪ As a diluent for IV administration of medications (2 1/2% to 10% solutions usually). ▪ A sclerosing solution (25% to 50% solution, 3 to 20 ml).

CONTRAINDICATIONS

Delirium tremens with dehydration; diabetic coma while blood sugar is excessive; hepatic coma intracranial or intraspinal hemorrhage; glucose-galactose malabsorption syndrome.

PRECAUTIONS

Use caution in severe kidney damage. ▪ 50% dextrose can be used as a sclerosing agent and will cause thrombosis. ▪ Use caution in infants of diabetic mothers, in patients with carbohydrate intolerance or sub-clinical or overt diabetes, and in patients receiving corticosteroids. ▪ Use hypertonic dextrose with extreme caution in low-birth-weight or septic infants. May cause severe hyperglycemia.

Monitor: Do not use as a diluent for blood or administer simultaneously through the same infusion set; dextrose in any dilution causes clumping of red blood cells unless sodium chloride is added. ▪ For concentrations over 12.5% (hypertonic) very large (central) veins and slow administration are absolutely necessary. ▪ Confirm patency of vein, avoid extravasation. ▪ Insulin requirements may be increased. Monitor blood glucose. ▪ Potassium and vitamins are readily depleted. Watch for any signs of beginning deficiency and replace as needed. Add other electrolytes and minerals as required by fluid and electrolyte status. ▪ Can cause fluid or solute overload. May result in dilution of serum electrolyte concentrations, overhydration, congested states or pulmonary edema. ▪ Rapid administration of hypertonic solutions will cause hyperglycemia (over 0.5 Gm/kg/hr) and may cause hyperosmolar syndrome. ▪ Concentrated dextrose solutions must not be withdrawn abruptly. Will cause reactive hypoglycemia. Reduce rate of administration gradually and then follow with administration of 5% or 10% dextrose solution.

Maternal/child: Pregnancy Category C: safety for use in pregnancy and lactation not established. Benefits must outweigh risks. ▪ Note Precautions.

DRUG/LAB INTERACTIONS

Note Monitor.

SIDE EFFECTS

Rare in small doses administered slowly: acidosis, alkalosis, fluid overload (congested states, pulmonary edema, overhydration, dilution of serum electrolyte concentrations), hyperglycemia (during infusion), hyperosmolar syndrome (mental confusion, loss of consciousness), hypokalemia, hypovitaminosis, reactive hypoglycemia (after infusion), thrombosis.

ANTIDOTE

Discontinue the drug and notify the physician of the side effect. Symptomatic treatment is probable.

DEZOCINE	Narcotic analgesic (Agonist-antagonist)
Dalgan	pH 4.0

USUAL DOSE

5 mg initially. Range is 2.5 to 10 mg. Repeat every 2 to 4 hours as necessary. Larger doses have been given IM.

DOSE ADJUSTMENTS

Reduce dose for the elderly or debilitated; in impaired liver or renal function; in patients with limited pulmonary reserve; and in the presence of other CNS depressants. ■ Note Drug/lab interactions.

DILUTION

May be given undiluted.

Storage: Use only clear solutions. Prior to use store at room temperature. Protect from light.

INCOMPATIBLE WITH

Specific information not available.

RATE OF ADMINISTRATION

Each 5 mg or fraction thereof evenly distributed over 2 to 3 minutes.

ACTIONS

A synthetic narcotic agonist-antagonist with a potent analgesic action. Analgesia similar to morphine or butorphanol is produced. Does produce respiratory depression, but this does not increase markedly with larger doses. Pain relief is effected within 15 minutes. Length of pain relief is related to the initial dose (i.e., 2 hours with a 5 mg dose and 3 to 4 hours with a 10 mg dose). Relief in some patients may last up to 6 hours. Metabolized in the liver. Primarily excreted in urine.

INDICATIONS AND USES

Relief of moderate to severe postoperative pain (e.g., abdominal, gynecologic, orthopedic).

CONTRAINDICATIONS

Hypersensitivity to dezocine or its components; contains sodium metabisulfite (can cause anaphylaxis from a sulfite sensitivity reaction).

PRECAUTIONS

Use caution in respiratory depression or difficulty from any source, head injury, increased intracranial pressure, biliary surgery, history of drug abuse, the elderly or debilitated, and in impaired liver or kidney function. Reduced doses may be indicated.

Monitor: Naloxone (Narcan), oxygen, and controlled ventilation equipment must be available. ■ Observe patient frequently and monitor vital signs. ■ Keep patient supine to minimize side effects; orthostatic hypotension and fainting may occur. Observe closely or assist during ambulation. ■ Pain control usually more effective with routinely administered doses. Determine appropriate interval through clinical assessment. ▪ Mild narcotic antagonist. May precipitate withdrawal symptoms in patients accustomed to narcotics.

Patient education: Avoid use of alcohol or other CNS depressants (e.g., antihistamines, diazepam [Valium]). ▪ Request assistance for ambulation. ▪ Use caution performing any tasks that require alertness; may cause dizziness, euphoria, and sedation. Do not drive or operate hazardous machinery until all effects have subsided. ▪ May be habit forming.

Maternal/child: Pregnancy Category C: use during pregnancy only if benefit justifies risk to the fetus and in labor and delivery only if the physician considers it essential. Safety not established. Not recommended for nursing mothers, or children under 18 years of age.

Elderly: Note Dose adjustments and Precautions. ▪ May be more sensitive to effects (e.g., respiratory depression, urinary retention, constipation, dizziness). ▪ Analgesia should be effective with lower dose. ▪ Consider age-related organ impairment.

DRUG/LAB INTERACTIONS

Use caution with cimetidine (Tagamet) and CNS depressants such as narcotic analgesics (e.g., morphine), general anesthetics, alcohol, anticholinergics (e.g., atropine), antihistamines (e.g., diphenhydramine [Benadryl]), barbiturates (e.g., phenobarbital), hypnotics, sedatives, psychotropic agents, MAO inhibitors (e.g., selegiline [Eldepryl]), and neuromuscular blocking agents (e.g., mivacurium [Mivacron]). Reduced doses of both drugs may be indicated. ▪ May decrease analgesic affects of other narcotics; avoid concurrent use.

SIDE EFFECTS

Dizziness, injection site reactions, nausea and vomiting are most common. Abdominal pain; allergic reactions including anaphylaxis or severe asthmatic episodes (especially in the sulfite-sensitive patient); atelectasis; blurred vision; chest pain; chills; confusion; constipation; crying; delirium; delusions; depression; diarrhea; diplopia, edema; erythema; flushing; headache; hiccups; hypertension; hypotension; irregular pulse; low hemoglobin; muscle pain; pallor; pruritus; rash; respiratory depression; sleep disturbances; slurred speech; sweating; tinnitus; thrombophlebitis; and urinary frequency, hesitancy, and retention have been reported.

ANTIDOTE

With increasing severity of any side effect or onset of symptoms of overdose (e.g., respiratory depression) or allergic reaction, discontinue the drug and notify the physician. Treat side effects symptomatically. Naloxone hydrochloride (Narcan) will reverse respiratory depression. A patent airway, artificial ventilation, oxygen therapy, and other symptomatic treatment must be instituted promptly. Treat anaphylaxis with epinephrine (Adrenalin), diphenhydramine (Benadryl), and corticosteroids as indicated.

DIAZEPAM

Benzodiazepine
Sedative-hypnotic
Antianxiety agent
Anticonvulsant
Amnestic
Skeletal muscle relaxant
(adjunct)

Dizac, Valium   pH 6.2 to 6.9

USUAL DOSE

Maximum dose except in status epilepticus is 30 mg in 8 hours.

Moderate anxiety disorder and symptoms of anxiety: 2 to 5 mg. Repeat in 3 to 4 hours if necessary.

Severe anxiety disorders and symptoms of anxiety: 5 to 10 mg. Repeat in 3 to 4 hours if necessary.

Acute alcohol withdrawal: 10 mg initially, then 5 to 10 mg in 3 to 4 hours if necessary.

Status epilepticus: 5 to 10 mg. May be repeated at intervals of 10 to 15 minutes up to a total dose of 30 mg. May repeat in 2 to 4 hours. Another source suggests 0.2 to 0.5 mg/kg every 15 to 30 minutes for 2 or 3 doses. Some specialists start with 20 mg and titrate the total dose over 10 minutes or until seizures stop. Maximum dose in 24 hours is 100 mg.

Cardioversion: 5 to 15 mg 5 to 10 minutes before procedure begins.

Endoscopy: 10 mg or less is usually effective given before procedure begins; titrate to desired sedation (e.g., slurred speech). Up to 20 mg may be indicated if a narcotic is not used.

Muscle spasm: 5 to 10 mg. Repeat in 3 to 4 hours if necessary. Larger doses may be required in tetanus.

PEDIATRIC DOSE

Sedative/muscle relaxant: 0.04 to 0.2 mg/kg every 2 to 4 hours. Maximum dose 0.6 mg/kg in 8 hours.

Tetanus in infants over 30 days: 1 to 2 mg every 3 to 4 hours.

Tetanus in children 5 years or older: 5 to 10 mg every 3 to 4 hours.

Status epilepticus in neonates: 0.3 to 0.75 mg/kg every 15 to 30 minutes for 2 to 3 doses. Maximum total dose is 5 mg. May repeat in 2 to 4 hours. Another source suggests 0.5 to 1 mg/kg/dose every 15 minutes for 2 or 3 doses to maximum 5 mg dose.

Status epilepticus in infants over 30 days: 0.2 to 0.5 mg every 2 to 5 minutes or 0.2 to 0.5 mg/kg every 15 to 30 minutes to maximum 5 mg dose. May repeat in 2 to 4 hours.

Status epilepticus in children 5 years or older: 0.5 to 1 mg every 2 to 5 minutes to maximum 10 mg dose. May repeat in 2 to 4 hours.

DOSE ADJUSTMENTS

Reduce dose by one-half for the elderly or debilitated, in impaired liver or renal function, in patients with limited pulmonary reserve, and in the presence of other CNS depressants. Begin with a small dose and increase in gradual increments. ■ Note Drug/lab interactions.

DILUTION

For all preparations, do not dilute or mix with any other drug; *not soluble in any solution.* Should be given directly into the vein. Inject into IV tubing close to vein site only when direct IV injection is not feasible. Some precipitation or absorption into plastic tubing may take place; dizac is incompatible with polyvinylchloride infusion sets. Consider heparin lock for frequent injection. Change site every 2 to 3 days. If dilution imperative, add diluent solution to diazepam, not diazepam to diluent. Consult pharmacist. Dizac is a new emulsified form that eliminates the use of nonphysiological, potentially irritating solvents. Direct IV administration is preferred but can be administered at a Y-tube injection site.

Storage: Dizac: Refrigerate, do not freeze. Protect from light. Note expiration date.

INCOMPATIBLE WITH

Manufacturers for all preparations recommend not mixing with any other drug or solution in syringe or solution. Precipitation can occur. Note dizac in Dilution.

RATE OF ADMINISTRATION

Adults: 5 mg (1 ml) or fraction thereof over 1 minute.

Infants and children: Give total dose over a minimum of 3 minutes but do not exceed a rate of 0.25 mg/kg over 3 min.

ACTIONS

A benzodiazepine that depresses the central, autonomic, and peripheral nervous systems in an undetermined manner. Exerts antianxiety, sedative/hypnotic, amnesic, anticonvulsant, skeletal muscle relaxant and antitremor effects. Diminishes patient recall. Metabolized in the liver; stays in the body in appreciable amounts for several days and is excreted very slowly in the urine. Crosses the placental barrier. Secreted in breast milk.

INDICATIONS AND USES

Management of moderate to severe anxiety disorders or short-term relief of symptoms of anxiety. ▪ Acute alcohol withdrawal. ▪ Acute stress reactions. ▪ Muscle spasm. ▪ Status epilepticus and severe recurrent convulsive seizures, including tetany. ▪ Preoperative medication, including endoscopic procedures. ▪ Cardioversion.

CONTRAINDICATIONS

Known hypersensitivity, open-angle glaucoma unless receiving appropriate therapy, shock, coma, acute alcoholic intoxication with depression of vital signs. Emulsion in Dizac contains soybean oil; do not use in patients with known hypersensitivity to soy protein.

PRECAUTIONS

Check label carefully. Some preparations are for IV use only (e.g., Dizac), others can be given IM/IV (e.g., Valium). ▪ Recently made available as a rectal gel. ▪ Drug of choice for initial treatment of status epilepticus or seizures resulting from drug overdose or poisoning. Some specialists administer phenytoin simultaneously to facilitate long-term control (onset of action is not as immediate as diazepam). Oral phenytoin or phenobarbital may be used for maintenance. ▪ May not be effective if seizures are due to acute brain lesions. ▪ Not recommended for treatment of petit mal or petit mal variant seizures; may cause tonic state epilepticus. ▪ Use caution in elderly, very ill, those with limited pulmonary reserve (e.g., chronic lung disease) or unstable cardiac status. ▪ Withdrawal symptoms will occur for several weeks after extended or large doses. ▪ Hypoalbuminemia may increase incidence of side effects. ▪ Intended for short-term use only.

Monitor: Note Dilution. ▪ To reduce incidence of thrombophlebitis, avoid smaller veins. Extravasation or arterial administration hazardous. ▪ Oxygen, respiratory assistance, and flumazenil (Romazicon) must always be available. ▪ Bed rest required for a minimum of 3 hours after IV injection.

Patient education: May produce drowsiness or dizziness. Request assistance with ambulation and use caution performing tasks that require alertness. Do not drive or operate hazardous machinery until all effects have subsided. ▪ Avoid use of alcohol or other CNS depressants (e.g., antihistamines, barbiturates). ▪ May be habit forming with long-term use or high-dose therapy. ▪ Has amnestic potential; may impair memory. ▪ Consider birth control options.

Maternal/child: Pregnancy Category D: has caused birth deformities, especially in the first trimester. ▪ Not recommended during pregnancy, childbirth or while breast feeding. ▪ Safety for use in neonates not established but is used. ▪ Use in infants and children is most frequent in tetany, status epilepticus, or allergic reactions. Not recommended but is used for other general indications.

Elderly: Note Dose adjustments. Start with a small dose and increase gradually based on response. ▪ More sensitive to therapeutic and adverse effects (e.g., ataxia, dizziness, oversedation). ▪ IV injection may be more likely to cause apnea, bradycardia, hypotention, and cardiac arrest. ▪ Note Precautions and Drug/lab interactions.

DRUG/LAB INTERACTIONS

Concurrent use with other CNS depressants (e.g., alcohol, antihistamines, barbiturates, MAO inhibitors [e.g., selegiline (Eldepryl)], narcotics [e.g., morphine, meperidine (Demerol), fentanyl], phenothiazines [e.g., prochlorperazine (Compazine)], tricyclic antidepressants [e.g., imipramine (Tofranil-PM)]) may result in additive effects for up to 48 hours. Reduced doses of both drugs may be indicated. ▪ May increase serum concentrations of digoxin and phenytoin (Dilantin); monitor digoxin and phenytoin serum levels. ▪ Ritonavir (Norvir) may increase risk of prolonged sedation and respiratory depression. Concurrent use not recommended. Benzodiazepines metabolized by alternate routes may be safer (e.g., lorazepam [Ativan], oxazepam [Serax], temazepam [Restoril]). ▪ Concurrent use with beta blockers (e.g., metoprolol [Lopressor], propranolol [Inderal]), cimetidine (Tagamet), estrogen containing oral contraceptives, disulfiram (Antabuse), fluoxetine (Prozac), isoniazid (Nydrazid), ketoconazole (Nizoral), omeprazole (Prilosec), probenicid, and valproic acid (Depakene), may inhibit hepatic metabolism resulting in increased plasma concentrations of benzodiazepines. ▪ Diazepam decreases clearance and increases toxicity of zidovudine (AZT). ▪ May increase clearance and decrease effectiveness of levodopa. ▪ Hypotensive effects of benzodiazepines may be increased by any agent that induces hypotension (e.g., antihypertensives, bretylium, CNS depressants, diuretics, lidocaine, paclitaxel). ▪ Use with rifampin (Rifadin) increases clearance and reduces effects of diazepam.

■ Theophyllines (Aminophylline) antagonize sedative effects of benzodiazepines. ■ Smoking increases metabolism and clearance of diazepam, decreasing plasma levels and sedative effects. ■ Clozapine (Leponiz) has caused respiratory distress or cardiac arrest in a few patients; use concurrently with extreme caution. ■ Decreased drowsiness may occur in cigarette smokers, especially if elderly.

SIDE EFFECTS

Apnea, ataxia, blurred vision, bradycardia, cardiac arrest, cardiovascular collapse, coma, confusion, coughing, depressed respiration, depression, diminished reflexes, drowsiness, dyspnea, headache, hiccups, hyperexcited states, hyperventilation, laryngospasm, neutropenia, nystagmus, somnolence, syncope, venous thrombosis and phlebitis at injection site, vertigo.

ANTIDOTE

Notify the physician of all side effects. Reduction of dosage may be required. Discontinue the drug for major side effects or paradoxical reactions including hyperexcitability, hallucinations, and acute rage. Flumazenil (Romazicon) will reverse all sedative effects of benzodiazepines. A patent airway, artificial ventilation, oxygen therapy, and other symptomatic treatment must be instituted promptly. May cause emesis; observe closely. Treat allergic reaction, or resuscitate as necessary.

DIAZOXIDE

Antihypertensive
(Vasodilator)

Hyperstat IV　　　　　　　　　　　　　　　　　　　pH 11.6

USUAL DOSE

1 to 3 mg/kg of body weight up to a maximum dose of 150 mg (10 ml). May be repeated in 5 to 15 minutes if an adequate response is not obtained. This second injection may effect a greater response. Repeat as indicated at intervals of 4 to 24 hours to maintain desired blood pressure. For short-term use until a regimen of oral antihypertensive medication is effective. Do not use for more than 10 days.

PEDIATRIC DOSE

1 to 3 mg/kg of body weight up to 150 mg/dose. See instructions in Usual dose.

DOSE ADJUSTMENTS

Note Drug/lab interactions.

DILUTION

Should be given undiluted.

Storage: Protect from light and freezing. Store at controlled room temperature.

INCOMPATIBLE WITH

Do not mix in syringe or solution with any other drug. Hydralazine (Apresoline), propranolol (Inderal).

RATE OF ADMINISTRATION

Rapidly as a single dose over 10 to 30 seconds. Not as effective when administered at a slower rate.

ACTIONS

A potent, rapid-acting antihypertensive agent. Produces vasodilation by relaxing the smooth muscle of peripheral arterioles. Increases cardiac output while maintaining coronary and cerebral blood flow. Effects on renal blood flow not significant. Effective in patients not responsive to other antihypertensive agents. Acts within 1 to 5 minutes with a duration of 2 to 12 hours (range is 30 minutes to 72 hours). Usually no further decrease in blood pressure after 30 minutes, but a gradual increase over the above duration to pretreatment levels. Crosses placental barrier; probably secreted in breast milk.

INDICATIONS AND USES

Severe hypertension (e.g., malignant and nonmalignant hypertensive emergencies).

CONTRAINDICATIONS

Compensatory hypertension (e.g., arteriovenous shunt or coarctation of the aorta), known sensitivity to thiazides or other sulfonamide-derived drugs (e.g., furosemide [Lasix], TMP-SMZ [Bactrim]), labor and delivery. Not effective in pheochromocytoma.

PRECAUTIONS

Avoid rapid decrease in blood pressure. Has caused angina and myocardial and cerebral infarction. ■ Use caution in patients with impaired cerebral or cardiac circulation.

Monitor: Give only into a peripheral vein, avoid extravasation. ■ Maintain patient in recumbent position during injection and for at least 1 hour after injection. ■ Check blood pressure every 5 minutes until stabilized and hourly thereafter. ■ Take blood pressure with patient in standing position before ambulation. ■ Use caution in diabetes; monitor blood glucose levels. May cause hyperglycemia; difficult to assess. ■ Diuresis may be required to reverse sodium and water retention before diazoxide can be effective. Causes sodium and water retention and may precipitate edema and CHF. ■ May cause hyperuricemia; difficult to assess. ■ Note Drug/lab interactions.

Maternal/child: Pregnancy Category C: safety for use in pregnancy, lactation, and children not established. ■ Note Contraindications. May stop uterine contractions if given during labor. Oxytoxics may be required. ■ May produce fetal or neonatal hyperbilirubinemia, thrombocytopenia, altered carbohydrate metabolism, and other adverse reactions if given before delivery. ■ Discontinue breast feeding.

DRUG/LAB INTERACTIONS

Potentiates coumarin and its derivatives; a reduced dose of anticoagulant may be required. ■ May increase hypotensive and hyperuricemic effects of thiazides and other diuretics. ■ May decrease phenytoin (Dilantin) levels reducing anticonvulsant effect. ■ Profound hypotension will result if used with peripheral vasodilators (e.g., hydralazine [Apresoline], nitroprusside sodium [Nipride]). ■ Use with sulfonyureas (e.g., tolbutamide [Orinase]) may cause hyperglycemia. ■ Interferes with assessment of hyperglycemia and hyperuricemia. ■ Will cause a false-negative insulin response to glucagon.

SIDE EFFECTS

Abdominal discomfort, cerebral ischemia, confusion, congestive heart failure, convulsions, edema, flushing, headache, hyperglycemia, hypotension (severe), ileus, lightheadedness, myocardial ischemia, nausea, orthostatic hypotension, palpitations, paralysis, sensations of warmth, sensitivity reactions, sodium and water retention, supraventricular tachycardia, sweating, vomiting, weakness.

ANTIDOTE

Notify the physician of all side effects. Some will subside spontaneously; others will require symptomatic treatment. Treat sensitivity reaction as indicated and resuscitate as necessary. If hypotension occurs, place patient in a Trendelenberg position. Treat undesirable hypotension with dopamine (Intropin) or norepinephrine (Levophed); if no response, diazoxide is probably not the cause of the hypotension. Excessive hyperglycemia may be treated with insulin. Hemodialysis or peritoneal dialysis may be required in overdose.

DIETHYLSTILBESTROL DIPHOSPHATE

Antineoplastic (Hormone/estrogen)

❦Honvol, Stilphostrol

pH 9.0 to 10.5

USUAL DOSE

Induction: 0.5 Gm/24 hr initially. Increase to 1 Gm/24 hr beginning with second day, and give 1 Gm/24 hr for 5 days or as indicated by patient response.

Maintenance dose: 0.25 to 0.5 Gm once or twice weekly. Usually given orally.

DOSE ADJUSTMENTS

May be required in impaired liver function.

DILUTION

A single daily dose must be diluted in 300 ml of D5W, D5/0.45NS, NS, 0.45S, or LR for infusion.

INCOMPATIBLE WITH

Sufficient information not available. Calcium gluconate.

RATE OF ADMINISTRATION

1 ml/min for the first 10 to 15 minutes; then increase rate to complete infusion within 1 hour of starting time.

ACTIONS

An estrogen hormone. In the diphosphate form there are fewer side effects, and large doses can be given. May be directly cytotoxic to malignant cells or may simply slow the growth. Does decrease the percentage of cells actively proliferating in a tumor mass. Metabolized in the liver. Excreted in the urine.

INDICATIONS AND USES

Palliative treatment of prostatic carcinoma. Particularly useful in advanced stages.

CONTRAINDICATIONS

Past history of or active thrombophlebitis, thromboembolic disorders or cerebral apoplexy, estrogen-dependent neoplasia. Not indicated for treatment of any disorder in females.

PRECAUTIONS

IV route used when oral route ineffective or not practical. ▪ Used with other antineoplastic drugs to achieve tumor remission. ▪ Feminization in the male is expected. ▪ Use caution in cardiac, liver, or renal disease and diabetes.

Monitor: Will cause salt and water retention. Monitor blood pressure, pulse, weight and encourage a low-salt diet.

Patient education: Consider birth control options.

Maternal/child: Pregnancy Category X: avoid pregnancy. ▪ Discontinue breast feeding. ▪ Safety for use in children not established.

DRUG/LAB INTERACTIONS

May decrease metabolism and increase toxicity of cyclosporine (Sandimmune). ▪ Risk of hepatotoxicity increased with other hepatotoxic agents (e.g., dantrolene [Dantrium], daunorubicin [Cerubidine]).

SIDE EFFECTS

Burning and local pain in the perineal region and metastatic sites are expected and last only a few moments. Other side effects are abdominal cramps, anemia, decreased libido, dizziness, elevated prothrombin time, headache, hypercalcemia, myocardial infarction, nausea, painful swelling of breasts, pulmonary embolism, thrombophlebitis, and vomiting. All side effects associated with estrogens are possible.

ANTIDOTE

Notify the physician of all side effects. Most will be treated symptomatically. Hypercalcemia is reversible when detected early (limit oral calcium, push fluids, record output, ambulate to keep calcium in the bones). There is no specific antidote. Supportive therapy as indicated will help sustain the patient in toxicity.

DIGOXIN IMMUNE FAB (OVINE)

Digibind

Antidote
(digitalis intoxication)

pH 6.0 to 8.0

USUAL DOSE

Acute toxicity in adults and children: Testing for sensitivity to sheep serum may be indicated before use (see Precautions/Monitor). Determine dose by symptoms and clinical findings. Serum concentration may not reflect actual toxicity for 6 to 12 hours.

Dose in numbers of vials based on ingested dose is calculated by dividing the body load of digoxin or digitoxin in milligrams by 0.5. Each vial contains 38 mg and will bind 0.5 mg digoxin or deslanoside. Dose may also be based on serum digoxin levels (see package insert, has charts for adults and children). One source indicates 1 or 2 vials are the average dose, with up to 20 vials used in serious cases, but the average dose in clinical trials was 10 vials. For an unknown ingestion or if serum digoxin level is not available, consider giving 10 vials (380 mg). Observe clinical response and repeat if indicated. 20 vials (760 mg) will bind approximately 50 (0.25 mg) tablets of Lanoxin and should provide adequate treatment of most life-threatening ingestions in adults and children. A single dose may be repeated in several hours if toxicity has not reversed or appears to recur. Febrile reactions are dose related.

Toxicity in chronic therapy: Adults: 6 vials (228 mg).

Children: less than 20 kg: 1 vial (38 mg).

DILUTION

Each vial (38 mg) must be diluted with 4 ml of sterile water for injection (9.5 mg/ml). Mix gently. May be given in this initial dilution or may be further diluted with any desired amount of NS (34 ml NS/vial yields 1 mg/ml). Consider volume overload in children when further diluting in NS. Administer to infants after initial dilution using a tuberculin syringe to deliver an accurate dose with less volume or for extremely small doses dilute to 1 mg/ml before administration.

Storage: Refrigerate unreconstituted vials. Use reconstituted solution promptly or store in refrigerator for up to 4 hours.

INCOMPATIBLE WITH

Specific information not available. Do not mix with any other drug in syringe or solution because of specific use.

RATE OF ADMINISTRATION

Must be given through a 0.22 micron membrane filter. A single dose as an IV infusion equally distributed over 15 to 30 minutes. May be given as an IV bolus injection if cardiac arrest is imminent. Be prepared to treat anaphylaxis.

ACTIONS

Antigen binding fragments (Fab) prepared from specific antidigoxin antibodies produced in sheep are isolated and purified. Fab fragments bind molecules of digoxin and make them unavailable for binding at their site of action. Freely distributed in extracellular space. Onset of action is prompt with improvement in symptoms of toxicity within 30 minutes. Excreted in urine.

INDICATIONS AND USES

Treatment of patients with life-threatening digitalis intoxication or overdose (digoxin or digitoxin). ▪ Also indicated when potassium concentrations are above 5 mEq/L with digitalis intoxication. ▪ Note Precautions and Maternal/child.

CONTRAINDICATIONS

None known when used for specific indications. If hypersensitivity exists and treatment is necessary, preload with corticosteroids and diphenhydramine, and prepare to treat anaphylaxis.

PRECAUTIONS

Cardiac arrest can result from ingestion of more than 10 mg digoxin by healthy adults, 4 mg digoxin by healthy children, or serum digoxin levels above 10 ng/ml. ▪ Larger doses of digoxin immune Fab act more quickly but increase the possibility of febrile or allergic reaction. ▪ Use caution in impaired cardiac function. Inability to use cardiac glycosides may endanger patient. Support with dopamine (Intropin) or vasodilators.

Monitor: Although allergy testing is not required before treating life-threatening digitalis toxicity, patients allergic to ovine proteins or those who have previously received antibodies or Fab fragments produced from sheep are at risk. Determine patient response to any previous injections of serum of any type and history of any allergic-type reactions. ▪ Test for sensitivity if indicated. Make a 1:100 solution by diluting 0.1 ml of initially diluted solution (10 mg/ml) with 9.9 ml sterile NS (100 mcg/ml).

Scratch test: Make a 1/4-inch skin scratch through a drop of 1:100 dilution in NS. Inspect the site in 20 minutes. An urticarial wheal surrounded by a zone of erythema is a positive reaction.

Skin test: Inject 0.1 ml (10 mcg) of 1:100 dilution intradermally. Inspect the site in 20 minutes. An urticarial wheal surrounded by a zone of erythema is a positive reaction. Concomitant use of antihistamines may interfere with sensitivity tests. If skin testing causes a systemic reaction, place a tourniquet above the testing site and treat anaphylaxis.

Monitor temperature, blood pressure, ECG, and potassium concentration frequently during and after drug administration. ▪ Consider that multiple drugs may have been used and are producing toxicity in suicide attempts. ▪ Obtain serum concentrations if possible. High margin of error will occur if drawn soon after ingestion. Six to eight hours is required after the last digitalis dose to obtain an accurate serum concentration. ▪ Potassium may be shifted from inside to outside the cell causing increased renal excretion. May appear to have hyperkalemia while there is a total body deficit of potassium. When the digitalis effect is reversed hypokalemia may develop rapidly. ▪ Do not redigitalize until all Fab fragments have been eliminated from the body. May take several days. May take longer in severe renal impairment, and reintoxication may occur by release of newly unbound digoxin into the blood. ▪ Note Drug/lab interactions.

Maternal/child: Pregnancy Category C: use only when clearly indicated

and benefits outweigh risks in pregnancy, lactation, and infants.
■ Should be used in infants and children if more than 0.3 mg of digoxin ingested, if serum digoxin levels ≥6.4 nmol/L, or there is underlying heart disease.

DRUG/LAB INTERACTIONS

Will cause a precipitous rise in total serum digoxin, but most will be bound to the Fab fragment. Will interfere with digitalis immunoassay measurements until Fab fragment is completely eliminated. ■ Catecholamines (e.g., epinephrine) may aggravate digitalis arrhythmias. ■ Note skin test in Monitor.

SIDE EFFECTS

Acute anaphylaxis with urticaria, respiratory distress, and vascular collapse are possible. Exacerbation of congestive heart failure and low cardiac output states and increased ventricular response in atrial fibrillation may occur due to withdrawal of digitalis effects. Hypokalemia may be life threatening.

ANTIDOTE

Notify the physician of all side effects. Discontinue the drug and treat anaphylaxis immediately. Corticosteroids, epinephrine (Adrenalin [note Drug/lab interactions]), diphenhydramine (Benadryl), oxygen, vasopressors (dopamine), and ventilation equipment must always be available. Resuscitate as necessary. Treat hypokalemia cautiously when necessary. Support exacerbated cardiac conditions as necessary.

DIGOXIN INJECTION

Cardiac glycoside
Antiarrhythmic
Inotropic agent

Lanoxin, Lanoxin pediatric

pH 6.8 to 7.2

USUAL DOSE

0.5 to 1 mg (2 to 4 ml) for digitalization. 0.25 to 0.5 mg (1 to 2 ml) as the initial dose, followed by 0.25 to 0.5 mg (1 to 2 ml) at 4- to 6-hour intervals until digitalized (approximately 4 to 6 hours). Assess clinical response before each additional dose. Maintenance dose is usually 0.125 to 0.5 mg daily.

PEDIATRIC DOSE

Use 0.1 mg/ml pediatric injection (100 mcg/ml).
Digitalizing dose: Give one half of total daily dose initially, then two doses of one fourth total daily dose at 8-hour intervals. Assess clinical response before each additional dose.

Usual Digitalizing and Maintenance Dosages

Age	Digitalizing dose (mcg/kg)*	Daily IV maintenance dose (mcg/kg)†
Premature	15–20	20%–30% of IV loading dose‡§
Full-term	20–30	

Age	Digitalizing dose (mcg/kg)*	Daily IV maintenance dose (mcg/kg)†
1–24 months	30–50	
2–5 years	25–35	25%–35% of IV loading dose‡
5–10 years	15–30	
Over 10 years	8–12	

*IV digitalizing doses are 80% of oral digitalizing doses.
‡Individual adjustments required.
‡Projected or actual digitalizing dose providing clinical response.
§Divided and given every 12 hours.

DOSE ADJUSTMENTS

Reduce dose in partially digitalized patients and patients with impaired renal function. ■ Dose reduction may be required before cardioversion. ■ Note Drug/lab interactions; adjustments may be required with numerous drugs. ■ Reduced doses may be indicated in advanced heart failure, myocardial infarction, severe carditis, or severe pulmonary disease. ■ Adjustments may be required in thyroid disease. ■ Note Precautions.

DILUTION

May be given undiluted or each 1 ml may be diluted in 4 ml sterile water, NS, D5W, or LR for injection. Less diluent will cause precipitation. Use diluted solution immediately. Give through Y-tube or three-way stopcock of IV infusion set.

INCOMPATIBLE WITH

Manufacturer recommends not mixing with any drug. Acids, alkalies, calcium chloride, calcium disodium edetate, calcium gluceptate, calcium gluconate, dobutamine (Dobutrex), doxapram (Dopram), fluconazole (Diflucan), foscarnet (Foscavir), insulin.

RATE OF ADMINISTRATION

Each single dose over a minimum of 5 minutes.

ACTIONS

A crystalline cardiac glycoside obtained from *Digitalis lanata,* this is a fast-acting hydrolytic product of lanatoside C. Onset of action is within 5 to 30 minutes and lasts 2 to 3 days. It has positive inotropic action, increasing the strength of myocardial contraction. It also alters the electric behavior of heart muscle through actions on myocardial automaticity, conduction velocity, and refraction. Results are a slower, stronger beat with increased cardiac output. Venous pressure falls, coronary circulation is increased, and heart size may become more normal. Widely distributed throughout the body and rapidly excreted in the urine. Secreted in breast milk.

INDICATIONS AND USES

Congestive heart failure. ■ Atrial fibrillation (note Precautions). ■ Atrial flutter. ■ Selected paroxysmal tachycardia or AV junctional rhythm. ■ Selected supraventricular tachycardias. ■ Cardiogenic shock. ■ Selected situations in myocardial infarction. ■ Preoperative, intraoperative, and postoperative need for digitalis because of stress on the heart.

CONTRAINDICATIONS

Beriberi heart disease, digitalis intoxication, or previous toxic response, hypersensitivity to digoxin, selected cases of hypersensitive carotid sinus syndrome, ventricular fibrillation, ventricular tachycardia unless heart failure occurs after a protracted episode and the etiology is not digitalis intoxication.

PRECAUTIONS

IV administration is the preferred parenteral route. Used only when oral therapy is not feasible or rapid therapeutic effect is necessary. ■ Diltiazem (Cardizem) or verapamil (Isotopin) generally preferred to treat atrial fibrillation; adenosine (Adenocard) preferred to treat PSVT. ■ Some clinicians suggest stopping digoxin 12 hours prior to surgery to reduce risk of perioperative arrhythmias in digitalized patients. The exception is patients with supraventricular tachyarrhythmias; they should receive a dose the morning of surgery. ■ Use with caution in patients with hypercalcemia or liver or kidney disease. ■ Hypocalcemia may nullify effect of digoxin. If calcium levels need to be restored to normal, give calcium slowly and in small amounts. Death has occurred in digitalized patients receiving calcium. ■ Plasma levels in thyroid disease are inversely proportional to thyroid status. Dose may be increased in thyrotoxic patients and decreased in patients with myxedema. ■ Use caution in patients with first- or second-degree heart block; may precipitate complete heart block. ■ Use caution in patients with advanced heart failure, myocardial infarction, severe carditis, or severe pulmonary disease. May be sensitive to digoxin-induced arrhythmia. Initiate therapy with lower doses. ■ If counter-shock is necessary (last-resort treatment of life-threatening arrhythmias), begin with low voltage levels and increase gradually to avoid ventricular arrhythmias. ■ Note Drug/lab interactions.

Monitor: Hypomagnesemia, hypokalemia, and hypercalcemia may predispose patient to digitalis toxicity. Monitor electrolytes frequently during therapy. Avoid rapid changes. Supplements indicated to maintain normal serum electrolyte levels. ■ Monitor HR and BP. ■ Baseline and periodic ECG monitoring suggested. ■ ECG monitoring recommended in children to avoid intoxication. ■ Monitor digoxin levels. Draw at least 6 to 8 hours after last dose; preferably just prior to next dose. ■ Monitor renal function. ■ Note Precautions and Drug/lab interactions.

Maternal/child: Pregnancy Category C: use only if clearly needed. ■ Has been used to treat fetal tachycardia. ■ Safety for use in nursing mothers not established.

Elderly: Monitor carefully. Reduced dose may be indicated. Consider reduced body mass and reduced kidney function.

DRUG/LAB INTERACTIONS

Monitor serum levels carefully and adjust doses as indicated. ■ Digoxin serum levels increased by amiodarone, benzodiazepines (e.g., diazepam [Valium]), calcium channel blockers (e.g., verapamil [Calan], diltiazem [Cardizem] to a lesser extent), cyclosporine (Sandimmune), esmolol (Brevibloc), flecanide (Tambocor), ibuprofen (Motrin), indomethacin (Indocin), nifedipine (Procardia), quinidine, tolbutamide, and many others; may increase therapeutic effects or cause toxicity. ■ Synergistic with beta blockers (e.g., Atenolol [Tenormin], metoprolol [Lopressor]); both drugs slow AV conduction and can cause complete heart block. ■ Digitalis toxicity may be precipitated by potassium-depleting corticosteroids and diuretics (e.g., furosemide [Lasix], chlorodiazide [Diuril]), calcium, sympathomimetic amines (e.g., epinephrine), reserpine, succinylcholine (Anectine), amphotericin B. ■ Increased risk of arrhythmias with nondepolarizing muscle relaxants (e.g., pancuronium [Pavulon]), reserpine, sympathomimetic amines (e.g., epinephrine), succinylcholine. ■ Initiation of thyroid treatment may require an increase in digoxin dose; treatment with thioamines (propylthiouracil [PTU]) may require a decreased dose. ■ Potassium-sparing diuretics (e.g., spironolactone), cimetidine (Tagamet) may increase or decrease toxic effects. ■ Serum levels may be reduced by barbiturates (e.g., phenobarbital), antineoplastic agents (e.g., cyclophosphamide, cytarabine, prednisone, vincristine), cholestyramine (Questran), hydantoins (phenytoin [Dilantin]), rifampin (Rifadin), and many others. When these drugs are discontinued, digitalis toxicity may occur. ■ Note Precautions and Monitor.

SIDE EFFECTS

Seldom last more than 3 days after drug is discontinued. Any form of digitalis may cause partial or AV block and almost any arrhythmia, including paroxysmal tachycardia, atrial tachycardia, fibrillation, or standstill. *First ECG signs of toxicity* are ST segment sagging, PR prolongation, and possible bigeminal rhythm. *Clinical signs of toxicity* are mostly abdominal discomfort or pain, anorexia, blurred vision, confusion, diarrhea, disturbed color (yellow) vision, headache, nausea, photopsia (points of light in peripheral vision), vomiting, and weakness.

ANTIDOTE

Discontinue the drug at the first sign of toxicity and notify the physician. Dosage may be decreased or discontinued. For severe toxicity, digoxin immune Fab is a specific antidote. Depending on symptoms, one or more of the following may be required: atropine, phenytoin (Dilantin), potassium salts (potassium chloride), procainamide (Pronestyl), or disodium edetate (EDTA disodium). Note Precautions. Peritoneal or hemodialysis not effective in overdose.

DIHYDROERGOTAMINE MESYLATE

Ergot alkaloid
Migraine agent

D.H.E. 45

pH 3.2 to 4.0

USUAL DOSE

Abort or prevent headaches: 1 mg (1 ml). May be repeated in 1 hour. No more than 2 doses (2 mg total) may be given IV in 24 hours. Do not exceed 6 mg in 1 week. Administration of an antiemetic (e.g. metoclopramide [Reglan] 10 mg) orally 1 hour before dihydroergotamine is recommended.

Chronic intractable headache: 0.5 mg (0.5 ml). Administer an antiemetic IV (e.g., metoclopramide) about 10 minutes before injection.

Prevention of orthostatic hypotension associated with spinal or epidural anesthesia (investigational): 0.5 mg (0.5 ml). Give a few minutes before the anesthetic.

PEDIATRIC DOSE

(See Maternal/child). Administration of an antiemetic (e.g., metoclopramide, prochlorperazine) usually orally 1 hour before dihydroergotamine is recommended.

Children 6 to 9 years of age: 100 to 150 mcg (0.1 to 0.15 mg).

Children 9 to 12 years of age: 200 mcg (0.2 mg).

Children 12 to 16 years of age: 250 to 500 mcg (0.25 to 0.5 mg).

For all age ranges, repeat up to 2 doses at 20 minute intervals if necessary. Another source suggests 250 mcg (0.25 mg) at the start of the attack. Repeat in 1 hour if necessary.

DILUTION

May be given undiluted.

Storage: Protect ampoules from light and heat.

INCOMPATIBLE WITH

Any other drug in syringe or solution.

RATE OF ADMINISTRATION

1 mg or fraction thereof over 1 minute.

ACTIONS

An alpha adrenergic blocking agent that causes constriction of both peripheral and cerebral blood vessels and produces depression of central vasomotor centers. Metabolized by the liver. Metabolites eliminated primarily in feces. Secreted in breast milk.

INDICATIONS AND USES

To abort or prevent vascular headaches (migraine, histamine cephalalgia). Used when rapid control is desired or other routes not feasible.
■ Treatment of chronic intractable headache.

Investigational use: To prevent orthostatic hypotension associated with spinal or epidural anesthesia. Use SC to enhance heparin effects in preventing postoperative deep vein thrombosis after abdominal, thoracic, or pelvic surgeries or total hip replacement and IM or SC to treat orthostatic hypotension.

CONTRAINDICATIONS

Coronary artery disease, hepatic or renal disease, hypersensitivity, uncontrolled hypertension, lactation, peripheral vascular disease, pregnancy or women who may become pregnant, sepsis.

PRECAUTIONS

IM use is preferred but may be given IV to obtain a more rapid effect.

Monitor: Monitor vital signs; observe closely. ▪ Note Drug/lab interactions.

Patient education: Consider birth control options. ▪ Take only as directed. ▪ Report ineffectiveness or an increase in frequency or severity of headaches. ▪ Report chest pain, increased heart rate, itching, muscle pain or weakness of arms or legs, numbness or tingling of extremities, or swelling.

Maternal/child: Pregnancy Category X: avoid pregnancy. Note Contraindications. ▪ Safety for use in children not established. Severe side effects (e.g., extrapyramidal reactions may occur). Pre-treatment with an antiemetic may be helpful. Limit pediatric use to patients who have not responded to less toxic treatment.

Elderly: Increased risk of hypothermia and ischemic complications (e.g., cardiac, peripheral). ▪ Consider age-related renal impairment.

DRUG/LAB INTERACTIONS

Opposes vasodilating effects of nitrates (e.g., nitroglycerin), decreasing their effectiveness. ▪ May cause hypertensive crisis in combination with other vasopressors (e.g., epinephrine). ▪ May cause peripheral vasoconstriction with ischemia and/or cyanosis with beta-adrenergic blockers (e.g., propranolol [Inderal]) or macrolide antibiotics (e.g., erythromycin, troleandomycin [TAO]), and nicotine.

SIDE EFFECTS

Rare in therapeutic doses, but may include angina pectoris, blindness, gangrene, muscle pains, muscle weakness, nausea, numbness and tingling of the fingers and toes, thirst, uterine bleeding, and vomiting.

ANTIDOTE

Discontinue the drug and notify the physician of any side effects. Another drug will probably be chosen if further treatment is indicated. Vasodilators (nitroprusside) and CNS stimulants (e.g., caffeine and sodium benzoate) are indicated as an antidote. Heparin and low-molecular-weight dextran may be used to reduce thrombosis due to excessive vasoconstriction. Hemodialysis may be indicated. Resuscitate as necessary.

DILTIAZEM HYDROCHLORIDE

Cardizem

Calcium channel blocker
Antiarrhythmic

pH 3.7 to 4.1

USUAL DOSE

0.25 mg/kg of body weight initially (20 mg for the average patient). A second dose of 0.35 mg/kg may be given in 15 minutes if needed to achieve heart rate reduction (25 mg for the average patient). Any additional bolus doses used to achieve an appropriate response must be individualized to each patient. Patients with PSVT will probably respond to bolus doses and may not require an infusion, but to maintain reduction in heart rate in patients with atrial fibrillation or atrial flutter, immediately follow with an intravenous infusion at an initial rate of 10 mg/hr. May only be used for up to 24 hours. Some patients may maintain response with an initial rate of 5 mg/hr. Infusion may be increased by 5 mg/hr increments to a maximum dose of 15 mg/hr. Discontinue infusion within 24 hours. Oral antiarrhythmic agents (e.g., digoxin, quinidine, procainamide, calcium channel blockers [e.g., diltiazem, verapamil], beta blockers [e.g., atenolol, metoprolol, propranolol]) to maintain reduced heart rate are usually started within 3 hours of initial bolus of diltiazem.

DOSE ADJUSTMENTS

Specific mg/kg dose must be used for patients with low body weights. ▪ Reduced dose may be indicated in impaired hepatic or renal function. ▪ Note Drug/lab interactions.

DILUTION

Available as a solution (25 mg vial [5 mg/ml]), as a powder with supplied diluent (Lyo-ject syringe [5 mg/ml]), and in a piggyback monovial containing 100 mg (with transfer needle set to facilitate preparation of an infusion).

CARDIZEM Injectable or CARDIZEM Lyo-Ject Syringe

Diluent volume	Quantity of cardizem (diltiazem) injection	Final concentration	Administration	
			Dose	Infusion rate
100 ml	125 mg (25 ml)	1.0 mg/ml	5 mg/hr 10 mg/hr 15 mg/hr	5 ml/hr 10 ml/hr 15 ml/hr
250 ml	250 mg (50 ml)	0.83 mg/ml	5 mg/hr 10 mg/hr 15 mg/hr	6 ml/hr 12 ml/hr 18 ml/hr
500 ml	250 mg (50 ml)	0.45 mg/ml	5 mg/hr 10 mg/hr 15 mg/hr	11 ml/hr 22 ml/hr 33 ml/hr

CARDIZEM Monovial

Diluent volume	Quantity of cardizem monovial to add	Final concentration	Administration	
			Dose*	Infusion rate
100 ml	100 mg (1 monovial)	1 mg/ml	10 mg/hr 15 mg/hr	10 ml/hr 15 ml/hr
250 ml	200 mg (2 monovials)	0.80 mg/ml	10 mg/hr 15 mg/hr	12.5 ml/hr 18.8 ml/hr
500 ml	200 mg (2 monovials)	0.40 mg/ml	10 mg/hr 15 mg/hr	25 ml/hr 37.5 ml/hr

*5 mg/hr may be appropriate for some patients.

Direct IV: May be given undiluted through Y-tube or three-way stopcock of tubing containing NS, D5W, or D5/0.45 NS.

Infusion: May be further diluted for infusion in any of the above solutions.

Storage: Vials may be stored at room temperature for up to 1 month, then discarded. Refrigeration before and after dilution preferred. Use within 24 hours of dilution. Discard unused medication and/or solution. Do not freeze.

INCOMPATIBLE WITH
Acetazolamide (Diamox), acyclovir (Zovirax), aminophylline, ampicillin (Polycillin-N), ampicillin/sulbactam (Unasyn), cefamandole (Mandol), cefoperazone (Cefobid), diazepam (Valium), furosemide (Lasix), heparin, hydrocortisone, (Solu-Cortef), insulin, methylprednisolone (Solu-Medrol), nafcillin (Unipen), phenytoin (Dilantin), rifampin (Rifadin), sodium bicarbonate.

COMPATIBLE WITH
Y-site: Cardizem monovial (1 mg/ml) in NS is considered compatible at a Y-site with aminophylline, ampicillin, ampicillin sodium/sulbactam sodium (Unasyn), cefamandole (Mandol), hydrocortisone (Solu-Cortef), regular insulin, methylprednisolone (Solu-Medrol), mezlocillin (Mezlin), nafcillin (Unipen), sodium bicarbonate.

RATE OF ADMINISTRATION
Direct IV: Each single dose equally distributed over 2 minutes.

Infusion: 5 mg to 15 mg/hr based on patient response. 125 mg diluted in 100 ml (1.0 mg/ml) yields 5 mg/hr at 5 ml/hr, 10 mg/hr at 10 ml/hr, and 15 mg/hr at 15 ml/hr. 250 mg diluted in 250 ml (0.83 mg/ml) yields 5 mg/hr at 6 ml/hr, 10 mg/hr at 12 ml/hr, and 15 mg/hr at 18 ml/hr. 250 mg diluted in 500 ml (0.45 mg/ml) yields 5 mg/hr at 11 ml/hr, 10 mg/hr at 22 ml/hr, and 15 mg/hr at 33 ml/hr. Use of a metriset (60 gtt/min) required; volumetric infusion pump preferred.

ACTIONS
Directly inhibits the influx of calcium ions through slow channels during membrane depolarization of cardiac and vascular smooth muscle. Effective in supraventricular tachycardias because it slows conduction through the AV node, prolongs the effective refractory period, reduces ventricular rates, and helps to prevent embolic complications. Prevents reentry phenomena through the AV node. Reduces

heart rate (10% with a single dose, 20% at peak effectiveness), systolic and diastolic blood pressure, systemic vascular resistance, pulmonary artery systolic and diastolic blood pressures, and coronary vascular resistance with no significant effect on contractility, left ventricular end diastolic pressure, right atrial pressure, or pulmonary capillary wedge pressure. Increases cardiac output and stroke volume. Has little or no effect on normal AV nodal conduction at normal heart rates. Produces less myocardial depression than verapamil. Effective within 3 minutes; maximum effect should occur within 7 to 11 minutes and last for 1 to 3 hours. 70% to 80% bound to plasma proteins. Metabolized in the liver. Excreted in urine and bile. Secreted in breast milk.

INDICATIONS AND USES

Temporary control of rapid ventricular rate in atrial fibrillation or atrial flutter unless associated with an accessory bypass tract (e.g., Wolff-Parkinson-White syndrome or short PR syndrome). ■ Rapid conversion of paroxysmal supraventricular tachycardia (PSVT) to normal sinus rhythm including AV nodal reentrant tachycardias and reciprocating tachycardias associated with an extranodal accessory pathway, (e.g., Wolff-Parkinson-White syndrome or short PR syndrome). ■ Narrow complex PSVT not responsive to adenosine (Adenocard).

Unlabeled use: Decrease refractory angina and pulse rates in unstable angina.

CONTRAINDICATIONS

■ Atrial fibrillation or flutter when associated with an accessory bypass tract (e.g., Wolff-Parkinson-White or short PR syndrome), cardiogenic shock, congestive heart failure (severe) unless secondary to supraventricular tachyarrhythmia treatable with diltiazem, known sensitivity to diltiazem, second- or third-degree AV block or sick sinus syndrome (unless functioning ventricular pacemaker in place), severe hypotension, patients receiving IV beta-adrenergic blocking agents (e.g., atenolol [Tenormin], propranolol [Inderal]) within 2 to 4 hours, ventricular tachycardia.

PRECAUTIONS

For short-term use only. ■ While diltiazem will effectively decrease heart rate, cardioversion will probably be required to convert atrial fibrillation or atrial flutter to a normal sinus rhythm. ■ Valsalva maneuver recommended before use of diltiazem in all paroxysmal supraventricular tachycardias if clinically appropriate. ■ Use IV diltiazem with caution in patients with preexisting impaired ventricular function (e.g., congestive heart failure, acute myocardial infarction or pulmonary congestion documented by x-ray); may exacerbate disease. Use of oral diltiazem in these patients is contraindicated. ■ May cause second- or third-degree AV block in sinus rhythm; discontinue diltiazem if AV block occurs. ■ Can cause life-threatening tachycardia with severe hypotension in atrial fibrillation or flutter in patients with an accessory bypass tract and periods of asystole in patients with sick sinus syndrome. ■ Use with caution in impaired renal or hepatic function. ■ Ventricular premature beats (VPBs) may occur on conversion of PSVT to sinus rhythm; considered to have no clinical significance. ■ Continue regular dosing on day of OR and thereafter unless otherwise specified by physician. If discontinued, may cause severe angina or MI.

Monitor: Accurate pretreatment diagnosis differentiating wide-complex QRS tachycardia of supraventricular origin from ventricular origin is imperative. ▪ ECG monitoring during administration preferred; must be available. ▪ Monitor blood pressure closely. ▪ Emergency resuscitation drugs and equipment must always be available. ▪ Note Drug/lab interactions.

Maternal/child: Pregnancy Category C: large doses (5 to 10 times mg/kg dose) have resulted in embryo and fetal death and skeletal abnormalities in animals. ▪ Discontinue breast feeding. ▪ Safety for use in children not established.

Elderly: Half-life may be prolonged. ▪ May cause tinnitus.

DRUG/LAB INTERACTIONS

Do not give concomitantly (within a few hours) with IV beta-adrenergic blocking agents (e.g., atenolol [Tenormin], propranolol [Inderal]) (see Contraindications). May result in bradycardia, AV block, and/or depression of contractility. Use extreme caution if these drugs are administered orally or if patient has received before admission; usually tolerated. ▪ May result in additive effects with any agent known to affect cardiac contractility and/or SA or AV node conduction (e.g., digoxin [Lanoxin], procainamide [Pronestyl], beta-blockers [e.g., propranolol], quinidine). ▪ Is used with digitalis, but monitor for excessive slowing of heart rate and/or AV block. ▪ May potentiate anesthetics; titrate both drugs carefully. ▪ Potentiates cyclosporine and carbamazepine; may potentiate theophyllines. ▪ May be potentiated by cimetidine (Tagamet) and ranitidine (Zantac). ▪ May cause severe hypotension with fentanyl (Sublimaze). ▪ Any drug metabolized in the liver may cause competitive inhibition of metabolism (e.g., insulin).

SIDE EFFECTS

Arrhythmia (junctional rhythm or isorhythmic dissociation), flushing, hypotension (asymptomatic and symptomatic), and injection site reactions (burning, itching) occurred most frequently and were most often mild and transient but could have serious potential. Amblyopia, asthenia, atrial flutter, AV block (first- or second-degree), bradycardia, chest pain, congestive heart failure, constipation, dizziness, dry mouth, dyspnea, edema, elevated alkaline phosphatase and AST (SGOT), headache, hyperuricemia, nausea, paresthesia, pruritus, sinus node dysfunction, sinus pause, sweating, syncope, ventricular arrhythmias, ventricular fibrillation, ventricular tachycardia, and vomiting have occurred.

ANTIDOTE

Discontinue diltiazem if a high-degree AV block occurs in sinus rhythm. Notify physician promptly of all side effects. Treatment will depend on clinical situation; maintain IV fluids as indicated. Rapid ventricular response in atrial flutter/fibrillation should respond to cardioversion, procainamide, and/or lidocaine. Treat bradycardia, AV block, and asystole with standard AHA protocol (atropine, isoproterenol, pacing). Treat cardiac failure with inotropic agents (isoproterenol, dopamaine, or dobutamine) and diuretics. Calcium chloride will reverse effects of verapamil; may be useful with diltiazem. Dopamine or norepinephrine (levarterenol) and Trendelenburg position should reverse hypotension. Treat allergic reactions or resuscitate as necessary.

DIPHENHYDRAMINE HYDROCHLORIDE

Antihistamine
Antidyskinetic/antiparkinsonism
Antiemetic
Antivertigo agent
Sedative-hypnotic

Bena-D 10/50, Benadryl, Benahist 10/50, Ben-Allergin-50, Bendylate, Benoject 10/50, Hyrexin-50, Nordryl, Wehdryl

pH 5.0 to 6.0

USUAL DOSE

10 to 50 mg. Up to 100 mg may be given. Individualize dose based on patient symptoms and response. Total dosage should not exceed 400 mg/24 hr.

PEDIATRIC DOSE

Children after neonatal period: 1.25 mg/kg/dose every 6 hours as needed or 150 mg/M^2/24 hr in equally divided doses given every 6 hours. Never exceed a total dosage of 300 mg/24 hr.

Anaphylaxis or phenothiazine overdose: 1 to 2 mg/kg IV slowly.

DOSE ADJUSTMENTS

Reduce dose for the elderly or debilitated. ■ Note Drug/lab interactions.

DILUTION

May be given undiluted.

INCOMPATIBLE WITH

Allopurinol (Zyloprim), amobarbital (Amytal), amphotericin B (Fungizone), cephalothin (Keflin), dexamethasone (Decadron), diatrizoate meglumine (Renografin-60), foscarnet (Foscavir), furosemide (Lasix), hydrocortisone (Solu-cortef), iodipamide meglumine (Cholografin), ioxaglate meglumine, methylprednisolone (Solu-Medrol), pentobarbital (Nembutal), phenobarbital (Luminal), phenytoin (Dilantin), secobarbital (Seconal), thiopental (Pentothal).

RATE OF ADMINISTRATION

25 mg or fraction thereof over 1 minute. Extend injection time in non-emergency situations and children (See Maternal/child)

ACTIONS

A potent antihistamine, it is capable of blocking the effects of histamines at various receptor sites, either eliminating allergic reaction or greatly modifying it. It also has anticholinergic (antispasmodic), antiemetic, and sedative effects. It has rapid onset of action and is widely distributed throughout the body. A portion of this drug is metabolized in the liver; the rest is excreted unchanged in the urine. Some secretion may occur in breast milk.

INDICATIONS AND USES

Allergic reactions to blood or plasma. ▪ Supplemental therapy to epinephrine in anaphylaxis and other uncomplicated allergic reactions requiring prompt treatment. ▪ Preoperative or generalized sedation. ▪ Management of parkinsonism including drug induced (e.g., phenothiazines [e.g., prochlorperazine (Compazine)]). ▪ Severe nausea and vomiting. ▪ Motion sickness. ▪ To replace oral therapy when it is impractical or contraindicated.

CONTRAINDICATIONS

Hypersensitivity to antihistamines, lactation, newborn or premature infants.

PRECAUTIONS

IV route used only in emergency situations. ▪ Avoid SC or perivascular injection. ▪ Use with extreme caution in infants, children, elderly or debilitated individuals, asthmatic attack, bladder neck obstruction, narrow-angle glaucoma, lower respiratory tract infections, prostatic hypertrophy, pyloroduodenal obstruction, and stenosing peptic ulcer.

Monitor: Will induce drowsiness. ▪ Monitor vital signs; observe closely. ▪ Note Drug/lab interactions.

Patient education: Do not drive or operate hazardous equipment until effects wear off. ▪ May cause drowsiness and dizziness; request help to ambulate. ▪ Avoid alcohol and other CNS depressants (e.g., diazepam [Valium], narcotics).

Maternal/child: Note Contraindications, Precautions/Monitor, and Side effects. ▪ Pregnancy category B. Use only when clearly needed. May increase risk of abnormalities during the first trimester. ▪ Use extreme caution in infants and children; may cause hallucinations, convulsions, or death. May also reduce mental alertness and cause excitation.

Elderly: Note Dose adjustments, Precautions/Monitor, and Side effects. ▪ May cause confusion, dizziness, hyperexcitability, hypotension and/or sedation. ▪ Sensitivity to cholinergic effects increased (e.g., dry mouth, urinary retention).

DRUG/LAB INTERACTIONS

Increases effectiveness of epinephrine and is often used in conjunction with it. ▪ Potentiates anticholinergics (e.g., Atropine); alcohol, hypnotics, sedatives, tranquilizers, and other CNS depressants (e.g., reserpine, antipyretics); thioridazine (Mellaril); procarbazine (Matulane); and others. Reduced dose of potentiated drug may be indicated. ▪ Anticholinergic and CNS sedative effects prolonged by MAO inhibitors (e.g., selegiline [Eldepryl]). Concurrent use not recommended. ▪ Effectiveness of many drugs is reduced in combination with diphenhydramine because of increased metabolism. ▪ May inhibit the wheal and flare reaction to antigen skin tests.

SIDE EFFECTS

Rare when used as indicated: anaphylaxis; blurring of vision; confusion; constipation; diarrhea; difficulty in urination; diplopia; drowsiness; drug rash; dryness of mouth, nose, and throat; epigastric distress; headache; hemolytic anemia; hypotension; insomnia; nasal stuffiness; nausea; nervousness; palpitations; photosensitivity; rapid pulse; restlessness; thickening of bronchial secretions; tightness of the chest and wheezing; tingling, heaviness, weakness of hands; urticaria; vertigo; vomiting. Overdose may cause convulsions, hallucinations, and death in children.

ANTIDOTE

For exaggerated drowsiness or other disturbing side effects, discontinue the drug and notify the physician. Side effects will usually subside within a few hours or may be treated symptomatically. Treat hypotension promptly; may lead to cardiovascular collapse. Use dopamine (Intropin), norepinephrine, or phenylephrine. Epinephrine is contraindicated for hypotension; further hypotension will occur. Propranolol (Inderal) is the drug of choice for ventricular arrhythmias. Treat convulsions with diazepam (Valium) 0.1 mg/kg IV slowly. Some central anticholinergic effects may require physostigmine. Avoid analeptics (e.g., caffeine); will cause convulsions. Epinephrine must be available to treat anaphylaxis. Resuscitate as necessary.

DIPHTHERIA
ANTITOXIN
Immunizing agent (active)

USUAL DOSE

Testing for sensitivity to horse serum required before use (See Precautions/Monitor) . Suggested ranges for adults and children to be given as a single dose.

Pharyngeal or laryngeal disease of 48 hours duration: 20,000 to 40,000 units.

Nasopharyngeal lesions: 40,000 to 60,000 units.

Extensive disease (3 or more days duration or anyone with brawny swelling of the neck): 80,000 to 120,000 units.

DILUTION

Each 1 ml should be diluted with 19 ml D5W or NS and given as an infusion. Warm to 32° to 35° C (90° to 95° F).

Storage: Refrigerate before dilution.

INCOMPATIBLE WITH

Specific information not available. Do not mix with any other drug in syringe or solution because of specific use.

RATE OF ADMINISTRATION

To be given as a slow IV infusion, 1 ml/min. Titrate carefully to patient reaction.

ACTIONS

A sterile solution of purified antitoxic substances prepared from the blood serum of horses immunized against diphtheria toxin. Neutralizes the toxins produced by *Corynebacterium diphtheriae*.

INDICATIONS AND USES

Passive transient protection against or treatment of patients with clinical symptoms of diphtheria.

CONTRAINDICATIONS

Hypersensitivity to horse serum unless only treatment available for a life-threatening situation. Several techniques including preload of antihistamines and/or desensitization may be considered (see literature).

PRECAUTIONS

In the United States, diphtheria antitoxin may be obtained from the CDC diphtheria duty officer. Call (404) 639-8255 during EST business hours or (404) 639-2888 during non-business hours. Read drug literature supplied with antitoxin completely before use. Essential to evaluate symptoms and individual status of each patient. ■ Determine patient response to any previous injections of serum of any type and history of any allergic-type reactions. ■ Hospitalize patient if possible. ■ Bacteriologic confirmation of the disease is not necessary to initiate treatment. Begin treatment as soon as possible. Each hour delay increases dosage requirements and decreases effectiveness.

Monitor: Test every patient without exception for sensitivity to horse serum (1 ml vial of 1:10 dilution horse serum supplied). Conjunctival test and skin test recommended for maximum safety. Always begin with the conjunctival test.

Conjunctival test: Instill 1 drop 1:10 horse serum into conjunctival sac for adults (1 drop 1:100 dilution for children). Itching, redness, burning, and/or lacrimation within 30 minutes is a positive reaction. A drop of normal saline in the opposite eye is used as a control and should be asymptomatic. Reverse adverse effects of positive reaction with 1 drop epinephrine ophthalmic solution.

Scratch test: Make a 1/4-inch skin scratch through a drop of 1:100 dilution in normal saline. Make a similar scratch through a drop of normal saline on a comparable skin site as a control. Compare sites in 20 minutes. An urticarial wheal surrounded by a zone of erythema is a positive reaction.

Skin test: Inject 0.02 to 0.1 ml of 1:100 horse serum intradermally. In patients with a history of allergies use a 1:1,000 solution. A like injection of normal saline can be used as a control. An urticarial wheal surrounded by a zone of erythema is a positive reaction. Compare in 20 minutes.

Other testing methods may be used. Use at least two. ■ Continue treatment until all symptoms controlled or bacteriologic confirmation of another disease entity confirmed. ■ Use of full therapeutic doses of antimicrobial agents recommended in conjunction with diphtheria antitoxin. ■ All contacts must be evaluated. Prophylactic antibiotics and immunization may be indicated. ■ Note Drug/lab interactions.

DRUG/LAB INTERACTIONS
Concomitant use of antihistamines may interfere with sensitivity tests.

SIDE EFFECTS
Acute anaphylaxis with urticaria, respiratory distress, and vascular collapse. Serum sickness may occur. Usually appears in 7 to 12 days. Local pain, local erythema, and urticaria without systemic reaction can occur.

ANTIDOTE
Discontinue the drug and notify the physician of all side effects. Treat anaphylaxis immediately. Epinephrine (Adrenalin) and diphenhydramine (Benadryl), oxygen, vasopressors (dopamine), corticosteroids, and ventilation equipment must always be available. Salicylates, antihistamines and/or corticosteroids may be useful in serum sickness. Resuscitate as necessary.

DIPYRIDAMOLE

Coronary vasodilator
Diagnostic agent
Platelet aggregation inhibitor

Persantine IV   pH 2.2 to 3.2

USUAL DOSE

Myocardial perfusion imaging: 0.57 mg/kg of body weight equally distributed over 4 minutes (0.142 mg/kg/min). A 70 kg adult would receive a total dose of 39.9 mg (10 mg/min). Never exceed 0.57 mg/kg dose. Thallium should be injected within 5 minutes following the 4-minute infusion of dipyridamole.

Platelet aggregation inhibitor (unlabeled use): 250 mg/24 hr as an infusion.

DILUTION

Each 1 ml (5 mg) must be diluted with a minimum of 2 ml D5W, D5/0.45 NS, or D5/NS. Total volume should range from a minimum of 20 ml to 50 ml (39.9 mg [8 ml] would be diluted in a minimum of 16 ml for a total infusion of 24 ml; additional diluent can be used to facilitate titration). May not be given undiluted; will cause local irritation.

Platelet aggregation inhibitor: Each 250 mg dose should be diluted with 250 ml D5W (1 mg/ml). Concentration may be increased if larger doses required.

Storage: Undiluted drug should be stored at controlled room temperature and protected from direct light; avoid freezing.

INCOMPATIBLE WITH

Specific information not available. Consider specific use.

RATE OF ADMINISTRATION

A single dose must be equally distributed over 4 minutes (0.142 mg/kg/min).

Platelet aggregation inhibitor: 10 mg/hr as a continuous infusion. Use of a microdrip (60 gtt/ml) or infusion pump recommended.

ACTIONS

A coronary vasodilator that will cause an increase in coronary blood flow velocity of from 3.8 to 7 times greater than resting velocity. Action may result from the inhibition of adenosine uptake. Peak velocity is reached in 2.5 to 8.7 minutes. Will cause a 20% increase in heart rate and a mild but significant decrease in systolic and diastolic blood pressure in the supine position. Vital signs may take up to 30 minutes to return to baseline measurements. Used in combination with thallium, visualization shows dilation with sustained enhanced flow of intact vessels, leaving reduced pressure and flow across areas of hemodynamically important coronary vascular constriction. Results achieved are comparable to exercise-induced thallium imaging. Metabolized in the liver. Excreted in bile. Secreted in breast milk.

INDICATIONS AND USES

An alternative to exercise in thallium myocardial perfusion imaging for the evaluation of coronary artery disease in patients who cannot exercise adequately.

Unlabeled use: Prophylactic inhibition of platelet aggregation in thromboembolism and myocardial infarction.

CONTRAINDICATIONS
Hypersensitivity to dipyridamole.

PRECAUTIONS
Administered by or under the direction of the cardiologist. ▪ Full facilities for treatment of any airway, allergic, or cardiac emergency, including laboratory analysis, must be available. ▪ Theophylline (aminophylline) and other emergency drugs must be immediately available. ▪ Patients with a history of unstable angina or a history of asthma may be at greater risk; use extreme caution. ▪ This drug has caused two fatal myocardial infarctions as well as other serious side effects in a small percentage of patients; clinical information to be gained must be weighed against risk to the patient.

Monitor: An IV line with a Y-tube or three-way stop-cock must be in place. ▪ Monitor vital signs continuously during infusion and for at least 15 minutes after or until return to baseline. ▪ ECG monitoring using at least 1 chest lead should be continuous. ▪ Patient is usually in a supine position, but tests have been conducted in a sitting position. Lower to supine with head tilted down (Trendelenburg) if hypotension occurs.

Maternal/child: Pregnancy Category B: safety for use during pregnancy not established. Use only if clearly needed. ▪ Temporarily discontinue nursing. ▪ Safety for use in children not established.

DRUG/LAB INTERACTIONS
May cause a false-negative thallium imaging result if the patient takes maintenance doses of theophylline.

SIDE EFFECTS
Average: Blood pressure lability, chest pain/angina pectoris, dizziness, dyspnea, ECG abnormalities (e.g., extrasystoles, ST-T changes, tachycardia), fatigue, flushing, headache, hypertension, hypotension, nausea, pain (unspecified), paresthesia. Numerous other side effects occur in less than 1% of patients.

Major: Bronchospasm, cerebral ischemia (transient), fatal and nonfatal myocardial infarction, ventricular fibrillation, ventricular tachycardia (symptomatic) occurred in 0.3% of patients.

ANTIDOTE
Physician will be present throughout test administration. Theophylline (aminophylline) is an adenosine receptor antagonist and will reverse the vasodilatory effect of dipyridamole. If bronchospasm or chest pain occur, administer 50 to 250 mg of theophylline at a rate not to exceed 50 mg over 30 seconds. If symptoms are not relieved by 250 mg of theophylline, sublingual nitroglycerin may be helpful. Persistent chest pain may indicate impending potentially fatal myocardial infarction. If patient condition permits, thallium may be injected and allowed to circulate for 1 minute before injection of theophylline (aminophylline); this will permit initial thallium perfusion imaging before reversal of vasodilatory effects of dipyridamole on coronary circulation. Use head-down supine position for hypotension before administering theophylline (aminophylline). After reversal of vasodilatory action, treat arrhythmias as indicated. Resuscitate as necessary.

DOBUTAMINE HYDROCHLORIDE

Inotropic agent
Cardiac stimulant

Dobutrex

pH 2.5 to 5.5

USUAL DOSE

2.5 to 15 mcg/kg of body weight/min initially. Adjust rate to effect desired response. Up to 40 mcg/kg/min has been used in some instances; increases potential for toxicity.

PEDIATRIC DOSE

2 to 20 mcg/kg/min initially. Adjust rate to effect desired response.

DOSE ADJUSTMENTS

Note Drug/lab interactions.

DILUTION

Now available prediluted in D5W. Each 250 mg (20 ml) vial must be further diluted to at least 50 ml. Any amount of infusion solution desired above 50 ml may be used. (250 mg in 1 L equals 250 mcg/ml; 250 mg in 500 ml equals 500 mcg/ml; 250 mg in 250 ml equals 1,000 mcg/ml). Adjust to fluid requirements of the patient. Compatible with D5W, D5/0.45 NS, D5/NS, D5/Isolyte M, Isolyte M, lactated Ringer's, D5/LR or Normosol-M in D5W; D10W; 20% Osmitrol in water; 0.45 NS, NS or sodium lactate.

Pediatric dilution: 6.0 mg/kg in 100 ml diluent. 1 ml/hr equals 1.0 mcg/kg/min.

Storage: When mixed in infusion solution, use within 24 hours. Pink coloring of solution does not affect potency; will crystallize if frozen.

INCOMPATIBLE WITH

Acyclovir (Zovirax), alkaline solutions (e.g., aminophylline, sodium bicarbonate), alteplase (tPA) bretylium (Bretylol), bumetanide (Bumex), calcium chloride, calcium gluconate, cefamandole (Mandol), cefazolin (Kefzol), cephalothin (Keflin), diazepam (Valium), digoxin, doxapram (Dopram), floxacillin (Floxapen), foscarnet (Foscavir), furosemide (Lasix), heparin, hydrocortisone, indomethacin (Indocin), insulin, magnesium sulfate, midazolam (Versed), penicillin, phenytoin (Dilantin), phytonadione (Aquamephyton), piperacillin/tazobactam (Zosyn), potassium chloride, potassium phosphate, sodium ethacrynate (Edecrin).

RATE OF ADMINISTRATION

Begin with recommended dose for body weight and seriousness of condition. Gradually increase to effect desired response. May take up to 10 minutes to achieve peak effect of a specific dose. Maintain at correct therapeutic level with microdrip (60 gtt/ml) or infusion pump. Half-life of dobutamine is only about 2 minutes.

Rates of Infusion for Dobutamine Concentrations of 250, 500, and 1,000 mcg/mL			
	Infusion delivery rate		
Drug delivery rate (mcg/kg/min)	250 mcg/mL* (mL/kg/min)	500 mcg/mL† (mL/kg/min)	1,000 mcg/mL‡ (mL/kg/min)
2.5	0.01	0.005	0.0025
5	0.02	0.01	0.005
7.5	0.03	0.015	0.0075
10	0.04	0.02	0.01
12.5	0.05	0.025	0.0125
15	0.06	0.03	0.015

*250 mcg/mL or 250 mg/1,000 mL of diluent.
†500 mcg/mL or 250 mg/500 mL of diluent.
‡1,000 mcg/mL or 250 mg/250 mL of diluent.

ACTIONS

A synthetic catecholamine chemically related to dopamine, it is a directacting inotropic agent possessing beta-stimulator activity. Induces short-term increases in cardiac output by improving stroke volume with minimum increases in rate and blood pressure, minimum rhythm disturbances, and decreased peripheral vascular resistance. Usually most effective for only a few hours. May improve atrioventricular conduction. Peak effect obtained in 2 to 10 minutes. Has a very short duration of action. Half-life is 2 minutes; may be up to 5 minutes in preterm infants. Metabolized in the liver and other tissues. Metabolites are primarily excreted in the urine.

INDICATIONS AND USES

Short-term inotropic support in cardiac decompensation resulting from depressed contractility (organic heart disease or cardiac surgical procedures).

Investigational use: Increase cardiac output in children with congenital heart disease undergoing cardiac catheterization.

CONTRAINDICATIONS

Hypersensitivity to any components (contains sulfites), idiopathic hypertrophic subaortic stenosis, shock without adequate fluid replacement.

PRECAUTIONS

Use extreme caution in myocardial infarction; increases in heart rate of more than 10% may increase myocardial ischemia and size of infarction. ■ Contains sulfites; use caution in patients with allergies. ■ Precipitous hypotension occurs rarely, usually reverses with a decrease in rate of administration. ■ Ineffective if marked mechanical obstruction (e.g., severe valvular aortic stenosis) is present.

Monitor: Correct hypovolemia and acidosis as indicated before initiating treatment. ■ Observe patient's response continuously, monitor heart rate, ectopic activity, blood pressure, and urine flow. Measure pulmonary wedge pressure, central venous pressure, and cardiac output if possible.

■ Use digitalis preparation before starting dobutamine in patients with atrial fibrillation with rapid ventricular response. ■ Compatible through common tubing with dopamine, lidocaine, tobramycin, nitroprusside, potassium chloride, and protamine sulfate. ■ Note Drug/lab interactions. *Maternal/child:* Pregnancy Category B; use only if benefits outweigh risks. Safety for use in pregnancy, lactation, and in children not established.

DRUG/LAB INTERACTIONS

May be ineffective if beta-blocking drugs (e.g., propranolol [Inderal]) have been given. ■ Produces higher cardiac output and lower pulmonary wedge pressure when given concomitantly with nitroprusside. ■ May cause serious arrhythmias in presence of cyclopropane or halogen anesthetics, severe hypertension with oxytocic drugs, or guanethidine (Ismelin). ■ Pressor response increased with tricyclic antidepressants (e.g., amitriptyline [Elavil]) and rauwolfia alkaloids (e.g., reserpine [Serpasil]); may cause hypertension. ■ May cause arrhythmias with bretylium.

SIDE EFFECTS

Anginal pain, chest pain, headache, hypertension, hypokalemia, increased ventricular ectopic activity, nausea, palpitations, shortness of breath, tachycardia.

Overdose: In addition to all of the above, overdose may cause anorexia, anxiety, excessive hypertension or hypotension, myocardial ischemia, tremor, ventricular tachycardia, and/or fibrillation.

ANTIDOTE

Notify physician of all side effects. Decrease infusion rate and notify physician immediately if number of PVCs increases or there is a marked increase in pulse rate (30 or more beats) or blood pressure (50 or more mm Hg systolic). For accidental overdose, reduce rate or temporarily discontinue until condition stabilizes. Note Precautions.

DOCETAXEL

Antineoplastic agent
(Miscellaneous)

Taxotere

USUAL DOSE

Premedication: Must be pretreated with oral corticosteroids, with or without diphenhydramine (Benadryl) and/or H_2 antagonists (e.g., famotidine [Pepcid], or ranitidine [Zantac]), to reduce the incidence and severity of fluid retention, hypersensitivity reactions, infection, stomatitis, and cutaneous toxicity. Usual regimen for dexamethasone (Decadron) is 8 mg twice a day for 5 days. Begin one day prior to each docetaxel infusion.

Breast cancer/non-small-cell lung cancer: 60 to 100 mg/M^2 as an infusion. Repeat every 3 weeks.

Ovarian/small-cell lung cancer (investigational): 100 mg/M^2 as an infusion. Repeat every 3 weeks.

PEDIATRIC DOSE

Safety for use in children not established.

DOSE ADJUSTMENTS

Withhold therapy if neutrophils below 1,500/mm^3 or platelets below 100,000 cells/mm^3. ■ Reduce dose to 75 mg/M^2 for patients initially dosed at 100 mg/M^2 who experience febrile neutropenia, severe neutropenia (neutrophils below 500/mm^3 for more than one week), severe or cumulative cutaneous reaction, or severe peripheral neuropathy. Further reduce to 55 mg/M^2 if any of the above reactions persist. ■ Reduce dose to 75 mg/M^2 in mild to moderate impaired liver function (e.g., ALT and/or AST greater than 1.5 times upper limit of normal range and increases in alkaline phosphatase greater than 2.5 times the upper limits of normal range); note Contraindications. ■ Patients receiving the lower dose of docetaxel (60 mg/M^2) may have the dose increased gradually if lower dose was well tolerated.

DILUTION

Specific techniques required; see Precautions. More than one vial of docetaxel and diluent may be required. Repeat procedure for reconstitution of each vial required. Allow vials to stand at room temperature for 5 minutes. Withdraw entire contents of diluent vial (provided by manufacturer) into a syringe and transfer to vial of docetaxel concentrate (10 mg/ml). Gently rotate docetaxel vial(s) at least 15 seconds to assure full mixture. Allow to stand for several minutes to allow most of the foam to dissipate. Total dose must be further diluted in a minimum of 250 ml of NS or D5W, manually rotated to mix thoroughly, and given as an infusion. Should be administered through polyethylene-lined administration sets. Desired concentration should be between 0.3 to 0.9 mg/ml (100 mg in 250 ml = 0.4 mg/ml). Solution should be clear.

Storage: Refrigerate unopened vials of docetaxel and diluent in cartons to protect from light. Reconstituted or diluted solutions should be used promptly. Fully diluted solutions are stable for up to 8 hours either refrigerated or at room temperature; glass or polypropylene bottles or plastic (polypropylene or polyolefin) bags are indicated to minimize patient exposure to leached DEHP.

INCOMPATIBLE WITH

Specific information not available. Consider toxicity and specific use.

RATE OF ADMINISTRATION

A single dose, properly diluted, equally distributed over 1 hour. Room temperature should be cool and lighting should be low. Extended infusion rates (e.g., 6 to 24 hours) or frequently repeated infusions (e.g., several days in a row) seem to increase the risk of dose-limiting mucositis.

ACTIONS

An antineoplastic. A novel semi-synthetic antimicrotubule agent derived from the needles of the yew plant. It inhibits cancer cell division by acting on the cells internal skeleton, which is made of elements called microtubules. Microtubules assemble and disassemble during the cell cycle. Docetaxel promotes the assembly and blocks the disassembly of microtubules, preventing the cancer cells from dividing. The end result is cancer cell death. May be up to twice as potent as paclitaxel; cross-resistance between docetaxel and paclitaxel does not occur consistently. Highly protein bound. Probably metabolized in the liver by isoenzymes of the P$_{450}$ family. Half-life is 11.1 hours. Eliminated primarily through feces and bile.

INDICATIONS AND USES

Treatment of locally advanced or metastatic breast cancer refractory to previous therapy which should have included an anthracycline (e.g., doxorubicin) unless contraindicated. ▪ Approved in Canada for treatment of locally advanced or metastatic non-small cell lung cancer after failure of platinum based chemotherapy (e.g., cisplatin).

Investigational uses: First line treatment in combination with other chemotherapy agents to treat breast or non-small cell lung cancers. ▪ Treatment of ovarian cancer, pancreatic cancer, stomach cancer, and soft tissue sarcoma.

CONTRAINDICATIONS

Baseline neutropenia < 1,500 cells/mm^3, history of hypersensitivity reactions to docetaxel or other drugs formulated with polysorbate 80, severe impaired liver function. In the U.S. docetaxel is not recommended for patients with a bilirubin in the upper limits of normal, or in patients with ALT and/or AST greater than 1.5 times upper limit of normal range and increases in alkaline phosphatase greater than 2.5 times the upper limits of normal range.

PRECAUTIONS

Follow guidelines for handling cytotoxic agents. See Appendix A. p. 893. ▪ Usually administered by or under the direction of the physician specialist. ▪ Adequate diagnostic and treatment facilities must be readily available. ▪ Patients hypersensitive to paclitaxel may also be hypersensitive to docetaxel. ▪ Myelosuppression may be more frequent and more severe in patients who have received prior cytotoxic drug therapy or radiation therapy. ▪ Incidence of mortality increased in patients with abnormal liver function and in those receiving higher doses. ▪ Use with caution in patients with pleural effusion; may be exacerbated by docetaxel-induced fluid retention. ▪ Note Drug/lab interactions.

Monitor: Obtain baseline CBC with differential and platelets, monitor frequently during therapy and before each dose. Note Dose adjustments. ▪ Obtain baseline bilirubin, AST, ALT, and alkaline phosphatase; monitor as indicated during therapy (recommended before each dose). ▪ Determine absolute patency of vein. A stinging or burning sensation indicates extravasation; severe cellulitis and tissue necrosis may result. Discontinue injection; use another vein. ▪ Monitor for hypersensitivity reactions, may occur within minutes. Discontinue docetaxel if severe (e.g., bronchospasm, hypotension, generalized rash/erythema). Continue to monitor for a minimum of 1 hour following the infusion, especially during the first two treatment cycles. ▪ Monitor for localized erythema of the palms of the hands and soles of the feet with or without desquamation. A reduced dose may be indicated if severe. ▪ Monitor for fluid retention. Severe salt restriction and treatment with oral diuretics may be indicated. ▪ Observe for signs of peripheral neurotoxicity. ▪ Observe for signs of infection. Use of prophylactic antibiotics may be indicated pending C/S in a febrile, neutorpenic patient. ▪ Prophylactic antiemetics may improve patient comfort.

Patient education: Avoid pregnancy; nonhormonal birth control recommended. ▪ Review of monitoring requirements and adverse events before therapy imperative. ▪ Report pain or burning at injection site, and any unusual or unexpected symptoms or side effects as soon as possible.

■ May produce significant hypotension. Effects may be additive with current medications. Review all medications (prescription and nonprescription) with nurse and/or physician. ■ See Appendix D, p. 900. ■ Obtain name and telephone number of a contact person for emergencies, questions, or problems. ■ Seek resources for counseling or supportive therapy.

Maternal/child: Category D, avoid pregnancy, may cause fetal harm. ■ Discontinue breast feeding. ■ Safety for use in children not established, but clinical studies have shown that the maximum tolerated dose is lower in children than in adults, especially if they have been treated with prior courses of chemotherapy. A colony-stimulating factor (e.g., filgrastim, sargramostim) has been used to reduce neutropenia and increase tolerance to the maximum dose.

Elderly: No specific recommendations at this time. Monitor hepatic function carefully.

DRUG/LAB INTERACTIONS

Metabolism inhibited and serum levels increased with ketoconazole (Nizoral). ■ Monitor drug profile carefully to avoid problems with other agents that may affect or be affected by cytochrome P_{450} processes (e.g., cyclosporine [Sandimmune], erythromycin, midazolam [Versed], terfenadine, testosterone, troleandomycin [TAO]). ■ Additive bone marrow depression may occur with radiation therapy and/or other bone marrow depressing agents (e.g., azathioprine [Imuran], chloramphenicol, melphalan [Alkeran]). Dose reduction may be required. ■ Risk of infection is increased with concurrent use of other immunosuppressants (e.g., azathioprine, chlorambucil [Leukeran], cyclophosphamide [Cytoxan], cyclosporine [Sandimmune], glucocorticoid corticosteroids [e.g., dexamethasone], muromonab CD-3 [Orthoclone], tacrolimus [Prograf]). ■ Docetaxel metabolism is inhibited by paclitaxel, and to a lesser extent paclitaxel may be inhibited by docetaxel. Docetaxel may also be inhibited by other agents metabolized by the CYP 3A isoenzyme. ■ Do not administer live vaccines to patients receiving antineoplastic agents.

SIDE EFFECTS

Generally reversible but can be fatal. Bone marrow suppression is dose dependent and can be dose limiting (leukopenia <4,000/mm^3 [97%], <1,000/mm^3 [27%], neutropenia <2,000/mm^3 [97%], <500/mm^3 [5%], thrombocytopenia <100,000/mm^3 [8%]). Alopecia (83%), anemia <11 Gm/dl (89%) <8 Gm/dl (10%), cardiac arrhythmias (2%), cutaneous (e.g., localized rash on hands, feet, arms, face, thorax) (65%) severe (9%), diarrhea (43%), increased ALT, AST (10%), and bilirubin (5%), infections (19%), febrile neutropenia (22%), fever without infection (36%), fluid retention (e.g., ascites, edema, pericardial effusion, pleural effusion) (47%) severe (9%), hypersensitivity reactions (e.g., back pain, chest tightness, chills, drug fever, dyspnea, flushing, pruritus, rash) (31%) severe with hypotension (7%), infusion site reactions (6%), nausea (45%), paresthesiae (e.g., pain, burning sensation) (48%), stomatitis (42%), vomiting (28%).

Overdose: Bone marrow suppression, mucositis, peripheral neurotoxicity.

ANTIDOTE

Keep physician informed of all side effects. Most will be treated symptomatically as indicated. Most hypersensitivity reactions will subside with temporary discontinuation of docetaxel, and incidence seems to decrease with subsequent doses. Severe reactions may require epinephrine (Adrenalin), antihistamines (e.g., diphenhydramine [Benadryl]), corticosteroids (e.g., dexamethasone [Decadron]), or bronchodilators (e.g., albuterol [Ventolin], theophylline [aminophylline]). Do not rechallenge. Neutropenia can be profound and the nadir usually occurs about day 8. Recovery is generally rapid and spontaneous but may be treated with filgrastim (G-CSF, Neupogen). Severe thrombocytopenia may require platelet transfusions or treatment with oprelvekin (Numega) may be indicated. Severe anemia (<8 Gm/dl) may require packed cell transfusions, moderate anemia (<11 Gm/dl) may be treated with epoetin alfa (Epogen). Hypotension and bradycardia do not usually occur at the same time except in hypersensitivity. Treat only if symptomatic. Treat any serious or symptomatic arrhythmia (e.g., conduction abnormalities, ventricular tachycardia) promptly and monitor continuously during subsequent doses. Serious cutaneous reactions with desquamation (rare), serious fluid retention (more frequent with cumulative doses of 1,300 mg/M^2), or severe liver impairment may require discontinuation of docetaxel. Cutaneous reactions (palmar-plantar erythrodysesthesia) that occur despite prophylaxis may respond to pyridoxine 50 mg three times a day. There is no specific antidote for overdose. Supportive therapy will help sustain the patient in toxicity. Resuscitate if indicated.

DOLASETRON MESYLATE

Anzemet

Antiemetic
(5 HT$_3$ Receptor antagonist)

pH 3.2 to 3.8

USUAL DOSE

Prevention of chemotherapy-induced nausea and vomiting: 1.8 mg/kg as a single dose 30 minutes before chemotherapy. Alternatively, a fixed dose of 100 mg may be used for most patients.

Prevention of postoperative nausea and/or vomiting: 12.5 mg as a single dose 15 minutes before cessation of anesthesia.

Treatment of postoperative nausea and/or vomiting: 12.5 mg as a single dose as soon as nausea or vomiting presents.

Radiotherapy-induced nausea and vomiting (unlabeled use): 40 mg or 0.3 mg/kg at time of treatment or when nausea or vomiting presents.

PEDIATRIC DOSE

Doses are those recommended for *pediatric patients 2 to 16 years of age.* Safety and effectiveness in children under 2 years of age have not been established. Dolasetron solution for injection may be mixed with apple or apple-grape juice for oral administration to pediatric patients.

Prevention of chemotherapy-induced nausea and vomiting: 1.8 mg/kg up to a maximum of 100 mg as a single dose 30 minutes before chemotherapy.

Prevention of postoperative nausea and/or vomiting: 0.35 mg/kg up to a maximum dose of 12.5 mg as a single dose 15 minutes before cessation of anesthesia.

Treatment of postoperative nausea and/or vomiting: 0.35 mg/kg up to a maximum dose of 12.5 mg as a single dose as soon as nausea or vomiting presents.

DOSE ADJUSTMENTS

No dose adjustments required for the elderly, renal failure, or impaired hepatic function.

DILUTION

IV injection: A single dose may be given undiluted.

IV infusion: A single dose may be further diluted up to 50 ml in NS, D5W, D5/0.45NS, D5/LR, LR, or 10% mannitol.

Storage: Store vials at CRT; protect from light. Stable after dilution at CRT for 24 hours or 48 hours if refrigerated.

INCOMPATIBLE WITH

Manufacturer states, "Should not be mixed with other drugs. Flush the infusion line with a compatible IV solution before and after administration."

RATE OF ADMINISTRATION

Flush infusion line before and after administration.

IV injection: A single dose over 30 seconds.

IV infusion: A single dose over up to 15 minutes.

ACTIONS

An antinauseant and antiemetic agent. A selective antagonist of specific serotonin receptors, similar to granisetron and ondansetron. Chemotherapeutic agents such as cisplatin increase the release of serotonin from specific cells in the GI tract, causing emesis. By antagonizing these receptors, chemotherapy-induced nausea and vomiting are prevented. Rapidly and completely metabolized to its active metabolite, hydrodolasetron. Hydrodolasetron is widely distributed throughout the body. Maximum concentration occurs 0.6 hours after injection or infusion. Average half-life is 7.3 hours. Plasma clearance increased and half-life reduced in children, more so in younger children. Excreted in urine and feces. Not known if dolasetron is secreted in breast milk.

INDICATIONS AND USES

Prevention of nausea and vomiting associated with initial and repeat courses of emetogenic cancer chemotherapy, including high-dose cisplatin. ▪ Prevention of postoperative nausea and vomiting when indicated. ▪ Treatment of postoperative nausea and/or vomiting. Also available in tablet form.

Unlabeled use: Prophylaxis and treatment of radiotherapy-induced nausea and vomiting.

CONTRAINDICATIONS

Known hypersensitivity to dolasetron.

PRECAUTIONS

Use with caution in patients who have or may develop prolongation of cardiac conduction intervals, particularly QT intervals (e.g., patients with hypokalemia, hypomagnesemia, congenital QT syndrome, cumultive high-dose anthracycline therapy [e.g., doxorubicin (Adriamycin)], patients taking diuretics with potential for inducing electrolyte abnormalities [e.g., furosemide, hydrochlorothiazide] or antiarrhythmic drugs or other drugs that lead to QT prolongation [amiodarone, procainamide, quinidine]). ▪ Available in tablet form. ▪ Note Drug/lab interactions and Side effects.

Monitor: Observe closely. Any patient found to have a second-degree or higher AV conduction block should be monitored continuously. ▪ Ambulate slowly to avoid orthostatic hypotension. ▪ Does not influence anesthesia recovery time.

Patient education: Request assistance for ambulation. ▪ Report promptly if nausea persists. ▪ Maintain adequate hydration. ▪ Review prescription medications with health care provider.

Maternal/child: Category B: no evidence of impaired fertility or harm to fetus. Use during pregnancy only if clearly needed. ▪ Use caution if required during lactation. ▪ Safety and effectiveness for use in children under 2 years of age have not been established. ▪ Plasma clearance increased and half-life reduced in children, more so in younger children.

Elderly: Response similar to other age groups. No dose adjustment required.

DRUG/LAB INTERACTIONS

Does not induce or inhibit the cytochrome P_{450} drug metabolizing system, but plasma levels increased when given concurrently with cimetidine (Tagamet [inhibitor of cytochrome P_{450}]), and decreased when given concurrently with rifampin (Rifadin [inducer of cytochrome P_{450}]); clinical significance not known. ▪ Clearance decreased when given concurrently with atenolol (Tenormin). ▪ Note precautions and use extreme caution with diuretics with potential for inducing electrolyte abnormalities (e.g., furosemide [Lasix], hydrochlorothiazide [Hydrodiuril]) or antiarrhythmic drugs or other drugs that lead to prolonged QT intervals (e.g., amiodarone [Cordarone], procainamide [Pronestyl], quinidine). ▪ Clearance not affected by ACE inhibitors (e.g., enalaprilat), calcium channel blockers (e.g., diltiazem [Cardizem], nifedipine [Procardia], verapamil [Isoptin]), glyburide (DiaBeta), propranolol (Inderal), and various chemotherapy agents. ▪ Has been safely coadministered with drugs used in chemotherapy and surgery (recovery time not affected). ▪ Has not inhibited the antitumor activity of cisplatin, 5-fluorouracil, doxorubicin, or cyclophosphamide in murine models.

SIDE EFFECTS

Can cause ECG interval changes (PR, QT, JT prolongation, and QRS widening). While these changes have rarely been reported, they may lead to cardiovascular consequences (e.g., cardiac arrhythmias, heart block). Usually self-limiting with declining blood levels, but may last as long as 24 hours.

Average dose: Abdominal pain, abnormal liver function tests (transient increased AST, ALT), chills, diarrhea, dizziness, fatigue, fever, headache, hypertension, pain, shivering. Numerous other side effects may occur in <2% of patients.

Overdose: Severe hypotension and dizziness.

ANTIDOTE

Most side effects will be treated symptomatically. Keep physician informed. Overdose in one patient was treated with plasma expanders (e.g., albumin, dextran), dopamine (Intropin), atropine, and continuous BP and ECG monitoring. Epinephrine, atropine, and/or cardiac pacing may be required to treat ECG interval changes. Prolonged QT interval may lead to VT or other ventricular arrhythmias. There is no specific antidote. Treat anaphylaxis and resuscitate as necessary.

DOPAMINE HYDROCHLORIDE

Inotropic agent
Cardiac stimulant
Vasopressor

Intropin, ✦Revimine

pH 2.5 to 5.0

USUAL DOSE

2 to 5 mcg/kg of body weight/min initially in patients likely to respond to minimum treatment. 5 to 10 mcg/kg/min may be required initially to correct hypotension in the seriously ill patient. Gradually increase by 5 to 10 mcg/kg/min at 10- to 30-minute intervals until optimum response occurs. Average dose is 20 mcg/kg/min; over 50 mcg/kg/min has been required in some instances but is not recommended. If more than 20 mcg/kg/min is required to maintain blood pressure, consider use of norepinephrine (Levophed) in addition. Doses over 20 mcg/kg/min decrease renal perfusion.

DOSE ADJUSTMENTS

Reduce dose to one tenth of the calculated amount for individuals being treated with MAO inhibitors (e.g., isocarboxazid [Marplan]) and drugs with MAO-inhibiting effects (e.g., furazolidone [Furoxone]).
■ Note Drug/lab interactions.

DILUTION

Each 5 or 10 ml (200 mg, 400 mg, or 800 mg) ampoule must be diluted in 250 to 500 ml of the following IV solutions and given as an infusion: NS, D5W, D5/NS, D5/0.45S, D5/LR, 1/6 molar sodium lactate, or lactated Ringer's injection.

Concentration of dopamine	40 mg/ml		80 mg/ml
Volume of dopamine	5 ml (200 mg)	10 ml (400 mg)	10 ml (800 mg)
250 ml diluent	800 mcg/ml	1,600 mcg/ml	3,200 mcg/ml
500 ml diluent	400 mcg/ml	800 mcg/ml	1,600 mcg/ml
1,000 ml diluent	200 mcg/ml	400 mcg/ml	800 mcg/ml

Available prediluted in 250 ml or 500 ml of D5W. Dopamine content varies: choose 0.8 mg/ml, 1.6 mg/ml, or 3.2 mg/ml. More concentrated solutions may be used if absolutely necessary to reduce fluid volume. Also available as 160 mg/ml to be added to 100 ml of diluent (1600 mcg/ml); may be used in patients with fluid retention or those requiring a very slow rate of infusion.
Pediatric dilution: 6.0 mg/kg in 100 ml D5W. 1 ml/hr equals 1.0 mcg/kg/min.
Storage: Discard diluted solution after 24 hours.

INCOMPATIBLE WITH

Acyclovir (Zovirax), alkaline solutions, alteplase (tPA), amphotericin B, ampicillin (Polycillin-N), cephalothin (Keflin), gentamicin (Garamycin), indomethacin (Indocin), insulin, penicillin, sodium bicarbonate.

RATE OF ADMINISTRATION

Begin with recommended dose for body weight and seriousness of condition. Gradually increase by 5 to 10 mcg/kg of body weight/min to effect desired response. Use slowest possible rate to maintain adequate or preset systolic blood pressure. Use a microdrip (60 gtt/ml) or an infusion pump for accuracy. Optimum urine flow determines correct evaluation of dosage. Decrease dose gradually; may cause marked hypotension if discontinued suddenly.

ACTIONS

Dopamine is a chemical precursor of norepinephrine, possessing alpha, beta, and dopaminergic-receptor-stimulating actions. Increases cardiac output with minimum increase in myocardial oxygen consumption. Dilates renal and mesenteric blood vessels at doses lower than those required to elevate systolic blood pressure. Therapeutic doses effect little change on diastolic blood pressure. Doses over 10 mcg/kg/min may cause peripheral vasoconstriction and marked increases in pulmonary occlusive pressure. Has short duration of action. Metabolized by monoamine oxidase (MAO) catechol-o-methyltransferase (COMT) to inactive metabolites and is promptly excreted in the urine.

INDICATIONS AND USES

To correct hemodynamic imbalances including hypotension resulting from shock syndrome of myocardial infarction, trauma, endotoxic septicemia, open heart surgery, renal failure, and chronic cardiac decompensation. ▪ Drug of choice for hypotension and shock.

Investigational uses: Chronic obstructive pulmonary disease (4 mcg/kg/min), congestive heart failure (2 to 5 mcg/kg/min), infant respiratory distress syndrome (begin at 5 mcg/kg/min).

CONTRAINDICATIONS

Hypersensitivity to any components (contains sulfites), pheochromocytoma, uncorrected tachyarrhythmias, ventricular fibrillation.

PRECAUTIONS

Some preparations contain sulfites; use caution in patients with allergies. ▪ Use caution in patients with a history of occlusive vascular disease.

Monitor: Recognition of signs and symptoms and prompt treatment with dopamine will improve prognosis. ▪ Check blood pressure every 2 minutes until stabilized at the desired level. Check every 5 minutes thereafter during therapy. Avoid hypertension. If possible check central venous pressure or pulmonary wedge pressure before administration and as ordered thereafter. ▪ Use larger veins (antecubital fossa) and avoid extravasation; may cause necrosis and sloughing of tissue. Central vein preferred for continuous infusions. ▪ If possible, correct hypovolemia with whole blood or plasma as indicated; correct acidosis if present. ▪ Monitor for decreased urine output, increased tachycardia, or new arrhythmias. ▪ With high dose administration, palpate pulses and monitor extremities for signs of peripheral vasoconstriction (e.g., coldness, paresthesias). ▪ Therapy may be continued until the patient can maintain hemodynamic and renal functions. ▪ Note Drug/lab interactions.

Maternal/ child: Pregnancy Category C: safety for use in pregnancy and lactation not established. If used benefits must outweigh risks. ■ Safety for use in children not established. Has been used, but experience is limited.

DRUG/LAB INTERACTIONS

Alkaline solutions, including sodium bicarbonate, inactivate dopamine. ■ May cause serious arrhythmias in presence of cyclopropane or halogen anesthetics, severe hypertension with oxytocic drugs (e.g., methylergonovine [Methergine] or oxytocin). ■ May cause hypertensive crisis with MAO inhibitors (e.g., selegiline [Eldepryl]). ■ Antagonizes effects of guanethidine (Ismelin). ■ Some effects may be antagonized by alpha- or beta-blocking agents (e.g., labetalol [Trandate], propranolol [Inderal]). ■ Pressor response may be decreased by tricyclic antidepressants; increased doses of dopamine may be required. ■ Will cause severe bradycardia and hypotension with phenytoin (Dilantin). ■ Note Dose adjustments.

SIDE EFFECTS

Aberrant conduction, anginal pain, azotemia, bradycardia, dyspnea, ectopic beats, headache, hypertension, hypotension, nausea, palpitation, piloerection, tachycardia, vasoconstriction, vomiting, widened QRS complex.

ANTIDOTE

Notify the physician of all side effects. Decrease infusion rate and notify the physician immediately for decrease in established urine flow rate, disproportionate rise in diastolic blood pressure, increasing tachycardia, or new arrhythmias. For accidental overdosage with hypertension, reduce rate or temporarily discontinue until condition stabilizes. Phentolamine may be required. To prevent sloughing and necrosis in areas where extravasation has occurred, with a fine hypodermic needle inject 5 to 10 mg of phentolamine (Regitine) diluted in 10 to 15 ml normal saline liberally throughout the tissue in the extravasated area. Begin as soon as extravasation recognized.

DOXACURIUM CHLORIDE

Nuromax

Neuromuscular blocking agent
(Nondepolarizing)
Anesthesia adjunct

pH 3.9 to 5.0

USUAL DOSE

Must be individualized based on age, weight/degree of obesity, renal, hepatic, and/or other diseases. Clinical duration varies greatly.

Adults under balanced anesthesia: 0.05 mg/kg of body weight to provide an average of 100 minutes of clinical relaxation (time to 25% recovery). Lower doses may result in a longer time for development of satisfactory conditions. In select situations where a very prolonged block is required, 0.08 mg/kg will provide an average of 160 minutes of clinical relaxation.

Following succinylcholine to facilitate intubation and with balanced anesthesia: 0.025 mg/kg to provide approximately 60 minutes of clinical relaxation. Use a larger initial dose to provide longer periods of relaxation.

Maintenance dose: 0.005 mg/kg to 0.01 mg/kg administered at 25% recovery will extend relaxation another 30 to 45 minutes. Determine need for maintenance dose based on beginning symptoms of neuromuscular blockade reversal determined by a peripheral nerve stimulator. Adjust dose based on desired duration. Repeated maintenance doses at 25% recovery usually do not produce a cumulative effect.

PEDIATRIC DOSE

Children over 2 years of age under halothane anesthesia: 0.03 mg/kg to 0.05 mg/kg to provide 30 to 45 minutes of clinical relaxation. Children require higher doses on a mg/kg basis than adults to achieve comparable levels of block. Time of onset and duration are shorter.

Maintenance dose: See adult mg/kg maintenance dose. Higher doses may be required in children receiving balanced anesthesia than those receiving halothane.

DOSE ADJUSTMENTS

In presence of inhalational anesthetics (e.g., isoflurane, enflurane, halothane) dose reduction by one-third should be considered. ■ Reduced dose based on ideal body weight required in obesity (30% or more over ideal body weight) Specific calculation required (males, [106 + (6 × inches in height above 5 feet) ÷ 2.2] = IBW in kg; females, [100 + (5 × inches in height above 5 feet) ÷ 2.2] = IBW in kg). ■ Reduced dose may be required in impaired renal function, the elderly, cachetic or debilitated patients, in patients with neuromuscular diseases, severe electrolyte abnormalities, or carcinomatosis. ■ Increased doses may be required in burn patients. ■ Impaired hepatic function may require an increased dose due to reduced sensitivity to effects. ■ Reduced dose may be required with other drugs that prolong neuromuscular blockade. ■ Note Drug/lab interactions.

DILUTION

Supplied as 1 mg/ml. May be further diluted in D5W or NS. Up to 10 ml diluent may be added to each 1 ml doxacurium (10 ml to 1 mg [1 ml] yields 0.1 mg/ml).

Storage: Stable for up to 24 hours aseptically diluted and stored in syringes at 5° to 25° C (41° to 77° F). Immediate use of diluted product is preferred; discard any unused portion after 8 hours.

INCOMPATIBLE WITH

Alkaline solutions with a pH over 8.5 (e.g., barbiturates). Use of a Y-site and irrigation with normal saline may be required.

COMPATIBLE WITH

D5W, NS, D5NS, D5LR, LR, alfentanil (Alfenta), fentanyl (Sublimaze), and sufetanil (Sufenta), through Y-site.

RATE OF ADMINISTRATION

A single dose over 5 to 15 seconds. Titrate to desired effect. Use a peripheral nerve stimulator to monitor response to doxacurium, avoid overdose, monitor need for additional relaxant, and monitor adequacy of spontaneous recovery or antagonism.

ACTIONS

A long-acting nondepolarizing neuromuscular blocking agent. Causes skeletal muscle relaxation and paralysis by competing for cholinergic receptors at the motor end-plate. Onset of action is dose dependent. Produces maximum neuromuscular blockade within 4 to 7 minutes and lasts from 1 to 2 hours. Length of action extended based on degree of renal impairment. 2.5 to 3 times more potent than pancuronium (Pavulon). It may take another 30 minutes or up to several hours before complete recovery occurs. Does not cause cardiovascular effects associated with other neuromuscular blocking agents (e.g., pancuronium [Pavulon]). Excreted mostly as unchanged drug in urine.

INDICATIONS AND USES

Recommended for use in procedures lasting 90 minutes or longer. Adjunct to general anesthesia, to facilitate endotracheal intubation and to provide skeletal muscle relaxation during surgery and mechanical ventilation.

Unlabeled use: Has had limited use in an ICU setting.

CONTRAINDICATIONS

Hypersensitivity to doxacurium.

PRECAUTIONS

For IV use only. ▪ Administered only by or under the direct observation of the anesthesiologist. ▪ Myasthenia gravis and other neuromuscular diseases increase sensitivity to drug. Can cause critical reactions. Shorteracting muscle relaxants (atracurium [Tracrium]) preferred. ▪ Resistance may develop in patients with burns, depending on the time elapsed since the initial injury and the size of the area involved. ▪ Acid-base or serum electrolyte abnormalities may potentiate or antagonize the action. ▪ Bradycardia may be more common because doxacurium has little effect on heart rate and will not counteract bradycardia caused by anesthetic agents or vagal stimulation. ▪ Use extreme caution in renal dysfunction; shorter-acting drugs (e.g., atracurium [Tracrium], vecuronium [Norcuron]) have a more predictable duration of action. Prolonged duration will occur in renal transplant patients. ▪ Variable onset and duration may occur in liver transplant patients and those with impaired hepatic function.

Monitor: This drug produces apnea. Controlled artificial ventilation with oxygen must be continuous and under direct observation at all times.

Maintain a patent airway. Neostigmine (Prostigmin) and antimuscarinic agents (e.g., atropine, glycopyrolate [Robinul]) must be available. ▪ Monitor all vital organ functions until adequate recovery. ▪ Use a peripheral nerve stimulator to monitor response and avoid overdose, monitor need for additional relaxant, and monitor adequacy of spontaneous recovery or antagonism. ▪ Patient may be conscious and completely unable to communicate by any means. Has no analgesic properties. ▪ Monitor for early signs of malignant hyperthermia; has not occurred but is a possibility. ▪ Review serum electrolytes and acid-base balance before administration. ▪ Note Drug/lab interactions.

Maternal/child: Category C: use during pregnancy only if benefits justify risks. ▪ Effects on neonate unknown, no studies available, duration of action exceeds duration of cesarean section. ▪ Safety for use during lactation not established. ▪ Not recommended for infants and children less than 2 years of age.

Elderly: Delay in onset time and prolonged duration occurs more frequently in the elderly; decrease dose, titrate, and allow more time for drug to achieve maximum effect.

DRUG/LAB INTERACTIONS

Prior administration of succinylcholine has no effect. ▪ Duration of action extended and recovery prolonged by inhalation anesthetics (e.g., enflurane, isoflurane, halothane). ▪ Prolongation of neuromuscular block may occur with many antibiotics (e.g., aminoglycosides [e.g., kanamycin (Kantrex), gentamicin (Garamycin)]), bacitracin, colistin (Coly-Mycin S), colistimethate (Coly-Mycin M), piperacillin, polymyxin-B (Aerosporin), tetracyclines, and with lithium, local anesthetics, diuretics, benzodiazepines (e.g., diazepam [Valium]) and other muscle relaxants, magnesium salts, procainamide (Pronestyl), and quinidine. ▪ Phenytoin (Dilantin) or carbamazepine (Tegretol) may lengthen time of onset and shorten duration of action. ▪ Potentiated by acidosis, inhibited by alkalosis. Electrolyte imbalance (acute [e.g., diarrhea] or chronic [e.g., adrenocortical insufficiency]) and acid-base imbalance are usually mixed; either reaction can occur.

SIDE EFFECTS

Prolonged action resulting in skeletal muscle weakness to profound and prolonged skeletal muscle paralysis with respiratory insufficiency or apnea is possible. Airway closure caused by relaxation of epiglottis, pharynx, and tongue muscles, cardiac arrhythmias, diplopia, fever, and injection site reaction can occur. Side effects associated with histamine release are very rare (e.g., bronchospasm, cutaneous flushing, hypotension, tachycardia, urticaria).

ANTIDOTE

All side effects resulting from prolonged action can be medical emergencies. Controlled ventilation must be continuous. Treat symptomatically and monitor continuously. Neostigmine (Prostigmin [usual dose, 0.06 mg/kg]) is the preferred antagonist but should not be given before spontaneous recovery has begun. Administer atropine or glycopyrolate (Robinul) a few minutes before neostigmine. Identify appropriate time for antagonism and monitor recovery with peripheral nerve stimulator. Evaluate 5-second head lift and grip strength. Time to recovery is based on level of residual neuromuscular block at time of dosing. The earlier an anticholinesterase is administered, the longer it will be to recovery. Action of antagonist may wear off before doxacurium.

DOXAPRAM HYDROCHLORIDE

Respiratory stimulant
Analeptic

Dopram

pH 3.5 to 5.0

USUAL DOSE

Post anesthesia respiratory depression: 0.5 to 1.0 mg/kg of body weight. Up to 1.5 mg/kg may be given as a single injection, or up to 2 mg/kg may be divided and given as several injections at 5-minute intervals. Maximum dosage equals 2 mg/kg. Repeat every 1 to 2 hours as necessary to maintain respiration or follow with an infusion. *Do not exceed 3 Gm/24 hr. Minimum effective dosage is recommended. Repetitive doses are to be used only if the initial dose elicits a positive response.*

Chronic obstructive pulmonary disease: 1 to 2 mg/min. Maximum dose is 3 mg/min (360 mg) over no more than 2 hours. Repeat doses not recommended.

DILUTION

May be given undiluted or diluted with equal parts of sterile water for injection; or dilute 250 mg (12.5 ml) in 250 ml D5W, D10W, D5/NS, D10/NS, or NS and give as an infusion.

Chronic obstructive pulmonary disease: Dilute 400 mg in 180 ml infusion fluid (2 mg/ml). May be given by injection or infusion.

INCOMPATIBLE WITH

Alkaline drugs, aminophylline, ascorbic acid, carbenicillin (Geopen), cefoperazone (Cefobid), cefotaxime (Claforan), cefotetan (Cefotan), cefuroxime (Zinacef), dexamethasone (Decadron), diazepam (Valium), digoxin, dobutamine (Dobutrex), folic acid (Folvite), furosemide (Lasix), hydrocortisone sodium phosphate (Hydrocortone), hydrocortisone sodium succinate (Solu-Cortef), ketamine (Ketalar), methylprednisolone (Solu-Medrol), minocycline (Minocin), pentobarbital (Nembutal), phenobarbital (Luminal), secobarbital (Seconal), sodium bicarbonate, thiopental (Pentothal), ticarcillin (Ticar).

RATE OF ADMINISTRATION

Post anesthesia respiratory depression: Total desired dose of undiluted medication over 5 minutes. Infusion rate may start at 5 mg/min, decrease to 1 to 3 mg/min with observance of respiratory response. If an infusion is used after the initial priming dose, rate may start at 1 to 3 mg/min depending on patient response. Discontinue use after 2 hours, wait 1 to 2 hours, and repeat entire process. Use an infusion pump or microdrip (60 gtt/ml) for accuracy. Note Precaution/Monitor.

Chronic obstructive pulmonary disease: Specific dose over a 2-hour period. Begin at 1 to 2 mg/min. May be titrated to response by injection or infusion. NEVER exceed 3 mg/min.

ACTIONS

An analeptic CNS stimulant. Affects medullary respiratory center to increase the depth of respiration and to slightly increase the rate. Achieves maximum effect in 2 minutes and lasts about 10 to 12 minutes with a single dose. Elevates blood pressure and heart rate. Rapidly metabolized.

INDICATIONS AND USES

Respiratory stimulation and return of protective reflexes (laryngopharyngeal) postanesthesia. ■ Chronic obstructive pulmonary disease with acute hypercapnia (to prevent Co_2 retention). ■ No longer recommended for CNS depressant drug overdose (except muscle relaxant and narcotic overdose) by some references; supportive therapy suggested.

CONTRAINDICATIONS

Cerebrovascular accidents, convulsive states of any etiology, coronary artery disease, head injury, severe hypertension, inadequate ventilation capacity, known hypersensitivity to doxapram, neonates, severe pulmonary dysfunction.

PRECAUTIONS

Not a muscle relaxant or narcotic antagonist. ■ Adjunctive therapy only. Does not inhibit depressant drug metabolism. ■ Stimulates systemic epinephrine increase. ■ Use care in agitation, asthma, cardiac arrhythmias or disease, cerebral edema, gastric surgery, hyperthyroidism, increased intracranial pressure, pheochromocytoma, tachycardia, and ulcers.

Monitor: Maintain an adequate airway at all times. Oxygen and facilities for controlled ventilation must be available. ■ Observe patient continuously and monitor blood pressure, pulse, and deep tendon reflexes during therapy until 1 hour after doxapram is discontinued. Adjust rate if indicated. ■ Arterial blood gas measurements are desirable to determine effective ventilation. ■ Failure to respond to treatment may indicate CNS source for sustained coma; requires neurologic evaluation; repeat doses are not indicated. ■ Confirm patency of vein; vascular extravasation and thrombophlebitis can result from extended use. ■ In chronic obstructive pulmonary disease, arterial blood gases before administration and every 30 minutes thereafter are mandatory; do not use in conjunction with mechanical ventilation. Adjust rate of infusion and oxygen delivery as indicated by arterial blood gases and patient response. Consider increased work of breathing. Observe for Co_2 retention and acidosis. Repeat infusions not recommended. ■ Note Drug/lab interactions.

Maternal/child: Pregnancy Category B: safety for use in pregnancy, lactation, and children under 12 years not established. ■ Note Contraindications.

DRUG/LAB INTERACTIONS

Sympathomimetics (e.g., epinephrine), MAO inhibitors (e.g., selegiline [Eldepryl]), and vasopressors (e.g., dobutamine, isoproterenol) may increase pressor effects when used concurrently with doxapram and produce excessive hypertension. ■ Delay administration for at least 10 minutes after inhalant anesthetics (e.g., cyclopropane, halothane) are discontinued. Doxapram may cause epinephrine release and anesthetics sensitize the myocardium to catecholamines (e.g., epinephrine); may cause cardiac arrhythmias.

SIDE EFFECTS

Confusion, cough, diaphoresis, dizziness, dyspnea, fever, hiccups, hyperactivity, nausea, salivation, urinary retention or urgency, vomiting, warmth.

Major: Aggravated deep tendon reflexes, bilateral Babinski sign, bronchospasm, convulsions, hypertension, hypotension, laryngospasm, PVCs, respiratory alkalosis, skeletal muscle spasm, tachycardia.

Chronic obstructive pulmonary disease: Acidosis and CO_2 retention.

ANTIDOTE

Notify the physician of any side effect. Depending on severity, physician may elect to continue the drug at a reduced rate of administration or discontinue it. Discontinue doxapram with onset of sudden hypotension or dyspnea. IV diazepam (Valium) or pentobarbital sodium (Nembutal) may be useful in overdose. Discontinue doxapram if blood gases deteriorate. Resuscitate as necessary.

DOXORUBICIN HYDROCHLORIDE/ DOXORUBICIN HYDROCHLORIDE LIPOSOME INJECTION

Antineoplastic
(Anthracycline antibiotic)

ADR, Adriamycin PFS, Adriamycin RDF, Rubex/Doxil

pH 3.8 to 6.5 / pH 6.5

USUAL DOSE

Conventional doxorubicin: 60 to 75 mg/M^2 once every 21 days. An alternate dose schedule is 30 mg/M^2 once each day for 3 days. Repeat every 4 weeks. Assessment required before dosing; note Precautions/ Monitor. Recent studies suggest that cardiotoxicity may be reduced and doses may be increased by administration of 20 mg/M^2 on a weekly basis or by giving larger doses (60 to 75 mg/M^2) as a prolonged infusion (48 to 96 hours). A central venous catheter or infuse-a-port would be necessary. Dexrazoxane (Zinecard) is now available to reduce the incidence and severity of cardiomyopathy for women with metastatic breast cancer who have received 300 mg/M^2 of doxorubicin (see product insert).

Doxil (liposome doxorubicin): 20 mg/M^2 once every 3 weeks. Continue as long as response is satisfactory and treatment is tolerated (20 mg/M^2 equals conventional doxorubicin equivalent).

PEDIATRIC DOSE

Conventional doxorubicin: 30 mg/M^2 once each day for 3 days. Repeat every 4 weeks. Note Maternal/child.

Doxil: Safety for use in children not established.

DOSE ADJUSTMENTS

All doxorubicins: Elevated serum bilirubin: Give 50% of above doses for serum bilirubin from 1.2 to 3.0 mg/ml and 25% for serum bilirubin above 3.0 mg/ml. ■ Note Precautions.

Conventional doxorubicin: Reduce dose in impaired liver and kidney function. ■ Lower-end doses are appropriate for the elderly (inadequate marrow reserves) and those with prior therapy or neoplastic marrow infiltration.

Doxil: Dose adjustments are required in hematological toxicity (see chart below), and in patients with stomatitis or palmar-plantar erythrodysethesia (see product literature for guidelines).

HEMATOLOGICAL TOXICITY			
Grade	ANC (cells/mm^3)	Platelets (cells/mm^3)	Modification
1	1500 – 1900	75,000 – 150,000	None
2	1000 – < 1500	50,000 – < 75,000	None

HEMATOLOGICAL TOXICITY			
3	500 – 999	25,000 – < 50,000	Wait until ANC ≥ 1,000 and/or platelets ≥ 50,000 then redose at 25% dose reduction
4	<500	<25,000	Wait until ANC ≥ 1,000 and/or platelets ≥ 50,000 then redose at 50% dose reduction

DILUTION

Specific techniques required; see Precautions.

Conventional doxorubicin: Each 10 mg must be diluted with 5 ml of NS. Do not use bacteriostatic diluent. An additional 5 ml of diluent for each 10 mg is recommended (2 mg/ml). Shake to dissolve completely. Also available in preservative-free solutions. May be further diluted in 50 ml or more D5W or NS and given as a continuous infusion through a central venous line.

Doxil: Each dose must be diluted in 250 ml D5W. Not a clear solution, but a translucent red liposomal dispersion. Do not use in-line filters. Maximum dose for dilution in 250 ml is 90 mg. Note Incompatible with.

Storage: Conventional doxorubicin: Refrigerate unopened vials; protect from light. Diluted solution stable 24 hours at room temperature, 48 hours if refrigerated; then discard. Protect from sunlight.

Doxil: Refrigerate unopened vials; avoid freezing for longer than 1 month. Refrigerate diluted solution and use within 24 hours.

INCOMPATIBLE WITH

Conventional doxorubicin: Aminophylline, cephalothin (Keflin), dexamethasone, diazepam (Valium), fluorouracil, furosemide (Lasix), gallium nitrate (Ganite), ganciclovir (Cytovene), heparin, hydrocortisone sodium succinate, methotrexate, piperacillin/tazobactam (Zosyn). Consider toxicity and specific use.

Doxil: Specific information not available. Manufacturer states, "Do not mix with other drugs. Do not use any other diluent (use D5W only). Do not use any bacteriostatic agents (e.g., benzyl alcohol)." May have actual incompatibilities similar to conventional formulations.

COMPATIBLE WITH

Conventional doxorubicin: May be compatible with bleomycin, cyclophosphamide, dacarbazine, vinblastine, and vincristine. Consult pharmacist.

RATE OF ADMINISTRATION

Conventional doxorubicin: Direct IV: A single dose of properly diluted medication over a minimum of 3 to 5 minutes. Should be given through Y-tube or three-way stopcock of a free-flowing infusion of NS or D5W. Slow injection rate further for erythematous streaking along the vein or facial flushing.

Continuous infusion: Central venous line required. Equally distributed over 24 hours.

Doxil: A single dose as an infusion evenly distributed over 30 min. Rapid infusion may increase risk of acute infusion- related reactions (e.g., back pain, chills, facial swelling, flushing, headache, hypotension, shortness of breath, tightness in the chest or throat). Primarily occurs during the first infusion; may resolve with a reduced rate or may take up to a day after infusion completed to resolve.

ACTIONS

Conventional doxorubicin: A highly toxic antibiotic antineoplastic agent that is cell cycle-specific for the S phase. Widely distributed and rapidly cleared from plasma, it interferes with cell division by binding with DNA to slow production of nucleic acid synthesis. Tissue levels remain constant for 7 to 10 days. Metabolized in the liver. Elimination half-life is 18 to 30 hours. Does not cross blood-brain barrier. Slowly excreted in bile and urine. Secreted in breast milk.

Doxil: Doxorubicin encapsulated in long-circulating STEALTH^R liposomes (phospholipids). The small size of these liposomes and their persistence in the circulation enable them to evade immune system detection and penetrate the often altered and/or compromised vasculature of tumors. Once distributed to tumor tissue, the doxorubicin is released by an unknown mechanism. It differs from conventional doxorubicin because it mostly confines itself to vascular fluid volume. Metabolized and eliminated renally. Plasma clearance is slower. Half-life is extended to 55 hours. Concentration in Kaposi's sarcoma lesions is much higher than in normal skin (range is 3 to 53 times higher).

INDICATIONS AND USES

Conventional doxorubicin: To suppress or retard neoplastic growth. Regression has been produced in soft tissue, osteogenic, and other sarcomas; Hodgkin's disease; non-Hodgkin's lymphomas; acute leukemias; breast, GU, thyroid, lung, and stomach carcinoma; neuroblastoma; and many other carcinomas.

Doxil: Currently approved only for the treatment of AIDS-related Kaposi's sarcoma in patients whose disease has progressed on prior combination chemotherapy or those who are intolerant to combination chemotherapy.

Investigational uses: Doxil: As a single agent in refractory drug-resistant ovarian cancer and in various combinations to treat late-stage malignancies.

CONTRAINDICATIONS

Conventional doxorubicin: Myelosuppression resulting from treatment with other antineoplastic agents, impaired cardiac function, or previous treatment with complete cumulative doses of doxorubicin and/or daunorubicin.

All doxorubicins: History of hypersensitivity to conventional or liposomal formulations of doxorubicin or to their components.

PRECAUTIONS

All doxorubicins: Follow guidelines for handling cytotoxic agents. See Appendix A, p. 893. ■ Usually administered by or under the direction of the physician specialist, with facilities for monitoring the patient and responding to any medical emergency. ■ For IV use only. Do not give

IM or SC. ▪ Use extreme caution in preexisting drug-induced bone marrow suppression, existing heart disease, previous treatment with other anthracyclines (e.g., daunorubicin), other cardiotoxic agents (e.g., bleomycin), or radiation therapy encompassing the heart; risk of cardiotoxicity increased. ▪ May have cross-sensitivity with lincomycin. ▪ All forms of doxorubicin may cause cardiotoxicity. The current recommended total cumulative dose is 550 mg/M^2. This dose recommendation is reduced to 400 mg/M^2 in patients who have received radiotherapy to the mediastinal area or concomitant therapy with other cardiotoxic agents (e.g., bleomycin, cyclophosphamide, daunorubicin, mitoxantrone, mitomycin C). These recommendations may change in specific situations now that dexrazoxane is available to reduce the incidence and severity of cardiomyopathy. ▪ Not considered effective in the treatment of brain tumors, cancers of the kidney or large bowel, CNS metastasis, or malignant melanoma. ▪ Note Side effects.

Conventional doxorubicin: Used cautiously with other antineoplastic drugs to achieve tumor remission.

Doxil: Benefits must outweigh risks if doxil is used in patients with a history of cardiovascular disease. ▪ Has caused palmar-plantar erythrodysesthesia in some Kaposi's sarcoma patients. Incidence may be increased with higher doses or increased frequency. May be severe and require discontinuation of Doxil. ▪ Severe additive myelosuppression may occur in Kaposi's sarcoma patients and may be dose limiting.

Monitor: All doxorubicins: Use only large veins. Avoid veins over joints or in extremities with compromised venous or lymphatic drainage. Determine absolute patency of vein. A stinging or burning sensation indicates extravasation; severe cellulitis and tissue necrosis will result. *Extravasation may occur with or without stinging or burning and even if blood returns well on aspiration of infusion needle.* Observe and touch site frequently to feel air and/or liquid under the skin. If extravasation occurs discontinue injection; use another vein. ▪ Monitoring of CBC including differential and platelet count, uric acid levels, liver function (AST, ALT, alkaline phosphatase, and bilirubin), kidney function, ECG, chest x-ray, and echocardiogram is necessary before and during therapy. At a minimum, recommended before each dose. ▪ Observe for S/S of cardiotoxicity (e.g., fast or irregular HR, shortness of breath, swelling of the feet or lower legs.) ▪ Endomyocardial biopsy or gated radionuclide scans have been used to monitor potential cardiac toxicity. ▪ Maintain adequate hydration. ▪ Allopurinol may prevent formation of uric acid crystals. ▪ Be alert for signs of bone marrow depression, bleeding, or infection. ▪ Use of prophylactic antibiotics may be indicated pending C/S in a febrile, neutropenic patient. ▪ Prophylactic antiemetics are indicated. ▪ Note Drug/lab interactions.

Patient education: All doxorubicins: Urine will be reddish for several days (from dye, not hematuria). ▪ Nonhormonal birth control recommended. ▪ Effects may be additive with current medications. Review all medications (prescription and nonprescription) with nurse and/or physician. Report promptly shortness of breath and/or swelling of the feet or lower legs. ▪ Report IV site burning, stinging, puffiness, or the feeling of liquid under the skin and any other side effects promptly. ▪ See Appendix D, p. 900.

Maternal/child: All doxorubicins: Category D: Avoid pregnancy; can cause fetal harm. ■ Has been used only when benefits outweigh risks. ■ Discontinue breast feeding. ■ Treatment during childhood may result in abnormal cardiac function, especially in females. Incidence of cardiotoxicity may increase in children under 2 years.

Elderly: All doxorubicins: Cardiotoxicity and myelotoxicity may be more severe in patients over 70 years of age.

DRUG/LAB INTERACTIONS

Studies not yet completed for Doxil; interactions may be similar to conventional doxorubicins. ■ May exacerbate cyclophosphamide-induced hemorrhagic cystitis or increase hepatotoxicity of 6-mercaptopurine. ■ May increase bone marrow toxicity of other chemotherapeutic agents. ■ Barbiturates increase clearance and decrease effects. ■ May decrease serum levels of digoxin. ■ May decrease serum levels of anticonvulsants (e.g., phenytoin [Dilantin], carbamazepine [Tegretol], valproate [Depacon]) when given concurrently with cisplatin. ■ Many drug interactions possible; observe patient closely. ■ Do not administer live vaccines to patients receiving antineoplastic drugs. ■ Increased toxicity, including skin redness and exfoliative changes, possible when given concurrently with or after radiation. ■ Dexrazoxane has recently been approved and is given with doxorubicin to reduce cardiotoxic effects. May also decrease antitumor effectiveness if given before a cumulative dose of doxorubicin 300 mg/M^2 is reached or other chemotherapeutic agents are included in the protocol (e.g., fluorouracil). ■ Note Precautions.

SIDE EFFECTS

All doxorubicins: Acute cardiac failure, allergic reactions, alopecia (complete), bone marrow depression (e.g., anemia, hypochromic anemia, neutropenia [ANC <1,000/mm^3], thrombocytopenia) may be dose limiting, depressed QRS voltage, diarrhea, esophagitis, fever, gonadal suppression, hyperpigmentation of nail beds and dermal creases, hyperuricemia, increase in alkaline phosphatase, nausea, oral moniliasis, stomatitis, weakness, vomiting.

Doxil: In addition to all of the above, acute infusion reactions, palmar-plantar erythrodysesthesia. Kaposi's sarcoma patients may be taking numerous other drugs that may confuse the overall side effect picture (e.g., didanosine [ddI], stavudine [D4T], trimethoprim-sulfamethoxazole [Bactrim], zalcitabine [ddC], zidovudine [AZT]).

Overdose (all doxorubicins): Increase in bone marrow suppression and mucositis.

ANTIDOTE

All doxorubicins: Most side effects will either be tolerated or treated symptomatically. Keep the physician informed. Hematopoietic toxicity may require cessation of therapy, antibiotics, platelet and granulocyte transfusions. Neutropenia may be treated with filgrastim (Neupogen) or sargramostim (Leukine). Oprelvekin (Numega) has been used to treat thrombocytopenia. Acute cardiac failure occurs suddenly (most common when total cumulative dosage approaches 550 mg/M^2) and frequently does not respond to currently available treatment (digoxin, diuretics [e.g., furosemide (Lasix)], peripheral vasodilators [e.g., papaverine]). Close monitoring of accumulated dosage, bone marrow, ECG, chest x-ray, echocardiography, and systolic ejection fraction may prevent most serious and potentially fatal cardiac side effects. There is no specific antidote. Supportive therapy as indicated will help sustain the patient in toxicity. Treat allergic reactions as required; discontinue therapy if severe. For extravasation flood the area with normal saline and inject long-acting dexamethasone (Decadron LA) or other injectable corticosteroid throughout extravasated tissue. Use a 27- or 25-gauge needle. Apply cold compresses, ice for 30 minutes, elevate extremity. Site should be observed promptly by a reconstructive surgeon.

Doxil: In addition to all of the above, treatment may have to be discontinued for severe palmar-plantar erythrodysesthesia or acute infusion reactions.

DOXYCYCLINE HYCLATE

Antibacterial (Tetracycline)

Doxy 100, Doxy 200, Doxychel hyclate, ♣Vibramycin, Vibramycin IV

pH 1.8 to 3.3

USUAL DOSE

Adults and children over 45 kg: 200 mg the first day in one or two infusions followed by 100 to 200 mg/24 hr on subsequent days in one or two infusions. Depends on severity of the infection.

Primary and secondary syphilis: 150 mg every 12 hours for at least 10 days.

PEDIATRIC DOSE

Children under 45 kg (but over 8 years): 4.4 mg/kg of body weight/24 hr in one or two equally divided doses. Follow with 2.2 mg/kg/24 hr given once daily or in two equally divided doses on subsequent days. Do not exceed adult dose.

DOSE ADJUSTMENTS

Reduction may be required in impaired liver function. ▪ Note Drug/lab interactions.

DILUTION

Check expiration date. Outdated ampoules may cause nephrotoxicity. Each 100 mg or fraction thereof is diluted with 10 ml of sterile water or normal saline for injection. Further dilute each 10 ml with 100 to 1,000 ml of a compatible infusion solution such as NS, D5W, R, LR, D5/LR, 10% invert sugar in water. Normosol-M or Normosol-R in 5% dextrose in water, or other compatible solutions (see literature). Recommended concentrations 0.1 to 1 mg/ml. 1,000 ml diluent equals 0.1 mg/ml, 100 ml equals 1 mg/ml. Protect from direct sunlight during infusion.

Storage: Store away from heat and light. After reconstitution, must be refrigerated and used within 72 hours.

INCOMPATIBLE WITH

Acid-sensitive additives (e.g., barbiturates, erythromycin, penicillins, sulfonamides), allopurinol (Zyloprim), cephalothin, piperacillin/tazobactam (Zosyn). Dilution in D5/LR or LR may present compatibility problems with some drugs. Administer separately.

RATE OF ADMINISTRATION

Each 100 mg or fraction thereof, properly diluted, over a minimum of 1 to 4 hours. 100 mg diluted in 100 ml equals 1 mg/ml and must be given over a minimum of 2 hours. 100 mg diluted in 200 ml equals 500 mcg/ml and can be given in 1 hour if absolutely necessary. Infusion must be completed in 6 hours when diluted in Ringer's lactate injection with or without dextrose 5% and in 12 hours when diluted in other compatible solutions.

ACTIONS

A broad-spectrum antibiotic, bacteriostatic against many gram-positive and gram-negative organisms and protozoa. Thought to interfere with the protein synthesis of microorganisms. Tetracyclines are well distributed in most body tissues and often bound to plasma protein. Doxycycline may penetrate normal meninges, the eye, and the prostate more easily than most tetracyclines. Partially metabolized in the liver and excreted in bile, urine, and feces. Crosses the placental barrier. Excreted in breast milk.

INDICATIONS AND USES

Infections caused by susceptible strains or organisms, such as rickettsiae, spirochetal agents, viruses, and many other gram-negative and gram-positive bacteria. ■ To substitute for contraindicated penicillin or sulfonamide therapy. ■ Drug of choice when a tetracycline is indicated for treatment of an extrarenal infection in patients with renal impairment. ■ Adjunct to amebicides in acute intestinal amebiasis.

CONTRAINDICATIONS

Known hypersensitivity to tetracyclines; pregnancy, lactation. Not recommended in children under 8 years.

PRECAUTIONS

Sensitivity studies indicated to determine susceptibility of the causative organism to doxycycline. ■ Continue for at least 2 to 3 days after all symptoms of infection subside. ■ Avoid prolonged use of drug; superinfection caused by overgrowth of nonsusceptible organisms may result. ■ Use caution in impaired liver function. Doxycycline serum concentrations and liver function tests are indicated. ■ Initiate oral therapy as soon as possible. ■ Organisms resistant to one tetracycline are usually resistant to others. ■ If syphilis is suspected, perform a darkfield examination before initiating tetracyclines. **Monitor:** Determine absolute patency of vein and avoid extravasation; thrombophlebitis may occur. ■ Monitor blood glucose; may reduce insulin requirements. ■ Note Drug/lab interactions. **Patient education:** Alert patient to photosensitive skin reaction. ■ Consider birth control options. **Maternal/child:** Pregnancy Category D: avoid pregnancy; note Contraindications. ■ May cause skeletal retardation in the fetus and infants and permanent tooth discoloration in children under 8 years, including in utero or through mother's milk. ■ Discontinue breast feeding.

DRUG/LAB INTERACTIONS

Inhibits oral contraceptives; may result in pregnancy or breakthrough bleeding. ■ May alter lithium levels. ■ Inhibits bactericidal action of all penicillins (e.g., ampicillin, oxacillin, methicillin). May be toxic with sulfonamides. ▪ May potentiate digoxin and anticoagulants; reduced dosage of these drugs may be necessary. ▪ Potentiated by alcohol and hepatotoxic drugs (e.g., methoxyflurane [Penthrane]); severe liver damage may result. ▪ Inhibited by barbiturates, carbamazepine (Tegretol), hydantoins (e.g., phenytoin), and others.

SIDE EFFECTS

Relatively nontoxic in average doses. More toxic in large doses or if given too rapidly.

Minor: Anogenital lesions, anorexia, blood dyscrasias, diarrhea, dysphagia, enterocolitis, nausea, skin rashes, vomiting.

Major: Hypersensitivity reactions including anaphylaxis; blurred vision and headache (benign intracranial hypertension); bulging fontanels in infants; liver damage, photosensitivity, systemic candidiasis; thrombophlebitis.

ANTIDOTE

Notify the physician of all side effects. If minor side effects are progressive or any major side effect occurs, discontinue the drug, treat allergic reaction, or resuscitate as necessary.

DROPERIDOL

Anesthesia adjunct
Tranquilizer
Antiemetic

Inapsine

pH 3.0 to 3.8

USUAL DOSE

Premedication: 2.5 to 10 mg 30 to 60 minutes preoperatively or before procedure. Repeat 1.25 to 2.5 mg as indicated.

Induction of anesthesia: 0.22 to 0.275 mg/kg of body weight. Given concomitantly with an analgesic and/or general anesthetic.

Maintenance of anesthesia: 1.25 to 2.5 mg as indicated.

General anesthetic in diagnostic procedures: 2.5 to 10 mg 30 to 60 minutes preoperatively or before procedure. Repeat 1.25 to 2.5 mg as indicated

Antiemetic (investigational): 0.5 mg every 4 hours. May increase dose if required. Often used in an antiemetic regimen with dexamethasone in chemotherapy.

PEDIATRIC DOSE

Premedication or induction of anesthesia in children 2 to 12 years: 0.088 to 0.165 mg/kg of body weight.

DOSE ADJUSTMENTS

Reduce dose of narcotics and all CNS depressants to one fourth or one third of usual dose before, during, and for 24 hours after injection of droperidol. ▪ If other CNS depressants (e.g., narcotics) have been given previously, reduce dose of droperidol. ▪ Reduce dose for elderly, debilitated, and poor-risk patients, and impaired kidney or liver function.

DILUTION

Given undiluted. Give through Y-tube or three-way stopcock of the infusion set. May be added to selected infusion solutions (D5W, NS, or LR). 20 mg in 1,000 ml equals 20 mcg/ml or 1 mg/50 ml.

INCOMPATIBLE WITH

Allopurinol (Zyloprim), barbiturates, epinephrine, fluorouracil (5-FU), foscarnet (Foscavir), furosemide (Lasix), heparin, leucovorin (Folinic acid), methotrexate, nafcillin, piperacillin/tazobactam (Zosyn).

COMPATIBLE WITH

Physically compatible for at least 15 minutes in a syringe with atropine, butorphanol (Stadol), chlorpromazine (Thorazine), diphenhydramine (Benadryl), fentanyl, glycopyrrolate (Robinul), hydroxyzine (Atarax [IM use only]), meperidine, morphine, perphenazine (Trilafon), promazine (Sparine), promethazine (Phenergan), and scopolamine. See each individual drug for requirements of administration.

RATE OF ADMINISTRATION

10 mg or fraction thereof over 1 minute. Infusion must be titrated by dose and desired patient response.

ACTIONS

An antianxiety agent that produces marked tranquilization and sedation. Has an antiemetic action also. It produces mild alpha adrenergic blockade and produces peripheral vascular dilation. May decrease an abnormally high pulmonary arterial pressure. Effective in 3 to 10 minutes with maximum results in 30 minutes. Lasts 2 to 4 hours. Some effects persist for 12 hours. Metabolized in the liver. Excreted in urine and feces. Crosses placental barrier very slowly.

INDICATIONS AND USES

Preoperative sedation. ▪ Induction and maintenance of anesthesia, regional or general. Frequently given concurrently with narcotic analgesics such as fentanyl (Sublimaze) to produce neuroleptanalgesia. ▪ Antiemetic, used in surgical and diagnostic procedures.

Investigational use: Antiemetic in cancer chemotherapy. ▪ Treatment of hyperemesis gravidarium. Used concurrently with diphenhydramine (Benadryl).

CONTRAINDICATIONS

Known hypersensitivity to droperidol.

PRECAUTIONS

Primarily used by or under direct observation of the anesthesiologist. ▪ Use caution with known Parkinson's disease. ▪ When used without a general anesthetic, topical anesthesia is still required when appropriate (e.g., bronchoscopy).

Monitor: A potent drug. Monitor the patient closely. Resuscitation equipment, a narcotic antagonist (if a narcotic has been used concurrently), IV infusion line, and drugs to manage hypotension must be readily available. ▪ Orthostatic hypotension is common; move and position patients with care. ▪ EEG pattern may be slow in returning to normal postoperatively.

Maternal/child: Pregnancy Category C: Safety for use during pregnancy not established; is rarely used. Exceptions are selected use during cesarean section and as a continuous infusion to treat hyperemesis gravidarum in the second and third trimester. ▪ Secretion in breast milk is unconfirmed; use caution in the nursing mother. ▪ Safety for use in children under 2 years not established.

Elderly: Note Dose adjustments.

DRUG/LAB INTERACTIONS
Note Dose adjustments.

SIDE EFFECTS
Minor: Abnormal EEG, chills, dizziness, hallucinations, hypotension, restlessness, shivering, tachycardia.

Major: Apnea, extrapyramidal symptoms, hypotension (severe), respiratory depression.

ANTIDOTE
Notify the physician of any side effect. Minor side effects will probably be transient; for major side effects discontinue the drug, treat symptomatically, and notify the physician. Treat hypotension with fluid therapy (rule out hypovolemia) and vasopressors such as dopamine hydrochloride (Intropin) or levarterenol (Levophed). Epinephrine is contraindicated for hypotension. Further hypotension will occur. Treat extrapyramidal symptoms with benztropine mesylate (Cogentin) or diphenhydramine hydrochloride (Benadryl). Resuscitate as necessary.

EDETATE CALCIUM DISODIUM

Antidote
Chelating agent
Lead mobilization

Calcium Disodium Edetate,
Calcium Disodium Versenate, Calcium EDTA

pH 6.5 to 8.0

USUAL DOSE

Asymptomatic adults and children with blood lead levels over 20 mcg/dl but under 70 mcg/dl: 1,000 mg/M^2/24 hr for 3 to 5 days. After a rest period of 2 to 4 days (preferably up to 2 weeks) to allow for redistribution of lead; repeat the process, if indicated, based on severity of lead toxicity and patient tolerance. Do not exceed 50 mg/kg/24 hr.

Symptomatic adults and children with blood levels over 70 mcg/dl: Dimercaprol (BAL) will be given IM in divided doses every 4 hours for 5 days. 4 hours after the first dose of BAL begin calcium disodium edetate 1,000 to 1,500 mg/M^2/24 hr (50 mg/kg/24 hr) for 5 days. BAL may be stopped after the first 3 days if the blood lead concentration has decreased to less than 50 mcg/dl. After a rest period of 7 to 14 days calcium disodium edetate should be repeated for blood lead concentrations above 45 mcg/dl.

DOSE ADJUSTMENTS

Reduce dose in preexisting renal disease and/or adults with lead nephropathy. In adults with lead nephropathy dose is based on serum creatine levels and repeated monthly until lead excretion is reduced towards normal.

Serum creatinine level	Dose
< 2 mg/dl	1,000 mg/M^2/24 hr for 5 days
2 to 3 mg/dl	500 mg/M^2/24 hr for 5 days
3 to 4 mg/dl	500 mg/M^2/48 hr for 3 doses
> than 4 mg/dl	500 mg/M^2/week

DILUTION

Add total daily dose to 250 to 500 ml of D5W or NS for infusion.

Storage: Prior to use, store at controlled room temperature.

INCOMPATIBLE WITH

Amphotericin B (Fungizone), hydralazine (Apresoline), D10W, 10% invert sugar in NS, lactate Ringer's, Ringer's solution, ⅙ molar lactate. Must be diluted in specific IV solutions (See Dilution).

RATE OF ADMINISTRATION

References vary greatly. Manufacturer recommends the total daily dose be evenly distributed over 8 to 12 hours. Others recommend infusing over 2 hours for symptomatic patients and over 1 hour for asymptomatic patients. Physician should order a specific rate. May cause hypocalcemic tetany and/or an increase in intracranial pressure with too rapid injection.

ACTIONS

Helps to remove metals, especially lead, from the body. Will form a stable chelate with metals that have the ability to displace calcium (e.g., lead, zinc, cadmium). These stable compounds are then excreted in urine; up to 50% in 1 hour and 95% in 24 hours. Mostly chelates from bone.

INDICATIONS AND USES

Acute and chronic lead poisoning and lead encephalopathy. ▪ Heavy metal poisoning. ▪ Removal of radioactive and nuclear fission products.

CONTRAINDICATIONS

Anuria, active renal disease, or hepatitus.

PRECAUTIONS

Patients with lead encephalopathy and cerebral edema may have a lethal increase in intracranial pressure with IV infusion; IM injection preferred. ▪ Usually given IM in children; unless given concurrently with BAL (insufficient IM injection sites). ▪ May produce toxic and fatal effects. Produces the same renal damage as lead poisoning (e.g., proteinuria and microscopic hematuria). ▪ Use with caution in mild renal disease; note Dose adjustments. ▪ The patient must be removed from the source of contamination promptly. ▪ Animal studies verify lead excretion from urine and decreased blood levels, but lead in the brain may increase due to internal redistribution. After a 5-day course of treatment, lead levels in animal brains did not decrease. ▪ Use for diagnosis of lead poisoning as a lead mobilization test is controversial; see literature. ▪ Do no confuse with edetate disodium (Endrate), which does not chelate lead but actually removes calcium from the body and can be very dangerous. ▪ Not effective in mercury, gold, or arsenic poisoning.

Monitor: Urine flow must be established before drug is administered. IV fluids may be used unless contraindicated (e.g., lead encelphalopathy, increased intracranial pressure). ▪ Monitor urinalysis, urine sediment, renal and hepatic function, and electrolyte levels before treatment; repeat daily in serious cases and on the second and fifth day in less serious cases. Daily urine specimens are recommended to determine status of renal function. ▪ Monitor ECG and vital signs. ▪ Excretion of calcium is not increased, but zinc excretion is; monitor and replace as indicated. ▪ Obtain specific fluid orders from the physician. ▪ Increased fluid intake is desirable except in the presence of cerebral edema or lead encephalopathy.

Patient education: If no urine output for 12 hours, report immediately.

Maternal/child: Pregnancy Category B: safety for use during pregnancy not established; benefits must outweigh risks. ▪ Use caution in nursing mothers.

Elderly: Consider age-related organ damage.

DRUG/LAB INTERACTIONS

Steroids will increase renal toxicity. ▪ Inhibits the action of zinc insulin preparations by chelating the zinc.

SIDE EFFECTS

Acute renal tubular necrosis, anemia, anorexia, cardiac rhythm irregularities, chills, excessive thirst, fever, headache, hematuria, hypercalcemia, hypersensitivity (e.g., sneezing, nasal congestion), hypotension, increases in liver function tests (mild), leg and other muscle cramps, malaise, nausea, numbness, proteinuria, tetany, tingling, transient bone marrow depression, tremors, vomiting, weakness, zinc deficiency.

ANTIDOTE

Notify the physicain of any side effects. Most will improve with a decrease in rate of the infusion or will be treated symptomatically. Discontinue if urine flow stops to avoid high tissue levels of the drug. Discontinue at the first sign of renal toxicity (e.g., presence of large renal epithelial cells or increasing numbers of red blood cells). Treat cerebral edema with repeated doses of mannitol.

EDETATE DISODIUM

Antihypercalcemic agent
Calcium chelating agent

Disotate, EDTA disodium, Endrate

pH 6.5 to 7.5

USUAL DOSE

50 mg/kg of body weight/24 hr or in equally divided doses every 12 hours. Total dose should not exceed 3 Gm/24 hr. Usually given for 5 days, held for 2 days. Regimen may be repeated to a total of 15 doses.

PEDIATRIC DOSE

40 mg/kg of body weight/24 hr in equally divided doses every 6 to 12 hours. Do not exceed 70 mg/kg/24 hr or adult dose, whichever is less. See instructions in Usual dose.

DILUTION

Recommended dose must be diluted in 500 ml D/5/W or NS and given as IV infusion. A 0.5% solution will reduce the risk of thrombophlebitis. Do not exceed cardiac reserve in any patient. Use less diluent if necessary in children. Must be diluted to at least a 3% solution.

Storage: Store at room temperature.

INCOMPATIBLE WITH

5% dextrose in 5% alcohol. Will chelate any metal. Not recommended to mix in syringe or solution with any other drug.

RATE OF ADMINISTRATION

Must not exceed more than 15 mg of actual medication over 1 minute. Total dose usually given over 3 to 4 hours. Reduce rate and further dilute solution for pain at injection site.

ACTIONS

A calcium-chelating agent. Attracts calcium ions immediately on injection and becomes calcium disodium edetate. Capable of severely depleting the body of calcium stores. Exerts a negative inotropic effect on the heart. It is well distributed in extracellular fluids and rapidly excreted in the urine.

INDICATIONS AND USES

Cardiac arrhythmias (atrial and ventricular, especially when caused by digitalis toxicity). ■ Hypercalcemia.

CONTRAINDICATIONS
Anuria, known sensitivity to edetate disodium, patients with seizures or intracranial lesions, renal disease.

PRECAUTIONS
Used only when the severity of disease indicates necessity. ■ May produce hypocalcemia quickly, especially if used for purposes other than chelating calcium. ■ Use repeatedly only with caution because of potential for nephrotoxicity and mobilization of extracirculatory calcium stores. ■ Use caution in cardiac disease (may adversely affect myocardial contractility), diabetes (lower blood sugar may require less insulin), severe renal disease, liver disease, congestive heart failure (1 Gm of sodium in each 5 Gm), and limited cardiac reserve.

Monitor: Monitor vital signs and ECG before and during therapy. ■ Confirm patency of vein, avoid extravasation; can cause tissue necrosis. ■ Routine electrolyte panel (potassium deficiency) and urine specimens for casts and cells necessary during therapy. Magnesium, zinc, and other trace element deficiencies can occur. ■ Keep patient in supine position during and after administration (15 to 30 minutes) to avoid postural hypotension. ■ Obtain blood for serum calcium levels just before beginning a new infusion; specific lab methods required. ■ Inhibits coagulation of blood (transient). ■ Note Drug/lab interactions.

Maternal/child: Pregnancy Category C: safety for use in pregnancy or lactation not established. Use with extreme caution and only if clearly needed.

DRUG/LAB INTERACTIONS
Inhibits mannitol. ■ Potentiates neuromuscular blocking antibiotics (e.g., gentamicin [Garamycin]). ■ Inhibits coagulation of blood (transient). ■ Obtain blood for serum calcium levels just before beginning a new infusion. Specific laboratory methods must be used for accurate evaluation.

SIDE EFFECTS
Minor: Anorexia, arthralgia, circumoral paresthesias, fatigue, fever, glycosuria, headache, hypotension, malaise, nasal congestion, nausea, sneezing, tearing, thirst, thrombophlebitis, urinary urgency, vomiting.

Major: Anaphylaxis, anemia, cardiac arrhythmias, dermatitis, hemorrhage, hypocalcemic tetany, prolonged QT interval, renal tubular destruction (reversible), seizures, death.

ANTIDOTE
Notify the physician of any side effect. For progression of minor side effects or any major side effect, discontinue drug immediately and notify the physician. Calcium gluconate is the antidote of choice and should be available for infusion at all times (use extreme caution if patient digitalized). Treat anaphylaxis and resuscitate as necessary.

EDROPHONIUM CHLORIDE

Cholinergic
Cholinesterase inhibitor
Antidote
Diagnostic agent

Enlon, Reversol, Tensilon

pH 5.4

USUAL DOSE

1 to 10 mg (0.1 to 1 ml) at specified intervals depending on usage. Maximum dose should never exceed 40 mg (4 doses of 10 mg each).

Myasthenia gravis diagnosis: 10 mg (1 ml) in tuberculin syringe. Give 2 mg (0.2 ml). If no reaction occurs in 45 seconds, give remaining 8 mg (0.8 ml). Test may be repeated after 30 minutes.

Myasthenia treatment evaluation: 1 to 2 mg (0.1 to 0.2 ml) 1 hour after oral intake of drug being used for treatment.

Myasthenia crisis evaluation: 2 mg (0.2 ml) in tuberculin syringe. Give 1 mg (0.1 ml). If the patient's condition does not deteriorate, give 1 mg (0.1 ml) after 60 seconds. Improvement in cardiac status and respiration should occur.

Antagonist to curare and other nondepolarizing muscle relaxants: 10 mg (1 ml). May be repeated as necessary up to 4 doses. (Available in combination with atropine [Enlon-Plus] for use in reversal of nondepolarizing muscle relaxants.)

Terminate paroxysmal atrial tachycardia (investigational): 5 to 10 mg as a bolus injection. Note Dose adjustments. Repeat once in 10 minutes if necessary.

Slow superventricular tachycardias (investigational): 2 mg as a test dose. Repeat 2 mg every 1 minute until arrhythmia controlled or total dose of 10 mg is given. If heart rate decreases, may begin an infusion of 0.25 mg/min. May be increased to 2 mg/min if necessary.

PEDIATRIC DOSE

Myasthenis gravis diagnosis: 0.1 mg for **neonates.** 0.5 mg for **infants.** 1 mg for **children under 34 kg;** if no response in 30 to 45 seconds give 1 mg every 30 to 45 seconds up to 5 mg. **Over 34 kg,** give 2 mg; if no response in 30 to 45 seconds, give 1 mg every 30 to 45 seconds up to 10 mg. Another source has the same dose for neonates but recommends 0.2 mg/kg/dose for **infants and children** with 20% of a dose given as a test dose slowly. If no response in 1 min, give in 1 mg increments to a maximum calculated dose or 10 mg, whichever is less.

DOSE ADJUSTMENTS

Reduce antiarrhythmic dose to 5 to 7 mg in the elderly.

DILUTION

May be given undiluted. In the treatment of myasthenia crisis, this drug may be diluted in D5W or NS and given as a continuous IV drip. Use an infusion pump or microdrip (60 gtt/ml).

INCOMPATIBLE WITH

An extremely specific drug. Should be considered incompatible in syringe or solution with any other drug.

RATE OF ADMINISTRATION

2 mg (0.2 ml) or fraction thereof over 15 to 30 seconds.
Curare antagonist: A single dose over 30 to 45 seconds.
Antiarrhythmic: See Usual dose.

ACTIONS

An anticholinesterase and antagonist of skeletal muscle relaxants. Inhibits the enzyme cholinesterase, allowing acetylcholine to accumulate at the myoneural junction. Restores normal transmission of nerve impulses. Acts within 30 to 60 seconds and has an extremely short duration of action, seldom exceeding 10 minutes. Produces vagal stimulation, shortens refractory period of atrial muscle, and slows conduction through the AV node.

INDICATIONS AND USES

Diagnosis of myasthenia gravis. ▪ Evaluation of adequate treatment of myasthenia gravis. ▪ Evaluation of emergency treatment of myasthenia crisis. ▪ An antagonist to nondepolarizing muscle relaxants (e.g., tubocurarine [Curare], gallamine triethiodide [Flaxedil], doxacurium [Nuromax]).
Investigational use: Termination of supraventricular tachycardia unresponsive to cardiac glycosides. Adenosine is the drug of choice. ▪ Diagnosis of supraventricular tachycardia ▪ Evaluate function of a demand pacemaker.

CONTRAINDICATIONS

Apnea, known hypersensitivity to anticholinesterase agents, mechanical intestinal and urinary obstructions, patients taking mecamylamine, pregnancy.

PRECAUTIONS

A physician should be present when this drug is used. ▪ Use caution in patients with bronchial asthma, cardiac arrhythmias, or myasthenia gravis treated with anticholine sterase drugs.
Monitor: Atropine 1 mg must be available and ready for injection at all times. ▪ Continuously observe patient reactions. ▪ Anticholinesterase insensitivity may develop; withhold drugs and support respiration as necessary. ▪ Note Drug/lab interactions.
Maternal/child: Note Contraindications. ▪ Discontinue breast feeding.

DRUG/LAB INTERACTIONS

Muscarinic effects antagonized by atropine (see Antidote) ▪ May be inhibited by corticosteroids and magnesium. ▪ May cause bradycardia with digitalis glycosides. ▪ Briefly antagonizes the effects of nondepolarizing neuromuscular blocking agents (e.g., atracurium, pancuronium, vecuronium). ▪ Prolongs muscle relaxant effect of succinylcholine chloride (Anectine).

SIDE EFFECTS

Abdominal cramps, anorexia, anxiety, bradycardia, bronchiolar spasm, cardiac arrhythmias and arrest, cold moist skin, contraction of the pupils, convulsions, diarrhea, dysphagia, fainting, increased lacrimation, increased pulmonary secretion, increased salivation, insomnia, irritability, laryngospasm, muscle weakness, nausea, perspiration, ptosis, respiratory arrest (either muscular or central), urinary frequency and incontinence, vomiting.

ANTIDOTE

If side effects occur, discontinue the drug and notify the physician. Atropine sulfate in doses of 0.4 to 0.5 mg IV will counteract most side effects and may be repeated every 3 to 10 minutes. Pralidoxime chloride 50 to 100 mg/min to 1 Gm may be used with extreme caution as a cholinesterase reactivator. Endotracheal intubation or tracheostomy is considered prophylactic in anesthesia or crises. Artificial ventilation, oxygen therapy, cardiac monitoring, adequate suctioning, and treatment of shock or convulsions must be instituted and maintained as necessary. Treat allergic reactions with epinephrine.

EDROPHONIUM CHLORIDE AND ATROPINE SULFATE

Cholinergic
Cholinesterase inhibitor
Antidote

Enlon-Plus

pH 4.4 to 4.6

USUAL DOSE

0.05 to 0.1 ml/kg (0.05 to 1.0 mg/kg of edrophonium with 0.007 to 0.014 mg/kg of atropine). Each 1 ml of prepared solution contains 10 mg edrophonium and 0.14 mg atropine. Must be administered at a point of at least 5% recovery of twitch response to neuromuscular stimulation. Use of peripheral nerve stimulator recommended. A total dose of 1.0 mg/kg of edrophonium is rarely exceeded. Length of action is usually sufficient to cover effects of commonly used short- and medium-acting nondepolarizing muscle relaxants (e.g., atracurium [Tracrium], mivacurium [Mivacron], vecuronium [Norcuron]).

DOSE ADJUSTMENTS

None required, even though elderly patients and those with impaired renal or hepatic function may have a prolonged half-life and reduced clearance.

DILUTION

May be given undiluted through Y-tube or three-way stopcock of infusion set.

Storage: Available in vials containing 5 ml or 15 ml. Store at room temperature 15° to 26° C (59° to 78° F).

INCOMPATIBLE WITH

An extremely specific drug. Should be considered incompatible in syringe or solution with any other drug. All incompatibilities of atropine are probable.

RATE OF ADMINISTRATION

A single dose over 45 to 60 seconds.

ACTIONS

A combination of anticholinesterase agent and a parasympatholytic (anticholinergic) drug. Edrophonium antagonizes the effect of nondepolarizing neuromuscular blocking agents by inhibiting or inactivating acetylcholinesterase. Acetylcholine is not hydrolyzed as rapidly by acetylcholinesterase and accumulates, improving transmission of impulses across the myoneural junction. Unavoidable accumulation of acetylcholine at muscarinic cholinergic sites may cause bradycardia, bronchoconstriction, increased secretions, and other parasympathomimetic effects. Magnitude of effects varies depending on vagal nerve activity present. Atropine counteracts these side effects. Edrophonium is effective immediately with maximum antagonism within 1 to 2 minutes and lasts for 70 minutes. Atropine affects heart rate immediately, peaks in 2 to 16 minutes, and lasts for over 2 hours. With this combination agent, full reversal is usually accomplished before patient leaves recovery, muscarinic effects are minimized, and patient evaluation can be accomplished in OR. Some hepatic metabolism. Primarily excreted in urine, with some excretion in bile.

INDICATIONS AND USES

Reversal agent or antagonist of non-depolarizing neuromuscular blocking agents. Not effective against depolarizing neuromuscular blocking agents (e.g., succinylcholine [Anectine]). ▪ Adjunctive treatment of respiratory depression of curare overdose.

CONTRAINDICATIONS

Acute glaucoma, adhesions between the iris and lens of the eye, known hypersensitivity to either component or sulfites, mechanical intestinal and urinary obstructions, and pyloric stenosis.

PRECAUTIONS

Administer only by or under the direct observation of the anesthesiologist. ▪ Use caution in patients with bronchial asthma, cardiac arrhythmias, myasthenia gravis (or symptoms of myasthenic weakness) treated with anticholinesterase drugs, prostatic hypertrophy, and debilitated patients with chronic lung disease. ▪ Recurarization has not been reported after satisfactory reversal obtained. ▪ Note Drug/lab interactions.

Monitor: An additional supply of atropine 1 mg must be available and ready for injection at all times. ▪ Continuously observe patient reactions and monitor responses. Monitor ECG, vital signs, and reversal with a peripheral nerve stimulator. Ventilation (assisted or controlled) must be secured. ▪ Anticholinesterase insensitivity may develop; reduce or withhold drugs and support respiration as necessary until sensitivity returns. ▪ Confirm patency of vein; will cause tissue irritation. ▪ Note Drug/lab interactions.

Maternal/Child: Category C: use during pregnancy only if benefits outweigh risks. ▪ Safety for use during lactation or in children not established. ▪ Pediatric patients may have increased vagal tone with greater variance in effects. ▪ Atropine rate of clearance decreased in children less than 2 years of age but dose adjustment not indicated.

Elderly: Prolonged plasma half-life and reduced clearance but dose adjustment not indicated; elimination of nondepolarizing muscle relaxants is similarly decreased.

DRUG/LAB INTERACTIONS

Never administer prior to any nondepolarizing muscle relaxant (e.g., mivacurium [Mivacron]). ▪ May cause symptoms of anticholinesterase overdose (cholinergic crisis) with anticholinesterase drugs (e.g., pyridostigmine [Mestinon], neostigmine [Prostigmin], glaucoma agents). ▪ Frequency and duration of bradycardia increased with nar-

cotic analgesics unless given with a potent inhalant anesthetic.
■ Excessive bradycardia may develop with beta-adrenergic blocking agents (e.g., atenolol [Tenormin], esmolol [Brevibloc], timolol [Timpotic]); atropine alone should be given prior to Enlon-Plus in these patients. ■ Bradycardia and first-degree heart block may be increased when muscle relaxants with no vagolytic effects (e.g., vecuronium [Norcuron]) are reversed. ■ Cardiac arrest has occurred in digitilized patients and jaundiced patients receiving anticholinesterase drugs (e.g., pyridostigmine [Mestinon], neostigmine [Prostigmin], glaucoma agents); all side effects could be additive. ■ Prolongs muscle relaxant effect of succinylcholine (Anectine). ■ Actions of atropine may interfere with absorption of other medications. ■ Concomitant use of atropine with other cholinergic drugs (e.g., antihistamines, antiparkinson agents, antipsychotics, tricyclic antidepressants) will increase mouth dryness and other side effects (e.g., decreased GI motility).

SIDE EFFECTS

Average dose: Allergic reactions including anaphylaxis; arrythmias in up to 10% of patients (e.g., bradycardia, first-, second-, and third-degree AV block, junctional rhythms, PACs, prolonged R-R interval, PVCs, P wave changes, tachycardia). All side effects of atropine and edrophonium can occur; refer to individual monographs.

Overdose: Cholinergic crisis due to overdose or concomitant use of other anticholinesterase drugs (bradycardia, diarrhea, increased bronchial and salivary secretions, nausea, sweating, vomiting); convulsions, delirium, fever, shock, tachycardia. In atropine poisoning (delirium, fever, tachycardia), death is usually due to medullary center paralysis.

ANTIDOTE

If side effects occur, discontinue the drug and notify the physician. Atropine sulfate in doses of 0.4 to 0.5 mg IV will counteract most side effects of edrophonium and may be repeated every 3 to 10 minutes. Endotracheal intubation or tracheostomy is considered prophylactic in anesthesia or crisis. In all situations treatment is symptomatic and includes artificial ventilation, oxygen therapy, cardiac monitoring, adequate suctioning, and treatment of fever, shock, or convulsions. Institute and maintain as necessary. Treat allergic reactions with diphenhydramine (Benadryl) and epinephrine (Adrenalin).

ENALAPRILAT

ACE inhibitor
Antihypertensive
Vasodilator

Vasotec IV

pH 6.5 to 7.5

USUAL DOSE

1.25 mg every 6 hours. Dosage is the same when converting from oral to IV therapy. Doses up to 5 mg every 6 hours have been tolerated for up to 36 hours, but clinical studies have not shown a need for dosage over 1.25 mg. Additional doses of 1.25 mg may be given every 6 hours except in dialysis patients.

PEDIATRIC DOSE

0.625 to 1.25 mg every 6 hours. See Maternal/child.

DOSE ADJUSTMENTS

Reduce initial dose to 0.625 mg in patients taking diuretics, patients with a creatinine clearance less than 30 ml/min (serum creatinine greater than 3 mg/dl), and dialysis patients. If the 0.625 dose is not clinically effective after 1 hour, it may be repeated. Reduce additional dose of 1.25 mg by one half for dialysis patients. ▪ Blood levels markedly increased in the elderly; reduced dose may be required. ▪ Note Drug/lab interactions and Precautions.

DILUTION

May be given undiluted through the port of a free-flowing infusion of NS, D5W, D5/NS, D5/LR; or Isolyte E. May also be diluted in up to 50 ml of any of the same solutions and given as an infusion.

Storage: Stable for up to 24 hours after dilution.

INCOMPATIBLE WITH

Must be diluted or infused with specific solutions; (See Dilution). Amphotericin B (Fungizone), phenytoin (Dilantin). Physically compatible with many drugs. Consult with pharmacist before mixing.

RATE OF ADMINISTRATION

A single dose must be evenly distributed over 5 minutes.

ACTIONS

An antihypertensive agent. An angiotensin-converting enzyme inhibitor that prevents conversion of angiotensin I to angiotensin II. Peripheral arterial resistance is reduced in hypertensive patients. In patients with heart failure, significant reduction in pulmonary capillary wedge pressure (preload), peripheral vascular resistance (afterload), blood pressure, and heart size occurs, as well as an increase in cardiac output (stroke index) and exercise tolerance time. Initial response may take 15 minutes to 1 hour. Peak blood pressure reduction occurs in 1 to 4 hours, and effects last up to 6 hours. Peak effects of subsequent doses may be greater than the initial dose. Excreted in bile and urine.

INDICATIONS AND USES

Hypertension. ▪ Heart failure not adequately responsive to diuretics and digitalis. Enalaprilat is used in addition to digitalis and diuretics. ▪ Hypertensive emergencies (effects are variable).

CONTRAINDICATIONS

Hypersensitivity to enalaprilat or its components.

PRECAUTIONS

Has been used IV for up to 7 days. ▪ Use caution in patients with aortic stenosis; afterload reduction may not be adequate. ▪ Use caution in surgery, with anesthesia, or with agents that produce hypotension. ▪ Average dose for conversion to oral therapy is 5 mg/day as a single dose. When a reduced dose of enalaprilat IV has been indicated (e.g., diuretics, impaired renal function, dialysis), reduce initial oral dose to 2.5 mg/day as a single dose. Adjust either by patient response. ▪ Patients sensitive to one ACE inhibitor may be sensitive to another.

Monitor: Monitor vital signs very frequently. May cause precipitous drop in blood pressure following the first dose. ▪ Use extreme caution in fluid-depleted patients. Patients with congestive heart failure may become hypotensive at any time. Arrhythmias or conduction defects may occur. ▪ Monitor BUN and serum creatinine. An increase in either may require a decrease in dose of enalaprilat or discontinuation of a diuretic. ▪ Diuretics given concomitantly may cause a precipitous drop in blood pressure within the first hour of the initial dose; observe the patient closely. Severe dietary salt restriction or dialysis will aggravate this effect. ▪ May cause oliguria or progressive azotemia in patients with severe congestive heart failure whose renal function is dependent on the activity of the renin-angiotensin-aldosterone system. Acute renal failure and death are possible. ▪ May cause hyperkalemia. May cause a significant increase in serum potassium with potassium-sparing diuretics or potassium supplements. Use with caution and only in documented hypokalemia. Use salt substitutes with caution. Monitor serum potassium levels. ▪ Note Drug/lab interactions.

Patient education: Consider birth control options.

Maternal/child: Avoid pregnancy; Category C (first trimester) and Category D (second and third trimester). Can cause fetal and neonatal morbidity and death. If pregnancy occurs, discontinue immediately; many alternate antihypertensive agents. ▪ Observe any infant with in utero exposure for hypotension, oliguria, and hyperkalemia. ▪ Has caused reversible acute renal failure in a premature infant whose mother received enalaprilat. ▪ Safety for use in lactation not established. ▪ Safety for use in children not established but has been used.

Elderly: Note Dose adjustments and Precautions/Monitor. ▪ Blood levels markedly increased in the elderly; may relate to decreased renal function or to increased sensitivity.

DRUG/LAB INTERACTIONS

Use caution in surgery, with anesthesia, or with any agents that produce hypotension. ▪ May be used concomitantly with other antihypertensive agents, (e.g., thiazide diuretics [chlorothiazide (Diuril)]). Effects are additive. ▪ Diuretics given concomitantly may cause a precipitous drop in blood pressure. ▪ Hypersensitivity reactions may increase in combination with allopurinol. ▪ May cause hyperkalemia with potassium-sparing diuretics (e.g., spironolactone) or potassium supplements. ▪ Use caution and consider lower doses when administering nitroglycerin, nitroprusside sodium, other nitrates, or other vasodilators (e.g., hydralazine). ▪ Potentiated by probenicid. ▪ May decrease hemoglobin and hematocrit slightly. ▪ See Precautions/Monitor.

SIDE EFFECTS

Abdominal pain, angioedema, atrial fibrillation, chest pain, cough (persistent dry), diarrhea, dizziness, dyspnea, fatigue, headache, hyperkalemia, hypotension (severe), impotence, insomnia, muscle cramps, nausea, palpitations, paresthesias, pruritus, pulmonary edema, pulmonary embolism and infarction, rash, somnolence, vomiting.

ANTIDOTE

For minor side effects, notify the physician. Most will be tolerated or treated symptomatically. If symptoms progress or any major side effect occurs (angioedema, precipitous hypotension, hyperkalemia), discontinue drug and notify the physician immediately. Hypotension should respond to IV fluids if the patient's condition allows their use.

Other drugs in the regimen may need to be discontinued or the dosage reduced. Use epinephrine immediately for angioedema. Maintain the patient as indicated. If cardiac arrhythmias occur, treat appropriately. Hemodialysis may be useful in toxicity.

EPHEDRINE SULFATE

Bronchodilator
Vasopressor

pH 4.5 to 7.0

USUAL DOSE

5 to 25 mg; may be repeated every 3 to 4 hours based on patient response. 150 mg/24 hr is the maximum total dose.

PEDIATRIC DOSE

3 mg/kg of body weight/24 hr or 25 to 100 mg/M^2/24 hr divided into four to six doses. Rarely used IV in children.

DOSE ADJUSTMENTS

Note Drug/lab interactions.

DILUTION

May be given undiluted. Not usually added to IV solutions. May be injected through Y-tube or three-way stopcock of infusion set.

INCOMPATIBLE WITH

Alkaline solutions, barbiturates (e.g., pentobarbital [Nembutal], phenobarbital [Luminal]), hydrocortisone (Solu-Cortef).

RATE OF ADMINISTRATION

Each 10 mg or fraction thereof over 1 minute.

ACTIONS

A sympathomimetic drug that stimulates both alpha and beta adrenergic receptors. It is less potent but longer acting than epinephrine. It has positive inotropic action, increasing the strength of myocardial contraction. It increases the heart rate and elevates the blood pressure. Some arteriolar vasoconstriction occurs. It stimulates the CNS, relaxes the smooth muscle of the bronchi and GI tract, and dilates the pupils. Metabolic rate and respiratory rate are increased. Widely distributed in body fluids, ephedrine crosses the blood-brain barrier. It is excreted in urine. Secreted in breast milk.

INDICATIONS AND USES

Bronchospasm. ■ Hypotension. ■ Bradycardia caused by atrioventricular block. ■ Pressor agent during spinal anesthesia. ■ Stokes-Adams syndrome. ■ Allergic disorders (epinephrine preferred). ■ Narcotic, barbiturate, and alcohol poisoning. Generally replaced by more effective agents for all uses.

CONTRAINDICATIONS

Hypersensitivity to ephedrine; labor and delivery if maternal blood pressure exceeds 130/80 mm Hg (may cause prolonged uterine atony with hemorrhage); narrow-angle glaucoma; psychoneurosis. Do not use to treat overdosage of phenothiazines (e.g., chlorpromazine [Thorazine]). A further drop in blood pressure and irreversible shock may result. One manufacturer states that it is contraindicated during anesthesia with halogenated anesthetics (e.g., halothane).

PRECAUTIONS

Note label; only specific solutions can be given IV. ■ Use caution in heart disease, angina, diabetes, hyperthyroidism, and prostatic hypertrophy. ■ Has a cumulative effect.

Monitor: Check blood pressure every 5 minutes. ■ Note Drug/lab interactions.

Maternal/child: Pregnancy Category C: may cause anoxia in fetus. ■ Safety for use in lactation not established. ■ Note Contraindications.

DRUG/LAB INTERACTIONS

Do not use concomitantly with other sympathomimetic agents (e.g., dopamine [Intropin], dobutamine [Dobutrex], epinephrine.) Additive effects may cause toxicity. ■ MAO inhibitors (e.g., selegiline [Eldepryl]) and furazolidone (Furoxone) increase pressor response and may cause hypertensive crisis and intracranial hemorrhage. ■ May cause severe hypertension with oxytocics (e.g., oxytocin [Pitocin]). ■ Cyclopropane or halogenated anesthetics (e.g., halothane, isoflurane) and digoxin may sensitize myocardium and increase risk of arrhythmias. ■ Reserpine (Hydropres), methyldopa (Aldomet), and tricyclic antidepressants (e.g., amytriptyline [Elavil]) may decrease pressor response and decrease effectiveness. ■ Atropine blocks reflex bradycardia enhancing pressor effect; observe for hypertension. ■ Antihypertensive effect of guanethidine (Ismelin) may be decreased; monitor carefully. ■ Urinary alkalinizers (e.g., acetazolamide, sodium bicarbonate) decrease ephedrine elimination and increase risk of toxicity with prolonged use. ■ Alpha- and beta-blocking drugs (e.g., phentolamine [Regitine], propranolol [Inderal]) antagonize effects of ephedrine. ■ Use with theophylline may increase CNS and GI side effects. ■ Interacts with many other drugs. ■ Note Contraindications.

SIDE EFFECTS

Rare in therapeutic doses; anorexia, cardiac arrhythmias, headache, insomnia, nausea, nervousness, painful urination, palpitations, precordial pain, sweating, tachycardia, urinary retention, vertigo, vomiting. Confusion, delirium, euphoria, and hallucinations may occur with higher doses. Convulsions, pulmonary edema, and respiratory failure may occur with overdose.

ANTIDOTE

If side effects occur, discontinue the drug and notify the physician. Side effects may be treated symptomatically. Treat hypotension with IV fluids; vasopressors (e.g., dopamine [Intropin]) are contraindicated. Treat hypertension with phentolamine (Regitine) and convulsions with diazepam (Valium). Treat cardiac arrhythmias with beta blockers (e.g., propranolol [Inderal]). Resuscitate as necessary.

EPINEPHRINE HYDROCHLORIDE

Cardiac stimulant
Bronchodilator
Antiallergic
Vasopressor

Adrenalin chloride

pH 2.5 to 5.0

USUAL DOSE

Start with a small dose, giving only as much as required to alleviate undesirable symptoms, and repeat as necessary, gradually increasing dose depending on need. 0.2 to 0.5 mg of 1:10,000 solution. May be repeated as necessary.

Cardiac arrest: 1 mg of 1:10,000 solution IV; may repeat every 3 to 5 minutes. Follow each dose with a 20 ml IV flush to ensure delivery to systemic circulation (See Incompatible with) . If the 1 mg dose is not effective, larger doses (up to 3 to 5 mg) are being used to treat ventricular fibrillation, pulseless ventricular tachycardia, asystole or electromechanical dissociation in patients under 65 years of age. JAMA recommends these approaches:

Intermediate: 2 to 5 mg every 3 to 5 min.

Escalating: 1 mg, 3 mg, 5 mg dosing 3 minutes apart.

High: 0.1 mg/kg of body weight every 3 to 5 min.

Endotracheal: A 1:10,000 solution may be given through the endotracheal tube before an IV is established. Dilute a 1:1,000 solution in 10 ml NS or SW for injection. Recent studies indicate a minimum of 2 to 2.5 times the IV dose may be needed.

Vasopressor or maintenance dose: 1 to 10 mcg/min titrated to desired response.

PEDIATRIC DOSE

Bradycardia: 0.01 mg/kg of 1:10,000 solution. (0.1 mg/kg 1:1000 diluted as above via ET).

Asystolic or pulseless arrest: 0.01 mg/kg of 1:10,000 solution initially; then 0.1 mg/kg. Up to 0.2 mg/kg may be required to be effective. Prepare an infusion and titrate from 0.1 to 1 mcg/kg/min to desired effect. Use upper dosing range if asystole present. With higher dose, be aware of preservative content to avoid toxicity.

DOSE ADJUSTMENTS

Note Drug/lab interactions. ■ Doses larger than 1 mg may not be indicated in patients over 65 years of age and patients in ventricular fibrillation.

DILUTION

Check label. Not all epinephrine solutions can be given IV.

Direct IV: Available prediluted (0.1 mg/ml [1:10,000 solution]) in 3 ml and 10 ml syringes. Each 1 mg (1 ml) of 1:1,000 solution must be diluted in at least 10 ml of NS to prepare a 1:10,000 solution. Available in a 30 ml vial (30 mg [1:1,000 solution]) to facilitate larger doses or continuous infusion.

Infusion: For occasional use as a vasopressor or for maintenance, epinephrine may be further diluted in 250 to 500 ml D5W. Give through Y-tube or three-way stopcock of infusion set.

Epinephrine Hcl infusion rates						
Desired dose	1 mg in 500 ml D5W (2 mcg/ml)			1 mg in 250 ml D5W 2 mg in 500 ml D5W (4 mcg/ml)		
mcg/min	mcg/hr	ml/min	ml/hr	mcg/hr	ml/min	ml/hr
1	60	0.5	30	60	0.25	15
2	120	1	60	120	0.5	30
3	180	1.5	90	180	0.75	45
4	240	2	120	240	1	60
5	300	2.5	150	300	1.25	75
6	360	3	180	360	1.5	90
7	420	3.5	210	420	1.75	105
8	480	4	240	480	2	120
Pediatric infusion: 0.6 mg/kg in 100 ml D5W - 1 ml/hr = 0.1 mcg/kg/min						

In *cardiac arrest,* 30 mg is sometimes added to 250 ml of NS or D5W (120 mcg/ml).

Storage: Do not use if brown or if a sediment is present. Deteriorates rapidly. Protect from light.

INCOMPATIBLE WITH

Any other drug in a syringe. Readily destroyed by alkalis alkaline solutions e.g., sodium bicarbonate and oxidizing agents. Unstable in any solution with a pH over 5.5, aminophylline, ampicillin, cephapirin (Cephadyl), mephentermine (Wyamine), sodium bicarbonate, warfarin (Coumadin).

RATE OF ADMINISTRATION

Direct IV: Each 1 mg or fraction thereof over 1 minute or longer. May be given more rapidly in cardiac resuscitation; follow with 20 ml IV flush.

Infusion: Vasopressor or maintenance: 1 to 10 mcg/min titrated to desired patient response.

Cardiac arrest: Titrated to deliver a single dose (1 to 3 mg) over 3 to 5 minutes based on patient response. Must be delivered by central venous access. Use an infusion pump to control rate.

ACTIONS

A naturally occurring hormone secreted by the adrenal glands. A sympathomimetic drug, it imitates almost all actions of the sympathetic nervous system. It is a vasoconstrictor and delays the absorption of many drugs; a potent cardiac stimulant, it strengthens the myocardial contraction (positive inotropic effect) and increases cardiac rate (positive chronotropic effect). Increases myocardial and cerebral blood flow during CPR. A potent dilator or relaxant of smooth muscle, especially bronchial muscle. Decreases blood supply to the abdomen and increases blood supply to skeletal muscles. Elevates systolic blood pressure, lowers diastolic pressure, and increases pulse pressure. Seldom used as a vasopressor because of its short duration of action. It is rapidly inactivated in the body by various enzymes and excreted in changed form in the urine. Crosses placental barrier. Secreted in breast milk.

INDICATIONS AND USES

Cardiac resuscitation. First-line drug of choice when initial CPR, intubation, ventilation, and initial defibrillation have failed to achieve response in ventricular fibrillation, ventricular tachycardia, asystole, or electromechanical dissociation. ▪ Drug of choice for anaphylactic shock. ▪ Antidote of choice for histamine overdose and allergic reactions including bronchial asthma, urticaria, and angioneurotic edema. ▪ Stokes-Adams syndrome. ▪ Occasionally used as a vasopressor (e.g., symptomatic bradycardia).

CONTRAINDICATIONS

Anesthesia with halogenated hydrocarbons or cyclopropane; cerebral arteriosclerosis, hypertension, labor and delivery if maternal blood pressure exceeds 130/80 mm Hg (may cause prolonged uterine atony with hemorrhage), hyperthyroidism, narrow-angle glaucoma, nervous instability, organic brain damage, patients receiving high doses of digitalis, shock. Do not use to treat overdosage of adrenergic blocking agents (e.g., phenoxybenzamine [Dibenzyline]), phenothiazines (e.g., chlorpromazine [Thorazine]), methotrimeprazine (Levoprome); a further drop in blood pressure will occur and irreversible shock may result. Do not use concurrently with esmolol (Brevibloc).

PRECAUTIONS

Usual route is SC except in cardiac resuscitation or as a vasopressor infusion. ▪ Give intracardiac only if no other route is available. ▪ Use caution in the elderly, diabetics, in hypotension (except in anaphylactic shock), patients receiving thyroid preparations, and those with long-term emphysema or bronchial asthma with degenerative heart disease. ▪ Often used with corticosteroids in treatment of anaphylactic shock. ▪ Larger doses in cardiac arrest are based on optimal response range of epinephrine (0.045 to 0.20 mg/kg). Data regarding effectiveness is not conclusive.

Monitor: Check blood pressure every 5 minutes. ▪ Vasoconstriction-induced tissue sloughing can occur. Avoid administering in areas of limited blood supply (e.g., fingers, toes) or if peripheral vascular disease is present. ▪ Infusion during cardiac arrest must be administered by central venous access to assure delivery to systemic circulation and to avoid extravasation. ▪ Intracardiac injection or IV injection in cardiac arrest must be accompanied by cardiac massage to perfuse drug into the myocardium and permit effective defibrillation. ▪ Note Drug/lab interactions.

Maternal/child: Pregnancy Category C: may cause anoxia in fetus. ▪ Discontinue breast feeding. ▪ Note Contraindications.

Elderly: Note Dose adjustments and Precautions.

DRUG/LAB INTERACTIONS

May be used alternately with isoproterenol (Isuprel), but they may not be used together. Both are direct cardiac stimulants and death may result. Adequate interval between doses must be maintained. ▪ Simultaneous use with oxytocics (e.g., ergonovine), MAO inhibitors (e.g., isocarboxazid [Marplan]), furazolidone (Furoxone), or guanethidine (Ismelin) may cause hypertensive crisis. ▪ Pressor response increased by anesthetics (e.g., halothane, cyclopropane), tricyclic antidepressants (e.g., amitriptyline [Elavil]), antihistamines (e.g., diphenhydramine [Benadryl]), rauwolfia alkaloids (e.g., reserpine [Serpasil]), sodium levothyroxine, and urinary alkalizers; may cause hypertension. ■ May cause hypertension with betaadrenergic blockers (e.g., propranolol [Inderal]) and alpha-adrenergic blockers (e.g., phentolamine [Regitine]). ■ Inhibited by ergot alkaloids and phenothiazines (e.g., prochlorperazine [Compazine]). ■ Inhibits insulin and oral hypoglycemic agents; increased dose may be required. ■ May cause arrhythmias with bretylium. ■ Interacts with many other drugs. ■ Note Contraindications for additional drug interactions.

SIDE EFFECTS

Often transitory; sometimes occur with average doses.

Average dose: Anxiety, dizziness, dyspnea, glycosuria, pallor, palpitations.

Overdose (frequently caused by too-rapid injection): Cerebrovascular hemorrhage, collapse (rapid), fibrillation, headache (severe), hypertension, hypotension (irreversible), pulmonary edema, pupillary dilation, restlessness, tachycardia, weakness, death.

ANTIDOTE

If side effects from the average dose become progressively worse, discontinue the drug and notify the physician. IM or SC route may be preferable. For a severe reaction caused by toxicity, treat the patient for shock and administer an antihypertensive agent such as phentolamine (Regitine) or nitroprusside (Nipride). Treat cardiac arrhythmias with a beta adrenergic blocker (propranolol [Inderal]). Resuscitate as necessary.

❦EPIRUBICIN HYDROCHLORIDE

Antineoplastic
(Anthracycline antibiotic)

❦Pharmorubicin PFS,
❦Pharmorubicin RDF

pH 4.0 to 5.5

USUAL DOSE

In combination therapies, epirubicin is used instead of doxorubicin in the combination regimen. Usually given on the same days and at the same intervals as the doxorubicin it replaces.

Metastatic Breast cancer: Single agent: 75 to 90 mg/M^2 once every 21 days. This dose may be divided and given on day 1 and day 2. An alternative weekly dose schedule of 12.5 to 25 mg/M^2 has been used and has been reported to produce less clinical toxicity than higher doses given every 3 weeks. *Combination therapy:* 50 mg/M^2. Used in combination with cyclophosphamide and fluorouracil.

Early stage breast cancer (Stage II-IIIA): 50 to 60 mg/M^2 given on days 1 and 8 every 4 weeks. Used in combination with cyclophosphamide and fluorouracil.

Small cell lung cancer: Single agent: 90 to 120 mg/M^2 once every 3 weeks. *Combination therapy:* 50 to 90 mg/M^2. Several combinations have been used (e.g., with either cisplatin or ifosfamide; with cyclophosphamide and vincristine; with cyclophosphamide and etoposide, or with cisplatin and etoposide).

Non–small cell lung cancer: Single agent: 120 to 150 mg/M^2 on day 1 every 3 to 4 weeks. *Combination therapy:* 90 to 120 mg/M^2 on day 1 every 3 to 4 weeks. Used in combination with cisplatin, etoposide, mitomycin, vinblastine, and vindesine.

Non-Hodgkin's lymphoma: Single agent: 75 to 90 mg/M^2 once every 3 weeks.

Combination therapy: 60 to 75 mg/M^2. Used in combination with cyclophosphamide, prednisone, and vincristine with or without bleomycin for the treatment of newly diagnosed non-Hodgkin's lymphoma.

Hodgkin's disease: Combination therapy: 35 mg/M^2 once every 2 weeks or 70 mg/M^2 once every 3 to 4 weeks. Used in combination with bleomycin, dacarbazine, and vinblastine.

Ovarian cancer: Single agent: 50 to 90 mg/M^2 once every 3 or 4 weeks in patients who have had prior therapy. *Combination therapy:* 50 to 90 mg/M^2 once every 3 or 4 weeks can be added to their regimen in patients who have had prior therapy; or the same dose in combination with cisplatin and cyclophosphamide is used for initial therapy of ovarian cancer.

Locally unresectable or metastatic gastric cancer: Single agent: 75 to 100 mg/M^2 once every 3 weeks. *Combination therapy:* 80 mg/M^2 once every 3 to 4 weeks. Used in combination with fluorouracil.

PEDIATRIC DOSE

Specific information on safety for use in children not available.

DOSE ADJUSTMENTS

Use lower dose in range for patients with inadequate marrow reserves due to old age, prior therapy, or neoplastic marrow infiltration. ▪ Reduced dose, delay, or suspension of epirubicin may be required based on hematologic toxicity; manufacturer provides no specific recommendations. ▪ *Elevated serum bilirubin:* Give 50% of a dose for serum bilirubin from 1.2 to 3.0 mg/ml and 25% of a dose for serum bilirubin above 3.0 mg/ml. ▪ No dose adjustment required in impaired renal function.

DILUTION

Specific techniques required; see Precautions. Epirubicin PFS available as 2 mg/ml in 5 ml, 25 ml, and 100 ml vials. Use of the 100 ml vial should be restricted to a pharmacy admixture program using a sterile transfer or dispensing device. Enter any vial only once and withdraw desired dose into a syringe. No further dilution is required.

Epirubicin RDF is available in 10, 20, 50, and 150 mg vials. Reconstitute each 10 mg with 5 ml NS (2 mg/ml). See comments above.

Storage: Store unopened RDF vials at controlled room temperature, PFS vials in refrigerator; keep in original cartons to protect from light. Use any filled syringe within 24 hours if stored at room temperature and within 48 hours if refrigerated. Syringes prepared from the pharmacy bulk vial must be used within 24 or 48 hours of the initial puncture of that vial based on method of storage. Once the transfer set has been inserted in the bulk vial, any remaining undispensed drug must be discarded in 8 hours.

INCOMPATIBLE WITH

Manufacturer recommends not mixing with other drugs until specific information is available. Consider toxicity and specific use.

RATE OF ADMINISTRATION

Direct IV: A single dose over a minimum of 3 to 5 minutes. Should be given through Y-tube or three-way stopcock of a free-flowing infusion of NS or D5W. Slow injection rate further for erythematous streaking along the vein or facial flushing.

ACTIONS

A semisynthetic anthracycline antineoplastic antibiotic agent. Rapidly penetrates cell and interferes with cell division by binding with DNA to slow production of nucleic acid synthesis. Metabolized in the liver, the process of glucuronidation distinguishes epirubicin from doxorubicin and may account for its faster elimination and reduced toxicity. It is less toxic and in particular less cardiotoxic than doxorubicin. Has the same antitumor effect at equal doses. Elimination half-life is 30 to 40 hours. Does not cross blood-brain barrier. Primarily excreted in bile; some excretion in urine.

INDICATIONS AND USES

Treatment of metastatic as well as early stage breast cancer, small cell lung cancer (both limited and extensive disease), advanced non-small cell lung cancer, non-Hodgkin's lymphoma, Hodgkin's disease, Stage III and IV ovarian cancer, and metastatic and locally unresectable gastric cancers. May be used as a single agent or in combination with other chemotherapeutic agents.

CONTRAINDICATIONS

History of severe cardiac disease, myelosuppression resulting from treatment with other antineoplastic agents or radiation therapy. Generally contraindicated in patients who have received previous treatment with maximum recommended cumulative doses of daunorubicin (Cerubidine), doxorubicin (Adriamycin), idarubicin (Idamycin), mitoxantrone (Novantrone), or mitomycin C.

PRECAUTIONS

■ Follow guidelines for handling cytotoxic agents. See Appendix A, p. 893. ■ Currently approved for use in Canada; application pending in the United States. ■ Administered by or under the direction of the physician specialist, with facilities for monitoring the patient and responding to any medical emergency. ■ For IV use only. Do not give IM or SC. ■ May cause serious, irreversible myocardial toxicity with congestive heart failure and/or cardiomyopathy as the cumulative dose approaches 1,000 mg/M^2. ■ Use extreme caution in preexisting drug-induced bone marrow suppression, existing heart disease, previous treatment with other anthracyclines (e.g., daunorubicin, doxorubicin, idarubicin), other cardiotoxic agents (e.g., bleomycin), or radiation therapy encompassing the heart; cardiac toxicity may occur at lower cumulative doses.

Monitor: Use only large veins. Avoid veins over joints or in extremities with compromised venous or lymphatic drainage. Determine absolute patency of vein. Extravasation may occur with or without stinging or burning along the injection site even if blood returns well on aspiration of the infusion needle. Observe site frequently. Extravasation can result in severe cellulitis and tissue necrosis; if it occurs, discontinue injection;

use another vein. ■ Obtain baseline CBC including differential and platelet count, uric acid level, liver function tests (AST, ALT, alkaline phosphatase, and serum bilirubin), ECG, chest x-ray, and echocardiogram. Monitor lab values during therapy especially before each dose. Monitor ECG, chest x-ray, echocardiogram, and/or radionuclide angiography in patients who have had mediastinal radiation, other anthracycline or anthracene therapy, those with preexisting cardiac disease, or those who have received prior epirubicin cumulative doses exceeding 650 mg/M^2. ■ Maintain adequate hydration. ■ Allopurinol may prevent formation of uric acid crystals. ■ Be alert for signs of bone marrow depression, bleeding, or infection. ■ Use of prophylactic antibiotics may be indicated pending C/S in a febrile, neutropenic patient. ■ Prophylactic antiemetics are indicated. ■ Note Drug/lab interactions.

Patient education: Urine will be reddish for several days (from drug, not hematuria). ■ Nonhormonal birth control recommended. ■ Report IV site burning, stinging, or puffiness promptly. ■ See Appendix D, p. 900.

Maternal/child: Can cause fetal harm. Avoid pregnancy. May cause testicular atrophy. ■ Discontinue breast feeding. ■ Information on safety for use in children not available.

Elderly: Cardiotoxicity and myelotoxicity may be more severe. ■ Note Dose adjustments.

DRUG/LAB INTERACTIONS

May increase bone marrow toxocity of other chemotherapeutic agents. ■ Increased toxicity including skin redness and exfoliative changes possible when given concurrently with or after radiation.

SIDE EFFECTS

Dose limiting toxicities are myelosuppression and cardiotoxicity. Severe cellulitis, vesication, local pain, and tissue necrosis can occur with extravasation. Venous sclerosis may result from injection into small veins or repeated injection into the same vein. Other side effects are alopecia, arrhythymias (transient), diarrhea, fever, malaise, mucositis (esophagitis, stomatitis), nausea and vomiting, phlebitis, recall of skin reaction associated with prior radiation.

Overdose: May cause an acute myocardial dysfunction within 24 hours. Pronounced mucositis, leukopenia and thrombocytopenia may occur within 7 to 14 days.

ANTIDOTE

Most side effects will either be tolerated or treated symptomatically. Keep the physician informed. Hematopoietic toxicity (leukopenia, thrombocytopenia) may require dose reduction or cessation of therapy, antibiotics, platelet and granulocyte transfusions, filgrastim (Neupogen), or sargramostim (Leukine). Acute cardiac failure occurs suddenly (most common when total cumulative doses approach 1,000 mg/M^2) and frequently does not respond to currently available treatment. Close monitoring of accumulated dose, bone marrow, ECG, chest x-ray, echocardiography, and systolic ejection fraction may prevent most serious and potentially fatal cardiac side effects. There is no specific antidote. Supportive therapy as indicated will help sustain the patient in toxicity. Dexrazoxane is currently available to prevent cardiotoxicity of doxorubicin in specific situations; in the future it may be considered with epirubicin. If extravasation occurs, attempt aspiration of the infiltrated epirubicin. Elevate the extremity and apply local intermittent ice compresses for up to 3 days. Observe the site frequently. Should be seen by a reconstructive surgeon if local pain persists or skin changes progress after 3 to 4 days. Ulceration may require early wide excision of the involved area.

EPOETIN ALFA

EPO, Epogen, Erythropoietin, Procrit

Recombinant human erythropoietin
Antianemic agent

pH 6.6 to 7.2

USUAL DOSE

In all situations rate of hematocrit increase is dose dependent and varies among patients. Availability of iron stores, baseline hematocrit, and concurrent medical problems affect the rate and extent of response. Note Precautions/Monitor.

Anemia of chronic renal failure: May be given by IV or SC injection. 50 to 100 units/kg of body weight 3 times a week initially. Range is from 15 to 500 units/kg/dose. Median dose is 75 to 100 units/kg. A 55 kg (120 lb) individual would receive 2,750 units at 50 units/kg, 4,125 units at 75 units/kg, and 5,500 units at 100 units/kg. Entire contents of a vial (2,000, 3,000, or 4,000 units) has been used instead of an exact calculated dose. Predialysis patients usually require doses in the average range, peritoneal dialysis patients respond rapidly to lower doses, and higher-end doses may be required, especially in dialysis patients (see literature). Reduce dose by 25 units/kg when the hemoglobin concentration reaches 10 Gm/dl or the hematocrit reaches the target range (30% to 36%) or rises more than 4 points in any 2-week period. Increase dose by 25 units/kg if the hematocrit does not increase by 5 to 6 points after 8 weeks of therapy and is below target range. Continue to increase by 25 units/kg/dose at 4- to 6-week intervals until target range is reached.

Maintenance dose: Individually titrated. After reaching target range, reduce by 25 units/kg. Median maintenance dose is 75 units/kg 3 times/week; range is 12.5 to 525 units/kg 3 times weekly. Adjust dose by 10 to 25 units/kg increments at 2- to 6-week intervals to keep hematocrit in target range. Evaluate iron stores if hematocrit falls (See Monitor).

Anemia in HIV-infected patients, including zidovudine-induced: May be given by IV or SC injection. 100 units/kg 3 times a week for 8 weeks. Obtain endogenous serum erythropoietin level (prior to transfusion) before initiating therapy (See Precautions/Monitor). After 8 weeks of therapy, the dose may be increased by 50 to 100 units/kg 3 times a week (total dose of 150 to 200 units/kg). Evaluate response every 4 to 8 weeks and adjust dose accordingly by 50 to 100 units/kg (total dose of 200 to 300 units/kg). Not likely to be effective if doses of 300 units/kg 3 times a week have not corrected the anemia.

Maintenance dose: When desired response is attained (i.e., reduced transfusion requirements or increased hematocrit) titrate dose to maintain the response. Consider variations in zidovudine (AZT) dose and presence of infectious or inflammatory episodes. If the hematocrit exceeds 40%, discontinue until the hematocrit drops to 36%. Reduce dose by 25% when treatment is resumed and titrate carefully to maintain desired hematocrit.

Anemia associated with cancer patients on chemotherapy: SC injection recommended. 100 to 150 units/kg 3 times a week. May be given with or without concomitant antineoplastic drug therapy. Obtain endogenous serum erythropoietin level (prior to transfusion) before initiating therapy (see Precautions/Monitor). If adequate response has not occurred after 8 weeks, increase the dose up to 300 units/kg 3 times a week. Not likely to be effective if doses of 300 units/kg 3 times a week have not corrected the anemia. If the hematocrit exceeds 40%, discontinue until the hematocrit drops to 36%. Reduce dose by 25% when treatment is resumed, and titrate carefully to maintain desired hematocrit.

Reduction of allogenic blood transfusions in surgery patients: SC injection recommended. Obtain hemoglobin before initiating therapy. Should be greater than 10 g/dl but less than 13 g/dl. 300 units/kg/day for 10 days before surgery, on the day of surgery, and for 4 days after surgery. Has been given concurrently with anticoagulant prophylaxis. An alternate dose schedule is 600 units/kg once each week on days 21, 14, and 7 before surgery and again on the day of surgery. Begin iron supplementaion no later than the beginning of treatment with epoetin alfa and continue throughout the course of therapy.

DOSE ADJUSTMENTS

Based on hematocrit. (See Usual dose) for each indication. ■ Dose based on average weight if edema is present. ■ Note Precautions/ Monitor.

DILUTION

Available in numerous concentrations; check dose on vial carefully. May be given undiluted as an IV bolus. Do not shake during preparation; will render it biologically inactive. Single-dose vial contains no preservatives. Use only 1 dose per vial, then discard. Never reenter vial. Now available in multidose vial with preservative; sterile technique imperative.

Storage: Refrigerate single and multidose vials prior to use; multidose vial after initial use. Discard in 21 days.

INCOMPATIBLE WITH

Any other drug in syringe or solution because of specific use and manufacturer's recommendation.

RATE OF ADMINISTRATION

A single dose over at least 1 minute.

ACTIONS

An amino acid glycoprotein manufactured by recombinant DNA technology. Has the same biologic effects as erythropoietin produced naturally by the kidneys. Stimulates bone marrow to produce red blood cells, increasing the reticulocyte count within 10 days and the red cell count, hemoglobin, and hematocrit within 2 to 6 weeks. Normal iron stores are necessary because it steps up red blood cell production to a rate above what the body usually makes. New cells need iron, which is quickly depleted. Detectable levels remain in plasma for up to 24 hours. Continued therapy will maintain improved red blood cell levels and decrease need for transfusions. Within 2 months most patients are transfusion independent. Considered replacement therapy as insulin is to diabetics.

INDICATIONS AND USES

To treat anemia associated with chronic renal failure and decrease the need for transfusions in patients receiving dialysis (end-stage renal disease) and those not receiving dialysis. ■ Treatment of anemias related to zidovudine (AZT, Retrovir) therapy in HIV-infected patients. ■ Treatment of anemia in cancer patients on chemotherapy. ■ Treament of anemic patients scheduled to undergo noncardiac, non-vascular surgery to reduce the need for allogenic blood transfusions, especially in patients at high risk for perioperative transfusions with significant anticipated blood loss. ■ Not indicated for anemic patients who are willing to donate autologous blood.

Investigational uses: Other drug-induced anemias; rheumatoid arthritis and other chronic inflammatory diseases; sickle cell anemia; and anemia of prematurity.

CONTRAINDICATIONS

Known hypersensitivity to albumin (human) or to mammalian cell-derived products, uncontrolled hypertension.

PRECAUTIONS

All patients: May be given IV or SC in patients not receiving dialysis. May be given to dialysis patients into the venous line at the end of the dialysis procedure to eliminate additional venous access. ■ In addition to low baseline hematocrit and inadequate iron stores, delayed or diminished response may result from concurrent medical problems (infections, inflammatory or malignant processes, occult blood loss, underlying hematologic disease, folic acid or vitamin B_{12} deficiency, hemolysis, aluminum intoxication, osteitis fibrosa cystica). ■ Not intended for use in anemias caused by iron or folate deficiencies, hemolysis, or GI bleeding. ■ Use caution in patients with prophyria; may exacerbate disease. ■ Not a substitute for emergency transfusion in patients requiring immediate correction of severe anemia. *Chronic renal failure:* 98% of previously transfusion-dependent patients are able to maintain a stable hematocrit greater than 30% with epoetin alfa therapy. ■ Epoetin alfa, with or without phlebotomy, has reduced iron and ferritin stores in hemodialysis patients with iron overload and associated hemosiderosis secondary to multiple red blood cell transfusions. ■ Some authorities believe epoetin should be discontinued 2 weeks before planned renal engraftment to prevent risk of excessive erythrocytosis and resultant adverse effects (renal artery thrombosis with loss of graft occurred in one patient). ■ Epoetin alfa reduces need for blood transfusions and decreases exposure to foreign histocompatibility; potential for finding a compatible graft may be increased. *HIV infection:* Epoetin has no effect on HIV disease process; primarily improves quality of life. ■ Used concomitantly with filgrastim (G-CSF, Neupogen) to control granulocytopenia; filgrastim increases the neutrophil count while epoetin alfa increases the hemoglobin concentration. Helps to maintain somewhat more normal counts in zidovudine therapy, but additional blood transfusions will probably be required. *Cancer patients on chemotherapy:* Treatment of patients with grossly elevated serum erythropoietin levels (e.g., greater than 200 mUnits/ml) is not recommended. *Surgery patients:* Safety established only for patients receiving anticoagulation prophylaxis.

Monitor: All patients: Hypertension must be controlled before initiation of therapy. Monitor blood pressure frequently and control aggressively; generally rises when hematocrit is increasing rapidly. 25% of renal patients require an increase in antihypertensive therapy and dietary restrictions. Exacerbation of hypertension has not been observed in patients being treated with epoetin alfa for other indicated anemias; however, any indication may require a decrease in dose of epoetin if blood pressure difficult to control or withhold epoetin until blood pressure is controlled. ▪ CBC with differential and platelet counts; BUN; uric acid; creatinine; phosphorus; and potassium are required before treatment is initiated and at regular intervals during therapy. Modest increases are expected. Changes in dialysis treatment may be required. ▪ Normal iron stores required to support epoetin-stimulated erythropoiesis. Transferrin saturation should be at least 20% and ferritin at least 100 ng/ml. Monitor before and during therapy. Supplemental iron (ferrous sulfate 325 mg orally 3 times a day) is usually required to increase and maintain transferrin saturation. ▪ Seizures rare, but more occur in the first 90 days. Observe blood pressure and neurologic symptoms. Caution against driving or operating heavy machinery. ▪ Monitor patients with preexisting vascular disease carefully (especially those with chronic renal failure); increase in hematocrit may precipitate a cerebrovascular accident, transient ischemic attack, or myocardial infarction. ▪ As anemia is corrected, elevated bleeding time decreases toward normal with epoetin treatment as it does with transfusion. ***Chronic renal failure:*** Can cause polycythemia. Base line hematocrit required. Repeat twice weekly until stabilization in the target range (30% to 36%). Continue monitoring at regular intervals. After any dose adjustment, twice-weekly hematocrit is required for 2 to 6 weeks to evaluate outcome and make further dose adjustments. If hematocrit exceeds 36%, withhold doses and check hematocrit twice weekly until it reaches 33%. Reduce dose as indicated in Usual dose. ▪ Dialysis patients may require additional anticoagulation with heparin to prevent clotting of artificial kidney or clotting of the vascular access (AV shunt) and to maintain efficiency of the dialysis procedure. ▪ Compliance with dialysis and/or dietary restrictions is mandatory. ▪ Monitor fluid and electrolyte balance carefully in patients not receiving dialysis. Improved sense of well-being may mask need for dialysis. ***HIV infection:*** ▪ Effectiveness in HIV-infected patients seems to be dependent on an endogenous serum erythropoietin level less than 500 mU/ml (normal levels are 4 to 26 mU/ml) and a dose of zidovudine (AZT, Retrovir) of less than 4,200 mg/wk. ***Cancer patients on chemotherapy:*** Monitor hematocrit weekly until stable. ***Surgery patients:*** Monitor iron supplementation and anticoagulant therapy.

Patient education: Risk of seizures, especially during first 90 days of therapy. Do not drive or operate heavy equipment. ▪ Menses may resume; possibility of pregnancy. Contraception may be indicated. ▪ Additional instruction (e.g., equipment, techniques) will be required in patients on home dialysis who will self-administer (manufacturer supplies brochure).

Maternal/child: Pregnancy Category C: may present risk to fetus; benefits must justify risk. ▪ Use caution in nursing mothers. ▪ Safety for use in children not established.

Elderly: Monitor blood chemistry and blood pressure carefully due to increased risk of renal and/or cardiovascular complications.

DRUG/LAB INTERACTIONS

Specific information not available.

SIDE EFFECTS

Generally well tolerated. Occur most frequently in patients with chronic renal failure. Increased hypertension is common, and hypertensive encephalopathy and seizures can occur. Clotted vascular access (AV shunt) and clotting of the artificial kidney may occur during dialysis. Too-rapid increase in hematocrit (over 4 points in 2 weeks) or a hematocrit over 36% (polycythemia) often occurs. Allergic reactions have been reported. Other reported side effects are those common to the underlying disease, and not necessarily attributable to epoetin and include: arthralgias, asthenia, bone marrow fibrosis, cerebrovascular accident or transient ischemic attack, chest pain, cough, CVA/TIA, diarrhea, dizziness, edema, fatigue, fever, headache, hyperkalemia, myocardial infarction, nausea, rash, respiratory congestion, shortness of breath, tachycardia, and vomiting.

ANTIDOTE

Notify physician of all side effects; most will be treated symptomatically. Excessive hypertension may require discontinuation of epoetin until blood pressure is controlled or may respond to reduction in dose of epoetin or to an increase in antihypertensive therapy. Reduce dose of epoetin in patients with an increase in hematocrit over 4 points in 2 weeks or any patient with a hematocrit over 36% (renal patients) to 40% (others). May need to withhold epoetin until hematocrit falls to 33%. Consider phlebotomy in toxicity. Additional heparin may be required during dialysis to prevent clotting. Treat minor allergic reactions symptomatically. Discontinue drug and treat anaphylaxis as indicated; resuscitate as necessary.

EPOPROSTENOL SODIUM

Flolan

Vasodilating agent

pH 10.2 to 10.8

USUAL DOSE

Acute dose ranging: May or may not take place during cardiac catheterization. May be administered through a peripheral line. Begin infusion at 2 ng/kg/min. Increase in increments of 2 ng/kg/min every 15 minutes or longer until dose-limiting pharmacologic effects occur. Flushing, headache, hypotension, nausea, vomiting are most common. See Side effects for others. Average mean dose range in trials before side effects occurred was 8.3 to 8.9 ng/kg/min. Usually given concomitantly with anticoagulant therapy; see Monitor.

Chronic continuous infusion: May be given through a peripheral line on a temporary basis until a central venous line is established. A central venous catheter should be in place as soon as possible and must be used for continuous long-term 24-hour administration with an ambulatory infusion pump. Begin at 4 ng/kg/min less than the maximum-tolerated infusion rate determined during acute dose ranging. If the maximum-tolerated rate is less than 5 ng/kg/min, begin at one half of that rate. Average mean dose range during trials was 5 ng/kg/min.

PEDIATRIC DOSE

Safety for use in children not established.

DOSE ADJUSTMENTS

Changes in the chronic infusion rate are to be expected. If symptoms of primary pulmonary hypertension (PPH) persist, recur, or worsen, increase infusion rate promptly by 1 to 2 ng/kg/min. Wait at least 15 minutes to assess clinical response. Observe patient for several hours to confirm patient tolerance and take BP and HR in supine and standing positions. In trials most patients progressed to a dose a little less than their acute dose-ranging intolerable dose within 12 weeks.
■ Occurrence of dose-related side effects that do not resolve may require a decrease in the chronic infusion rate. Begin with 2 ng/kg/min and wait at least 15 minutes to assess clinical response. Use extreme caution if decreasing the dose; abrupt withdrawal or sudden large reductions may cause a rapid return of PPH symptoms and may precipitate death. ■ In patients receiving lung transplants, doses were tapered after the initiation of cardiopulmonary bypass. ■ Dose selection for the elderly should be cautious. ■ Note Precautions.

DILUTION

Infusion pump required. It must be small and lightweight; able to adjust infusion rates in 2-ng/kg/min increments; have occlusion, end of infusion, and low battery alarms; be accurate to ±6% of the programmed rate; be positive-pressure driven (continuous or pulsatile) with intervals between pulses not exceeding 3 minutes at rates required to deliver drug; and have a disposable reservoir cassette made of polyvinyl chloride, polypropylene, or glass with a capacity of at least 100 ml. Pumps used during trials were manufactured by Pharmacia Deltec, Medfusion, INC. and Baxter Health Care. Sterile diluent for epoprostenol is provided by the manufacturer. Do not use any other diluent. Concentration will be determined by desired dose/kg/min and parameters of ambulatory infusion pump to be used. See Rate of administration. Two vials of provided sterile diluent will be required to prepare each 24-hour dose in each of the concentrations in the chart below:

To make 100 ml of solution with final concentration (ng/ml) of:	Directions
3,000 ng/ml	Dissolve contents of one 0.5-mg vial with 5 ml of STERILE DILUENT for FLOLAN. Withdraw 3 ml and add to sufficient STERILE DILUENT for FLOLAN to make a total of 100 ml.
5,000 ng/ml	Dissolve contents of one 0.5-mg vial with 5 ml of STERILE DILUENT for FLOLAN. Withdraw entire vial contents and add sufficient STERILE DILUENT for FLOLAN to make a total of 100 ml.
10,000 ng/ml	Dissolve contents of two 0.5-mg vials each with 5 ml of STERILE DILUENT for FLOLAN. Withdraw entire vial contents and add sufficient STERILE DILUENT for FLOLAN to make a total of 100 ml.
15,000 ng/ml	Dissolve contents of one 1.5-mg vial with 5 ml of STERILE DILUENT for FLOLAN. Withdraw entire vial contents and add sufficient STERILE DILUENT for FLOLAN to make a total of 100 ml.

Acute dose-ranging may require more than one solution strength. 3,000 ng/ml and 10,000 ng/ml concentrations should be satisfactory to deliver between 2 and 16 ng/kg/min in adults. A maximum 2-day supply can be diluted at one time (200 ml). For use at room temperature withdraw 33.3 ml and deposit in pump reservoir cassette or sterile infusion bag for each 8-hour period. If used with cold pouches and frozen gel packs, 100 ml can be placed in the pump reservoir cassette or a 100-ml sterile infusion bag for each 24-hour period. Frozen gel packs must be changed every 12 hours. Reservoir cassettes are disposable. Most patients prepare a 24-hour dose in a new reservoir cassette before a new dose is required and use cold pouches to maintain temperature.

Storage: Unopened vials of epoprostenol may be stored at controlled room temperature in the carton to protect from light. Diluent may be stored at controlled room temperature. Protection from light not required. Note expiration dates on both. Prior to use, reconstituted solutions must be refrigerated and protected from light. Do not freeze. Reconstituted solution must be discarded after 48 hours or if accidentally frozen. While in use, must not be exposed to direct sunlight or temperatures above 25° C (77° F) or below 0° C (32° F). Stable in pump reservoir for only 8 hours at controlled room temperature. Use of cold pouches with frozen gel packs can extend reservoir life to 24 hours. Time stored in refrigerator and in reservoir of pump must be included in maximum 48-hour time frame.

INCOMPATIBLE WITH

Manufacturer states, "Must not be reconstituted or mixed with any other drug or solution prior to or during administration."

RATE OF ADMINISTRATION

Administered by a continuous IV infusion based on rate determined for acute dose-ranging, continuous chronic infusion, or dose adjustments. Flow must not be interrupted for longer than 2 to 3 minutes. Time to completion of administration must never exceed more than 8 hours at room temperature, more than 24 hours with use of cold pouches and changing frozen gel packs every 12 hours, or more than 48 hours from time of initial reconstitution. The infusion rate may be calculated using the following formula:

$$\text{Infusion rate (ml/hr)} = \frac{\text{Dose (ng/kg/min)} \times \text{Weight in kg} \times 60 \text{ min/hr}}{\text{Final concentration (ng/ml)}}$$

The following table may be used for infusion rates at a final concentration of 3,000 ng/ml. See package insert for tables at additional concentrations:

Infusion rates for epoprostenol at a concentration of 3,000 ng/ml								
	Dose or Drug Delivery Rate (ml/hr)							
Patient Weight (kg)	2	4	6	8	10	12	14	16
	Infusion Delivery Rate (ml/hr)							
10	—	—	1.2	1.6	2	2.4	2.8	3.2
20	—	1.6	2.4	3.2	4	4.8	5.6	6.4
30	1.2	2.4	3.6	4.8	6	7.2	8.4	9.6
40	1.6	3.2	4.8	6.4	8	9.6	11.2	12.8
50	2	4	6	8	10	12	14	16
60	2.4	4.8	7.2	9.6	12	14.4	16.8	19.2
70	2.8	5.6	8.4	11.2	14	16.8	19.6	22.4
80	3.2	6.4	9.6	12.8	16	19.2	22.4	25.6
90	3.6	7.2	10.8	14.4	18	21.6	25.2	28.8
100	4	8	12	16	20	24	28	32

ACTIONS

A naturally occuring prostaglandin. It directly vasodilates pulmonary and systemic arterial vascular beds and inhibits platelet aggregation. Right and left ventricle afterload is reduced, and cardiac output and stroke volume are increased. Effect on heart rate is dose related. Produces dose-related increases in cardiac index and stroke volume and dose-related decreases in pulmonary vascular resistance, total pulmonary resistance, and mean systemic arterial pressure. Has been shown to increase exercise capacity, improve hemodynamic status, and extend survival. Onset of action is immediate but lasts for only 6 minutes at body pH of 7.4. Metabolized to two primary metabolites by rapid hydrolyzation and enzymatic degradation.

INDICATIONS AND USES

Long-term IV treatment of primary pulmonary hpertension (PPH) for patients with New York Heart Association Class III and IV PPH disease.

CONTRAINDICATIONS

Congestive heart failure due to severe left ventricular systolic dysfunction, known hypersensitivity to epoprostenol or related compounds (e.g., alprostadil [Prostin VR Pediatric], prostaglandin E_1 [Alprostadil]).

PRECAUTIONS

Administered by or under the direction of the physician specialist.
■ During dose-ranging, facilities for monitoring the patient and responding to any medical emergency must be available. ■ Causes of secondary pulmonary hypertension should be eliminated and diagnosis of PPH carefully established. ■ Abrupt withdrawal, interruptions in drug delivery, or sudden large reductions in dose may result in rebound pulmonary hypertension, including dyspnea, dizziness, and weakness. Death of one patient was attributed to these causes. Backup medication and equipment must always be available. ■ Use of a multilumen catheter should be considered if other IV therapy is used.
■ Not recommended for patients who develop pulmonary edema during acute dose-ranging; may develop pulmonary veno-occlusive disease. ■ Asymptomatic increases in pulmonary artery pressure with increases in cardiac output may occur during acute dose-ranging; consider dose adjustment. ■ Cardiac catheterization used during trials for acute dose-ranging, but is not necessary; consider benefit versus risk.
■ Note Monitor, Patient education, Drug/lab interactions.

Monitor: ECG monitoring and frequent monitoring of vital signs recommended during acute dose-ranging. ■ Observe for dose-limiting side effects. ■ To reduce the risk of pulmonary thromboembolism or systemic embolism, anticoagulant therapy is recommended concomitantly unless contraindicated. ■ Therapy may be required for months or years; consideration must be given to the ability of the patient and family to manage this care. ■ Monitor standing and supine HR and BP for several hours after any adjustment. ■ Thorough patient teaching and continued support services are imperative to facilitate a good clinical outcome. ■ Note Precautions, Patient education, Drug/lab interactions.

Patient education: After initial dose titration and training, this is a self-administered drug. Must assume responsibility for drug reconstitution, drug administration, and care of the permanent central venous catheter. ■ Aseptic technique during reconstitution and with routine care of permanent indwelling central venous catheter is imperative to prevent infection. ■ Delivery of medication cannot be interrupted. Interruption will cause a rapid return of PPH symptoms. ■ Should have access to a backup infusion pump and intravenous infusion sets to avoid potential interruption in drug delivery. ■ Dose adjustments should be made only under the direction of the physician except in an emergency situation (e.g., unconsciousness, collapse).

Maternal/child: Pregnancy category B: Use only if clearly needed. No evidence of fetal harm in animal studies to date. ▪ Safety for use during labor and delivery not established. ▪ Use caution in nursing mothers; safety not established. ▪ Safety for use in children not established.

Elderly: Note Dose adjustments. Decreased organ function (cardiac, hepatic, renal), concomitant disease, and other drug therapy may cause concern.

DRUG/LAB INTERACTIONS

Hypotension may be increased with diuretics, antihypertensive agents, or other vasodilators. ▪ Risk of bleeding may be increased with anti-platelet agents or anticoagulants.

SIDE EFFECT

Acute dose-ranging: Flushing, headache, hypotension, nausea, and vomiting are most common and are dose-limiting. Abdominal pain, anxiety/nervousness, back pain, bradycardia, chest pain, constipation, dizziness, dyspnea, dyspepsia, musculoskeletal pain, paresthesia, sweating, tachycardia, and many other side effects may occur.

Chronic continuous infusion: Any of the above and chills, diarrhea, fever, flu-like symptoms, infection (may be local at site of catheter insertion), jaw pain.

ANTIDOTE

Continuous maintenance of drug flow imperative. Keep physician informed of all side effects. Most will be treated with dose reduction; some may require symptomatic treatment. Marketed through Glaxo Wellcome Inc. Flolan Lifeline Services program. Call 1-800-9-FLOLAN for drug or pump problems.

ERGONOVINE MALEATE

Uterine stimulant
(Oxytocic)
Diagnostic agent

Ergotrate maleate

pH 2.7 to 3.5

USUAL DOSE

Uterine stimulant: 1 ml (0.2 mg or gr 1/300). Repeat in 2 to 4 hours if necessary. A maximum of 5 doses is usually not exceeded.

Diagnosis of Prinzmetal's angina (investigational): 0.05 mg IV during coronary angiography (See Precautions). Repeat every 5 minutes until onset of chest pain or a total dose of 0.4 mg.

DILUTION

May be given undiluted. Some clinicians recommend dilution with 5 ml of NS. Do not add to IV solutions. Give through Y-tube or three-way stopcock of infusion set.

Storage: Should be refrigerated; may not be stored at room temperature more than 60 days. Check expiration date on vial; deteriorates with age.

INCOMPATIBLE WITH

Amobarbital (Amytal), ampicillin (Polycillin), cephalothin (Keflin), chloramphenicol (Chloromycetin), chlortetracycline (Aureomycin), epinephrine (Adrenalin), heparin, methicillin (Staphcillin), pentobarbital (Nembutal), thiopental (Pentothal), warfarin (Coumadin).

RATE OF ADMINISTRATION

0.2 mg or fraction thereof over 1 minute. Too-rapid injection may cause severe nausea and vomiting.

ACTIONS

An oxytocic, it exerts a direct stimulation on the smooth muscle of the uterus, causing contraction of the uterus. Produces vasoconstriction, increases central venous pressure, elevates BP, and may rarely produce peripheral ischemia. In therapeutic doses the prolonged initial contraction is followed by periods of relaxation and contraction. Effective within 1 minute for up to 3 hours. The least toxic of the ergot derivatives, it is probably metabolized in the liver and excreted in feces. Secreted in breast milk.

INDICATIONS AND USES

Prevents or controls postpartum or postabortal hemorrhage.

Investigational use: Diagnosis of Prinzmetal's angina.

CONTRAINDICATIONS

Known hypersensitivity to ergot alkaloids; pregnancy prior to the third stage of labor (delivery of placenta).

PRECAUTIONS

Not recommended for use before the delivery of the placenta. ▪ IV administration is for emergency use only. IM or PO route is preferred and should be used after the initial IV dose. ▪ Use caution in patients with cardiac, renal, or liver disease and in febrile or septic states. ▪ Simulates spontaneous coronary arterial spasms responsible for Prinzmetal's angina when injected during coronary arteriography. These spasms are reversible with nitroglycerin. This use has precipitated arrhythmias including ventricular tachycardia and myocardial infarction.

Monitor: Monitor blood pressure, pulse, and uterine response. Observe for vaginal bleeding and frequent periods of uterine relaxation. ▪ Uterine response may be poor in calcium-deficient patients and will require calcium replacement for effective response. Avoid or use extreme caution if calcium replacement is needed in patients taking digoxin. ▪ Note Drug/lab interactions.

Maternal/child: Note Contraindications. Do not administer before delivery of the placenta; it may cause hypoxia and intracranial hemorrhage in the infant, captivation of the placenta, or missed diagnosis of a second infant. ▪ May decrease prolactin levels and inhibit lactation.

DRUG/LAB INTERACTIONS

Severe hypertension and cerebrovascular accidents can result with ephedrine, epinephrine, methoxamine (Vasoxyl), and other vasopressors. Chlorpromazine (Thorazine) IV will reduce this hypertension.

SIDE EFFECTS

Rare in therapeutic doses, but may include the following:

Average dose: Allergic phenomena, blindness, chest pain, confusion, diarrhea, dilated pupils, dizziness, headache, hypertension, hypotension, nausea, numb and/or cold extremities, ringing in the ears, shortness of breath, vomiting, weakness.

Overdose: Abortion, convulsions, excitement, gangrene, hypercoagulability, severe nausea and vomiting, shock, tachycardia, thirst, tremor, uterine bleeding.

ANTIDOTE

Discontinue the drug immediately at the onset of any side effect and notify the physician. Most side effects are transient unless there is severe toxicity and will be treated symptomatically. Use antiemetics (e.g., prochlorperazine [Compazine], ondansetron [Zofran]) for nausea and vomiting. Treat cardiac ischemia with nitroglycerin, seizures with diazepam (Valium) or phenytoin (Dilantin). Treat peripheral ischemia with nitroprusside, tolazoline (Priscoline), or phentolamine (Regitine). Treat hypertension with nitroprusside, chlorpromazine (Thorazine), or hydralazine (Apresoline). Severe poisoning is treated with vasodilator drugs, sedatives, calcium gluconate to relieve muscular pain, and other supportive treatment. Heparin is used to control hypercoagulability.

ERYTHROMYCIN GLUCEPTATE/ ERYTHROMYCIN LACTOBIONATE

Antibacterial (Macrolide)

Erythrocin IV, Ilotycin gluceptate

pH 6.5 to 7.7

USUAL DOSE

Antibacterial: 15 to 20 mg/kg of body weight/24 hr in equally divided doses every 6 hours (350 to 500 mg every 6 hours). Continuous infusion over 24 hours is preferred. Up to 4 Gm/24 hr has been given.

Legionnaires' disease: 1 Gm every 6 hours as a continuous infusion.

Pelvic inflammatory disease: 500 mg every 6 hours as a continuous infusion for 3 days. Follow with oral erythromycin 250 mg every 6 hours for 7 days.

PEDIATRIC DOSE

15 to 20 mg/kg of body weight/24 hr in equally divided doses every 6 hours is recommended. Another source recommends 20 to 50 mg/kg/24 hr in equally divided doses every 6 hours.

DOSE ADJUSTMENTS

Reduced dose may be required in impaired liver function.

DILUTION

Each 500 mg or fraction thereof must be diluted with 10 ml of sterile water for injection without preservatives to form a 5% solution and avoid precipitation. Shake well to ensure dilution.

Erythromycin gluceptate: *Continuous infusion (preferred):* Further dilute each 1 Gm in 1,000 ml of D5W or NS (1 mg/ml). Not stable if final pH less than 5.5. Give within 4 hours or use 1 ml Neut to 100 ml solution to stabilize.

Intermittent infusion: Dilute each 1-Gm dose of reconstituted solution in 100 to 250 ml of D5W or NS.

Erythromycin lactobionate: *Continuous infusion (preferred):* Further dilute to a 1- to 5-mg/ml solution (e.g., each 1 Gm in 200 to 1,000 ml of NS, LR, or other electrolyte solution). If a dextrose solution is used, add sodium bicarbonate (Neut) 1 ml for each 100 ml of solution.

Intermittent infusion: Dilute to a maximum concentration of 5 mg/ml (1 Gm in 200 ml).

Storage: Erythromycin gluceptate: Reconstituted solution stable for 7 days if refrigerated. Use diluted and/or buffered solution within 24 hours.

Erythromycin lactobionate: Reconstituted solution stable for 14 days if refrigerated or for 24 hours at room temperature. Diluted and/or buffered solution stable for 8 hours at CRT or 24 hours if refrigerated.

INCOMPATIBLE WITH

Do not add any drug to solution unless effects on chemical and physical stability are determined. Amikacin (Amikin), aminophylline, ampicillin (Polycillin-N), ascorbic acid, cefazolin (Kefzol), cephalothin (Keflin), cephapirin (Cefadyl), chloramphenicol (Chloromycetin), colistimethate (Coly-Mycin M), fluconazole (Diflucan), furosemide (Lasix), heparin, lincomycin (Lincocin), metaraminol (Aramine), metoclopramide (Reglan), pentobarbital (Nembutal), phenobarbital (Luminal), phenytoin (Dilantin), prochlorperazine (Compazine), secobarbital (Seconal), sodium chloride solutions until after initial dilution, sodium salts, streptomycin, thiopental (Pentothal), vancomycin (Vancocin), warfarin (Coumadin).

RATE OF ADMINISTRATION

Administer with a volume control set. 1 Gm or fraction thereof in at least 100 ml over 20 to 60 minutes. Slow infusion rate for pain along injection site. IV infusion of a 0.1% to 0.2% solution by continuous drip over 6 hours is preferable.

ACTIONS

Macrolide antibiotic, bactericidal and bacteriostatic, used as a substitute for penicillin or tetracyclines. Effective against a number of gram-positive and some gram-negative organisms as well as chlamydia trachomatis, mycoplasmas, and spirochetes. Metabolized by the liver and excreted in urine and bile. Crosses placental barrier. Secreted in breast milk.

INDICATIONS AND USES

Treatment of mild to moderate infections of the upper and lower respiratory tract, skin and skin structures and gynecologic infections caused by susceptible organisms. ■ Alternative treatment in several sexually transmitted diseases in females with a history of penicillin sensitivity. ■ Legionnaires' disease.

CONTRAINDICATIONS

Known erythromycin sensitivity.

PRECAUTIONS

Sensitivity studies indicated to determine susceptibility of the causative organism to erythromycin. ■ Begin oral therapy as soon as practical. ■ Superinfection caused by overgrowth of nonsusceptible organisms is rare unless this drug is given in combination with other antibacterial agents. ■ Use caution in impaired liver function or a history of cardiac disease (may induce torsades de pointes).

Monitor: Monitor vital signs. ■ Note Drug/lab interactions.

Maternal/child: Pregnancy category B: Use only if clearly needed. ■ Considered safe for use in lactation; use caution. ■ Some products contain benzyl alcohol; not recommended for use in neonates.

DRUG/LAB INTERACTIONS

Bacterial activity is antagonized by coadministration of clindamycin. ■ May inhibit penicillins. ■ Will increase serum levels and potentiate effects of alfentanil, anticoagulants (e.g., warfarin [Coumadin]), astemizole (Hismanal), bromocriptine (Parlodel), carbamazepine (Tegretol), cisapride (Propulsid), cyclosporine (Sandimmune), digoxin, disopyramide (Norpace), ergot alkaloids (e.g., Hydergine), lovastatin (Mevacor), methylprednisolone, midazolam (Versed), phenytoin (Dilantin), terfenadine (Seldane), theophyllines, and triazolam (Halcion); serious toxicity may result. ■ Concomitant administration with astemizole (Hismanal), cisapride, or terfenadine is contraindicated. May cause serious cardiotoxicity. ■ Severe vinblastine toxicity has been reported in conjunction with erythromycin.

SIDE EFFECTS

Relatively free from side effects when given as directed. Nausea and vomiting, urticaria and mild local venous discomfort. Increased incidence of usually reversible ototoxicity with larger doses. Anaphylaxis may occur.

ANTIDOTE

Notify the physician of early or mild symptoms. For severe symptoms, discontinue the drug, treat allergic reactions, or resuscitate as necessary and notify physician.

ESMOLOL HYDROCHLORIDE

Beta-adrenergic blocking agent
Antiarrhythmic

Brevibloc

pH 3.5 to 5.5

USUAL DOSE

Supraventricular tachycardia: 100 mcg/kg of body weight/min is an average dose. Range is 50 to 200 mcg/kg/min. Dosage must be individualized by titration. Each step in the process consists of a loading dose followed by a maintenance dose. Begin with a **loading dose** of 500 mcg/kg/min for 1 minute only. Follow with a **maintenance infusion** of 50 mcg/kg/min for 4 minutes. If desired therapeutic effect has not occurred, repeat the loading dose and increase the maintenance infusion to 100 mcg/kg/min. Continue this two-step process by repeating the same loading dose while increasing the maintenance infusion by 50 mcg/kg/min. As the desired heart rate is approached or a safety end-point (decreasing blood pressure) occurs, omit the loading dose and titrate the maintenance dose up or down in 25- to 50-mcg/kg/min increments to desired heart rate. Interval between titration steps may be increased from 5 to 10 minutes if desired. Hypotension is common and is dose related. Doses greater than 200 mcg/kg/min are not recommended.

Intraoperative and postoperative tachycardia and/or hypertension: For immediate control 80 mg (~1 mg/kg) over 30 seconds. Follow with an infusion of 150 mcg/kg/minute if necessary. Adjust as required up to 300 mcg/kg/min to maintain desired HR and/or BP. For gradual control, use procedure listed for SVT. Higher doses (250 to 300 mcg/kg/min) may be required to control BP. Another source recommends 250 to 500 mcg (0.25 to 0.5 mg) over 1 minute as a loading dose, followed with a maintenance dose of 50 mcg/kg/min for 4 minutes. Repeat loading dose and increase maintenance dose by 50 mcg/kg/min.

PEDIATRIC DOSE

Safety for use in children not established. 50 mcg/kg/min, titrate every 10 minutes in 25 to 50 mcg/kg/min increments up to 300 mcg/kg/min. Another source recommends a loading dose of 100 to 500 mcg/kg administered over 1 minute. Follow with a maintenance infusion of 25 to 100 mcg/kg/min. If inadequate response, repeat loading dose and/or increase maintenance dose in 25- to 50-mcg/kg/min increments every 5 to 10 minutes. Titrate to individual desired response. Usual range may be from 50 to 500 mcg/kg/min.

DOSE ADJUSTMENTS

Reduced dose may be required in impaired renal function. ■ Reduction required with transfer to alternate agent; ssee Precautions/Monitor. ■ Note Drug/lab interactions.

DILUTION

10 mg/ml preparation (10-ml vial) may be given direct IV without further dilution. May be further diluted by removing 20 ml from a 500-ml bottle of one of the following solutions; D5W, D5/R, D5/LR, D5/NS, D5½NS, NS, LR, or ½NS. Add 5 Gm (two 10-ml

ampoules [250 mg/ml]) to the remaining 480 ml of solution to produce a final concentration of 10 mg/ml.

Storage: Stable at room temperature for 24 hours.

INCOMPATIBLE WITH

Manufacturer recommends not mixing with any other drug before full dilution in a compatible infusion solution. Diazepam (Valium), furosemide (Lasix), procainamide (Pronestyl), sodium bicarbonate, thiopental (Pentothal).

RATE OF ADMINISTRATION

Titrate infusion according to procedure outlined in Usual dose.

ACTIONS

A short-acting B_1 selective adrenergic blocking gent with antiarrhythmic effects. Decreases heart rate and BP in a dose-related titratable manner. Hemodynamically similar to propranolol, but vascular resistance is not increased. Onset of action occurs within 1 to 2 minutes and lasts about 20 to 30 minutes. Metabolized via esterases in RBCs and excreted in urine.

INDICATIONS AND USES

Management of supraventricular tachycardia (atrial fibrillation or atrial flutter) in situations requiring short-term control of ventricular rate with a short-acting agent (perioperative, postoperative, or other emergent circumstances). ▪ Management of noncompensatory tachycardia when heart rate requires specific intervention. ▪ Management of intraoperative and postoperative tachycardia and/or hypertension.

CONTRAINDICATIONS

Not intended for use in chronic settings when transfer to another agent is anticipated. Do not use concurrently with epinephrine. Bradycardia; cardiogenic shock; congestive heart failure not secondary to a tachycardia responsive to beta-adrenergic blockers; overt cardiac failure; second- or third-degree heart block.

PRECAUTIONS

Use with extreme caution in asthmatics, diabetics, impaired renal function, or patients with a history of hypoglycemia. ▪ If patient is scheduled for surgery, administer esmolol before, during, and after without interruption. May cause arrhythmia, angina, MI, or death if stopped abruptly. ▪ Although it has not been a problem with esmolol, it is recommended that the dose of beta-adrenergic blockers be reduced gradually to avoid rebound angina, MI, or ventricular dysrhythmias. Use caution, especially in patients with coronary artery disease.

Monitor: Continuous observation of the patient and ECG and blood pressure monitoring are mandatory during administration. Hypotension should reverse within 30 minutes after decreasing the infusion rate or discontinuing the drug. ▪ Well tolerated if administered through a central vein. Incidence of infusion site inflammation. Incidence of inflammation or thrombophlebitis increases with dilutions greater than 10 mg/ml. ▪ Intended for short-term use only. Transfer to an alternative antiarrhythmic agent (e.g., propranolol [Inderal], digoxin [Lanoxin], verapamil [Calan]) is required after stable clinical status and heart rate control are obtained. Thirty minutes after first dose of alternative agent, reduce dose of esmolol by 50%. Monitor patient carefully. One hour after the second dose of alternative agent, discontinue esmolol infusion if condition remains satisfactory. ▪ May cause hypoglycemia and mask the symptoms. ▪ Note Drug/lab interactions and Contraindications.

Maternal/child: Pregnancy category C: Safety for use in pregnancy, lactation, and children not established. Use only when clearly indicated. Has caused fetal problems during delivery.

Elderly: Potential risk of increased cardiac depression, monitor and reduce dose if indicated.

DRUG/LAB INTERACTIONS

Increases digoxin blood levels, synergistic with digoxin; both drugs slow AV conduction. ▪ IV morphine increases esmolol steady-state levels by 50%. ▪ Epinephrine concurrently is contraindicated. ▪ Esmolol should not be used in patients receiving drugs that are vasoconstrictive or inotropic (e.g., dopamine [Intropin], epinephrine, norepinephrine [Levophed], digoxin) because of the potential for blocked cardiac contractility when the supraventricular rate is high. ▪ Concomitant use with catecholamine-depleting drugs (e.g., reserpine [Serpasil]) may produce additive effects. Monitor for hypotension and bradycardia. ▪ May prolong neuromuscular blockade produced by succinylcholine (Anectine). ▪ Use with verapamil may potentiate both drugs and result in severe depression of myocardium and AV conduction. ▪ Warfarin (Coumadin) may increase esmolol concentrations. Warfarin is not affected. ▪ May mask S/S of developing hypoglycemia in patients on insulin or oral antidiabetic agents. ▪ Concurrent use with xanthines (e.g., aminophylline, theophyllines) may result in mutual inhibition of therapeutic effect. ▪ Note Contraindications.

SIDE EFFECTS

Hypotension and inflammation or induration of the infusion site are the major side effects. Asthenia, bronchospasm, congestive heart failure, confusion, fever, flushing, lightheadedness, midscapular pain, nausea and vomiting, pallor, paresthesia, rhonchi, somnolence, speech disorders, taste disorders, and urinary retention have occurred. One grand mal seizure has been reported.

ANTIDOTE

Notify the physician of all side effects. Decrease rate or discontinue drug if hypotension occurs, and notify physician immediately. Hypotension should reverse within 30 minutes. Trendelenburg position may be appropriate. May require treatment with IV fluids or vasopressors (e.g., dopamine [Intropin], norepinephrine [levarterenol]), but protracted severe hypotension may result. Unresponsive hypotension and bradycardia may be reversed by glucagon 5 to 10 mg over 30 seconds followed by a continuous infusion of 5 mg/hr. Reduce rate as condition improves. Use atropine for bradycardia; digitalis and diuretics for cardiac failure. Treat other side effects symptomatically and resuscitate as necessary.

ETIDRONATE DISODIUM

Antihypercalcemic (Bisphosphonate)

Didronel IV

pH 4.0 to 5.5

USUAL DOSE

7.5 mg/kg of body weight/24 hr daily for 3 days. In selected situations, patients have been treated for 7 days during the first course of therapy. If hypercalcemia recurs, a second course of therapy limited to 3 days may be given. Begin at least 7 days after completion of first course. The day after the last infusion, begin follow-up treatment with oral etidronate 20 mg/kg/day. Usually continues for 30 days but may be extended up to 90 days if serum calcium levels remain normal or within clinically acceptable parameters. Note Precautions/Monitor.

DOSE ADJUSTMENTS

Reduce dose in patients with a serum creatinine between 2.5 to 4.9 mg/dl (see Contraindications).

DILUTION

Must be diluted in 250 ml or more of NS and given as an infusion. One source states, "May be diluted in D5W" (Note Incompatible with).

Storage: Stable at room temperature for 48 hours.

INCOMPATIBLE WITH

Specific information not available. Consider specific use and required dilution in normal saline.

RATE OF ADMINISTRATION

250 ml of diluted solution over a minimum of 2 hours. Extend infusion time if larger amounts of fluid are used.

ACTIONS

A bisphosphonate, reduces normal and abnormal bone resorption and bone formation. Does not appear to alter renal tubular reabsorption of calcium. Not effective in hyperparathyroidism where increased renal tubular reabsorption may contribute to the cause of hypercalcemia. In hypercalcemia of malignancy the renal tubules become less able to concentrate urine, and this reduces the ability of the kidneys to eliminate excess calcium. By reducing excess bone resorption, etidronate interrupts this process. Not metabolized. Within 24 hours about one half of this drug is chemically absorbed to bone and the remainder is excreted in the urine. Half-life in bone is 3 to 6 months.

INDICATIONS AND USES

Hypercalcemia of malignancy inadequately managed by dietary modification or oral hydration or persisting after adequate hydration has been restored. ■ Oral form has other uses. ■ Newer antihypercalcemic agents available (e.g., gallium nitrate [Ganite], pamidronate disodium [Aredia]).

CONTRAINDICATIONS

Hypersensitivity to bisphosphonates (e.g., pamidronate [Aredia]), serum creatinine greater than 5 mg/dl.

PRECAUTIONS

Use caution in patients with enterocolitis. ▪ Delay treatment in patients with fractures until callus is evident (especially fractures of long bones). ▪ Hypercalcemia of hyperparathyroidism may coexist in patients with malignancy. Etidronate will probably not be effective.

Monitor: Increased risk of hypocalcemia in patients treated over 3 days IV. ▪ Monitor serum calcium and albumin. ▪ Monitor renal function with serum creatinine. ▪ Must be adequately hydrated and have adequate urine output. Pretreatment and simultaneous treatment with IV saline and loop diuretics (e.g., furosemide [Lasix]) is recommended and will increase calcium excretion. Rate of renal calcium excretion is directly related to renal sodium excretion. ▪ Avoid overhydration in the elderly and in cardiac failure. ▪ Maintain adequate nutrition including calcium and vitamin D.

Patient education: Regular visits and assessment of lab tests imperative. ▪ Restriction of dietary calcium and vitamin D may be required. ▪ Take only prescribed medications. ▪ Report abdominal cramps, chills, confusion, muscle spasms, sore throat, and/or any new medical problems promptly.

Maternal/child: Pregnancy category C: Safety for use in pregnancy or lactation not established. Use only when clearly indicated. ▪ Safety for use in children not established.

Elderly: Note Precautions/Monitor.

DRUG/LAB INTERACTIONS

Renal toxicity may be potentiated by nephrotoxic drugs (e.g., aminoglycosides [gentamicin].

SIDE EFFECTS

Diarrhea, elevated serum creatinine and BUN, hypersensitivity reactions (angioedema, pruritus, rash, urticaria), hypocalcemia, loss of taste or metallic taste (temporary), nausea, renal insufficiency. Bleeding and ECG changes have occurred in animals with too-rapid injection or excessive doses (27 mg/kg).

ANTIDOTE

Notify the physician of any side effect. May respond to symptomatic treatment or to decrease in rate of infusion. Hypocalcemia is rare but can be treated with IV calcium gluconate. Treatment is symptomatic and supportive. Resuscitate as necessary.

ETOPOSIDE

Antineoplastic
(Mitotic inhibitor)

Etopophos, etoposide phosphate,
❦Novopharm, Toposar, VePesid, VP-16-213

pH 2.9 to 4.0

USUAL DOSE

Testicular cancer: 50 to 100 mg/M^2 daily for 5 days or 100 mg/M^2/day on days 1, 3, and 5. Repeat at 3- to 4-week intervals.

Small cell lung cancer: 35 mg/M^2/day for 4 days to 50 mg/M^2/day for 5 days. Repeat at 3- to 4-week intervals. Note Precautions/Monitor.

Investigational uses: High-dose regimens of 400 to 800 mg/M^2/day for 3 days have been given for one or two courses and have been used prior to bone marrow transplantation.

DOSE ADJUSTMENTS

Modify dose if indicated based on myelosuppressive effects of other drugs administered in combination and any previous radiation therapy or chemotherapy (compromised bone marrow reserve). Frequently given in combination with cisplatin, bleomycin, and doxorubicin. ▪ Withhold dose if platelets less than 50,000/mm^3 or absolute neutrophil count less than 500/mm^3. Do not restart until adequate recovery. Reduce dose by 25% if CrCl is 15 to 50 ml/minute. ▪ Dose reduction may be required in impaired hepatic function.

DILUTION

Specific techniques required; see Precautions. Non-phosphate products (e.g., VePesid): Each 100 mg (5 ml) must be diluted in at least 250 ml of D5W or NS and given as an infusion (0.4 mg/ml). 500 ml of solution will yield 0.2 mg/ml. Maximum concentration to prevent precipitation is 0.4 mg/ml. Monitor closely for precipitation from dilution to completion of infusion. Undiluted etoposide has caused acrylic or ABS plastic devices to crack and leak; handle carefully during dilution process.

Phosphate product (e.g., Etopophos): Reconstitute each 100-mg vial with 5 or 10 ml of SW, D5W, or NS (with or without benzyl alcohol). 5 ml of diluent will yield 20 mg/ml, 10 ml will yield 10 mg/ml. May be given without further dilution (to reduce possibility of fluid overload) or may be further diluted to concentrations as low as 0.1 mg/ml with D5W or NS. A 1-mg/ml solution has a pH of 2.9. The water solubility of etopophos decreases the potential for precipitation following dilution and during administration.

Storage: Non-phosphate products (e.g., VePesid): May be stored at room temperature before dilution. Stable after dilution at room temperature for 96 hours (0.2 mg/ml solution) or 48 hours (0.4 mg/ml). *Phosphate product (e.g., Etopophos):* Refrigerate in carton until use. Store reconstituted or diluted solutions in glass or plastic containers at controlled room temperature or refrigerate for up to 24 hours. When returned to room temperature from refrigeration, use etopophos solutions immediately.

INCOMPATIBLE WITH

Non-phosphate products (e.g., VePesid): Filgrastim (Neupogen), gallium nitrate (Ganite), idarubicin (Idamycin). Hydrolysis may occur in alkaline solutions. Consider toxicity and specific use. *Phosphate products (e.g., Etopophos):* Specific information is not available.

COMPATIBLE WITH

May be compatible with carboplatin, cisplatin (Platinol), cytarabine (ARA-c), daunorubicin, mesna, mannitol, and/or potassium chloride. Consult pharmacist.

RATE OF ADMINISTRATION

Non-phosphate products (e.g., VePesid): Total desired dose, properly diluted (0.2 to 0.4 mg/ml) and evenly distributed over at least 30 to 60 minutes. Rapid infusion may cause marked hypotension. May be extended if fluid volume is a concern.

Phosphate products (e.g., Etopophos): Total desired dose, properly reconstituted or diluted may be given evenly distributed over as little as 5 minutes or up to 210 minutes.

ACTIONS

A semisynthetic derivative of podophyllotoxin. Cell cycle specific for the G_2 phase, it inhibits DNA synthesis. Etopophos (phosphate) is a water-soluble ester of etoposide that promptly converts to etoposide in plasma. Half-life is from 1.5 to 11 hours. Highly protein bound to human plasma proteins. Metabolized in the liver. Primarily excreted through urine and feces.

INDICATIONS AND USES

To suppress or retard neoplastic growth in refractory testicular tumors (used in combination with other agents after previous surgery, chemotherapy, and radiotherapy). ▪ Suppress or retard small cell lung cancer (used in combination with other chemotherapeutic agents as first-line treatment).

Investigational uses: High-dose regimens before bone marrow transplantation. Treatment of acute nonlymphocytic leukemias, Hodgkin's disease, non-Hodgkin's lymphomas, carcinoma of the breast, Kaposi's sarcoma, and neuroblastoma. Additional tumors have shown up to 20% response. Used alone or in combination with other agents.

CONTRAINDICATIONS

Hypersensitivity to etoposide, etoposide phosphate, or any other component of the formulations.

PRECAUTIONS

Follow guidelines for handling cytotoxic agents. See Appendix A, p. 893. ▪ Usually administered by or under the direction of the physician specialist. ▪ A low serum albumin may result in a decreased clearance of etoposide, resulting in an increased risk of toxicity. Occurs more frequently in children. ▪ Oral dose of non-phosphate product (e.g., etoposide) is usually twice the IV dose.

Monitor: Determine absolute patency and quality of vein and adequate circulation of extremity. Avoid extravasation. ▪ Use caution to prevent bone marrow depression. Platelet count, hemoglobin, white blood cell count, and differential must be completed before start of therapy and before each dose. Note Dose adjustments. Monitor between courses also. ▪ Examine patient's mouth for ulceration before each dose. ▪ Monitor hepatic and renal function before and during therapy. ▪ Bone marrow recovery from a course is usually complete within 20 days. No cumulative toxicity has been reported as yet. ▪ Be alert for signs of bone marrow depression or infection. ▪ Prophylactic antibiotics may be indicated pending results of C/S in a febrile neutropenic patient. ▪ Maintain adequate hydration. ▪ Prophylactic antiemetics may increase patient comfort.

Patient education: Nonhormonal birth control recommended ▪ Report IV site burning or stinging promptly. ▪ Report chills, difficult breathing, fever, and rapid heartbeat promptly. See Appendix D, p. 900.

Maternal/child: Pregnancy category D: Avoid pregnancy. Can cause fetal harm. ▪ Discontinue breast feeding. ▪ Has been used in children but safety and effectiveness not established, anaphylactic reactions have been reported. Note Precautions.

Elderly: Monitor renal, hepatic, and hematologic function closely.

DRUG/LAB INTERACTIONS

All products: Do not administer vaccine or chloroquine to patients receiving antineoplastic drugs. ▪ *Non-phosphate products (e.g., VePesid)* may potentiate warfarin; monitor prothrombin time. ***Phosphate product (e.g., Etopophos):*** Use caution with drugs that are known to inhibit phosphatase activities (e.g., levamisole [Ergamisol]).

SIDE EFFECTS

Bone marrow toxicity (e.g., leukopenia, neutropenia, thrombocytopenia) can be severe, is dose related, and may be dose limiting. Side effects are usually reversible: abdominal pain, alopecia, anaphylactic reactions (bronchospasm, chills, dyspnea, fever, hypotension), anemia, anorexia, constipation, diarrhea, dizziness, hypertension or hypotension, mucositis, nausea, neuritic pain, paralytic ileus, peripheral neurotoxicity, stomatitis, thrombophlebitis, vomiting. Hepatic toxicity and metabolic acidosis have occurred with higher than recommended doses.

ANTIDOTE

Notify the physician of all side effects; symptomatic treatment is often indicated, dose reduction may be necessary. For extravasation, discontinue the drug immediately and administer into another vein. Consider injection of long-acting dexamethasone (Decadron LA) throughout extravasated tissue. Use a 27- or 25-gauge needle. Elevate extremity; moist heat may be helpful. Hypotension is usually due to a rapid infusion rate. Discontinue infusion. Trendelenburg position and IV fluids should reverse the hypotension; vasopressors (e.g., dopamine [Intropin]) may be required. After recovery, restart at slower rate. Oprelvekin (Numega) has been used to treat thrombocytopenia. Discontinue infusion at first sign of allergic reaction; resuscitate as necessary.

FACTOR IX (HUMAN)/
FACTOR IX COMPLEX (HUMAN)

Antihemorrhagic

AlphaNine, AlphaNine SD, Mononine/
Konyne 80, Profinine HT, Proplex T

pH 7.0 to 7.4 / pH 7.0 to 7.4

USUAL DOSE

Completely individualized based on patient's circumstances, condition, degree of deficiency, and desired blood level percentage. Specific products may be indicated or preferred in some situations; see Indications and uses. Range is 10 to 75 IU/kg of body weight. May be repeated every 12 hours in some situations, required only every 2 or 3 days in others. Actual number of international units contained shown on each bottle or vial. Units required to raise blood level percentages can be calculated as follows:

Body weight (kg) × Desired increase (% of normal) × 1 Unit/kg

(70 kg × 40% increase × 1 IU/kg equals 2,800 IU]). To maintain levels above 25%, calculate each dose to raise level to 40% to 60% of normal.
Minor hemorrhage: A single injection calculated to increase plasma level to 20% to 30%. May be repeated in 24 hours if indicated.
Major trauma or surgery: Increase plasma level to 25% to 50% and maintain at that level for a minimum of 1 week or as indicated. May require daily injections (every 18 to 30 hours).
Dental extraction: Increase plasma level to 50% before procedure; repeat if indicated.
Reversal of coumarin effect: Factor IX Complex: 15 IU/kg.
Prophylaxis: 10 to 20 IU/kg once or twice a week or increase plasma level to 20% to 30%.

DILUTION

Diluent usually provided. Some preparations also supply double-ended needles for dilution and filter needle for aspiration into a syringe. Sterile technique imperative. Confirm expiration date. Use plastic syringes to prevent binding to glass surfaces. Factor IX and diluent should be at room temperature. Direct diluent from above to side of vial to gently moisten all contents. Swirl gently to dissolve; avoid foaming. Do not shake. May take 1 to 5 minutes. Should be clear and colorless. Must be used within 3 hours to avoid bacterial contamination. The addition of 2 to 3 units of heparin/ml factor IX complex may reduce the incidence of thrombosis. May be given through an IV administration set (often provided) if multiple vials are required. Discard any unused contents. Discard all administration equipment after single use; do not attempt to resterilize.
AlphaNine: Follow general directions above. After diluent is drawn through double-ended needle, remove diluent bottle first; then remove double-ended needle. *Do not invert concentrate vial until ready to withdraw contents!* Air from syringe into vial required to withdraw contents. Withdraw through filter.

Mononine: Follow general directions above. After diluent is drawn through double-ended needle, remove diluent bottle first; then remove double-ended needle. *Use only the provided self-venting filter spike to transfer Mononine to a syringe! Do not inject any air into Mononine vial; could cause product loss.* Discard filter and use only provided wing needle and micropore tubing to administer.

Storage: Store lyophilized powder at 2° to 8° C (36° to 46° F); do not freeze. Do not refrigerate after dilution. *Mononine* may be stored at room temperature before dilution for up to 30 days.

INCOMPATIBLE WITH

All protein precipitants. Sufficient information not available.

RATE OF ADMINISTRATION

Average rate is 2 to 3 ml or 100 units/min. Completely individualized according to patient's condition. Decrease rate of administration for side effects such as burning or pain at injection site, chills, fever, flushing, headache, tingling, or changes in blood pressure or pulse. Never exceed 10 ml/min.

ACTIONS

A lyophilized concentrate of human coagulation factors: IX (plasma thromboplastin and antihemophilic factor B), II (prothrombin), VII (proconvertin), X (Stuart-Prower factor). In contrast to other products, AlphaNine and Mononine are highly purified factor IX and contain only minimal amounts of the other factors. All products are obtained from fresh human plasma and prepared, irradiated, and dried by specific processes. Konyne 80 is dry heat-treated at 80° C for 72 hours. Additional processes are used to prepare AlphaNine and Mononine that markedly reduce the possibility of viral contamination. Concentration of 25 units/ml is 25 times greater than normal plasma. Preparations contain varying amounts of total protein in each vial. Half-life extends beyond 24 hours.

INDICATIONS AND USES

All Factor IX products: Prevention and control of bleeding in patients with Factor IX deficiency due to hemophilia B. May be required to correct or prevent a dangerous bleeding episode or to perform surgery. ■ Prophylaxis to prevent spontaneous bleeding in patients with proven specific congenital deficiency (hemophilia B). *Factor IX (human)* is preferred for surgical coverage, treatment of crush injuries, treatment of large IM hemorrhages requiring several days of replacement therapy, and treatment in neonates, individuals with severe hepatocellular dysfunction, or those with a history of thrombotic complications associated with factor IX complex. *Factor IX Complex:* Prevention and control of bleeding in patients with hemophilia A who have inhibitors to Factor VIII. ■ Reversal of coumarin effect (fresh-frozen plasma preferred unless risk of hepatitis transfer would be life threatening). ■ Hemorrhage caused by hepatitis-induced lack of production of liver-dependent coagulation factors. ■ Proplex T is used for prevention or control of bleeding episodes in patients with Factor VII deficiency.

CONTRAINDICATIONS

Factor IX Complex: Known liver disease with suspicion of intravascular coagulation or fibrinolysis. ■ Factor VII deficiency except for Proplex T. *Mononine:* Known hypersensitivity to mouse protein. ■ No other known contraindications for **AlphaNine or Konyne 80.** ■ **AlphaNine, Alpha-Nine SD, and Mononine** are not indicated for replacement of any other coagulation factors.

PRECAUTIONS

Used when plasma infusions would result in hypervolemia and/or pro-teinemia or when blood volume or red blood cell replacement is not indicated. ■ Use extreme caution in newborns, infants, postoperative patients, and patients with liver disease. Factor IX (human) (e.g., Alpha-Nine, Mononine) would be preferred because studies show no incidence of thrombin generation. ■ Fresh-frozen plasma may be required in addi-tion to factor IX complex when prompt reversal is required. ■ Danger of thromboembolic episodes (DIC, myocardial infarction, pulmonary em-bolism, venous thrombosis) increases with plasma levels over 50%.
■ Large or frequently repeated doses of factor IX complex may cause intravascular hemolysis in patients with type A, B, or AB blood.

Monitor: Monitor the patient's levels of coagulation factors before, after, and between administrations. *Do not overdose* (see Side effects).
■ AIDS or hepatitis is possible for the recipient. Health professionals should exercise caution in handling. Possibility markedly reduced with additional preparation process of AlphaNine, AlphaNine SD, Konyne 80, and Mononine. ■ Observe for signs and symptoms of postoperative thrombosis or disseminated intravascular coagulation (DIC). Risk multiplies with repeated administrations except for AlphaNine, Alpha-Nine SD, and Mononine.

Patient education: Alert to possible risk of HIV virus and hepatitis.
■ Report early signs of hypersensitivity promptly (burning or pain along injection site, hives, rash, tightness of chest, wheezing). ■ Notify physician if medication seems less effective. May be developing antibodies to factor IX. ■ Carry identification card. ■ Proper prepara-tion and administration imperative if given in home.

Maternal/child: Pregnancy category C: Safety for use during pregnancy not established; use only if clearly indicated. Note Precautions. ■ Use extreme caution in neonates with hepatitis; high rate of morbidity.

DRUG/LAB INTERACTIONS

Concurrent use of aminocaproic acid (Amicar) may increase risk of thrombosis.

SIDE EFFECT

Minor: Burning or pain along injection site, changes in blood pressure, chills, fever, flushing, headache, nausea, tingling, urticaria, vomiting.

Major: Anaphylaxis, DIC, hepatitis, myocardial infarction, postoperative thrombosis (rare with pure factor IX [Human] products), pulmonary embolism. Consider risk potential of contracting AIDS and hepatitis; markedly reduced with pure factor IX (Human) products, (AlphaNine, AlphaNine SD, Mononine) and Konyne 80.

ANTIDOTE

Temporarily discontinue or decrease rate of administration for minor side effects. If any major symptoms appear, discontinue drug and notify physician. Treat allergic reactions as indicated; a different lot may not cause the reaction. For thrombosis or DIC, anticoagulation with heparin may be indicated.

FACTOR IX (RECOMBINANT)

BeneFIX

Antihemorrhagic

USUAL DOSE

Adults and children: Completely individualized based on the degree of deficiency, location and extent of bleeding, and the patient's clinical condition, age, and recovery of factor IX. All doses should be titrated to the patient's clinical response. Actual number of international units contained shown on each bottle or vial. Units required to raise blood level percentages are somewhat increased with this recombinant product compared to other factor IX products and can be calculated as follows:

number of factor IX IU required =
body weight (in kg) × desired factor IX increase (%) × 1.2 IU/kg

In the presence of an inhibitor, higher doses may be required.
The following chart may be used to guide dosing in bleeding episodes and surgery:

Type of Hemorrhage	Circulating Factor IX Activity Required (%)	Frequency of Doses (hours)	Duration of Therapy (days)
Minor Uncomplicated hemarthroses, superficial muscle, or soft tissue	20-30	12-24	1-2
Moderate Intramuscle or soft tissue with dissection, mucous membranes, dental extractions, or hematuria	25-50	12-24	Treat until bleeding stops and healing begins, about 2 to 7 days
Major Pharynx, retropharynx, retroperitoneum, CNS, surgery	50-100	12-24	7-10
Source: Roberts and Eberst			

DILUTION

Sterile diluent, double-ended needle, filter spike, and infusion set provided. Sterile technique imperative. Confirm expiration date. Use plastic syringes to prevent binding to glass surfaces. Factor IX and diluent should be at room temperature. After removing the vial caps on Factor IX and diluent, wipe with antiseptic and allow to dry. Insert short end of the double-ended needle into the diluent vial. Insert long end into the Factor IX vial with the tip directed to the side of the wall to prevent excessive foaming. Fully invert the diluent vial to a vertical position and allow the diluent to run completely into the Factor IX vial. If the diluent does not transfer completely, **do not use** (a very small amount remaining is permissible). Remove transfer needle. Gently rotate the vial to dissolve. Should be clear and colorless. Attach filter spike to the plastic syringe and insert into the reconstituted solution; invert and withdraw contents. **Do not** inject air into the vial; may cause partial loss of product. Multiple vials may be drawn into the same syringe, but a new sterile filter spike must be used for each vial. Must be used within 3 hours of reconstitution.

Storage: Refrigerate packaged product (2° to 8° C [36° to 46° F]). Packaged product may be stored at room temperature not exceeding 25° C (77° F) for up to 6 months (mark date removed from refrigerator on carton). Avoid freezing. Do not use after the expiration date.

INCOMPATIBLE WITH

Specific information not available. Consider incompatible in syringe or solution with any drug based on specific use.

RATE OF ADMINISTRATION

A single dose over several minutes. Average rate during studies was 50 units/kg infused over 10 minutes. Individualized according to patient's condition and comfort level. Decrease rate for side effects such as burning or pain at injection site, chills, fever, flushing, headache, tingling, or changes in blood pressure or pulse.

ACTIONS

An antihemorrhagic. A purified protein produced by recombinant DNA technology for use in the treatment of factor IX deficiency. Its primary amino acid sequence is identical to a form of plasma-derived factor IX, and it has structural and functional characteristics similar to those of endogenous factor IX. Inherently free from the risk of transmission of human bloodborne pathogens such as HIV, hepatitis viruses, and parvovirus. Factor IX is the specific clotting factor deficient in patients with hemophilia B and in patients with acquired factor IX deficiencies. Factor IX (Recombinant) increases plasma levels of factor IX and can temporarily correct the coagulation defect in these patients. Half-life ranges from 11 to 26 hours.

INDICATIONS AND USES

Control and prevention of hemorrhagic episodes in patients with hemophilia B (congenital factor IX deficiency or Christmas disease), including control and prevention of bleeding in surgical settings.

CONTRAINDICATIONS

Known history of hypersensitivity to hamster protein. ▪ Not indicated for the treatment of other factor deficiencies (e.g., factors II, VII, and X). ▪ Not indicated for the treatment of hemophilia A patients with inhibitors to factor VIII. ▪ Not indicated for the reversal of coumarin-induced anticoagulation. ▪ Not indicated for the treatment of bleeding due to low levels of liver-dependent coagulation factors.

PRECAUTIONS

Usually administered under the supervision of a physician experienced in the treatment of hemophilia B. ▪ Allergic type hypersensitivity reactions are possible. ▪ BeneFIX contains only coagulation factor IX, but thromboembolic episodes (e.g., disseminated intravascular coagulation [DIC], myocardial infarction, pulmonary embolism, venous thrombosis) have been reported with other factor IX concentrates. These episodes increase with plasma levels over 50%. May be hazardous in patients with signs of fibrinolysis or DIC. ▪ Because of potential thromboembolic problems, use caution in patients with liver disease, patients in the postoperative period, neonates, or in patients at risk of thromboembolic phenomena or DIC. Benefit must be weighed against risk.

Monitor: To ensure desired factor IX activity levels, precise monitoring using the Factor IX activity assay is recommended, especially during surgical intervention. *Do not overdose* (see Side effects). ▪ Monitor for development of factor IX inhibitors. Patients dosed with high-purity factor IX products who develop inhibitors are at increased risk of anaphylaxis with repeat doses.

Patient education: Allergic reactions can occur. Report difficulty breathing, hives, itching, tightness of the chest, and/or wheezing promptly. If self-administering, discontinue use and contact physician immediately.

Maternal/child: Category C: use during pregnancy or during lactation only if clearly indicated. ▪ To this date, no adverse reactions related to treatment have been reported in children.

Elderly: Response similar to other age groups.

DRUG/LAB INTERACTIONS
Specific information not available.

SIDE EFFECTS
Minor: Allergic rhinitis, altered taste, burning or pain along injection site, burning sensation in jaw and skull, changes in blood pressure, chills, dizziness, drowsiness, dry cough, fever, flushing, headache, lethargy, lightheadedness, nausea, phlebitis at injection site, rash, tightness in the chest, tingling, urticaria, vomiting.

Major: Anaphylaxis, DIC, myocardial infarction, postoperative thrombosis (rare with pure factor IX products), pulmonary embolism.

ANTIDOTE
Temporarily discontinue or decrease rate of administration for minor side effects. If any major symptoms appear, discontinue drug and notify physician. Treat allergic reactions as indicated. For thrombosis or DIC, anticoagulation with heparin may be indicated.

FAMOTIDINE

Antiulcer agent
(H₂ antagonist)
Gastric acid inhibitor

Pepcid IV

pH 5.0 to 5.6

USUAL DOSE
20 mg (2 ml) every 12 hours. Increase frequency of dose, not amount, if necessary for pain relief.

PEDIATRIC DOSE
0.6 to 0.8 mg/kg/24 hr as equally divided doses every 12 hours. May need to reduce interval to every 8 hours because of increased elimination. Maximum dose is 40 mg/24 hr.

DOSE ADJUSTMENTS
Increase intervals between injections or lower doses to achieve pain relief in severe renal dysfunction. Half-life may exceed 20 hours if creatinine clearance less than 10 ml/min.

DILUTION
Direct IV: Each 20 mg must be diluted with 5 to 10 ml of NS or other compatible infusion solutions for injection (e.g., D5W, D10W, LR, 5% sodium bicarbonate). Available premixed 20 mg in 50 ml diluent.

Intermittent infusion: Each 20 mg may be diluted in 100 ml of D5W or other compatible infusion solution and given piggyback.

Storage: Refrigerate before dilution. Stable at room temperature for 48 hours after dilution or up to 14 days refrigerated in polyvinyl minibags.

INCOMPATIBLE WITH
Piperacillin/tazobactam (Zosyn). Physically compatible with many drugs for limited time frames; consult pharmacist.

RATE OF ADMINISTRATION
Direct IV: Each 20 mg or fraction thereof over at least 2 minutes.

Intermittent infusion: Each 20-mg dose over 15 to 30 minutes.

ACTIONS
A histamine H₂ antagonist, it inhibits both daytime and nocturnal basal gastric acid secretion. It also inhibits gastric acid secretion stimulated by food and pentagastrin. Onset of action occurs within 30 minutes and lasts for 10 to 12 hours. No cumulative effect with repeated doses. 30 to 60 times more potent than cimetidine. Eliminated by renal and other metabolic routes. Crosses placental barrier. May be secreted in breast milk.

INDICATIONS AND USES
Short-term treatment of active duodenal ulcers, benign gastric ulcers, and pathologic hypersecretory conditions in hospitalized patients or in patients unable to take oral medication. ■ Used orally for short-term treatment of gastroesophageal reflux disease (GERD) including erosive or ulcerative esophagitis. IV dose recommendations not yet available.

Investigational uses: GI bleeding. ■ Stress ulcer prophylaxis.

CONTRAINDICATIONS
Known hypersensitivity to famotidine or its components.

PRECAUTIONS

Gastric malignancy may be present even though patient is asymptomatic. ■ Effects maintained with oral dosage. Total treatment usually discontinued after 4 to 8 weeks.

Monitor: Use antacids concomitantly to relieve pain. ■ Note Precautions.

Patient education: Stop smoking or at least avoid smoking after last dose of the day. ■ Gastric pain and ulceration may recur after medication stopped.

Maternal/child: Pregnancy category B: Use during pregnancy only when clearly needed. ■ Advisable to discontinue breast feeding. ■ Safety for use in children not established but has been used.

DRUG/LAB INTERACTIONS

May inhibit gastric absorption of ketoconazole (Nizoral). ■ May decrease cyclosporine serum levels when famotidine is given concurrently with ketoconazole and cyclosporine.

SIDE EFFECTS

Constipation, diarrhea, dizziness, and headache are the most common side effects. Allergic reactions (bronchospasm, fever, pruritus, rash, eosinophilia) can occur. Abdominal discomfort, agitation, alopecia, anorexia, anxiety, arthralgias, confusion, decreased libido, depression, dry mouth, dry skin, elevated ALT (SGPT), flushing, grand mal seizure, hallucinations, insomnia, malaise, muscular pain, nausea and vomiting, orbital edema, palpitations, paresthesias, somnolence, taste disorder, thrombocytopenia, and tinnitus have been reported.

ANTIDOTE

Notify physician of all side effects. May be treated symptomatically or may respond to decrease in frequency of dosage. Resuscitate as necessary for overdosage.

FAT EMULSION, INTRAVENOUS

Nutritional supplement (Fatty acid)

Intralipid 10%, 20%, & 30%, Liposyn II 10% & 20%, Liposyn III 10%, 20%, & 30%

pH 6.0 to 9.0

USUAL DOSE

Total parenteral nutrition component: 500 ml of 10% or 250 ml of 20% on the first day. Increase dose gradually each day. Do not exceed 60% of the patient's total caloric intake or 2.5 to 3 Gm/kg of body weight.

Fatty acid deficiency: Supply 8% to 10% of the total caloric intake each 24 hours.

PEDIATRIC DOSE

Total parenteral nutrition component: Up to 1 Gm/kg of body weight. Increase dose gradually each day. Do not exceed 60% of total caloric intake or 3 to 4 Gm/kg.

Premature infants: Begin with 0.5 Gm fat/kg/24 hr. Note comments under Pediatric dose.

DOSE ADJUSTMENTS

Normal renal function required. Reduced dose may be indicated.

DILUTION

Must be given as prepared by manufacturer. Note Precautions. Use only freshly opened solutions; discard remainder of partial dose. Do not use if there appears to be an oiling out of the emulsion. *Intralipid 30% is not to be given by direct IV infusion.* Packaged for bulk use in a pharmacy admixture program. Must be specifically combined with dextrose solutions and amino acids (TPN) so total fat content does not exceed 20%. Prepared for an individual patient in the pharmacy. Lipids may extract phthalates from phthalate-plasticized PVC. Non-phthalate infusion sets recommended; available with most commercial products.

Storage: Must be stored at temperatures not exceeding 25° C (77° F) or refrigerated. Specific storage conditions required (see literature). Do not freeze. Manufacturer recommends admixtures (3 in 1) be refrigerated for no more than 24 hours after mixing. In actual practice a 7-day supply in individual containers for daily adminstration is frequently prepared and refrigerated for home use.

INCOMPATIBLE WITH

Manufacturer recommends not mixing with any electrolyte or other nutrient solution. No additives or medications are to be placed in bottle or tubing (see Precautions). In actual practice, carbohydrates, amino acids, and fat emulsion are being mixed in specific percentages and in a specific order to meet individual total parenteral nutritional needs but should be prepared in the pharmacy. Any addition of supplemental vitamins, minerals, or electrolytes (e.g., calcium, magnesium, phosphates) may cause a precipitate unless a specific order is followed.

RATE OF ADMINISTRATION

May be administered via a Y-tube or three-way stopcock near the infusion site. Rates of both solutions (fat emulsion and amino acid products) should be controlled by infusion pumps. Keep fat emulsion line higher than all other lines (has low specific gravity and could run up into other lines). Do not use filters; will disturb emulsion. FDA suggests use of a 1.2 micron filter for admixtures containing lipids (e.g., 3 in 1); precipitates difficult to detect in lipids.

Adult: 10%: 1 ml/min or 0.1 Gm fat/min for the first 15 to 30 minutes. If no untoward effects, increase rate to administer 500 ml equally distributed over 4 to 6 hours or 0.2 Gm fat/min.

20%: 0.5 ml/min or 0.1 Gm fat/min for the first 15 to 30 minutes. If no untoward effects, increase rate to administer 250 ml equally distributed over 4 to 6 hours or 0.2 Gm fat/min.

Pediatric: 10%: 0.1 ml/min for the first 10 to 15 minutes. Reduce initial rate to 0.05 ml/min for a *20%* solution. If no untoward effects, increase rate to administer 1 Gm/kg of body weight (total usual dose) equally distributed over 4 hours. An infusion pump is recommended. Do not exceed a rate of 50 ml/hr (20%) or 100 ml/hr (10%).

ACTIONS

An isotonic nutrient. Contains emulsified fat particles about 0.4 to 0.5 micron in size. Total caloric value (fat, phospholipid, and glycerol) is 1.1 cal/ml for the 10% emulsion and 2 cal/ml for the 20% emulsion. Metabolized and used as a source of energy. Increases heat production and oxygen consumption. Decreases respiratory quotient. Cleared from the bloodstream by a process not fully understood.

INDICATIONS AND USES
To provide additional calories and essential fatty acids for patients requiring parenteral nutrition whose caloric requirements cannot be met by glucose or who will be receiving parenteral nutrition over extended periods (over 5 days usually). ▪ Prevent essential fatty acid deficiency.

CONTRAINDICATIONS
Any condition that disturbs normal fat metabolism, such as pathologic hyperlipemia, lipoid nephrosis, and acute pancreatitis with hyperlipemia; severe egg allergies.

PRECAUTIONS
Isotonic; may be administered by a peripheral vein or central venous infusion. ▪ Infuse separately from any other IV solution or medication. Do not disturb emulsion. Heparin 1 to 2 units/ml is the exception. It may be added before administration (activates lipoprotein lipase). ▪ Fatty acids displace bilirubin bound to albumin. Use caution in jaundiced or premature infants. ▪ Use caution in pulmonary disease, liver disease, anemia, or blood coagulation disorders, or when there is any danger of fat embolism. ▪ Note Maternal/child.

Monitor: Monitor lipids before each infusion; lipemia should clear daily. ▪ Monitor hemogram, blood coagulation, liver function tests, plasma lipid profile, and platelet count, especially in neonates. Discontinue use for significant abnormality.

Maternal/child: Pregnancy category C: Use in pregnancy only when clearly needed; safety not established. ▪ Use extreme caution in neonates; death from intravascular fat accumulation in the lungs has occurred.

DRUG/LAB INTERACTIONS
No specific information available (note Dilution).

SIDE EFFECTS
Anaphylaxis, back pain, chest pain, cyanosis, dizziness, dyspnea, elevated temperature, flushing, headache, hypercoagulability, hyperlipemia, nausea and vomiting, pressure over eyes, sepsis (from contamination of IV catheter), sleepiness, sweating, thrombophlebitis (from concurrent hyperalimentation fluids), a delayed overloading syndrome (focal seizures, fever, leukocytosis, splenomegaly, shock), and many others.

ANTIDOTE
Notify physician of all side effects. Many will be treated symptomatically. Treat allergic reaction promptly and resuscitate as necessary. For accidental overdose, stop the infusion. Obtain blood sample for inspection of plasma, triglyceride concentration, and measurement of plasma light-scattering activity by nephelometry. Repeat blood samples until the lipid has cleared. Stop infusion immediately for any signs of acute respiratory distress. May represent pulmonary embolus or interstitial pneumonitis, which may be caused by an unseen precipitate of electrolytes (e.g., calcium and phosphates) in the solution.

FENOLDOPAM MESYLATE

Corlopam

Antihypertensive
Vasodilator

USUAL DOSE

Choose an initial dose from within the ranges given in the charts below that produce the desired magnitude and rate of blood pressure reduction for either mild to moderate hypertension or hypertensive emergency. Note indications; FDA approval is limited to severe hypertension, including malignant hypertension. Must be given as a continuous infusion. Avoid hypotension and rapid decreases in BP. Doses below 0.1 mcg/kg/min have modest effects and may have minimal use. Initial doses of 0.03 to 0.1 mcg/kg/min have been associated with less reflex tachycardia than initial doses of >0.3 mcg/kg/min. As the dose increases, there is a greater and more rapid reduction in blood pressure. Doses ranging from 0.01 o 1.6 mcg/kg/min were studied in clinical trials. Maximum effect of each range usually attained within 15 minutes.

Titrate initial dose upward or downward in increments of 0.05 to 0.1 mcg/kg/min no more frequently than every 15 to 20 minutes. Extend duration of intervals as desired BP goal is approached. Note Precautions, Monitor, and Drug/lab interactions.

The following charts are from the clinical trials that evaluated fenoldopam. The manufacturer states that the initial dose may be chosen from the appropriate table. Select a dose that corresponds to the desired magnitude and rate of blood pressure reduction.

Mild to moderate hypertension: Doses ranging from 0.04, 0.1, 0.4, to 0.8 mcg/kg/min have been used.

Time Point and Mean Change From Time Zero ± SE	Infusion Rate (µg/kg/min)				
	Placebo n = 7	0.04 n = 7	0.1 n = 7	0.4 n = 5	0.8 n = 6
15 Minutes of Infusion* Systolic BP	0 ± 6	−15 ± 6	−19 ± 8	−14 ± 4	−24 ± 6
Diastolic BP	0 ± 2	−5 ± 3	−12 ± 4	−15 ± 3	−20 ± 4
Heart rate	+2 ± 2	+3 ± 2	+5 ± 1	+16 ± 3	+19 ± 3
30 Minutes of Infusion* Systolic BP	−6 ± 5	−17 ± 6	−18 ± 6	−14 ± 8	−26 ± 6
Diastolic BP	−6 ± 3	−7 ± 3	−16 ± 4	−14 ± 3	−20 ± 2
Heart rate	+2 ± 2	+3 ± 2	+10 ± 2	+18 ± 3	+23 ± 3

Continued

Time Point and Mean Change From Time Zero ± SE	Infusion Rate (μg/kg/min)				
	Placebo n = 7	0.04 n = 7	0.1 n = 7	0.4 n = 5	0.8 n = 6
1 Hour of Infusion* Systolic BP	−15 ± 4	−22 ± 7	−22 ± 7	−26 ± 9	−22 ± 9
Diastolic BP	−5 ± 3	−9 ± 2	−18 ± 4	−19 ± 4	−21 ± 1
Heart rate	+1 ± 3	+5 ± 2	+12 ± 3	+19 ± 4	+25 ± 4
4 Hours of Infusion* Systolic BP	−14 ± 5	−16 ± 9	−31 ± 15	−22 ± 11	−25 ± 7
Diastolic BP	−14 ± 8	−8 ± 4	−19 ± 9	−25 ± 3	−20 ± 1
Heart rate	+5 ± 3	+6 ± 3	+10 ± 4	+21 ± 2	+27 ± 7
24 Hours of Infusion* Systolic BP	−20 ± 6	−23 ± 8	−35 ± 7	−22 ± 6	−23 ± 11
Diastolic BP	−11 ± 6	−11 ± 5	−23 ± 10	−22 ± 5	−13 ± 3
Heart rate	+6 ± 3	+5 ± 3	+13 ± 2	+17 ± 4	+15 ± 3
48 Hours of Infusion* Systolic BP	−12 ± 8	−31 ± 6	−22 ± 8	−9 ± 6	−14 ± 10
Diastolic BP	−9 ± 5	−10 ± 6	−9 ± 7	−9 ± 2	−9 ± 3
Heart rate	+1 ± 2	0 ± 4	+1 ± 4	+12 ± 3	+8 ± 3
*Mean change from time zero ± S.E.					

Hypertensive emergency: Doses ranging from 0.01, 0.03, 0.1, to 0.3 mcg/kg/min have been used. Several sources suggest an initial dose of 0.1 mcg/kg/min to a maximum recommended dose of 1.7 mcg/kg/min (average effective dose 0.3 mcg/kg/min). Note all statements under Usual dose.

Time Point and Pharmacodynamic Parameters	Infusion Rate (μg/kg/min)			
	0.01 n = 25	0.03 n = 24	0.1 n = 22	0.3 n = 23
Preinfusion Baseline Systolic BP—mean ± SE	210 ± 21	208 ± 26	205 ± 24	211 ± 17
Diastolic BP—mean ± SE	136 ± 16	135 ± 11	133 ± 14	136 ± 15
Heart rate—mean ± SE	87 ± 20	84 ± 14	81 ± 19	80 ± 14
15 minutes of Infusion* Systolic BP	−5 ± 4	−7 ± 4	−16 ± 4	−19 ± 4
Diastolic BP	−5 ± 3	−8 ± 3	−12 ± 2	−21 ± 2
Heart rate	−2 ± 3	+1 ± 1	+2 ± 1	+11 ± 2

Continued

Time Point and Pharmacodynamic Parameters	Infusion Rate (µg/kg/min)			
	0.01 n = 25	0.03 n = 24	0.1 n = 22	0.3 n = 23
30 Minutes of Infusion* Systolic BP	−6 ± 4	−11 ± 4	−21 ± 3	−16 ± 4
Diastolic BP	−10 ± 3	−12 ± 3	−17 ± 3	−20 ± 2
Heart rate	−2 ± 3	−1 ± 1	+3 ± 2	+12 ± 3
1 Hour of Infusion* Systolic BP	−5 ± 3	−9 ± 4	−19 ± 4	−22 ± 4
Diastolic BP	−8 ± 3	−13 ± 3	−18 ± 2	−23 ± 2
Heart rate	−1 ± 3	0 ± 2	+3 ± 2	+11 ± 3
4 Hours of Infusion* Systolic BP	−14 ± 4	−20 ± 5	−23 ± 4	−37 ± 4
Diastolic BP	−12 ± 3	−18 ± 3	−21 ± 3	−29 ± 3
Heart rate	−2 ± 4	0 ± 2	+4 ± 2	+11 ± 2

*Mean change from baseline ± S.E.

PEDIATRIC DOSE

Safety and effectiveness for use in children not established.

DOSE ADJUSTMENTS

Dose adjustment is not required in end-stage renal disease; in patients on continuous ambulatory peritoneal dialysis (CAPD); in severe hepatic failure; or by age, gender, or race. Effects of hemodialysis have not been evaluated.

DILUTION

Each 10 mg (1 ml) must be diluted with 250 ml of NS or D5W and given as a continuous infusion. (10 mg in 250 ml, 20 mg in 500 ml, or 40 mg in 1,000 ml all yield 40 mcg/ml.)

Storage: Diluted solution is stable at CRT and normal light conditions for 24 hours. Discard any solution not used within 24 hours of preparation.

INCOMPATIBLE WITH

Specific information not available. Consider specific use and need for continuous adjustment.

RATE OF ADMINISTRATION

Do not given as a bolus injection; must be given as an infusion. Use of a calibrated, mechanical infusion pump is recommended for accurate, reliable delivery of desired infusion rate. Avoid hypotension and rapid decreases in BP. Infusion may be abruptly discontinued or gradually tapered as indicated by patient condition and/or use of other antihypertensive agents. See chart on page 383 for desired infusion rates:

Body Weight (kg)	Drug Dose Rate				
	0.025 μg/kg/min	0.05 μg/kg/min	0.1 μg/kg/min	0.2 μg/kg/min	0.3 μg/kg/min
	Infusion Rates (mL/min)				
40	0.025	0.05	0.1	0.2	0.3
50	0.031	0.06	0.13	0.25	0.38
60	0.038	0.08	0.15	0.3	0.45
70	0.044	0.09	0.18	0.35	0.53
80	0.05	0.1	0.2	0.4	0.6
90	0.056	0.11	0.23	0.45	0.68
100	0.063	0.13	0.25	0.5	0.75
110	0.069	0.14	0.28	0.55	0.83
120	0.075	0.15	0.3	0.6	0.9
130	0.081	0.16	0.33	0.65	0.98
140	0.088	0.18	0.35	0.7	1.05
150	0.094	0.19	0.38	0.75	1.13

ACTIONS

A peripherally acting rapid-acting vasoldilator. Causes a dose-dependent fall in systolic and diastolic blood pressure. May cause a reflex increase in heart rate. Onset of action begins within 5 minutes, and with continuous infusion, steady state concentrations (peak effects) are reached in 15 to 20 minutes. Maintains or increases glomerular filtration rate (GFR) in normotensive or hypertensive patients with or without renal insufficiency. Increases renal blood flow by dilating both afferent and efferent arterioles. Increases sodium excretion and decreases sodium reabsorption. Increases potassium, calcium, and phosphate excretion, with or without an increase in GFR. Elimination half-life is about 5 minutes. Metabolized in the liver primarily by conjugation (without cytochrome P_{450} enzymes). Primarily eliminated in urine; some excretion in feces.

INDICATIONS AND USES

In-hospital, short-term (up to 48 hours) management of severe hypertension when rapid, but quickly reversible, emergency reduction of blood pressure is indicated including malignant hypertension with deteriorating end-organ function.

CONTRAINDICATIONS

Manufacturer states "none known."

PRECAUTIONS

Use limited to the hospital. Adequate personnel and appropriate equipment must be available for continuous monitoring. ■ Use extreme caution in patients with glaucoma or intraocular hypertension. Has caused a dose-dependent increase in intraocular pressure. ■ Causes a dose-related tachycardia with infusion rates above 0.1 mcg/kg. May diminish over time but is consistent at higher doses. Has not been reported, but could lead to ischemic cardiac events or worsened heart failure. ■ Although hypotension should be avoided in all patients, use extreme caution in patients with an acute cerebral infarction or hemmorrhage. ▪ Rapidly decreases serum potassium leading to hypokalemia; note Monitor. ▪ Use caution; contains sulfites. Sulfite sensitivity is seen more frequently in asthmatic than nonasthmatic individuals. ▪ Note Drug/lab interactions.

Monitor: Determine patency of vein; avoid extravasation. Monitor BP and HR at least every 15 minutes. Avoid hypotension. More frequent monitoring may be required, but intraarterial blood pressure monitoring has not been required. ▪ Monitor serum electrolytes frequently; monitoring of serum potassium is recommended every 6 hours. Has reduced serum potassium values to less than 3 mEq/L in less than 6 hours. Oral or intravenous supplements are required. ▪ Transfer to oral antihypertensive agents when BP is stable. May be added during fenoldopam infusion or following its discontinuation; monitor effects carefully. ▪ Note Precautions and Drug/lab interactions.

Patient education: Report IV site burning or stinging promptly. ▪ Request assistance to ambulate.

Maternal/child: Category B: use only if clearly needed. ▪ Use caution during lactation; not known if fenoldopam is secreted in breast milk (is secreted in milk of rats). ▪ Safety and effectiveness for use in children not established.

Elderly: Reponse similar to other age gropus.

DRUG/LAB INTERACTIONS

No specific drug interaction studies have been conducted. ▪ Concurrent use not recommended with beta-adrenergic blocking aents (e.g., atenolol [Tenormin], esmolol [Brevibloc], metoprolol [Lopressor], propranolol [Inderal]). May cause unexpected hypotension from beta-blocker inhibition of the reflex response to fenoldopam. ▪ Has been given safely with digitalis and sublingual nitroglycerin. ▪ Limited experience with concomitant use of other antihypertensive agents (e.g., ACE inhibitors [e.g., enalaprilat (Vasotec)], calcium channel blockers [e.g., diltiazem (Cardizem), verapamil (Isoptin)], or thiazide or loop diuretics [e.g., chlorothiazide (Diuril), furosemide (Lasix), torsemide (Demadex)]).

SIDE EFFECTS

Abdominal pain or fullness, anxiety, back pain, constipation, diaphoresis, diarrhea, dizziness, flushing, headache, increased serum creatinine, injection site reaction, insomnia, nasal congestion, nausea, postural hypotension, urinary infection, and vomiting occurred in up to 5% of patients. Additional side effects have been reported in 0.5% to 5% of patients (see literature).

Major: Cardiac arrhythmias (e.g., bradycardia, extrasystoles, ST-T wave abnormalities, tachycardia), hypotension, hypokalemia, and myocardial infarction can occur with average doses.

ANTIDOTE

Keep physician informed of all side effects. Most will be treated symptomatically. Use oral and/or intravenous potassium to treat hypokalemia. Reduce dose gradually as desired BP is reached. Discontinue fenoldopam immediately for execessive hypotension. Half-life is short. Recovery should begin within 5 to 15 minutes; support patient as indicated (e.g., Trendelenburg position, IV fluids if appropriate). With short half-life the need for vasopressors in unlikely. Discontinue fenoldopam and treat life-threatening arrhythmias as indicated.

FENTANYL CITRATE

Narcotic analgesic
(agonist)
Anesthesia adjunct

Fentanyl, Fentanyl citrate PF, Sublimaze

pH 4.0 to 7.5

USUAL DOSE

Adjunct to regional anesthesia: 50 to 100 mcg (0.05 to 0.1 mg).
Adjunct to general anesthesia: Low dose: 2 mcg/kg of body weight.
Moderate dose: 2 to 20 mcg/kg of body weight. Additional doses of 25 to 100 mcg may be administered as needed. *High dose:* 20 to 50 mcg/kg of body weight. Additional doses of 25 mcg to one half the initial loading dose may be administered as needed.
General anesthetic: 50 to 100 mcg/kg of body weight administered with oxygen and a muscle relaxant.
In all situations, use smallest effective dose at maximum intervals.

PEDIATRIC DOSE

1 to 2 mcg/kg/dose over 3 to 5 minutes. May repeat in 30 to 60 minutes. To give as an infusion, begin with 1 mcg/kg/hr and titrate to effect. Maximum dose is 3 mcg/kg/hr.

DOSE ADJUSTMENTS

Reduce dose in patients receiving other CNS depressants, such as general anesthetics, alcohol, anticholinergics, antihistamines, barbiturates, cimetidine (Tagamet), hypnotics, sedatives, psychotropic agents, and narcotic analgesics. When administered with narcotics, reduce initial narcotic dose to one fourth to one third of normal. ■ Reduce dose or increase intervals for elderly, debilitated, and poor-risk patients or those with impaired pulmonary, hepatic, or renal function. ■ Note Drug/lab interactions.

DILUTION

May be given undiluted by the anesthesiologist. In other situations dilution with at least 5 ml of SW or NS for injection is preferred to facilitate titration. Other IV solutions may be used. May be given through Y-tube or three-way stopcock of infusion set.
Storage: Store at room temperature and protect from light before dilution. Use promptly.

INCOMPATIBLE WITH

Diazepam (Valium), methohexitol (Brevitol), pentobarbital (Nembutal), phenytoin (Dilantin), sodium bicarbonate, thiopental (Pentothal). Physically compatible with many other drugs for at least 15 minutes.

RATE OF ADMINISTRATION

Administer over a minimum of 3 to 5 minutes. Rapid administration may result in apnea or respiratory paralysis. Rate must be titrated by desired dose and patient response.

ACTIONS

An opium derivative, narcotic analgesic, which is a descending CNS depressant. Approximately 100 times more potent than morphine milligram for milligram. It has definite respiratory depressant actions that outlast its analgesic effect. In healthy individuals, respiratory rate returns to normal more quickly than with other opiates. Effective within one circulation time and lasts about 30 minutes. Effects are cumulative with repeat doses. Has little hypnotic activity, and histamine release rarely occurs. Cardiovascular system remains stable. Depresses many other senses or reflexes. Metabolized in the liver and excreted in the urine. Crosses the placental barrier. May be secreted in breast milk.

INDICATIONS AND USES

Adjunct to general and regional anesthesia. ▪ Short-term analgesia during perioperative period. ▪ Useful in short-duration minor surgery in outpatients and in diagnostic procedures or treatments that require the patient to be awake or very lightly anesthetized (e.g., bronchoscopy, radiological studies, burn dressings, cystoscopy). ▪ For administration with a neuroleptic such as droperidol as an anesthetic premedication, for the induction of anesthesia, and as an adjunct in the maintenance of general and regional anesthesia. ▪ For use as an anesthetic agent with oxygen in selected high-risk patients, such as those undergoing open heart surgery or certain complicated neurological or orthopedic procedures.

CONTRAINDICATIONS

Patients with known intolerance to fentanyl.

PRECAUTIONS

▪ Primarily used by or under the direct observation of the anesthesiologist. ▪ Use caution in the elderly, in patients with impaired hepatic or renal function, and in patients with pulmonary disease; reduced dose may be indicated. ▪ Use extreme caution in craniotomy, head injury, and increased intracranial pressure. ▪ Respiratory depression may cause an increased P_{CO_2}, cerebral vasodilation, and increased intracranial pressure. Clinical course of head injury may be obscured. ▪ Symptoms of acute abdominal conditions may be masked. ▪ Use caution in patients with bradyarrhythmias. ▪ Cough reflex is suppressed. ▪ Use caution in patients with benign prostatic hypertrophy, diarrhea resulting from poisoning until toxic material is eliminated, hypersensitivity to opiates, and in premature infants or labor and delivery of premature infants.

Monitor: Oxygen, controlled respiratory equipment, naloxone (Narcan), and neuromuscular blocking agents (e.g., succinylcholine [Anectine]) must always be available. May cause rigidity of respiratory muscles; may require a muscle relaxant to permit artificial ventilation. ▪ Observe patient frequently and monitor vital signs. Patient will appear to be asleep and may forget to breathe unless commanded to do so. ▪ Keep patient supine; orthostatic hypotension and fainting may occur. ▪ Note Precautions.

Patient education: Avoid alcohol or other CNS depressants (e.g., antihistamines, diazepam [Valium]). ▪ Blurred vision, dizziness, drowsiness, or lightheadedness may occur; use caution. ▪ Review all medications for interactions.

Maternal/child: Pregnancy category C: Safety for use in pregnancy not established; has impaired fertility and had embryocidal effects in rats. ▪ Postpone breast feeding for at least 4 to 6 hours after use of fentanyl. ▪ Safety for use in children under 2 years not established; has caused chest wall rigidity in neonates and may be associated with methemoglobinemia and hypotension in premature neonates (see Precautions).

Elderly: Note Dose adjustments and Precautions. ▪ May markedly decrease pulmonary ventilation. ▪ May be more sensitive to effects (e.g., respiratory depression, urinary retention, constipation). ▪ Analgesia should be effective with lower doses. ▪ Consider age-related organ impairment; may delay postop recovery.

DRUG/LAB INTERACTIONS

Higher doses may cause prolonged hypotension with diazepam (Valium). ▪ Potentiated by phenothiazines (e.g., chlorpromazine [Thorazine]); MAO inhibitors (e.g., selegiline [Eldepryl]); neuromuscular blocking agents (e.g., tubocurarine) and beta-adrenergic blocking agents (e.g., propranolol [Inderal]). Reduced dose of both drugs may be indicated. ▪ Cardiovascular depression may result from concurrent use of nitrous oxide and high-dose fentanyl.

SIDE EFFECTS

Average dose: Bradycardia, diaphoresis, hypersensitivity reactions, hypertension, hypotension, hypothermia, increased intracranial pressure, nausea, orthostatic hypotension, respiratory depression (slight), respiratory muscle rigidity, urinary retention, vomiting.

Overdose: Anaphylaxis, apnea, cardiac arrest, circulatory collapse, coma, excitation, hypotension (severe), inverted T wave on ECG, myocardial depression (severe), pinpoint pupils, respiratory depression (severe), tachycardia, death.

ANTIDOTE

Buprenorphine is sometimes used prior to the end of surgery to reverse fentanyl-induced anesthesia. With increasing severity of any side effect or onset of symptoms of overdose, discontinue the drug and notify the physician. Naloxone (Narcan) will reverse serious respiratory depression. A patent airway, artificial ventilation, oxygen therapy, and other symptomatic treatment must be instituted promptly. A fast-acting muscle relaxant (e.g., succinylcholine [Anectine]) may be required to facilitate ventilation. Use atropine to treat bradycardia. Resuscitate as necessary.

FILGRASTIM

Colony-stimulating factor
Antineutropenic

G-CSF, Human granulocyte colony-stimulating factor, Neupogen

pH 4.0

USUAL DOSE

Myelosuppressive chemotherapy: 5 mcg/kg/24 hr as a single daily dose for 2 to 4 weeks based on specific chemotherapy protocol and post nadir absolute neutrophil count (ANC). May be given IV by intermittent or continuous infusion, by SC injection, or as a 24-hour SC infusion. May be increased by 5-mcg/kg/24 hr increments for each chemotherapy cycle. Should not be used 24 hours before to 24 hours after the administration of cytotoxic chemotherapy because of the potential sensitivity of rapidly dividing myeloid cells to cytotoxic chemotherapy. Expect a transient increase in neutrophil counts in the first several days after initiation of therapy. Neutrophil response may not be adequate and dose increases as outlined may be required in heavily pretreated patients, those who have received prior radiation therapy to a significant portion of their medullary bone marrow (e.g., pelvis), bone marrow transplant patients, and/or those receiving dose-intensified chemotherapy. Maximum tolerated dose not identified. Up to 115 mcg/kg/24 hr has been used. For a sustained therapeutic response, therapy must be continued until the post nadir ANC is 10,000/mm^3 after the expected chemotherapy nadir (lowest point) has passed. Usually discontinued when this point is reached. (Average is 2 weeks or less.) In patients receiving dose-intensified chemotherapy, continue filgrastim until 2 consecutive ANCs $\geq$ 10,000 cells/mm^3 are documented. (Range is 6 to 28 days.) Note Precautions/Monitor.

Bone marrow transplant (BMT): 10 mcg/kg/24 hr as an IV infusion over 4 to 24 hours or as a continuous 24-hour SC infusion. Give the first dose at least 24 hours after cytotoxic chemotherapy and 24 hours after bone marrow infusion.

DOSE ADJUSTMENTS

Reduce dose or discontinue filgrastim if ANC> 10,000/mm^3 for three days. ■ During neutrophil recovery after BMT titrate the daily dose as follows based on daily or three consecutive-day evaluations:

Absolute Neutrophil Count (ANC)	Filgrastim dose
ANC > 1,000/mm^3 × 3 days	↓ to 5 mcg/kg/24 hr
ANC remains > 1,000/mm^3 × 3 more days on 5 mcg/kg/24 hr	DC filgrastim
ANC < 1,000/mm^3	Resume at 5 mcg/kg/24 hr
ANC < 1,000/mm^3 on 5 mcg/kg/24 hr	↑ to 10 mcg/kg/24 hr

DILUTION

Available as a ready-to-use single-dose vial with either 300 mcg/ml or 480 mcg/1.6 ml. Remove from refrigerator to allow to warm to room temperature (never longer than 24 hours). Confirm expiration date to ensure valid product. Avoid shaking. Contains no preservatives; use sterile technique, entering vial only once to withdraw a single dose. Dilute with 10 to 50 ml D5W to concentrations of 15 mcg/ml or greater. With concentrations from 5 to 15 mcg/ml, the addition of 2 ml of 5% albumin to each 50 ml D5W is required before adding filgrastim. Protects from adsorption to plastics and glass. Discard any unused portion. Should be clear and colorless. Do not dilute to <5 mcg/ml.

Storage: Store in refrigerator before use. Do not allow to freeze. Do not expose to direct sunlight. Stable undiluted in a syringe for 24 hours at controlled room temperature or up to 7 days if refrigerated. Refrigerate diluted solutions and use within 24 hours.

INCOMPATIBLE WITH

Any solution other than D5W.

Y-site: Amphotericin B (Fungizone), cefonicid (Monocid), cefoperazone (Cefobid), cefotaxime (Claforan), cefoxitin (Mefoxin), ceftizoxime (Cefizox), ceftriaxone (Rocephon), cefuroxime (Zinacef), clindamycin (Cleocin), dactinomycin (Cosmegen), etoposide (VePesid), fluorouracil (5FU), furosemide (Lasix), heparin, mannitol, methylprednisolone (Solu-medrol), metronidazole (Flagyl IV), mezlocillin (Mezlin), mitomycin (Mutamycin), normal saline, piperacillin (Pipracil), prochlorperazine (Compazine), thiotepa (Tespa).

RATE OF ADMINISTRATION

Recent studies suggest that an extended infusion time (intermittent or continuous) promotes increased recovery of neutrophils.

Intermittent infusion: A single dose over 15 to 30 minutes.

Continuous infusion: A single dose over 4 to 24 hours. In all situations flush IV line with D5W before and after administration.

ACTIONS

Colony-stimulating factors are glycoproteins that bind to specific hematopoietic cell surface receptors and stimulate proliferation, differentiation commitment, and some end-cell functional activation. Endogenous granulocyte colony-stimulating factors are produced by monocytes, fibroblasts, and endothelial cells. They are lineage-specific with selectivity for the neutrophil lineage. With recombinant DNA technology, filgrastim is produced by specifically prepared *Escherichia coli* bacteria inserted with the human G-CSF gene. It regulates the production of neutrophils within the bone marrow. Although not species specific, it mimics the actions of endogenous glycoprotein. By accelerating the recovery of neutrophil counts following a variety of chemotherapy regimens, it decreases infections manifested by febrile neutropenia, need for hospitalization, and IV antibiotic usage. May also cause some increase in lymphocyte counts. Increase in circulating neutrophils is dose-dependent, and a return to baseline occurs shortly after discontinuation (50% of baseline in 1 to 2 days and to pretreatment levels in 1 to 7 days).

INDICATIONS AND USES

Decrease the incidence of infection (febrile neutropenia) in patients with nonmyeloid malignancies receiving myelosuppressive anticancer drugs associated with a significant incidence of severe neutropenia with fever. ■ Decrease duration of neutropenia and related clinical problems (e.g., febrile neutropenia) in patients with nonmyeloid malignancies receiving myeloablative chemotherapy followed by BMT. ■ Used SC to treat severe chronic neutropenia (e.g., congenital, cyclic, or idiopathic) after all diseases associated with neutropenia have been ruled out. ■ Used SC or as a 24° SC infusion to mobilize hematopoietic progenitor cells into the peripheral blood for collection by leukapheresis with transplantation after myeloablative chemotherapy.

Investigational uses: Filgrastim-mobilized peripheral blood progenitor cells (PBPCs) are being used in place of BMT because they provide more rapid recovery of the patient's WBCs (neutrophils), RBCs, and platelets. ■ Increase neutrophil count in adults with myelodysplastic syndrome (MDS). May accelerate progression to usually fatal acute myelogenous leukemia (AML); relationship unclear. ■ Increase neutrophil count in aplastic anemia. ■ Increase neutrophil count in hairy cell leukemia and acute leukemias. ■ Treat granulocytopenia in HIV-infected patients receiving zidovudine. May be used concomitantly with epoetin-alfa.

CONTRAINDICATIONS
Hypersensitivity to *E. coli*-derived proteins.

PRECAUTIONS
Should be administered under the direction of a physician knowledgeable about appropriate use for each indication (e.g., expert in bone marrow transplantation). ■ Frequently given by SC injection or SC continuous infusion. ■ Effective in patients receiving chemotherapy with protocols containing cisplatin, cyclophosphamide, doxorubicin, etoposide, ifosfamide, mesna, methotrexate, vinblastine, and similar antineoplastic agents. ■ Effectiveness has not been evaluated in patients receiving chemotherapy associated with delayed myelosuppression (e.g., nitrosoureas [carmustine]), with mitomycin C, or with myelosuppressive doses of antimetabolites (e.g., 5-fluorouracil or cytosine arabinoside). ■ Use extreme caution in any malignancy with myeloid characteristics; can act as a growth factor for any tumor type, particularly myeloid malignancies. ■ Adult respiratory distress syndrome may occur in septic patients. ■ Use caution in patients with preexisting cardiac disease; cardiac events (e.g., myocardial infarction) have occurred but the relationship to filgrastim is unclear. ■ Chronic use at varying doses over several years may cause subclinical splenomegaly in adults and children.

Monitor: Obtain a CBC and platelet count before chemotherapy begins and twice weekly thereafter to monitor the neutrophil count and to avoid leukocytosis. Following cytotoxic chemotherapy, the neutrophil nadir occurs earlier during cycles when filgrastim is used, duration of severe neutropenia is reduced, and white blood cell differentials may have a left shift. ■ Increase monitoring of CBC and platelet count to 3 times a week after bone marrow infusion. ■ Because higher doses of chemotherapy may be tolerated, side effects associated with the chemotherapeutic drug may be more pronounced; observe carefully. ■ Use caution with any additional drugs known to lower the platelet count. ■ Note Precautions.

Patient education: Promptly report any symptoms of infection (e.g., fever)

or allergic reaction (itching, redness, swelling at the injection site).
■ May be self-injected SC by the patient at home; requires instruction.
Literature includes a patient handout.

Maternal/child: Pregnancy category C: Safety for use during pregnancy
not established. Very large doses have caused fetal damage and death in
rabbits. Use only if benefit justifies the potential risk to the fetus.
■ Secretion through breast milk not established; use caution during
lactation. ■ Has been used in over 100 children from 3 months to 18
years of age with similar experience to the adult population, even though
literature says safety not established. May cause bone pain, fever, or rash.

DRUG/LAB INTERACTIONS

Interaction with other drugs has not been evaluated. ■ Use with
caution any drug that may potentiate the release of neutrophils (e.g.,
lithium). ■ Concurrent use with vincristine (Oncovin) may cause a
severe atypical neuropathy (foot pain, severe motor weakness).

SIDE EFFECTS

No serious adverse reactions that would limit the use of the product
have been reported. Allergic reactions (itching, redness, swelling at
the injection site) have occurred; anaphylaxis has not occurred but is
possible. Complaints of dose-related bone pain are common and may
require analgesics. With doses above 5 mcg/kg/day, leukocytosis
(white blood cell counts greater than $100,000/mm^3$) has occurred in
5% of patients with no adverse effects reported. Cutaneous vasculitis
has occurred in a few patients. Reduced dose may be indicated with
subsequent treatment.

ANTIDOTE

Notify physician promptly if any signs of infection (fever) or other
potential side effects occur. Monitor potential leukocytosis with twice-
weekly CBCs. Discontinue therapy after ANC surpasses $10,000/mm^3$
and the chemotherapy nadir has occurred. Discontinue filgrastim and
notify physician immediately if a generalized allergic reaction should
occur. Treat allergic reactions as indicated.

FLUCONAZOLE

Antifungal

Diflucan

pH 4.0 to 8.0

USUAL DOSE

IV dose has been used for a maximum of 14 days. Plasma levels are similar with IV or oral, so oral dose can replace IV dose at any time. Note Precautions/Monitor.

Oropharyngeal candidiasis: Initial dose of 200 mg followed by 100 mg daily for a minimum of 14 days. Oral maintenance therapy usually required in patients with AIDS to prevent relapse.

Esophageal candidiasis: Initial dose of 200 mg followed by 100 mg daily for a minimum of 21 days and for at least 2 weeks after symptoms subside. Up to 400 mg/24 hr may be used.

Urinary tract or peritoneal candidiasis: 50 to 200 mg daily has been used.

Systemic candidiasis: Initial dose of 400 mg followed by 200 mg daily for a minimum of 28 days and for at least 2 weeks after symptoms subside. Another source suggests optimal dose and duration of therapy has not been established. Doses up to 400 mg daily have been used.

Acute cryptococcal meningitis: Initial dose of 400 mg followed by 200 mg daily for a minimum of 10 to 12 weeks after CSF culture becomes negative. Oral maintenance therapy of 200 mg daily usually required in patients with AIDS to prevent relapse.

Prevention of candidiasis in bone marrow transplant: 400 mg once daily. If severe neutropenia ($< 500/mm^3$) is expected, begin fluconazole prophylaxis several days ahead of expected neutropenia. Continue for 7 days after neutrophils reach $1,000/mm^3$.

PEDIATRIC DOSE

Ages 3 to 13 years: 10 mg/kg as a loading dose. Maintain with 3 to 6 mg/kg of body weight daily. Begin 24 hours after loading dose. Experience with children is limited. A second source recommends the dosing guidelines specific for each indication as follows:

Oropharyngeal candidiasis: Initial dose of 6 mg/kg of body weight followed by 3 mg/kg daily.

Esophageal candidiasis: Initial dose of 6 mg/kg of body weight followed by 3 mg/kg daily. Up to 12 mg/kg has been used.

Systemic candidiasis: 6 to 12 mg/kg of body weight daily.

Acute cryptococcal meningitis: Initial dose of 12 mg/kg of body weight followed by 6 mg/kg daily.

Duration of therapy for each indication is the same as that listed in Usual dose.

DOSE ADJUSTMENTS

In all adult situations the infecting organism and response to therapy may justify increased doses up to 400 mg daily. ■ In impaired renal function, dose should be adjusted according to creatinine clearance and/or dialysis schedule (see literature). ■ Note Drug/lab interactions.

DILUTION

Packaged prediluted and ready for use as an iso-osmotic solution containing 2 mg/ml in both glass bottles and Viaflex Plus plastic containers. Do not remove moisture barrier overwrap of plastic container until ready for use. Tear overwrap down side at slit to open, and remove sterile inner bag. Plastic may appear somewhat opaque due to sterilization process but will clear. Squeeze inner bag firmly to check for leaks. Discard if leakage noted; sterility is impaired. Do not use if cloudy or precipitated.

Storage: Store glass bottles between 5° C (41° F) and 30° C (86° F); store plastic containers between 5° C (41° F) and 25° C (77° F). Protect both from freezing.

INCOMPATIBLE WITH

Manufacturer states "do not add supplementary medication."

Y-site: Amphotericin B (Fungizone), ampicillin (Polycillin-N), calcium gluconate, cefotaxime (Claforan), ceftazidime (Tazicef), ceftriaxone (Rocephin), cefuroxime (Zinacef), chloramphenicol, clindamycin (Cleocin), diazepam (Valium), digoxin (Lanoxin), erythromycin (Erythrocin IV), furosemide (Lasix), haloperidol (Haldol), hydroxyzine (Vistaril), imipenem-cilastin (Primaxin), pentamidine (Pentam 300), piperacillin (Pipracil), ticarcillin (Ticar), trimethoprim-sulfamethoxazole.

Additive: trimethoprim-sulfamethoxazole (Bactrim).

RATE OF ADMINISTRATION

A single dose as a continuous infusion at a rate not to exceed 200 mg/hr. Do not use plastic containers in series connections; air embolism could result.

ACTIONS

A synthetic broad-spectrum bis-Triazole antifungal agent. Inhibits fungal growth of *Candida* and *Cryptococcus neoformans* by acting on a key enzyme and depriving the fungus of ergosterol; the cell membrane becomes unstable and can no longer function normally. Human sterol synthesis is not affected. Has shown some effectiveness against *Aspergillus flavus, Aspergillus fumigatus, Blastomyces dermatitidis*, and *Coccidoides immitis* in laboratory mice. Peak action achieved in 1 to 2 hours; half-life extends for 30 hours. Initial double dose results in steady state plasma concentration by day 2 when given IV or orally. Penetrates into all body fluids in similar and effective concentrations and remains constant with daily single dose administration. 80% excreted as unchanged drug through the kidneys. Secreted in breast milk.

INDICATIONS AND USES

Oropharyngeal and esophageal candidiasis. ▪ Serious systemic candidal infections including GU tract infections, peritonitis, and pneumonia. ▪ Cryptococcal meningitis including maintenance to prevent relapse. ▪ Prevention of candidiasis in bone marrow transplant patients.

CONTRAINDICATIONS

Hypersensitivity to fluconazole or any of its components. Use caution in patients hypersensitive to other azoles (e.g., ketoconazole).

PRECAUTIONS

For IV use only; do not give IM.

Monitor: Specimens for fungal culture, serology, and histopathology should be obtained before therapy to isolate and identify causative organisms. Therapy may begin as soon as all specimens are obtained and before results are known. ▪ Inadequate treatment may lead to recurrence of active infection; continue treatment until clinical parameters or laboratory tests indicate that active fungal infection has subsided. Note specific recommendations in Usual dose. ■ Serious hepatotoxicity may occur. Causal relationship uncertain but many patients are taking hepatotoxic drugs for treatment of malignancies and AIDS. Note any increase in liver function tests (e.g., AST [SGOT]). If any clinical signs and symptoms that are consistent with liver disease develop, discontinue drug. Has caused deaths. ■ Exfoliative skin disorders have been reported. ■ Note Drug/lab interactions.

Maternal/child: Pregnancy category C: Safety for use in pregnancy and lactation and in children not established. Use in pregnancy only if potential benefits outweigh risk to fetus. ■ Use in nursing mothers is not recommended.

DRUG/LAB INTERACTIONS

Hepatoxicity increased if used concurrently with ketoconazole (Nizoral). ■ Potentiated by hydrochlorothiazide (HydroDIURIL); decreases renal clearance of fluconazole. ■ Potentiates cyclosporine, phenytoin, and theophyllines; careful monitoring of their plasma levels is required. ■ Potentiates coumarin-type anticoagulants (e.g., warfarin); monitor prothrombin times. Potentiates oral hypoglycemic agents (e.g., tolbutamide); monitor blood glucose levels. In all of these situations dose reductions of the above drugs may be indicated. ■ Rifampin increases metabolism; fluconazole dose may need to be increased. ■ Increases serum levels of zidovudine (Retrovir, AZT). ■ Studies have not been completed on interactions with pentamidine (Pentam 300). ■ Use with astemizole (Hismanal) and terfenadine (Seldane) may cause serious cardiotoxicity. ■ Use with cisapride (Propulsid) may increase cisapride levels and cause cardiac arrhythmias; concurrent use not recommended.

SIDE EFFECTS

More frequent in HIV-infected patients.

Average dose: Abdominal pain, diarrhea, dizziness, dry mouth, exfoliative skin disorders, headache, hepatic reactions, increased appetite, increased sweating, nausea, pallor, rash, taste perversion, tremor, vomiting.

Overdose: Cyanosis, decreased motility, decreased respirations, lacrimation, loss of balance, salivation, urinary incontinence. Clonic convulsions preceded death in experimental animals.

ANTIDOTE

Notify physician of all side effects; most will be treated symptomatically. Discontinue drug and notify physician of abnormal liver function tests progressing to clinical signs and symptoms of liver disease. Rash may be the first sign of an exfoliative skin disorder in immunocompromised patients; discontinue drug and notify physician. In overdose a 3-hour dialysis session will decrease plasma levels by 50%. Treat anaphylaxis or resuscitate if indicated.

FLUDARABINE PHOSPHATE

Antineoplastic (Antimetabolite)

Fludara

pH 7.2 to 8.2

USUAL DOSE

25 mg/M^2 daily for 5 consecutive days. Repeat every 4 weeks. Optimum duration of treatment not established. If there is no major toxicity, treat until maximum response achieved, then administer three additional complete cycles.

DOSE ADJUSTMENTS

Decreased or delayed based on evidence of hematologic or nonhematologic toxicity. Increased toxicity may occur in the elderly and in patients with renal insufficiency or bone marrow impairment.

DILUTION

Specific techniques required; see Precautions. Each 50 mg must be initially diluted with 2 ml of SW for injection (25 mg/ml). Should dissolve within 15 seconds. Further dilute a single dose in 100 to 125 ml of NS or D5W and give as an infusion.

Storage: Refrigerate between 2° and 8° C (36° to 46° F) before dilution. No preservative; use within 8 hours of dilution.

INCOMPATIBLE WITH

Consider toxicity and specific use. *Y-site:* Acyclovir (Zovirax), amphotericin B (Fungizone), chlorpromazine (Thorazine), daunorubicin (Cerubidine), ganciclovir (Cytovene), hydroxyzine (Vistaril), miconazole (Monistat IV), prochlorperazine (Compazine).

RATE OF ADMINISTRATION

Single daily dose properly diluted for infusion over 30 minutes.

ACTIONS

A potent antineoplastic agent. A fluorinated nucleotide analog of the antiviral agent vidarabine. Rapidly converts to the active metabolite 2-fluoro-ara-ATP and interferes with the synthesis of DNA. Actual mechanism of action unknown and may be multifaceted. Median time to response in studies of patients with refractory chronic lymphocytic leukemia (CLL) was 7 to 21 weeks (range 1 to 68 weeks). Elimination half-life is 9 to 10 hours. Probably excreted in urine.

INDICATIONS AND USES

Treatment of patients with B-cell CLL who have not responded to or progressed during treatment with at least one standard alkylating-agent-containing regimen.

Investigational uses: Treatment of non-Hodgkin's lymphoma, macroglobulinemic lymphoma, prolymphocytic leukemia or prolymphocytoid variant of CLL, mycosis fungoides, hairy-cell leukemia, and Hodgkin's disease. Dose and/or efficacy not established.

CONTRAINDICATIONS

Hypersensitivity to fludarabine or its components (e.g., mannitol and sodium hydroxide).

PRECAUTIONS

Follow guidelines for handling cytotoxic agents. See Appendix A, p. 893. ■ Administered by or under the direction of the physician specialist. ▪ Use with caution in advanced age, renal insufficiency, or bone marrow impairment. ▪ Most patients have hematologic impairment at base line because of disease or prior myelosuppressive therapy. Myelosuppression may be severe and cumulative. ▪ Response can occur within 1 week. Use caution in patients with large tumor burdens; may cause tumor lysis syndrome.

Monitor: Observe closely for signs of toxicity, both hematologic and non-hematologic. ▪ Obtain baseline CBC and differential and repeat regularly to monitor hematopoietic suppression (especially neutrophils and platelets). ▪ Observe closely for all signs of infection and any fever of unknown origin. ▪ Prophylactic antibiotics may be indicated pending results of C/S in a febrile neutropenic patient. ▪ Nausea and vomiting usually less severe than many antineoplastics; prophylactic administration of antiemetics may be indicated.

Patient education: Nonhormonal birth control recommended. ▪ See Appendix D, p. 900.

Maternal/child: Pregnancy category D: Avoid pregnancy; may cause fetal harm. ▪ Discontinue breast feeding. ▪ Safety for use in children not established.

Elderly: Note Precautions and Dose adjustments.

DRUG/LAB INTERACTIONS

Do not use with pentostatin (Nipent); may increase risk of fatal pulmonary toxicity.

SIDE EFFECTS

Are frequent, may be dose limiting, and may cause death.

Average dose: Agitation, anorexia (21%), chills (15%), coma, confusion, diarrhea (14%), edema (17%), GI bleeding (8%), infection (both opportunistic [39%] and pneumonia [19%]), fatigue (24%), fever (65%), malaise (7%), myelosuppression (anemia [60%], neutropenia [59%], thrombocytopenia [55%]), nausea and vomiting (34%), pain (21%), peripheral neuropathy (8%), pulmonary hypersensitivity (cough [27%], dyspnea [16%], interstitial pulmonary infiltrate [1%]), rashes (15%), stomatitis (4%), visual disturbances (9%), weakness (37%). Onset of flank pain and hematuria may indicate tumor lysis syndrome (hyperkalemia, hyperphosphatemia, hyperuricemia, hypocalcemia, metabolic acidosis, urate crystalluria, and renal failure); one reported.

Overdose: Severe bone marrow suppression (neutropenia and thrombocytopenia). Severe neurologic toxicity including delayed blindness, coma, and death occurred from 21 to 60 days after the last dose in 36% of patients treated with doses only 4 times greater than the recommended dose. Has occurred (0.2%) with average doses.

ANTIDOTE

Notify the physician of all side effects. Most will be treated symptomatically. Some toxicity is necessary to produce remission. Delay or discontinue the drug for serious hematologic depression. Restart as soon as signs of bone marrow recovery occur. Delay or discontinue if neurotoxicity occurs. There is no specific antidote; supportive therapy as indicated will help sustain the patient in toxicity.

FLUMAZENIL

Benzodiazepine antagonist
Antidote

Romazicon   pH 4.0

USUAL DOSE

Reversal of conscious sedation or in general anesthesia: 0.2 mg (2 ml) as an initial dose. Assess level of consciousness. May be repeated at 1-minute intervals, assessing level of consciousness between each dose, until desired level of consciousness achieved or a total cumulative dose of 1 mg (10 ml) has been given (average dose to awakening is 0.6 mg to 1 mg). If resedation occurs (may occur if flumazenil wears off before the benzodiazepine) the above process may be repeated at 20-minute intervals as indicated. Do not give more than a cumulative dose of 1 mg in a 20-minute period or 3 mg in any 1 hour.

Management of suspected benzodiazepine overdose: 0.2 mg (2 ml) as an initial dose. Assess level of consciousness. If results inadequate, give an additional dose of 0.3 mg (3 ml) in 1 minute. If results are still inadequate, 0.5 mg (5 ml) may be repeated at 1-minute intervals. Assess level of consciousness between each dose until desired level of consciousness achieved or a total cumulative dose of 3 mg (30 ml) has been given (average dose to awakening is 1 mg to 3 mg). If a partial response is achieved with 3 mg, continue dosing in 0.5-mg increments until awakening or a cumulative dose of 5 mg is reached (rarely required). If patient has not responded to a cumulative dose of 5 mg within 5 minutes, benzodiazepines are not the major cause of sedation; discontinue use. If desired results are achieved and resedation occurs (expected), no more than 1 mg given in 0.5-mg increments may be given in any 20-minute period and no more than a cumulative total dose of 3 mg in any 1 hour.

PEDIATRIC DOSE

Not recommended for use in children (to reverse sedation, manage overdose, or resuscitate newborn) because no clinical studies have been done. However, it is being used. One source suggests from 10 mcg (0.01 mg)/kg for reversing sedation to 100 mcg (0.1 mg)/kg in a life-threatening overdose to a maximum cumulative dose of 1 mg. Has been given as an infusion at 5 to 10 mcg (0.005 to 0.01 mg)/kg/hr. Another source suggests 0.3 mg (3 ml) as an initial dose. Procedure same as adult except all subsequent doses are also 0.3 mg to a maximum dose of 3 mg.

DOSE ADJUSTMENTS

Not required for the elderly. ■ Reduce dose and extend intervals after the initial dose in impaired liver function. ■ In high-risk patients, administer the smallest amount that is effective and wait for peak effect (6 to 10 minutes). Slower titration rates and lower total doses may be especially important in these patients (see Precautions) to reduce emergent confusion and agitation and evaluate effect.

DILUTION

May be given undiluted through a free-flowing IV into a large vein (to minimize pain at injection site). Compatible with D5W, D21/2W,

LR, 0.45NS, and NS if further dilution required by a specific situation. Discard in 24 hours if drawn undiluted into a syringe or diluted in any solution.

INCOMPATIBLE WITH

Limited information available.

RATE OF ADMINISTRATION

Series of small injections allows control of the reversal of sedation to desired endpoint, avoids abrupt awakening, and minimizes the possibility of adverse effects.

Reversal of conscious sedation or in general anesthesia: Each single dose (0.2 mg [2 ml]) over 15 seconds.

Management of suspected benzodiazepine overdose: Each single dose (0.2 mg [2 ml], 0.3 mg [3 ml], or 0.5 mg [5 ml] respectively) over 30 seconds.

ACTIONS

A benzodiazepine antagonist. Competes with benzodiazepines, inhibiting their effect at benzodiazepine receptor sites. Action is very specific and reverses the sedative effects of benzodiazepines only. Duration and degree of reversal are dose and plasma content related (both for amount of benzodiazepine and amount of flumazenil). Onset of action usually occurs within 1 to 2 minutes of reaching the appropriate dose, with peak effect at 6 to 10 minutes. Enables the physician to control the duration of action of benzodiazepines, helps to evaluate the patient's postoperative condition much earlier than waiting for effect to wear off on its own, and may facilitate the postprocedural course. In overdose, it allows the physician to communicate sooner with patients who have taken an excessive dose. Extensively metabolized in the liver. Excreted in changed form in urine.

INDICATIONS AND USES

Complete or partial reversal of the effects of general anesthesia induced and/or maintained with benzodiazepines (e.g., diazepam [Valium], midazolam [Versed]). ■ Complete or partial reversal of the sedative effects of benzodiazepines used to produce and/or maintain sedation for diagnostic and therapeutic procedures. ■ Adjunct to conventional treatment in managing benzodiazepine overdose (e.g., chlordiazepoxide [Librium], diazepam [Valium], lorazepam [Ativan], midazolam [Versed]).

CONTRAINDICATIONS

Known hypersensitivity to flumazenil or any benzodiazepine, patients who are on benzodiazepine therapy for control of a potentially life-threatening conditions (e.g., control of intracranial pressure, status epilepticus), and patients showing signs of serious cyclic antidepressant overdose. ■ Use in treatment of benzodiazepine dependence is not recommended.

PRECAUTIONS

Excess administration increases risk of side effects and decreases desired therapeutics of benzodiazepines. ■ Will not reverse the central nervous system (CNS) effects of drugs such as alcohol, analgesics, antidepressants, barbiturates, and narcotics. In overdose, will bring the patient to a conscious state only if a benzodiazepine is responsible for the sedation. Has reversed benzodiazepine-induced hypotension and bradycardia unresponsive to other measures (e.g., IV fluids, atropine, dopamine). ■ Convulsions may occur, especially in patients who rely on benzodiazepines to control seizures, are physically dependent on benzodiazepines for long-term sedation, in overdose cases where large doses of other drugs have been ingested, in patients showing signs of serious cyclic antidepressant overdose (some clinicians recommend a diagnostic ECG or quantitative analytical testing before use—see Contraindications), or in ICU patients who may have an unrecognized dependence on benzodiazepines because of frequent use as a sedative (can occur with only 3 to 5 days of benzodiazepine administration). Intubation with ventilatory and circulatory support may be the treatment of choice for these high-risk patients (see Dose adjustments) ▪ Risk of adverse reactions increased in patients with a history of alcohol, benzodiazepine, or sedative use (increased frequency of benzodiazepine tolerance and dependence). Can precipitate benzodiazepine withdrawal (also high-risk, see Dose adjustments). ▪ Use extreme caution in head injury (may alter cerebral blood flow or cause convulsions). ▪ Do not use until effects of neuromuscular blockade have been fully reversed. ▪ May cause panic attacks in patients with a history of panic disorder. ▪ Additional ventilatory support may be required in patients with serious lung disease. ▪ Half-life prolonged based on amount of hepatic impairment. ▪ Ingestion of food increases clearance of flumazenil.

Monitor: Secure airway, ventilation, and IV access prior to administration. ▪ Monitor BP, HR, and respirations closely. ECG monitoring and oxygenation determination by pulse oximetry is recommended. ▪ Emergency equipment and supplies including drugs for seizure control (See Antidote) must always be available. ▪ Observe continuously for resedation, respiratory depression, preseizure activity, or other residual benzodiazepine effects for an appropriate period (2 or more hours). ▪ Extend observation time for larger doses, in presence of long-acting benzodiazepines (e.g., diazepam [Valium]), or large doses of short-acting benzodiazepines (e.g., more than 10 mg of midazolam [Versed]). ▪ Observe ambulatory patients for a minimum of 2 hours after a 1-mg dose; resedation after 2 hours is unlikely. Extend observation time as above. ▪ Awake patients may require pain medication sooner than those without benzodiazepine reversal. ▪ All postprocedural instructions must be given to the patient verbally and in writing; does not reverse benzodiazepine amnesia. ▪ Note Drug/lab interactions.

Patient education: Effects of benzodiazepines may recur, for 24 to 48 hours memory and judgment may be impaired. ▪ All instructions should be in writing. ▪ Do not drive, operate hazardous machinery, or engage in activities that require alertness. ▪ Do not take alcohol, other CNS depressants (e.g., antihistamines, barbiturates), or nonprescription drugs for 24 hours.

Maternal/child: Pregnancy category C: Use only if benefit justifies risk. ▪ Not recommended during labor and delivery because effect on newborn unknown. ▪ Safety for use in lactation not established. ▪ Not recommended for use in children.

Elderly: Note Dose adjustments. ▪ Monitor carefully; benzodiazepine-induced sedation may be deeper and more prolonged.

DRUG/LAB INTERACTIONS

May cause cardiac arrhythmias or convulsions in cases of mixed drug overdose. These toxic effects may emerge (especially with cyclic antidepressants [e.g., amitriptyline (Elavil)], imipramine (Tofranil)]) with reversal of benzodiazepine effect (note Precautions). May reverse sedative and anticonvulsant effects. ▪ May precipitate withdrawal symptoms if given to chronic benzodiazepine users. ▪ No specific deleterious interactions noted when flumazenil administered after narcotics, inhalational anesthetics, muscle relaxants, and muscle relaxant antagonists administered in conjunction with sedation or anesthesia. ▪ Lab test interactions have not been evaluated.

SIDE EFFECTS

Most common at doses above 1.0 mg and/or with abrupt reversal.

Average dose: Abnormal vision, agitation, anxiety, dizziness, dry mouth, dyspnea, emotional lability, fatigue, flushing, headache, hot flashes, hypertension, hyperventilation, insomnia, involuntary movements, irritability, muscle tension, nausea, pain or reaction (rash, thrombophlebitis) at the injection site, palpitations, panic, paresthesia, sweating, tachycardia, tinnitus, tremors, and vomiting. Convulsions may occur (note Precautions).

Overdose: Agitation, anxiety, arrhythmias, convulsions, hyperesthesia, increased muscle tone.

ANTIDOTE

Notify the physician of any side effect. Treat symptoms of benzodiazepine withdrawal (agitation, confusion, dizziness, emotional lability, or sensory distortions) with a barbiturate, benzodiazepine, or other sedative. Larger doses may be required because of presence of flumazenil. Treat convulsions from overdose with barbiturates, benzodiazepines, and phenytoin (Dilantin). Maintain an adequate airway, adequate ventilation, and IV access at all times. Hemodialysis not effective in overdose if 1 hour has passed since administration.

FLUOROURACIL

Antineoplastic
(Antimetabolite)

Adrucil, 5-FU, 5-Fluorouracil

pH 9.2

USUAL DOSE

12 mg/kg of body weight/24 hr for 4 days. Total dose should not exceed 800 mg/24 hr. If no toxicity is observed, one-half dose (6 mg/kg) is given on the even days for 4 additional doses. No medication is given on the odd days following the initial 4 doses. Note Precautions/Monitor. The most common form of maintenance therapy is to repeat the entire course of therapy beginning 30 days after the previous course is completed and any toxicity has subsided or to give a single dose of 10 to 15 mg/kg/week; not to exceed 1 Gm. Adjustments are made depending on side effects and tolerance.

Advanced colorectal cancer: Many protocols have been used. Examples are: 425 mg/M^2 preceded by 20 mg/M^2 of leucovorin calcium or 370 mg/M^2 preceded by 200 mg/M^2 leucovorin, daily for 5 days. Repeat at 4-week intervals twice, then repeat every 28 to 35 days based on complete recovery from toxic effects. Do not initiate or continue in any patient with GI toxicity until completely subsided. Reduce 5-FU dose based on tolerance to previous course; 20% for moderate hematologic or GI toxicity, 30% for severe. Increase 5-FU dose 10% if no toxicity. Leucovorin dose not adjusted.

DOSE ADJUSTMENTS

For poor-risk patients or those in a poor nutritional state; either reduce dose by one half or more throughout a course of therapy or give 6 mg/kg/day for 3 days. If no toxicity observed, give 3 mg/kg on days 5, 7, and 9. Give nothing on day 4, 6, or 8. Do not exceed 400 mg/day. ■ Dose based on ideal body weight in presence of edema, ascites, or obesity. ■ Used with other antineoplastic drugs in reduced doses to achieve tumor remission. ■ See Usual dose.

DILUTION

Specific techniques required; See Precautions. May be slightly discolored without affecting safety and potency. Dissolve any precipitate by heating to 60° C (140° F) and shaking vigorously. Cool to body temperature before using.

Direct IV: May be given undiluted. May inject through Y-tube or three-way stopcock of a free-flowing infusion.

Infusion: May be further diluted with D5W or NS and given as an infusion. Doses up to 2 Gm are being given with extreme caution under the specific supervision of experienced specialists. Leucovorin has been mixed into the solution with fluorouracil.

Storage: Store at room temperature; protect from light.

INCOMPATIBLE WITH

Usually not mixed with IV additives or other chemotherapeutic agents; give separately. Carboplatin (Paraplatin), cisplatin, cytarabine (ARA-C), daunorubicin, diazepam (Valium), doxorubicin (Adriamycin), droperidol (Inapsine), filgrastim (Neupogen), gallium nitrate (Ganite), methotrexate (Folex), ondansetron (Zofran), vinorelbine tartrate.

COMPATIBLE WITH

May be compatible leucovorin with magnesium sulfate, methotrexate, potassium chloride, vincristine (Oncovin). Consult pharmacist.

RATE OF ADMINISTRATION

Direct IV: A single dose over 1 to 3 minutes.

Infusion: A single dose is usually administered over 24 hours. Toxicity may be lessened by extended administration.

ACTIONS

An antimetabolite. A fluorinated pyrimidine antagonist, cell cycle specific, that interferes with the synthesis of DNA and RNA. Through various chemical processes this deprivation acts more quickly on rapidly growing cells and causes their death. Distributes into tumors, intestinal mucosa, bone marrow, liver, and readily crosses the blood-brain barrier into cerebrospinal fluid and brain tissue. Metabolized by the liver within 3 hours. Excretion is through the urine and as respiratory Co_2.

INDICATIONS AND USES

To suppress or retard neoplastic growth. Response has been experienced in carcinoma of the colon, rectum, breast, ovary, head and neck, urinary bladder, stomach, and pancreas, either alone or in combination with other drugs.

CONTRAINDICATIONS

Potentially serious infections, depressed bone marrow function, poor nutritional state, hypersensitivity, major surgery within the previous month.

PRECAUTIONS

Follow guidelines for handling cytotoxic agents. See Appendix A, p. 893. ■ Administered by or under the direction of the physician specialist. First dose should be given in a hospital. ■ Use caution in patients who have had high-dose pelvic irradiation, previous alkylating agents (e.g., cisplatin), other antimetabolic drugs (e.g., methotrexate), metastatic tumor involvement of the bone marrow, impaired hepatic or renal function, or dihydropyrimidine dehydrogenase deficiency.

Monitor: Confirm patency of vein. Avoid extravasation. Change peripheral injection site every 48 hours. ■ Obtain a complete blood cell count with differential and platelet count before each dose. When given with leucovorin, repeat weekly the first two courses and then at the time of anticipated WBC nadir in following courses. Electrolytes and liver function test should be done prior to the first three courses, then every other course. ■ Be alert for signs of bone marrow depression or infection. Prophylactic antibiotics may be indicated pending results of C/S in a febrile neutropenic patient. ■ Examine mouth and lips daily for sores or other signs of stomatitis. ■ Prophylactic antiemetics may reduce nausea and vomiting and increase patient comfort. ■ Toxicity increased by any form of therapy that adds to stress, poor nutrition, and bone marrow depression. ■ Note Drug/lab interactions.

Patient education: Nonhormonal birth control recommended. ■ See Appendix D, p. 900. ■ Report IV site burning and stinging promptly. ■ Drink at least 2 liters of fluid each day.

Maternal/child: Pregnancy category D: Avoid pregnancy; can cause fetal harm. ■ Safety for use in children not established.

Elderly: Toxicity may be increased. At greater risk for GI toxicity and severe diarrhea, especially in combination with leucovorin. ■ Note Dose adjustments.

DRUG/LAB INTERACTIONS

Potentiates anticoagulants. ■ Do not administer live vaccines to patients receiving antineoplastic drugs. ■ Cimetidine (Tagamet), interferon alfa, and leucovorin may increase toxicity. ■ Allopurinol may decrease effectiveness. ■ Methotrexate 1 hour before fluorouracil increases fluorouracil toxicity less than methotrexate 24 hours before. ■ Metabolism inhibited and toxicity significantly increased by halogenated antiviral drugs (e.g., sorivudine [Bravanir], netivudine). ■ May increase alkaline phosphatase, AST (SGOT), serum bilirubin, and lactic dehydrogenase (LDH).

SIDE EFFECTS

Abnormal Bromsulphalein (BSP), prothrombin, total protein, sed rate; alopecia (reversible), anaphylaxis, anemia, bleeding, bone marrow depression (agranulocytosis, leukopenia, pancytopenia, thrombocytopenia), cerebellar syndrome, cramps, dermatitis, diarrhea, disorientation, dry lips, erythema, esophagopharyngitis and stomatitis (may lead to sloughing and ulceration), euphoria, frequent stools, GI ulceration and bleeding, headache, hemorrhage from any site, increased skin pigmentation, lacrimal duct stenosis, mouth soreness and ulceration, nail changes, nausea, photophobia, photosensitivity, thrombophlebitis, visual changes, vomiting (intractable). Diarrhea and stomatitis are most common and may be more severe with a prolonged duration in patients on combination therapy.

ANTIDOTE

Keep physician informed of any side effects. Discontinue the drug and notify physician promptly at the first sign of toxicity (e.g., bleeding, diarrhea, esophagopharyngitis, gastritis, intractable vomiting, rapidly falling white count, sores in or around the lips or mouth, stomatitis). Discontinue the drug if the white blood cell count is less than 3,500/mm^3 or platelets are less than 100,000/mm^3; should reach 4,000/mm^3 and 130,000/mm^3 respectively in 2 weeks; if they do not, discontinue treatment. Oprelvekin (Numega) has been used to treat thrombocytopenia. In either situation, continue to monitor for 4 weeks. Death may occur from the progression of many side effects. There is no specific antidote; supportive therapy as indicated will help sustain the patient in toxicity.

FOLIC ACID

Nutritional supplement
(vitamin)
Antianemic

Folvite

pH 8.0 to 11.0

USUAL DOSE

Therapeutic dose: 0.25 to 1 mg daily. Larger doses may be required.

Maintenance dose: 0.4 mg daily, 0.8 mg daily in *pregnant or lactating females.*

PEDIATRIC DOSE

Therapeutic dose: 0.25 to 1 mg daily.

Maintenance dose: Infants: 0.1 mg daily. *Under 4 years:* up to 0.3 mg daily. *Over 4 years:* same as adult.

DOSE ADJUSTMENTS

Increased initial and maintenance doses may be required in alcoholism, hemolytic, anemia, anticonvulsant therapy, or chronic infection.

DILUTION

Each dose (up to 5 mg) should be diluted in at least 50 ml of SW, D5W, NS. May be added to most IV solutions and given as an infusion.

Storage: Protect from light and freezing.

INCOMPATIBLE WITH

Calcium salts, chlorpromazine (Thorazine), dextrose in 40% or greater concentrations, doxapram (Dopram), heavy metal ions, iron sulfate, oxidizing agents, reducing agents.

RATE OF ADMINISTRATION

5 mg or fraction thereof over 1 minute in undiluted form.

ACTIONS

Folic acid (pteroylglutamic acid) is part of the vitamin B complex. In humans, exogenous folate is required for nucleoprotein synthesis and the maintenance of normal erythropoiesis. It is the precursor of tetrahydrofolic acid, an important cofactor involved in the synthesis of amino acids and DNA. Stimulates the production of red blood cells, white blood cells, and platelets. Metabolized in the liver and excreted in the urine. Crosses the placental barrier. Secreted in breast milk.

INDICATIONS AND USES

For prevention and treatment of folic acid deficiency. Megaloblastic anemias resulting from folic acid deficiency may be seen in sprue, anemias of malnutrition, pregnancy, infancy, and childhood, developmental or surgical anomalies of the GI tract, as well as other conditions.

CONTRAINDICATIONS

Pernicious anemia unless used in combination with diagnostic testing.

PRECAUTIONS

Folic acid is not commonly administered by the IV route. Oral or IM administration provides adequate absorption in most cases.
■ Obscures the peripheral blood picture and prevents the diagnosis of pernicious anemia. May actually aggravate the neurologic symptoms.

Monitor: Obtain CBC before and during therapy.

Maternal/child: Pregnancy category A: An important vitamin before and during pregnancy. Folate-deficient mothers have a higher incidence of fetal anomalies and complications of pregnancy. ■ Safe for use during lactation; infant may require supplementation if mother is folate deficient. ■ Some products contain benzyl alcohol as a preservative. Avoid use in neonates.

Elderly: More likely to have folate deficiency.

DRUG/LAB INTERACTIONS

Toxic effects of antineoplastic folic acid antagonists are blocked by folinic acid (leucovorin) but not by folic acid IV. ■ Increases hydantoin metabolism (e.g., phenytoin [Dilantin]), seizures may result. ■ Inhibited by dihydrofolate reductase inhibitors (e.g., methotrexate, trimethoprim), pyrimethamine, and triamterene and by depressed hematopoiesis, alcoholism, and deficiencies of vitamins B_6, B_{12}, C, and E. ■ Aminosalicylic acid (Pamisyl) or sulfasalazine (Azulfidine) may decrease serum folate levels. ■ Oral contraceptives may inhibit folate metabolism.

SIDE EFFECTS

Almost nonexistent. Some slight flushing or feeling of warmth; anaphylaxis can occur.

ANTIDOTE

If anaphylaxis occurs, discontinue drug, treat anaphylaxis, and notify physician. Resuscitate as necessary.

FOMEPIZOLE INJECTION

Antidote

Antizol

USUAL DOSE

Ethylene glycol is the main component of antifreeze and coolants. Begin fomepizole treatment immediately upon suspicion of ethylene glycol ingestion based on patient history and/or anion gap metabolic acidosis, increased osmolar gap, oxalate crystals in the urine, or a documented serum ethylene glycol level greater than 20 mg/dL.

Adults with blood levels over 20 mg/dL but less than 50 mg/dL: Administer a loading dose of 15 mg/kg as a slow intravenous infusion. Follow with 10 mg/kg every 12 hours times 4 doses, then 15 mg/kg every 12 hours until ethylene glycol levels have been reduced below 20 mg/dL.

Adults with blood levels over 50 mg/dL, renal failure, or significant or worsening metabolic acidosis: In addition to dosing as above, dialysis should be considered to correct metabolic abnormalities and to lower the ethylene glycol levels below 50 mg/dL.

Dosage with Renal Dialysis: Amount of loading dose and following doses (mg/kg) remains the same, but fomepizole is dialyzable and the frequency of dosing should be increased to every 4 hours during hemodialysis. Base frequency on the following chart:

DOSE AT THE BEGINNING OF HEMODIALYSIS	
If <6 hours since last fomepizole dose	If ≥6 hours since last fomepizole dose
Do not administer dose	Administer next scheduled dose
DOSING DURING HEMODIALYSIS	
Dose every 4 hours	
DOSING AT THE TIME HEMODIALYSIS IS COMPLETED	
Time between last dose and the end of the hemodialysis	
< 1 hour	Do not administer dose at the end of hemodialysis
1-3 hours	Administer ½ of next scheduled dose
>3 hours	Administer next scheduled dose
MAINTENANCE DOSING OFF HEMODIALYSIS	
Give next scheduled dose 12 hours from last dose administered	

PEDIATRIC DOSE

Safety and effectiveness for use in pediatric patients has not been established.

DOSE ADJUSTMENTS

Fomepizole has not been studied sufficiently to determine whether the pharmacokinetics differ for the elderly (note Precautions/elderly), children, between genders, in renal insufficiency (excreted renally), or in hepatic insufficiency (metabolized by the liver).

DILUTION

Fomepizole solidifies at temperatures less than 25° C (77° F). If it is solidified, liquefy by running the vial under warm water or by holding in the hand. Solidification does not affect the efficacy, safety, or stability. Withdraw the appropriate dose. Each single dose must be diluted in at least 100 ml of NS or D5W and given as an infusion. Mix well.

Storage: Store vials at CRT 20° to 25° C (68° to 77° F). Diluted solutions are stable refrigerated or at CRT for 24 hours. Must be used within 24 hours of dilution.

INCOMPATIBLE WITH

Specific information not available. Consider specific use and short duration of infusion.

RATE OF ADMINISTRATION

Each single dose must be given as a slow intravenous infusion equally distributed over 30 minutes. *Do not given undiluted or by bolus injection;* has caused serious venous irritation and phlebosclerosis.

ACTIONS

A synthetic alcohol dehydrogenase inhibitor. Effectively blocks formation of toxic ethylene glycol metabolites, which are responsible for metabolic acidosis and renal damage. Has shown minimal CNS depressant effects. Plasma half-life varies with dose and has not been calculated. Rapidly distributes to total body water. Metabolized in the liver by the P_{450} mixed-function oxidase system. Significant increases in the elimination rate occur after 30 to 40 hours. Excreted in urine.

INDICATIONS AND USES

An antidote for ethylene glycol (antifreeze) poisoning, or for use in suspected ethylene glycol ingestion.

CONTRAINDICATIONS

Known serious hypersensitivity to fomepizole or other pyrazoles (e.g., sulfinpyrazone [Anturane]).

PRECAUTIONS

Acute ethylene glycol poisoning is a medical emergency that is characterized by a syndrome that can include CNS depression, severe metabolic acidosis, renal failure, and coma. Can be lethal if left untreated or when treatment is delayed due to delayed diagnosis. The lethal dose of ethylene glycol is approximately 1.4 ml/kg. ▪ If ethylene glycol poisoning is left untreated, the natural progression of the poisoning leads to accumulation of toxic metabolites, including glycolic and oxalic acids. These metabolites can induce metabolic acidosis, nausea and vomiting, seizures, stupor, coma, calcium oxaluria, acute tubular necrosis, and death. The diagnosis of these poisonings may be difficult because ethylene glycol levels diminish in the blood as it is metabolized to glycolate. Both the ethylene glycol levels and the acid-base balance, as determined by serum electrolyte (anion gap) and/or arterial blood gas analysis, should be frequently monitored and used to guide treatment. ■ Has caused minor allergic reactions (mild rash, eosinophilia).

Monitor: Patients must be managed for metabolic acidosis, acute renal failure, adult respiratory distress syndrome, and hypocalcemia. Fluid therapy and sodium bicarbonate administration may be required as supportive therapies. Potassium and calcium supplementation and oxygen administration are usually necessary. ■ Hemodialysis is necessary in the anuric patient or in patients with severe metabolic acidosis or azotemia. ■ ECG should be continuous to monitor for cardiac irregularities. ■ EEG may be required in the comatose patient. ■ The effective inhibition of alcohol dehydrogenase requires fomepizole plasma concentrations in the range of 100 to 300 micromol/L (8.6 to 24.6 mg/L). ■ To assess treatment success, obtain baseline and frequently monitor measurements of blood gases, pH, electrolytes, BUN, creatinine, and urinalysis in addition to other laboratory tests as indicated by each patient's condition. ■ To assess the status of ethylene glycol and metabolite clearance, obtain baseline ethylene glycol plasma and urine concentrations and presence of urinary oxalate crystals and monitor frequently. ■ Obtain baseline and monitor hepatic enzymes and WBC counts during treatment; transient increases in serum transaminase levels and eosinophilia have been noted with repeated fomepizole dosing. ■ Monitor for signs of allergic reactions; see Precautions.

Patient education: Monitoring of urine output imperative. ■ Cooperation with adequate hydration and frequent laboratory analysis required. ■ Request assistance with ambulation.

Maternal/child: Category C: Use during pregnancy only if clearly needed. ■ Use caution during lactation; not known if fomepizole is secreted in breast milk. ■ Safety and effectiveness for use in children not established.

Elderly: Risk of toxic reactions may be greater in patients with impaired renal function. Dose adjustment may be indicated.

DRUG/LAB INTERACTIONS

Has not been studied, but reciprocal interactions (increasing or decreasing clearance, effects, or toxicity) may occur with concomitant use of drugs that induce or inhibit the cytochrome P_{450} system (e.g., carbamazepine [Tegretol], cimetidine [Tagamet], ketoconazole [Nizoral], phenytoin [Dilantin]. Oral fomepizole significantly reduced the rate of elimination of ethanol (by 40%) in healthy subjects. Ethanol decreased the rate of elimination of fomepizole (by 50%).

SIDE EFFECTS

Most common side effects are dizziness, headache, and nausea. Abdominal pain, abnormal smell, allergic reactions (e.g., mild rash, eosinophilia), anemia, anorexia, arrhythmias (bradycardia, tachycardia), back pain (lower), blurred vision, decreased awareness of surroundings, diarrhea, feeling of drunkenness, fever, hangover, heartburn, hiccups, hypotension, injection site reaction, lightheadedness, lymphangitis, nystagmus, pharyngitis, phlebosclerosis, siezure, slurred speech, somnolence, taste changes (bad or metallic), vertigo, visual problems, vomiting occurred in up to 6% of patients.

Overdose: Dizziness, nausea, and vertigo occurred in healthy volunteers given 3 to 6 times the recommended dose.

ANTIDOTE

Keep physician informed of all side effects, laboratory results, and concurrent medical problems. Dialysis may be indicated for changes in patient condition (e.g., renal failure, significant or worsening metabolic acidosis, or a measured ethylene glycol level of greater than 50 mg/dL) or in the treatment of overdose. Treat side effects symptomatically as indicated. Resuscitate as necessary.

FOSCARNET SODIUM

Foscavir

Antiviral

pH 7.4

USUAL DOSE

CMV Retinitis: 90 mg/kg every 12 hours or 60 mg/kg every 8 hours for 14 to 21 days. Length of induction treatment based on clinical response. Begin a maintenance dose of 90 mg/kg/day the next day (day 15 to 22). If retinitis progresses during the maintenance regimen, re-treat with the induction and maintenance regimens. Maintenance dose may be increased to 120 mg/kg/day in patients who show excellent tolerance to foscarnet or those who require early reinduction because of retinitis progression. Normal renal function required. Adequate hydration and specific testing required (See Precautions/Monitor)

CMV retinitis combination therapy (foscarnet and ganciclovir) for patients who have relapsed after monotherapy with either drug: In patients who have received foscarnet induction with 90 mg/kg every 12 hours followed by 120 mg/kg/day maintenance, continue their present therapy (e.g., foscarnet 120 mg/kg/day) and begin ganciclovir induction with 5 mg/kg every 12 hours for 14 to 21 days followed immediately by maintenance doses of foscarnet 90 mg/kg/day and ganciclovir 5 mg/kg/day (see ganciclovir monograph). Monitor renal function very closely with this combination regimen.

Acyclovir-resistant HSV patients: 40 mg/kg every 8 or 12 hours for 2 to 3 weeks or until healed.

DOSE ADJUSTMENTS

Must be reduced and individualized according to patient's renal function. May be required during treatment even if patient had normal renal function initially. Specific calculation and testing required (see literature).

DILUTION

Central venous catheter: Standard 24-mg/ml solution may be given undiluted.

Peripheral vein: Each 1 ml of a calculated dose must be diluted with 1 ml of D5W or NS (yields a 12-mg/ml solution). To avoid any possibility of overdose in either situation, only the calculated dose should be in the infusion bottle. Discard any excess before administration.

INCOMPATIBLE WITH

Manufacturer states "no other drug or supplement should be administered concurrently via the same catheter." Because of chelating properties, a precipitate can occur. Acyclovir (Zovirax), amphotericin B (Fungizone), diazepam (Valium), diphenhydramine (Benadryl), digoxin (Lanoxin), dobutamine (Dobutrex), droperidol (Inapsine), *ganciclovir (Cytovene),* haloperidol (Haldol), leucovorin (folinic acid), lorazepam (Ativan), midazolam (Versed), pentamidine (Pentam 300), phenytoin (Dilantin), prochlorperazine (Compazine), promethazine (Phenergan), trimethoprim/sulfamethoxazole (Bactrim), trimetrexate glucuronate, vancomycin (Vancocin).

RATE OF ADMINISTRATION

Infusion pump required to deliver accurate dose evenly distributed over specific time frame. Excessive plasma levels and toxicity (including hypocalcemia) will occur with too-rapid rate of infusion. Advisable to clear tubing with normal saline if possible before and after administration through Y-tube or three-way stopcock. Never exceed 1 mg/kg/min.

CMV Retinitis: Induction doses: Each 60-mg dose equally distributed over a minimum of 1 hour. Increase to 1½ to 2 hours for 90-mg dose.

Maintenance dose: Each dose equally distributed over a minimum of 2 hours.

Acyclovir-resistant HSV: Each dose equally distributed over a minimum of 1 hour.

ACTIONS

An antiviral agent capable of inhibiting replication of all known herpesviruses, including cytomegalovirus (CMV), herpes simplex virus types 1 and 2 (HSV-1, HSV-2), human herpesvirus 6 (HHV-6), Epstein-Barr (EBV), and varicella-zoster virus (VZV). Does not destroy existing viruses but stops them from reproducing and invading healthy cells. Also capable of chelating metal ions (e.g., calcium, magnesium). CMV strains resistant to ganciclovir may be sensitive to foscarnet. Half-life averages 3 hours and increases markedly with renal impairment. Some penetration into bone and cerebrospinal fluid. Probably secreted in breast milk. Excreted unchanged in urine.

INDICATIONS AND USES

Treatment of CMV retinitis in patients with AIDS. Most frequently used in patients who do not tolerate or are resistant to ganciclovir. ■ Combination therapy (foscarnet and ganciclovir) may be indicated with progressive retinitis refractory to single therapy. ■ Treatment of acyclovir-resistant mucocutaneous HSV infections in immunocompromised patients.

CONTRAINDICATIONS

Hypersensitivity to foscarnet.

PRECAUTIONS

For IV use only. ■ May cause potentially life-threatening changes in renal function with cumulative exposure. Careful monitoring of renal function and dose adjustment is imperative. Changes can occur at any time, most likely during second week of therapy. ■ Confirm diagnosis of CMV retinitis by indirect ophthalmoscopy. Diagnosis may be supported by cultures of CMV from urine, blood, throat, etc.; negative culture does not rule out CMV retinitis. ▪ Use caution in patients with a history of impaired renal function, altered calcium or other electrolyte levels, neurologic or cardiac abnormalities, a low baseline absolute neutrophil count (ANC), and those receiving other drugs known to influence minerals and electrolytes (See Drug/lab interactions) . Has caused hyperphosphatemia, hypocalcemia, hypokalemia, hypomagnesemia, and hypophosphatemia, resulting in cardiac disturbances, seizures, and tetany. ▪ Foscarnet was superior to vidarabine (ARA-A) for treatment of acyclovir-resistant HSV. ▪ Resistance has been reported to develop. May be higher in patients treated for a prolonged period. ▪ Sensitivity testing for viral isolate is recommended before repeat treatment and/or to evaluate sensitivity versus development of resistance. ▪ Cidofovir is a newly approved agent for treatment of CMV retinitis.

Monitor: Baseline 24-hour creatinine clearance verified by creatinine index; baseline serum creatinine, calcium, magnesium, potassium, phosphorus, and electrolytes required before treatment begins. Correct any deficiencies. ▪ Repeat entire testing process 2 to 3 times a week during induction therapy and a minimum of every 2 weeks during maintenance therapy. Foscarnet dose must be adjusted as indicated by test results. More frequent testing may be indicated in specific patients. ▪ To minimize renal toxicity, hydration adequate to establish diuresis is recommended before and during treatment unless contraindicated. Give 750 to 1,000 ml NS or D5W before the first foscarnet infusion to establish diuresis. With subsequent infusions, give 750 to 1,000 ml concurrently with 90 to 120 mg/kg foscarnet and a minimum of 500 ml concurrently with 40 to 60 mg/kg. ▪ Discontinue foscarnet if creatinine clearance drops below 0.4 ml/min/kg or serum creatinine is greater than 2.8 mg/100 ml (1 dL). Monitor patient daily until resolution of renal impairment is ensured. Safety for use in these patients has not been studied. ▪ Anemia may be severe enough to require transfusion. ▪ Phlebitis or pain may occur at site of infusion; confirm patency of vein and use large veins to ensure adequate blood flow for rapid dilution and distribution. ▪ Note Drug/lab interactions.

Patient education: Not a cure. Retinitis may recur during maintenance or after treatment; regular ophthalmologic exams imperative. ▪ Complete healing of HSV infections may occur, but most relapse. ▪ Perioral tingling, numbness in the extremities or paresthesias indicate electrolyte abnormalities; report immediately. ▪ Adequate hydration and increased personal hygiene may minimize some side effects. ▪ Dose modification or discontinuation may be required for major side effects.

Maternal/child: Pregnancy category C: Use only if clearly needed; has caused skeletal anomalies in animals. ▪ Excreted at three times maternal blood concentrations in lactating rats; human data not available. ▪ Safety for use in children not established; deposited in teeth and bones, and deposition greater in young animals. Use only if benefits outweigh risks.

Elderly: Safety not established; assessment of renal function even more imperative because of potential for reduced glomerular filtration.

DRUG/LAB INTERACTIONS

Because of physical incompatibilities, foscarnet sodium and ganciclovir sodium must never be mixed. ▪ Coadministration with any other drugs could theoretically alter its antiviral activity, toxicity, or pharmacokinetics. ▪ Has caused hypocalcemia with parenteral pentamidine. ▪ Capable of causing calcium or electrolyte disorders. Use caution when administering any drug known to influence minerals or electrolytes (e.g., hypocalcemic agents [gallium nitrate (Ganite)], diuretics [furosemide (Lasix), mannitol], adrenocortical steroids). ▪ Elimination of foscarnet may be impaired and toxicity increased by drugs that inhibit renal tubular secretion (e.g., probenecid). ▪ Avoid concomitant use with other nephrotoxic drugs (e.g., aminoglycosides [e.g., gentamicin (Garamycin)], amphotericin B [Fungizone], cyclosporine [Sandimmune], pentamidine) unless benefits outweigh risks. ▪ Anemia may be additive with zidovudine (AZT). ▪ Use with ciprofloxacin (Cipro IV) may cause seizures; monitor patient carefully.

SIDE EFFECTS

Impaired renal function, alterations in plasma minerals and electrolytes, and seizures are major side effects and are dose limiting. Abnormal renal function including acute renal failure, decreased creatinine clearance and increased serum creatinine (27%); anemia (33%); bone marrow suppression (10%); diarrhea (30%); fever (65%); headache (26%); hyperphosphatemia; hypocalcemia (perioral tingling, numbness in extremities, paresthesias, tetany); hypokalemia; hypomagnesemia; hypophosphatemia; irritation at injection site; irritation and ulcerations of penile and vaginal epithelium; nausea (47%); seizure (10%); vomiting (26%); and death (14%) have occurred. All deaths could not be directly related to foscarnet. Abdominal pain, anorexia, anxiety, asthenia, confusion, coughing, depression, dizziness, dyspnea, hypoesthesia, granulocytopenia, infection, involuntary muscle contractions, leukopenia, malaise, neuropathy, pain, rash, sweating, and vision abnormalities have occurred in 5% of patients. Numerous other side effects have occurred in less than 5% of patients.

ANTIDOTE

There is no specific antidote. Keep physician informed. Adequate hydration and careful monitoring will help reduce potential for renal impairment and may minimize other side effects. Elevations in serum creatinine are usually reversible (within 1 week) with dose adjustment or discontinuation but have caused death. Discontinue foscarnet if creatinine clearance falls below 0.4 ml/min/kg or serum creatinine greater than 2.8 mg/100 ml. Monitor daily until resolution of renal impairment is ensured. Discontinue foscarnet if perioral tingling, numbness in the extremities, or paresthesias occur during or after infusion; evaluate calcium and electrolyte levels (decrease in ionized serum calcium may not be reflected in total serum calcium); notify physician. Administration of foscarnet can be resumed following seizures or cardiac disturbances after treatment of underlying disease, electrolyte disturbance, or after dose adjustment. Overdose can occur with too-rapid rate of infusion. Hemodialysis and hydration are useful in overdose. Treat anaphylaxis and resuscitate as indicated.

FOSPHENYTOIN SODIUM

Anticonvulsant
(Hydantoin)

Cerebyx

pH 8.6 to 9.0

USUAL DOSE

In all situations, dose of fosphenytoin is expressed as phenytoin sodium equivalents (PE).

Status epilepticus: Adult loading dose: 15 to 20 mg PE/kg. Full effect is not immediate; concomitant administration of an IV benzodiazepine (e.g., diazepam [Valium]) is usually necessary to control status epilepticus. If seizures are not controlled, consider other anticonvulsants and other measures as needed (e.g., barbiturates or anesthesia). *Maintenance dose:* 4 to 6 mg PE/kg/24 hr. *Elderly loading dose:* 14 mg PE/kg. Note all comments under adult dose. Note Rate of administration.

Nonemergent indications: Loading dose: 10 to 20 mg PE/kg. *Maintenance dose:* 4 to 6 mg PE/kg/24 hr.

Substitute for oral phenytoin: May be substituted at the same total daily dose (due to a 10% increase in bioavailability [IV/IM to oral], plasma levels with the IV/IM product may be increased slightly).

PEDIATRIC DOSE

Status epilepticus: 15 to 20 mg PE/kg at a rate of up to 3 mg PE/kg/min. Safety for use in children not established. Limited data available; no significant differences apparent to this date.

DOSE ADJUSTMENTS

Reduced doses may be required in the elderly (see Usual dose), in impaired renal or hepatic function, or in patients with hypoalbuminemia. ■ Note Precautions, Monitor, Drug/lab interactions, and Antidote.

DILUTION

Use only clear solutions. Should be diluted in D5W or NS to a concentration of 1.5 to 25 mg PE/ml. Supplied solution is 75 mg PE/ml. Dilute each milliliter of fosphenytoin with 2 ml of diluent to equal 25 mg PE/ml. Dilute a 1,500-mg dose in 100 ml diluent to equal 15 mg PE/ml and in 1,000 ml diluent to equal 1.5 mg PE/ml.

Storage: Keep refrigerated; do not store at room temperature for more than 48 hours. After dilution, solutions are stable at room temperature for 8 hours and for 24 hours if refrigerated.

INCOMPATIBLE WITH

Specific information not available.

RATE OF ADMINISTRATION

Each 100 to 150 mg PE or fraction thereof over a minimum of 1 minute. Risk of hypotension increased if this rate is exceeded. Slow or temporarily stop rate of infusion for burning, itching, numbness, or pain along injection site.

Elderly rate: Do not exceed 37.5 mg PE/min (equivalent to 25 mg/min of phenytoin). A rate of 7.5 mg PE/min to 12.5 mg PE/min is preferred (equivalent to 5 to 10 mg/min of phenytoin). Risk of toxic serum concentrations is increased because metabolism of hydantoins is slow and serum albumin may be low (see Precautions).

Pediatric rate: 0.5 to 3 mg PE/kg/min has been suggested for neonates and pediatric patients (equivalent to 0.33 to 2 mg/kg/min of phenytoin). Another source suggests a rate of 1.6 mg PE/kg/min (1 mg/kg/min phenytoin). Do not exceed a rate of 37.5 mg PE/min (25 mg/min phenytoin).

ACTIONS

A water-soluble prodrug of phenytoin. Converts to phenytoin, phosphate, and formate within 15 minutes of IV/IM administration. An anticonvulsant, chemically related to barbiturates. Selectively stabilizes seizure threshold and depresses seizure activity in the motor cortex. Also exerts a depressant effect on the myocardium by selectively elevating the excitability threshold of the cell, reducing the cell's response to stimuli. Peak levels of fosphenytoin are achieved by the end of an infusion, but conversion to therapeutic serum levels of phenytoin takes longer. Extensively bound to protein, fosphenytoin displaces phenytoin from protein binding sites and increases free phenytoin (dose and rate dependent). Phenytoin is metabolized in the liver by hepatic cytochrome P^{450} enzymes and excreted in urine. Crosses the placental barrier. Secreted in breast milk. Advantages of fosphenytoin over present phenytoin products include solubility in IV solutions, improved infusion site tolerance, more rapid rate of injection, and well-tolerated IM option.

INDICATIONS AND USES

Treatment and control of generalized convulsive status epilepticus. ▪ Treatment or prophylaxis of seizures in neurosurgical patients. ▪ Substitute for oral phenytoin when oral administration is not feasible or prompt increases in antiepileptic drug levels are needed.

CONTRAINDICATIONS

Hypersensitivity to fosphenytoin, any of its components, phenytoin, or other hydantoins. ▪ Sinus bradycardia, sinoatrial block, second- and third-degree AV block, and Adams-Stokes syndrome.

PRECAUTIONS

Doses of fosphenytoin are expressed as phenytoin equivalents; no adjustment required when substituting fosphenytoin or vice versa. ▪ IV route indicated in emergency situations (e.g., status epilepticus). May be given IM in nonemergency situations. ▪ Intended for short-term parenteral use (up to 5 days). ▪ Transfer to oral phenytoin therapy as soon as feasible. ▪ Abrupt withdrawal may cause increased seizure activity. Gradually reduce dose, discontinue, or substitute alternative antiepileptic agents. ▪ Discontinue immediately for hypersensitivity reactions; with caution substitute a nonhydantoin anticonvulsant (e.g., phenobarbital [Luminal], valproate sodium [Depacon]). ▪ May cause severe cardiovascular depression (e.g., bradycardia, various degrees of AV block, ventricular fibrillation (VF); use extreme caution in elderly or seriously ill patients. ▪ Use with caution in patients with hypotension or severe myocardial insufficiency. ▪ May exacerbate porphyria. ▪ May cause acute phenytoin hepatotoxicity (e.g., elevated liver function tests, fever, jaundice, lymphadenopathy, skin eruptions). Discontinue immediately and substitute alternate anticonvulsant therapy. ▪ Has caused lymphadenopathy and hemopoietic complications (e.g., agranulocytosis, granulocytopenia, leukopenia, thrombocytopenia, or pancytopenia with or without bone marrow suppression). If lymphadenopathy occurs with or without signs of serum sickness (e.g., fever, rash, hepatotoxicity), substitute alternate anticonvulsant therapy. ■ Use caution with low serum albumin levels, and adjust dose as indicated. Phenytoin is highly bound to serum protein, and a reduced albumin causes an increase in free drug availability and may increase toxicity. ■ Not effective for petit mal seizures; combined therapy required if both conditions present. ■ Inhibits insulin release and may increase serum glucose; monitoring indicated in diabetics. ■ May lower serum folate levels.

Monitor: Monitor ECG, BP, and respirations continuously during loading dose and for at least 30 minutes after infusion complete. ■ Allow fosphenytoin time to convert to phenytoin; accurate serum levels are not available until 2 hours after the end of an IV infusion or 4 hours after IM injection. Narrow margin of error between therapeutic and toxic dose. Plasma levels above 10 mcg/ml usually control seizure activity. The acceptable range is 5 to 20 mcg/ml. Toxicity begins with nystagmus at levels exceeding 20 mcg/ml. ■ Observe for rash and discontinue if one appears. If rash is mild, fosphenytoin may be resumed when the rash has completely disappeared. If the mild rash occurs again or the initial rash is serious in nature (e.g., exfoliative, purpuric, bullous) or lupus erythematous, Stevens-Johnson syndrome, or toxic epidermal necrolysis is suspected, discontinue fosphenytoin. Do not resume; consider alternative therapy. ■ Contains phosphates; monitor in patients who require phosphate restriction (e.g., renal impairment). ■ Monitor closely patients who are gravely ill, have impaired liver function, or are elderly. May show early signs of toxicity. ■ Determine absolute patency of vein; avoid extravasation. Not as alkaline as phenytoin.

Patient education: Report burning, itching, numbness, pain, or rash. ■ Consider birth control options; nonhormonal birth control recommended.

Maternal/child: Pregnancy category D: Avoid pregnancy. Risk of serious congenital malformations triple that of the general population. ■ An increase in seizure frequency may occur during pregnancy; monitoring of plasma phenytoin levels may be helpful. ■ Newborns whose mothers received phenytoin during pregnancy may develop a life-threatening bleeding disorder that can be prevented by giving vitamin K to the mother before delivery and to the neonate after birth. ■ Discontinue breast feeding.

Elderly: Note Dose adjustments and Rate of administration. ■ Sensitivity and/or toxicity may be increased because serum concentrations may be elevated due to reduced clearance, or low serum albumin may cause a decrease in protein binding and an increase in free phenytoin.

DRUG/LAB INTERACTIONS

No drugs are known to interfere with the conversion of fosphenytoin to phenytoin, although phosphatase activity may have an impact. ■ Capable of innumerable catastrophic drug interactions; review of drug profile by pharmacist imperative. In all situations, monitoring of phenytoin serum levels may be indicated. ■ Serum levels and toxicity of phenytoin may be increased by alcohol (acute intake), amiodarone (Cordarone), anticonvulsants (e.g., succinimides [ethosuximide (Zarontin)]), antidepressants (e.g., fluoxetine [Prozac], trazodone [Deseryl]), antifungal agents (e.g., fluconazole, miconazole, ketoconazole), chloramphenicol, chlordiazepoxide (Librium) H_2 antagonists (e.g., cimetidine [Tagamet]), diazepam (Valium), dicumarol, disulfiram (Antabuse), estrogens, halothane, isoniazid (Nydrazid), methylphenidate (Ritalin), phenothiazines (e.g., prochlorperazine [Compazine]), phenylbutazone (Butazolidin), salicylates (aspirin), sulfonamides (e.g., sulfisoxazole), tolbutamide (Orinase). ■ Serum levels and effectiveness of phenytoin may be decreased by carbamazepine (Tegretol), chronic alcohol abuse, doxorubicin (with cisplatin), leucovorin, and reserpine (Serpasil). ■ Serum levels of phenytoin may be increased or decreased by phenobarbital (Luminal), valproate sodium (Depacon), valproic acid (Depakene). ■ Tricyclic antidepressants (e.g., amitriptyline [Elavil]) may precipitate seizures in susceptible patients or phenytoin may increase metabolism of antidepressants. Dose adjustment may be indicated for either or both drugs. ■ Phenytoin will inhibit effects of anticoagulants (e.g., warfarin [Coumadin]), corticosteroids, cardiac glycosides (e.g., digoxin) doxycycline, estrogens, furosemide (Lasix), itraconazole (Sporanox), oral contraceptives, rifampin (Rifadin), quinidine, theophylline, vitamin D. ■ In one case report, a patient stabilized on phenytoin and valproic acid experienced seizures and a reduction in antiepileptic drug serum concentration when acyclovir was added to the regimen. ■ Alters some clinical laboratory tests (e.g., may decrease T_4 increase glucose, alkaline phosphatase, and GGT may produce low results in dexamethasone or metyrapone tests).

SIDE EFFECTS

Ataxia, dizziness, headache, nystagmus, and somnolence are most common signs of impending toxicity. Coma, hyperreflexia, hypotension, lethargy, nausea, slurred speech, tremor, and vomiting are also signs of increased toxicity. Paresthesia and pruritus are dose and rate related, occur within several minutes of the start of the infusion, and usually resolve within 10 minutes of completion. Fosphenytoin breaks down into formate and phosphate metabolites that may cause formate toxicity (hypocalcemia, metabolic acidosis, muscle spasms, paresthesia, and seizures).

Major: Bradycardia, cardiac arrest, heart block, hypotension, respiratory arrest, tonic seizures, ventricular fibrillation.

ANTIDOTE

Notify the physician of any side effects. Obtain serum plasma levels at first signs of toxicity; reduce dose. If symptoms persist or major side effects appear, discontinue fosphenytoin and notify the physician. Treat symptomatically, maintain a patent airway, and resuscitate as necessary. Symptoms of bradycardia or heart block may be reversed with IV atropine. Epinephrine may also be useful. One source says hemodialysis may be helpful in overdose. Another source says hemodialysis, peritoneal dialysis, forced fluid diuresis, exchange transfusions, and plasmapheresis are ineffective. In overdose, measure ionized free calcium levels to guide treatment in phosphate toxicity.

FUROSEMIDE

Diuretic (loop)
Antihypertensive
Antihypercalcemic

Lasix, ✹Uritol

pH 8.0 to 9.3

USUAL DOSE

Edema/congestive heart failure: 20 to 40 mg. May be repeated in 1 to 2 hours. If necessary, increase dosage by 20-mg increments (under close medical supervision and no sooner than 2 hours after previous dose) until desired diuresis is obtained. IV bolus dose should not exceed 1 Gm/day. If larger doses are required, give as an infusion. In severe refractory congestive heart failure, doses up to 4 Gm/24 hr have been given with extreme caution. After the initial diuresis the minimum effective dose may be given once or twice every 24 hours as required for maintenance.

Hypertension: Up to 40 mg twice daily. If this dose does not reduce hypertension, the addition of other antihypertensive agents is recommended instead of larger doses of furosemide.

Hypertensive crisis: 40 to 80 mg concomitantly with other antihypertensive agents.

Acute pulmonary edema or post-cardiac arrest cerebral edema: 40 mg. If no response in 1 hour, increase to 80 mg. An alternate regimen is 0.5 to 1.0 mg/kg (JAMA recommendation).

Acute or chronic renal failure: Initial dose required can range from 100 mg to 2 Gm. Higher doses are well tolerated in these patients. Increase dose as needed to achieve desired effect. IV bolus dose should not exceed 1 Gm/day. If larger doses are required, give as an infusion. Has been doubled at 2- to 24-hour intervals in some studies. One protocol calls for an infusion of 250 mg over 1 hour. If urine output insufficient in 1 hour, increase to 500 mg infused over 2 hours. If urine output still insufficient after the first hour, increase to 1 Gm over 4 hours. For high-dose infusions, individualize dose and titrate to maximum therapeutic effect from the lowest dose. Highest total IV dose was 6 Gm.

Hypercalcemia: 80 to 100 mg at 1- to 2-hour intervals. Given concomitantly with NS. Total IV dose required has ranged from 160 mg to 3.2 Gm.

PEDIATRIC DOSE

Acute pulmonary edema or edema associated with congestive heart failure or renal disease: 1 mg/kg of body weight. After 2 hours increase by 1-mg/kg increments to effect desired response. Effective dose may be given every 6 to 12 hours. Do not exceed 6 mg/kg.

DOSE ADJUSTMENTS

Higher doses may be required in renal insufficiency and acute or chronic renal failure. ■ Reduced dose or extended intervals may be appropriate in the elderly. ■ Note Drug/lab interactions.

DILUTION

May be given undiluted. May be given through Y-tube or three-way stopcock of infusion set. Not usually added to IV solutions, but large doses may be added to NS, LR, D5W, D5/NS and given as an infusion. pH of solution must be over 5.5. If obtaining large doses from ampules, use of a filter is recommended to eliminate possible pieces of glass.

Storage: If diluted for infusion, discard after 24 hours.

INCOMPATIBLE WITH

Acidic solutions, amiodarone (Cordarone), ascorbic acid, buprenorphine (Buprenex), chlorpromazine (Thorazine), ciprofloxacin (Cipro IV), corticosteroids, diazepam (Valium), diltiazem (Cardizem), diphenhydramine (Benadryl), dobutamine (Dobutrex), doxapram (Dopram), doxorubicin (Adriamycin), droperidol (Inapsine), esmolol (Brevibloc), epinephrine (Adrenalin), erythromycin (Erytrocin IV), filgrastim (Neupogen), fluconazole (Diflucan), labetalol (Normodyne), gentamicin (Garamycin), hydralazine (Apresoline), hydrocortisone sodium (Solucortef), idarubicin (Idamycin), isoproterenol (Isuprel), levarterenol (Levophed), meperidine (Demerol), metoclopromide (Reglan), midazolam (Versed), milrinone (Primacor), morphine, netilmicin (Netromycin), ondansetron (Zofran), opium alkaloids, prochlorperazine (Compazine), promethazine (Phenergan), quinidine, reserpine, spironolactone hydrochlorothiazide (Aldactazide), tetracyclines, vinblastine (Velban), vincristine (Oncovin), vinorelbine (Navelbine), any drug in a syringe.

RATE OF ADMINISTRATION

Direct IV: Each 40 mg or fraction thereof should be given over 1 to 2 minutes. A 1-Gm bolus must be given over at least 30 minutes, up to 3 hours is preferred. In oliguric or anuric patients the total dose (undiluted) should be infused at a rate of 4 mg/min. Constant rate infusion pump required.

Infusion: High-dose therapy in an infusion should not exceed a rate of 4 mg/min. A 1-Gm dose should take at least 3 hours to prevent ototoxicity.

ACTIONS

A sulfonamide-type diuretic, related to the thiazides. Extremely potent and has a rapid onset of action. Effectiveness is noted within 5 minutes and may last for 2 hours. Apparently acts on the proximal and distal ends of the tubule and the ascending limb of the loop of Henle to excrete water, sodium, chlorides, and potassium. Will produce diuresis in alkalosis or acidosis. Highly protein bound. Metabolized and excreted in the urine. Crosses the placental barrier. Secreted in breast milk.

INDICATIONS AND USES

Edema associated with congestive heart failure, cirrhosis of the liver with ascites, and renal disease including the nephrotic syndrome. ▪ Acute pulmonary edema. ▪ Edema unresponsive to other diuretic agents. ▪ Hypercalcemia. ▪ Hypertension. ▪ Post-cardiac arrest cerebral edema.

CONTRAINDICATIONS

Anuria, severe progressive renal disease with increasing azotemia and oliguria; rarely used in children, pregnancy, and lactation.

PRECAUTIONS

May be used concurrently with aldosterone antagonists (e.g., spironolactone [Aldactone]) for more effective diuresis and to prevent excessive potassium loss. ▪ Use caution and improve basic condition first in hepatic coma, electrolyte depletion, and advanced cirrhosis of the liver. ▪ May increase risk of gastric hemorrhage during corticosteroid therapy. ▪ Use extreme caution in known sulfonamide sensitivity. ▪ Risk of ototoxicity increases with higher doses, rapid injection, decreased renal function, or concurrent use with other ototoxic drugs (see Drug/lab interactions). ▪ May activate or exacerbate systemic lupus erythematosus.

Monitor: Discontinue at least 2 days before elective surgery. ▪ Monitor blood pressure frequently, especially during initial therapy. ▪ May precipitate excessive diuresis with water and electrolyte depletion. Routine checks on electrolyte panel, Co_2, and BUN are necessary during therapy. Potassium chloride replacement may be required. ▪ May increase blood glucose and has precipitated diabetes mellitus. ▪ May lower serum calcium level; may cause tetany. ▪ Rarely precipitates an acute attack of gout. ▪ Note Drug/lab interactions.

Patient education: Hypotension may cause dizziness; request assistance with ambulation. ▪ Report cramps, dizziness, muscle weakness, or nausea promptly. ▪ May cause a decrease in potassium levels and require a supplement. ▪ Skin may become photosensitive; avoid unprotected exposure to sun.

Maternal/child: Pregnancy category B: Safety for use in pregnancy not established. ▪ Discontinue breast feeding. ▪ Safety for use in children not established. ▪ Note Contraindications.

Elderly: Consider increased sensitivity to hypotensive and electrolyte effects. ▪ May be more susceptible to dehydration; observe carefully. ▪ Avoid rapid contraction of plasma volume and hemoconcentration. May cause thromboembolic episodes (e.g., CVA, pulmonary emboli).

DRUG/LAB INTERACTIONS

Causes excessive potassium depletion with corticosteroids, thiazide diuretics (e.g., hydrochlorothiazide [HydroDIURIL]), amphotericin B (Fungizone). ▪ Potentiates antihypertensive drugs (e.g., nitroglycerin, nitroprusside); reduced dose of the antihypertensive agent or both drugs may be indicated. ▪ May cause transient or permanent deafness with doses exceeding the usual or when given in conjunction with other ototoxic drugs (e.g., cisplatin, aminoglycosides [e.g., gentamicin]). ▪ May increase activity of anticoagulants; monitor PT. ▪ May increase serum levels of beta blockers (e.g., propranolol [Inderal]) and of lithium (may cause toxicity). ▪ May cause cardiac arrhythmias with digitalis (potassium depletion). ▪ Risk of cardiotoxicity increased with pimozide (Orap) and sparfloxacin (Zagam); concurrent use not recommended. ▪ May enhance or inhibit actions of non-depolarizing muscle relaxant (e.g., mivacurium [Mivacron]) or theophyllines. ▪ May cause hyperglycemia with sulfonylureas (e.g., tolbutamide) by decreasing glucose tolerance. ▪ Effects may be inhibited by ACE inhibitors (e.g., captopril [Capoten]), NSAIDs (e.g., ibuprofen [Motrin]), probenecid, or in patients with cirrhosis and ascites on salicylates. ▪ May cause profound diuresis and serious electrolyte abnormalities with thiazide diuretics (e.g., chlorothiazide [Diuril]) because of synergistic effects. ▪ Clofibrate (Atromid-S) may cause increased diuresis. ▪ May be inhibited by phenytoin (Dilantin). ▪ Do not use concomitantly with ethacrynic acid (Edecrin); risk of ototoxicity markedly increased. ▪ Smoking may increase secretion of ADH-decreasing diuretic effects and cardiac output. ▪ Note Precautions.

SIDE EFFECTS

Usually occur in prolonged therapy, seriously ill patients, or following large doses.

Minor: Anemia, anorexia, blurring of vision, deafness (reversible), diarrhea, dizziness, hyperglycemia, hyperuricemia, hypokalemia, leg cramps, lethargy, leukopenia, mental confusion, paresthesia, postural hypotension, pruritus, tinnitus, urinary frequency, urticaria, vomiting, weakness.

Major: Anaphylactic shock, blood volume reduction, circulatory collapse, dehydration, excessive diuresis, hypokalemia, metabolic acidosis, vascular thrombosis, and embolism.

ANTIDOTE

If minor side effects are noted, discontinue the drug and notify the physician, who may treat the side effects symptomatically and continue the drug. If side effects are progressive or any major side effect occurs, discontinue the drug immediately and notify the physician. Treatment of major side effects is symptomatic and aggressive. Resuscitate as necessary.

GALLIUM NITRATE

Ganite

Antihypercalcemic

pH 6.0 to 7.0

USUAL DOSE

200 mg/M^2 daily for 5 consecutive days. Must be administered as an IV infusion. Discontinue treatment at any time the serum calcium levels are lowered into the normal range (8.5 to 10.5 mg/100 ml, corrected for serum albumin). Safety and effectiveness of retreatment not established. Note Precautions/Monitor.

DOSE ADJUSTMENTS

Consider reduction to 100 mg/M^2/day for 5 days in patients with mild hypercalcemia (12 mg/100 ml range corrected for serum albumin) and few symptoms. ■ Reduced dose may be required in impaired renal function based on creatinine clearance (2.0 to 2.5 mg/100 ml). (See Contraindications).

DILUTION

A single daily dose must be diluted in 1000 ml NS (preferred) or D5W. Less diluent may be used if absolutely necessary in patients with compromised cardiovascular status.

Storage: Store at controlled room temperature prior to dilution. Stable after dilution for 48 hours at controlled room temperature and for 7 days if refrigerated.

INCOMPATIBLE WITH

Consider specific use and controlled rate of infusion. *Y-site:* Cisplatin (Platinol), cytarabine (ARA-C), doxorubicin (Adriamycin), etoposide (VePesid), fluorouracil (5FU), haloperidol (Haldol), hydromorphone (Dilaudid), ifosfamide (Ifex), imipenem-cilastatin (Primaxin), lorazepam (Ativan), morphine, prochlorperazine (Compazine).

RATE OF ADMINISTRATION

A single daily dose equally distributed over 24 hours as an IV infusion. Use of a microdrip (60 gtt/ml) or an infusion pump recommended for even distribution. Too-rapid injection rate may lead to overdose.

ACTIONS

A hypocalcemic agent that inhibits calcium resorption from bone. Thought to act by reducing increased bone turnover. Does not have cytotoxic effects on bone cells. Plasma levels achieve a steady state 24 to 48 hours after infusion initiated. In one study it normalized serum calcium in 75% of patients who began treatment with a serum calcium corrected for albumin greater than 12 mg/100 ml. Maintains duration of normocalcemia/hypocalcemia longer than calcitonin. Route of metabolism is unknown. Significant excretion occurs through the kidneys.

INDICATIONS AND USES

Treatment of clearly symptomatic cancer-related hypercalcemia that has not responded to adequate hydration. Serum calcium above 12 mg/100 ml corrected for serum albumin. Symptoms may include anorexia, cardiac arrest, coma, confusion, constipation, dehydration, depression, fatigue, muscle weakness, nausea and vomiting.

CONTRAINDICATIONS

- Severe renal impairment (serum creatinine over 2.5 mg/100 ml).

PRECAUTIONS

Calcium is bound to serum protein; concentration fluctuates with changes in blood volume. Changes in serum calcium (especially during rehydration) may not reflect true plasma levels. All calcium measurement should be corrected for albumin to establish a basis for treatment and evaluation of treatment. ■ Mild or asymptomatic hypercalcemia will be treated with conservative measures (e.g., saline hydration, with or without diuretics). Consider patient's cardiovascular status. Corticosteroids may be indicated if the underlying cancer is sensitive (e.g., hematologic cancers).

Monitor: Baseline measurements of serum calcium corrected for serum albumin, serum phosphorus, electrolytes, plasma pH, serum creatinine and BUN are required. Monitor calcium daily, phosphorus twice weekly, and electrolytes, plasma pH, creatinine, and BUN closely as indicated by baseline results (may be daily). ■ Patients with cancer-related hypercalcemia are frequently dehydrated. Must be adequately hydrated orally and/or intravenously before treatment is initiated. Hydration with saline is preferred to facilitate renal excretion of calcium and correct dehydration. A pretreatment urine output of 2 L/day is recommended. ■ Avoid overhydration in patients with compromised cardiovascular status. Observe frequently for signs of fluid overload. Correct hypovolemia before using diuretics. ■ Maintain adequate hydration and urine output throughout treatment.

Patient education: Regular visits and assessments of lab tests imperative. ■ Restriction of dietary calcium and vitamin D may be required. ■ Take only prescribed medications. ■ Report abdominal cramps, chills, confusion, fever, muscle spasms, sore throat, and/or any new medical problem promptly.

Maternal/child: Pregnancy category C: Use in pregnancy has not been studied; use only if clearly needed. ■ Discontinue nursing or do not use gallium nitrate. Consider importance of drug to mother. ■ Safety for use in children not established.

DRUG/LAB INTERACTIONS

Nephrotoxicity may be increased with other nephrotoxic drugs (e.g., aminoglycosides [gentamicin], amphotericin B [Fungizone], Edecrin).

SIDE EFFECTS

Average dose: Acute renal failure, anemia, asymptomatic decrease in blood pressure, fluid overload, hearing loss, optic neuritis (acute), respiratory alkalosis, tinnitus. Many other side effects, possibly from underlying disease, have occurred in less than 1% of patients.

Overdose: Acute renal failure, anemia, hypocalcemia, hypophosphatemia, nausea, vomiting.

ANTIDOTE

Discontinue drug if creatinine clearance reaches 2.5 mg/100 ml at any time during treatment. Discontinue drug for any symptoms of overdose. Monitor serum calcium; use vigorous IV hydration, with or without diuretics for 2 to 3 days. Monitor intake and output to ensure adequacy and balance. For asymptomatic or mild to moderate hypocalcemia (6.5 to 8.0 mg/100 ml corrected for serum albumin), short-term calcium therapy may be indicated. Oral phosphorus may be required for hypophosphatemia. Red blood cell transfusions may be required in anemia. Keep physician informed. Some side effects may respond to symptomatic treatment. Treat anaphylaxis and resuscitate as indicated.

GANCICLOVIR SODIUM

Cytovene IV, DHPG

Antiviral

pH 9.0 to 11.0

USUAL DOSE

CMV retinitis: Adults and children over 3 months: 5 mg/kg of body weight every 12 hours or 2 to 5 mg/kg every 8 hours for 14 to 21 days. Begin a maintenance dose the next day (day 15 to 22) of 5 mg/kg daily for 7 days each week or 6 mg/kg daily for 5 days each week. Note Precautions/ Monitor. After IV induction and when retinitis is stable, Cytovene capsules may be used for maintenance therapy. If retinitis progresses during the maintenance regimen, initiate the twice-daily program again. Treatment continues as long as the patient is immunocompromised, perhaps months or years. Do not exceed recommended dosage or frequency.

CMV retinitis combination therapy (ganciclovir and foscarnet) for patients who have relapsed after monotherapy with either drug: In patients who have received ganciclovir induction with 5 mg/kg every 12 hours followed by 5 mg/kg/day maintenance, continue their present therapy (e.g., ganciclovir 5 mg/kg/day) and begin foscarnet induction with 90 mg/kg every 12 hours for 14 to 21 days followed immediately by maintenance doses of ganciclovir 5 mg/kg/day and foscarnet 90 mg/kg/day (see foscarnet monograph). Monitor renal function very closely with this combination regimen.

Prevention of CMV disease in transplant recipients: 5 mg/kg every 12 hours for 7 to 14 days. Follow with maintenance regimen as outlined in CMV retinitis. Length of treatment based on immunosuppression degree and duration; 3 to 4 months or longer is common. CMV disease may occur if treatment stopped prematurely.

DOSE ADJUSTMENTS

With impaired renal function, dose may need to be reduced up to 50% or dosing interval may be adjusted. ▪ Assess renal function before administration to elderly patients and adjust dose appropriately. ▪ Note Drug/lab interactions.

DILUTION

Specific techniques required; see Precautions. Initially dissolve the 500-mg vial with 10 ml SW (50 mg/ml). Do not use bacteriostatic water containing parabens; will cause precipitation. Shake well to dissolve completely. Discard if particulate matter or discoloration observed. Withdraw desired dose and further dilute with NS, D5/R, or LR to provide a concentration less than 10 mg/ml (70-kg adult at 5 mg/kg equals 350 mg; dissolved in 100 ml of solution equals 3.5 mg/ml).

Storage: Use reconstituted solution within 12 hours. Do not refrigerate. Solution fully diluted for administration must be refrigerated and used within 24 hours to reduce incidence of bacterial contamination.

INCOMPATIBLE WITH

Any other drug in syringe or solution because of alkaline pH. Precipitation may occur if pH is altered. Advisable to clear tubing with normal saline if possible before and after administration through Y-tube or three-way stopcock. Because of physical incompatibilities, ganciclovir sodium and **foscarnet sodium** must never be mixed. Aldesleukin (Proleukin), amifostine (Ethyol).

Y-site: Cytarabine (ARA-C), doxorubicin (Adriamycin), fludarabine (Fludara), foscarnet (Foscavir), ondansetron (Zofran), parabens, piperacillin/tazobactam (Zosyn), sargramostim (Leukine), TPN (selected), vinorelbine.

RATE OF ADMINISTRATION

A single dose must be administered at a constant rate over 1 hour as an infusion. Use of an infusion pump or microdrip (60 gtt/ml) recommended. Excessive plasma levels and toxicity will occur with too-rapid rate of injection. Advisable to clear tubing with NS before and after administration through Y-tube or three-way stopcock.

ACTIONS

An antiviral agent that stops cytomegalovirus (CMV) from multiplying. Does not destroy existing viruses but stops them from reproducing and invading healthy cells. May allow a weakened immune system to defend the body against the CMV infection. May also be inhibitory against herpes simplex virus 1 and 2, Epstein-Barr virus, and varicella zoster virus, but clinical studies have not been done. Onset of action is prompt, and therapeutic levels are maintained for 3 to 6 hours with some drug remaining 11 hours after infusion. Widely distributed in tissues and body fluids. Probably crosses the placental barrier. Suspected to be secreted in breast milk. Over 90% excreted unchanged in urine by glomerular filtration in patients with normal renal function.

INDICATIONS AND USES

Treatment of CMV retinitis in immunocompromised individuals, including patients with AIDS. ■ Combination therapy (ganciclovir and foscarnet) may be indicated with progressive retinitis refractory to single therapy. ■ CMV disease prevention in at-risk transplant patients. ■ Now available as an ophthalmic surgical aid (intravitreal implant) to treat CMV retinitis. ■ Capsules are used for prevention of CMV retinitis in at-risk patients with advanced HIV infection and in the prevention of CMV disease in solid organ transplant recipients.

CONTRAINDICATIONS

Hypersensitivity to ganciclovir or acyclovir; patients with a neutrophil count less than 500 cells/mm^3 or a platelet count less than 25,000 cells/mm^3; patients receiving zidovudine (Retrovir), since both drugs cause granulocytopenia.

PRECAUTIONS

■ A nucleoside analog; follow guidelines for handling and disposal of cytotoxic agents. See Appendix A, p. 893. ■ For IV use only; IM or SC administration will cause severe tissue irritation. ■ Resistance has been reported to develop. May be higher in patients treated for a prolonged period. ■ Cidofovir is a newly approved agent for treatment of CMV retinitis.

Monitor: Confirm diagnosis of CMV retinitis by indirect ophthalmoscopy. Diagnosis may be supported by cultures of CMV from urine, blood, throat, etc.; negative culture does not rule out CMV retinitis. ■ CBC with differential and platelet counts, serum creatinine, and creatinine clearance are required before treatment initiated. Monitor neutrophil and platelet counts every 2 days during twice-daily dosing and weekly thereafter. Monitor daily in patients with previous leukopenia from nucleoside analogs or those with neutrophils less than 1000 cells/mm^3 at beginning of treatment. Withhold dose if neutrophils less than 500 cells/mm^3 or platelets less than 25,000 cells/mm^3. Monitor serum creatinine or creatinine clearance every 2 weeks. ■ Maintain adequate hydration and urine flow before and during infusion. ■ Phlebitis or pain may occur at site of infusion; confirm patency of vein and use small needles and large veins to ensure adequate blood flow for rapid dilution and distribution. ■ Note Drug/lab interactions.

Patient education: Must use effective birth control throughout treatment. Men should continue barrier contraception for at least 90 days. ■ Not a cure; retinitis may still progress. Frequent ophthalmoscopic examinations important. ■ Cooperation for close monitoring of blood counts is imperative to control side effects. ■ Patients with AIDS receiving zidovudine (Retrovir) may not tolerate ganciclovir. ■ High frequency of impaired renal function increased with concomitant use of nephrotoxic agents (e.g., cyclosporine, amphotericin); high risk for transplant recipients.

Maternal/child: Pregnancy category C: Avoid pregnancy. A potential carcinogen. Teratogenic and embryotoxic; will cause birth defects. Do not use during pregnancy unless risk is justified. May cause temporary or permanent infertility in men and women. ■ Discontinue nursing during treatment; do not resume until at least 72 hours after final dose of ganciclovir. ■ Use extreme caution in children under 12 years of age. Long-term carcinogenicity and reproductive toxicity are probable.

Elderly: Note Dose adjustments.

DRUG/LAB INTERACTIONS

Because of physical incompatibilities, ganciclovir and foscarnet must never be mixed. ▪ Additive toxicity may occur with concomitant use of other drugs that inhibit replication of rapidly dividing cell populations (e.g., dapsone, pentamidine [Pentam 300], flucytosine [Ancobon], vincristine [Oncovin], vinblastine [Velban], doxorubicin [Adriamycin], amphotericin B [Fungizone], trimethoprim/sulfamethoxazole [Bactrim]). ▪ May cause severe granulocytopenia with zidovudine (Retrovir). Combination used in patients with AIDS is rarely tolerated. ▪ Concurrent treatment with didanosine (Videx) may cause increased didanosine levels. ▪ May cause seizures with imipenem-cilastatin (Primaxin). ▪ Potentiated by probenecid and other drugs that may reduce renal clearance; will increase toxicity. ▪ Impaired renal function markedly increased with other nephrotoxic agents (e.g., cyclosporine, amphotericin B). ▪ Note Contraindications.

SIDE EFFECTS

Granulocytopenia and thrombocytopenia are the most common and are generally reversible if treatment discontinued. Anemia, fever, infection, pain at injection site, phlebitis, rash, and abnormal liver function tests occur in some patients. Fewer than 1% of patients experienced abdominal pain, alopecia, ataxia, chills, coma, confusion, day dreaming, diarrhea, dreams, dizziness, dyspnea, dysrhythmias, edema, eosinophilia, headache, hematuria, hemorrhage, hypertension, hypoglycemia, hypotension, increased BUN and creatinine clearance, malaise, nausea, nervousness, paresthesia, pruritus, psychosis, retinal detachment, somnolence, tremor, and urticaria.

Overdose: Anorexia, bloody diarrhea, cytopenia, hypersalivation, increased BUN and liver function tests, testicular atrophy, vomiting, death.

ANTIDOTE

Notify physician of all side effects, most will be treated symptomatically. Discontinue drug if neutrophils fall below 500 cells/mm^3 or platelets fall below 25,000 cells/mm^3. Hydration and hemodialysis (up to 50% removal) are useful in overdose. Treat anaphylaxis and resuscitate as necessary.

GEMCITABINE HYDROCHLORIDE

Antineoplastic
(Miscellaneous)

Gemzar

pH 2.7 to 3.3

USUAL DOSE

Pancreatic cancer: 1,000 mg/M^2 once each week for up to 7 weeks (or until toxicity necessitates reducing or holding a dose). Follow with a week of rest. In subsequent cycles, 1,000 mg/M^2 or appropriate reduced or increased dose once each week for 3 consecutive weeks. Follow with a week of rest.

Non-small cell lung cancer (investigational): 1,000 mg/M^2 as an infusion once each week for 3 weeks, follow with a 1-week rest.

DOSE ADJUSTMENTS

Reduce dose based on the degree of hematologic toxicity. See chart below:

Gemcitabine Dosage Reduction Guidelines			
Absolute granulocyte count		Platelet count	% of full dose
≥1,000/mm^3	and	≥100,000/mm^3	100
500 to 999/mm^3	or	50,000 to 99,000/mm^3	75
<500/mm^3	or	<50,000/mm^3	hold

Dose may be increased by 25% (to 1,250 mg/M^2) in patients who complete an entire 7-week initial cycle or a subsequent 3-week cycle at a dose of 1,000 mg/M^2. Absolute granulocyte count nadir must exceed 1,500/mm^3 and platelet nadir must exceed 100,000/mm^3. Nonhematologic toxicity should not be greater than WHO Grade 1 (some examples are: able to eat, reasonable intake, no more than one emesis in 24 hours, asymptomatic heart and lungs, mild paresthesia). If this cycle is tolerated, dose for the next cycle may be increased to 1,500 mg/M^2 providing the same criteria have been met (e.g., granulocyte nadir, platelet nadir, nonhematologic toxicity).

DILUTION

Specific techniques required; see Precautions: Each 200 mg must be reconstituted with 5 ml NS without preservatives (25 ml NS for 1 Gm). Yields 40 mg/ml. Shake to dissolve. Do not use less solution to reconstitute; dissolution will be incomplete. The appropriate dose may be given without further dilution or may be further diluted with NS to concentrations as low as 0.1 mg/ml. 1,500 mg diluted in 250 ml yields 6 mg/ml. 750 mg in 100 ml yields 7.5 mg/ml.

Storage: Store unopened vials at controlled room temperature. Reconstituted or diluted solutions are stable at controlled room temperature for 24 hours. Do not refrigerate in any form; may crystallize. Discard unused portion.

INCOMPATIBLE WITH

Compatibility with other drugs has not been studied. Should be considered incompatible in syringe or solution with any other drug until specific information is available because of toxicity and specific use.

RATE OF ADMINISTRATION

A single dose as an infusion equally distributed over 30 minutes. Do not extend infusion time beyond 60 minutes; will increase toxicity.

ACTIONS

A nucleoside analogue with antineoplastic activity. Metabolized intracellularly to two active nucleosides. Cell phase specific, these nucleosides induce internucleosomal DNA fragmentation, primarily killing cells undergoing DNA synthesis (S-phase) and also blocking the progression of cells through the G_1/S-phase boundary. Very little is bound to plasma protein. Volume of distribution is increased by infusion length. Half-life is shorter (32 to 94 minutes) with a short infusion (<70 minutes), and longer (245 to 638 minutes) with a long infusion (>70 minutes). Half-life is slightly longer and rate of clearance is lower in women and in the elderly, resulting in higher concentrations for any given dose. Primarily excreted in urine.

INDICATIONS AND USES

First-line treatment for patients with nonresectable or metastatic cancer of the pancreas and for patients previously treated for cancer of the pancreas with fluorouracil.

Investigational uses: As a single agent or in combination with cisplatin for the palliative treatment of locally advanced or metastatic non-small cell lung cancer.

CONTRAINDICATIONS

Hypersensitivity to gemcitabine or any of its components.

PRECAUTIONS

Follow guidelines for handling cytotoxic agents. See Appendix A, p. 893.
■ Administered by or under the direction of the physician specialist.
■ Adequate diagnostic and treatment facilities must be available. ■ For IV use only. ■ Prolongation of the infusion time beyond 60 minutes and more frequent than weekly dosing have been shown to increase toxicity.
■ Clearance in women and the elderly is reduced; women, especially older women, were more likely not to proceed to a subsequent cycle and to experience grade 3 or 4 neutropenia and thrombocytopenia. No age or gender dose adjustments recommended. ■ Use with caution in impaired renal or hepatic function. ■ Gemcitabine is a potent radiosensitizer. Depending on the site being radiated, concurrent use with gemcitabine may cause severe, life-threatening esophagitis and pneumonitis. ■ If gemcitabine-induced pneumonitis is confirmed or suspected, discontinue permanently. ■ Use caution in patients who have had previous cytotoxic chemotherapy or radiation therapy.

Monitor: Use caution to prevent bone marrow depression; myelosuppression is the dose-limiting toxicity. Note Dose adjustments. ■ Obtain a CBC, including differential and platelet count, before each dose.
■ Obtain baseline renal function (e.g., serum creatinine) and liver function tests (e.g., AST [SGOT], AKT [SGPT]) and repeat periodically.
■ Monitor vital signs ■ Maintain adequate hydration. ■ Nausea and vomiting are frequent and were severe in 15% of patients; prophylactic

administration of antiemetics will increase patient comfort. ▪ Observe closely for S/S of infection. May cause fever in the absence of infection or prophylactic antibiotics may be indicated pending results of C/S in a febrile or nonfebrile patient. ▪ Not a vesicant, but monitor injection site for inflammation an/or extravasation.

Patient education: Nonhormonal birth control recommended. ▪ See Appendix D, p. 900. ▪ Report any unusual or unexpected symptoms or side effects as soon as possible.

Maternal/child: Pregnancy category D: Avoid pregnancy. May cause fetal harm. ▪ Discontinue breast feeding. ▪ Safety and effectiveness for use in children not established.

Elderly: Clearance reduced in the elderly; they are more likely to experience grade 3 or 4 thrombocytopenia. Usual dose adjustments based on toxicity are considered appropriate. Age-related impaired renal function may further reduce clearance and increase toxicity.

DRUG/LAB INTERACTIONS

Interaction of gemcitabine with other drugs has not been adequately studied. ▪ Additive bone marrow depression may occur with radiation therapy, other bone marrow depressing agents (e.g., amphotericin B [traditional and lipid], azathioprine [Imuran], chloramphenicol, melphelan [Alkeran]), and/or immunosuppressants (e.g., azathioprine, chlorambucil [Leukeran], cyclophosphamide [Cytoxan], cyclosporine [Sandimmune], glucocorticoid corticosteroids [e.g., dexamethasone], muromonab CD-3 [Orthoclone], tacrolimus [Prograf]; dose reduction may be required. ▪ Do not administer live vaccines to patients receiving antineoplastic agents.

SIDE EFFECTS

Alopecia (15%), bone marrow toxicity (e.g., anemia [68%], leukopenia [62%], neutropenia [63%], thrombocytopenia [24%]), bronchospasm, constipation, diarrhea, dyspnea, edema, elevated lab tests (e.g., alkaline phosphatase, bilirubin, BUN, creatinine, hematuria, proteinuria), fever, flu syndrome (e.g., anorexia, chills, cough, headache, myalgia, weakness), hemorrhage, infection, nausea and vomiting (69%), pain, paresthesias, pneumonitis (rare), pruritus, rash, somnolence, stomatitis, transient increases in AST (SGOT), ALT (SGPT). Anaphylaxis and hemolytic uremic syndrome have been reported.

ANTIDOTE

Keep physician informed of all side effects. Symptomatic and supportive treatment is indicated. Reduce dose or withhold gemcitabine until myelosuppression improves to specific criteria; see Dose adjustments. If gemcitabine-induced pneumonitis or esophagitis is confirmed or suspected, discontinue permanently (in one study severe stomatitis and pharyngeal damage required patients to be fed by feeding tube for up to 12 months after receiving doses of 300 mg/M^2 [25% of the usual dose]). Anemia may require RBC transfusions. Most side effects are reversible with dose reduction or temporary withholding of gemcitabine. No known antidote for overdose. If hemolytic uremic syndrome occurs, renal failure may not be reversible even with discontinuation of therapy and dialysis may be required. Treat allergic reactions with oxygen, epinephrine, corticosteroids, and antihistamines.

GENTAMICIN SULFATE

Antibacterial
(Aminoglycoside)

🍁Cidomycin, Garamycin, Jenamicin

pH 3.0 to 5.5

USUAL DOSE

3 mg/kg of body weight/24 hr equally divided into 3 or 4 doses. Up to 5 mg/kg/24 hr may be given if indicated. Reduce to usual dose as soon as feasible. A loading dose of 1 to 2 mg/kg is commonly used. Dosage based on ideal body weight. Recent studies suggest that a total daily dose administered as a single dose (instead of divided into 2 to 3 doses) may provide higher peak levels and enhance drug effectiveness while actually reducing or having no adverse effects on risk of toxicity. Monitor with trough levels. Note Precautions/Monitor.

Prevention of bacterial endocarditis in dental, respiratory tract, GI or GU tract surgery or instrumentation: 1.5 mg/kg 30 minutes before procedure. Do not exceed 80 mg. Repeat in 8 hours. Given concurrently with ampicillin or vancomycin and amoxicillin.

Pelvic inflammatory disease: 2 mg/kg as an initial dose. Follow with 1.5 mg/kg every 8 hours for 4 days or 48 hours after patient improves. Given concurrently with clindamycin.

PEDIATRIC DOSE

6 to 7.5 mg/kg of body weight/24 hr (2 to 2.5 mg/kg every 8 hours).

Prevention of bacterial endocarditis in dental, respiratory tract, GI or GU tract surgery or instrumentation: 2 mg/kg. See Adult dose for instructions.

NEONATAL DOSE

2.5 mg/kg.

0 to 7 days of age: less than 28 weeks gestation: Every 24 hours. *28 to 34 weeks gestation:* Every 18 hours. *Over 34 weeks gestation:* Every 12 hours. *Over 7 days of age: less than 28 weeks gestation:* Every 18 hours. *28 to 34 weeks gestation:* Every 12 hours. *Over 34 weeks gestation:* Every 8 hours.

DOSE ADJUSTMENTS

Reduce daily dose commensurate with amount of renal impairment and/or increase intervals between injections. ■ Reduced dose or extended intervals may be indicated in the elderly. ■ Note Precautions/ Monitor and Drug/lab interactions.

DILUTION

Prepared solutions equal 10 or 40 mg/ml. Further dilute each single dose in 50 to 200 ml of IV NS or D5W. Decrease volume of diluent for children. Commercially diluted solutions available.

INCOMPATIBLE WITH

Administer separately. Inactivated in solution with carbenicillin, other penicillins, and most cephalosporins. Allopurinol (Zyloprim), amphotericin B, ampicillin, cefamandole (Mandol), cefuroxime (Zinacef), cephalothin (Keflin), cephapirin (Cefadyl), clindamycin (Cleocin), cytarabine (ARA-C), dopamine (Intropin), furosemide (Lasix), heparin, hetastarch (Hespan), idarubicin (Idamycin), iodipamide meglumine, indomethacin (Indocin), nafcillin (Unipen), ticarcillin (Ticar).

RATE OF ADMINISTRATION

Each single dose, properly diluted, over 30 to 60 minutes, up to 2 hours in children. Recent studies suggest bolus dosing (versus infusion over 30 minutes) may produce an earlier bactericidal effect, which is sustained. No dose, dilution, or rate recommendations are available at this time.

ACTIONS

An aminoglycoside antibiotic with neuromuscular blocking action. Bactericidal against specific gram-negative bacilli, including *Escherichia coli, Klebsiella, Proteus,* and *Pseudomonas.* Not effective for fungi or viral infections. Well distributed throughout all body fluids; serum and urine levels remain adequate for 6 to 12 hours. Usual half-life is 2 hours. Half-life is prolonged in infants, postpartum females, fever, liver disease and ascites, spinal cord injury, cystic fibrosis, and the elderly; shorter in severe burns. Crosses the placental barrier. Excreted through the kidneys.

INDICATIONS AND USES

Treatment of serious infections of the GI (peritonitis), respiratory, and urinary tracts, CNS (meningitis), skin, bone, soft tissue (burns), septicemia, and bacterial neonatal sepsis. ■ Primarily used when penicillin and other less toxic antibiotics are ineffective or contraindicated. ■ Prevention of bacterial endocarditis in dental, respiratory tract, GI or GU surgery or instrumentation. ■ Used concurrently with clindamycin to treat pelvic inflammatory disease. ■ Considered initial therapy after culture and sensitivity is drawn in suspected or confirmed gram-negative infections or other serious infections. ■ Treat suspected infection in the immunosuppressed patient. ■ May be used synergistically in gram-positive infections. ■ Used concurrently with penicillin for endocarditis and neonatal sepsis.

CONTRAINDICATIONS

Known gentamicin or aminoglycoside sensitivity, renal failure. Sulfite sensitivity may be a contraindication.

PRECAUTIONS

Sensitivity studies indicated to determine susceptibility of the causative organism to gentamicin. ■ Use extreme caution if therapy is required over 7 to 10 days. ■ Superinfection may occur from overgrowth of nonsusceptible organisms. ■ Use caution in infants, children, and the elderly. ■ May contain sulfites; use caution in patients with asthma. ■ Use extreme caution in patients with end-stage renal disease.

Monitor: Narrow range between toxic and therapeutic levels. Periodically monitor peak and trough concentrations. Therapeutic level is between 4 and 8 mcg/ml. Monitor frequently in patients with impaired renal function. ■ Watch for decrease in urine output and rising BUN and serum creatinine. May require decreased dose. ■ Routine serum levels and evaluation of hearing are recommended. ■ Maintain good hydration. ■ Monitor serum calcium, magnesium, sodium, and potassium; levels may decline. Depressed levels have caused mental confusion, paresthesia, positive Chvostek and Trousseau signs (provoked spasm of facial muscles and other muscles; occurs in tetany), and tetany in adults; muscle weakness and tetany in infants. ■ In extended treatment, monitoring of serum levels, electrolytes, renal, auditory, and vestibular functions is recommended daily. ■ Note Drug/lab interactions.

Patient education: Report promptly: dizziness, hearing loss, weakness, or any changes in balance. ■ Consider birth control options.

Maternal/child: Pregnancy category D: Avoid pregnancy. Potential hazard to fetus. ■ Safety for use during lactation not established; use extreme caution. ■ Peak concentrations are generally lower in infants and young children.

Elderly: Consider less toxic alternatives. ■ Half-life prolonged. Longer intervals between doses may be more important than reduced doses. ■ Monitor renal function and drug levels carefully. Measurement of creatinine clearance more useful than BUN or serum creatinine to assess renal function. ■ Note Precautions.

DRUG/LAB INTERACTIONS

Inactivated in solution with penicillins but is synergistic when used in combination with beta-lactam antibiotics (e.g., sulbactam sodium, clavulanate potassium, cephalosporins, penicillins) and vancomycin. Dose adjustment and appropriate spacing required because of physical incompatibilities and interactions. Synergism may be inconsistent; measure aminoglycoside levels. ■ Concurrent use topically or systemically with any other ototoxic or nephrotoxic agents should be avoided. May have dangerous additive effects with anesthetics (e.g., enflurane), other neuromuscular blocking antibiotics (e.g., kanamycin, streptomycin), beta-lactam antibiotics (e.g., cephalosporins), diuretics (e.g., furosemide [Lasix]), vancomycin, and many others. ■ Neuromuscular blocking muscle relaxants (e.g., doxacurium [Nuromax], succinylcholine [Anectine]) are potentiated by aminoglycosides. *Apnea can occur.* ■ Aminoglycosides are also potentiated by anticholinesterases (e.g., edrophonium), antineoplastics (e.g., nitrogen mustard, cisplatin). ■ May be antagonized by bacteriostatic antibiotics (e.g., chloramphenicol, erythromycin, tetracyclines); bactericidal action may be impacted.

SIDE EFFECTS

Occur more frequently with impaired renal function, higher doses, or prolonged administration, in dehydrated or elderly patients, and in patients receiving other ototoxic or nephrotoxic drugs.

Minor: Anorexia, burning, dizziness, fever, headache, hypertension, hypotension, itching, lethargy, muscle twitching, nausea, numbness, rash, roaring in ears, tingling sensation, tinnitus, urticaria, vomiting, weight loss.

Major: Acute organic brain syndrome, blood dyscrasias, convulsions, elevated bilirubin, BUN, serum creatinine, AST (SGOT), and ALT (SGPT); hearing loss, laryngeal edema; neuromuscular blockade; oliguria; respiratory depression or arrest.

ANTIDOTE

Notify the physician of all side effects. If minor side effects persist or any major symptom appears, discontinue the drug and notify the physician. Treatment is symptomatic. In overdose, hemodialysis may be indicated. Monitor fluid balance, creatinine clearance, and plasma levels carefully. Complexation with ticarcillin or carbenicillin (12 to 30 Gm/day) may be as effective as hemodialysis. Consider exchange transfusion in the newborn. Calcium salts or neostigmine may reverse neuromuscular blockade. Resuscitate as necessary.

GLUCAGON HYDROCHLORIDE

Antihypoglycemic
Diagnostic agent
Antidote

pH 2.5 to 3.0

USUAL DOSE

Hypoglycemia: 0.5 to 1 mg. May be repeated in 20 minutes for 2 doses if indicated. Up to 2 mg has been given as initial dose.

Diagnostic aid: 0.25 to 2 mg.

Reverse effects of beta blockade: 3 to 10 mg or 50 to 150 mcg/kg of body weight. Follow either dose regimen with a continuous infusion of 1 to 5 mg/hr. Specific process required; (See Dilution).

PEDIATRIC DOSE

0.03 to 0.1 mg/kg every 5 to 20 minutes until adequate response. Maximum single dose is 1 mg.

NEONATAL DOSE

Less than 10 kg: 0.1 mg/kg up to 1 mg every 30 minutes until adequate response. *Over 10 kg:* 1 mg every 30 minutes until adequate response.

DILUTION

Dilute 1 unit (1 mg) of glucagon powder with 1 ml of its own diluting solution. Do not add to IV solutions. May be given through Y-tube or three-way stopcock of infusion set if a dextrose solution is infusing. A 2-mg dose may be diluted with an equal amount of SW for injection.

Reverse effects of beta blockade: Provided diluent contains phenol, which can be toxic. Reconstitute with NS or D5W for these larger doses. For *continuous infusion* this reconstituted solution may be further diluted in D5W to deliver 1 to 5 mg/hr.

Storage: Store at controlled room temperature prior to reconstitution. Immediate use after reconstitution is preferred. May refrigerate for up to 48 hours if necessary.

INCOMPATIBLE WITH

Any other drug in the syringe; solutions containing sodium chloride, potassium chloride, or calcium chloride. Not soluble in any solution with a pH range of 3 to 9.5.

RATE OF ADMINISTRATION

1 unit (1 mg) or fraction thereof over 1 minute.

Reverse effects of beta blockade: A single dose (10 mg) over 1 minute. Follow with an infusion of 1 to 5 mg/hr. Titrate to patient response.

ACTIONS

A pancreatic polypeptide hormone from the alpha cells of the islets of Langerhans. Blood glucose is raised by activating phosphorylase, which converts glycogen to glucose in the liver. Glucagon acts only on liver glycogen. Has a half-life of 3 to 6 minutes. Produces relaxation of the smooth muscle of the stomach, duodenum, small bowel, and colon.

INDICATIONS AND USES

Treatment of hypoglycemic reactions during insulin therapy in the management of diabetes mellitus and in induced insulin shock during psychiatric therapy. ■ Induction of a hypotonic state and smooth muscle relaxation in the radiologic examination of the stomach, duodenum, small bowel, and colon.

Investigational uses: May be helpful in reversing adverse beta-blockade of beta-adrenergic blocking agents (e.g., propranolol [Inderal]) and calcium channel blockers (e.g., diltiazem [Cardizem], verapamil [Calan]) or may be used to enhance digitalis effects in heart failure.

CONTRAINDICATIONS

Known hypersensitivity to protein compounds.

PRECAUTIONS

Easily absorbed IM or SC. ▪ If glucagon and glucose do not awaken the patient, coma is probably caused by a condition other than hypoglycemia. ▪ Not as effective in the juvenile diabetic patient; supplement with carbohydrate as soon as possible. ▪ Use caution in patients with insulinoma and/or pheochromocytoma. ▪ As a smooth muscle relaxant, it is as effective as anticholinergic drugs and has fewer side effects.

Monitor: Should awaken the patient in 5 to 20 minutes. Prolonged hypoglycemic reactions may result in severe cortical damage. ▪ Emesis on awakening is common. Prevent aspiration by turning the patient face down. ▪ Dose may be repeated if necessary. Supplement with IV glucose (50%) to precipitate awakening. Utilize oral sugars after awakening to prevent secondary hypoglycemia.

Patient education: Eat some form of sugar if hypoglycemia recurs. ▪ Report episodes of hypoglycemia and glucagon use at home. ▪ Teach patient and family proper preparation of glucagon from kits. Include signs of hypoglycemia and procedures to be followed after administration to an unconscious patient.

Maternal/child: Pregnancy category B: Safety for use in pregnancy and lactation not established.

DRUG/LAB INTERACTIONS

Potentiates oral anticoagulants.

SIDE EFFECTS

Rare in recommended doses: anaphylaxis, hyperglycemia (excessive dosage), hypersensitivity reactions, hypertension (rare), hypotension (rare), nausea, vomiting. Larger doses cause nausea and vomiting and may cause hyperglycemia, hypocalcemia, and hypokalemia.

ANTIDOTE

Nausea and vomiting are tolerable and do occur in hypoglycemia. Antiemetics are indicated when larger doses are given. For any other side effects, discontinue the drug and notify the physician. Treat allergic reactions and resuscitate as necessary. Insulin administration may be indicated in acute overdose.

GLYCOPYRROLATE

Robinul

Anticholinergic
Antidote

pH 2.0 to 3.0

USUAL DOSE

Peptic ulcer: 0.1 to 0.2 mg at 4-hour intervals 3 to 4 times/day.

Reversal of neuromuscular blockade: 0.2 mg for each 1 mg neostigmine or 5 mg of pyridostigmine. Administer IV simultaneously. May be mixed in the same syringe.

Intraoperative medication: 0.1 mg as needed, may repeat every 2 to 3 minutes. Maximum dose 0.8 mg/24 hr.

Respiratory antisecretory: 0.1 to 0.2 mg every 4 to 8 hours. Maximum single dose 0.2 mg. Maximum in 24 hours is 0.8 mg.

PEDIATRIC DOSE

Intraoperative medication: 0.004 mg/kg of body weight. Do not exceed 0.1 mg as a single dose. May repeat every 2 to 3 minutes. Maximum dose 0.8 mg/24 hr.

Reversal of neuromuscular blockade: Same as adult dose.

Respiratory antisecretory: 0.004 to 0.01 mg/kg every 4 to 8 hours. Do not exceed adult dose.

DOSE ADJUSTMENTS

Note Drug/lab interactions.

DILUTION

May be given undiluted. Administer through Y-tube or three-way stopcock of infusion tubing.

INCOMPATIBLE WITH

Alkaline solutions, chloramphenicol, dexamethasone (Decadron), diazepam (Valium), dimenhydrinate (Dramamine), methohexital (Brevital), methylprednisolone (Solu-Medrol), pentazocine (Talwin), pentobarbital (Nembutal), phenothiazines (e.g., Compazine), secobarbital (Seconal), sodium bicarbonate, thiopental (Pentothal).

RATE OF ADMINISTRATION

0.2 mg or fraction thereof over 1 to 2 minutes.

ACTIONS

A synthetic anticholinergic agent. It inhibits the action of acetylcholine. It reduces the volume and free acidity of gastric secretions and controls excessive pharyngeal, tracheal, and bronchial secretions. Antagonizes cholinergic drugs. Onset of action is within 1 minute. Some effects last 2 to 3 hours.

INDICATIONS AND USES

Adjunctive therapy in peptic ulcer. ■ Reversal of neuromuscular blockade (usually intraoperatively). ■ Reduction of salivary, tracheobronchial, and pharyngeal secretion preoperatively. ■ Reduction of volume and free acidity of gastric secretions. ■ Other intraoperative uses controlled by the anesthesiologist (counteract drug-induced or vagal traction reflexes and associated arrhythmias).

CONTRAINDICATIONS

Known hypersensitivity to glycopyrrolate. May be contraindicated in patients with glaucoma, obstructive uropathy, obstructive disease of the GI tract, paralytic ileus, unstable cardiovascular status in acute hemorrhage, severe ulcerative colitis, megacolon, and myasthenia gravis, when used for treatment of peptic ulcer disease because of long duration of therapy.

PRECAUTIONS

Use IV only when immediate drug effect is essential. ■ Not recommended for peptic ulcer therapy in children under 12 years of age. ■ Use extreme caution in autonomic neuropathy, asthma, glaucoma, pregnancy, lactation, cardiac arrhythmias, congestive heart failure, coronary artery disease, hepatic or renal disease, hiatal hernia, hypertension, hyperthyroidism, and ulcerative colitis.

Monitor: Urinary retention can be avoided if the patient voids just prior to each dose. ■ Note Drug/lab interactions.

Patient education: Use caution if a task requires alertness; may cause blurred vision, dizziness, or drowsiness. ■ Report constipation, difficulty urinating, dry mouth, flushing, increased light sensitivity, or skin rash promptly.

Maternal/child: Pregnancy category B: Safety for use in pregnancy not established. ■ It is not known whether this drug is secreted in breast milk; use caution.

Elderly: May produce excitement, agitation, confusion or drowsiness in the elderly. ■ May precipitate undiagnosed glaucoma. ■ Risk of urinary retention and constipation increased. ■ May increase memory impairment.

DRUG/LAB INTERACTIONS

Potentiated by alkalinizing agents, amantadine, synthetic narcotic analgesics, tricyclic antidepressants (e.g., amitriptyline [Elavil]), antihistamines, phenothiazines (e.g., chlorpromazine [Thorazine]), and many others. Reduced dose of either or both drugs may be indicated. ■ May decrease antipsychotic effects of phenothiazines. Dose adjustment may be required. ■ Risk of ventricular arrhythmias increased when given in presence of cyclopropane. ■ Potentiates atenolol (Tenormin) and digoxin.

SIDE EFFECTS

Anaphylaxis, anticholinergic psychosis, blurred vision, constipation, decreased sweating, dizziness, drowsiness, dry mouth, heat prostration, impotence, increased ocular tension, loss of taste, muscular weakness, nervousness, paralysis, tachycardia, urinary hesitancy and retention.

ANTIDOTE

Notify physician of all side effects. May be treated symptomatically or drug may be discontinued. Neostigmine, in 0.25-mg increments, may be used to counteract peripheral anticholinergic effects. May repeat every 5 to 10 minutes to a maximum dose of 2.5 mg. Physostigmine, in increments of 0.5 to 2 mg, may be used to counteract CNS effects. May repeat as needed to a maximum dose of 5 mg. Proportionately smaller doses should be used in children. Resuscitate as necessary.

GONADORELIN ACETATE

Hormone
(Gonad stimulating)

Lutrepulse

USUAL DOSE

5 mcg every 90 minutes (range is 1 to 20 mcg). Usually administered over a period of 21 days. Response to Lutrepulse usually occurs within 2 to 3 weeks. When ovulation occurs during this time, therapy is continued for another 2 weeks to maintain the corpus luteum. Note Precautions/Monitor.

DOSE ADJUSTMENTS

Are usually indicated if no ovulation occurs after 3 cycles and may need to be made cautiously in a stepwise fashion based upon response. See manufacturer's literature for specific dose adjustment process.

DILUTION

All necessary supplies for administration and dilution provided in Lutrepulse kit and Lutrepulse pump kit. Add 8 ml of provided diluent to both the 0.8- or 3.2-mg vials. Sterile technique essential. Provides 5 mcg/50 mcl with the 0.8-mg vial and 20 mcg/50 mcl with the 3.2-mg vial. Shake for a few seconds until solution is clear, colorless, and free of particulate matter. Prepare immediately before use and transfer to the plastic reservoir following specific instructions for the Lutrepulse pump. 8 ml of solution provides an adequate supply for 7 days.

Storage: Store dry powder between 15° to 30° C (59° to 86° F).

INCOMPATIBLE WITH

Specific information not available. Heparin was used in reservoir in some studies. Consider specific use.

RATE OF ADMINISTRATION

Each dose must be delivered via pulsatile IV injection with the Lutrepulse pump, which delivers a single dose over a pulse period of 1 minute at a pulse frequency of 90 minutes. Pump should be set at 25 or 50 mcl of solution based on desired dose and dilution and is capable of delivering 2.5, 5, 10, or 20 mcg every 90 minutes.

ACTIONS

A synthetic hormone that is identical in amino acid sequence to endogenous gonadotropin-releasing hormone (GnRH). When released by pulsatile IV injection through the Lutrepulse pump, it causes normal pulsatile releases of pituitary gonadotropins. Luteinizing and follicle-stimulating hormones are synthesized and released and stimulate the gonads to produce steroids instrumental in regulating reproductive hormonal status. Actually replaces defective hypothalamic secretion of GnRH. Initial and terminal half-life ranges from 2 to 10 minutes to 10 to 40 minutes. Rapidly metabolized to peptide fragments and excreted in urine. Half-life prolonged with renal impairment.

INDICATIONS AND USES

Induction of ovulation in women with primary hypothalamic amenorrhea.

CONTRAINDICATIONS

History of sensitivity to gonadorelin acetate or any of its components or to gonadorelin hydrochloride (Factrel); ovarian cysts or other causes of anovulation other than hypothalamic origin; pituitary prolactinoma; hormonally dependent tumors or any other condition that could be exacerbated or worsened by pregnancy or reproductive hormones.

PRECAUTIONS

Must be administered under the direction of a physician familiar with pulsatile GnRH delivery and clinical ramifications of ovarian induction. ▪ Specific diagnosis of hypothalamic amenorrhea or hypogonadism due to a deficiency in quantity or pulsing of endogenous GnRH must be established. Generally based on the exclusion of other causes of the dysfunction (e.g., disorders of general health, reproductive organs, anterior pituitary, and central nervous system). ▪ IV pulsatile injection results in more pregnancies than SC injection, reduces overall costs, and has a limited risk of infection with appropriate technique and care. ▪ Does not increase risk of abnormalities when administered during the first trimester but should be used during pregnancy only to maintain the corpus luteum in ovulation induction cycles. ▪ Spontaneous termination of pregnancy has been reported.

Monitor: Ovarian ultrasound is required as a baseline and on therapy days 7 and 14. Obtain a midluteal phase serum progesterone. At each scheduled visit the infusion site must be observed closely and a physical exam, including a pelvic, performed. ▪ Evidence of ascites, pleural effusion, fluid or electrolyte imbalance, hemoconcentration, or complaints of lower abdominal pain may indicate possible ovarian hyperstimulation; notify physician immediately. Risk of ovarian hyperstimulation may be increased with spontaneous variations in GnRH secretions. ▪ Monitoring follicle formation with ovarian ultrasound will minimize multiple pregnancies. ▪ Scrupulous aseptic technique in preparation, insertion of catheter, and care of the continuous IV site is required, including changing at 48-hour intervals.

Patient education: Instruct in use of the pump, and signs, symptoms of infection (e.g., fever, inflammation, or redness at the catheter site). ▪ Inform of potential for multiple pregnancy. ▪ All information included with kit.

Maternal/child: Potential for secretion in breast milk unknown; no indication for use in a nursing woman. ▪ Safety or efficacy for use in children under the age of 18 not established.

DRUG/LAB INTERACTIONS

Should not be used concomitantly with other ovulation-stimulating drugs (e.g., clomiphene [Clomid]).

SIDE EFFECTS

Equipment related: Hematoma, infection, inflammation, or mild phlebitis at IV site; infusion set malfunction; interruption of infusion.

Gonadorelin related: Anaphylaxis reported with related drug (gonadorelin hydrochloride [Factrel]); multiple pregnancy; ovarian hyperstimulation syndrome (e.g., ascites, cyst rupture, fluid and electrolyte imbalance, hemoconcentration, sudden ovarian enlargement with or without pain and/or pleural effusion); pregnancy termination.

ANTIDOTE

Discontinue drug and notify physician immediately for symptoms of ovarian hyperstimulation syndrome. Restart IV in another site for any signs of inflammation. Continuous infusion (versus pulsatile) from pump malfunction or accidental administration of entire dose can temporarily reduce pituitary responsiveness. Keep physician informed, and manage other side effects as indicated by severity. Treat allergic reactions and resuscitate as necessary.

GONADORELIN HYDROCHLORIDE

**Hormone
(Gonad stimulating)
Diagnostic agent**

Factrel

USUAL DOSE

100 mcg. In females administer during the early follicular phase (day 1 through 7 of the menstrual cycle). Specific procedure required (see Precautions and manufacturer's literature).

PEDIATRIC DOSE

Over 12 years of age: 100 mcg.

DILUTION

Diluent provided, 1 ml for 100 mcg and 2 ml for 500 mcg. Best to prepare immediately before use but may be kept at room temperature and must be used within 1 day of dilution.

Storage: Store below 40° C.

INCOMPATIBLE WITH

Specific information not available. Consider specific use.

RATE OF ADMINISTRATION

A single dose over 15 to 30 seconds.

ACTIONS

This synthetic hormone is structurally identical to natural luteinizing hormone-releasing hormone (LH-RH). It has gonadotropin-releasing effects on the anterior pituitary, causing synthesis and release of luteinizing hormone, and, to a lesser extent, follicle stimulating hormone. Terminal half-life is 10 to 40 minutes. Rapidly metabolized. Inactive metabolites are renally eliminated.

INDICATIONS AND USES

Evaluating hypothalamic-pituitary gonadotropic function in patients with suspected deficiency or following removal of a pituitary tumor by surgery and/or irradiation.

Investigational uses: Ovulation inhibition. ▪ Treatment of precocious puberty.

CONTRAINDICATIONS

Hypersensitivity to gonadorelin or any of its components.

PRECAUTIONS

Results of test should be interpreted by a physician familiar with hypothalamic-pituitary-gonadal physiology. ▪ Collection and assay methods and thus results vary with each laboratory performing this test. Coordinate process and confirm desired method for collecting blood samples.

Monitor: Blood samples are analyzed for luteinizing hormone concentrations. Draw venous blood samples 15 minutes and immediately before gonadorelin administration. Draw additional blood samples at 15, 30, 45, 60, and 120 minutes after administration. ■ Patient must not be receiving any other drugs that affect pituitary secretion of the gonadotropins (e.g., androgens, estrogens, progestins, or glucocorticoids).

Maternal/child: Pregnancy category B: Safety for use during pregnancy not established.

DRUG/LAB INTERACTIONS
Incorrect results may be caused by spironolactone, levodopa, oral contraceptives, digoxin, phenothiazines and dopamine antagonists (e.g., metoclopramide [Reglan]).

SIDE EFFECTS
Abdominal discomfort, flushed sensation, headache, lightheadedness, nausea.

ANTIDOTE
Notify physician and manage side effects as indicated by severity. Treat allergic reactions and resuscitate as necessary.

GRANISETRON HYDROCHLORIDE

Antiemetic
(5 HT$_3$ Receptor antagonist)

Kytril

pH 4.7 to 7.3

USUAL DOSE
A single dose of 10 mcg/kg of body weight as an injection or as an infusion. Begin within 30 minutes before giving emetogenic cancer chemotherapy (e.g., cisplatin, carboplatin) and only on the day(s) chemotherapy is given. Clinical trials used doses up to 40 mcg/kg with effects similar to the recommended 10-mcg/kg dose. Recent studies question the effectiveness of a 10-mcg/kg dose. Repeat doses are frequently required to prevent nausea with chemotherapy. Oral granisetron is now available.

Unlabeled use: Acute nausea and vomiting post-op: 1 to 3 mg IV.

PEDIATRIC DOSE
Children 2 to 16 years of age: Identical to adult dose.

DOSE ADJUSTMENTS
No dose adjustment required for the elderly or in renal failure or impaired hepatic function.

DILUTION
A single dose may be given undiluted by IV injection or further diluted to a total volume of 20 to 50 ml with NS or D5W and given as an infusion.

Storage: Store vials at controlled room temperature or below. Do not freeze, protect from light. Should be administered after dilution (preservative free) but is stable up to 24 hours at room temperature.

INCOMPATIBLE WITH

Manufacturer recommends not mixing in solution with other drugs as a general precaution. In practice, granisetron is being mixed with other agents (e.g., dexamethasone) as an additive (given over 30 minutes) or at the Y-site. See Compatible with.

COMPATIBLE WITH

Additive: dexamethasone (Decadron), mannitol (Osmitrol), methylprednisolone (Solu-Medrol).

Y-site: Compatible only if the following drugs are in specific concentrations, consult pharmacist: dexamethasone (Decadron), mannitol (Osmitrol), cyclophosphamide (Cytoxan), cytarabine (ARA-C), dacarbazine (DTIC), doxorubicin (Adriamycin), fluorouracil (5FU), furosemide (Lasix), ifosfamide (Ifex), magnesium sulfate, methotrexate (Folex), potassium chloride (KCl). Manufacturer has extensive information on Y-site compatibility at specific mg/ml.

RATE OF ADMINISTRATION

IV injection: A single dose over 30 seconds.

Intermittent infusion: A single dose equally distributed over 5 minutes.

ACTIONS

An antinauseant and antiemetic agent. A selective antagonist of specific serotonin receptors. Chemotherapeutic agents such as cisplatin increase the release of serotonin from specific cells in the GI tract, causing emesis. By antagonizing these receptors, chemotherapy-induced nausea and vomiting are prevented. Has little effect on blood pressure, heart rate, ECG, plasma prolactin or aldosterone concentrations. Moderately bound to protein (65%). Distributes freely between plasma and red blood cells. Metabolized in the liver by hepatic cytochrome P_{450} enzymes. Excreted in urine and feces.

INDICATIONS AND USES

Prevention of nausea and vomiting associated with initial and repeat courses of emetogenic cancer therapy, including high-dose cisplatin. Has been shown to be effective with most emetogenic antineoplastic agents.

Unlabeled use: Acute nausea and vomiting following surgery.

CONTRAINDICATIONS

Known hypersensitivity to granisetron.

PRECAUTIONS

Sterile technique imperative when withdrawing a single dose from the new multidose vial. ■ Stool softeners or laxatives may be required to prevent constipation. ■ Note Drug/lab interactions. ■ Related to an increased incidence of hepatocellular carcinomas and adenomas in rat studies with large doses. Exceeding maximum suggested dose is not recommended.

Monitor: Ambulate slowly to avoid orthostatic hypotension.

Patient education: Request assistance for ambulation. ■ Report promptly if nausea persists for more than 10 minutes. ■ Maintain adequate hydration. ■ Stool softeners may be required to avoid constipation.

Maternal/child: Pregnancy category B: No evidence of impaired fertility or harm to fetus. Use during pregnancy only if benefits justify risks. ■ Use caution if required during lactation. ■ Safety and effectiveness for use in children under 2 years of age have not been established. ■ Response rates seem somewhat less effective in children when compared with those in adults.

Elderly: Response similar to other age groups. ▪ Clearance lower and half-life prolonged but has no clinical significance.

DRUG/LAB INTERACTIONS

Metabolism may by inhibited by ketoconazole (Nizoral). ▪ Does not induce or inhibit the cytochrome P_{450} drug metabolizing system, but definitive interaction studies have not been done. Its clearance and half-life may be affected by inducers or inhibitors of these enzymes (e.g., cimetidine [Tagamet]). ▪ Has been safely administered with benzodiazepines (e.g., lorazepam [Ativan], midazolam [Versed]), neuroleptics (e.g., chlordiazepoxide [Librium]), and antiulcer drugs (e.g., ranitidine [Zantac]) commonly prescribed with antiemetic treatment. ▪ Does not appear to interact with emetogenic cancer chemotherapies.

SIDE EFFECTS

Constipation (3%), diarrhea (4%), headache (14%), somnolence (4%), and weakness (5%) occur most frequently. Allergic reactions including anaphylaxis (rare) have occurred. Transient elevation of AST (SGOT) or ALT (SGPT) may occur. Other side effects have occurred in fewer than 2% of patients but could not be clearly associated with granisetron.

ANTIDOTE

Most side effects will be treated symptomatically. Keep physician informed as indicated. Overdose of up to 38.5 mg has not caused significant problems. There is no specific antidote. Treat anaphylaxis and resuscitate as necessary.

HALOPERIDOL LACTATE

Antipsychotic
Sedative/tranquilizer
Antiemetic

Haldol

pH 3.0 to 3.6

USUAL DOSE

All IV doses are unlabeled.

Treatment of agitation and delirium: Initial dose based on degree of agitation. 2 to 5 mg is average. Range is 0.5 to 10 mg.

Acute psychosis: 2 to 50 mg.

In all situations observe for effectiveness. Several sources suggest repeating the initial dose as needed every 30 to 60 minutes and extending internals to 4 to 8 hours as symptoms are controlled. Another source suggests the following regimen: If agitation persists in 20 to 30 minutes, either repeat the first dose one time or give a second dose double the size of the first dose because repeat administration of a dose that does not sedate is ineffective. Continue doubling the dose every 20 to 30 minutes until the patient begins to calm down. The dose given when calming begins is the appropriate dose for that particular patient and may be repeated every hour if necessary. Titrate repeat doses to beginning signs of agitation, observe carefully, and give repeat doses at regular intervals to prevent recurrence of agitation.

Maintenance dose: On succeeding days the total required daily dose is divided and given at specific intervals for that patient (300 mg in 24 hours may be 12.5 mg every 1 hour or 50 mg every 4 hours). IV dosing has been used for up to several days until the source of agitation subsides or is removed. Most patients can then be treated with lower doses of oral haloperidol at less frequent intervals.

Treatment of pain and agitation in cancer patients: 100 to 480 mg/24 hr of haloperidol concurrently with 36 to 480 mg/24 hr of lorazepam has been used in critically ill cancer patients. May be given as a continuous infusion.

Control agitation in critically ill patients requiring mechanical ventilation: 3 to 25 mg/hr as a continuous infusion.

Antiemetic or treatment of intractable hiccups: 2 to 5 mg every 2 hours for 5 to 7 doses. May be used in an antiemetic regimen with dexamethasone in chemotherapy.

DOSE ADJUSTMENTS

Lower initial doses and more gradual adjustments are recommended in the elderly or debilitated.

DILUTION

Check vial carefully; only haloperidol lactate can be used IV. May be given undiluted. Give through Y-tube or three-way stopcock of the infusion set. Flush with at least 2 ml of NS before and after administration of haloperidol. A single dose may be added to 30 to 50 ml of most infusion solutions (D5W preferred) and given as an infusion.

Storage: Store below 40° C; protect from light. Do not freeze.

INCOMPATIBLE WITH

Y-site: Allopurinol (Zyloprim), fluconazole (Diflucan), foscarnet (Foscavir), gallium nitrate (Ganite), heparin, NS (concentrations above 1 Gm/L), phenytoin, piperacillin/tazobactam (Zosyn), sargramostim (Leukine), and sodium nitroprusside. IV line must be flushed with 2 ml of NS or D5W before and after administration. One manufacturer recommends that haloperidol not be mixed in syringe or solution with any other drug.

RATE OF ADMINISTRATION

Direct IV: 5 mg/min. When using multiple drugs, each individual drug should be given at correct rate. (Review text of each drug before administration.)

Intermittent IV: A single dose over 30 minutes.

Infusion: Up to 25 mg/hr has been used. Must be titrated by desired dose and patient response.

ACTIONS

An antipsychotic agent structurally similar to the neuroleptic droperidol with effects similar to selected phenothiazines (e.g., prochlorperazine [Compazine], perphenazine [Trilafon]). A potent dopamine blocker, it produces marked tranquilization and sedation and has a potent antiemetic action. Has minimum effect on cardiac, pulmonary, renal, hepatic, or hematopoietic functions. Peak plasma concentrations occur within 10 to 20 minutes. Half-life is 14 hours. Metabolized in the liver and excreted in urine and feces.

INDICATIONS AND USES

All IV uses are unlabeled. Control acute delirium, especially in emergency situations involving psychotic patients. ■ Control of agitation or acute delirium interfering with appropriate treatment of cancer, cardiac, surgical, respiratory, and medical patients in intensive care units. ■ May be given concurrently with lorazepam (Ativan) or midazolam (Versed). Both haloperidol and lorazepam have been given concurrently with morphine in agitation or hydromorphone (Dilaudid) in cancer patients. ■ Antiemetic in cancer chemotherapy and in surgery patients. ■ Treatment of intractable hiccups.

CONTRAINDICATIONS

Severe toxic CNS depression or comatose states from any cause. ■ Hypersensitivity to haloperidol. ■ Patients with Parkinson's diseases.

PRECAUTIONS

Not FDA approved for IV use but is being used. Check vial carefully: only haloperidol lactate can be used IV. Haloperidol decanoate contains sesame oil and is for IM use only. ■ Use should be restricted to closely monitored patients. ■ Rule out other possible causes of agitation (e.g., metabolic and systemic abnormalities, drug toxicity, drug withdrawal) before initiating haloperidol. ■ Use caution with known history of seizures or EEG abnormalities; may lower seizure threshold. Maintain adequate anticonvulsant therapy. ■ Use caution in the presence of severe cardiovascular disorders. ■ May cause severe neurotoxicity in patients with thyrotoxicosis; use caution. ■ Development of tardive dyskinesia, usually associated with chronic therapy, has been reported after brief treatment periods at low doses. ■ Neuroleptic malignant syndrome, a rare syndrome manifested by hyperpyrexia, muscle rigidity, autonomic instability and altered mental status, may develop hours to months after drug initiation. ■ Antiemetic effects may obscure signs of toxicity of other drugs or mask symptoms of another disease. ■ May potentiate Parkinson's disease; note Contraindications.

Monitor: A potent drug. Monitor the patient constantly. Resuscitation equipment, a narcotic antagonist (if a narcotic has been used concurrently), IV infusion line, and drugs to manage hypotension, cardiac arrhythmias, and extrapyramidal symptoms must be readily available.

Maternal/child: Safety for use in pregnancy, lactation, and children under 12 years not established.

Elderly: Note Dose adjustments. ■ May have increased serum levels. Sensitivity to postural hypotension, anticholinergic, and sedative effects increased. ■ Risk of extrapyramidal side effects (e.g., tardive dyskinesia) increased.

DRUG/LAB INTERACTIONS

May cause life-threatening hypotension and bradycardia with propranolol (Inderal). ■ Concurrent use with epinephrine may result in severe hypotension and tachycardia. ■ May potentiate CNS depressants (e.g., anesthetics, narcotics, alcohol). CNS and respiratory depression, as well as hypotensive effects, may all be potentiated. ■ May cause increased intraocular pressure with anticholinergic drugs (e.g., atropine), including antiparkinsonian agents. ■ Note Dose adjustments.

SIDE EFFECTS

Considered to have a good range of safety, even in large total daily doses.

Minor: Hypotension (mild), muscle twitching, prolongation of corrected QT interval, tremors, tachycardia.

Major: Apnea, cardiac arrest, excessive sedation, extrapyramidal symptoms (rare), hypotension (severe), impaired vision, jaundice, neuroleptic malignant syndrome, respiratory depression. Numerous other side effects common to phenothiazines and neuroleptic drugs are possible but not common with IV use.

ANTIDOTE

Notify the physician of any side effect. If minor side effects progress or major side effects occur, discontinue the drug, support the patient, treat symptomatically, and notify the physician. Rule out hypovolemia, other hypotensive agents, low cardiac output, and sepsis as causes of hypotension. Then, if indicated, treat hypotension with fluid therapy or vasopressors such as metaraminol (Aramine) or phenylephrine (Neo-Synephrine). Epinephrine is contraindicated for hypotension. Further hypotension will occur. Monitor ECG for QT prolongation or torsades de pointes. Treat cardiac arrhythmias as indicated. Treat extrapyramidal symptoms with benztropine mesylate (Cogentin) or diphenhydramine hydrochloride (Benadryl). Dialysis is not effective in overdose. Resuscitate as necessary.

HEMIN
Porphyrin inhibitor

Panhematin

USUAL DOSE
A single dose of 1 to 4 mg/kg of body weight/24 hr of hematin for 3 to 14 days. This dose could be repeated in 12 hours for severe cases. Never exceed a total dose of 6 mg/kg/24 hr. Length of treatment dependent on severity of symptoms and clinical response. Note Precautions.

DILUTION
Each vial containing 313 mg of hemin must be diluted with 43 ml of SW for injection (provides 301 mg of hematin). Shake well for 2 to 3 minutes to ensure dissolution. Each 1 ml contains 7 mg hematin. Each 0.14 ml contains 1 mg hematin. May be given directly from vial as an infusion or through Y-tube or three-way stopcock of infusion set. Use of a 0.45-micron or smaller filter recommended.

Storage: Store in refrigerator at 2° to 8° C. Contains no preservative, decomposes rapidly; discard unused solution.

INCOMPATIBLE WITH
Specific information not available. Do not mix with other drugs.

RATE OF ADMINISTRATION
A single dose evenly distributed over 10 to 15 minutes.

ACTIONS
An iron-containing metalloporphyrin enzyme inhibitor extracted from red blood cells. Inhibits rate of porphyria/heme biosynthesis in the liver and bone marrow by an unknown mechanism. Induces remission of symptoms only; not curative. Some excretion occurs in urine and feces.

INDICATIONS AND USES
To control symptoms of recurrent attacks of acute intermittent porphyria in selected patients (often related to the menstrual cycle in susceptible women).

CONTRAINDICATIONS
Hypersensitivity to hemin; porphyria cutanea tarda.

PRECAUTIONS
Confirm diagnosis of acute porphyria before use (positive Watson-Schwartz or Hoechst test). ■ Alternate therapy of 400 Gm glucose/24 hr for 1 to 2 days should be tried before use of hemin initiated. ■ Give as early as possible with onset of attack to achieve the most benefit. ■ Must be given before irreversible neuronal damage of porphyria has begun.

Monitor: Use of a large arm vein or central venous catheter recommended to avoid phlebitis. ■ Effectiveness monitored by decrease in urine concentration of S-aminolevulinic acid (ALA), uroporphyrinogen (UPG), or porphobilinogen (PBG).

Maternal/child: Pregnancy category C: Safety for use during pregnancy, lactation, and in children not established.

DRUG/LAB INTERACTIONS

Action inhibited by estrogens, barbiturates, and steroid metabolites. Avoid concurrent use. ■ Has anticoagulant effects. Avoid concurrent use with anticoagulants (e.g., heparin, warfarin [Coumadin]).

SIDE EFFECTS

Almost nonexistent with usual dosage and appropriate technique; fever, phlebitis. Reversible renal shutdown has been reported with excessive doses.

ANTIDOTE

Discontinue temporarily if known or questionable side effect appears, and notify physician. Renal shutdown of overdose has responded to ethacrynic acid (Edecrin) and mannitol. Treat anaphylaxis (antihistamines, epinephrine, corticosteroids) and resuscitate as necessary.

HEPARIN SODIUM   Anticoagulant

🍁Hepalean, Heparin Lock-Flush,
Hep-Lock, Hep-Lock PF, Hep-Lock U/P,
Liquaemin sodium, Liquaemin sodium
Preservative Free
                                                          pH 5.0 to 8.0

USUAL DOSE

Intermittent injection: 10,000 units initially. Dosage is repeated every 4 to 6 hours and adjusted according to clotting time. Usually 5,000 to 10,000 units.

IV infusion: 20,000 to 40,000 units/24 hr in normal saline or other compatible infusion solution. Available premixed, 12,500 units/250 ml or 25,000 units/250 or 500 ml. An initial bolus dose of 5,000 units is required.

Open heart surgery: 150 to 400 units/kg of body weight during surgical procedure.

Maintain patency of infusion needle, catheter, or implanted port: 1,000 to 1,500 units to each 1,000 ml IV fluid.

Additive to TPN and IV fat emulsion: 1 to 2 units/ml.

Maintain patency of central venous lines and selected peripheral lines: 10 to 500 units diluted in sufficient milliliters of NS to reach the tip of the needle, catheter, or implanted port. Use after each medication injection or every 8 to 24 hours.

Blood transfusion: 400 to 600 units/100 ml whole blood.

Treatment of ulcerative colitis (investigational): 30,000 to 36,000 units IV daily or 10,000 units SC twice daily. Concomitant administration of sulfasalazine (Azulfidine) is recommended (heparin treatment ineffective without sulfasalazine). Maintain with SC heparin. Improvement should be noted in 1 to 16 weeks. Treatment may continue for more than 6 months.

Reduce incidence of thrombophlebitis from TPN infusions in peripheral lines (investigational): 1,500 U and hydrocortisone 15 mg as IV additives to TPN solution. A 5-mg nitroglycerin transdermal patch is applied to the catheter insertion site and changed daily.

PEDIATRIC DOSE

Intermittent IV: An initial dose of 50 units/kg of body weight is followed by a maintenance dose of 50 to 100 units/kg every 4 hours adjusted to coagulation tests, or 20,000 units/M^2/24 hr as a continuous infusion.

DOSE ADJUSTMENTS

Reduction of initial dose indicated in low-birth-weight infants and may be indicated in patients 60 years of age and older (especially women). Dose is based on coagulation tests (see Monitor).

■ Increased dose may be required in smokers (half-life shortened and elimination rate increased).

DILUTION

May be given undiluted or diluted in any given amount of normal saline, dextrose, or Ringer's solution for infusion and given direct IV or as an intermittent IV injection or continuous IV infusion. Invert container a minimum of 6 times to ensure adequate mixing of heparin with solution in all situations. Available premixed for all uses in suitable dilutions.

Blood transfusion: Add 7,500 units heparin to 100 ml NS injection. Add 6 to 8 ml of this sterile solution to each 100 ml of whole blood.

INCOMPATIBLE WITH

Alteplase (tPA), amikacin (Amikin), amiodarone (Cordarone), ampicillin (Amcill), atracurium (Tracrium), atropine, cephalothin (Keflin), chlordiazepoxide (Librium), chlorpromazine (Thorazine), ciprofloxacin (Cipro IV), codeine, cytarabine (ARA-C), dacarbazine (DTIC), daunorubicin (Cerubidine), diazepam (Valium), diltiazem (Cardizem), dobutamine (Dobutrex), doxorubicin (Adriamycin), droperidol (Inapsine), erythromycin (Ilotycin, Erythrocin), ergonovine, fentanyl/droperidol (Innovar), filgrastim (Neupogen), gentamicin (Garamycin), haloperidol (Haldol), hyaluronidase, hydrocortisone (Solu-Cortef), hydroxyzine (Vistaril), idarubicin (Idamycin), insulin (aqueous), kanamycin (Kantrex), labetalol (Trandate), levorphanol (Levo-Dromoran), meperidine (Demerol), metaraminol (Aramine), methadone, methicillin (Staphcillin), methylprednisone (Solu-Medrol), morphine sulfate, netilmicin (Netromycin), penicillin G, pentazocine (Talwin), phenytoin (Dilantin), polymyxin B (Aerosporin), procainamide (Pronestyl), prochlorperazine (Compazine), promazine (Sparine), promethazine (Phenergan), quinidine, streptomycin, tobramycin (Nebcin), vancomycin (Vancocin), vinblastine (Velban).

RATE OF ADMINISTRATION

First 1,000 units or fraction thereof over 1 minute. After this test dose, any single injection (5,000 units or fraction thereof) may be given over 1 minute. A continuous IV infusion may be given over 4 to 24 hours, depending on specific dosage of heparin required, amount of heparin added, and amount of infusion fluid used as a diluent. Continuous IV infusion is the preferred method of administration. Use an infusion pump for accuracy.

Treatment of ulcerative colitis: A daily dose as a continuous infusion over 24 hours.

ACTIONS

An anticoagulant with immediate and predictable effects on the blood. Heparin combines with other factors in the blood to inhibit the conversion of prothrombin to thrombin and fibrinogen to fibrin. Adhesiveness of platelets is reduced. Well-established clots are not dissolved, but growth is prevented and newer clots may be dissolved. Duration of action is short, about 4 to 6 hours. Average half-life is 30 to 180 minutes. The half-life is prolonged by higher doses and in liver or kidney disease and shortened in patients with pulmonary embolism. Does not cross the placental barrier. Metabolized in the liver and excreted by the kidneys. Has a wide margin of safety.

INDICATIONS AND USES

Prevention and/or treatment of all types of thromboses and emboli including deep vein thrombosis (DVT), pulmonary emboli (PE), and embolization associated with atrial fibrillation (AF). ▪ Diagnosis and treatment of disseminated intravascular coagulation (DIC). ▪ Prevention of clotting in surgery of the heart or blood vessels, during blood transfusion, and hemodialysis. ▪ Adjunct in treatment of coronary occlusion with acute myocardial infarction (MI). ▪ Prevention of rethrombosis or reocclusion during MI after thrombolytic therapy (e.g., alteplase, anistreplase, streptokinase). ▪ Maintain patency of needle, catheter, or implanted port during prolonged IV infusion. ▪ Maintain patency of heparin lock needle for intermittent medication injection or vein access. ▪ Additive to TPN to decrease incidence of subclavian vein thrombosis and to IV fat emulsion to activate lipoprotein lipase system and improve clearance of emulsion from bloodstream.

Unlabeled uses: Prevention of left ventricular thrombi and cerebrovascular accidents after MI. ▪ Continuous infusion for treatment of myocardial ischemia in unstable angina refractory to conventional treatment. ▪ Prevention of cerebral thrombosis in the evolving stroke.

Investigational use: Treatment of chronic, refractory, symptomatic ulcerative colitis. ▪ Reduce incidence of thrombophlebitis with peripheral TPN. Used concurrently with hydrocortisone and NTG transdermal patch.

CONTRAINDICATIONS

Blood dyscrasias (e.g., severe thrombocytopenia), hypersensitivity to heparin (derived from animal protein), inadequate laboratory facilities, uncontrolled bleeding except in DIC.

PRECAUTIONS

Read label carefully. Comes in many strengths. ▪ Unit to milligram conversions are not consistent. ▪ Use extreme caution in any disease state where risk of hemorrhage may be increased (i.e., subacute bacterial endocarditis); arterial sclerosis; aneurysm; severe hypertension; during or following spinal tap, spinal anesthesia, or major surgery; hemophilia; thrombocytopenia; ulcerative lesions; diverticulitis; ulcerative colitis; continuous tube drainage of the stomach or small intestine; threatened abortion; menstruation; alcohol abuse; tuberculosis; visceral carcinoma; and severe biliary, liver, or renal disease. ▪ Resistance to heparin increased in cancer, fever, infections with thrombosing tendencies, MI, postoperative states, thrombophlebitis, and thrombosis. ▪ Use caution if administering ACD-converted blood (variable). ▪ Some products contain the preservative benzyl alcohol associated with gasping syndrome in premature infants.

Monitor: Recent studies show a small reduction in phlebitis when longer IV catheters (30 cm) versus short (3 to 4 cm) are used for heparin infusion. ▪ Whole blood clotting time (WBCT), activated coagulation time (ACT), or activated partial thromboplastin time (aPTT) must be done before initial injection. Often done before each injection on the first day of treatment or every 4 hours with a continuous infusion. Usually repeated daily thereafter during IV therapy and more often if indicated. Depending on the test chosen the desired therapeutic level is approximately one and one half to three times greater than the control level. Confirm desired control level with physician. Obtain test just before next dose due in intermittent injection. Notify the physician if aPTT, ACT, or WBCT is above therapeutic level. ■ Decrease dosage gradually. Abrupt withdrawal may precipitate increased coagulability. ■ Monitor platelet count. Discontinue heparin if it falls below 100,000 or a thrombosis forms. Early or delayed thrombocytopenia can occur and may be dose related. May develop white clot syndrome, which may lead to skin necrosis, gangrene, MI, pulmonary embolism, and stroke. ■ Monitor hematocrit and occult blood in stool also. ■ May cause an increase in free fatty acid serum levels. Patients with dysbetalipoproteinemia cannot catabolize lipid fragments; will result in hyperlipidemia. ■ May cause hyperkalemia in patients with diabetes or renal insufficiency. ■ To avoid precipitation, irrigate heparin plug catheters with NS before and after injecting acidic or incompatible solutions. ■ Use extensive precautionary methods to prevent bleeding if patient requires IM injection, arterial puncture, or venipuncture.

Patient education: Report all episodes of bleeding and apply local pressure if indicated. ■ Report tarry stools. ■ Compliance with all measures to minimize bleeding is very important (e.g., avoid use of razors, toothbrushes, other sharp items). ■ Use caution while moving to avoid excess bumping.

Maternal/child: Pregnancy category C: Preferred anticoagulant in pregnancy but must be used with caution. Hemorrhage most likely to occur during the last trimester or postpartum. Has caused stillbirths and prematurity. ■ Not secreted in breast milk. ■ Risk of intraventricular hemorrhage four times greater in low-birth-weight infants. ■ Use heparin lock flush with caution in infants with diseases with an increased risk of hemorrhage. Use minimal doses and monitor carefully. ■ Note Dose adjustments and Precautions.

Elderly: Higher incidence of bleeding in patients 60 years of age and older (especially women).

DRUG/LAB INTERACTIONS

Nitroglycerin IV may cause heparin resistance; monitor coagulation status and adjust heparin dose if indicated. ■ Increased risk of bleeding with ACD-converted blood, adrenal cortical steroids (especially chronic therapeutic use), some cephalosporins (e.g., cefamandole [Mandol], ceforperazone [Cefobid], cefotetan, moxalactam [Moxam]), dextran, penicillins, platelet inhibitors (e.g., dipyridamole [Persantine], ticlopidine [Ticlid], phenylbutazone [Butazolidine]), hydroxychloroquine (Chloroquine), NSAIDs (e.g., ibuprofen [Motrin], indomethacin [Indocin], ketorolac [Toradol]), plicamycin (Mithracin), salicylates (e.g., aspirin), other thrombolytic agents (e.g., alteplase, anistreplase [Eminase], streptokinase), thyroid agents (e.g., methimazole [Tapazole], propylthiouracil), valproic acid (Depakote), or any drug that may cause hypothrombinemia, thrombocytopenia, GI ulceration, or hemorrhage. ■ Anticoagulant effect may be prolonged by Probenecid. ■ Resistance to heparin anticoagulation may occur following administration of streptokinase as a systemic thrombolytic agent, adjust dose of heparin based on more frequent aPTTs. ▪ Half-life may be decreased and elimination increased in smokers, reducing thrombolytic effect. ▪ Inhibited by antihistamines, digitalis, hydroxyzine (Vistaril), nicotine, tetracyclines, and others; may counteract anticoagulant action of heparin. ▪ Potentiates oral anticoagulants. ▪ Note Precautions/Monitor. ▪ Use caution when administered after other anticoagulants. Lab data may not provide an accurate baseline. ▪ Blood gas sample errors will occur if heparin is 10% or more of sample volume. ▪ Numerous lab values (e.g., imaging studies, thyroid, AST [SGOT], ALT [SGPT], free fatty acid, triglycerides, cholesterol) may be altered. Notify lab of heparin use. Diagnostic results may not be attainable.

SIDE EFFECTS

Bruising, epistaxis, hematuria, hemorrhage (10%), prolonged coagulation time (in excess of two to three times the control level), tarry stools or any other signs of bleeding, thrombocytopenia, white clot syndrome (platelet aggregation, arterial clotting). Allergic reactions, including anaphylaxis, do occur. Vasospastic reactions resulting in a painful, ischemic, cyanotic limb may develop. Alopecia, arthralgias, chest pain, cutaneous necrosis, headache, hypertension, itching on the plantar surface of the feet, osteoporosis, priapism (painful penile erection), rebound hyperlipidemia, and suppressed aldosterone synthesis have been reported. Several studies have shown that moderately high doses of heparin can cause excessive internal bleeding that may lead to paralyzing or lethal strokes. Fewer side effects occur with controlled continuous IV infusion as compared to intermittent.

ANTIDOTE

Discontinue the drug and notify the physician of any side effects. Protamine sulfate is a heparin antagonist and specifically indicated in overdose or desired heparin reversal. Each milligram of protamine neutralizes approximately 100 units heparin. Whole blood transfusion may be indicated. If thrombocytopenia or white clot syndrome occurs, a coumarin anticoagulant may be indicated.

HETASTARCH
Hespan

Plasma volume expander

pH 5.5

USUAL DOSE

Shock: Variable, depending on amount of fluid loss and resultant hemoconcentration. Initially 500 ml (30 Gm). Total dose should not exceed 1,500 ml/24 hr or 20 ml/kg of body weight; however, higher doses have been used in postoperative and trauma patients who have had severe blood loss.

Leukapheresis: 250 to 700 ml in continuous flow centrifugation procedures.

DILUTION

Available as a 6% solution in 500 ml containers properly diluted in NS and ready for use. Calculated osmolarity is approximately 310 mOsm/L.

Storage: Store at controlled room temperature. Do not freeze. Do not use if color is a turbid deep brown or a crystalline precipitate is visible.

INCOMPATIBLE WITH

Amikacin (Amikin), ampicillin, cefamandole (Mandol), cefazolin (Kefzol), cefonicid (Monocid), cefoperazone (Cefobid), cefotaxime (Claforan), cefoxitin (Mefoxin), cephalothin (Keflin), gentamicin (Garamycin), ranitidine (Zantac), theophylline, tobramycin (Nebcin).

RATE OF ADMINISTRATION

Variable, depending on indication, present blood volume, and patient response. Initial 500 ml may be given at rates approaching 20 ml/kg of body weight per hour. Reduce rate in burns or septic shock. If additional hydroxyethyl starch is required, reduce flow to lowest rate possible to maintain hemodynamic status. If pressure infusion is used (flexible containers), withdraw all air through medication port before infusing.

Leukapheresis: Usually infused at a constant ratio to venous whole blood, (i.e., 1:8).

ACTIONS

A synthetic polymer with properties similar to dextran. Approximates colloidal properties of human albumin. Provides hemodynamically significant plasma volume expansion in excess of the amount infused for about 24 hours. Dilutes total serum protein and hematocrit values. Increases erythrocyte sedimentation rate. Granulocyte collection by centrifuging becomes more efficient. Enzymatically degraded to molecules small enough to be excreted through the kidneys attached to glucose units.

INDICATIONS AND USES

As an adjunct in treatment of shock due to burns, hemorrhage, sepsis, surgery, or trauma. ▪ Adjunct in leukapheresis to improve harvesting and increase yield of granulocytes.

CONTRAINDICATIONS

Severe bleeding disorders, severe congestive heart failure, hypersensitivity to hetastarch, renal failure with oliguria or anuria.

PRECAUTIONS

For IV use only. ▪ Not a substitute for whole blood or plasma proteins. ▪ Use caution in heart disease, renal shutdown, congestive heart failure, pulmonary edema, and liver disease. ▪ Does not interfere with blood typing or cross-matching. ▪ Anaphylactic reactions have occurred. Patients allergic to corn may also be allergic to hetastarch.

Monitor: Monitor pulse, blood pressure, central venous pressure, and urine output every 5 to 15 minutes for the first hour and hourly thereafter while indicated. ▪ Maintain adequate hydration of patient with additional IV fluids. ▪ Change IV tubing or flush with NS before imposing blood. ▪ May reduce coagulability of the circulating blood. Observe patient for increased bleeding and/or circulatory overload. ▪ Hemoglobin, hematocrit, electrolyte, and serum protein evaluation are necessary during therapy. During leukapheresis also monitor leukocyte and platelet count, leukocyte differential, prothrombin time (PT), and partial thromboplastin time (PTT). ▪ Observe frequent donors carefully; may have a marked decline in platelet count and hemoglobin levels resulting from hemodilution by hetastarch and saline. Temporary declines in total protein, albumin, calcium, and fibrinogen may also be present.

Maternal/child: Pregnancy category C: No data available pertaining to use in pregnant women or in children. Not recommended for use in pregnancy, especially early pregnancy.

DRUG/LAB INTERACTIONS

May increase indirect bilirubin levels. Total bilirubin remained normal.

SIDE EFFECTS

Chills, circulatory overload, fever, headache, itching, muscle pains, peripheral edema, pulmonary edema, submaxillary and parotid glandular enlargement, urticaria, and vomiting. Anaphylaxis can occur.

ANTIDOTE

Notify the physician of any side effect. Discontinue the drug immediately at the first sign of an allergic reaction, provided other means of sustaining the circulation are available. Antihistamines such as diphenhydramine (Benadryl) are helpful. Ephedrine or epinephrine (Adrenalin) may also be indicated. Resuscitate as necessary.

HYDRALAZINE HYDROCHLORIDE
Antihypertensive
Vasodilator

Apresoline
pH 3.4 to 4.0

USUAL DOSE

10 to 40 mg. Begin with a low dose. Increase gradually as indicated. Repeat every 3 to 6 hours as necessary. Maximum dose is 300 to 400 mg/24 hr.

Eclampsia: 5 to 10 mg every 20 minutes. If no effect after a total dose of 20 mg, use another agent.

PEDIATRIC DOSE

0.1 to 0.2 mg/kg every 4 to 6 hours. Do not exceed 20 mg.

DOSE ADJUSTMENTS

Reduced dose may be required with advanced renal disease and in the elderly. ▪ Note Drug/lab interactions.

DILUTION

May be given undiluted. Do not add to IV solutions. May be given through Y-tube or three-way stopcock of infusion set. Color changes occur in most 10% dextrose solutions and after drawing through a metal filter. Use immediately after drawing up solution.

INCOMPATIBLE WITH

Aminophylline, ampicillin, calcium disodium edetate, chlorothiazide (Diuril), diazoxide (Hyperstat), ethacrynic acid (Edecrin), furosemide (Lasix), hydrocortisone (Solu-Cortef), mephentermine (Wyamine), methohexital (Brevital), nitroglycerin, phenobarbital (Luminal), verapamil (Calan), 10% fructose, 10% dextrose in lactated Ringer's injection.

RATE OF ADMINISTRATION
A single dose over 1 minute.

ACTIONS
A potent antihypertensive drug. It lowers blood pressure by direct relaxation of smooth muscle of arteries and arterioles. Peripheral vasodilation and decreased peripheral vascular resistance result. Heart rate, cardiac output, and strobe volume are all increased. Renal blood flow increased in some cases, while cerebral blood flow maintained. Onset of action is 10 to 20 minutes. Average duration of action is 2 to 4 hours. Metabolized by the liver and excreted in urine. Crosses placental barrier. Secreted in breast milk.

INDICATIONS AND USES
Severe essential hypertension. ■ Vasodilation in cardiogenic shock. ■ Drug of choice for pregnancy-induced hypertension (eclampsia).

CONTRAINDICATIONS
Hypersensitivity to hydralazine, coronary artery disease, mitral valvular rheumatic heart disease.

PRECAUTIONS
IV use recommended only when the oral route is not feasible. ■ Rarely the drug of choice for hypertension unless used in combination (effectiveness increased and side effects decreased) with spironolactone (Aldactone), reserpine (Serpasil), guanethidine (Ismelin), and thiazide diuretics. ■ Tolerance is easily developed but subsides about 7 days after the drug is discontinued. ■ Use caution in advanced renal disease, cerebrovascular accidents, congestive heart failure, coronary insufficiency, headache, increased intracranial pressure, and tachycardia. ■ Use in pregnancy should be limited to treatment of eclampsia.

Monitor: Check blood pressure every 5 minutes until stabilized at the desired level. Check every 15 minutes thereafter throughout crisis. Average maximum decrease occurs in 10 to 80 minutes. ■ Withdraw drug gradually to avoid rebound hypertension.

Patient education: Report chest pain, fatigue, fever, joint or muscle pain promptly.

Maternal/child: Pregnancy category C: Can cause fetal abnormalities (see Indications and Precautions). ■ Safety for use in children not established. ■ May be used in lactating women.

Elderly: Increased risk of hypotension ■ Consider age-related renal impairment.

DRUG/LAB INTERACTIONS
Sometimes used with a beta-adrenergic blocking drug (e.g., propranolol [Inderal]) or diuretics (e.g., hydrochlorothiazide [Aldactazide]); use caution, may potentiate effects. ■ Potentiated by anesthetics, MAO inhibitors (e.g., selegiline [Eldepryl]), and other antihypertensive agents. ■ Inhibits epinephrine, levarterenol (Levophed). ■ Use with diazoxide (Hyperstat IV) can cause profound hypotension. ■ NSAIDs (e.g., ibuprofen [Motrin]) may decrease antihypotensive effect.

SIDE EFFECTS
May often be minimized by initiating therapy with a small dose and increasing the dose gradually.

Minor: Anxiety, depression, dry mouth, flushing, headache, nausea, numbness, palpitations, paresthesia, postural hypotension, tachycardia, tingling, unpleasant taste, vomiting.

Major: Angina, blood dyscrasias, chills, coronary insufficiency, delirium, dependent edema, fever, ileus, lupus erythematosus (simulated), myocardial ischemia and infarction, rheumatoid syndrome (simulated), toxic psychosis.

ANTIDOTE

If minor side effects occur, notify the physician, who will probably treat them symptomatically. Beta-adrenergic blocking agents (e.g., propranolol [Inderal]) will control tachycardia. Pyridoxine will relieve numbness, tingling, and paresthesia. Antihistamines, barbiturates, and salicylates may be required. Treat hypotension with a vasopressor that is least likely to precipitate cardiac arrhythmias (methoxamine [Vasoxyl]). If side effects are progressive or any major side effects occur, discontinue the drug immediately and notify the physician. Treatment is symptomatic. Resuscitate as necessary. Occasionally methyldopa (Aldomet) will be used as a substitute, since it is effective for the same indications but has fewer side effects.

HYDROCORTISONE SODIUM PHOSPHATE / HYDROCORTISONE SODIUM SUCCINATE

Hormone
(Adrenocorticoid glucocorticoid)
Antiinflammatory
Antiemetic

Hydrocortone phosphate/
A-hydrocort, Solu-Cortef

pH 7.5 to 8.5 / 7.0 to 8.0

USUAL DOSE

The IV route is usually used in an emergency situation or when oral dosing is not feasible. Larger doses may be justified by patient condition. Repeat until adequate response, then decrease dose as indicated. Doses must be individualized and are not always reduced for children. High dose treatment is utilized until patient condition stabilizes, usually no longer than 48 to 72 hours.

Hydrocortisone phosphate: Average dose range is 15 to 240 mg repeated as necessary every 4 to 6 hours. Another source suggests 100 to 500 mg repeated every 2 to 6 hours. Total dose usually does not exceed 1 Gm/24 hr but may be higher in acute disease.

Acute adrenal insufficiency: 1 to 2 mg/kg initially, follow with 25 to 250 mg/24 hr in equally divided doses every 8 to 12 hours. Another source suggests 100 mg initially. Repeat every 8 to 12 hours in IV fluids.

Hydrocortisone sodium succinate: Average dose range is 100 to 500 mg repeated as necessary every 2 to 10 hours. For severe shock, doses up to 2 Gm or more every 2 to 4 hours have been given. Maximum dose is 8 Gm/24 hr. Never give less than 25 mg/24 hr.

Acute asthma: 100 to 500 mg every 6 hr.

Life-threatening shock: 50 mg/kg initially. Repeat in 4 hours and/or every

24 hours as needed or

0.5 to 2 Gm initially. Repeat every 2 to 6 hours as needed.

Physiological replacement: 0.25 to 0.35 mg/kg daily (usually given IM).

PEDIATRIC DOSE

Hydrocortisone phosphate:

0.16 to 1 mg/kg of body weight/24 hr or 6 to 30 mg/M^2. May be given as a single dose or equally divided and given every 12 hours. Dose varies with disease.

Adrenal insufficiency: 0.19 to 0.28 mg/kg/24 hr equally divided and given every 8 hours.

Hydrocortisone sodium succinate:

Acute asthma: 1 to 2 mg/kg/dose every 6 hours for 24 hours; then 2 to 4 mg/kg/24 hr in equally divided doses every 6 hours. For status asthmaticus another source suggests a *loading dose* of 4 to 8 mg/kg up to a maximum dose of 250 mg. *Maintenance dose:* 8 mg/kg/24 hr in equally divided doses every 6 hours.

Antiinflammatory: 0.8 to 4 mg/kg/24 hr in equally divided doses every 6 hours.

DOSE ADJUSTMENTS

Reduced dose may be required in the elderly. ▪ Note Drug/lab interactions.

DILUTION

Hydrocortisone phosphate: May be given without mixing or dilution. Always use a separate syringe for hydrocortisone. May be added to normal saline or dextrose solutions and given by IV infusion. Solution must be used within 24 hours of dilution. Sensitive to heat.

Hydrocortisone sodium succinate: Available in Act-O-Vials and Univials, which are reconstituted by removing the protective cap, turning the rubber stopper a quarter turn, and pressing down, allowing the diluent into the lower chamber. Agitate gently. Using sterile techniques, a needle can be easily inserted through the center of the rubber stopper to withdraw the solution. Also available in flip top vials. For these other preparations, reconstitute each 250 mg or fraction thereof with 2 ml bacteriostatic water for injection. Agitate gently to mix solution. May be given direct IV, or each 100 mg (250 mg, 500 mg, etc.) may be further diluted in at least 100 ml (250 ml, 500 ml, etc.) but not more than 1,000 ml of D5W, NS, or D5/NS. Sensitive to heat and light. Discard unused solutions after 3 days. If fluid restriction is necessary 100 to 500 mg may be diluted in 50 ml of the above solutions. Stable for 4 hours.

INCOMPATIBLE WITH

Hydrocortisone phosphate: Amobarbital (Amytal), calcium gluconate, cephalothin (Keflin), chloramphenicol (Chloromycetin), doxapram (Dopram), erythromycin, heparin, kanamycin (Kantrex), metaraminol (Aramine), methicillin (Staphcillin), nitrofurantoin (Ivadantin), pentobarbital (Nembutal), phenobarbital (Luminal), phytonadione (Aquamephyton), prochlorperazine (Compazine), promazine (Sparine), sargramostin (Leukine), vancomycin (Vancocin), warfarin (Coumadin).

Hydrocortisone sodium succinate: Aminophylline, amobarbital (Amytal), ampicillin, bleomycin (Blenoxane), chlorpromazine (Thorazine), ciprofloxacin (Cipro-IV), colistimethate (Coly-Mycin M), cytarabine (ARA-C), diazepam (Valium), dimenhydrinate (Dramanate), diphenhydramine (Benadryl), doxapram (Dopram), doxorubicin (Adriamycin), ephedrine, ergotamine, furosemide (Lasix), heparin, hyaluronidase, hydralazine (Apresoline), hydroxyzine (Vistaril), idarubicin (Idamycin), kanamycin (Kantrex), lidocaine, lobeline, magnesium sulfate, meperidine (Demerol), metaraminol (Aramine), methicillin (Staphcillin), methylprednisolone (Solu-Medrol), midazolam (Versed), nafcillin (Unipen), netilmicin (Netromycin), pentobarbital (Nembutal), phenobarbital (Luminal), phenytoin (Dilantin), prochlorperazine (Compazine), promazine (Sparine), promethazine (Phenergan), sargramostim (Leukine), secobarbital (Seconal), thiamylal (Surital), tolazoline (Priscoline), vancomycin (Vancocin).

RATE OF ADMINISTRATION

Hydrocortisone phosphate: Direct IV: 25 mg or fraction thereof over 1 minute. Decrease rate of injection if any complaints of burning or tingling along injection site.

Hydrocortisone sodium succinate: Direct IV: Each 500 mg or fraction there-of over 30 seconds to 1 minute. Extend to 10 minutes for larger doses. Direct IV is usually the route of choice and eliminates the possibility of overloading the patient with IV fluids. At the discretion of the physician, a continuous infusion may be given, properly diluted over the specified time desired.

ACTIONS

Both agents contain the principal hormone secreted by the adrenal cortex and have both glucocorticoid and mineralocorticoid properties. Have potent metabolic, antiinflammatory, and innumerable other effects. Peak plasma levels achieved promptly. Metabolized in the liver and excreted as inactive metabolites in the urine. Crosses placental barrier. Secreted in breast milk.

INDICATIONS AND USES

Agents of choice for adrenocortical insufficiency; total, relative, and operative. ■ Agents of choice for acute exacerbation of disease for patients on steroid therapy. ■ Occasionally used for asthma or shock, but non-mineralocorticoid steroids are preferred (e.g., dexamethasone, methylprednisolone).

Investigational use: Hydrocortisone 15 mg and heparin 1,500 units as additives to TPN to reduce thrombophlebitis in peripheral lines. A 5-mg transdermal patch of NTG is applied to the catheter insertion site and changed daily.

CONTRAINDICATIONS

Absolute contraindications except in life-threatening situations: Hypersensitivity to any product component including sulfites; systemic fungal infections.

Relative contraindications: Active or latent peptic ulcer, active or healed tuberculosis, acute psychoses, chickenpox, congestive heart failure, diabetes mellitus, diverticulitis, fresh intestinal anastomoses, hypertension, myasthenia gravis, ocular herpes simplex, osteoporosis, pregnancy, psychotic tendencies, renal insufficiency, thromboembolic tendencies, vaccinia.

PRECAUTIONS

To avoid relative adrenocortical insufficiency, do not stop therapy abruptly. Taper off. Patient is observed carefully, especially under stress, for up to 2 years. The exception is very short-term therapy. ■ Prophylactic antacids may prevent peptic ulcer complications.

Monitor: Monitor electrolytes. May cause sodium retention and potassium and calcium excretion. May cause hypertension secondary to fluid and electrolyte disturbances. ■ May mask signs of infection. ■ May increase insulin needs in diabetes. ■ Administer before 9 AM to reduce suppression of individual's own adrenocortical activity. ■ Periodic ophthalmic exams may be necessary with prolonged treatment. ■ Note Drug/lab interactions.

Patient education: Report edema, tarry stools, or weight gain promptly. Anorexia, diarrhea, dizziness, fatigue, low blood sugar, nausea, weakness, weight loss, and vomiting may indicate adrenal insufficiency after dose reduction or discontinuing therapy; report any of these symptoms. ■ May mask signs of infection and/or decrease resistance. ■ Diabetics may have an increased requirement for insulin or oral hypoglycemics. ■ Avoid immunization with live vaccines. ■ Carry ID stating steroid dependent if receiving prolonged therapy.

Maternal/child: Pregnancy category C: Could produce fetal abnormalities. ■ Discontinue breast feeding. ■ Observe newborn for hypoadrenalism if mother has received large doses. ■ Some preparations contain benzyl alcohol; do not use in neonates. ■ Observe growth and development in long-term use in children.

Elderly: Reduced muscle mass and plasma volume may require a reduced dose. ■ Monitor blood pressure, blood glucose, and electrolytes carefully; increased risk of hypertension. ■ Higher risk of glucocorticoid induced osteoporosis. ■ Avoid aluminum-based antacids (risk of Alzheimer's disease).

DRUG/LAB INTERACTIONS

Aminoglutethimide (Cytadren) and mitotane (Lysodren) suppress adrenal function of corticosteroids. Monitor carefully if concurrent use is necessary. ■ Metabolism increased and effects reduced by hepatic enzyme inducing agents (e.g., alcohol, barbiturates [e.g., phenobarbital], hydantoins [e.g., phenytoin (Dilantin)], and rifampin [Rifadin]); dose adjustment may be required when adding or deleting from drug profile. ■ Risk of hypokalemia increased with amphotericin B, or potassium-depleting diuretics (e.g., thiazides, furosemide, ethacrynic acid). Monitor potassium levels and cardiac function. Increased risk of digitalis (e.g., digoxin), toxicity secondary to hypokalemia. ■ May also decrease effectiveness of potassium supplements; monitor serum potassium. ■ Diuretics decrease sodium and fluid retention effects of corticosteroids; corticosteroids decrease sodium excretion and diuretic effects of diuretics. ■ May antagonize effects of anticholinesterases (e.g., neostigmine), isoniazid, salicylates, and somatrem; dose adjustments may be required. ■ Clearance decreased and effects increased with estrogens, oral contraceptives, and ketoconazole (Nizoral). ■ May interact with anticoagulants, nondepolarizing muscle relaxants (e.g., doxacurium [Nuromax]), or theophyllines; may inhibit or potentiate action. ■ Monitor patients receiving insulin or thyroid hormones carefully; dose adjustments of either or both agents may be required. ■ Use with ritodrine (Yutopar) has caused pulmonary edema in the mother, discontinue both agents with onset of S/S of pulmonary edema. ■ Do not vaccinate with attenuated-virus vaccines (e.g., smallpox) during therapy. ■ Altered protein-binding capacity will impact effectiveness of this drug. ■ Note Dose adjustments.

SIDE EFFECTS

Do occur but are usually reversible: alteration of glucose metabolism including hyperglycemia and glycosuria; Cushing's syndrome (moon face, fat pads, etc.); electrolyte and calcium imbalance; euphoria or other psychic disturbances; hypersensitivity reactions including anaphylaxis; increased blood pressure; increased intracranial pressure; masking of infection; menstrual irregularities; perforation and hemorrhage from aggravation of peptic ulcer; protein catabolism with negative nitrogen balance; spontaneous fractures; sweating, headache, or weakness; thromboembolism; transitory burning or tingling; and many others.

ANTIDOTE

Notify the physician of any side effect. Will probably treat the side effect if necessary. Resuscitate as necessary for anaphylaxis and notify physician. Keep epinephrine immediately available.

HYDROMORPHONE HYDROCHLORIDE

Dilaudid

Narcotic analgesic
(agonist)

pH 4.0 to 5.5

USUAL DOSE

Older children and adults: Direct IV: 1 to 4 mg every 4 to 6 hours.

Infusion: In selected terminally ill cancer patients hydromorphone may be administered in doses as high as 2 to 9 mg/hr. Must be administered through a controlled infusion device that may be patient activated. The initial loading dose, the continuous background infusion to provide a level of pain relief and maintain patency of the vein, additional patient-activated doses with specific time interval, additional health professional-provided boluses with specific time interval, and the total dose allowed per hour must be determined by the physician specialist and individualized for each patient. When seeking the required dose to achieve pain relief for an individual patient, increases in increments of at least 25% of the previous dose are suggested. May lower slightly if pain controlled but patient is too drowsy; or lower dose and increase frequency.

DOSE ADJUSTMENTS

Reduced dose or extended intervals may be required in impaired renal or hepatic function and in the elderly or debilitated patients. ■ Note Drug/lab interactions.

DILUTION

Direct IV: To facilitate titration, each dose should be diluted with 5 ml of SW or NS. May give through Y-tube or three-way stopcock of infusion set.

Infusion: Each 0.1 to 1 mg is usually diluted in 1 ml NS to provide 0.1 to 1 mg/ml for use in a narcotic syringe infusor system. Available in 1-, 2-, 4-, or 10-mg/ml ampoules. Use concentrated preparations for larger doses. May be diluted in larger amounts of D5W, D5/NS, D5/1/2NS, or

NS (concentration is usually 1 mg/ml) for infusion and given through a standard infusion pump (requires very close titration).

Storage: Store below 40° C and protect from light.

INCOMPATIBLE WITH

Alkalies, ampicillin (Polycillin-N), bromides, cefazolin (Kefzol), dexamethasone (selected), diazepam (Valium), gallium nitrate (Ganite), iodides, minocycline (Minocin), pentobarbital (Nembutal), phenobarbital (Luminal), phenytoin (Dilantin), prochlorperazine (Compazine), sargramostim (Leukine), sodium bicarbonate, thiopental (Pentothal).

RATE OF ADMINISTRATION

Direct IV: 2 mg or fraction thereof properly diluted solution over 2 to 5 minutes. Frequently titrated according to symptom relief and respiratory rate.

Infusion: All parameters (outlined in Usual dose) should be ordered by the physician. Any dose requiring a controlled infusion device requires accurate titration and close monitoring.

ACTIONS

An opium derivative narcotic analgesic closely related to morphine. Provides potent analgesia without hypnotic effects. Six times more potent than morphine milligram for milligram. Onset of action is 10 to 15 minutes and lasts 2 to 3 hours. Hydromorphone is metabolized in the liver and excreted in the urine. Crosses placental barrier. May be secreted in breast milk.

INDICATIONS AND USES

Moderate to severe, acute or chronic pain, especially in situations in which a hypnotic effect is not desirable, such as postoperatively or in some malignancies.

CONTRAINDICATIONS

Acute bronchial asthma, diarrhea caused by poisoning until toxic material eliminated, known hypersensitivity to opiates, pulmonary edema caused by chemical respiratory irritant, respiratory depression, status asthmaticus, upper airway obstruction.

PRECAUTIONS

Use caution in the elderly or debilitated and in patients with impaired hepatic or renal function, pulmonary disease, or concurrent anticoagulation therapy. ■ Use extreme caution in craniotomy, head injury, and increased intracranial pressure. Respiratory depression may cause an increased PCO_2, cerebral vasodilation, and increased intracranial pressure. Clinical course of head injury may be obscured. ■ Symptoms of acute abdominal conditions may be masked. ■ Cough reflex may be suppressed. ■ May cause apnea in the asthmatic. ■ Tolerance to hydromorphone gradually increases. A marked increase in dose may precipitate seizures in presence of a history of convulsive disorders. ■ Physical dependence can develop but is not a factor in the presence of chronic pain of malignancy.

Monitor: Oxygen, controlled respiratory equipment, and naloxone (Narcan) must be available. ■ Monitor vital signs and observe patient frequently to continuously based on amount of dose. Keep patient supine; orthostatic hypotension and fainting may occur; less likely with continuous low doses, but observe closely during ambulation. ■ Uncontrolled pain causes sleep deprivation, decreases pain threshold, and increases pain. When pain is finally controlled, expect the patient to sleep more until recovery from sleep deprivation. ■ Stool softeners and/or laxatives will be required to avoid constipation and fecal impaction, especially with increased doses and extended use. Maintain adequate hydration. ■ Symptoms of acute abdominal conditions may be masked. ■ May increase ventricular response rate in presence of supraventricular tachycardias. ■ Cough reflex is suppressed.

Patient education: Avoid alcohol or other CNS depressants (e.g., barbiturates, benzodiazepines [e.g., diazepam (Valium)]). ■ May cause blurred vision, drowsiness, or dizziness; use caution in tasks that require alertness. ■ May be habit forming.

Maternal/child: Pregnancy category C: Safety for use during pregnancy or lactation not established. Benefits must outweigh risks. ■ Note Contraindications.

Elderly: Note Precautions. ■ May be more susceptible to effects (e.g., respiratory depression, urinary retention, constipation). ■ Analgesia should be effective with lower doses. ■ Consider-age related organ impairment.

DRUG/LAB INTERACTIONS

Potentiated by phenothiazines and other CNS depressants such as narcotic analgesics, alcohol, anticholinergics, antihistamines, barbiturates, hypnotics, sedatives, MAO inhibitors (e.g., selegiline [Eldepryl]), neuromuscular blocking agents (e.g., tubocurarine) and psychotropic agents. Reduced dosages of both drugs may be indicated.

SIDE EFFECTS

Nausea, vomiting, and drowsiness are less frequent than with morphine.

Minor: Anorexia, constipation, dizziness, skin rash, urinary retention, urticaria.

Major: Anaphylaxis, hypotension, respiratory depression, somnolence.

ANTIDOTE

Notify the physician of any side effect. If minor side effects progress or any major side effect occurs, discontinue the drug and notify the physician. Treat anaphylaxis as indicated or resuscitate as necessary. Naloxone (Narcan) will reverse serious respiratory depression.

L-HYOSCYAMINE SULFATE

Anticholinergic
GI antispasmodic
Diagnostic agent

Levsin   pH 3.0 to 6.5

USUAL DOSE

GI disorders: 0.25 to 0.5 mg (0.5 to 1.0 ml) at 4-hour intervals 2 to 4 times/day.

Hypotonic duodenography: 0.25 to 0.5 mg 5 to 10 minutes prior to the diagnostic procedure.

Reversal of neuromuscular blockade: 0.2 mg for each 1 mg of neostigmine or equivalent dose of physostigmine and pyridostigmine.

Adjunct to anesthesia: 5 mcg/kg (0.005 mg/kg) 30 to 60 minutes prior to anesthesia.

Antiarrhythmic: 0.125 mg as needed.

PEDIATRIC DOSE

Adjunct to anesthesia (children over 2 years of age): 5 mcg/kg (0.005 mg/kg) 30 to 60 minutes prior to anesthesia.

DOSE ADJUSTMENTS

Note Drug/lab interactions.

DILUTION

May be given undiluted. Administer through Y-tube or three-way stopcock of infusion tubing.

Storage: Store below 40° C.

INCOMPATIBLE WITH

Specific information not available.

RATE OF ADMINISTRATION

A single dose over at least 1 minute.

ACTIONS

A chemically pure anticholinergic/antispasmodic component of belladonna alkaloids. Affects peripheral cholinergic receptors in autonomic effector cells of smooth muscle, cardiac muscle, sinoatrial node, atrioventricular node, and exocrine glands. Does not affect autonomic ganglia. Inhibits GI motility, reduces gastric secretions, and controls excessive pharyngeal, tracheal, and bronchial secretions. Onset of action is 2 to 3 minutes and lasts 4 to 6 hours. Metabolized, to a small extent, in the liver and excreted in urine. Crosses placental barrier. Traces occur in breast milk.

INDICATIONS AND USES

Adjunctive therapy in GI disorders. ■ Hypotonic duodenography. ■ Adjunct to anesthesia, reducing secretions and blocking vagal inhibitory reflexes. ■ To improve radiographic visibility of the kidneys. ■ Reduction of drug-induced bradycardia during surgery. ■ Antidote for overdose of anticholinesterase agents (reversal of neuromuscular blockade).

CONTRAINDICATIONS

Glaucoma, hypersensitivity, intestinal atony of the elderly or debilitated, toxic megacolon, myasthenia gravis, obstructive disease of the GI tract, obstructive uropathy, paralytic ileus, ulcerative colitis, unstable cardiovascular status in acute hemorrhage.

PRECAUTIONS

Use caution in autonomic neuropathy, cardiac arrhythmias (especially tachycardia), congestive heart failure, coronary artery disease, dehydration, hypertension, hyperthyroidism, and renal disease.

Monitor: Urinary retention can be avoided if the patient voids just before each dose.

Patient education: Use caution in any task requiring alertness. ■ Report persistent constipation, difficulty in urination, dry mouth, and increased sensitivity to light.

Maternal/child: Pregnancy category C: Safety not established; benefits must outweigh risks. ■ May cause toxicity to infant during lactation or reduce milk production.

Elderly: May cause agitation, confusion, drowsiness, or excitement. ■ Increased risk of constipation, dryness of mouth, urinary retention.

■ May precipitate undiagnosed glaucoma. ■ May increase memory impairment.

DRUG/LAB INTERACTIONS

Potentiated by alkalinizing agents, amantadine, synthetic narcotic analgesics, tricyclic antidepressants (e.g., amitriptyline [Elavil]), antihistamines, haloperidol, MAO inhibitors (e.g., selegiline [Eldepryl]), phenothiazines (e.g., chlorpromazine [Thorazine]), and many others. Reduced dose of either or both drugs may be indicated. ■ Antagonized by histamine, reserpine, and others. ■ Use caution with digoxin, cholinergics, diphenhydramine (Benadryl), levodopa, and neostigmine. May cause adverse effects. ■ Will cause cardiac arrhythmias with cyclopropane anesthesia.

SIDE EFFECTS

Anaphylaxis, blurred vision, cycloplegia, decreased sweating, drowsiness, dry mouth, headache, heat prostration, increased ocular tension, mydriasis, nervousness, palpitations, suppression of lactation, tachycardia, urinary hesitancy and retention, urticaria, weakness.

ANTIDOTE

Notify the physician of all side effects. May be treated symptomatically or the drug may be discontinued. For overdose, physostigmine 0.5 to 2 mg IV up to 4 mg may be used; however, it may cause profound bradycardia, seizures, or asystole. Thiopental sodium 2% may be required to decrease excitement. Mechanical ventilation equipment must be available. Treat fever with cooling measures. Treat anaphylaxis and resuscitate as necessary.

IBUTILIDE FUMARATE   Antiarrhythmic

Corvert   pH 4.6

USUAL DOSE

Patient Weight	Initial Infusion (over 10 minutes)	Second Infusion
60 kg (132 lb) or more	1 mg ibutilide fumarate (one vial [10 ml])	If the arrhythmia does not terminate within 10 minutes after the end of the initial infusion, a second 10-minute infusion of equal strength may be administered 10 minutes after completion of the first infusion.
Less than 60 kg (132 lb)	0.01 mg/kg ibutilide fumarate (0.1 ml/kg)	

Discontinue infusion promptly when the presenting arrhythmia is terminated (desired effect). Must also be discontinued immediately if sustained or nonsustained ventricular tachycardia or marked prolongation of QT or QTc occur (adverse effects). Post-conversion treatment with appropriate antiarrhythmics (e.g., digoxin, verapamil [Calan], or propranolol [Inderal]) is usually required.

PEDIATRIC DOSE

Safety and effectiveness for use in children under 18 years old not established.

DOSE ADJUSTMENTS

No adjustments required in patients with impaired hepatic or renal function or in the elderly (note Monitor).

DILUTION

May be given undiluted or may be diluted in 50 ml of NS or D5W and given as an infusion. 1 mg (10 ml of a 0.1-mg/ml solution) of ibutilide in 50 ml diluent yields 0.017 mg/ml.

Storage: Store at controlled room temperature in carton until use. Stable after dilution for 24 hours at room temperature, 48 hours if refrigerated.

INCOMPATIBLE WITH

Sufficient information not available. Is compatible with NS and D5W packaged in glass, polyvinyl chloride, or polyolefin infusion containers.

RATE OF ADMINISTRATION

A single dose by injection or infusion over 10 minutes.

ACTIONS

A class III antiarrhythmic agent that produces mild slowing of the sinus rate and atrioventricular conduction. Delays repolarization by activation of a slow inward current (sodium) rather than blocking outward potassium currents. Prolonged atrial and ventricular action potential duration and refractoriness result. Produces dose-related prolongation of the QT interval (may result from dose of ibutilide or rate of injection). Conversion of atrial flutter/fibrillation usually occurs within 30 minutes but may take up to 90 minutes after the start of the infusion. Most patients remain in normal sinus rhythm (NSR) for 24 hours. At recommended doses, ibutilide has no clinically significant effects on cardiac output, mean pulmonary arterial pressure, or pulmonary capillary wedge pressure. Rapidly distributed and metabolized. Elimination half-life is 6 hours (range 2 to 12 hours). Primarily excreted in urine (7% as unchanged drug). Excreted in small amounts in feces.

INDICATIONS AND USES

Rapid conversion of recent onset atrial fibrillation or atrial flutter to sinus rhythm. Patients with more recent onset of arrhythmia have a higher rate of conversion. Effectiveness was less in those with a longer-duration arrhythmia.

CONTRAINDICATIONS

Known hypersensitivity to ibutilide or any of its components. ■ Not recommended in patients who have had a previous polymorphic ventricular tachycardia (e.g., torsades de pointes). ■ Note Drug/lab interactions.

PRECAUTIONS

Usually administered by or under the direction of the physician specialist. ■ Skilled personnel and proper equipment (e.g., cardiac monitors, intracardiac pacing facilities, cardioverter/defibrillator, emergency drugs) must be immediately available. ■ May cause life-threatening arrhythmias (e.g., torsades de pointes) with or without documented

QT prolongation. ▪ Correct hypokalemia and hypomagnesemia before use; may exaggerate a prolonged QT and cause arrhythmias. ▪ Adequate anticoagulation (usually at least 2 weeks) is required for any patient with atrial fibrillation of more than 2 to 3 days' duration. ▪ Select patients carefully; benefits (potential for maintaining sinus rhythm) must outweigh risks. Patients with chronic atrial fibrillation are more likely to revert back to atrial fibrillation after conversion to sinus rhythm. Patients with a QTc interval >440 msec or a serum potassium <4.0 mEq/L are at very high risk to develop life-threatening arrhythmias. ▪ Patients with a history of CHF may be more susceptible to sustained polymorphic VT. ▪ Slightly more effective in atrial flutter than atrial fibrillation. ▪ Note Drug/lab interactions.

Monitor: Obtain weight, baseline vital signs, and ECG before administration. Continuous ECG monitoring during and after infusion indicated to observe for arrhythmias. Watch for QT or QTc prolongation; may cause arrhythmia (torsades de pointes) with or without QT prolongation. ▪ Monitor BP and HR. Bradycardia, a varying heart rate, and/or hypokalemia may increase risk of arrhythmia. ▪ Arrhythmia occurs most frequently within 40 minutes of completion of infusion but may occur for up to 3 hours after infusion. Monitor ECG for a minimum of 4 hours or until QTc has returned to baseline. Monitor longer if there are any episodes of arrhythmias or if the patient has impaired liver function.

Patient education: Report promptly any feeling of faintness, difficulty breathing, or pain or stinging along injection site.

Maternal/child: Pregnancy category C: Benefits must outweigh risks. Caused birth defects and was embryocidal in rats. ▪ Temporarily discontinue breast feeding. ▪ Safety and effectiveness for children under 18 years not established.

Elderly: No age-related differences observed. Median age in clinical trials was 65 years.

DRUG/LAB INTERACTIONS

Should not be given concurrently with Class Ia antiarrhythmics (e.g., disopyramide [Norpace], procainamide [Pronestyl], quinidine) or other Class III antiarrhythmics (e.g., amiodarone [Cordarone], sotalol [betapace]). Withhold any of these agents for at least 5 half-lives prior to ibutilide infusion and for 4 hours after. ▪ Incidence of arrhythmia may be increased with other drugs that prolong the QT interval (e.g., phenothiazines [e.g., promethazine (Phenergan)], tricyclic antidepressants [e.g., amitriptyline (Elavil)], tetracyclic antidepressants [e.g., maprotiline (Ludiomil)], specific H_1 receptor antagonists [e.g., antihistamines including astemizole (Hismanal), terfenadine (Seldane)]). ▪ Monitor serum digoxin levels to avoid digoxin toxicity. ▪ Use with digoxin, beta blockers, or calcium channel blockers does not alter safety or effectiveness of ibutilide. However, sotalol is a beta-blocker and its use with ibutilide is restricted because it has Class III antiarrhythmic activity; see above.

SIDE EFFECTS

Sustained polymorphic VT (1.7%) and nonsustained polymorphic VT (2.7%) can deteriorate into ventricular fibrillation and be fatal. May cause many other arrhythmias (e.g., first-, second, or third-degree AV block [1.5%], bradycardia [1.2%], bundle branch block [1.9%], nonsustained monomorphic VT [4.9%], prolonged QT segment [1.2%], PVCs [5.1%], tachycardia [2.7%]), CHF (0.5%), headache (3.6%), hypertension (1.2%), hypotension (2%), nausea (1.9%), palpitation (1%).

Overdose: Side effects exaggerated with overdose in humans. Acute overdose in animals resulted in CNS depression, rapid gasping breathing, convulsions.

ANTIDOTE

If proarrhythmias occur; discontinue ibutilide; correct electrolyte abnormalities (e.g., potassium and magnesium). Overdrive cardiac pacing, electrical cardioversion, or defibrillation may be required. Infusions of magnesium sulfate may be helpful. Avoid treatment with antiarrhythmic agents. VT that deteriorates to VF will require immediate defibrillation.

IDARUBICIN HYDROCHLORIDE

Antineoplastic
(Antibiotic)

Idamycin, Idamycin PFS, IDR

pH 5.0 to 7.0

USUAL DOSE

Adult acute myeloid leukemia (AML) induction therapy: 12 mg/M^2 daily for 3 days. Used in combination with cytarabine (ARA-C) as an infusion of 100 mg/M^2 daily for 7 days. An alternate schedule is 25 mg/M^2 daily for 2 days in combination with an infusion of cytarabine 200 mg/M^2 daily for 5 days. Note Precautions/Monitor. If unequivocal evidence of leukemia remains after the first course a second course may be given. Maintenance with idarubicin not recommended because of toxicity.

DOSE ADJUSTMENTS

Delay second course until full recovery if mucositis has occurred and reduce dose by 25%. ▪ Consider dose reductions in impaired liver and kidney function based on bilirubin and/or creatinine levels above the normal range. Do not administer if bilirubin above 5 mg/dl.

DILUTION

Specific techniques required; see Precautions. Idamycin PFS is a liquid formulation; each 5 mg of powdered idamycin must be reconstituted with 5 ml of nonbacteriostatic NS for injection (1 mg/ml). Use extreme caution inserting the needle; vial contents are under negative pressure. Avoid any possibility of inhalation from aerosol or any skin contamination.

Storage: PFS product must be refrigerated. Reconstituted idamycin is stable for 7 days under refrigeration (2° to 8° C [36° to 46° F]) or 3 days (72 hours) at room temperature (15° to 30° C [59° to 86° F]). Discard unused solution appropriately.

INCOMPATIBLE WITH

Consider toxicity and specific use. Prolonged contact with solution of an alkaline pH (e.g., sodium lactate, sodium bicarbonate) will result in degradation of idarubicin. Acyclovir (Zovirax), allopurinol (Zyloprim), ampicillin sodium/sulbactam sodium (Unasyn), cefazolin (Kefzol), ceftazidime (Ceptaz), clindamycin (Cleocin), dexamethasone (Decadron), etoposide (VePesid), fluorouracil, furosemide (Lasix), gentamicin (Garamycin), heparin, hydrocortisone sodium succinate (Solu-Cortef), lorezapam (Ativan), meperidine (Demerol), methotrexate (Folex), mezlocillin (Mezlin), piperacillin/tazobactam (Zosyn), sodium bicarbonate, vancomycin (Vancocin), vincristine (Oncovin). May be compatible at Y-site with cytarabine; consult pharmacist.

RATE OF ADMINISTRATION
A single dose of properly diluted medication over 10 to 15 minutes through Y-tube or three-way stopcock of a free-flowing infusion of D5W or NS.

ACTIONS
A highly toxic synthetic antibiotic antineoplastic agent. An analog of daunorubicin. Rapidly cleared from plasma; has an increased rate of cellular uptake compared to other anthracyclines. It inhibits synthesis of DNA and interacts with the enzyme topoisomerase II. Results in a greater number of remissions and longer survival than previous protocols (daunorubicin and cytarabine). Extensive extrahepatic metabolism. It is severely immunosuppressive. Half-life averages 20 to 22 hours. Slowly excreted in bile and urine.

INDICATIONS AND USES
Treatment of acute myeloid leukemia (AML) in adults in combination with other approved antileukemic drugs.

CONTRAINDICATIONS
Not absolute; preexisting bone marrow suppression, impaired cardiac function, preexisting infection (See Precautions/Monitor)

PRECAUTIONS
Follow guidelines for handling cytotoxic agents. See Appendix A, p. 893. ■ Administered by or under the direction of the physician specialist, with facilities for monitoring the patient and responding to any medical emergency. ■ For IV use only. Do not give IM or SC. ■ Use extreme caution in preexisting drug-induced bone marrow suppression, existing heart disease, previous treatment with other anthracyclines (e.g., daunorubicin), other cardiotoxic agents (e.g., bleomycin), or radiation therapy encompassing the heart. ■ Myocardial toxicity may cause potentially fatal acute congestive heart failure, acute life-threatening arrhythmias, or other cardiomyopathies.

Monitor: Determine absolute patency of vein. A stinging or burning sensation indicates extravasation, but extravasation may occur without stinging or burning; severe cellulitis and tissue necrosis will result. Discontinue injection; use another vein. ■ Monitoring of white blood cells, red blood cells, platelet count, liver function, kidney function, ECG, chest x-ray, echocardiography, and systolic ejection fraction indicated before and during therapy. ■ Severe myelosuppression occurs with effective therapeutic doses. Observe closely for all signs of infection or bleeding. ■ Prophylactic antibiotics may be indicated pending results of C/S in a febrile neutropenic patient. ■ Prophylactic antiemetics may reduce nausea and vomiting and increase patient comfort. ■ Monitor uric acid levels; maintain hydration; allopurinol may be indicated. ■ Note Precautions.

Patient education: Nonhormonal birth control recommended. ■ Report IV site burning or stinging promptly. ■ See Appendix D, p. 900.

Maternal/child: Category D: avoid pregnancy. May produce teratogenic effects on the fetus. Contraceptive measures indicated during childbearing years. ■ Discontinue nursing before taking idarubicin. ■ Safety and efficacy for use in children not established.

Elderly: Cardiotoxicity or myelotoxicity may be more severe. ■ Monitor renal, hepatic, and hematologic functions closely.

DRUG/LAB INTERACTIONS

Do not administer any live vaccines to patients receiving antineoplastic drugs. ■ Note Precautions/ Monitor.

SIDE EFFECTS

Acute congestive heart failure, alopecia (reversible), arrhythmias, bone marrow suppression (marked with average doses), cramping, decrease in systolic ejection fraction, depressed QRS voltage, diarrhea, erythema and tissue necrosis (if extravasation occurs), fever, headache, hemorrhage (severe), hepatic function changes, mucositis, myocarditis, nausea, pericarditis, renal function changes, skin rash, urticaria (local), vomiting.

ANTIDOTE

Most side effects will be tolerated or treated symptomatically. Keep physician informed. Close monitoring of bone marrow, ECG, chest x-ray, echocardiography, and systolic ejection fraction may prevent most serious and potentially fatal side effects. There is no specific antidote, but adequate supportive care including platelet transfusions, antibiotics, and symptomatic treatment of mucositis is required. For extravasation, elevate the extremity and apply intermittent ice packs over the area immediately and 4 times a day for ½ hour. Continue for 3 days. Consider aspiration of as much infiltrated drug as possible, flooding of the site with NS, and injection of hydrocortisone sodium succinate (Solu-Cortef) or hyaluronidase (Wydase) throughout extravasated tissue. Use a 27- or 25-gauge needle. Site should be observed promptly by a reconstructive surgeon. If ulceration begins or there is severe persistent pain at the site, early wide excision of the involved area will be considered. Hemodialysis or peritoneal dialysis probably not effective in overdose.

IFOSFAMIDE

Ifex

Antineoplastic
(Alkylating agent/nitrogen mustard)

pH 6.0

USUAL DOSE

1.2 Gm/M^2/day for 5 consecutive days. Repeat every 3 weeks as hematologic recovery permits. To initiate this protocol, platelets must be above 100,000/mm^3 and white blood cells must be above 4,000/mm^3. To prevent hemorrhagic cystitis, a protector such as mesna should be administered with every dose. Ifosfamide dose has been mixed with the initial mesna dose each day in the same solution. Appears to be compatible.

DOSE ADJUSTMENTS

Reduced dose may be required for adrenalectomized patients and in renal or hepatic impairment. Adequate data not available. ■ Severe myelosuppression is frequent, especially when ifosfamide is given with other chemotherapeutic agents. Dose adjustments of all agents may be required.

DILUTION

Specific techniques required; see Precautions. Each 1 Gm must be diluted with 20 ml sterile water or bacteriostatic water for injection (parabens or benzyl alcohol preserved only). Shake solution to dissolve. May be further diluted with D5W, NS, LR, or sterile water for injection. 1 Gm in 20 ml equals 50 mg/ml, 1 Gm in 50 ml equals 20 mg/ml, 1 Gm in 200 ml equals 5 mg/ml (additional diluent recommended by some researchers to reduce side effects).

Storage: Store dry powder at room temperature, never above 40° C (104° F). Diluted solution may be stored at room temperature up to 1 week except solutions prepared with sterile water for injection without preservatives. These must be refrigerated and used within 6 hours.

INCOMPATIBLE WITH

Limited information available. Note Precautions. Give separately except as indicated in usual dose.

COMPATIBLE WITH

Additive: with carboplatin (Paraplatin), cisplatin (Platinol), etoposide (VePesid), fluorouracil (5FU).

Y-site: with carboplatin (Paraplatin), cisplatin (Platinol), etoposide (VePesid), fluorouracil (5FU), allopurinol (Zyloprim), filgrastim (Neupogen), fludarabine (Fludara), gallium nitrate (Ganite), melphalan (Alkeran), ondanseton (Zofran), paclitaxel (Taxol), piperacillin/tazobactam (Zosyn), sargramostim (Leukine), vinorelbine (Navelbine). Consult with pharmacist.

RATE OF ADMINISTRATION

A single dose over a minimum of 30 minutes as an infusion. Extend administration time based on amount of diluent and patient condition.

ACTIONS

An alkylating agent. A synthetic analog of cyclophosphamide chemically related to the nitrogen mustard group. An inert compound; metabolic activation by microsomal liver enzymes is required to produce biologically active metabolites. These alkylated metabolites interact with DNA to effect regression in the size of malignant tumors. Elimination half-life for a usual dose is 7 to 15 hours. Larger doses extend half-life. Extensively metabolized (considerable individual variation); this drug or its metabolites are excreted in urine. Secreted in breast milk.

INDICATIONS AND USES
In combination with other specific antineoplastic agents to suppress or retard neoplastic growth in germ cell testicular cancer. Usually used after other chemotherapy protocols have failed.
Unlabeled uses: Lung, breast, ovarian, pancreatic, and gastric cancer; sarcomas; acute leukemias (except acute myelogenous); malignant lymphomas.

CONTRAINDICATIONS
Hypersensitivity to ifosfamide; patients with severely depressed bone marrow function.

PRECAUTIONS
Follow guidelines for handling cytotoxic agents. See Appendix A, p. 893. ■ Usually administered by or under the direction of the physician specialist. ■ Use caution in impaired renal function; may increase CNS toxicity. Use caution in patients with compromised bone marrow reserve (e.g., leukopenia, granulocytopenia, extensive bone marrow metastases, prior radiation therapy, treatment with other cytotoxic agents) and patients with severe hepatic or renal disease. ■ May interfere with normal wound healing. Consider waiting 5 to 7 days or more after a major surgical procedure before beginning treatment.
Monitor: Urinalysis before each dose recommended. Withhold drug if red blood cells in urine exceed 10 per high-powered field. Reinstitute after complete resolution. Mesna given concurrently should prevent hemorrhagic cystitis. ■ Differential WBC, platelet count, and hemoglobin are recommended before each daily dose and as clinically indicated. White blood cells must be above 2,000/mm^3 and platelet count above 50,000/mm^3. ■ Observe constantly for signs of infection (e.g., fever, sore throat, tiredness) or unusual bleeding or bruising. ■ Prophylactic antibiotics may be indicated pending results of C/S in a febrile neutropenic patient. ■ Adequate hydration required; encourage fluid intake (minimum of 2 L/day) and frequent voiding to prevent cystitis. Bladder irrigation with acetylcysteine (2,000 ml/day) has also been used to prevent hematuria. ■ Prophylactic administration of antiemetics recommended.
Patient education: Nonhormonal birth control recommended. ■ See Appendix D, p. 900.
Maternal/child: Category D: avoid pregnancy. Embryotoxic and teratogenic to the fetus. ■ Discontinue breast feeding. ■ Safety and effectiveness for use in children not established.
Elderly: Monitor renal, hepatic, and hematologic functions closely.

DRUG/LAB INTERACTIONS
Note Dose adjustments. ■ Because it is a synthetic analog of cyclophosphamide, ifosfamide may share similar interactions with numerous drugs, including allopurinol, antidiabetics, barbiturates, chloramphenicol, corticosteroids, succinylcholine (Anectine), thiazide diuretics, and other alkylating agents to produce potentially serious

reactions. ■ Do not administer live vaccine to patients receiving anti-neoplastic drugs.

SIDE EFFECTS
Hematuria, hemorrhagic cystitis, and myelosuppression are dose-limiting side effects. Alopecia, anorexia, confusion, constipation, diarrhea, depressive psychosis with hallucinations, nausea, somnolence, and vomiting occur frequently. Allergic reactions, cardiotoxicity, coagulopathy, coma, cranial nerve dysfunction, dermatitis, dizziness, disorientation, fatigue, fever of unknown origin, hematuria, hemorrhagic cystitis, hypertension, hypotension, infection, liver dysfunction, leukopenia, malaise, neutropenia, phlebitis, polyneuropathy, pulmonary symptoms, thrombocytopenia, or seizures may occur.

ANTIDOTE
Minor side effects will be treated symptomatically if necessary. Discontinue ifosfamide and notify physician immediately if hematuria, hemorrhagic cystitis, confusion, coma, white blood cells below 2,000/mm^3, or platelets below 50,000 mm^3 occur. Oprelvekin (Numega) has been used to treat thrombocytopenia. There is no specific antidote. Supportive therapy as indicated will help sustain the patient in toxicity. May respond to hemodialysis.

IMIGLUCERASE	Enzyme replenisher (Glucocerebrosidase)
Cerezyme	pH 6.1

USUAL DOSE
Adults and Children: Individualized to each patient based on the severity of illness and patient response. The average initial dose is 15 to 60 units/kg/infusion every 2 weeks. However, the dose may range from 2.5 units/kg 3 times a week up to 60 units/kg at weekly intervals or as infrequently as once every 4 weeks. Imiglucerase should be given at least every 4 weeks or symptoms and condition may relapse to pretreatment status. Patients beginning imiglucerase therapy are usually given higher-range initial doses for a limited time to stabilize their disease. Patients with very severe Gaucher's disease also may require higher-range initial doses and/or increased frequency because they have accumulated more lipid throughout their bodies, requiring more enzyme to remove the excess stored lipid and bring their disease under control. Some clinicians recommend a test dose; see Rate of administration.

DOSE ADJUSTMENTS
To utilize each bottle fully and reduce waste, a single dose may be increased or decreased slightly as long as the total monthly dose remains unaltered. ■ After patient response is well established (disease symptoms lessen and the accumulated lipid is reduced), the dose may be adjusted downward to achieve the optimal individualized maintenance dose. Usually progressively lowered at 3- to 6-month

intervals while response parameters are closely monitored. Optimal goal is to establish the lowest dose that is effective in maintaining control of the disease and preventing recurrence of symptoms for each patient.

DILUTION

weight in kg × dose/kg desired ÷ 200 (units/vial) = # of vials required

Adjust number of vials up or down within monthly dose requirement to fully utilize each vial. Manufacturer has a large plasticized dosing chart/kg to determine vials required for various desired doses. After patient is weighed and appropriate dose is calculated, remove sufficient vials (200 units/vial) from refrigerator and warm to room temperature. Each vial must be diluted with 5.1 ml of sterile water without preservatives (40 units/ml). Gently swirl to mix the solution. Do not shake. Let stand for several minutes to allow product to dissolve and bubbles to dissipate. A total dose must be further diluted with NS to a volume of 100 to 200 ml. Minimum adequate dilution requires at least 1 or more ml diluent to each 1 ml of imiglucerase. Do not use if discolored or particulate matter present. Note that the concentration of imiglucerase (200 units/5 ml) is one half that of alglucerase (400 units/5 ml) and requires twice as many vials for the same dose.

Storage: Refrigerate prior to use. Do not use after expiration date on bottle. Return of unsuitable vials (reconstituted, prior to reconstitution, or expired) may be authorized; call 1-800-745-4447. Contains no preservative; do not store opened vials for future use.

INCOMPATIBLE WITH

Do not use as an additive with any other drug. Do not mix in any solution other than NS.

RATE OF ADMINISTRATION

Use of an inline 0.5 or 0.2 micron filter is recommended. Use of a microdrip (60 gtt/ml) or an infusion pump helpful. Flush the IV line with NS at the end of the infusion to assure the total dose is received.

Test dose: Administer at prescribed rate (0.5 to 1 unit/kg/min for 5 minutes. Take vital signs and assess patient for symptoms of allergic reaction.

Full dose: A single dose equally distributed over 1 to 2 hours. One reference says the maximum rate is 1 unit/kg/min; another recommends one-half that rate or a maximum of 30 unit/kg/hr.

ACTIONS

An analog of the human enzyme, beta-glucocerebrosidase produced by recombinant DNA technology. Gaucher's disease is characterized by a functional deficiency in beta-glucocerebrosidase enzymatic activity and the resultant accumulation of lipid glucocerebroside in tissue macrophages (Gaucher's cells). These cells are found in the liver, spleen, bone marrow and occasionally in the lung, kidney, and intestine. Imiglucerase acts like glucocerebrosidase to facilitate the release of the lipid glucocerebrosides. Effective in controlling and actually reversing disease symptoms. Increase in appetite and energy level and improvement in hemoglobin are often the first observable effects and may occur in 2 to 4 months. Cachexia and wasting in children are reduced. Within 6 months splenomegaly and hepatomegaly are significantly reduced, and hemoglobin, hematocrit, erythrocyte, and platelet counts improved. Replenishment of bone marrow and improving mineralization of bone may take several years.

INDICATIONS AND USES

Long-term enzyme replacement therapy for patients with confirmed diagnosis of type I Gaucher's disease, with signs and symptons severe enough to result in one or more of the following conditions: moderate-to-severe anemia, thrombocytopenia, bone disease, hepatomegaly, or splenomegaly. As availability through increased production improves, imiglucerase will eventually replace alglucerase (Ceredase). Studies are being conducted to see if dose can be lowered without decreasing effectiveness. Treatment costs (>$150,000/yr) could be markedly reduced with lower doses.

CONTRAINDICATIONS

None known. Reevaluate if there is significant clinical evidence of hypersensitivity to imiglucerase.

PRECAUTIONS

Effective only via IV route. ■ Should be used under the direction of a physician knowledgeable in the management of Gaucher's disease. ■ A recombinant product; risk of transmission of any bacterial, mycoplasmal, fungal, or viral agent is remote. ■ A few patients have developed IgG antibodies, but to date only one patient developed a transient rash. Potential for allergic reaction must always be considered. ■ Use caution in patients who have had hypersensitivity reaction to alglucerase (Ceredase).

Monitor: Evaluation of hemoglobin, hematocrit, platelets, WBC, acid phophatase (AP), plasma glucocerebroside, liver and/or spleen size, and bone changes are required before and during therapy. Frequency determined by patient response; more frequent when determining response to initial dose and when dose is being adjusted (i.e., every 3 to 6 months). Blood tests will be done more frequently, since anemia is the first symptom to improve. ■ Monitor weight prior to each dose (used to calculate dose) and monitor vital signs. ■ MRI provides the best evaluation of liver and spleen. ■ Standard x-rays provide adequate evaluation of bone changes. ■ Observe patient closely for signs of improvement (e.g., increased energy, reduced bleeding tendency, reduction in size of liver and/or spleen, reduced joint swelling, reduced bone pain).

Patient education: Treatment required for life. No longer than 1 month should elapse between treatments, or symptoms and condition may relapse to the pretreatment state.

Maternal/child: Category C: use in pregnancy only if clearly needed. No studies available on fetal harm or reproductive capacity. ■ Safety for use during lactation not established. Not known if imiglucerase is secreted in breast milk.

Elderly: Specific information not available in product information.

DRUG/LAB INTERACTIONS

None indicated. Limited information available.

SIDE EFFECTS

Have been transient and did not occur frequently: Abdominal discomfort, decreased urinary frequency, dizziness, headache, hypotension (mild), nausea, pruritus, and rash. A protein immune reaction may develop. Side effects may improve with continued therapy because antibody levels decrease.

ANTIDOTE

Keep physician informed of side effects; may be treated symptomatically if indicated. Discontinue imiglucerase for clinical evidence of hypersensitivity. Treat anaphylaxsis as necessary.

IMIPENEM-CILASTATIN

Primaxin

**Antibacterial
(Carbapenem)**

pH 6.5 to 7.5

USUAL DOSE

Range is from 250 mg to 1 Gm every 6 to 8 hours. Dosage based on severity of disease, susceptibility of pathogens, condition of the patient, age, weight, and creatinine clearance. Do not exceed the lower of 50 mg/kg of body weight/24 hr or 4 Gm/24 hr. Continue for at least 2 days after all symptoms of infection subside.

PEDIATRIC DOSE

Children over 12 years: 50 to 100 mg/kg/24 hours in equally divided doses every 6 to 8 hours. Follow Usual dose information.

DOSE ADJUSTMENTS

Reduce total daily dose if renal function impaired. Calculated according to degree of impairment (see literature). ■ Note Monitor and Drug/lab interactions.

DILUTION

Dilute each single dose with 10 ml of compatible infusion solutions (e.g., D5W, D10W, NS [see chart on back cover or literature]). Must be further diluted in 100 ml of the same infusion solution and given as an intermittent infusion. Agitate until clear. Also available in ADD-Vantage vials for use with ADD-Vantage diluent containers and in 120 ml infusion bottles for one-step dilution.

Storage: Stable at room temperature for 4 hours after preparation or 24 hours if refrigerated. Do not freeze.

INCOMPATIBLE WITH

All aminoglycosides (e.g., kanamycin [Kantrex]), all solutions except those recommended for dilution by manufacturer: fluconazole (Diflucan), gallium nitrate (Ganite), lorazepam (Ativan), meperidine (Demerol), midazolam (Versed), sargramostim (Leukine), sodium bicarbonate. Should be considered incompatible in syringe or solution with any other bacteriostatic agent.

RATE OF ADMINISTRATION

Intermittent IV: Each 500 mg or fraction thereof over 20 to 30 minutes. Slow infusion rate if patient develops nausea. May be given through Y-tube or three-way stopcock of infusion set.

ACTIONS

A potent broad-spectrum antibacterial agent. Imipenem is a thienamycin antibiotic, and cilastatin sodium inhibits its renal metabolism. Both components are present in equal amounts. Bactericidal to many gram-negative, gram-positive, and anaerobic organisms. Effective against many otherwise resistant organisms. Rapidly and widely distributed into many body fluids and tissues. Excreted in the urine. May cross the placental barrier.

INDICATIONS AND USES

Treatment of serious lower respiratory tract, urinary tract, skin and skin structure, bone and joint, gynecologic, intraabdominal, and polymicrobic infections; bacterial septicemia, and endocarditis. Most effective against specific organisms (see literature).

CONTRAINDICATIONS

Known sensitivity to any component of this product.

PRECAUTIONS

Specific sensitivity studies are indicated to determine susceptibility of the causative organism to imipenem-cilastatin. ■ Use extreme caution in patients with a history of allergic reactions, especially to other beta lactam antibiotics. Cross sensitivity is possible. ■ Avoid prolonged use of drug; superinfection caused by overgrowth of nonsusceptible organisms may result. ■ CNS adverse effects, including seizures, have been reported. Incidence increases with higher doses, compromised renal function, or preexisting CNS disorders.

Monitor: May cause thrombophlebitis. Use small needles and large veins, and rotate infusion sites. ■ Electrolyte imbalance and cardiac irregularities resulting from sodium content are possible. Contains 3.2 mEq of sodium/Gm. ■ Monitor renal, hepatic, and hemopoietic systems in prolonged therapy. ■ Note Drug/lab interactions.

Maternal/child: Pregnancy Category C: use only if absolutely necessary in pregnancy and lactation. ■ Safety for use in infants and children under 12 years of age not established.

DRUG/LAB INTERACTIONS

May be used concomitantly with aminoglycosides and other antibiotics, but these drugs must never be mixed in the same infusion or given concurrently. ■ Use with ganciclovir (Cytovene) may cause generalized seizures. Use only if benefit outweighs risk. ■ Half-life and plasma levels slightly increased by probenecid. Avoid concurrent use.

SIDE EFFECTS

Full scope of allergic reactions including anaphylaxis. Abdominal pain; abnormal clotting time; altered CBC and electrolytes; anuria; burning, discomfort, and pain at injection site; confusion; diarrhea; dizziness; dyspnea; elevated alkaline phosphotase, AST (SGOT), ALT (SGPT), bilirubin, creatinine, BUN, and LDH; fever; gastroenteritis; glossitis; headache; heartburn; hemorrhagic colitis; hyperventilation; hypotension; increased salivation; myoclonus; nausea and vomiting; paresthesia; pharyngeal pain; polyarthralgia; polyuria; positive direct Coombs' test; presence of white or red blood cells, protein, casts, bilirubin, or urobilinogen in urine; pseudomembranous colitis; seizures; somnolence; thrombophlebitis; tinnitus; tongue papillar hypertrophy; transient hearing loss in the hearing impaired; vertigo; and many others.

ANTIDOTE

Notify physician of any side effects. Discontinue the drug if indicated. Treat allergic reaction as indicated and resuscitate as necessary. Begin anticonvulsants if focal tremors, myoclonus, or seizures occur. If symptoms continue, decrease dose or discontinue the drug. Mild cases of colitis may respond to discontinuation of drug. Oral vancomycin or metronidazole (Flagyl) are the treatment of choice for antibiotic-related pseudomembranous colitis. Hemodialysis may be useful in overdose.

IMMUNE GLOBULIN INTRAVENOUS

Immunizing agent (passive)
Platelet count stimulator
Antibacterial
Antiviral
Antipolyneuropathy agent

Gamimune N, Gammagard SD, Gammar P-IV,
IGIV, Iveegam, Polygam SD, Sandoglobulin,
Venoglobulin-1, Venoglobulin-S, Veno-S

pH 4.0 to 7.2

USUAL DOSE

Immunodeficiency syndrome:

Gamimune N: 100 to 200 mg/kg (2 to 4 ml/kg) as a single-dose IV infusion. May be repeated monthly if indicated. If adequate IgG levels in the circulation or clinical response not achieved, may be increased to 400 mg/kg (8 ml/kg), or a lesser dose may be given more frequently.

Gammagard SD/Polygam SD: 200 to 400 mg/kg of body weight as a single-dose IV infusion. Repeat at least 100 mg/kg monthly.

Gammar P-IV: 200 to 400 mg/kg as a single-dose IV infusion every 3 to 4 weeks. Up to 600 mg/kg may be required. High-end doses may be given initially and for several doses at more frequent intervals based on individual patient response and adequate IgG levels. Reduce dose 100 to 200 mg/kg and/or interval when therapeutic IgG levels are achieved.

Iveegam: 200 mg/kg/month as a single-dose IV infusion. If adequate IgG levels in the circulation or clinical response not achieved, may be increased up to 800 mg/kg or intervals shortened. Do not exceed 800 mg/kg/month.

Sandoglobulin: 200 mg/kg as a single-dose IV infusion. May be repeated monthly if indicated. If adequate IgG levels in the circulation or clinical response not achieved, may be increased to 300 mg/kg or a lesser dose may be given more frequently.

Venoglobulin-1/Venoglobulin-S: 200 mg/kg monthly. If adequate IgG levels in the circulation or clinical response not achieved, increase to 300 to 400 mg/kg monthly, or a lesser dose may be given more frequently.

Idiopathic thrombocytopenic purpura:

Gamimune N: 400 mg/kg for 2 to 5 consecutive days. 1 Gm/kg may be given as an alternate regimen for induction therapy. Do not use in expanded fluid volume or when fluid volume is a concern. May be repeated the next day only if an adequate increase in the platelet count does not occur from the initial dose. If clinically significant bleeding occurs or the platelet count falls below 30,000/mm^3, 400 mg/kg may be given as a single infusion. If response inadequate, increase to 800 to 1,000 mg/kg. May be given intermittently to maintain platelet count.

Gammagard SD/Polygam SD: 1,000 mg/kg. Up to 3 doses can be given on alternate days based on clinical response and platelet count.

Sandoglobulin: 400 mg/kg for 2 to 5 consecutive days. Maintenance dose same as Gamimune N above.

Venoglobulin-1: 500 mg/kg for 2 to 7 consecutive days to a total dose of

2,000 mg/kg. If clinically significant bleeding occurs or the platelet count falls below 30,000/mm³, 500 to 2,000 mg/kg may be given as a single IV infusion every 2 weeks or less. Maintain platelet count above 20,000/mm³ in adults and 30,000/mm³ in children.

Venoglobulin-S: Total dose of 2,000 mg/kg distributed over 5 days. Maintenance dose is 1,000 mg/kg as needed to maintain parameters as above.

B-cell chronic lymphocytic leukemia (CLL):
Gammagard SD/Polygam SD: 400 mg/kg every 3 to 4 weeks.

Prevention of infection in bone marrow transplant patients over 20 years of age:
Gamimune-N: 500 mg/kg of IGIV on day 7 and day 2 pretransplant (or at time conditioning therapy for transplant is begun). Give the same dose once each week through day 90 post-transplant.

Prevention of bacterial infections in HIV-infected children and adults:
Gamimune-N: 400 mg/kg every 28 days.

Kawasaki disease:
Gammagard SD, Gamimune-N, Sandoglobulin: 2 Gm/kg as a single dose over 10 to 12 hours or 1 Gm/kg for 2 days.

Iveegam: 400 mg/kg/day for 4 days or a single dose of 2,000 mg/kg given over a minimum of 10 hours. Initiate within 10 days of onset of disease. Concomitantly give aspirin 100 mg/kg daily for 14 days, then 3 to 5 mg/kg/day for 5 weeks.

DILUTION

Absolute sterile technique required at all steps of reconstitution process for each formulation. Complete dilution may take up to 20 minutes or longer. For all preparations, filtration is required as drawn into a syringe for administration or as administered through IV tubing. Check each brand for specific equipment.

Gamimune N: May be given undiluted (a 5% solution) or may be further diluted with a given amount of D5W to facilitate slow and accurate rate of infusion. Available in 10, 50, and 100 ml single-dose vials as a 5% solution and in 50, 100, and 200 ml vials as a 10% solution. pH 4.0 to 4.5

Gammagard SD/Polygam SD: Must be warmed to room temperature prior to dilution. Diluent (sterile water for injection), transfer device, administration set with integral airway, and filter provided with each single-use vial. Available in 2.5, 5, and 10 Gm single-dose vials with diluent. Use full amount of diluent (50, 96, 192 ml) to prepare a 5% solution (50 mg/ml) or one half the amount of diluent (25, 48, 96 ml) to prepare a 10% solution (100 mg/ml). Must be used within 2 hours of dilution. pH 6.4 to 7.2.

Gammar P-IV: Must be warmed to room temperature prior to dilution. Diluent (sterile water for injection), transfer device (plastic piercing pin to diluent vial; metal needle to product vial), administration set with integral airway, and filter provided with each single-use vial. Available in 1, 2.5, 5, and 10 Gm single-dose vials with diluent (50 mg/ml). Do not shake to dissolve; rotate or agitate vial. Must be used within 3 hours of dilution. pH 6.4 to 7.2.

Iveegam: Diluent (sterile water for injection), transfer device, administration set with integral airway, and filter provided with each single-use vial. Available in 0.5, 1, 2.5, and 5 Gm vials with 10, 20, 50, or 100 ml diluent providing 50 mg/ml. Do not shake to dissolve; rotate or agitate vial. Use immediately after dilution. May be further diluted with a given amount of D5W or NS.

Sandoglobulin: Must be warmed to room temperature prior to dilution. Dilute with NS diluent provided. Makes a 3% solution. Invert so that diluent flows into the IV bottle. Available as 1 (3 or 6) Gm with 33 (100 or 200) ml diluent. For a 6% solution use one half diluent provided. pH 6.4 to 6.8.

Venoglobulin-1: Must be warmed to room temperature prior to dilution. Diluent (sterile water for injection), reconstitution kit, and transfer device usually provided. Available in 0.5, 2.5, 5, and 10 Gm vials. If diluent not provided, dilute with 10, 20, 50, or 100 ml sterile water for injection respectively (50 mg/ml). Use promptly. pH 6.8. May be given through Y-site if primary IV is NS or if line is flushed with NS.

Venoglobulin-S: Ready for use as 5% or 10% immune globulin IV in 50, 100, and 200 ml with sterile administration set. pH 5.2 to 5.8. May be temporarily unavailable from manufacturer.

Storage: Store Gammagard SD, Gammar P-IV, Polygam SD, Sandoglobulin, Venoglobulin-1, and Venoglobulin-S 5% at controlled room temperature. Refrigerate Gamimune-N, Iveegam, and Venoglobulin-S 10%. Discard partially used vials. Do not use if turbid or has been frozen.

INCOMPATIBLE WITH

Should be considered incompatible in syringe or solution with any other drug or solution because of specific use, potential for anaphylaxis, and manufacturer's recommendation. Exceptions noted in Dilution.

Venoglobulin-1: Dextrose solutions.

RATE OF ADMINISTRATION

In all situations, slow rate of infusion at onset of patient discomfort or any adverse reactions. Administer via a separate IV tubing with filter or filter needle (provided by most manufacturers). Do not mix with other drugs or IV solutions. An infusion pump will facilitate an accurate rate of administration.

Gamimune N: 0.01 to 0.02 ml/kg/min for the first 30 minutes (0.7 to 1.4 ml/min of undiluted drug for a 70 kg individual). If no discomfort or adverse effects, may be increased to 0.08 ml/kg/min.

Gammagard SD/Polygam SD: 5% solution 0.5 ml/kg/hr. May be gradually increased to 4 ml/kg/hr if no discomfort or adverse effects. If 5% solution well tolerated at 4 ml/kg/hr, a 10% solution can be used. Begin with 0.5 ml/kg/hr. If no adverse effects, gradually increase to 8 ml/kg/hr.

Gammar P-IV: 0.01 ml/kg/min. May be increased to 0.02 ml/kg/min after 15 to 30 min. May be gradually increased to 0.03 to 0.06 ml/kg/min if no discomfort or adverse effects.

Iveegam: 1 ml/min. May be increased to a maximum of 2 ml/min in the standard 5% solution. Rate may be adjusted proportionately with further dilution. Note rate for single-dose regimen in Kawasaki disease.

Sandoglobulin: 0.5 to 1 ml/min for 15 to 30 minutes. May then be increased to 1.5 to 2.5 ml/min. After the first infusion, the rate may be initiated at 2 to 2.5 ml/min. After the first dose, a 6% solution may be used to facilitate the administration of larger doses. Begin at 1 to 1.5 ml/min and increase in 15 to 30 minutes to 2 to 2.5 ml/min.

Venoglobulin-1/Venoglobulin-S: 0.01 to 0.02 ml/kg/min for 30 minutes. May be gradually increased to 0.04 ml/kg/min if no discomfort or adverse effects. Subsequent infusions may be given at the higher rate.

ACTIONS

An immune serum containing immune globulin. Obtained, purified, and standardized from human serum or plasma. Specific methods (e.g., detergents, solvents) inactivate blood-borne viruses (e.g., hepatitis). Provides immediate antibody levels. Half-life approximately 3 weeks.

INDICATIONS AND USES

Maintenance and treatment of individuals unable to produce adequate amounts of IgG antibodies, especially in the following situations: need for immediate increase in intravascular immunoglobulin levels, small muscle mass or bleeding tendencies that contraindicate IM injection, and selected disease states (congenital agammaglobulinemia, common variable hypogammaglobulinemia, or combined immunodeficiency). ■ Temporary increase in platelet counts in patients with idiopathic thrombocytopenic purpura and with thrombocytopenia associated with bone marrow transplant. ■ Gammagard SD/Polygam SD is used to prevent bacterial infections in patients with hypogammaglobulinemia or recurrent bacterial infection associated with B-cell CLL. ■ Infection prophylaxis or control and to improve immunologic parameters in patients with symptomatic AIDS or ARC, children with HIV, low-birth-weight neonates, or patients with iatrogenically induced or disease-associated immunosuppression (major surgery [e.g., bone marrow or cardiac transplants], hematologic malignancies, extensive burns, or collagen-vascular diseases). ■ Reduce graft-vs-host disease in bone marrow patients. ■ Supportive treatment in tetanus (tetanus antitoxin for IV use is no longer available in the United States).

Unlabeled uses: Autoimmune neutropenia, chronic fatigue syndrome, myasthenia gravis, rheumatoid arthritis, polymyositis, children with type I diabetes. ■ Prevention of recurrent bacterial infections in patients with IgG subclass deficiences (e.g., allergies, HIV). ■ Treatment of quinidine-induced thrombocytopenia (400 mg/kg/24 hr for 2 to 5 days).

CONTRAINDICATIONS

Individuals known to have allergic response to gamma globulin or thiomerosol; patients with isolated IgA deficiency or preexisting anti-IgA antibodies.

PRECAUTIONS

Gammagard and Polygam were withdrawn worldwide because of postinfusion hepatitis C in a few patients. They have been replaced by Gammagard SD and Polygam SD. An additional purification process deactivates the hepatitis C virus. ■ Check label; must state for IV use. ■ Do not use IM or SC. Do not skin test. Will cause a localized chemical skin reaction. ■ Use extreme caution in individuals with a history of prior systemic allergic reactions. Incidence of anaphylaxis may be increased, especially with repeated injections. ■ May cause aseptic meningitis syndrome (AMS), especially with 2 Gm doses. May begin from 2 hours to 2 days after treatment. Symptoms are drowsiness, fever, headache (severe), nausea and vomiting, nuchal rigidity, painful eye movements, and photophobia.

Monitor: Use of larger veins (e.g., antecubital) recommended to reduce infusion site discomfort, especially with 10% solutions. ■ Monitor vital signs and observe patient continuously during infusion. A precipitous drop in blood pressure or anaphylaxis can occur at any time. Emergency equipment and supplies must be at bedside. ■ Minimal serum level of IgG after infusion should exceed 300 mg/dl.

Patient education: Report a burning sensation in the head, chills, cyanosis, diaphoresis, dyspnea, faintness or lightheadedness, fatigue, fever, tachycardia, wheezing.

Maternal/child: Category C: use with caution in pregnancy; no adverse effects documented, but adequate studies are not available. ■ Safety for use in lactation not established. ■ Response in children usually exceeds response in adults. ■ Gammimune-N contains maltose and may cause osmotic diuresis.

DRUG/LAB INTERACTIONS

Do not administer live-virus vaccines from 2 weeks before to at least 3 months after immune globulin IV. ■ Provides immediate antibody levels that last for about 3 weeks. In selected patients, may have an immunemodulating effect that may alter their response to corticosteroids or antineoplastic agents.

SIDE EFFECTS

Full range of allergic symptoms including anaphylaxis is possible. Angioedema, erythema, fever, and urticaria are most frequently observed. Backache, chills, fatigue, flushing, headache, hypertension (slight), leg cramps, lightheadedness, nausea, rash, and vomiting have been reported. Is made from human plasma; process attempts to eliminate risk of hepatitis or HIV infection. A precipitous hypotensive reaction can occur and is most frequently associated with too-rapid rate of injection. Aseptic meningitis syndrome occurs infrequently; note Precautions.

ANTIDOTE

Reduce rate immediately for patient discomfort or any sign of adverse reaction. Discontinue the drug if symptoms persist and notify the physician. May be treated symptomatically, and infusion resumed at slower rate if symptoms subside. Treat anaphylaxis immediately. Epinephrine (Adrenalin), diphenhydramine (Benadryl), oxygen, vasopressors (e.g., dopamine [Intropin]), corticosteroids, and ventilation equipment must always be available. Resuscitate as necessary.

INDIUM IN-111 PENTETREOTIDE

OctreoScan

Diagnostic radiopharmaceutical

pH 3.8 to 4.3

USUAL DOSE

Labeling yield of reconsitiuted solution must be checked before administration; above 90% radioactivity required.

Planar imaging: 111 MBq (3 mCi) prepared from 1 OctreoScan kit.

Imaging obtained at 4 and 24 hours post injection. Additional views may be required including one at 48 hours (to differentiate between neuroendocrine tumor and normal bowel uptake).

Spect imaging: 222 MBq (6 mCi) prepared from 2 OctreoScan kits. Imaging obtained at 24 hours post injection. Recommended for small neuroendocrine tumors poorly visualized by planar imaging due to overprojection by other tissues and organs.

DILUTION

Supplied as a kit containing a vial with a 10 mcg pellet of lyophilized pentetreotide, a vial of 1.1 ml of 111 MBq/ml indium in-111 chloride, a needle, and a label. **Two vials must be combined; do not administer as separate agents.** Dilution, labeling yield, and assay, should be accomplished by specifically trained personnel. Requires the use of a lead dispensing shield with lid, shielded sterile syringe, and other specialized equipment including protective clothing and waterproof gloves. Aseptic technique required. See literature for specific process. The indium in-111 chloride solution is injected into the vial of pentetreotide. Swirl gently until the pellet is completely dissolved. Allow to stand at controlled room temperature for at least 30 minutes to assure adequate labeling of the mixture. Visually inspect using proper shielding to assure a clear colorless solution free of particulate matter. Labeling yield must be confirmed prior to administration using a specific process and a suitably calibrated ionization chamber. May be further diluted with NS to a maximum volume of 3 ml immediately before injection. Administered in a shielded, sterile syringe.

Storage: Kits are refrigerated until use. After reconstitution, must be used within 6 hours. Discard in an appropriate manner if not suitable for administration (e.g., particulate matter, coloring, radiochemical purity less than 90%).

INCOMPATIBLE WITH

Do not administer in TPN solution or through the same IV line; will form a precipitate.

RATE OF ADMINISTRATION

A single dose over several seconds.

ACTIONS

Pentetreotide is a subtherapeutic octapeptide analog of octreotide. When combined with radiolabeled indium in-111, it binds to somatostatin receptors present in tissues throughout the body, concentrating in tumors that contain a high density of somatostatin receptors, primarily neuroendocrine tumors (e.g., GI tract [carcinoids], pancreas [islet cell carcinomas such as gastrinoma, glucagonoma, insulinoma, VIPoma], pituitary adenomas [GH-secreting, TSH-secreting, ACTH-secreting, prolactin-secreting, and nonfunctioning tumors], lung [carcinoids, small cell lung cancers], CNS [chemodectoma, meningioma, neuroblastoma paragangliomas], adrenal medulla [pheochromocytomas], thyroid [medullary thyroid carcinomas]). Rapidly distributes from plasma to extravascular body tissues to concentrate in these tumors. After background clearance, visualization of somatostatin receptor-rich tissue is possible, allowing sensitive visualization of primary neuroendocrine tumors and their metastases. In addition to somatostatin receptor-rich tumors, the normal pituitary gland, thyroid gland, liver, spleen, and urinary bladder also are visualized in most patients, as is the bowel to a lesser extent. Only one third of a dose remains in plasma after 10 minutes. Biologic half-life is 6 hours, physical half-life (decays by electron capture) is 2.8 days. Excreted primarily in the kidneys (50% within 6 hours, 90% within 48 hours); a very small amount excreted in feces.

INDICATIONS AND USES

Scintigraphic localization of primary and metastatic neuroendocrine tumors bearing somatostatin receptors. Helps to accurately determine extent of a patient's disease and may decrease the need for multiple invasive procedures (e.g., biopsy, angiography). May accelerate the initiation of appropriate treatment (e.g., resection, drug therapy). May be used for patient follow-up to monitor effects of surgery, radiotherapy, or chemotherapy. Also provides a functional assessment that may promote selection of optimal therapy based on tumor biochemistry.

CONTRAINDICATIONS

Hypersensitivity to indium in-111 pentetreotide or its components.

PRECAUTIONS

Radiopharmaceuticals usually administered by or under the direction of the physician specialist whose experience and training have been approved by the appropriate government agency. ■ Follow specific guidelines for handling radioactive agents to ensure minimal radiation exposure to patients and occupational workers consistent with appropriate patient management. Contact radiation safety officer. ■ If a splash occurs, flush eyes for at least 15 minutes; for skin contact, wash affected areas thoroughly with soap and water, blot dry, do not abrade skin. In both situations, notify the radiation safety officer and continue process until no more radiation can be detected. ■ Notify radiation safety officer immediately if any ingestion occurs (inhalation not expected to be a problem). ■ Sensitivity of scintigraphy may vary with different tumors based on the concentration of somatostatin receptors. ■ Other radio-pharmaceuticals may better identify pheochromocytomas. ■ May cause severe hypoglycemia in patients with insulinomas. If insulinoma is suspected, establish an IV line and administer a glucose solution just before and during administration. Observe carefully. ■ Use with caution in impaired renal function. Primary excretion is renal; delayed excretion may cause unnecessary radiation to the GU tract. ■ Cold or flu may cause accumulation of radioactivity in the nasal area and lung hili. ■ External radiation of the lung may cause local pulmonary accumulation of radioactivity. ■ Radioactivity may accumulate at recent surgical sites. ■ May cause cholelithiasis (not probable with a single dose). ■ Note Drug/lab interactions.

Monitor: To reduce unnecessary radiation exposure to vital organs (e.g., thyroid, kidneys, bladder), patients must be well hydrated before, during, and for at least 1 day after administration. Encourage fluid intake and frequent voiding. ■ Use of a mild laxative (e.g., bisacodyl [Dulcolax], lactulose [Constilac]) as a bowel prep is recommended before and for 48 hours after administration; cleans the bowel to enhance tumor visualization and then promotes excretion of radioactive material. ■ If therapeutic doses of octreotide (Sandostatin) have been suspended, monitor the patient for any signs of withdrawal (e.g., diarrhea, flushing, sweating, weakenss). ■ Note Precautions.

Patient education: Explain importance of increased fluid intake, frequent voiding, and use of mild laxatives to promote excretion of radioactive materials.

Maternal/child: Pregnancy Category C: safety for use during pregnancy not established; benefits must outweigh risk to fetus from radiation. ■ Safety for use during lactation not established. Consider witholding breast milk for 24 to 48 hours or longer until estimated radiation exposure to infant is within safe limits. ■ Safety for use in children not established.

Elderly: Consider age-related impaired organ function. May have difficulty drinking adequate fluids, difficulty voiding, delayed renal excretion (see Precautions), or an inadequate or increased response to laxatives.

DRUG/LAB INTERACTIONS

Sensitivity of scintigraphy may be reduced with therapeutic dose of octreotide (Sandostatin). Best to temporarily suspend octreotide therapy 12 to 24 hours pre test, if possible. ■ Bleomycin may cause local pulmonary accumulation of indium in-111 pentetreotide.

SIDE EFFECTS

Occurred in only a few patients and most were attributed to patient's disease and/or withdrawal from octreotide therapy. Dizziness, fever, flushing, headache, hypotension, joint pain, nausea, sweating, weakness. Severe hypoglycemia is possible in insulinoma patients; see Precautions.

ANTIDOTE

Keep physician informed of patient status. IV fluids may be indicated in patients unable to take adequate fluids.

INDOMETHACIN SODIUM TRIHYDRATE

**Prostaglandin inhibitor
(Patent ductus arteriosus adjunct)**

Indocin IV   **pH 6.0 to 7.5**

USUAL DOSE

Neonates: Three IV doses, specific to age at first dose, given at 12- to 24-hour intervals constitute a course of therapy.

Less than 48 hours of age: First dose (0.2 mg/kg of body weight), second dose (0.1 mg/kg), third dose (0.1 mg/kg).

2 to 7 days of age: 0.2 mg/kg for each of 3 doses.

Over 7 days of age: First dose (0.2 mg/kg), then 0.25 mg/kg for the next 2 doses. A second course of 1 to 3 doses may be repeated one time at 12- to 24-hour intervals as above if the ductus arteriosus reopens.

DOSE ADJUSTMENTS

If urinary output is less than 0.6 ml/hr at any time a dose is to be given, withhold dose until lab studies confirm normal renal function.

DILUTION

Each 1 mg must be diluted with at least 1 ml NS or SW for injection without preservatives (0.1 mg/0.1 ml); may be diluted with 2 ml diluent (0.05 mg/0.1 ml). The preservative benzyl alcohol is toxic in neonates. Prepare a fresh solution for each dose. Discard any unused portion.

INCOMPATIBLE WITH

Any other drug in a syringe. Dilute only with stated preparations. Further dilution with IV infusion solutions not recommended. Dextrose solutions (selected), dobutamine (Dobutrex), dopamine (Intropin), gentamicin (Garamycin), tobramycin (Nebcin).

RATE OF ADMINISTRATION

A single dose properly diluted direct IV over 5 to 10 seconds.

ACTIONS

A potent inhibitor of prostaglandin synthesis. Through an unconfirmed method of action (thought to be inhibition of prostaglandin synthesis), it causes closure of a patent ductus arteriosus 75% to 80% of the time, eliminating the need for surgical intervention. Plasma half-life varies inversely with postnatal age and weight and ranges from 12 to 20 hours. Metabolized in the liver and eventually excreted in urine and bile.

INDICATIONS AND USES

Closure of a hemodynamically significant patent ductus arteriosus in premature infants weighing between 500 and 1,750 Gm if usual medical management (e.g., fluid restriction, diuretics, digitalis, respiratory support) has not been effective after 48 hours.

CONTRAINDICATIONS

Bleeding, especially active intracranial hemorrhage or GI bleeding; coagulation defects; necrotizing enterocolitis; infants with congenital heart disease (e.g., pulmonary atresia, severe coarctation of the aorta, severe tetralogy of Fallot) who require patency of the ductus arteriosus for satisfactory pulmonary or systemic blood flow; proven or suspected untreated infection; significant renal impairment; thrombocytopenia.

PRECAUTIONS

Clinical evidence of a hemodynamically significant patent ductus arteriosus (respiratory distress, a continuous murmur, a hyperactive precordium, cardiomegaly and pulmonary plethora on chest x-ray) should be present before use is considered. ▪ For use only in a highly supervised setting such as an intensive care nursery. ▪ May increase potential for GI or intraventricular bleeding. ▪ Use caution in presence of existing controlled infection; may mask signs and symptoms of exacerbation. ▪ For IV use only. ▪ Surgery is indicated if condition is not responsive to two courses of therapy.

Monitor: Vital signs, oxygenation, acid-base status, fluid and electrolyte balance, and kidney function must be monitored and maintained. ▪ Can cause marked reduction in urine output (over 50%), increase BUN and creatinine, and reduce glomerular filtration rate and creatinine clearance. These symptoms usually disappear when therapy completed but may cause acute renal failure, especially in infants with impaired renal function from other causes. ▪ Discontinue drug if signs of impaired liver function appear. ▪ Confirm absolute patency of vein. Avoid extravasation; will irritate tissue. ▪ Note Drug/lab interactions.

DRUG/LAB INTERACTIONS

May increase serum levels of aminoglycosides (e.g., gentamicin [Garamycin]) and digitalis. ■ Use with furosemide (Lasix) may help to maintain renal function.

SIDE EFFECTS

Abdominal distention; acidosis; alkalosis; apnea; bleeding into the GI tract (gross or microscopic); bradycardia; DIC; elevated BUN or creatinine; exacerbation of preexisting pulmonary infection; fluid retention; hyperkalemia; hypoglycemia; hyponatremia; intracranial bleeding; necrotizing enterocolitis; oliguria; oozing from needle puncture sites; pulmonary hemorrhage; pulmonary hypertension; reduced urine sodium, chloride, potassium, urine osmolality, free water clearance or glomerular filtration rate; retrolental fibroplasia; uremia; transient ileus; vomiting.

ANTIDOTE

Discontinue the drug and notify the physician of all side effects. Based on severity, side effects may be treated symptomatically or drug will be completely discontinued in favor of surgical intervention. Resuscitate as necessary.

INSULIN INJECTION (REGULAR)

Hormone
Antidiabetic agent

✤Actrapid McPork, Humulin R, Novolin R, ✤ Novolin-Toronto, Pork Regular Iletin II, Purified Regular Pork Insulin, Regular Iletin I, Velosulin

pH 7.0 to 7.8

USUAL DOSE

Varies greatly. Range is from 2 to 100 units/hr as indicated by patient's condition and response. It is imperative that dosing is individualized and adjusted based on blood and urine glucose determinations because of the marked loss of insulin from adsorption to glass and plastic infusion containers and tubing (see Precautions).

Low-dose treatment in ketoacidosis or diabetic coma is preferred: 10 to 30 units initially, then 2 to 12 units/hr. Note Precautions.

Diagnosis of growth hormone deficiency (unlabeled use): 0.05 to 0.15 units/kg of body weight as a rapid, one-time injection.

PEDIATRIC DOSE

Ketoacidosis: One reference recommends 10 to 20 units followed by 0.1 unit/kg/hour.

DOSE ADJUSTMENTS

A reduced dose of insulin may be indicated when infusions are discontinued and SC administration is indicated. As in Usual dose, base on blood and urine determinations and patient's response to therapy.

DILUTION

Use only if water clear. May be given undiluted either directly into the vein or through a Y-tube or three-way stopcock. Insulin is compatible with commonly used IV solutions and may be given as an infusion. Usually diluted in 0.9% (normal) or 0.45% saline for infusion. Fifty units of insulin added to 500 ml of infusion solution given at a rate of 1 ml/min will deliver 6 units/hr. Another regimen adds 100 units of insulin to 100 ml of normal saline. This solution is given at a rate of 0.1 unit/kg of body weight/hr.

Storage: Store unopened vials in refrigerator; vial that is in use may be stored in a cool, dark room. Discard any open vial not used for several weeks.

INCOMPATIBLE WITH

Aminophylline, amobarbital (Amytal), chlorothiazide (Diuril), cytarabine (ARA-C), digoxin (Lanoxin), diltiazem (Cardizem), dobutamine (Dobutrex), dopamine (Intropin), heparin, nafcillin (Unipen), norepinephrine (Levophed), penicillin G potassium, pentobarbital (Nembutal), phenobarbital (Luminal), phenytoin (Dilantin), secobarbital (Seconal), sodium bicarbonate, thiopental (Pentothal).

RATE OF ADMINISTRATION

Each 50 units or fraction thereof over 1 minute. When given in an IV infusion, the rate should be ordered by the physician and will depend on insulin and fluid needs (see Dilution for example). Decrease rate when plasma glucose falls to 250 mg/dL.

ACTIONS

A hormone produced by the pancreas. Responsible for storage, metabolism, and uptake of carbohydrates, proteins, and fat. Stimulates protein and free fatty acid synthesis and promotes conversion of glucose to glycogen. Rapidly and widely distributed. Half-life is 5 to 6 minutes. Eliminated to some extent renally. Does not cross the placenta. Not found in breast milk.

INDICATIONS AND USES

Treatment of diabetes mellitus (Type I, Type II, and gestational) ▪ Diabetic coma. ▪ Ketoacidosis. ▪ In combination with glucose to treat hyperkalemia. ▪ Induction of insulin shock for psychotherapy. ▪ Add to total parenteral nutrition to control hyperglycemia.

Unlabeled uses: Diagnosis of growth hormone deficiency. Continuous intravenous infusions administered via a special pump have been used to treat severe brittle diabetics who have failed more conventional therapy.

CONTRAINDICATIONS

There are no contraindications when insulin is indicated as a lifesaving measure.

PRECAUTIONS

Regular insulin only may be given IV. Humulin R is one of the newest products (recombinant DNA origin). All insulin is standardized at 100 units/ml. ▪ Insulin potency may be reduced by at least 20% and possibly up to 80% via the glass or plastic infusion container and plastic IV tubing before it actually reaches the venous system in an infusion. The percentage adsorbed is inversely proportional to the concentration of insulin (the larger the dose, the less adsorption) and takes place within 30 to 60 minutes. Albumin is sometimes added to reduce this adsorption. Other additives (e.g., electrolytes, other drugs, vitamins) may also reduce adsorption. Other methods of compensation for insulin loss include the addition of added insulin to saturate binding sites or the use of a syringe pump (instead of infusion containers) to reduce surface area for adsorption. ▪ In low-dose treatment of diabetic coma or ketoacidosis, an initial priming dose of 10 units followed by 2 to 12 units/hr has achieved normal plasma levels of 100 to 200 microunits/ml of blood more quickly than previously used large doses. ▪ Circulating levels of insulin may be increased in patients with renal or hepatic failure.

Monitor: Response to insulin measured by blood glucose, blood pH, acetone, BUN, sodium, potassium, chloride, and Co_2 levels. Monitor patient carefully in all situations. Use frequent blood glucose and ketone monitoring. ▪ Hypovolemia is a common complication of diabetic acidosis. ▪ Note Drug/lab interactions. ▪ Insulin is inactivated at pH above 7.5.

Patient education: Monitor blood glucose as directed. ▪ Adhere to consistent diet and exercise programs. ▪ Avoid alcohol.

Maternal/child: Category B. Human insulin is drug of choice for control of diabetes in pregnancy. Additional insulin may be required to control serum glucose and avoid ketoacidosis. Monitor carefully; insulin requirements may drop immediately postpartum. Normal prepregnancy dose should be achieved within 6 weeks. Patients with gestational diabetes usually do not require insulin therapy following childbirth. ▪ Breast feeding may decrease insulin requirements. ▪ Inadequately controlled maternal blood glucose late in pregnancy may cause increased insulin production in the fetus. Monitor and treat neonatal hypoglycemia postpartum.

DRUG/LAB INTERACTIONS

Combination of insulin and MAO inhibitors (e.g., selegiline [Eldepryl]) or alcohol is hazardous and may be lethal. ▪ Hypoglycemic effect is potentiated by beta-adrenergic blockers (e.g., propranolol [Inderal]), anabolic steroids (e.g., nandrolone [Durabolin]), guanethidine, isoniazid, pyrazolone compounds (e.g., phenylbutazone [Butazolidin]), salicylates, sulfonamides, tetracyclines, and many others. ▪ Inhibited by corticosteroids, thiazide diuretics, dobutamine (Dobutrex), epinephrine (Adrenalin), furosemide (Lasix), oral contraceptives, thyroid preparations, and others. ▪ Hypoglycemic effects may be decreased in smokers; dose adjustment may be required. ▪ Will affect serum potassium levels; use caution in patients taking digitalis products. ▪ Octreotide (Sandostatin) may alter insulin, glucagon, and growth hormone secretion, resulting in hypoglycemia or hyperglycemia. Monitor serum glucose, and adjust insulin dose as indicated. ▪ Pentamidine is toxic to the beta cells of the pancreas. Patients may develop hypoglycemia initially as insulin is released. This may be followed by hypoinsulinemia and hyperglycemia with continued pentamidine therapy. ▪ Octreotide (Sandostatin) markedly increases adsorption of insulin to glass and plastic and reduces availability.

SIDE EFFECTS

Hypoglycemia with overdose. **Early:** Ashen color, clammy skin, drowsiness, faintness, fatigue, headache, hunger, nausea, nervousness, sweating, tremors, weakness. **Advanced:** Coma, convulsions, disorientation, hypokalemia (with ECG changes), psychic disturbances, unconsciousness, hypersensitivity reactions including anaphylaxis; death is rare.

ANTIDOTE

Discontinue the drug immediately and notify physician. **Glucagon** is specific antidote for insulin overdose. It may be supplemented by glucose 50% IV and/or oral carbohydrates such as orange juice. Oral carbohydrates may be sufficient to combat early symptoms of hypoglycemia. Allergic reactions usually respond to symptomatic treatment.

INTERFERON ALFA-2b, RECOMBINANT

Biological response modifier
Antineoplastic

Intron A   pH 6.9 to 7.5

USUAL DOSE

Malignant melanoma: Induction: 20,000,000 IU/M^2 as an infusion each day for 5 consecutive days per week for 4 weeks. Begin therapy within 56 days of surgical resection.

Maintenance: Follow with 10,000,000 IU/M^2 as a SC injection three times each week for 48 weeks.

Total treatment regimen lasts for 1 year and should be completed unless there is progression of disease or the drug is discontinued because of specific side effects.

PEDIATRIC DOSE

Safety for use in children under 18 years of age not established.

DOSE ADJUSTMENTS

Temporarily discontinued for serious adverse reactions, if granulocytes decrease to <500/mm^3 or ALT (SGPT)/AST (SGOT) increases to >5 times upper limit of normal. When adverse reactions subside or improvement of granulocytes or liver function tests occur, treatment can be restarted at 50% of the previous dose. Discontinue permanently if serious adverse reactions persist, if granulocytes decrease to <250/mm^3, or if ALT/AST increases to >10 times upper limit of normal.

DILUTION

Prepare immediately prior to use. Only the sterile powder is suitable for dilution for IV use. Do not use different brands of interferon in any single treatment regimen; variations exist and may adversely affect dosage and response to treatment. Available in 3, 5, 10, 18, 25, and 50 million IU vials; select one most appropriate for desired dose. Reconstitute with the diluent provided. Withdraw desired dose and inject into 100 ml of NS. Final concentration should be at least 10 million IU/100 ml.

Storage: Unopened vials of powder for injection should be refrigerated; stable at room temperature for up to 7 days. Refrigerate reconstitued solution if not used immediately; stable for 1 month.

INCOMPATIBLE WITH

Specific information not available. Consider toxicity and specific use.

RATE OF ADMINISTRATION

A single dose equally distributed over 20 minutes. Administration at bedtime and the use of acetaminophen may prevent or partially reduce common side effects (e.g., fever, headache, "flu-like" symptoms).

ACTIONS

A naturally occurring small protein and glycoprotein of the interferon family produced by recombinant DNA techniques. It binds to specific membrane receptors on the cell surface and initiates a complex sequence of intracellular events (e.g., induction of specific enzymes, suppression of cell proliferation, immunomodulating activities [e.g., enhancement of phagocytic activity of macrophages, augmentation of the specific cytotoxicity of lymphocytes for target cells, inhibition of virus replication in virus-infected cells]). Peak concentration achieved within 30 minutes. Half-life about 2 hours, undetectable 4 hours after infusion. Has produced a significant increase in relapse-free and overall survival in patients with malignant melanoma. The kidney may be the site of interferon catabolism.

INDICATIONS AND USES

Adjuvant to surgical treatment in patients with malignant melanoma who are free of disease but at high risk for systemic recurrence. ■ Used IM or SC to treat hairy cell leukemia, AIDS-related Kaposi's sarcoma, chronic hepatitis non-A, non-B/C, chronic hepatitis B, and intralesionally to treat condylomata acuminata.

CONTRAINDICATIONS

Hypersensitivity to interferon alfa or any of its components (benzyl alcohol, glycine, human albumin, and sodium phosphate dibasic and monobasic). Not recommended for patients with a preexisting psychiatric condition, especially depression or a history of severe psychiatric disorder. Not recommended for patients with preexisting thyroid abnormalities if they cannot be maintained within the normal range with medication.

PRECAUTIONS

Use cautiously in patients with a history of pulmonary disease (e.g., COPD), diabetes mellitus prone to ketoacidosis, coagulation disorders (e.g., thrombophlebitis, pulmonary embolism) or severe myelosuppression. ■ Use cautiously in patients with a history of cardiovascular disease (e.g., unstable angina, uncontrolled CHF, recent MI, and previous or current arrhythmic disorder). ■ May cause depression and suicidal behavior. ■ Use caution in patients with psoriasis; may exacerbate disease. ■ Serum neutralizing antibiodies have been detected in some patients; clinical significance unknown.

Monitor: Obtain baseline CBC including differential and platelet count, blood chemistries (electrolytes, liver function tests, and TSH), chest x-ray. Obtain baseline eye exam for patients with diabetes or hypertension. Obtain baseline ECG if there is a history of cardiovascular disease and/or patient is in advanced stages of cancer. Monitor all tests periodically during therapy. ■ Monitor differential WBC and liver function tests weekly during the induction phase and monthly during maintenance. Dose adjustments will be determined by results or drug may be discontinued. ■ Closely monitor any patient with a history of cardiovascular disease (note Precautions), arrhythmias including tachycardia, hypotension and transient reversible cardiomyopathy have occurred. ■ Hypotension may occur during administration or up to 2 days posttherapy; monitor frequently, may require fluid replacement. ■ Maintain adequate hydration, particularly during initial states of treatment. ■ Monitor for signs of depression and/or suicidal behavior. ■ Use of narcotics, hypnotics, or sedatives may be required to manage adverse effects; use with caution and monitor carefully. ■ Monitor thyroid function; abnormalities not normalized by medication may require discontinuing interferon.

■ Determine cause of persistent fever. ■ Repeat chest x-ray if cough, dyspnea, fever, or other respiratory symptoms occur. Monitor closely if pulmonary infiltrates or evidence of pulmonary function impairment is present; may require discontinuing interferon. ■ Obtain an eye exam for any patient who complains of changes in visual acuity, visual fields, or other ophthalmologic symptoms; retinal hemorrhages, cotton-wool spots, and retinal artery or vein obstruction have been observed rarely.

Patient education: Must use effective birth control throughout treatment; nonhormonal birth control preferred. ■ Cooperation for close monitoring and reporting of side effects is imperative. ■ Manufacturer provides a patient information sheet. ■ Home use may require extensive patient education. ■ See Appendix D, p. 900. ■ Do not change brands of interferon without medical consultation. ■ Do not drive or operate machinery; mental alertness may be impaired. ■ Administration at bedtime and/or use of acetaminophen may be helpful to prevent the most common "flu-like" side effects. ■ Side effects may decrease in severity as treatment continues. Avoid excessive sunlight or artificial ultraviolet light. Potential for photosensitivity; wear protective clothing, sunscreens, and sunglasses.

Maternal/child: Pregnancy category C: has abortifacient effects, should be used only if benefits justify risks. ■ Discontinue breast feeding. ■ Safety for use in children under age 18 not established.

Elderly: Incidence of obtundation and coma has occurred, especially at higher doses.

DRUG/LAB INTERACTIONS

Specific information not available. Use caution with any other potenially myelosuppressive agent (e.g., cisplatin [Platinol], zidovudine [AZT]). ■ May increase serum levels of aminophylline; monitoring of aminophylline levels recommended. ■ May have synergistic additive effects with zidovudine (AZT) and increase incidence of neutropenia; monitor WBC closely.

SIDE EFFECTS

Occur in high percentages of patients and may be serious enough to require a decreased dose or discontinuation of drug. Usually rapidly reversible after therapy discontinued, but may require up to 3 weeks to resolve. Alopecia, anemia, anorexia, arrhythmias, bleeding, coughing, depression, diarrhea, dizziness, dyspnea, "flu-like" symptoms (e.g., chills, fatigue, fever, headache, myalgia), granulocytopenia, increased AST and/or ALT, leukopenia, nausea, pain (variable), paresthesia, rash, taste alteration, thrombocytopenia. Many other side effects may occur. Acute serious hypersensitivity reactions (e.g., anaphylaxis, angioedema, bronchoconstriction, urticaria) are rare but have occurred.

ANTIDOTE

Keep physician informed of all side effects. Some will be tolerated or treated symptomatically. Discontinue interferon immediately for any acute serious hypersensitivity reactions and treat as appropriate. Discontinue drug for any patient developing severe depression or other psychiatric disorder, myelosuppression that persists after dose reduction, thyroid abnormalities not normalized by medication, serious liver function abnormalities, serious pulmonary function impairment, or pulmonary infiltrates. Resuscitate as necessary.

IRINOTECAN HYDROCHLORIDE

Antineoplastic
(Topoisomerase 1 inhibitor)

Camptosar   pH 3.0 to 3.8

USUAL DOSE

Premedication with antiemetics recommended. Dexamethasone 10 mg and a 5-HT_3 blocker (e.g., ondansetron or granisetron) should be given on the day of treatment. Begin at least 30 minutes before giving irinotecan.

Irinotecan: Administer 125 mg/M^2 as an infusion once each week for 4 weeks, followed by a 2-week rest period. After adequate recovery additional doses may be repeated in a similar 6-week cycle and continued indefinitely in patients who attain a response or in those whose disease remains stable. A new course of therapy should not begin until the granulocyte count has recovered to $\geq$ 1500 mm³, the platelet count has recovered to $\geq$100,000/mm³, and treatment-related diarrhea is fully resolved. Treatment should be delayed 1 to 2 weeks to allow for recovery from treatment-related toxicities. If the patient has not recovered after a 2-week delay, consideration should be given to discontinuing irinotecan.

DOSE ADJUSTMENTS

Discontinue if neutropenic fever occurs or absolute neutrophil count drops below 500/mm³. ■ Reduce dose if total WBC is <2,000/mm³, neutrophil count is <1,000/mm³, hemoglobin is <8 Gm/dL, or platelets are <100,000/mm³ (see table below). ■ Dose may be increased to 150 mg/M^2 or decreased to as low as 50 mg/M^2 based on individual patient tolerance (see table). Most common reasons for dose reduction are late diarrhea, neutropenia, and leukopenia. ■ Dose reduction may be required in the elderly and in patients who have previously received pelvic/abdominal irradiation.

Toxicity NCI Grade* (Value)	During a Course of Therapy†	At the Start of the Next Courses of Therapy† (After Adequate Recovery), Compared to the Starting Dose in the Previous Course
No toxicity	Maintain dose level	↑25 mg/m² up to a maximum dose of 150 mg/m²
Neutropenia 1 (1500 to 1900/.mm³) 2 (1000 to 1400/mm³) 3 (500 to 900/mm³) 4 (<500/mm³)	Maintain dose level ↓25 mg/m² Omit dose, then ↓25 mg/m² when resolved to ≤grade 2 Omit dose, then ↓50 mg/m² when resolved to ≤grade 2	Maintain dose level Maintain dose level ↓25 mg/m² ↓50 mg/m²
Neutropenic fever- (grade 4 neutropenia & ≥grade 2 fever)	Omit dose, then ↓50 mg/m² when resolved	↓50 mg/m²

Continued

Toxicity NCI Grade* (Value) *continued*	During a Course of Therapy† *continued*	At the Start of the Next Courses of Therapy† (After Adequate Recovery), Compared to the Starting Dose in the Previous Course *continued*
Other hematologic toxicities	Dose modifications for leukopenia, thrombocytopenia, and anemia during a course of therapy and at the start of subsequent courses of therapy are also based on NCI toxicity criteria and are the same as recommended for neutropenia above.	
Diarrhea 1 (2-3 stools/day > pretx)	Maintain dose level	Maintain dose level
2 (4-6 stools/day > pretx)	↓25 mg/m2	Maintain, if the only grade 2 toxicity
3 (7-9 stools/day > pretx)	Omit dose, then ↓25 mg/m² when resolved to ≤ grade 2	↓25 mg/m², if the only grade 3 toxicity
4 (≥10 stools/day > pretx)	Omit dose, then ↓50 mg/m² when resolved to ≤ grade 2	↓50 mg/m²
Other nonhematologic toxicities 1	Maintain dose level	Maintain dose level
2	↓25 mg/m²	↓25 mg/m²
3	Omit dose, then ↓25 mg/m² when resolved to ≤ grade 2	↓50 mg/m²
4	Omit dose, then ↓50 mg/m² when resolved to ≤ grade 2	↓50 mg/m²

*National Cancer Institute Common Toxicity Criteria.
†All dose modifications should be based on the worst preceding toxicity.

DILUTION
Specific techniques required: see Precautions. Must be diluted for infusion with D5W (preferred) or NS to concentrations between 0.12 to 1.1 mg/ml. Usually diluted in 500 ml D5W.

Storage: Packaged in a blister pack to protect against accidental breakage and leakage. Store in carton protected from light at controlled room temperature. Do not freeze. If damaged, incinerate the unopened package. Recommended that diluted solution be used within 24 hours if refrigerated, within 6 hours if kept at controlled room temperature. However, when mixed with D5W, is stable for 48 hours if refrigerated and 24 hours at CRT. Do not refrigerate if mixed with NS; a precipitate may form. Stable for 24 hours at CRT.

INCOMPATIBLE WITH
Manufacturer states, "Other drugs should not be added to the infusion solution."

RATE OF ADMINISTRATION
A single dose as an infusion equally distributed over 90 minutes.

ACTIONS
An alkaloid extract from plants such as *Camptotheca acuminata*. A new class of antineoplastic agent that inhibits the enzyme topoisomerase I required for DNA replication. Together with its active metabolite SN-38 it causes cell death by damaging DNA produced during the S-phase of cell synthesis. Maximum plasma SN-38 levels are reached within 1 hour of infusion end. Extensively distributed to body tissues. Terminal half-life of irinotecan is about 6 hours; SN-38 is 10 hours. Irinotecan is moderately bound to plasma proteins (35%), but SN-38

is highly bound (95%). Metabolic conversion of irinotecan to SN-38 primarily occurs in the liver. Approximately 25% to 50% excreted through bile and urine.

INDICATIONS AND USES

Treatment of metastatic carcinoma of the colon or rectum that has recurred or progressed following treatment with fluorouracil.

CONTRAINDICATIONS

Hypersensitivity to irinotecan or any of its components.

PRECAUTIONS

Follow guidelines for handling cytotoxic agents. See Appendix A, p. 893. ▪ Administered by or under the direction of the physician specialist. ▪ Adequate diagnostic and treatment facilities must be available. ▪ Must have normal biliary function. Hepatic dysfunction may impair the metabolism of both irinotecan and SN-38. ▪ Use caution in the elderly (may have an increased incidence and severity of diarrhea) and in patients with previous pelvic/abdominal irradiation (likely to have an increased incidence and severity of myelosuppression). Monitor closely. ▪ Use caution in patients with a history of allergies. ▪ Use caution in patients with pleural effusions and/or with impaired pulmonary function. ▪ Note Monitor.

Monitor: Obtain an accurate bowel history to evaluate changes in bowel habits after administration of irinotecan. ▪ Obtain a WBC with differential, hemoglobin, and platelet count before each dose. ▪ Prophylactic antiemetics are recommended; (See Usual dose). To reduce nausea and vomiting and increase patient comfort after initial dosing, additional antiemetics should be available (e.g., prochlorperazine [Compazine]). ▪ Consider obtaining baseline electrolytes and liver function tests. ▪ Not a vesicant, but monitor injection site for inflammation and/or extravasation. ▪ Monitor vital signs. ▪ Monitor for "early" diarrhea. Occurs during or within 24 hours of irinotecan administration; is primarily cholinergic (e.g., abdominal cramping, diaphoresis, severe, usually transient, diarrhea). At the first indication, treat with atropine 0.25 to 1 mg IV unless clinically contraindicated. ▪ Monitor for "late" diarrhea (more than 24 hours after irinotecan administration), which probably results from cytotoxic effects on GI epithelium. May be prolonged, cause dehydration and electrolyte imbalances, and can be life threatening. At first onset give loperamide (Imodium) 4 mg; give 2 mg every 2 hours (4 mg every 4 hours during the night) until diarrhea-free for a minimum of 12 hours. Monitor carefully; replace fluids and electrolytes as needed. Premedication or prophylaxis with loperamide is not recommended. ▪ Use of laxatives is not recommended; however, they may be used in patients requiring them for constipation caused by narcotics. Close supervision is required. ▪ Maintain adequate hydration. ▪ Be alert for signs of bone marrow suppression or infection. Prophylactic antibiotics may be indicated pending results of C/S in a febrile or nonfebrile neutropenic patient. ▪ Patients who have a cholinergic reaciton to irinotecan will probably have similar reactions to susbsequent doses. Atropine may be considered for prophylactic use. No studies available. ▪ Expected nadir for platelets is 14 days, 21 days for hemoglobin, neutrophils, and leukocytes. ▪ Note Dose adjustments.

Patient education: Manufacturer provides a patient education brochure, "Important Facts About Your Chemotherapy." ▪ Report any unusual or unexpected symptoms or side effects as soon as possible. ▪ Report diarrhea, dry mouth, fainting, fever or chills, infections, urine changes or vomiting immediately; each must be treated promptly. ▪ Compliance with regimen imperative (e.g., taking temperature, obtaining lab work, adequate rest, nourishment, and fluids). ▪ Nonhormonal birth control recommended. ▪ Inform health care professionals of any problems with previous treatments. ▪ See Appendix D, p. 900.

Maternal/child: Category D: Avoid pregnancy. May cause fetal harm. ▪ Discontinue breast-feeding. ▪ Safety and effectiveness for use in children not established.

Elderly: Half-life slightly extended; no dose adjustment routinely recommended. ▪ Monitor carefully; may dehydrate more quickly from diarrhea. Begin loperamide therapy promptly. Avoid laxatives.

DRUG/LAB INTERACTIONS

Interaction of irinotecan with other drugs has not been adequately studied. ▪ Toxicity (e.g., myelosuppression, diarrhea) may be increased by other antineoplastic agents with similar side effects (e.g., fluorouracil). ▪ Concurrent administration with irradiation is not recommended. ▪ Dexamethasone for antiemetic prophylaxis may increase lymphocytopenia and may contribute to hyperglycemia in patients with diabetes. ▪ Use caution or withhold diuretics (e.g., furosemide [Lasix]) and laxatives during treatment; may increase risk of dehydration secondary to vomiting and/or diarrhea. ▪ Do not administer live vaccines to patients receiving antineoplastic drugs.

SIDE EFFECTS

Myelosuppression (anemia, leukopenia, neutropenia) and diarrhea ("early" [e.g., abdominal cramping or pain, diaphoresis] or "late") occur in patients and are the most common dose-limiting toxicities. Nausea and vomiting occur in most patients and can be severe. Abdominal bloating, alopecia, anorexia, back pain, chills, constipation, coughing, dehydration, dizziness, dyspepsia, dyspnea, edema, fever, flatulence, flushing, headache, increased alkaline phosphatase and AST (SGOT), infection, insomnia, rash, rhinitis, stomatitis, and weight loss may occur. Death was preceeded by cyanosis, tremors, respiratory distress, and convulsions.

ANTIDOTE

Keep physician informed of all side effects and monitor carefully. Adjust or omit dose as indicated for toxicity; see Dose adjustments. Treat diarrhea immediately; see Monitor. Myelosuppression may require whole blood or platelet transfusion. G-CSF (Filgrastim) may be indicated during neutropenia episodes. Death may occur from the progression of many side effects. No known antidote for overdose. Maximum supportive care (e.g., to prevent dehydration due to diarrhea and to treat any infectious complications) will help to sustain patient in toxicity. If extravasation occurs, flush site with sterile water, elevate the extremity, and apply ice.

IRON DEXTRAN INJECTION

Antianemic
Iron supplement

Dexferrum, ✵Dexlron, InFed, Proferdex

pH 5.2 to 6.5

USUAL DOSE

0.5 ml (25 mg) on the first day as a test dose. Wait 1 hour. If no adverse reactions, may be increased gradually to 2 ml (100 mg)/24 hr and repeated daily until results achieved or maximum calculated dosage reached (see literature). A total calculated dose has been given as an infusion. Though not FDA approved, this method is preferred to multiple small-dose infusions or injections by some.

PEDIATRIC DOSE

0.5 ml (25 mg) on the first day as a test dose. Wait 1 hour. If no adverse reactions, may give remainder of daily dose. The following daily doses have been recommended by one source: <5 kg: 25mg. 5-10 kg: 50 mg. >10 kg: 100 mg. Repeat daily until results achieved or maximum calculated dosage reached (see literature).

DILUTION

Check vial carefully; must state "for IV use." Given undiluted, or up to the total desired dose may be further diluted in 50 to 1,000 ml NS for infusion. D5W may cause additional local pain and phlebitis.

INCOMPATIBLE WITH

Any other drug in syringe or solution. Has been added to TPN (2 in 1 solutions). However, this is not recommended by the manufacturer.

RATE OF ADMINISTRATION

Direct IV: 1 ml (50 mg) or fraction thereof over 1 minute or more.

Infusion: Test dose of 25 mg over 5 minutes. If no adverse reactions, infuse remaining dose over 1 to 8 hours (based on amount of dose, amount of diluent, and patient comfort). Discontinue IV infusion solutions during administration of iron dextran injection.

ACTIONS

The iron-dextran complex is separated into smaller molecules by cellular systems in the bone marrow, liver, spleen, etc. By chemical processes usable iron can then be absorbed into the hemoglobin. After hemoglobin needs of the blood are met, iron is stored in the body for reserve use. Small amounts of unabsorbed iron are excreted in the urine, feces, and bile. Crosses the placental barrier. Trace amounts of unmetabolized iron dextran are excreted in breast milk.

INDICATIONS AND USES

Iron-deficiency anemia in patients for whom oral administration is unsatisfactory or impossible; identify and treat the cause of the anemia.

Unlabeled use: Iron supplementation for patients taking epoetin (Epogen, Procrit).

CONTRAINDICATIONS

Manifestation of allergic reaction, any anemia other than iron deficiency.

PRECAUTIONS

Use only when truly indicated to avoid excess storage of iron.
■ Increases joint pain and swelling in patients with rheumatoid arthritis. ■ Use caution with history of asthma or allergies. ■ Allergic reactions are often delayed, are more frequent with certain batches, and may happen at any time during an infusion even if no reaction from test dose. ■ Use only if absolutely necessary in liver disease. ■ Do not use during acute phase of an infectious kidney disease.

Monitor: Keep patient lying down after injection to prevent postural hypotension. ■ Observe continuously for an allergic reaction during an infusion. Monitor vital signs. ■ Monitor serum ferritin assays in prolonged therapy. Consider possibility of false results for months after injection caused by delayed utilization.

Maternal/child: Pregnancy Category C: use only if absolutely necessary in pregnancy, lactation, or childbearing years. Known hazard to fetus. ■ Not recommended in infants younger than 4 months of age.

DRUG/LAB INTERACTIONS

Inhibited by chloramphenicol. ■ May cause a false elevated bilirubin, false decreased calcium, or affect numerous other tests or scans. ■ Note Monitor.

SIDE EFFECTS

Minor: Backache, dizziness, headache, itching, local phlebitis at injection site, malaise, nausea, rash, shivering, transitory paresthesias.

Major: Anaphylaxis; arthritic reactivation; dyspnea; febrile episodes; hypotension; leukocytosis; local phlebitis; lymphadenopathy; peripheral vascular flushing, especially with too-rapid injection; urticaria; tachycardia; shock (severe iron toxicity increases vasodilation and venous pooling and decreases circulating blood volume. Results in decreased cardiac output, hypotension, increased peripheral vascular resistance, and shock).

ANTIDOTE

Discontinue the drug and notify the physician of early symptoms. For severe symptoms, discontinue drug, treat allergic reactions or resuscitate as necessary, and notify physician. Epinephrine (Adrenalin) and diphenhydramine (Benadryl) should always be available.

ISOPROTERENOL HYDROCHLORIDE

Cardiac stimulant (inotropic/chronotropic) Bronchodilator Antiarrhythmic

Isuprel hydrochloride

pH 3.5 to 4.5

USUAL DOSE

Asthma unresponsive to inhalation therapy: 0.01 to 0.02 mg (0.5 to 1 ml of a 1:50,000 dilution). Repeat as necessary.

Control bronchospasm during anesthesia: 0.01 to 0.02 mg (0.5 to 1 ml of a 1:50,000 dilution). Repeat as necessary.

Atropine-resistant hemodynamically significant bradycardia: 0.02 to 0.06 mg (1 to 3 ml of a 1:50,000 dilution) as an initial dose. Subsequent doses may range from 0.01 to 0.2 mg (0.5 to 10 ml of a 1:50,000 dilution) or may be maintained with an infusion. 5 mcg/min (1.25 ml of a 1:250,000 dilution) is the average initial dose. Range is 2 to 20 mcg/minute. JAMA recommendation is 2 to 10 mcg/min.

Complete heart block following closure of ventricular septal defects: 0.04 to 0.06 mg (2 to 3 ml of a 1:50,000 dilution) as a bolus injection. May maintain a sinus rhythm with a heart rate above 90 to 100/min or may relapse into complete heart block again.

Shock: 0.5 to 5 mcg/min as an infusion (0.25 to 2.5 ml of a 1:500,000 dilution [2 mcg/ml]). Titrate to patient response (e.g., heart rate, central venous pressure, blood pressure, urine output). Up to 30 mcg/min have been used in advanced stages of shock. Administer only for 1 hour or less in patients with septic shock.

Diagnosis of mitral regurgitation: 4 mcg/min as an infusion (1 ml/min of a 1:250,000 dilution).

Diagnosis of coronary artery disease or lesions: 1 to 3 mcg/min as an infusion (0.25 to 0.75 ml/min of a 1:250,000 dilution).

Intracardiac: 0.02 mg (0.1 ml) of a 1:5,000 dilution (rarely used).

PEDIATRIC DOSE

Status asthmaticus: 0.08 to 1.7 mcg/kg/min as an infusion. Begin with 0.1 mcg/kg/min and increase every 5 to 10 minutes by 0.1 mcg/kg/min until desired effect. Reduce rate for tachycardia over 180 or if arrhythmia occurs.

Atropine-resistant hemodynamically significant bradycardia: Begin with 0.1 mcg/kg/min as an infusion. Increase by 0.1 mcg/kg/min until desired effect. Titrate to patient response and monitor cardiac status carefully. Maximum dose is 1 mcg/kg/min.

Complete heart block after closure of ventricular septal defects in infants: 0.01 to 0.03 mg (0.5 to 1.5 ml of a 1:50,000 dilution) as a bolus injection. See comments in Adult dose.

DILUTION

IV injection: Available in a 1:50,000 solution or dilute 0.2 mg (1 ml) of a 1:5,000 solution with 9 ml NS for injection (1:50,000 solution).

Infusion: 1 mg (5 ml) of a 1:5,000 solution in 250 ml (2 mg [10 ml] in

500 ml) of D5W. 1 ml equals 4 mcg in this 1:250,000 solution. Dilute 1 mg in 500 ml (1:500,000 soluton [2 mcg/ml) to treat shock. Use an infusion pump or microdrip (60 gtt equals 1 ml) to administer. Less diluent may be used to reduce fluid intake.

Pediatric infusion: 0.6 mg/kg isoproterenol in 100 ml D5W. 1 ml/hr equals 0.1 mcg/kg/min.

Intracardiac: 1:5,000 solution undiluted. (Rarely used). No longer recommended as an acceptable route for bradycardia or cardiac arrest. Do not use if pink or brown in color or contains a precipitate.

INCOMPATIBLE WITH

Aminophylline, barbiturates, carbenicillin (Geopen), diazepam (Valium), epinephrine (Adrenalin), furosemide (Lasix), lidocaine, sodium bicarbonate.

RATE OF ADMINISTRATION

Infusion: Titrate to desired dose, heart rate and rhythm. Decrease rate of infusion as necessary. Ventricular rate generally should not exceed 110 beats/min.

Isoproterenol (Isuprel) infusion rates						
Desired dose	1 mg in 500 ml D5W (2 mcg/ml)			1 mg in 250 ml D5W 2 mg in 500 ml D5W (4 mcg/ml)		
mcg/min	mcg/hr	ml/min	ml/hr	mcg/hr	ml/min	ml/hr
2	120	1	60	120	0.5	30
5	300	2.5	150	300	1.25	75
10	600	5	300	600	2.5	150
15	900	7.5	450	900	3.75	225
20	1200	10	600	1200	5	300
25	1500	12.5	750	1500	6.25	375
30	1800	15	900	1800	7.5	450
Pediatric infusion: 0.6 mg/kg in 100 ml D5W 1 ml/hr = 0.1 mcg/kg/min.						

IV injection: Each 1 ml of a 1:50,000 (0.02 mg) solution or fraction thereof over 1 minute. Follow with a 20 ml flush of NS if indicated to assure distribution to circulation.

Intracardiac: Each 0.1 ml of a 1:5,000 solution over 1 second. See note in Dilution for this route.

ACTIONS

A synthetic cardiac beta receptor stimulant (sympathomimetic amine) similar to epinephrine and norepinephrine. Has positive inotropic and chronotropic actions more potent than those of epinephrine. It increases cardiac output, cardiac work, coronary flow, and venous return. Improves atrioventricular conduction. Stimulates only the higher ventricular foci, allowing a more normal cardiac pacemaker to take over, thus suppressing ectopic pacemaker activity. Decreases peripheral vascular resistance by relaxing arterial smooth muscle and is a most effective bronchial smooth muscle relaxant. Onset of action is immediate and lasts 1 to 2 hours. Excreted in the urine.

INDICATIONS AND USES

Atrioventricular heart block and Stokes-Adams syndrome. ■ Some ventricular arrhythmias due to AV nodal block. ■ Treatment of refractory torsades de pointes until pacemaker implanted. ■ Temporary control of symptomatic bradycardia in denervated hearts of heart transplant patients until pacemaker implanted. ■ Bronchospasm during anesthesia. ■ Management of shock (cardiogenic, CHF, hypoperfusion [low cardiac output], hypovolemic, septic). Adequate fluid and electrolyte replacement required. ■ Pulmonary embolism, to increase pulmonary blood volume and decrease pulmonary arterial pressure and vascular resistance. ■ Cardiac arrest only until pacemaker available or if pacemaker fails. No longer recommended by JAMA or AHA. ■ Cardiac catheterization to simulate exercise. ■ On occasion as an antidote to reverse severe hypotension caused by tricyclic antidepressants (e.g., amitriptyline [Elavil]).

CONTRAINDICATIONS

Tachyarrhythmias, patients with tachycardia or heart block caused by digitalis intoxication, angina pectoris, ventricular arrhythmias that require inotropic therapy.

PRECAUTIONS

Intracardiac or IV injection in cardiac standstill must be accompanied by cardiac massage to perfuse drug into the myocardium. Current JAMA recommendations do not include isoproterenol in the treatment of cardiac arrest or hypotension. ■ Fourth-line agent for bradycardia; considered possibly helpful but may be harmful. ■ Can cause a severe drop in blood pressure and can be very harmful in bradycardia. ■ Use extreme caution when inhalant anesthetics (e.g., cyclopropane) are being administered and supplementary to digitalis administration. ■ Use caution in coronary insufficiency, diabetes, hyperthyroidism, known sensitivity to sympathomimetic amines, and preexisting cardiac arrhythmias with tachycardia. ■ Increased cardiac output and work can increase ischemia and worsen arrhythmias. ■ Contains sulfites; use caution in allergic patients.

Monitor: Decrease rate of infusion as necessary. Ventricular rate generally should not exceed 110 beats/min. Maintain adequate blood volume and correct acidosis. ■ Continuous cardiac monitoring, central venous pressure readings, blood pressure, and urine flow measurements are advisable during therapy with isoproterenol. ■ Note Drug/lab interactions.

Maternal/ child: Pregnancy Category C: safety for use in pregnancy or lactation not established. Benefits must outweigh risks.

DRUG/LAB INTERACTIONS

May be used alternately with epinephrine (Adrenalin), but they may not be used together. Both are direct cardiac stimulants; serious arrhythmias and death may result. An adequate interval between doses must be maintained. ■ Simultaneous use with oxytoxics may cause hypertensive crisis. ■ May cause hypertension with guanethidine (Ismelin). ■ May cause arrhythmia with bretylium. ■ Halogenated hydrocarbon anesthetics (e.g., halothane) may sensitize myocardium and cause serious arrhythmias. ■ Antagonized by propranolol (Inderal). May be used to treat tachycardia caused by isoproterenol, but tachycardia and hypotension secondary to peripheral vasodilation may occur. ■ Potentiated by tricyclic antidepressants. ■ Severe hypotension and bradycardia may occur with hydantoins (e.g., phenyoin [Dilantin]).

SIDE EFFECTS

Anginal pain, cardiac arrhythmias, flushing, headache, nausea, nervousness, palpitations, sweating, tachycardia, vomiting. Cardiac dilation, marked hypotension, pulmonary edema, and death may occur with prolonged use or overdose.

ANTIDOTE

Notify the physician of any side effect. Treatment will probably be symptomatic. For ventricular rate over 110 beats/min, PVCs, or ECG changes, decrease rate of infusion or discontinue drug. For accidental overdose, discontinue drug immediately, resuscitate and sustain patient, and notify physician.

KANAMYCIN SULFATE

♣Anamid, Kantrex

Antibacterial
(Aminoglycoside)

pH 4.5

USUAL DOSE

Up to 15 mg/kg of body weight/24 hr equally divided into 2 or 3 doses. Dosage based on ideal body weight. Do not exceed a total adult dose of 1.5 Gm by all routes in 24 hours. Recent studies suggest that a total daily dose administered as a single dose (instead of divided into 2 or 3 doses) may provide higher peak levels and enhance drug effectiveness while actually reducing or having no adverse effects on risk of toxicity. Monitor with trough levels.

Mycobacterium avium *complex:* 11 to 13 mg/kg/24 hr in equally divided doses every 8 to 12 hours (part of a 3 to 5 agent regimen).

Tuberculosis: 15 to 30 mg/kg to maximum dose of 1 Gm daily.

PEDIATRIC DOSE

15 to 30 mg/kg/24 hr in equally divided doses every 12 hours. Maximum dose is 1.5 Gm.

NEONATAL DOSE

Less than 2,000 Gm; under 7 days of age: 7.5 mg/kg every 12 hours. *Over 7 days of age:* 6.67 mg/kg every 8 hours.

Over 2,000 Gm; under 7 days of age: 10 mg/kg every 12 hours. *Over 7 days of age:* 10 mg/kg every 8 hours.

DOSE ADJUSTMENTS

Reduce daily dose for renal impairment or increase intervals between injections. ■ Reduced dose or extended intervals may be required in the elderly. ■ Note Monitor and Drug/lab interactions.

DILUTION

Each 500 mg or fraction thereof must be diluted with at least 100 ml of D5W, D5/NS, or NS for infusion. Discard partially used vials after 48 hours.

INCOMPATIBLE WITH

Administer separately. Incompatible with amphotericin B, ampicillin, carbenicillin (Geopen), cefoxitin (Mefoxin), cephalothin (Keflin), cephapirin (Cefadyl), chlorpheniramine (Chlor-Trimeton), colistimethate (Coly-Mycin M), heparin, hydrocortisone (Solu-Cortef), methohexital (Brevital), penicillins.

RATE OF ADMINISTRATION

Do not exceed a rate of 3 to 4 ml/min diluted solution. Give total dose over 30 to 60 minutes.

ACTIONS

An aminoglycoside antibiotic with neuromuscular blocking action. Bactericidal against many gram-negative organisms resistant to other antibiotics. Well distributed through all body fluids; crosses the placental barrier. Usual half-life is 2 to 3 hours. Half-life is prolonged in infants, postpartum females, fever, liver disease and ascites, spinal cord injury, cystic fibrosis, and the elderly; shorter in severe burns. Excreted in high concentrations through the kidneys. Secreted in breast milk. Cross-allergenicity does occur between aminoglycosides.

INDICATIONS AND USES

Short-term treatment of serious infections caused by susceptible organisms. ▪ Concurrent therapy with a penicillin or cephalosporin sometimes indicated. ▪ Treatment of tuberculosis. ▪ Primarily used when penicillin and other less toxic antibiotics are ineffective or contraindicated.

Unlabeled uses: Treatment of *Mycobacterium avium* complex, a common infection in AIDS (part of a multiple drug [3 to 5] regimen).

CONTRAINDICATIONS

Known kanamycin or aminoglycoside sensitivity, prior hearing damage by kanamycin or other ototoxic agents unless infection is life threatening. Sulfite sensitivity may be a contraindication.

PRECAUTIONS

Most frequently given IM. ▪ Use extreme caution if therapy is required over 7 to 10 days. ▪ Sensitivity studies necessary to determine susceptibility of the causative organism to kanamycin. ▪ Superinfection may occur from overgrowth of nonsusceptible organisms. ▪ Use caution in children and the elderly. ▪ May cause "malabsorption syndrome" (increase in fecal fat, decrease in serum carotene and xylose absorption); most common in prolonged therapy. ▪ May contain sulfites; use caution in patients with asthma.

Monitor: Routine evaluation of hearing is necessary. Watch for decrease in urine output, rising BUN and serum creatinine, and declining creatinine clearance levels. Dose may need to be decreased. ▪ Narrow range between toxic and therapeutic levels. Periodically monitor peak and trough concentrations to avoid peak serum concentrations above 30 mcg/ml and trough concentrations above 5 mcg/ml. ▪ Maintain good hydration. ▪ Monitor serum calcium, magnesium, potassium, and sodium; levels may decline. ▪ In extended treatment, daily monitoring of serum levels, electrolytes, renal, auditory, and vestibular functions is recommended. ▪ Note Drug/lab interactions.

Patient education: Report promptly dizziness, hearing loss, weakness, or any changes in balance. ▪ Consider birth control options.

Maternal/child: Category D: avoid pregnancy; use during pregnancy and

lactation only when absolutely necessary. Potential hazard to fetus.
■ Rarely used IV in infants; use extreme caution in premature infants and neonates; immature kidney function will result in prolonged half-life.

Elderly: Consider less toxic alternatives. ■ Half-life prolonged. ■ Longer intervals between doses may be more important than reduced doses. ■ Monitor renal function and drug levels carefully. Measurement of creatinine clearance more useful than BUN or serum creatinine to assess renal function. ■ Note Precautions.

DRUG/LAB INTERACTIONS

Inactivated in solution with penicillin but is synergistic when used in combination with beta-lactam antibiotics (e.g., sulbactam sodium, clavulanate potassium, cephalosporins, penicillins), and vancomycin. Dose adjustment and appropriate spacing required because of physical incompatibilities and interactions. Synergism may be inconsistent; measure aminoglycoside levels. ■ Concurrent use topically or systemically with any other ototoxic or nephrotoxic agents should be avoided. May have dangerous additive effects with anesthetics (e.g., enflurane), other neuromuscular blocking antibiotics (e.g., gentamicin), diuretics (e.g., furosemide [Lasix]), beta-lactam antibiotics (e.g., cephalosporins), vancomycin, and many others. ■ Neuromuscular blocking muscle relaxants (e.g., doxacurium [Nuromax], succinylcholine [Anectine]) are potentiated by aminoglycosides. *Apnea can occur.* ■ Aminoglycosides are also potentiated by anticholinesterases (e.g., edrophonium), antineoplastics (e.g., nitrogen mustard, cisplatin). ■ Digoxin dose may need adjustment. ■ May be antagonized by bacteriostatic antibiotics (e.g., chloramphenicol, erythomicin, and tetracyclines); bactericidal action may be impacted.

SIDE EFFECTS

Occur more frequently with impaired renal function, higher doses, prolonged administration, in dehydrated or elderly patients, and in patients receiving other ototoxic or nephrotoxic drugs.

Minor: Fever, headache, paresthesias, skin rash, thrombophlebitis.

Major: Apnea; azotemia; elevated BUN, nonprotein nitrogen, creatinine; granular casts; hearing loss; malabsorption syndrome; neuromuscular blockade; oliguria; proteinuria; tinnitus; vertigo.

ANTIDOTE

Notify the physician of all side effects. If minor symptoms persist or any major symptom appears, discontinue the drug and notify the physician. Treatment is symptomatic, or a reduction in dose may be required. In overdose, hemodialysis may be indicated. Monitor fluid balance, creatinine clearance, and plasma levels carefully. Complexation with ticarcillin or carbenicillin (12 to 30 Gm/day) may be as effective as hemodialysis. Consider exchange transfusion in the newborn. Calcium salts or neostigmine may reverse neuromuscular blockade. Resuscitate as necessary.

KETOROLAC TROMETHAMINE

Analgesic
(NSAID)

Toradol

pH 6.9 to 7.9

USUAL DOSE

Adults less than 65 years: 30 mg. May repeat every 6 hours. Maximum dose is 120 mg in 24 hours. Do not increase the dose or frequency for breakthrough pain. Consider alternating with low doses of opioids (e.g., morphine or meperidine). Ketorolac oral may be used only as continuation therapy to parenteral dosing. Maximum oral dose is 40 mg/24 hours. Do not administer for longer than 5 days (IV/IM alone or combined use with oral).

Adults over 65 years, impaired renal function, and/or patients under 50 kg (110 lb): 15 mg. May repeat every 6 hours. Maximum dose is 60 mg in 24 hours. Note all restrictions for adults less than 65 years outlined above.

DOSE ADJUSTMENTS

Required for patients under 50 kg (110 lb); over 65 years of age; and those with reduced renal function, (See Usual dose). Further dose reductions may be required with high-dose salicylates (See Drug/lab interactions)

DILUTION

May be given undiluted through Y-tube or three-way stopcock of infusion set. Administration through a free-flowing IV is preferred.

Storage: Store at controlled room temperature, protect from light.

INCOMPATIBLE WITH

Syringe: Diazepam (Valuim), Hydroxyzine (Vistaril), meperidine (Demerol), nalbuphine (Nubain), prochlorperazine (Compazine), promethazine (Phenergan).

RATE OF ADMINISTRATION

A single dose over a minimum of 15 seconds, evenly distributed over 1 to 2 minutes is preferred.

ACTIONS

A nonsteroidal antiinflammatory drug (NSAID) with peripheral analgesic, antiinflammatory, and antipyretic actions. Inhibits prostaglandin synthesis. 30 to 60 mg produces analgesia similar to morphine 12 mg or demerol 100 mg. Studies reflect less drowsiness, nausea, and vomiting. Not a narcotic agonist or antagonist. Cardiac and hemodynamic parameters are not altered. Onset of action is 30 to 60 minutes. Half-life varies from 3.8 to 8.6 hours based on age and clinical status. Relief in some patients may last 6 to 8 hours. Excreted primarily in urine. Secreted in breast milk.

INDICATIONS AND USES

Short-term management of moderately severe, acute pain (no longer than 5 days).

CONTRAINDICATIONS

Hypersensitivity to ketorolac or its components, labor and delivery, lactation, preoperative or intraoperative medication, patients currently receiving ASA or NSAIDs, active peptic ulcer disease, recent GI bleeding or perforation, patients with a history of peptic ulcer disease or GI bleeding, suspected or confirmed cerebrovascular bleeding, hemorrhagic diathesis, incomplete hemostasis, high risk of bleeding, advanced renal impairment. Do not use for epidural or intrathecal administration, contains alcohol. Note Drug/lab interactions.

PRECAUTIONS

Inhibits platelet aggregation and may prolong bleeding time. ▪ May cause serious GI ulceration and bleeding without warning. ▪ In addition to the usual caution in patients with reduced hepatic or renal function, ketoralac may also cause a dose-dependent reduction in renal prostaglandin formation. Can precipitate renal failure in patients with impaired renal function, heart failure, or liver dysfunction; in the elderly or in patients receiving diuretics. ▪ Use caution in patients with cardiac decompensation, hypertension, or similar conditions; may cause fluid retention and edema.

Monitor: Correct hypovolemia before giving ketorolac and maintain adequate hydration. ▪ Observe patient frequently, especially for heartburn or signs and symptoms of GI upset or bleeding, and monitor vital signs. ▪ Observe closely during ambulation. ▪ Low doses of narcotics may be required to treat breakthrough pain.

Patient education: Side effects have resulted in extended hospitalization and could be fatal. ▪ Discard any remaining oral ketorolac at end of 5 day total cumulative maximum time for use.

Maternal/child: Note Contraindications. ▪ Pregnancy Category C: safety for use not established, use only if other alternatives are not available. ▪ Discontinue breast feeding. ▪ Not recommended for use in children under 16 years of age.

Elderly: Note Dose Adjustments and Precautions. ▪ More sensitive to side effects. ▪ Incidence of GI bleeding and acute renal failure increases with age.

DRUG/LAB INTERACTIONS

Probenecid inhibits clearance and may triple plasma levels of ketorolac. Concomitant use is contraindicated. ▪ Potentiated by salicylates (especially high-dose regimens). May double plasma levels of ketorolac. Reduce dose of ketorolac by half. ▪ May decrease clearance and increase toxicity of methotrexate. ▪ Additive if used with other NSAIDs (e.g., indomethacin); side effects may increase markedly. ▪ May potentiate lithium levels. ▪ May increase risk of bleeding, especially from the GI tract, when given concomitantly with anticoagulants (e.g., warfarin [Coumadin], heparin). ▪ May increase risk of bleeding when given with agents that may cause hypoprothrombinema or inhibit platelet aggregation (e.g., cefamandole [Mandol], cefaperazone [Cefobid]). ▪ Can precipitate renal failure concomitantly with diuretics (e.g., furosemide [Lasix]); note Precautions. ▪ Can reduce response to furosemide (Lasix) in normovolemic healthy individuals. ▪ May increase risk of renal impairment with ACE inhibitors (e.g., enalapril [Vasotec]). ▪ Nephrotoxicity of both agents may be increased with cyclosporine (Sandimmune). ▪ May potentiate nondepolarizing muscle relaxants (e.g., doxacurium [Nuromax]). ▪ Has caused seizures in a few patients taking antiepileptics (e.g., phenytoin [Dilantin], carbamazepine [Tegretol]). ▪ May cause hallucinations with antipsychotics (e.g, thiothixene [Navane]), antidepressants (e.g., fluoxetine [Prozac]). ■ May cause elevations of liver function tests AST (SGOT), ALT (SGPT).

SIDE EFFECTS

Average dose: Diarrhea, dizziness, dyspepsia, drowsiness, edema, GI bleeding, GI pain, headache, injection site pain, nausea, and sweating are most common. Capable of all side effects of other NSAIDs, especially with extended use: abnormal taste, abnormal vision, asthenia, asthma, confusion, constipation, depression, dry mouth, dypsnea, euphoria, excessive thirst, flatulence, inability to concentrate, insomnia, liver function abnormalities, melena, myalgia, nervousness, oliguria, pallor, paresthesia, peptic ulcer, rectal bleeding, stimulation, stomatitis, pruritus, purpura, urinary frequency, urticaria, vasodilation, vertigo, vomiting.

Overdose: Abdominal pain, diarrhea, labored breathing, metabolic acidosis, pallor, peptic ulcer, rales, vomiting.

ANTIDOTE

With increasing severity of any side effect or onset of symptoms of overdose, discontinue the drug and notify the physician. A patent airway, artificial ventilation, oxygen therapy, and other symptomatic treatment must be instituted promptly if indicated. Treat anaphylaxis with epinephrine (Adrenalin), diphenhydramine (Benadryl), and corticosteroids as indicated. Not significantly cleared by dialysis.

LABETALOL HYDROCHLORIDE

Alpha/beta-adrenergic blocking agent
Antihypertensive

Normodyne, Trandate

pH 3.0 to 4.0

USUAL DOSE

20 mg as an initial dose direct IV. May repeat with injections of 40 to 80 mg at 10-minute intervals until desired blood pressure is achieved, or may be diluted and given as a continuous infusion. Usually effective with 50 to 200 mg. Do not exceed a total dose of 300 mg. Initiate oral labetalol after desired blood pressure has been achieved and the supine diastolic pressure starts to rise. See literature for dose regimen.

DOSE ADJUSTMENTS

Note Precautions and Drug/lab interactions.

DILUTION

Direct IV: May be given undiluted.

Continuous infusion: May be diluted in most commonly used IV solutions; (i.e., Ringer's injection; LR, D5W, NS, D5/0.2%S, D5/0.33%S, or D5/NS; and D2.5/0.45%S). Addition of 200 mg (40 ml) to 160 ml solution yields 1 mg/ml, 300 mg (60 ml) to 240 ml yields 1 mg/ml, or 200 mg (40 ml) to 250 ml yields 2 mg/3 ml. Amount of solution may be decreased if required by fluid restrictions of the patient.

Storage: Stable after dilution for 24 hours at room temperature.

INCOMPATIBLE WITH

Cefoperazone (Cefobid), furosemide (Lasix), heparin, nafcillin (Unipen), sodium bicarbonate. Mixing with any other drug in syringe or solution not recommended. Consider special use and need for adjustment of rate.

RATE OF ADMINISTRATION

Direct IV: Each 20 mg or fraction thereof over at least 2 minutes.

Continuous infusion: Begin at 2 mg/min. Adjust according to orders of physician and blood pressure response. Use of a microdrip (60 gtt/ml) or an infusion pump may be helpful.

ACTIONS

Labetalol is an alpha/beta-adrenergic blocking agent. Causes dose-related falls in blood pressure without reflex tachycardia or significant reduction in heart rate. Maximum effect of each dose is reached in 5 minutes. Half-life is about 5 hours, but some effects last up to 16 hours. Metabolized and excreted as metabolites in urine and through bile to feces. Crosses the placental barrier. Present in small amounts in breast milk.

INDICATIONS AND USES

Control of blood pressure in severe hypertension.

Unlabeled uses: Treatment of clonidine withdrawal hypertension. ■ Decrease BP and relieve symptoms in patients with pheochromocytoma.

CONTRAINDICATIONS

Bronchial asthma, cardiogenic shock, greater than first-degree heart block, overt cardiac failure, severe bradycardia, and hypersensitivity to labetalol or its components.

PRECAUTIONS

Use caution in impaired liver function. ■ Use extreme caution in patients with any degree of cardiac failure; may further depress myocardial contractility. Does not alter effectiveness of digitalis on heart muscle. ■ Effective in lowering blood pressure in pheochromocytoma, but may cause a paradoxical hypertensive response. ■ Use with extreme caution in diabetics or patients with a history of hypoglycemia. May mask the symptoms of hypoglycemia. ■ Some authorities recommend that drugs with beta-adrenergic properties be discontinued 48 hours before major surgery (beta blockade interferes with cardiac response to reflex stimuli). ■ Note Drug/lab interactions.

Monitor: Keep patient supine. Postural hypotension can occur for several hours after administration. Ambulate with care and assistance. ■ Monitor blood pressure before and 5 and 10 minutes after each direct IV injection. Monitor at least every 5 minutes during infusion. Avoid rapid or excessive falls in either systolic or diastolic blood pressure. When severely elevated blood pressure drops too rapidly, catastrophic reactions can occur (e.g., cerebral infarction, optic nerve infarction, angina, ischemic ECG changes). ■ Although rebound angina, myocardial infarction, or ventricular dysrhythmias have not been a problem with labetalol, it is recommended that the dose of beta-adrenergic blockers be reduced gradually to avoid these conditions. ■ Note Drug/lab interactions.

Patient education: Report cough, dizziness, irregular pulse, or shortness of breath promptly. ■ May cause dizziness or fainting; request assistance with ambulation.

Maternal/child: Category C: use in pregnancy only when clearly indicated and benefit outweighs risk. Has been used during labor and delivery. ▪ Use caution during lactation. ▪ Safety for use in children not established.

Elderly: Use with caution in age-related peripheral vascular disease; risk of hypothermia increased. ▪ May exacerbate mental impairment.

DRUG/LAB INTERACTIONS

May potentiate tricyclic antidepressants (e.g., imipramine [Tofranil]). ▪ Inhibits beta agonist bronchodilators (e.g., epinephrine); increased doses may be required, especially in asthmatics. ▪ Synergistic with halothane anesthesia. Notify anesthesiologist that patient is receiving labetalol. ▪ Potentiated by cimetidine (Tagamet). ▪ May cause further hypotension with nitroglycerin. ▪ May decrease insulin availability; dose of antidiabetics may need to be adjusted. ▪ May interfere with lab tests in diagnosis of pheochromocytoma.

SIDE EFFECTS

Diaphoresis, dizziness, flushing, moderate hypotension, numbness, severe postural hypotension, somnolence, tingling of scalp, and ventricular dysrhythmias (e.g., intensified atrioventricular block) occur most frequently.

ANTIDOTE

Notify the physician of all side effects. Decrease rate or discontinue drug if hypotension occurs. Notify physician immediately. Trendelenburg position may be appropriate. May require treatment with IV fluids or vasopressors (e.g., norepinephrine [levarterenol], dopamine [Intropin]). Use atropine for severe bradycardia; digitalis and diuretics for cardiac failure. Unresponsive hypotension and bradycardia may be reversed by glucagon 5 to 10 mg over 30 seconds followed by a continuous infusion of 5 mg/hr. Reduce rate as condition improves. Treat other side effects symptomatically and resuscitate as necessary. Hemodialysis is not effective.

LEUCOVORIN CALCIUM

Antidote
Antineoplastic adjunct

Citrovorum factor, folinic acid

pH 6.0 to 8.1

USUAL DOSE

Delayed excretion or overdose of methotrexate (MTX): 10 mg/M^2 every 6 hours until the serum MTX level is less than 0.05 micromolar. Milligram for milligram or greater than the dose of MTX is common. Administer within the first hour (or as soon as possible) in overdose or within 24 hours of MTX dose if there is delayed excretion. At least every 24 hours, obtain a serum creatinine and MTX level. If serum creatinine is more than 50% above pretreatment level, increase the leucovorin dose to 100 mg/M^2 every 3 hours until the serum MTX level is less than 0.05 micromolar.

Leucovorin rescue after high-dose MTX therapy: With high-dose methotrexate (12 to 15 gm/M^2 as an infusion over 4 hr); begin leucovorin 15 mg ($\approx$ 10 mg/M^2) 24 hours after MTX infusion started. Repeat every 6 hours times 10 doses. If MTX elimination is delayed, extend every 6 hour dosing until MTX levels less than 0.05 micromolar. If there is evidence of acute renal injury, increase leucovorin to 150 mg every 3 hours until MTX level is less than 1 micromolar, then 15 mg every 3 hours until MTX level is less than 0.05 micromolar. In both situations obtain serum creatinine and MTX level at least every 24 hours. Other protocols are in use. Amount of leucovorin is dependent on MTX dose, MTX serum levels, and serum creatinine.

Megaloblastic anemia: Up to 1 mg daily.

Advanced colorectal cancer: 200 mg/M^2 followed by fluorouracil (5-FU) 370 mg/M^2 or 20 mg/M^2 followed by 5-FU 425 mg/M^2 daily for 5 days. Repeat at 4 week intervals twice, then repeat every 28 to 35 days based on complete recovery from toxic effects. Reduce 5-FU dose based on tolerance to previous course, 20% for moderate hematologic or GI toxicity, 30% for severe. Leucovorin doses remain the same. Increase 5-FU dose 10% if no toxicity.

DOSE ADJUSTMENTS

Note adjustments in Usual dose; larger reductions may be required in the elderly, especially in combination with fluorouracil. ■ Note Precautions/Monitor.

DILUTION

Each 50 mg, 100 mg, or 350 mg vial should be diluted to a 10 mg to 20 mg/ml solution. For total doses less than 10 mg/M^2, dilute with bacteriostatic water for injection (contains benzyl alcohol as a preservative). Use sterile water for injection without a preservative for any dose 10 mg/M^2 or greater. May be further diluted in 100 to 500 ml of D5W, D10W, NS, R, or LR. 1 ml (3 mg) ampoules may be given undiluted (contain benzyl alcohol).

Storage: If prepared without a preservative, use immediately; stable up to 7 days with a preservative.

INCOMPATIBLE WITH

Droperidol (Inspsine), foscarnet (Foscavir). Consider incompatible in syringe or solution with any other drug because of specific use.

RATE OF ADMINISTRATION

Because of calcium content, do not exceed a rate of 160 mg/min (16 ml of a 10 mg/ml or 8 ml of a 20 mg/ml solution). May be given more slowly. Large doses may be infused equally distributed over 1 to 6 hours. Never exceed above limits.

ACTIONS

Potent agent for neutralizing immediate toxic effects of methotrexate (and other folic acid antagonists) on the hematopoietic system. Preferentially rescues normal cells without reversing the oncolytic effect of methotrexate. Also enhances the therapeutic and toxic effects of fluoropyrimidines (e.g., fluorouracil [5-FU]).

INDICATIONS AND USES

Treatment of accidental folic acid antagonist (e.g., methotrexate) overdose or delayed excretion of MTX. ■ Folinic acid rescue to prevent or decrease the toxicity of massive MTX doses used to treat resistant neoplasms. ■ Treatment of megaloblastic anemia due to folic acid deficiency when oral therapy not appropriate. ■ In combination with fluorouracil to prolong survival in palliative treatment of advanced colorectal cancer.

CONTRAINDICATIONS

Pernicious anemia and other megaloblastic anemias secondary to lack of vitamin B_{12}. None when used as indicated for other specific uses.

PRECAUTIONS

Usually administered in the hospital by or under the direction of the physician specialist. ■ Permits use of massive doses of methotrexate. ■ Do not discontinue leucovorin until methotrexate serum levels fall below toxic levels. ■ Much less effective in accidental overdose after a 1-hour delay. ■ Delayed MTX excretion may occur from third-space fluid accumulation (ascites, pleural effusion), renal insufficiency, or inadequate hydration. ■ All doses over 25 mg should be given IM or IV (no more than 25 mg can be absorbed orally). ■ IM or IV dosing required in presence of GI toxicity, nausea, or vomiting. ■ Benzyl alcohol associated with gasping syndrome in premature infants.

Monitor: Monitor serum blood levels of MTX and serum creatinine levels at least daily until level is less than 0.05 micromolar. Death can occur in 5 to 10 days if MTX remains at toxic levels longer than 48 hours. ■ Minimum fluid intake of 3 L/24 hr and alkalinization of urine to a pH of 7 or more with oral sodium bicarbonate recommended. Begin 12 hours before MTX dose and continue for 48 hours after final dose in each sequence. Does not reduce nephrotoxicity of MTX from drug or metabolite precipitation in the kidney. ■ See methotrexate or fluorouracil monograph.

Maternal/child: Pregnancy Category C: safety for use in pregnancy and lactation not established. Benefits must outweigh risks.

Elderly: At greater risk for GI toxicity and severe diarrhea in combination with fluorouracil. ■ Note Dose adjustments.

DRUG/LAB INTERACTIONS

May inhibit phenytoins (e.g., Dilantin), phenobarbital and primidone; may cause increased frequency of seizures. ■ Toxicity of fluorouracil increased. ■ When given with MTX avoid any drug that may interfere with MTX elimination or binding to serum albumin (e.g., NSAIDs [e.g., indomethacin, ketoprofen, naproxen], probenecid, procarbazine [Matulane], salicylates, sulfonamides). Consider as possible cause of toxicity.

SIDE EFFECTS

Allergic reactions including analyphylaxis have occurred rarely. Methotrexate or fluorouracil may cause many serious and dose-limiting side effects; see individual monographs.

ANTIDOTE

Keep physician informed of patient's condition. Symptomatic treatment indicated.

LEVOCARNITINE

L-carnitine, Carnitor

Nutritional supplement

pH 6.0 to 8.0

USUAL DOSE

50 mg/kg/24 hr in equally divided doses every 3 to 4 hours (preferred). Intervals between administration must never exceed 6 hours. Repeat daily and adjust dose as indicated by clinical response or as therapy may require. In **severe metabolic crisis** an initial loading dose of 50 mg/kg may be given followed by an equivalent dose (50 mg/kg) in equally divided doses every 3 to 4 hr over 24 hr. Then give 50 mg/kg/day. Up to 300 mg/kg/24 hr has been given.

Pediatric cardiomyopathy: Dose same as in Usual dose. Cardiomyopathy may be part of a carnitine deficiency or be idiopathic. May have a dramatic response; in some cases the heart has returned to normal size within 72 hours.

DILUTION

May be given direct IV or added to NS or LR for infusion.

Storage: Store ampoules at controlled room temperature in carton to protect from light. Discard any unused portion; contains no preservative. Infusion solution stable at room temperature for 36 hours, 7 days if refrigerated.

INCOMPATIBLE WITH

IV solution compatibility studies not yet available.

RATE OF ADMINISTRATION

Direct IV: A single dose equally distributed over 2 to 3 minutes.

Infusion: Give at rate ordered for primary infusion. Do not exceed direct IV rate.

ACTIONS

A synthetic version of a naturally occurring amino acid derivative. Promotes the excretion of excess organic or fatty acids in patients with defects in fatty acid metabolism and/or specific organic acidopathies that bioaccumulate acyl CoA esters. Can correct acidosis from these specific causes, which can be life threatening. Clears toxic organic acids by forming acyl carnitine, which is excreted primarily in the urine.

INDICATIONS AND USES

Acute and chronic treatment of patients (including infants and children) with an inborn error of metabolism that results in secondary carnitine deficiency (e.g., glutaric aciduria II, methyl malonic aciduria, propionic acidemia, medium chain fatty acyl CoA dehydrogenase deficiency). ▪ Treatment of pediatric cardiomyopathy (orphan designation).

Investigational uses: Modify abnormal plasma lipoprotein patterns (e.g., loss of plasma L-carnitine during hemodialysis). ▪ Valproate toxicity.

CONTRAINDICATIONS

None known at this time when used as directed for specific indications.

PRECAUTIONS

Oral dose form used to treat primary carnitine deficiency and when feasible in secondary deificency. ▪ Note Drug/lab interactions.

Monitor: Obtain base line plasma carnitine levels before treatment and monitor weekly and then monthly based on response (normal range is 35 to 60 micromoles/L). ▪ Monitor blood chemistries, vital signs, and over-all clinical condition before treatment, as indicated during acute phase, and weekly to monthly thereafter.

Patient education: Stress importance of follow-up evaluation and treatment.

Maternal/ child: Pregnancy Category B: no adequate studies; use only if clearly needed. ▪ Carnitine is a normal component of breast milk. Highly probable that L-carnitine is secreted in breast milk also; discontinue breast feeding.

DRUG/LAB INTERACTIONS

Vitamin B_T (D, L-carnitine) sold in health food stores, competitively inhibits L-carnitine and can cause a secondary deficiency.

SIDE EFFECTS

Diarrhea, gastritis, and transient nausea and vomiting may occur; most common with oral dosing. Drug-related body odor (11%).

ANTIDOTE

Keep physician informed. If clinically appropriate, dose reduction may decrease or eliminate body odor and GI symptoms. No reports of toxicity, but treatment would be supportive.

LEVOFLOXACIN

Antibacterial
(Fluoroquinolone)

Levaquin

pH 3.8 to 5.8

USUAL DOSE

250 to 500 mg once every 24 hours. Dose and duration of treatment are based on degree of infection and specific diagnosis. Creatinine clearance ≥ 50 ml/min is required. Dose and serum levels similar by oral or IV route. Transfer to oral dose as soon as practical.

Acute bacterial exacerbation of chronic bronchitis: 500 mg once each day for 7 days.

Community acquired pneumonia: 500 mg once each day for 7 to 14 days.

Acute maxillary sinusitis: 500 mg once each day for 10 to 14 days.

Uncomplicated skin and skin structure infections: 500 mg once each day for 7 to 10 days.

Complicated urinary tract infections: 250 mg once each day for 10 days.

Acute pyelonephritis: 250 mg once each day for 10 days.

DOSE ADJUSTMENTS

Clearance is reduced and half-life is prolonged in patients with a creatinine clearance (CrCl) ≤ 80 ml/min. ▪ In patients with reduced CrCl, the initial dose remains the same as it is in Usual dose for all indications with an initial dose of 500 mg. Reduce subsequent doses to 250 mg once each day for CrCl from 20 to 49 ml/min; 250 mg every 48 hours for CrCl from 10 to 19 ml/min and for patient receiving hemodialysis or CAPD. In complicated UTI or acute pyelonephritis, reduce subsequent doses to 250 mg every 48 hours for CrCl from 10 to 19 ml/min. Consult package insert for formula to convert serum creatinine to creatinine clearance. ▪ Supplemental doses are not required after hemodialysis or peritoneal dialysis. ▪ No dose adjustment is required specifically for age, gender, race, or in impaired hepatic function.

DILUTION

Available in single-use vials and as pre-diluted, ready-to-use infusions.

Single-use vials: Withdraw desired dose from single-use vial (10 ml for 250 mg, 20 ml for 500 mg). Each 10 ml (250 mg) must be further diluted with a minimum of 40 ml NS, D5W, D5/NS, D5/LR, D5/plasma-Lyte 56, D5/0.45NS with 0.15 KCL, or 1/6 molar sodium lactate. Desired concentration is 5 mg/ml. No preservatives; enter vial only once to prepare either one 500 mg dose or two doses of 250 mg each.

Pre-mix flexible containers: No further dilution necessary. Available as 250 mg in 50 ml or 500 mg in 100 ml D5W. Instructions for access to and use of pre-mix flexible containers are on its storage carton. Do not use flexible containers in series connections.

Storage: Store vials at controlled room temperature; protect from light. Store pre-mix at or below 25° C (77° F); protect from freezing, light, and excessive heat. Both are stable to expiration date. Solutions diluted from vials are stable at controlled room temperature for 3 days, up to 14 days if refrigerated. May be frozen for up to 6 months. Do not force thaw (e.g., microwave or water bath) and do not refreeze. Discard any unused portion of premixed solutions and/or opened vials.

INCOMPATIBLE WITH

Manufacturer recommends levofloxacin be administered separately. Never administer in the same IV or through the same tubing with any solution containing multivalent cations (e.g., magnesium calcium). Always flush line with compatible solution before and after administration of any other drug through the same IV line.

RATE OF ADMINISTRATION

A single dose must be equally distributed over 60 minutes as an infusion. Too-rapid administration may cause hypotension. May be given through a Y-tube or three-way stopcock of infusion set. Temporarily discontinue other solutions infusing at the same site and flush tubing with compatible solutions before and after levofloxacin.

ACTIONS

A synthetic, broad-spectrum, fluoroquinolone antibacterial agent. First once-daily anti-infective indicated to treat all three of the most difficult to treat bacterial respiratory infections in adults. Bactericidal to a wide range of aerobic gram-negative and gram-positive organisms as well as some anaerobic organisms through interference with an enzyme (topoisomerase II) needed for synthesis of bacterial DNA. Onset of action is prompt, and serum levels are dose related. Mean terminal half-life is 6 to 8 hours. Steady state is achieved within 48 hours. Widely distributed into body tissues, including blister fluid, and lung tissues. Moderately bound to serum protein (24% to 38%). May be active against bacteria resistant to beta-lactam antibiotics. Metabolism is minimal; primarily excreted as unchanged drug in urine. Very small amounts found in bile and feces. May cross placental barrier. May be secreted in breast milk.

INDICATIONS AND USES

Treatment of adults with mild, moderate, and severe infections caused by susceptible strains of microorganisms in conditions including acute maxillary sinusitis, acute bacterial exacerbation of chronic bronchitis, and community-acquired pneumonia. ■ Treatment of mild to moderate uncomplicated skin and skin structure infections, complicated urinary tract infections, and acute pyelonephritis. ■ Not recommended for use in complicated skin and skin structure infections.

CONTRAINDICATIONS

History of hypersensitivity to levofloxacin, its components, or any other quinolone antimicrobial agents (e.g., ciprofloxacin [Cipro], norfloxacin [Noroxin], ofloxacin [Floxin]).

PRECAUTIONS

For IV use only. ■ Culture and sensitivity studies indicated to determine susceptibility of the causative organism to levofloxacin. ■ *Pseudomonas aeruginosa* may develop resistance during treatment. Ongoing culture and sensitivity studies indicated. ■ Prolonged use may cause superinfection because of overgrowth of nonsusceptible organisms. ■ Use with caution in patients with known CNS disorders that predispose to seizures or alter seizure threshhold (e.g., epilepsy, severe cerebral arteriosclerosis, concomitant drug therapy). Convulsions, toxic psychosis, increased intracranial pressure, and CNS stimulation have been reported. ■ Use caution in patients with impaired renal function; note Dose adjustments. ■ May be used by patients who are allergic to penicillin or intolerant of macrolides (e.g., erythromycin). ▪ Cross-resistance may occur with other fluoroquinolones, but some microorganisms resistant to other fluoroquinolones may be susceptible to levofloxacin. ▪ Rupture of shoulder, hand, and achilles tendons has been reported in patients receiving quinolones.

Monitor: Hypersensitivity reactions including anaphylaxis with the first or succeeding doses has been reported in patients receiving quinolones, even in those without known hypersensitivity. Emergency equipment must always be available. ▪ Obtain baseline CBC with differential, creatinine clearance, and blood glucose. Periodic monitoring of organ systems, including hematopoietic, hepatic, and renal, is recommended. ▪ Maintain adequate hydration to prevent concentrated urine throughout treatment. Other quinolones have formed crystals. ▪ Monitor infusion site for inflammation and/or extravasation. ▪ Symptomatic hyperglycemia or hypoglycemia may occur, usually in diabetic patients receiving oral hypoglycemic agents (e.g., glyburide) or insulin. Monitor blood glucose closely. ▪ Note Drug/lab interactions and Antidote.

Patient education: Drink fluids liberally. ▪ Report skin rash or any other hypersensitivity reaction promptly. ▪ Photosensitivity has occurred in a minimal number of patients, but it is best to avoid excessive sunlight or artificial ultraviolet light. May cause severe sunburn, use sunscreen; wear dark glasses outdoors. ▪ Dizziness or lightheadedness may interfere with ambulation and motor coordination. ▪ Effects of caffeine or theophylline preparations may be increased; monitor if use necessary. ▪ Report tendon pain or inflammation promptly. ▪ Note Precautions, Monitor, Drug/lab interactions, and Antidote.

Maternal/ child: Category C: Safety for use in pregnancy not established; benefits must outweigh risks. ▪ Discontinue breast feeding. ▪ Safety for use in children and adolescents under 18 years of age not established. Quinolones have caused arthropathy and osteochondrosis in juvenile animals.

Elderly: Half-life may be slightly extended due to age-related renal impairment. Dose reduction required only in the elderly with CrCl $\leq$ 50 ml/min.

DRUG/LAB INTERACTIONS

Risk of CNS stimulation and convulsive seizures increased with NSAIDs (e.g., ibuprofen [Motrin]). ▪ May cause hyperglycemia and hypoglycemia with concurrent administration of antidiabetic agents (e.g., metformin [Glucophage], insulin); monitoring of blood glucose recommended. ▪ Concomitant administration with cimetidine or probenecid reduces levofloxacin renal clearance by 24% and 35% respectively, but dose adjustment is not required. ▪ Interactions with theophylline that occur with other quinolones have not been noted, but monitoring of theophylline levels is recommended with concomitant use. ▪ Interactions with warfarin that occur with other quinolones have not been noted, but monitoring of PT is recommended with concomitant use. ▪ No dose adjustment required for either drug when levofloxacin is administered concomitantly with cyclosporine or digoxin.

SIDE EFFECTS

Minor: Abdominal pain (0.3%), anorexia (0.1%), anxiety (0.1%), constipation (0.1%), decreased glucose (1.9%), decreased lymphocytes

(1.9%), diarrhea (1.2%), dizziness (0.3%), dyspepsia (0.3%), edema (0.1%), fatigue (0.1%), flatulence (0.5%), genital moniliasis (0.3%), headache (0.1%), injection site reaction (5.6%), insomnia (0.3%), leukorrhea (0.1%), malaise (0.1%), nausea (1.2%), phototoxicity (sun sensitivity [0.1%]), pruritus (0.5%), rash (0.3%), sweating (0.1%), taste disturbances (0.2%), tremor (0.1%), urticaria (0.1%), vaginitis (0.8%), vomiting (0.2%). Capable of numerous other reactions in less than 1% of patients.

Major: Allergic reactions (e.g., anaphylaxis, cardiovascular collapse, death, dyspnea, edema [facial, laryngeal, or pharyngeal]); CNS stimulation (e.g., anxiety, confusion, depression, hallucinations), convulsions, increased intracranial pressure, and toxic psychoses; fever, rash, and severe dermatologic reactions (e.g., toxic epidermal necrolysis, Stevens-Johnson syndrome); hypoglycemic reactions; pseudomembranous colitis; and pain, inflammation, and ruptures of the shoulder, hand, and Achilles tendons have all been reported in patients receiving quinolones.

ANTIDOTE

Keep physician informed of all side effects. Most minor side effects will be treated symptomatically; monitor closely. Discontinue levofloxacin at the first sign of any major side effect (hypersensitivity, CNS symptoms, dermatologic reactions, hypoglycemic reactions, pseudomembranous colitis, tendon rupture) or phototoxicity. Treat allergic reactions as indicated with epinephrine, airway management, oxygen, IV fluids, antihistamines (e.g., diphenhydramine [Benadryl]), corticosteroids (e.g., Solu-Cortef), and pressor amines (e.g., dopamine [Intropin]). Treat CNS symptoms as indicated; may require diazepam (Valium) for seizures. Mild cases of colitis may respond to discontinuation of levofloxacin. Oral vancomycin (Vancocin) or metronidazole (Flagyl) is the treatment of choice for antibiotic-related pseudomembranous colitis. Adequate hydration and supplementation of electrolytes and proteins usually indicated. Complete rest is indicated for an affected tendon until treatment is available. Maintain hydration in overdose. No specific antidote; not removed by hemodialysis or peritoneal dialysis. Maintain patient until drug is excreted and symptoms subside.

LEVORPHANOL TARTRATE

Narcotic analgesic (agonist)

Levo-Dromoran

pH 4.3

USUAL DOSE

1 to 2 mg every 6 to 8 hours.

When seeking the required dose to achieve pain relief for an individual patient, increases in increments of at least 25% of the previous dose are suggested. Lower slightly if pain is controlled but patient is too drowsy; or lower dose and increase frequency.

DOSE ADJUSTMENTS

Reduced dose may be required with hepatic or renal disease. ■ Note Drug/lab interactions.

DILUTION

Each dose should be diluted with 5 ml of sterile water or NS for injection. Do not add to IV solutions. May give through Y-tube or three-way stopcock of infusion set.

Storage: Store below 40° C.

INCOMPATIBLE WITH

Aminophylline, ammonium chloride, amobarbital (Amytal), chlorothiazide (Diuril), heparin, methicillin (Staphcillin), pentobarbital (Nembutal), phenobarbital (Luminal), phenytoin (Dilantin), secobarbital (Seconal), sodium bicarbonate, sodium iodide, thiopental (Pentothal).

RATE OF ADMINISTRATION

2 mg or fraction thereof properly diluted solution over 4 to 5 minutes.

ACTIONS

A synthetic narcotic analgesic and CNS depressant closely related to morphine. Five times more potent than morphine milligram for milligram. Onset of action is immediate and lasts 6 to 8 hours. Levorphanol is metabolized in the liver and excreted in the urine. Crosses the placental barrier. May be secreted in breast milk.

INDICATIONS AND USES

Relief of moderate to severe, acute or chronic pain such as pain of biliary or renal colic, cancer, myocardial infarction, severe trauma, or postoperatively. ■ Preanesthetic sedation.

CONTRAINDICATIONS

Acute alcoholism, anoxia, bronchial asthma, diarrhea caused by poisoning until toxic material eliminated, increased intracranial pressure, known hypersensitivity to levorphanol, respiratory depression, upper air-way obstruction.

PRECAUTIONS

IV is not the route of choice. Usually given SC. ■ Tolerance to levorphanol gradually increases. ■ Use caution in the elderly, in patients with impaired hepatic or renal function, pulmonary disease, and concurrent anticoagulation therapy. ■ Use caution during pregnancy or delivery, especially during labor and delivery of premature infants. Enters fetal circulation readily; will cause respiratory depression. ■ Use extreme caution in craniotomy, head injury, and increased intracranial pressure; respiratory depression and intracranial pressure may be further increased. ■ May cause apnea in the asthmatic. ■ Symptoms of acute abdominal conditions may be masked. ■ May increase ventricular response rate in presence of supraventricular tachycardias. ■ Cough reflex is suppressed.

Monitor: Oxygen, controlled respiratory equipment, and naloxone (Narcan) must be available. ■ Observe patient frequently and monitor vital signs. Keep patient supine; orthostatic hypotension and fainting may occur. ■ Uncontrolled pain causes sleep deprivation, decreases pain threshold, and increases pain. When pain is finally controlled, expect the patient to sleep more until recovery from sleep deprivation. ■ Note Precautions and Drug/lab interactions.

Patient education: Avoid alcohol or other CNS depressants (e.g., barbiturates, benzodiazepines [e.g., diazepam (Valium)]). ■ May cause blurred vision, dizziness, or drowsiness; use caution in tasks that require alertness. ■ May be habit forming.

Maternal/child: Pregnancy Category C: safety for use in pregnancy or lactation not established. Benefits must outweigh risks. ■ Note Precautions.

Elderly: Note Precautions. ■ May be more sensitive to effects (e.g., respiratory depression, constipation, urinary retention). ■ Analgesia should be effective with lower doses. ■ Consider age-related organ impairment.

DRUG/LAB INTERACTIONS

Potentiated by phenothiazines (e.g., chlorpromazine [Thorazine]) and other CNS depressants, such as narcotic analgesics, alcohol, anticholinergics, antihistamines, barbiturates, hypnotics, sedatives, MAO inhibitors (e.g., selegiline [Eldepryl]), neuromuscular blocking agents (e.g., tubocurarine), and psychotropic agents. Reduced dosage of both drugs may be indicated.

SIDE EFFECTS

Nausea, vomiting, and constipation are less frequent than with morphine.

Minor: Dizziness, skin rash, urinary retention, urticaria.

Major: Anaphylaxis, cardiac arrhythmias, hypotension, respiratory depression.

ANTIDOTE

With increasing severity of any side effect or onset of symptoms of overdose, discontinue the drug and notify the physician. Naloxone (Narcan) will reverse serious respiratory depression. A patent airway, artificial ventilation, oxygen therapy, and other symptomatic treatment must be instituted promptly. Resuscitate as necessary.

LEVOTHYROXINE SODIUM

Hormone
(Thyroid)

Levothroid, Levoxine, Synthroid, T_4, L-thyroxine

USUAL DOSE

When oral ingestion is not practical, IV dose should be ½ of any previously established oral dose. Adjust in small increments as indicated. Initiate oral treatment as soon as possible. 0.05 to 0.06 mg (50 to 60 mcg) equals approximately 60 mg (gr 1) thyroid hormone.

Hypothyroidism: Usual IV starting dose would be 25 mcg/day. Increase in increments of 12.5 to 25 mcg. Average maintenance dose is 50 to 100 mcg/day.

Myxedema coma: 400 mcg as initial dose. Range is 200 to 500 mcg. 100 to 300 mcg may be repeated the next day unless considerable improvement has occurred, as indicated by patient response or serum protein-bound iodine levels. Maintenance dose ranges from 50 to 200 mcg. Note Precautions. Liothyronine (Triostat) is the drug of choice for myxedema coma.

Thyroid suppression therapy: 1.3 mcg/kg/day for 7 to 10 days. Usually yield normal serum T_4 and T_3 levels and lack of response to TSH.

PEDIATRIC DOSE

Given orally (may be crushed in food or liquid). Note Precautions. Any IV dose should be 75% of oral dose. Size of **oral** dose is inversely proportional to age from 8 to 10 mcg/kg/24 hours at 0 to 6 months to 2 to 3 mcg/kg/24 hours over 12 years.

DOSE ADJUSTMENTS

Note Drug/lab interactions. Reduce dose in elderly, functional or ECG evidence of cardiovascular disease including angina, long-standing thyroid disease, other endocrinopathies, and severe hypothyroidism.

DILUTION

Each 100 mcg of lyophilized powder is diluted with 1 ml of NS for injection (without preservatives). Shake well to dissolve completely. 1 ml equals 100 mcg. More diluent may be added to Synthroid (5 ml to 200 mcg yields 40 mcg/ml) and bacteriostatic normal saline may be used. Do not add to IV solutions. May be given through Y-tube or three-way stopcock of infusion set. Must be used immediately after dilution; any remaining solution is discarded.

INCOMPATIBLE WITH

No specific references available. Should be considered incompatible in the syringe with any other drug.

RATE OF ADMINISTRATION

100 mcg or fraction thereof over 1 minute.

ACTIONS

A synthetic thyroid hormone. Effective replacement for decreased or absent thyroid function. Requires peripheral metabolic conversion to active hormone T_3 to be effective. Process inhibited by illness or stress. Onset of action is slow. Up to 5 or 6 hours is required before any noticeable improvements occur, and 24 hours may be required to note full benefits. Thyroid hormone is essential to many body functions, including rate of metabolism.

INDICATIONS AND USES

Hypothyroid states due to any cause. ▪ An emergency measure in myxedema coma. ▪ Thyroid suppression therapy.

CONTRAINDICATIONS

Hypersensitivity to levothyroxine, myocardial infarction, thyrotoxicosis.

PRECAUTIONS

Correct adrenocortical insufficiency before administration or acute adrenal crisis and death may result. ▪ Corticosteroid therapy is also required concomitantly to prevent acute adrenal insufficiency in myxedema coma or any preexisting manifestation of adrenal insufficiency. ▪ Use caution in diabetes and cardiovascular disease. ▪ Larger doses (e.g., 0.3 to 0.4 mg) may cause cardiovascular side effects; use with extreme caution.

Monitor: Observe patient continuously and monitor vital signs. ▪ Monitor thyroid function tests (e.g., free T_4 index, TSH).

Maternal/child: Category A: may be used during pregnancy. ▪ Presumed safe in lactation; use caution and observe infant. ▪ Avoid excessive dose in children; can cause brain damage in thyrotoxicosis during infancy. Can also accelerate bone age and cause craniosynotosis (premature closing of sutures in the skull).

Elderly: Note Dose adjustments, more sensitive to effects.

DRUG/LAB INTERACTIONS

Increases rate of metabolism and requires dose adjustment for anticoagulants, antidepressants, oral antidiabetics, barbiturates, digitalis, catecholamines (e.g., epinephrine), beta adrenergic blockers (e.g., propranolol), insulin, estrogens, theophylline, and others. Cardiac arrhythmias, hypoglycemia, and bleeding can occur with unadjusted dose of some of these drugs.

SIDE EFFECTS

Chest pain, diarrhea, heart palpitations, muscle cramps, nervousness, perspiration, tachycardia, vomiting.

ANTIDOTE

Notify the physician of any side effect. A reduction in dose will usually decrease symptoms. In massive overdose control fever, hypoglycemia, and fluid loss. Digitalis may be indicated for CHF; propranolol (Inderal) has been used to treat increased sympathetic activity (1 to 3 mg IV over 10 minutes). Adrenal insufficiency may be unrecognized.

LIDOCAINE HYDROCHLORIDE

Xylocaine, ✤Xylocard

Antiarrhythmic

pH 5.0 to 7.0

USUAL DOSE

1 to 1.5 mg/kg of body weight (50 to 100 mg) as a loading dose. May repeat 0.5 to 1.5 mg/kg every 5 to 10 minutes to desired effect, up to a total of 3 mg/kg. Should not exceed 200 to 300 mg/hr. 1.5 mg/kg loading dose, repeat doses of 0.5 to 1.5 mg/kg, and bolus therapy indicated in *ventricular fibrillation and pulseless ventricular tachycardia when defibrillation and epinephrine have failed.*

Maintenance dose: With return of perfusion, initiate an infusion of 1 to 4 mg/min (20 to 50 mcg/kg/min). *Do not exceed 4 mg/min rate.* If arrhythmias occur during an infusion, give a small bolus of 0.5 mg/kg to increase plasma concentration.

Prophylactic dose: Initiate a keep-open IV of D5W. Begin with a bolus dose of 0.5 mg/kg. Repeat 0.5 mg/kg bolus every 5 minutes to a total dose of 2 mg/kg if ventricular ectopic activity is present. Not recommended in uncomplicated acute MI or ischemia without PVCs.

Status epilepticus (investigational): 1 mg/kg as a loading dose. If seizure does not terminate in 2 minutes, give an additional 0.5 mg/kg to prevent recurrences, a maintenance infusion of 30 mcg/kg/min has been used. Another source suggests a loading dose of 100 mg. Give an additional 50 mg in 20 minutes. Follow with a maintenance infusion of 1 to 3 mg/minute. Reduce infusion rate gradually based on patient response. Complete withdrawal may take several days.

PEDIATRIC DOSE

1 mg/kg IV or intratracheally. May repeat in 10 to 15 minutes times 2 if indicated. Maximum total dose is 3 to 4.5 mg/kg/hr. Follow with an infusion of 20 to 50 mcg/kg/min.

DOSE ADJUSTMENTS

Reduce loading dose in digitalis toxicity with AV block. ▪ Consider loading dose reduction (not universally recommended) in congestive heart failure, reduced cardiac output, liver disease, and the elderly. ▪ Reduce maintenance dose by one-half in presence of decreased cardiac output (e.g., acute MI, congestive heart failure, or shock from any cause), impaired liver function, the elderly (over 65), and in patients receiving drugs that may decrease clearance of lidocaine or decrease liver blood flow (e.g., beta-blockers [propranolol (Inderal), cimetidine (Tagamet)]). ▪ Reduce maintenance dose after 24 hours or monitor blood levels; half-life of lidocaine increases with prolonged administration.

DILUTION

Label must state "for IV use" and be preservative free. Bolus dose may be given undiluted.

Infusion: Add 1 Gm of lidocaine to 500 or 250 ml of D5W (preferred), D5/1/2NS, D5/NS, or RL. Solution gives 2 or 4 mg/ml of lidocaine. Available prediluted (2, 4, or 8 mg/ml). Titrate to desired response.

Pediatric infusion: Add 120 mg of lidocaine to 100 ml of diluent (1200 mcg/ml). 1 to 2.5 ml/kg/hr will deliver 20 to 50 mcg/kg/min or add 6.0 mg/kg to 100 ml diluent. 1 ml/hr equals 1.0 mcg/kg/min.

Storage: Discard diluted solution after 24 hours.

INCOMPATIBLE WITH

Ampicillin, cefazolin (Kefzol), methohexital (Brevital), phenytoin. Do not add lidocaine to blood transfusion tubings (Dilantin). Physically compatible with many drugs. However, combination is not practical because of extensive individualized rate adjustments to achieve desired effects.

RATE OF ADMINISTRATION

Bolus dose: 25 to 50 mg or fraction thereof over 1 minute. Too-rapid injection may cause seizures.

Infusion: Using a microdrip (60 gtt/ml) or an infusion pump delivers lidocaine in recommended doses. Adjust as indicated by progress in patient's condition. Note Dose adjustments.

Lidocaine infusion rates						
Desired dose	1 gm in 500 ml diluent (2 mg/ml)			1 gm in 250 ml diluent (4 mg/ml)		
mg/min	mg/hr	ml/min	ml/hr	mg/hr	ml/min	ml/hr
1	60	0.5	30	60	0.25	15
2	120	1	60	120	0.5	30
3	180	1.5	90	180	0.75	45
4	240	2	120	240	1	60

Pediatric infusion: 120 mg to 100 ml diluent = 1200 mcg/ml
1 to 2.5 ml/kg/hr = 20 to 50 mcg/kg/min or
6 mg/kg to 100 ml diluent 1 ml/hr = 1 mcg/kg/min

ACTIONS

A local anesthetic agent. Exerts an antiarrhythmic effect similar to procainamide but is more potent. Decreases ventricular excitability without depressing the force of ventricular contractions by increasing the stimulation threshold of the ventricle during diastole. Decreases cell membrane permeability and prevents loss of sodium and potassium ions. Onset of action should occur within 2 minutes and last approximately 10 to 20 minutes. Crosses placental barrier. Metabolized in the liver and excreted in the urine.

INDICATIONS AND USES

Drug of choice for treatment of ventricular arrhythmias (e.g., PVCs, ventricular tachycardia [VT], ventricular fibrillation [VF]) occurring during acute myocardial infarction and during cardiac and other surgery. ■ Wide complex tachycardia of uncertain origin. ■ Wide complex PSVT. ■ Prophylactic administration to reduce incidence of primary VF in acute MI.

Investigational uses: Status epilepticus.

Unlabeled use: Pediatric cardiac arrest.

CONTRAINDICATIONS

Known sensitivity to lidocaine or any other local anesthetic of the amide type; Wolff-Parkinson-White syndrome, Stokes-Adams syndrome or any other severe first-, second-, or third-degree heart block without an artificial pacemaker in place.

PRECAUTIONS

Oral antiarrhythmic drugs are preferred for maintenance. ■ Use caution in severe liver or renal disease, hypovolemia, shock, all forms of heart block, and untreated bradycardia. ■ Acceleration of ventricular rate may occur in patients with atrial flutter or fibrillation.

Monitor: Monitor IV flow rate and the patient's ECG continuously. Therapeutic serum levels range from 1.5 to 5 mcg/ml; above 6 mcg/ml is usually toxic. ■ Half-life increases over time. Reduce dose of continuous infusion after 24 hours and monitor blood levels. ■ Keep patient lying down to reduce hypotensive effects. ■ Discontinue lidocaine when patient's cardiac condition is stable or any signs of toxicity become apparent. ■ Keep a bolus dose, 100 mg (5 ml), available at all times for emergency use in myocardial infarction.

Patient education: May cause dizziness; remain at bed rest; request assistance if ambulation permitted.

Maternal/child: Pregnancy Category C: safety not established. Benefits must outweigh risks. ■ Safety for use in lactation and children not established.

Elderly: Note Dose adjustments. ■ Increased sensitivity to adverse effects. ■ Consider age-related hepatic impairment.

DRUG/LAB INTERACTIONS

Cross-sensitivity and/or potentiation may occur with other antiarrhythmics (e.g., procainamide or quinidine); may cause conduction abnormalities. ■ Potentiated by amiodarone (Cordarone), beta-adrenergic blockers (e.g., propranolol [Inderal]), and cimetidine (Tagamet); toxicity can occur. Monitor cardiac function. ■ May produce excessive cardiac depression with phenytoin (Dilantin). ■ Potentiates neuromuscular blockade of muscle relaxants (e.g., tubocurarine, succinylcholine [Anectine]) and aminoglycoside antibiotics (e.g., polymyxin B). ■ Effects may be altered by smoking; monitor carefully.

SIDE EFFECTS

Transient because of short duration of action of lidocaine.

Minor: Apprehension, blurred vision, confusion, dizziness, "doom" anxiety, drowsiness, edema, euphoria, hallucinations, lightheadedness, mood changes, nervousness, sensations of heat, cold, and numbness, slurred speech, tinnitus, urticaria, vomiting.

Major: Anaphylaxis, bradycardia, cardiac arrest, cardiovascular collapse, convulsions, hypotension, malignant hyperthermia (tachycardia, tachypnea, metabolic acidosis, fever), PR interval prolonged, QRS complex widening, respiratory depression, tremors, twitching, unconsciousness.

ANTIDOTE

Notify the physician of any side effects. For major side effects, discontinue the drug immediately and institute appropriate measures. For anaphylactic shock use epinephrine and corticosteroids, etc. To correct CNS stimulation use diazepam (Valium), rapid ultra-short-acting barbiturates (e.g., thiopental [Pentothal]); or if under anesthesia, muscle relaxants (e.g., succinylcholine [Anectine]). Use vasopresssors (e.g., dopamine [Intropin]) and IV fluids to correct hypotension. Maintain and support patient; resuscitate as necessary.

LIOTHYRONINE SODIUM

Hormone
(Thyroid)

T$_3$, Triostat

pH 9.5 to 11.5

USUAL DOSE

Initial and subsequent doses must be determined on the basis of continuous monitoring of clinical condition and response to liothyronine therapy. An adequate dose is important in determining clinical outcome.

Myxedema coma: 25 to 50 mcg as an initial dose. At least 4 hours but no more than 12 hours should elapse between doses; allows sufficient time to evaluate response and avoids fluctuation in hormone levels. Myxedametous patients have an increased sensitivity to thyroid hormones. Begin with lower doses and increase gradually. Use caution in adjusting dose to avoid large changes that may precipitate adverse cardiovascular events. A total daily dose of 65 mcg/day in the initial days of treatment has decreased mortality. Experience with doses above 100 mcg/day is limited. Preadministration testing and adjunctive therapy with corticosteroids required; see Precautions/Monitor.

Transfer to oral therapy: Initiate oral therapy as soon as condition is stabilized and patient is able to take oral medications. With oral liothyronine, discontinue IV liothyronine and begin with low doses. Increase gradually based on response. If L-thyroxine (Synthyroid, T$_4$) is used, discontinue IV therapy gradually to compensate for several-day delay in effectiveness of oral L-thyroxine.

DOSE ADJUSTMENTS

Reduce initial dose to 10 to 20 mcg in known or suspected cardiovascular disease. ■ Begin with lower doses in the elderly. ■ Note Drug/lab interactions.

DILUTION

May be given undiluted. Available as 10 mcg/ml in 1 ml vials.

Storage: Must be refrigerated until administration. Discard unused portion.

INCOMPATIBLE WITH

No specific references available.

RATE OF ADMINISTRATION

Each 10 mcg or fraction thereof over 1 minute.

ACTIONS

A synthetic form of the natural thyroid hormone triiodothyronine (T$_3$). Enters peripheral tissues readily and binds to specific nuclear receptor(s) to initiate hormonal, metabolic effects. Affinity for these receptors is 10-fold higher than prohormone T$_4$ (levothyroxine) and no additional conversion (T$_4$ to T$_3$) is required. Increases metabolic rate and reverses the loss of consciousness, hypothermia, lactic acidosis, and other symptoms of myxedema coma. Thyroid hormones have many beneficial effects on general metabolism and the cardiovascular system. Liothyronine produces a detectable metabolic response in 2 to

4 hours. Achieves maximum therapeutic response within 48 hours. Has a rapid cutoff of activity, permitting quick dose adjustments and/or control of overdose. Metabolized in the liver to an inactive metabolite. Does not readily cross the placental barrier. Minimal secretion in breast milk.

INDICATIONS AND USES

Treatment of myxedema coma and precoma (patient not completely unconscious). ▪ May be used in patients allergic to desiccated thyroid or thyroid extract derived from pork or beef.

CONTRAINDICATIONS

Concomitant use with artificial patient rewarming; generally contraindicated in diagnosed but uncorrected adrenal cortical insufficiency or untreated thyroxicosis; hypersensitivity to any components (no documented evidence of true allergic idiosyncratic reactions). Not justified for use in treatment of obesity or male or female infertility without hypothyroidism.

PRECAUTIONS

For IV use only. ▪ Myxedema coma is a medical emergency usually precipitated in a hypothyroid patient by illness, sedatives, or anesthetics. Has a 50% to 70% mortality rate even with aggressive therapy. ▪ Use with caution in presence of any compromised cardiac function or cardiac disease, particularly of the coronary arteries. ▪ May precipitate a hyperthyroid state or may aggravate existing hyperthyroidism. ▪ Due to the rarity of myxedema coma and precoma, no systematic studies have been performed with IV liothyronine.

Monitor: Confirm diagnosis with serum TSH (>60 mcU/ml), serum total T_4 and free T_4 (low), and serum total T_3 and free T_3 (normal or low). Repeat as indicated to evaluate response to treatment. ▪ ECG, chest x-ray, CBC, AST (SGOT), CPK, LDH, lipids, serum electrolytes, serum cortisol, cerebrospinal fluid examination, and EEG are helpful before dose administration. Monitor progress by repeat evaluations at selected intervals. ▪ Correct adrenocortical insufficiency before administration or acute adrenal crisis and death may result. Corticosteroids (e.g., dexamethasone [Decadron], methylprednisolone [Solu-Medrol]) should be administered routinely in the initial emergency treatment of all myxedema coma patients; required before starting liothyronine or simultaneously with administration in pituitary myxedema; recommended in primary myxedema. During therapy metabolism increases at a greater rate than adrenocortical activity; can precipitate adrenocortical insufficiency and shock; corticosteroids may be needed throughout therapy. ▪ In any patient with compromised cardiac function, monitoring of cardiac function is required. ▪ Assisted or artificial ventilation may be required. ▪ Treatment should correct electrolyte disturbances, possible infection, or other illness. ▪ IV fluids will be required, but use caution to prevent cardiac decompensation and be alert for water intoxication from inappropriate secretion of ADH. ▪ Do not rewarm patient artificially; may further decrease circulation to vital internal organs and increase shock. Normal body temperature can be restored in 24 to 48 hours by preventing heat loss. Keep patient covered with blankets in a warm room. ▪ Note Drug/lab interactions.

Maternal/child: Category A: clinical experience does not indicate adverse effect on fetus. ▪ Observe infant carefully for any adverse symptoms if breast feeding; minimal amounts secreted in breast milk. ▪ Experience with children under 18 is limited; safety and effectiveness not established.

Elderly: Evaluate carefully for any occult cardiac disease (note Precautions/Monitor). ▪ Note Dose adjustments; more sensitive to effects.

DRUG/LAB INTERACTIONS

Metabolic requirements are markedly reduced in hypothyroid patients. Concomitant use with vasopressors (e.g., epinephrine, dopamine [Intropin]) may increase risk of coronary insufficiency, arrhythmias, or circulatory collapse. Use lower doses and extreme caution. ▪ Observe any patient previously stabilized on anticoagulants carefully; dose reduction may be required. Monitor prothrombin time. ▪ Increased doses of insulin or oral hypoglycemics may be required. ▪ Higher doses of levothyroxine may be required with estrogens or estrogen-containing oral contraceptives in the patient with a nonfunctioning thyroid. ▪ May cause transient cardiac arrthymias with tricylic antidepressants (e.g., imipramine [Tofranil]). ▪ May potentiate toxic effects of digitalis, while increased metabolism may require a higher digitalis dose. ▪ Hypertension and tachycardia are probable with ketamine anesthesia. Be prepared to treat promptly. ▪ Pregnancy as well as many drugs (e.g., androgens, corticosteroids, estrogens, estrogen oral contraceptives, iodine preparations, salicylates) in combination with thyroid preparations interfere with accurate interpretation of lab tests. Consult with lab personnel.

SIDE EFFECTS

Average dose: Arrhythmia (6%), cardiopulmonary arrest (2%), hypotension (2%), myocardial infarction (2%), tachycardia (3%). Angina, congestive heart failure, fever, hypertension, phlebitis, and twitching occurred in 1% or less.

Overdose: Acute myocardial infarction, angina pectoris, arrhythmia, congestive heart failure, headache, increased bowel motility, irritability, menstrual irregularities, nervousness, shock, sweating, tachycardia, thyroid storm, tremor.

ANTIDOTE

Keep physician informed of all side effects. If side effects progress or overdose occurs, reduce or temporarily discontinue liothyronine. Restart at lower doses when feasible. Treatment is symptomatic and supportive. Oxygen and artificial ventilation may be required. Treat increased sympathetic activity with beta-adrenergic antagonists (e.g., esmolol [Brevibloc]). Monitor fever, hypoglycemia, and fluid loss and treat as needed. Digoxin (Lanoxin) may be required in congestive heart failure.

LORAZEPAM

Benzodiazepine
Sedative-hypnotic
Antianxiety agent
Anticonvulsant
Amnestic
Skeletal muscle relaxant
Antiemetic

Ativan

USUAL DOSE

2 mg or 0.044 mg/kg of body weight, whichever is smaller, 15 to 20 minutes before procedure. For greater lack of recall 0.05 mg/kg up to 4 mg may be given. 2 mg is usually the maximum dose for patients over 50 years of age.

Sedation: 2 mg as the initial dose (may not be necessary if patient is receiving intermittent benzodiazepines (e.g., diazepam, midazolam). Follow with an infusion 0.5 to 1 mg/hr (0.25 to 0.5 mg/hr if less agitated or has cardiorespiratory problems). Titrate to achieve adequate sedation. Increase in 1 mg/hr increments. Up to 5 to 10 mg/hr has been used. When sedation is adequate, reduce to lowest amount needed.

Status epilepticus: 4 mg as the initial dose. May repeat once in 10 to 15 minutes if seizures continue. Experience with further doses is very limited. Another source suggests 0.05 mg/kg of body weight to a total dose of 4 mg. May repeat once in 10 to 15 min. If still not effective, use another anticonvulsant agent (e.g., diazepam, phenytoin). Do not exceed a total dose of 8 mg in 12 hours.

High-dose therapy for refractory status epilepticus (investigational): With continuous EEG monitoring, begin a continuous infusion of lorazepam at 1 mg/hr. Increase by 1 mg/hr at 15-minute intervals until patient is seizure free. Maintain seizure-free state with lorazepam for 24 hours. Use therapeutic doses of phenytoin and phenobarbital in addition to lorazepam. At the end of 24 hours, begin to reduce the lorazepam by 1 mg/hr at hourly intervals. Observe closely and monitor EEG for signs of recurrent seizures. Repeat process if seizures recur.

Control of acute agitated delirium in combination with haloperidol (unlabeled): Range is from 0.5 to 10 mg lorazepam every hour until agitation subsides. Repeat successful dose as needed for agitation. Consult haloperidol monograph.

Treatment of pain and agitation in critically ill cancer patients in combination with haloperidol and hydromorphone [Dilaudid] (unlabeled): Range is from 0.5 to 10 mg lorazepam every 20 to 30 minutes. Begin with a small dose and increase gradually until agitation subsides, then discontinue lorazepam. Consult haloperidol monograph and hydromorphone monograph.

Management of emetic-inducing chemotherapy (unlabeled): 1.5 mg/M^2 (up to a maximum of 3 mg/M^2) over 5 minutes. Administer 30 to 45 minutes before administration of antineoplastic agent. May be given in combination with metoclopramide and dexamethasone. Repeat every 4 hours as needed.

PEDIATRIC DOSE

Sedation: 0.05 mg/kg every 4 to 8 hours.

Status epilepticus; infants and children (investigational): 0.1 mg/kg up to a maximum of 4 mg/dose. May repeat 0.05 mg/kg once in 5 to 10 min if needed. *Neonates:* 0.05 to 0.1 mg/kg dose over 2 to 3 min.

DOSE ADJUSTMENTS

Reduce dose by one half for the elderly or debilitated, in impaired liver or renal function, in patients with limited pulmonary reserves, and in the presence of other CNS depressants. ■ Note Drug/lab interactions.

DILUTION

Direct IV: Dilute immediately before use with an equal volume of sterile water, D5W, or NS. May be given direct IV or through Y-tube or three-way stopcock of infusion tubing.

Infusion: Not an approved method but is being diluted in D5W or NS and given as an infusion. Best solubility is in concentrations of 0.1 mg/ml or 0.2 mg/ml.

Base concentration	2 mg/ml		4 mg/ml	
Desired concentration	0.1 mg/ml	0.2 mg/ml	0.1 mg/ml	0.2 mg/ml
Volume of diluent required for each 1 ml lorazepam	19 ml	9 ml	39 ml	19 ml

Very viscous; mix well and observe for crystallization. Crystallization does occur and is thought to be due to propylene glycol preservative. May occur more frequently in NS than in D5W and with 4 mg/ml vials of lorazepam base than with 2 mg/ml vials. Prepare only enough to last for 12 hours. If necessary for fluid restriction, a 2 mg/ml vial has been stable for 24 hours when diluted in a 1 mg (lorazepam base) to 1 ml diluent (D5W preferred). Monitor carefully.

Storage: Refrigerate before dilution; protect from light. Use only freshly prepared solutions; discard if discolored or precipitate forms. Infusions stable at room temperature for 12 hours in plastic, 24 hours in glass.

INCOMPATIBLE WITH

Aldesleukin (Proleukin), foscarnet (Foscavir), gallium nitrate (Ganite), idarubicin (Idamycin), imipenem-cilastin (Primaxin), ondansetron (Zofran), sargramostim (Leukine).

RATE OF ADMINISTRATION

Each 2 mg or fraction thereof over 1 minute. Use a microdrip or infusion pump for accuracy to deliver desired dose and/or titrate to desired level of sedation.

Antiemetic: See Usual dose.

Pediatric rate: 1 mg or fraction thereof over 1 minute.

ACTIONS

A benzodiazepine that relieves anxiety, produces sedation, and inhibits ability to recall events. Effective in 15 to 30 minutes. Lasts up to 12 to 24 hours. Widely distributed in body fluids. Metabolized by the liver to inactive metabolites; some is slowly excreted in urine. Crosses the placental barrier. Excreted in breast milk.

INDICATIONS AND USES

Preanesthetic medication for adult patients. ■ Produce sedation, relieve anxiety, and provide anterograde amnesia.

Investigational uses: Management of status epilepticus, especially in children. ■ Treatment of severe agitation concurrently with haloperidol. ■ Treatment of pain and agitation in critically ill cancer patients concurrently with haloperidol and hydromorphone or morphine sulfate. ■ High-dose therapy for status epilepticus clinically or EEG diagnosed as refractory to high doses of phenytoin and phenobarbital. ■ Management of emetic-inducing chemotherapy.

CONTRAINDICATIONS

Hypersensitivity to benzodiazepines (diazepam [Valium], chlordiazepoxide [Librium], etc.), glycols, or benzyl alcohol. Acute narrowangle glaucoma.

PRECAUTIONS

Rapidly and completely absorbed IM. ■ Patient is able to respond to simple instructions. ■ Airway support, emergency drugs, and equipment must be immediately available. ■ Dependence is possible with prolonged use or high dose. ■ Use with extreme caution in the elderly, the very ill, or patients with limited pulmonary reserve.

Monitor: Bed rest required for a minimum of 3 hours after IV injection and assistance required for up to 8 hours. ■ To reduce incidence of thrombophlebitis, avoid smaller veins. Extravasation is hazardous; arterial administration may cause arteriospasms and gangrene and/or require amputation. ■ Maintain patent airway. Respiratory assistance and flumazenil (Romazicon) must be available.

Patient education: May produce drowsiness or dizziness; request assistance with ambulation and use caution performing tasks that require alertness. ■ Avoid use of alcohol or other CNS depressants (e.g., antihistamines, barbiturates). ■ May be habit-forming with long-term use or high-dose therapy. ■ Has amnestic potential; may impair memory. ■ Consider birth control options.

Maternal/child: Category D: avoid pregnancy. Not recommended during pregnancy, labor and delivery, lactation, or in children under 12 years of age. Has FDA approval for treatment of status epilepticus in adults over 18 years of age, but is used in status epilepticus in neonates, infants, and children.

Elderly: Note Usual dose and Dose adjustments. Start with a small dose and increase gradually based on response. ■ More sensitive to therapeutic and adverse effects (e.g., ataxia, dizziness, oversedation). ■ IV injection may be more likely to cause apnea, bradycardia, hypotension, and cardiac arrest. ■ Note Precautions and Drug/lab interactions.

DRUG/LAB INTERACTIONS

Concurrent use with other CNS depressants (e.g., alcohol, antihistamines, barbiturates, MAO inhibitors [e.g., selegiline (Eldepryl)], narcotics [e.g., morphine, meperidine (Demerol), fentanyl], phenothiazines [e.g., prochlorperazine (Compazine)], and tricyclic antidepressants [e.g., imipramine (Tofanil-PM)]) may result in additive effects for up to 48 hours. Reduced dose may be indicated. ■ May increase serum concentrations of digoxin and phenytoin (Dilantin);

monitor digoxin and phenytoin serum levels. ■ Benzodiazepines decrease clearance and increase toxicity of zidovudine (AZT). ■ Hypotensive effects of benzodiazepines may be increased by any agent that induces hypotension (e.g., antihypertensives, bretylium, CNS depressants, diuretics, lidocaine, paclitaxel). ■ Use with rifampin (Rifadin) increases clearance and reduces effects of benzodiazepines. ■ Theophyllines (Aminophylline) antagonize sedative effects of benzodiazepines. ■ Clozapine (Leponix) has caused respiratory distress or cardiac arrest in a few patients; use concurrently with extreme caution. ■ Estrogen-containing oral contraceptives increase clearance and decrease effects. ■ Scopolamine increases sedation, hallucinations, and irrational behavior. ■ Inhibits antiparkinson effectiveness of levodopa. ■ Smoking increases metabolism and clearance of lorazepam, decreasing plasma levels and effectiveness.

SIDE EFFECTS

Airway obstruction, apnea, blurred vision, confusion, crying, delirium, depression, excessive drowsiness, hallucinations, restlessness.

ANTIDOTE

Notify physician of all symptoms. Reduction of dose may be required. Treat hypotension with dopamine (Intropin) or norepinephrine (Levophed). In overdose, flumazenil (Romazicon) will reverse all sedative effects of benzodiazepines. A patent airway, artificial ventilation, oxygen therapy, and other symptomatic and supportive treatment must be instituted promptly.

LYMPHOCYTE IMMUNE GLOBULIN

Immunosuppressant

Anti-Thymocyte Globulin [Equine], Atgam

pH 6.8

USUAL DOSE

Range is 10 to 30 mg/kg of body weight/24 hr. Actual potency and activity may vary from lot to lot. Given concomitantly with other immunosuppressive therapy (antimetabolites such as azathioprine [Imuran] and corticosteroids). Skin test required (See Precautions/ Monitor)

Delay onset of renal allograft rejection: 15 mg/kg/24 hr for 14 days, then every other day for 7 more doses. Initial dose should be given 24 hours before or after the transplant.

Treat allograft rejection: 10 to 15 mg/kg/24 hr for 14 days, then every other day for 7 more doses (optional). Initial dose should be given when first rejection episode is diagnosed.

Aplastic anemia: 10 to 20 mg/kg/24 hr for 8 to 14 days. Additional alternate-day therapy up to a total of 21 doses may be given.

PEDIATRIC DOSE

Range is 5 to 25 mg/kg/24 hr.

DILUTION

Total daily dose must be further diluted with NS, D5/0.2 NS, or D5/0.45 NS for infusion. Invert solution while injecting drug so contact is not made with air in infusion bottle. Gently rotate diluted solution. Do not shake. Concentration should not exceed 4 mg/ml. May be infused into a vascular shunt, AV fistula, or high-flow central vein. Use of a 0.2 to 1.0 micron filter recommended.

Storage: Keep refrigerated before and after dilution. Discard diluted solution after 24 hours.

INCOMPATIBLE WITH

Should be considered incompatible in syringe or solution with any other drug or solution (except solutions listed in Dilution) because of specific use. Will precipitate with D5W or other acid infusion solutions.

RATE OF ADMINISTRATION

A total daily dose equally distributed over a minimum of 4 hours.

ACTIONS

A lymphocyte-selective immunosuppressant. Reduces the number of thymus-dependent lymphocytes and contains low concentrations of antibodies against other formed elements in blood. Effective without causing severe lymphopenia. Supports an increase in the frequency of resolution of an acute rejection episode. Has a serum half-life of 5 to 8 days.

INDICATIONS AND USES

Management of allograft rejection in renal transplant patients. ■ Adjunctive to other immunosuppressive therapy to delay onset of initial rejection episode. ■ Treatment of moderate to severe aplastic anemia in patients who are not candidates for bone marrow transplant.

CONTRAINDICATIONS

Systemic hypersensitivity reaction to previous injection of lymphocyte immune globulin or any other equine gamma globulin preparation.

PRECAUTIONS

Administered only under the direction of a physician experienced in immunosuppressive therapy and management of renal transplant patients in a facility with adequate laboratory and supportive medical resources. ■ Use caution in repeated courses of therapy; observe for signs of allergic reaction.

Monitor: Intradermal skin test required before administration. Use 0.1 ml of a 1:1,000 dilution in normal saline and a saline control. If a systemic reaction (rash, dyspnea) occurs, do not administer. If a limited reaction (10 mm wheal or erythema) occurs, proceed with extreme caution. Anaphylaxis can occur even if skin test is negative. ■ Will cause chemical phlebitis in peripheral veins. ■ Monitor carefully for signs of infection, leukopenia, or thrombocytopenia. Thrombocytopenia is usually transient in renal transplant patients. Platelet transfusions may be necessary in patients with aplastic anemia. Notify physician immediately so prompt treatment can be instituted and/or drug discontinued. ■ Prophylactic antibiotics may be indicated pending results of C/S in a febrile neutropenic patient. ■ Masked reactions may occur as dose of corticosteroids and antimetabolites is decreased. Observe carefully. ■ Antihistamines (e.g., diphenhydramine [Benadryl]) may be required to control itching. ▪ Anaphylaxis can occur at any time. Emergency equipment and supplies must be at bedside.

Patient education: See Appendix D, p. 900.

Maternal/child: Pregnancy Category C: No studies conducted in pregnant patients. Use caution. ▪ Safety for use in lactation not established. Limited experience on use in children.

DRUG/LAB INTERACTIONS

Note Monitor.

SIDE EFFECTS

Full range of allergic symptoms including anaphylaxis is possible. Arthralgia, back pain, chest pain, chills, clotted AV fistula, diarrhea, dyspnea, fever, headache, hypotension, infusion site pain, leukopenia, nausea, night sweats, pruritus, rash, stomatitis, thrombocytopenia, thrombophlebitis, urticaria, vomiting, wheal and flare.

ANTIDOTE

Notify physician of all side effects. Discontinue if anaphylaxis, severe and unremitting thrombocytopenia, and/or severe and unremitting leukopenia occur (note Monitor). May be discontinued if infection or hemolysis present even if appropriately treated. Clinically significant hemolysis may require erythrocyte transfusion, IV mannitol, furosemide, sodium bicarbonate, and fluids. Prophylactic or therapeutic antihistamines (e.g., diphenhydramine [Benadryl]) or corticosteroids should control chills caused by release of endogenous leukocyte pyrogens. Treat anaphylaxis immediately. Epinephrine (Adrenalin), diphenhydramine (Benadryl), oxygen, vasopressors (e.g., dopamine [Intropin]), corticosteroids, and ventilation equipment must always be available. Resuscitate as necessary.

MAGNESIUM SULFATE

Electrolyte replenisher
Anticonvulsant
Antiarrhythmic
Uterine relaxant

pH 5.5 to 7.0

USUAL DOSE

Convulsive states: 1 to 4 Gm (8 to 32 mEq [10 to 40 ml of a 10% solution]). Repeat as indicated, observing all necessary precautions. An alternate regimen is 4 Gm diluted in 250 ml of D5W infused at a rate not to exceed 3 ml/min. In severe **preeclampsia or eclampsia,** a total dose of 8 to 15 Gm may be required depending on body weight. Repeat doses are frequently given IM or an infusion of 1 to 2 Gm/hr is initiated.

Hypomagnesemia (mild): 1 Gm every 6 hours for 4 doses.

Hypomagnesemia (severe): 5 Gm (40 mEq) in 1,000 ml D5W or NS as an infusion evenly distributed over 3 hours.

Hyperalimentation: Adults, 8 to 24 mEq/24 hr. Infants, 2 to 10 mEq/24 hr.

Torsades de pointes, ventricular tachycardia/ventricular fibrillation (VT/VF): 1 to 2 Gm (8 to 16 mEq) in 100 ml D5W over 1 to 2 min. 2 to 6 Gm has been used with extreme caution over several minutes followed by an infusion of 3 to 20 mg/min for 5 to 48 hours.

Reduce incidence of postinfarction arrhythmias associated with hypo-magnesemia: Loading dose: 1 to 2 Gm (8 to 16 mEq) in 50 to 100 ml D5W over 5 to 60 minutes. Follow with an infusion of 0.5 to 1.0 Gm (4 to 8 mEq) per hour for up to 24 hours. Base rate and duration on level of hypomagnesemia. 3 to 4 Gm (30 to 40 ml) of a 10% solution has been used with extreme caution over 30 seconds in the management of paroxysmal tachycardia.

Alternative to thrombolytic therapy post MI (investigational): 22 Gm equally distributed over 48 hours. Effectively decreases incidence of arrhythmias in acute MI patients who cannot receive thrombolytic therapy. Does not decrease incidence of CHF or conduction disturbances.

Alleviate bronchospasm in acute asthma (investigational): 2 Gm. Usually given concurrently with inhaled albuterol (Proventil).

PEDIATRIC DOSE

Hypomagnesemia or hypocalcemia: 25 to 50 mg/kg of body weight. May repeat at 4- to 6-hour. intervals for 3 or 4 doses. Maintain with 30 to 60 mg/kg/24 hr (approximately 0.25 to 0.5 mEq/kg/24 hr). Maximum dose is 1 Gm/24 hr.

Acute nephritis in children: 100 to 200 mg/kg as a 1% to 3% solution (1 Gm in 100 ml=1% solution, 3 Gm in 100 ml=3%). One-half dose should be given over 15 to 20 minutes. Complete balance of dose within 1 hour.

DOSE ADJUSTMENTS

Reduce dose of other CNS depressants (e.g., narcotics, barbiturates) when given in conjunction with magnesium sulfate. ■ Reduce dose in impaired renal function and in the elderly.

DILUTION

Available as a 10%, 12.5%, 20%, and 50% solution. Recently made available (Abbott) as a 1% solution (10 mg/ml) in 100 or 1,000 ml

D5W, a 2% solution (20 mg/ml) in 500 or 1,000 ml D5W, a 4% solution (40 mg/ml) and an 8% solution (80 mg/ml) in sterile water (osmolality will not cause hemolysis). The 8% is in 50 ml, the 4% in 100, 500, or 1,000 ml. Must be diluted to at least a 20% solution. (See Usual dose) for specific dilutions. May be given through Y-tube or three-way stopcock of infusion set.

INCOMPATIBLE WITH

Alcohol, alkalies (bicarbonates, carbonates, and hydroxides), amphotericin B (Fungizone), arsenates, calcium gluconate, calcium gluceptate, chlorpromazine (Thorazine), ciprofloxacin (Cipro IV), clindamycin (Cleocin), cyclosporine (Sandimmune), dobutamine (Dobutrex), hydrocortisone (Solu-Cortef), IV fat emulsion 10%, phosphates, polymyxin B (Aerosporin), phytonadione (Aquamephyton), procaine (Novocaine), salicylates, sodium bicarbonate, strontium, tartrates, tobramycin (Nebcin).

RATE OF ADMINISTRATION

Direct IV: 1.5 ml of a 10% solution or its equivalent over at least 1 minute or as directed in Usual dose. Too-rapid administration may cause hypotension and asystole.

IV infusion: As directed in Usual dose.

ACTIONS

A CNS depressant and a depressant of smooth, skeletal, and cardiac muscle. It also possesses a mild diuretic effect and vasodilating effect. Can reverse refractory VF caused by hypomagnesemia and help replenishment of intracellular potassium. Onset of action is immediate and effective for about 30 minutes. Excreted in the urine. Secreted in breast milk. Crosses the placental barrier.

INDICATIONS AND USES

Prevention and control of convulsive states (eclampsia, glomerulonephritis, hypoparathyroidism). ■ Severe hypomagnesemia. ■ Nutritional supplementation in hyperalimentation. ■ Cerebral edema. ■ Uterine tetany, especially after large doses of oxytocin. ■ Treatment of choice in torsades de pointes, recurrent and refractory ventricular tachycardia, and ventricular fibrillation (VT/VF). ■ Reduce the incidence of postinfarction arrhythmias by counteracting postinfarction hypomagnesemia (given on admission to CCU of a patient with suspected myocardial infarction). ■ Counteract muscle-stimulating effects of barium poisoning. ■ Acute nephritis in children to control hypertension, encephalopathy, and convulsions.

Investigational use: Inhibit premature labor. ■ Treatment of alcohol withdrawal ■ Adjunctive to alleviate bronchospasm in acute asthma. ■ Alternative to thrombolytic therapy in post myocardial infarction patients. ■ Chronic fatigue syndrome. ■ Adjunctive therapy with digoxin in treatment of new-onset atrial fibrillation. ■ Decrease complications during premature labor and/or decrease incidence of cerebral palsy.

CONTRAINDICATIONS

Presence of heart block or myocardial damage; within 2 hours of delivery.

PRECAUTIONS

Do not administer during the 2 hours preceding delivery of the toxemic patient. May cause magnesium toxicity in the newborn requiring assisted ventilation and calcium administration. ■ Each 1 Gm contains 8.12 mEq of magnesium. A normal adult body contains 20 to 30 Gm of magnesium. ■ Use caution in impaired renal function and in patients receiving digitalis. Even in normal renal function, use caution to prevent exceeding renal excretory capacity. ■ Hypomagnesemia can precipitate refractory VF and hinder potassium replacement.

Monitor: Discontinue IV administration when the desired therapeutic effect is obtained. ■ Test knee jerks and observe respirations before each additional dose. If the knee jerk is absent or respirations are less than 16/min, do not give additional magnesium sulfate. ■ Equipment to maintain artificial ventilation must be available at all times. Patient must be continuously observed. Maintain minimum of 100 ml of urine output every 4 hours. ■ Closely monitor patients with suspected or probable MI for hypotension or asystole and measure magnesium levels.

Maternal/child: Note Precautions. ■ Category A: appears to be safe for use during pregnancy except for the last 2 hours before delivery (See Contraindications) ■ A continuous infusion given to control convulsions in toxemic mothers before delivery (especially in the 24 hours preceding) may cause signs of magnesium toxicity in the newborn (e.g., respiratory depression). ■ Some literature indicates possible harm to the fetus during pregnancy if mother is not toxic. ■ Use caution during lactation. ■ Safety for children not established.

Elderly: Note Dose adjustments.

DRUG/LAB INTERACTIONS

Note Dose adjustments and Monitor. ■ Potentiates neuromuscular blocking agents (e.g., tubocurarine [Curare], vecuronium [Norcuron], succinylcholine [Anectine]).

SIDE EFFECTS

Usually the result of magnesium intoxication; absence of knee jerk reflex, cardiac arrest, circulatory collapse, CNS depression, complete heart block, flaccid paralysis, flushing, hypocalcemia with signs of tetany, hypotension, hypothermia, increased PR interval, increased QRS complex, prolonged QT interval, respiratory depression, paralysis, and failure; stupor, sweating.

ANTIDOTE

Discontinue the drug and notify the physician of the occurrence of any side effect. Calcium gluconate and calcium gluceptate are specific antidotes; 5 to 10 mEq should reverse respiratory depression and heart block. Physostigmine 0.5 to 1.0 mg SC may be helpful. Treat hypotension with dopamine (Intropin). Employ artificial ventilation as necessary and resuscitate as necessary. Peritoneal dialysis or hemodialysis are effective in overdose. *Newborn resuscitation* will require endotracheal intubation, assisted ventilation, and calcium 1 mEq as an antidote.

MANNITOL

Osmitrol

Diuretic
(osmotic)

pH 4.5 to 7.0

USUAL DOSE

Test dose may be required; see Precautions/Monitor.

1 to 2 Gm/kg of body weight or 20 to 200 Gm/24 hr. Very flexible. 1 Gm equal to approximately 5.5 mOsm.

Available as:

25% solution (12.5 Gm/50ml) (1,375 mOsm/L)

20% solution (50 Gm/250 ml, 100 Gm/500 ml) (1,100 mOsm/L)

15% solution (22.5 Gm/150 ml, 75 Gm/500 ml) (825 mOsm/L)

10% solution (50 Gm/500 ml, 100 Gm/L) (550 mOsm/L)

5% solution (50 Gm/L) (275 mOsm/L)

Prevention of oliguric phase of acute renal failure: 50 to 100 Gm as a 5% to 25% solution.

Treatment of oliguria: 300 to 400 mg/kg of body weight of a 15% to 25% solution or 50 to 100 Gm of a 15% to 25% solution.

Reduction of intracranial pressure and brain mass: 0.25 to 2.0 Gm/kg of body weight as a 15% to 25% solution.

Reduction of intraocular pressure: 0.25 to 2 Gm/kg of body weight as a 15%, 20%, or 25% solution. May be used 60 to 90 minutes before surgery.

Promote diuresis in intoxication: 50 to 200 Gm. Discontinue if no benefit derived from this dose.

Measurement of glomerular filtration rate: see Rate of Administration.

PEDIATRIC DOSE

Test dose may be required; see Precautions/Monitor.

0.25 to 2 Gm/kg of body weight or 30 to 60 Gm/M^2 of body surface as a 15% to 20% solution. Start with low dose and increase gradually based on clinical situation.

Promote diuresis in intoxication: Use a 5% or 10% solution in the above dose.

Anuria/oliguria: 0.5 to 1.0 Gm/kg as an initial dose. Maintain with 0.25 to 0.5 Gm/kg every 4 to 6 hours.

Cerebral edema: 0.25 Gm/kg. May repeat every 5 minutes as indicated. May give furosemide (Lasix) 1 mg/kg 5 minutes before or concurrently. May gradually increase dose to 1 Gm/kg to effect satisfactory response.

Preop for neurosurgery: 1.5 to 2.0 Gm/kg over 30 to 60 min.

DOSE ADJUSTMENTS

Reduce dose by one half for small or debilitated patients. ■ Reduced dose may be required in oliguria or impaired renal function; note Monitor.

DILUTION

No further dilution is necessary; however, if there are any crystals present in the solution, they must be completely dissolved before administration. Warm ampoule or bottle in hot water (to 50° C [122° F]) and shake vigorously at intervals. Cool to at least body temperature before administration. Use an in-line filter for 15%, 20%, and 25% solutions. Discard unused portions.

Glomerular filtration rate: (See Rate of Administration).

Storage: Store below 40° C.

INCOMPATIBLE WITH

Filgrastim (Neupogen), imipenem-cilastin (Primaxin), potassium chloride, sodium chloride, strongly acidic or alkaline solutions, whole blood. Mixing with whole blood may cause agglutination and irreversible crenation.

RATE OF ADMINISTRATION

A single dose should be given over 30 to 90 minutes. Up to 3 Gm/kg have been given over this time span. A test dose (see Precautions) or loading doses may be given over 3 to 5 minutes.

Oliguria: A single dose over 90 minutes to several hours.

Reduction of intracranial pressure and brain mass: A single dose over 30 to 60 minutes.

Treatment of edema or ascites in pediatric patients: A single dose over 2 to 6 hours.

Glomerular filtration rate: 100 ml of a 20% solution (20 Gm) diluted with 180 ml of NS should be infused at a rate of 20 ml/min. Collect urine and plasma samples as ordered.

ACTIONS

A sugar alcohol and most effective osmotic diuretic. It is a stable, inert, nontoxic solution. Distribution in the body is limited to extracellular compartments. Mannitol is not reabsorbed by the tubules of the kidneys. It is excreted almost completely in the urine along with water, sodium, and chloride. Onset of diuresis is 1 to 3 hours. Reduction in cerebrospinal and intraocular fluid occurs within 15 minutes and lasts 4 to 8 hours. Rebound may occur within 12 hours.

INDICATIONS AND USES

Prophylaxis of acute renal failure (cardiovascular procedures, severe trauma, surgery in presence of jaundice, and hemolytic transfusion reactions). ■ Reduction of intracranial pressure and brain mass before and after surgery. ■ Reduction of extremely high intraocular pressure. ■ Promotion of excretion of toxic substances. ■ Kidney function test (glomerular filtration rate). ■ Reduction of generalized edema and ascites. ■ Oliguric phase of acute renal failure.

CONTRAINDICATIONS

Anuria, edema associated with capillary fragility of membrane permeability, fluid and electrolyte depletion, intracranial bleeding except during craniotomy, some cases of metabolic edema, severe congestive heart failure, severe dehydration, severe pulmonary congestion or frank pulmonary edema, severe renal impairment or progressive renal dysfunction, including increasing azotemia or oliguria.

PRECAUTIONS

Evaluate cardiac status to avoid fulminating congestive heart failure.

Monitor: Test dose should be used in patients with marked oliguria or impaired renal functions. Give 200 mg/kg of body weight over 3 to 5 minutes. 40 ml of urine should be produced in 1 hour. If adequate urine not produced, repeat once. If still ineffective, reevaluate patient. ■ Observe urine output continuously; should exceed 30 to 50 ml/hr. Insert Foley catheter if necessary. ■ Electrolyte depletion may occur.

Check with laboratory studies and replace as necessary. ■ Observe infusion site to prevent infiltration. ■ Maintain hydration; may obscure signs of inadequate hydration or hypovolemia. ■ Before attempting to reduce intracranial pressure and brain mass, evaluate circulatory and renal reserve, fluid and electrolyte balance, body weight, and total input and output before and after mannitol infusion. Reduced cerebrospinal fluid pressure must be observed within 15 minutes after starting infusion. *Maternal/child:* Category C: safety for use in pregnancy not established. Benefits must outweigh risks. ■ Use caution in lactation. ■ Doses for children under 12 years not established but are used clinically.

DRUG/LAB INTERACTIONS

May increase lithium excretion, thereby decreasing its effectiveness. ■ Mannitol-induced hypokalemia may increase the potential for digoxin toxicity.

SIDE EFFECTS

Rare when used as directed but may include backache, blurred vision, chest pain, chills, convulsions, decreased chloride levels, decreased sodium levels, dehydration, diuresis, dizziness, dryness of mouth, edema, fever, fulminating congestive heart failure, headache, hyperosmolality, hypertension, hypotension, nausea, polyuria then oliguria, pulmonary edema, rhinitis, tachycardia, thirst, thrombophlebitis, and urinary retention.

ANTIDOTE

If minor side effects persist, notify the physician. For all major side effects or if urine output is under 30 to 50 ml/hr, discontinue the drug and notify the physician. Treatment will be supportive to correct fluid and electrolyte imbalances. Hemodialysis may be used to clear mannitol and reduce serum osmolality.

MECHLORETHAMINE HYDROCHLORIDE

Antineoplastic
(Alkylating agent/nitrogen mustard)

HN$_2$, Mustargen, nitrogen mustard

pH 3.0 to 5.0

USUAL DOSE

0.4 mg/kg of body weight as a single dose is preferred, or may be divided into 2 to 4 equal doses and given daily for 2 to 4 days. Allow about 3 to 6 weeks between courses of therapy. Confirm bone marrow recovery. Results with subsequent courses are rarely as satisfactory as the initial course.

Hodgkin's disease: 6 mg/M^2 on day 1 and 8 of a monthly treatment cycle.

DOSE ADJUSTMENTS

Dose based on average weight in presence of ascites or edema. ■ Used in reduced doses with other chemotherapeutic agents to produce tumor remission. ■ Note Drug/lab interactions.

DILUTION

Specific techniques required; see Precautions. Mix solution immediately before use. Very unstable. Dilute each 10 mg vial with 10 ml of sterile water or NS. Do not remove needle and syringe. Hold securely and shake vial to dissolve completely. Withdraw desired dose. Contains 1 mg/ml. Do not use if solution is discolored or if droplets of water remain isolated in the vial. May be given direct IV, but administration through a Y-tube or three-way stopcock of a free-flowing infusion is preferred. Neutralize unused portion with equal volume 5% sodium thiosulfate-5% sodium bicarbonate solution and let stand 45 minutes, then discard appropriately.

INCOMPATIBLE WITH

Any other drug in syringe or solution, very unstable.

COMPATIBLE WITH

Y-site with filgrastim (Neupogen), fludarabine (Fludara), melphalan (Alkeran), ondansetron (Zofran), sargramostim (Leukine), vinorelbine (Navelbine).

RATE OF ADMINISTRATION

Total daily dose equally distributed over 3 to 5 minutes.

ACTIONS

An alkylating agent, cell cycle phase nonspecific, with antitumor activity. It has a selective cytotoxic effect on rapidly growing cells. Palliative, not curative, in its effects; regression in the size of malignant tumor may occur; pain and fever subside; appetite, strength, and a sense of well-being are increased. Rapidly metabolized. Excreted in changed form in the urine.

INDICATIONS AND USES

To suppress or retard neoplastic growth. Good response is inconsistent but has been experienced in Hodgkin's disease, lymphosarcoma, bronchogenic carcinoma, specific types of chronic leukemia, polycythemia vera, and mycosis fungoides. Used in generalized metastasis and in patients refractory to radiation therapy.

CONTRAINDICATIONS

Not recommended in patients with infectious disease, previous anaphylactic reactions, or in terminal stages of malignancy.

PRECAUTIONS

Follow guidelines for handling cytotoxic agents. See Appendix A, p. 893. ▪ Administered by or under the direction of the physician specialist. ▪ Highly toxic; must not be inhaled or come into contact with skin or any mucous membrane, especially the eyes, at any stage of mixing, administration, or destruction. For accidental contact, copious irrigation with water for at least 15 minutes is indicated. Follow with rinse of 2% sodium thiosulfate. Use an isotonic ophthalmic irrigation solution if eye contamination occurs. ▪ Use precaution with radiation therapy, other chemotherapy, severe leukopenia, thrombocytopenia, anemia, and bone marrow infiltrated with malignant cells. ▪ Specific tissue can be protected from the effects of this agent by temporary interruption of its blood supply during and immediately after injection. ▪ In the presence of acute or chronic suppurative inflammation, do not use nitrogen mustard. May cause rapid development of amyloidosis.

Monitor: Extremely narrow margin of safety; dose is individual, and frequent blood examinations are mandatory. ▪ Extravasation into surrounding tissue can cause sloughing and possible necrosis. ▪ Often given in the late evening with antiemetics and sedatives to promote patient comfort. ▪ Maintain adequate hydration. ▪ Allopurinol may prevent formation of uric acid crystals. ▪ Observe closely for all signs of infection. Prophylactic antibiotics may be indicated pending results of C/S in a febrile neutropenic patient.

Patient education: Report IV site burning or stinging promptly ▪ Non-hormonal birth control recommended. ▪ See Appendix D, p. 900.

Maternal/child: Category D: avoid pregnancy. May produce teratogenic effects on the fetus. Has mutagenic potential. ▪ Discontinue breast feeding. ▪ Limited use in children; safety not established.

DRUG/LAB INTERACTIONS

Alkalating agents interact with radiation therapy, other antineoplastics, and other bone marrow depressants (e.g., doxorubicin [Adriamycin], vincristine [Oncovin]) to produce serious reaction. ▪ Do not administer live vaccines to patients receiving antineoplastic drugs.

SIDE EFFECTS

Alopecia, anaphylaxsis, anorexia, bleeding, bone marrow depression, cerebrovascular accidents, delayed catamenia, depression of formed elements in circulating blood, diarrhea, hemolytic anemia, hyperuricemia, jaundice, leukopenia, nausea, petechiae, sloughing, susceptibility to infection, tinnitus, thrombophlebitis, vertigo, vomiting, weakness, death.

ANTIDOTE

For external contact and cleaning purposes, use a 2% sodium thiosulfate solution. ▪ To prevent sloughing and necrosis in areas where extravasation has occurred, inject isotonic sodium thiosulfate with a fine hypodermic needle into the indurated area. Apply ice compress for 6 to 12 hours. Elevate extremity. ▪ Use chlorpromazine (Thorazine) or other phenothiazines to control nausea and sodium pentobarbital (Nembutal) to produce sedation. ▪ Notify physician of any side effect. Discontinue the drug and use supportive therapy, including blood transfusion, as necessary to sustain the patient in toxicity.

MELPHALAN HYDROCHLORIDE

Antineoplastic
(Alkylating agent/nitrogen mustard)

Alkeran, L-PAM, L-Sarcolysin,
phenylalanine mustard

pH 6.5 to 7.0

USUAL DOSE

16 mg/M^2 every 2 weeks for 4 doses. After recovery from toxicity, repeat a dose every 4 weeks. Prednisone is administered concurrently (0.6 mg/kg daily with dose reductions every 2 weeks). WBC should be above 4,000/mm^3 and platelets above 100,000/mm^3. Other similar regimens are in use. No exact dosage conversion from oral to parenteral or parenteral to oral.

PEDIATRIC DOSE

See Investigational uses.

DOSE ADJUSTMENTS

Reduce dose by 50% if BUN above 30 mg/dl or serum creatinine above 1.5 mg/dl. ■ Reduce dose based on myelotoxicity; by 25% if WBC between 3,000 to 4,000/mm^3 and platelets between 75,000 to 100,000/mm^3; by 50% if WBC between 2,000 and 3,000/mm^3 and platelets between 50,000 to 75,000/mm^3. Withhold dose for WBC below 2,000/mm^3 and platelets below 50,000/mm^3. ■ Somewhat reduced dose may be appropriate for patients undergoing hemodialysis.

DILUTION

Specific techniques required; see Precautions.

Reconstitution to completion of administration must take place within 60 minutes due to instability of melphalan (rapid hydrolysis). Rapidly inject 10 ml of supplied diluent into vial. Shake vigorously until a clear solution results (5 mg/ml). Use only clear solutions. Has been given without further dilution. Usually further diluted in NS to a concentration of 0.1 to 0.45 mg/ml (45 mg in 100 ml equals 0.45 mg/ml). Must always be further diluted for use in peripheral lines.

Storage: Protect from light and store at room temperature before reconstitution. Reconstituted solution is stable for only 90 minutes maximum. Stable at a concentration of 0.1 to 0.45mg/ml for only 60 minutes. Will precipitate if refrigerated.

INCOMPATIBLE WITH

Consider toxicity and specific use. Very unstable. Amphotericin B (Fungizone), chlorpromazine (Thorazine). May be compatible at *Y-site* with numerous drugs; consult with pharmacist.

RATE OF ADMINISTRATION

Direct IV: A single dose less than 23 mg/M^2 over 2 to 5 minutes via a peripheral vein; up to 200 mg/M^2 over 2 to 20 minutes via a central line.
Intravenous infusion: A single dose over 15 minutes.

ACTIONS

A phenylalanine derivative of nitrogen mustard that is a bifunctional alkylating antineoplastic agent. Cytotoxicity is related to the extent of its interstrand cross-linking with DNA. Not dependent on cell cycle phase. Active against both resting and dividing tumor cells. Eliminated from plasma primarily by chemical hydrolysis rather than metabolism. 30% bound to plasma protein. Distribution to terminal half-life is 10 to 75 minutes. About 10% excreted as unchanged drug in urine.

INDICATIONS AND USES

Palliative treatment of patients with multiple myeloma when oral therapy is not appropriate.

Investigational uses: Treatment of multiple myeloma in combination with other cytotoxic agents. ▪ Treatment of refractory multiple myeloma (high-dose melphalan [100 to 140 mg/M^2] in combination with prednisone [MP], vincristine, doxorubicin [Adriamycin], and dexamethasone [Decadron], [VAD], and bone marrow support). ▪ Treatment of newly diagnosed aggressive multiple myeloma in combination with other cytotoxic agents and interferon. ▪ High doses (above 100 mg/M^2) with bone marrow reinfusion or colony-stimulating factor (e.g., filgrastim [GCSF]) to treat poor-prognosis Hodgkin's and non-Hodgkin's lymphoma, leukemia, multiple myeloma, and neuroblastoma. ▪ High-dose melphalan (180 to 220 mg/M^2) with bone marrow rescue to treat neuroblastoma, Ewing's sarcoma and soft tissue sarcoma, leukemia, and lymphoma in children over 1 year. May be combined with other cytotoxic agents, surgery, and/or total body irradiation. ▪ Intraarterial injection (hyperthermic isolated limb perfusion) is used with surgery for extremity melanoma and as a palliative treatment with locally advanced, unresectable malignant melanoma of the extremity. ▪ Intraperitoneal route used to treat advanced ovarian cancers.

CONTRAINDICATIONS

Prior resistance to or hypersensitivity to melphalan.

PRECAUTIONS

Follow guidelines for handling cytotoxic agents. See Appendix A, p. 893. ▪ Administered by or under the direction of the physician specialist, with facilities for monitoring the patient and responding to any medical emergency. ▪ Use extreme caution in patients whose bone marrow is compromised by or recovering from previous radiation or chemotherapy. ▪ Severe myelotoxicity (WBC below 1,000/mm^3 and platelets below 25,000/mm^3) is more common with IV dosing. ▪ Do not abandon treatment prematurely. Improvement may continue slowly over many months with repeated courses. ▪ Patients with an elevated BUN had a greater incidence of severe leukemia.

Monitor: Determine absolute patency of vein. A stinging or burning sensation indicates extravasation; cellulitis and tissue necrosis may result. Discontinue injection; use another vein. ▪ Monitor platelet count, hemoglobin, white blood count, and differential frequently. Indicated before each dose as well as between doses to determine optimal dose and avoid toxicity. Nadirs occur 2 to 3 weeks after treatment, recovery should occur in 4 to 5 weeks. ▪ Monitor kidney function before and during therapy. ▪ Severe myelosuppression can occur with effective doses. Withhold further doses until blood counts have recovered if thrombocytopenia and/or leukopenia occur. ▪ Hypersensitivity reactions may occur with initial treatment but frequently are delayed and occur after multiple courses. Observe closely, anaphylaxis and death have occurred. ■ Observe closely for all signs of infection or bleeding. Prophylactic antibiotics may be indicated pending results of C/S in a febrile neutropenic patient. ■ Prophylactic antiemetics may reduce nausea and vomiting and increase patient comfort. ■ Some facilities are using ice pops to help prevent stomatitis. ■ Note Drug/lab interactions.

Patient education: Avoid pregnancy; nonhormonal birth control recommended. ■ Report IV site burning or stinging promptly. ■ See Appendix D, p. 900.

Maternal/child: Category D: avoid pregnancy. Can cause chromosomal damage and severe birth defects in the fetus and impairment of fertility in men and women. ■ Discontinue breast feeding. ■ Safety and effectiveness for use in children not established (See Investigational uses)

Elderly: No differences in response from younger patients. Consider age-related organ impairment and history of previous disease or drug therapy.

DRUG/LAB INTERACTIONS

Coadministration with cyclosporine (Sandimmune) may result in acute renal failure. May occur after the first dose of each drug. renal toxicity. ■ Renal dysfunction and increased toxicity may occur with concurrent cisplatin. ■ Lung toxicity associated with carmustine (BCNU) may be increased with concurrent use. ■ Interferon alfa may decrease seurm concentrations of melphalan. ■ Use with nalidixic acid (NegGram) may cause severe hemorrhagic necrotic enterocolitis in pediatric patients.

SIDE EFFECTS

Reversible bone marrow suppression is dose-limiting. Irreversible bone marrow failure has been reported. Alopecia, diarrhea, hemolytic anemia, hepatic toxicity (including veno-occlusive disease), hypersensitivity reactions (2% [e.g., anaphylaxis, bronchospasm, dyspnea, edema, hypotension, pruritus, urticaria, tachycardia]), interstitial pneumonitis, nausea and vomiting, oral ulceration, pulmonary fibrosis, secondary malignancies (long-term use), skin ulceration at injection site, vasculitis.

Overdose: Severe bone marrow depression, cholinomimetic effects (e.g., bradycardia, increased peristalsis and salivation, incontinence), convulsions, decreased consciousness, hyponatremia (inappropriate secretion of ADH), muscular paralysis, severe nausea and vomiting.

ANTIDOTE

Keep physician informed of all side effects. Close monitoring of bone marrow may prevent most serious and potentially fatal side effects. White blood cell and platelet count nadirs occur 2 to 3 weeks after treatment with recovery in 4 to 5 weeks. Withhold further doses until blood counts have recovered if leukopenia or thrombocytopenia occur. There is no specific antidote, but adequate supportive care including administration of autologous bone marrow or filgrastim (G-CSF) may shorten the period of pancytopenia. Appropriate blood transfusions and antibiotics may be indicated. Monitor closely until recovery (6 weeks or more). Discontinue the infusion and treat allergic reactions with antihistamines, corticosteroids, pressor agents, or volume expanders, do not readminister melphalan (IV or oral). Hemodialysis probably not effective in overdose. For extravasation, elevate the extremity and apply intermittent ice packs over the area immediately and 4 times daily for 1/2 hour. Continue for several days.

MEPERIDINE HYDROCHLORIDE

Narcotic analgesic (agonist)

Demerol, Demerol hydrochloride

pH 3.5 to 6.0

USUAL DOSE

Direct IV: 10 to 50 mg. Repeat every 2 to 4 hours as necessary. When seeking the required dose to achieve pain relief for an individual patient, increases in increments of at least 25% of the previous ineffective dose are suggested. Lower slightly if pain controlled but patient is too drowsy; or lower dose and increase frequency.

Infusion: Must be administered through a controlled infusion device. May be patient activated. Based on a 10 mg/ml dilution an initial loading dose of 20 to 25 mg (2 to 2.5 ml) is average. The continuous background infusion to provide a level of pain relief and maintain patency of the vein may range from 10 to 15 mg/hr (1 to 1.5 ml/hr). Additional doses of 5 to 10 mg (0.5 to 1 ml) may be activated by the patient at selected intervals every 3 to 60 minutes (averaging 10 to 15 minutes). Additional boluses (averaging 5 to 10 mg [0.5 to 1 ml]) may be given by health care professionals (e.g., every 30 min prn). In selected patients all of these doses may be somewhat higher.

Supplement anesthesia: 1 mg/ml dilution given as a continuous infusion under the direct observation and control of the anesthesiologist.

Control of postoperative pain: 600 mg/liter diluent. Infuse at 0.5 ml (0.3 mg)/kg/hr.

Treatment or prevention of shaking chills (investigational): 0.5 mg/kg 20 minutes before shaking chills are expected to begin or 50 mg after onset of chills. Up to 150 mg have been required within 30 minutes if administered after onset.

PEDIATRIC DOSE

1 to 1.5 mg/kg/dose. May repeat every 3 to 4 hours. Maximum dose 100 mg. See Maternal/child.

DOSE ADJUSTMENTS

Reduced dose may be required in the elderly or debilitated, in hepatic or renal disease, or in numerous other disease entities; see Precautions. ■ Note Drug/lab interactions.

DILUTION

Direct IV: Should be diluted in at least 5 ml of sterile water, NS, or other IV solutions.

Infusion: Available as 10, 25, 50, 75, or 100 mg/ml for infusion. Each 10 mg must be diluted in at least 1 ml of NS, D5W, D5/NS, or other compatible infusion solution. Usually diluted in NS for use in narcotic syringe infusor systems, but may be added to larger amounts and given as an infusion.

INCOMPATIBLE WITH

Acylovir (Zovirax), allopurinol (Zyloprim), aminophylline, amobarbital (Amytal), cefoperazone (Cefobid), furosemide (Lasix), heparin, hydrocortisone sodium succinate (Solu-Cortef), idarubicin (Idamycin), imipenem-cilastatin (Primaxin), methicillin (Staphcillin), methylprednisolone (Solu-Medrol), mezlocillin (Mezlin), minocycline (Minocin), morphine, Nafcillin (Nafcill), pentobarbital (Nembutal), phenobarbital (Luminal), phenytoin (Dilantin), secobarbital (Seconal), sodium bicarbonate, sodium iodide, thiopental (Pentothal).

RATE OF ADMINISTRATION

Direct IV: A single dose over 4 to 5 minutes. Frequently titrated according to symptom relief and respiratory rate.

Infusion: Must be administered through a controlled infusion device. May be patient activated. Initial loading dose, basal rate (continuous rate of infusion), patient self-administered dose and interval, additional boluses permitted and total dose for 1 hour should be ordered by physician. Do not exceed direct IV rate. For continuous infusion note range of mg/hr under Usual dose; distribute evenly via infusion device.

ACTIONS

A synthetic narcotic analgesic and descending CNS depressant, similar to but slightly less potent than morphine. Onset of action occurs in about 5 minutes and lasts for about 2 hours. Pain threshold is elevated, and the reaction of the individual to the painful experience is altered. Crosses the placental barrier. Readily absorbed and distributed throughout the body. Metabolized to normeperidine in the liver, its extended half-life (15 to 30 hours) may lead to cumulative effects. Excreted in the urine. Secreted in breast milk.

INDICATIONS AND USES

Short-term relief of most moderate to severe pain. ■ Preoperative medication. ■ Support of anesthesia. ■ Obstetric analgesia. ■ Restoration of uterine tone and contractions in a uterus made hyperactive by oxytocics.

Investigational uses: Treatment or prevention of shaking chills (rigors) caused by some medications (e.g., amphotericin B [Fungizone], aldesleukin [Proleukin]).

CONTRAINDICATIONS

Acute bronchial asthma, hypersensitivity to meperidine, patients who have received MAO inhibitors (e.g., selegiline [Eldepryl]) in the previous 2 weeks, diarrhea resulting from poisoning until toxic material eliminated, pregnancy before labor, premature infants or labor and delivery of premature infants, pulmonary edema caused by chemical respiratory irritant, upper airway obstruction.

PRECAUTIONS

Use with caution in glaucoma, head injuries, increased intracranial pressure (elevates spinal fluid pressure), asthma, chronic obstructive pulmonary disease, decreased respiratory reserve or respiratory depression, supraventricular tachycardia, convulsions, acute abdominal conditions before diagnosis, the elderly and debilitated, and hepatic or renal insufficiency. ■ Cough reflex is suppressed. ■ Morphine is usually preferred for pain during cardiac arrhythmias. ■ IM route frequently used. Frequent IM injections may lead to severe fibrosis of muscle tissue. ■ Do not use in patients in cycle cell crisis or for any long-term pain relief (e.g., cancer).

Monitor: Oxygen, controlled respiratory equipment, and naloxone (Narcan) must always be available. ■ Observe patient frequently to continuously based on amount of dose and monitor vital signs. ■ Keep patient supine; orthostatic hypotension and fainting may occur; less likely with continuous low doses, but observe closely during ambulation. ■ Uncontrolled pain causes sleep deprivation, decreases pain threshold, and increases pain. When pain is finally controlled, expect the patient to sleep more until recovery from sleep deprivation. ■ With use the active metabolite normeperidine accumulates to toxic levels; will decrease renal function and lower seizure threshhold. Monitor for twitching, jerking, shaky hands, tremors; may lead to grand mal seizure. ■ Stool softeners and/or laxatives may be required to avoid constipation and fecal impaction. Maintain adequate hydration.

Patient education: Avoid alcohol or other CNS depressants (e.g., barbiturates, benzodiazepines [e.g., diazepam (Valium)]). ■ May cause blurred vision, dizziness, or drowsiness; use caution in tasks that require alertness. ■ May be habit forming.

Maternal/child: Pregnancy Category C: note Contraindications. ■ Use caution during lactation. Levels are low, but best to wait 4 to 6 hours before breast feeding. ■ Not recommended for IV use in children but is used.

Elderly: Note Dose Adjustments, Precautions. ■ May be more sensitive to effects (e.g., respiratory depression, constipation, urinary retention). ■ Analgesia should be effective with lower doses. ■ Consider age-related renal impairment.

DRUG/LAB INTERACTIONS

Potentiated by antacids, anticholinergics, cimetidine (Tagamet), tricyclic antidepressants (e.g., amitriptyline [Elavil]), isoniazid (Nydrazid), neostigmine (Prostigmin), neuromuscular blocking agents, (e.g., tubocurarine), oral contraceptives, phenothiazines (e.g., promazine [Sparine]), general anesthetics, other narcotic analgesics, and CNS depressants including alcohol. Reduced dosage of both drugs may be indicated. ■ Do not use with MAO inhibitors (e.g., selegiline [Eldepryl]), may cause cardiovascular collapse. ■ Concurrent use with ritonavir (Norvir) not recommended. May increase risk of side effects, including seizures and cardiac arrhythmias. ■ Inhibited by hydantoins (e.g., phenytoin [Dilantin]). ■ Metabolism increased and analgesic effects may be decreased or delayed in smokers.

SIDE EFFECTS

Minor: Dizziness, flushing, lightheadedness, nausea, postural hypotension, rash, restlessness, sedation, sweating, syncope, vomiting.

Major: Allergic reactions, apnea, cardiac arrest, cardiovascular collapse, cold and clammy skin, convulsions, dilated pupils, normeperidine toxicity (jerking, tremor, twitching, shaky hands, grand mal seizure), respiratory depression, shock, tremor.

ANTIDOTE

With increasing severity of minor side effects or onset of any major side effect, discontinue the drug and notify the physician. Naloxone hydrochloride (Narcan) will reverse serious respiratory depression. A patent airway, artificial respiration, oxygen therapy, and other symptomatic treatment must be instituted promptly. Resuscitate as necessary.

MEROPENEM

Antibacterial
(Carbapenem)

Merrem I.V.   pH 7.3 to 8.3

USUAL DOSE

Intra-abdominal infections in adults and children over 50 kg: 1 Gm every 8 hours.

PEDIATRIC DOSE

Intra-abdominal infections in children over 3 months of age and under 50 kg: 20 mg/kg every 8 hours.

Meningitis in children over 3 months of age and under 50 kg: 40 mg/kg every 8 hours.

Meningitis in children over 50 kg: 2 Gm every 8 hours.

DOSE ADJUSTMENTS

Reduce dose required if creatinine clearance ≤ 51 ml/min based on table below:

Recommended Meropenem IV Dosage Schedule for Adults with Impaired Renal Function		
Creatinine clearance (ml/min)	Dose (dependent on type of infection)	Dosing interval
26 to 50	recommended dose (1000 mg)	every 12 hours
10 to 25	one half recommended dose	every 12 hours
< 10	one half recommended dose	every 24 hours

Consult package insert or front matter of this text for formula to convert serum creatinine to creatinine clearance. ■ No dose adjustment necessary in impaired hepatic function or in the elderly with a creatinine clearance ≥ 51 ml/min.

DILUTION

Available as vials for injection, vials for infusion, and ADD-Vantage vials for infusion.

Vials for injection: Reconstitute each 500 mg with 10 ml SW (1 Gm with 20 ml). Yields 50 mg/ml. Shake to dissolve and let stand until clear. May be given as an IV injection or further diluted with 50 to 250 ml of compatible infusion solutions (e.g., NS, D5W, D10W, D5/NS, D5/0.2NS, Ringer's, Ringer's Lactate; see package insert for complete listing).

Vials for infusion: Reconstitute with 50 to 100 ml of compatible infusion solutions above.

ADD-Vantage vials for infusion: Must be reconstituted only with 50, 100, or 250 ml of D5W, 0.45 NS, or NS. Instructions for preparation and use on packaging. Do not use flexible containers in series connections.

Storage: Store unopened vials at controlled room temperature. Use of freshly prepared solutions preferred. Vials for injection stable at room temperature for 2 hours after reconstitution. Stability of all other dilutions dependent on diluent and room temperature or refrigeration. Range is from 1 hour to 24 hours; see package insert or consult pharmacist. Do not freeze.

INCOMPATIBLE WITH

Manufacturer states, "Meropenem should not be mixed or physically added to solutions containing other drugs." Specific studies have not been done.

RATE OF ADMINISTRATION

Same rate is used for adults and children over 3 months of age.

IV injection: A single dose (up to 20 ml after dilution) over 3 to 5 minutes.

Intermittent infusion: A single dose over 15 to 30 minutes.

ACTIONS

A synthetic, broad-spectrum, carbapenem antibiotic. Bactericidal to selected gram-negative, gram-positive, and anaerobic organisms. Bactericidal activity results from the inhibition of cell wall synthesis. Readily penetrates the cell wall of susceptible organisms to reach penicillin-binding protein targets. Peak plasma concentrations reached by the end of an infusion. Penetrates well into most body fluids and tissues, including cerebrospinal fluid. Peak fluid and tissue concentrations reached in 0.5 to 1.5 hours. Minimal protein binding. Elimination half-life averages 1 hour in adults, 1.5 hours in children age 3 months to 2 years. 70% recovered as unchanged drug in urine within 12 hours. Not yet known if it crosses the placental barrier or is secreted in breast milk.

INDICATIONS AND USES

Treatment of intra-abdominal infections (e.g., complicated appendicitis, peritonitis) in adults and children caused by specific susceptible organisms (e.g., viridans group streptococci). ▪ Treatment of bacterial meningitis in children 3 months of age and older caused by specific susceptible organisms.

CONTRAINDICATIONS

History of hypersensitivity to meropenem, its components, any other carbapenem antibiotic (e.g., imipenem-cilastin [Premaxin], or patients with hypersensitivity to beta-lactams.

PRECAUTIONS

Specific sensitivity studies are indicated to determine susceptibility of the causative organism to meropenem. ▪ Use extreme caution in patients with a history of allergic reactions to penicillins, cephalosporins, and other allergens. ▪ May cause seizures in patients with a history of CNS disorders (e.g., brain lesions, history of seizures) or with bacterial meningitis and/or compromised renal function. Use extreme caution; continue administration of anticonvulsants in patients with known seizure disorders. ▪ Use with caution in patients with impaired renal function (see Dose adjustment); thrombocytopenia may occur. ▪ Staphylococci resistant to methicillin/oxacillin must be considered resistant to meropenem. ▪ May have cross-resistance with strains resistant to other carbapenems (e.g., imipenem-cilastatin [Primaxin]). ▪ Has been found to eliminate concurrent bacteremia associated with bacterial meningitis. ▪ Avoid prolonged use of drug; superinfection caused by overgrowth of nonsusceptible organisms may result. ▪ Pseudomembranous colitis has been reported; see Antidote.

Monitor: Anaphylaxis has been reported. Emergency equipment must always be available. ▪ Monitor infusion site for inflammation and/or extravasation. May cause thrombophlebitis. ▪ Monitor for S/S of CNS reactions (e.g., focal tremors, myoclonus, seizures). ▪ Monitor renal, hepatic, and hemopoietic systems in prolonged therapy. ▪ Each 1 Gm contains 3.92 mEq of sodium; monitoring of electrolytes may be indicated. ▪ Note Side effects.

Patient education: Report any diarrhea, itching, rash, shortness of breath, or twitching sensation immediately. ▪ Report any burning, pain, or stinging at injection site.

Maternal/child: Category B: Safety for use in pregnancy not established; use only if clearly needed. ▪ Use caution during lactation; not known if meropenem is secreted in breast milk, safety not established. ▪ Approved only for use in infants and children over 3 months of age.

Elderly: Dose adjustments not indicated unless the creatinine clearance is ≤ 51 ml/min.

DRUG/LAB INTERACTIONS

Probenecid inhibits renal excretion and increases serum levels of meropenem extending its half-life and increasing systemic exposure; coadministration is not recommended. ▪ May be synergistic with aminoglycosides against some isolates of *Pseudomonas aeruginosa.* ▪ Additional drug interaction studies have not been conducted to date.

SIDE EFFECTS

Toxicity rate is usually low. *Children:* Diarrhea (4.3%), diaper area moniliasis (3.5%), glossitis (1%), oral moniliasis (2%), rash (1.4%), vomiting (1%). *Adults:* Constipation (1.2%), diarrhea (5%), headache (2.8%), nausea and vomiting (3.9%), rash (1.7%). Injection site reactions (e.g., edema, inflammation, pain, phlebitis [3%], pruritus [1.6%]), are most common. Many other side effects including increases or decreases in hematologic, hepatic, and renal lab tests may occur in less than 1% of patients. *Adults and children:* Full scope of allergic reactions including anaphylaxis have occurred in a few patients. Bleeding events (e.g., GI bleeding, epistaxis), pseudomembranous colitis, seizures, and thrombocytopenia can occur.

ANTIDOTE

Notify physician of all side effects. Most will be treated symptomatically. Discontinue immediately if an allergic reaction occurs. Treat allergic reaction as indicated (e.g., oxygen, epinephrine, corticosteroids, diphenhydramine, vasopressors). If focal tremors, myoclonus, or seizures occur, evaluate neurologically, initiate anticonvulsant therapy, and decide whether to decrease or discontinue meropenem. Mild cases of colitis may respond to discontinuation of meropenem. Oral vancomycin (Vancocin) or metronidazole (Flagyl) is the treatment of choice for antibiotic-related pseudomembranous colitis. Adequate hydration and supplementation of electrolytes and proteins usually indicated. Hemodialysis may be helpful in overdose.

MESNA

Antidote
Antineoplastic adjunct
Prophylactic for hemorrhagic cystitis

Mesnex, ♦Uromitexan   pH 6.5 to 8.5

USUAL DOSE

Total daily dose is 60% of the ifosfamide dose equally divided into 3 doses. A single dose of mesna equal to 20% of the ifosfamide dose is given at the time of the ifosfamide injection and repeated 4 hours and 8 hours later. (e.g., ifosfamide 1.2 Gm/M^2 would require mesna 240 mg/M^2 with the ifosfamide, 240 mg/M^2 in 4 hours, and again at 8 hours). The initial mesna dose each day may be mixed with the ifosfamide. Appears to be compatible.

DOSE ADJUSTMENTS

Dose of mesna must be repeated each day ifosfamide is administered and adjusted with each increase or decrease of the ifosfamide dose.

DILUTION

Each 100 mg (1 ml) must be diluted in a minimum of 4 ml D5W, D5/NS, D5/1/2NS, NS, or LR. Desired concentration is 20 mg/ml.

Storage: Refrigerate diluted solutions and use within 6 hours. Discard any unused drug from the ampoule. Mesna oxidizes to disulfide dimesna when exposed to oxygen.

INCOMPATIBLE WITH

Carboplatin (Paraplatin), cisplatin (Platinol).

RATE OF ADMINISTRATION

A single dose over a minimum of 1 minute given as a single agent. Administer at rate for ifosfamide if given together.

ACTIONS

A detoxifying agent. Reacts chemically in the kidney with urotoxic ifosfamide metabolites to detoxify them and inhibit hemorrhagic cystitis. Remains in the intravascular compartment and much of a single dose is excreted within 4 hours in urine.

INDICATIONS AND USES

A prophylactic agent used to reduce the incidence of hemorrhagic cystitis caused by ifosfamide.

Unlabeled uses: May reduce the incidence of hemorrhagic cystitis caused by cyclophosphamide.

CONTRAINDICATIONS

Hypersensitivity to mesna or other thiol compounds.

PRECAUTIONS

Repeated doses are required to maintain adequate levels of mesna in the kidneys and bladder to detoxify urotoxic ifosfamide metabolites. ■ Hemorrhagic cystitis caused by ifosfamide is dose dependent. Mesna is most effective when ifosfamide dose is less than 1.2 $Gm/M^2/24$ hr. Somewhat less effective when ifosfamide dose 2 to 4 $Gm/M^2/24$ hr. If hematuria develops with appropriate doses of mesna, ifosfamide dose may need to be reduced or discontinued. ■ Does not inhibit any other side effects or toxicities caused by ifosfamide therapy. ■ Not effective in preventing hematuria caused by other conditions (e.g., thrombocytopenia).

Maternal/child: Category B: use during pregnancy only if benefits clearly outweigh risks. ■ Discontinue nursing.

DRUG/LAB INTERACTIONS

May cause a false-positive reaction for urinary ketones. If a red-violet color develops, glacial acetic acid returns the coloring to violet.

SIDE EFFECTS

Average dose: Bad taste in the mouth, diarrhea, nausea, soft stool, vomiting.

Overdose: Allergic reactions, diarrhea, fatigue, headache, hematuria, hypotension, limb pain, nausea.

ANTIDOTE

No specific antidote. Keep physician informed of all side effects. Notify promptly if signs of overdose occur. Resuscitate as necessary.

METARAMINOL BITARTRATE

Aramine

Vasopressor

pH 3.5 to 4.5

USUAL DOSE

0.5 to 5 mg direct IV only in severe shock. 15 to 100 mg in 500 ml of specific infusion solution. 150 to 500 mg/500 ml of infusion solution has been used at an extremely slow rate. Adjust to desired clinical fluid volume. Titrate to maintain blood pressure at desired level. Allow at least 10 minutes before increasing any dose.

Unlabeled dose/route of administration: 5 mg has been given via an endotracheal tube if an IV route is not available. Dilute to 10 ml and ventilate patient at least 5 times before and after injection.

PEDIATRIC DOSE

0.01 mg/kg of body weight as a single dose or as a solution of 1 mg/25 ml in dextrose or saline for infusion. Note Maternal/child.

DILUTION

Single dose up to 5 mg may be given undiluted. Should be diluted in at least 500 ml of NS or D5W and administered as an IV infusion.

Storage: Store below 40° C. Use infusion solutions within 24 hours.

INCOMPATIBLE WITH

Amphotericin B (Fungizone), ampicillin, cephalothin (Keflin), dexamethasone (Decadron), erythromycin (Erythrocin), heparin, hydrocortisone phosphate, hydrocortisone sodium succinate, Solu-Cortef invert sugar, levarterenol (Levophed), methicillin (Staphcillin), methylprednisolone (Solu-Medrol), oxacillin (Prostaphlin), oxytetracycline (Terramycin), penicillin G potassium or sodium, pentobarbital (Nembutal), phenytoin (Dilantin), prednisolone (Hydeltrasol), Rantidine (Zantac), sodium bicarbonate, sodium lactate injection, thiopental (Pentothal), warfarin (Coumadin), whole blood.

RATE OF ADMINISTRATION

Direct IV administration, 5 mg or fraction thereof over 1 minute. In solution use slowest possible flow rate to correct hypotension gradually and maintain adequate or preset blood pressure. Use of a micro-drip (60 gtt/ml) or an infusion pump helpful.

ACTIONS

A potent sympathomimetic amine, but less potent than norepinephrine. Produces gradual action with long effect. It constricts blood vessels, increasing peripheral resistance, and elevating systolic and diastolic pressure. Increases cardiac contractility and cerebral, coronary, and renal blood flow. May cause reflex bradycardia. Inactivated in the body and excreted in the urine. Effective within 1 to 2 minutes. Maximum effect may take 10 minutes and lasts 20 minutes to 1 hour. Metabolic fate and route of excretion are not clearly understood.

INDICATIONS AND USES

Acute hypotensive states resulting from spinal anesthesia, hemorrhage, medication reaction, and shock associated with brain damage due to trauma or tumor. ▪ May be useful as an adjunct in the treatment of hypotension due to cardiogenic shock or septicemia.

CONTRAINDICATIONS

Hypersensitivity to any component, including sulfites. Do not use with cyclopropane or halothane anesthesia.

PRECAUTIONS

Whole blood or plasma should be given in a separate IV site. Is not a replacement for blood, plasma, fluid, or electrolytes when loss has occurred. ▪ Avoid hypertension; pulmonary edema, arrhythmia, and cardiac arrest may result. ▪ Cumulative effect is possible. Hypertension may remain even after drug is discontinued. ▪ Use care in liver, heart, and thyroid disease and in hypertension or diabetes. ▪ May cause a relapse of malaria. ▪ Discontinue slowly; rebound effect may occur if stopped abruptly.

Monitor: Hypovolemia must be corrected to receive adequate response. Note Precautions. ▪ Check blood pressure every 5 minutes until stabilized at the desired level. Check every 15 minutes thereafter throughout therapy. ▪ Use a large vein and confirm patency. Discontinue IV administration if vein infiltrates or is thrombosed; can result in tissue necrosis and sloughing.

Maternal/child: Pregnancy Category C: benefits must outweigh risks. ▪ Use caution in lactation. ▪ Safety and effectiveness in children not established.

DRUG/LAB INTERACTIONS

MAO inhibitors (e.g., selegiline [Eldepryl]), guanethedine (Ismelin), oxytocic drugs (e.g., oxytocin), and tricyclic antidepressants potentiate metaraminol and can cause an acute hypertensive crisis. ▪ May cause severe hypertension and stroke with ergot alkaloids. ▪ May cause arrhythmias with digitalis. ▪ Atropine blocks reflex bradycardia and will further increase BP (pressor effect).

SIDE EFFECTS

May occur with average doses; cardiac arrest, cardiac arrhythmias, dizziness, headache, hypertension, nervousness, sweating, tachycardia, and tremor.

ANTIDOTE

Notify the physician of any side effects. Most will be treated symptomatically or dosage of metaraminol will be decreased. Should a sudden or uncontrolled hypertensive state occur, discontinue metaraminol, notify the physician, and treat with an alpha-adrenergic blocking agent (e.g., phentolamine [Regitine]). Beta-blockers (e.g., propranolol [Inderal]) may be useful in the treatment of arrhythmias. Resuscitate as necessary. To prevent sloughing and necrosis in areas where extravasation has occurred, with a fine hypodermic needle inject 5 to 10 mg of phentolamine diluted in 10 to 15 ml of NS liberally throughout the tissue in the extravasated area.

METHOCARBAMOL

Skeletal muscle relaxant
(Central acting)

Robaxin   pH 4.0 to 5.0

USUAL DOSE
1 Gm (10 ml) every 8 hours for no more than 3 days. May be repeated after an additional 2 days (days 6, 7, and 8) if indicated. In tetanus treatment, dose may be as high as 3 Gm every 6 hours. Initiate with 1 to 2 Gm direct IV. Give balance of dose by infusion.

PEDIATRIC DOSE
Not recommended for children under 12 years of age except in tetanus.

In tetanus: 15 mg/kg of body weight initially. Repeat every 6 hours as indicated.

DILUTION
May be given undiluted, or a single dose may be given as an IV infusion diluted in no more than 250 ml NS or D5W.

Storage: Store below 40° C. Do not refrigerate after dilution.

INCOMPATIBLE WITH
Physically compatible with many drugs. Sufficient information not available. Note Precautions and Contraindications.

RATE OF ADMINISTRATION
300 mg (3 ml) or fraction thereof over 1 minute or longer. Adjust infusion rate for patient comfort.

ACTIONS
A skeletal muscle relaxant. Action may be due to general CNS depression. Diminishes skeletal muscle hyperactivity without altering normal muscle tone. Widely distributed throughout the body. Metabolized in the liver and excreted in the urine.

INDICATIONS AND USES
Relief of discomfort from acute, painful musculoskeletal conditions. Adjunctive to other measures (e.g., rest, physical therapy). ■ Treatment of neuromuscular manifestations of tetanus. Adjunctive to other measures (e.g., tetanus antitoxin, fluid and electrolyte replacement). While FDA approved, this use is generally replaced by diazepam (Valium) or, in very severe cases, neuromuscular blocking agents (e.g., pancuronium [Pavulon]).

CONTRAINDICATIONS
Hypersensitivity to methocarbamol, known or suspected renal pathology.

PRECAUTIONS

Blood aspirated into syringe will not mix with medication; an expected phenomenon. ▪ Use caution in known or suspected epileptic patients. ▪ Maintenance doses should be oral even if the pills are crushed and given through a nasogastric tube.

Monitor: Observe site of injection continuously. A hypertonic solution; extravasation may cause thrombophlebitis or sloughing. ▪ Keep patient in recumbent position for at least 15 minutes to avoid postural hypotension. ▪ Monitor renal function if duration of treatment is 3 or more days. ▪ Note Drug/lab interactions.

Patient education: Avoid alcohol or other CNS depressants (e.g., barbiturates, benzodiazepines [e.g., diazepam (Valium)]). ▪ May cause dizziness, drowsiness, and visual disturbances. Request assistance for ambulation. ▪ Use caution in any task that requires alertness. ▪ Report fever, itching, nasal congestion, or rash promptly. ▪ Urine may discolor to very dark green.

Maternal/child: Use caution in pregnancy and lactation. Safety for use not established. American Academy of Pediatrics considers it compatible with breast feeding.

Elderly: Males may have sensitivity to anticholinergic effects (e.g., dry mouth, urinary retention). ▪ Consider age-related renal impairment; may preclude use.

DRUG/LAB INTERACTIONS

Potentiated by alcohol, CNS depressants, MAO inhibitors (e.g., selegiline [Eldepryl]), and phenothiazines (e.g., chlorpromazine [Thorazine]). ▪ May interfere with some laboratory tests (5-HIAA, VMA).

SIDE EFFECTS

Infrequent but more often associated with too-rapid injection.

Minor: Blurred vision, conjunctivitis, diplopia, dizziness, drowsiness, fainting, fever, flushing, headache, hypotension, GI upset, lightheadedness, metallic taste, muscular incoordination, nasal congestion, nystagmus, pruritus, rash, urticaria, vertigo.

Major: Anaphylactic reaction, bradycardia, convulsions, pain at injection site, sloughing at injection site, syncope, thrombophlebitis.

ANTIDOTE

Notify the physician of minor side effects. If these side effects progress or major side effects occur, discontinue the drug, notify the physician, and treat symptomatically. Epinephrine, steroids, and antihistamines should be readily available. Resuscitate as necessary.

METHOTREXATE SODIUM

Antineoplastic
(Antimetabolite)
Antipsoriatic
Antirheumatic

Amethopterin, Folex, Folex PFS,
Methotrexate LPF, MTX

pH 8.5

USUAL DOSE

Many dose limitations based on patient condition, renal and hepatic function, and concomitant drugs; (See Precautions/Monitor). Part of numerous protocols. Doses vary from 20 to 50 mg/M^2 every 1 to 2 weeks for treatment of solid tumors to 200 to 500 mg/M^2 every 2 to 4 weeks for treatment of leukemias or lymphomas. Any dose over 80 mg/week should be accompanied by leucovorin rescue. Other examples outside of these dose ranges include:

Ewing's sarcoma: 12 mg/M^2 on days 1 to 3 and days 42 to 44. Given with bleomycin, cyclophosphamide, dactinomycin, doxorubicin, leucovorin, and vincristine.

Gastric cancers: 1.5 Gm/M^2 on day 1. Given with doxorubicin, fluorouracil, and leucovorin.

Acute lymphoblastic leukemia: 690 mg/M^2 over a 42 hour period with leucovorin.

Trophoblastic neoplasms: 15 to 30 mg/24 hr for 5 days. Repeat course of therapy 3 to 5 times with rest periods of 7 to 12 days unless contraindicated by toxicity. Usually given orally or IM.

Leukemia: 3.3 mg/M^2 with prednisone 60 mg/M^2. Give daily if tolerated, and continue for up to 8 weeks or until satisfactory response (usually 4 to 6 weeks). Maintenance dose individualized; 30 mg/M^2 (or 2.5 mg/kg) every 14 days has been used IV, IM, or orally.

Psoriasis and rheumatoid arthritis: 10 to 25 mg once a week. Do not exceed 50 mg. Use smallest effective dose. Usually given orally or IM.

Osteosarcoma: One regimen recommends 12 Gm/M^2 as a single dose. Begin the 4th week after surgery and repeat weekly at weeks 5, 6, 7, 11, 12, 15, 16, 29, 30, 44, and 45. A peak serum concentration of 1,000 micromolars/L at the end of the infusion is desired. Dose may be increased to 15 Gm/M^2 if required. Must be accompanied by leucovorin rescue; begin 24 hours after start of methotrexate infusion and give 15 mg every 6 hours times 10 doses. Additional doses may be required. Usually given orally. Osteosarcoma also requires combination chemotherapy. Protocols vary but may include doxorubicin, cisplatin, bleomycin, cyclophosphamide, dactinomycin and vincristine. These massive doses are highly individualized, require exacting calculations, and constant patient monitoring (see Precautions/Monitor).

DOSE ADJUSTMENTS

Reduce dose by 25% if bilirubin is between 3 and 5 or asparate aminotransferase (AST) above 180; if bilirubin above 5, omit dose.
■ Often used with other antineoplastic drugs to achieve tumor remission. ■ Reduced dose may be required with impaired renal function,

in the very young or very elderly, the debilitated, and in other diseases (note Precautions). ▪ Note Drug/lab interactions.

DILUTION

Specific techniques required; see Precautions. 25 mg/ml is the maximum concentration that can be given IV. Reconstitution of each 5 mg with 2 ml of preservative-free D5W or NS is preferred. Each milliliter equals 2.5 mg of methotrexate. Available in preservative-free solutions. Do not use formulations or diluents with preservatives (e.g., bacteriostatic) for experimental high-dose therapy or intrathecal injection. 1 Gm vial available for high-dose use with appropriate dilution. Not usually added to IV solutions when given in standard doses. Discard solution if a precipitate forms. May be given through Y-tube or three-way stopcock of a free-flowing IV.

A single dose may be further diluted with D5W or NS immediately before use as an infusion with high methotrexate doses.

Storage: If prepared without a preservative, use immediately. May be stable up to 14 days with a preservative.

INCOMPATIBLE WITH

Note Precautions and Contraindications. Bleomycin (Blenoxane), chlorpromazine (Thorazine), doxorubicin (Adriamycin), droperidol (Inapsine), idarubicin (Idamycin), metoclopramide (Reglan), prednisolone (Hydeltrasol), ranitidine (Zantac).

COMPATIBLE WITH

Consult pharmacist. May be compatible with amino acids, cephalothin (Keflin), cytarabine, dacarbazine, fluorouracil, furosemide (Lasix), hydrocortisone, idarubicin (Idamycin), leucovorin, mercaptopurine, metoclopramide (Reglan), promethazine (Phenergan), sodium bicarbonate, vincristine (Oncovin). *Y-site:* Cisplatin, fluorouracil, and heparin.

RATE OF ADMINISTRATION

Direct IV: Each 10 mg or fraction thereof over 1 minute.

Infusion: A single dose equally distributed over 30 minutes to 4 hours or as prescribed by protocol.

ACTIONS

An antimetabolite and folic acid antagonist. Cell cycle specific for the S phase, it interrupts the mitotic process during nucleic acid synthesis. Rapidly proliferating malignant cells are inhibited by a cytostatic effect. Widely distributed, average doses of methotrexate are excreted unchanged in the urine within 24 hours. Clearance rates decrease with higher doses. Does not cross blood-brain barrier. Secreted in breast milk.

INDICATIONS AND USES

Treatment of trophoblastic disease (e.g., uterine choriocarcinoma), acute lymphocytic leukemia, lymphosarcoma, osteogenic sarcoma, malignancies of the breast, testis, head, neck, and lung and many others. ▪ Severe disabling psoriasis or rheumatoid arthritis unresponsive to other treatment. ▪ High-dose regimen for treatment of osteosarcoma. ▪ Given orally or IM for mycosis fungoides and other diagnoses and intrathecally for meningeal leukemia.

CONTRAINDICATIONS

Hypersensitivity to methotrexate; nursing mothers. Not absolute, but methotrexate is not recommended during pregnancy or with hepatic, renal, or bone marrow damage.

PRECAUTIONS

Follow guidelines for handling cytotoxic agents. See Appendix A, p. 893. ▪ Administered by or under the direction of the physician specialist. ▪ Evacuate excess fluid from ascites and pleural effusions before treatment. ▪ Use with extreme caution in patients with infection, impaired renal or liver function, peptic ulcer, or ulcerative colitis; in debilitated patients; and in the very young or very elderly.

Monitor: Close patient observation is mandatory. Course of therapy is not repeated until all signs of toxicity from the previous course subside. ▪ Complete blood cell counts with platelets, chest x-ray, and renal and liver function tests before, during, and after therapy are essential to comprehensive treatment. Liver biopsy and bone marrow studies may be indicated in high dose or long-term therapy. ▪ Monitor renal function closely; verify by creatinine clearance levels. Maintain adequate hydration and urine alkalinization. ▪ Monitor serum methotrexate levels. ▪ Use prophylactic antiemetics to reduce nausea and vomiting and increase patient comfort. ▪ Observe closely for signs of infection. Prophylactic antibiotics may be indicated pending results of C/S in a febrile neutropenic patient. ▪ Administration of high-dose methotrexate requires a white blood cell count above 1,500 mm^3; neutrophil count above 200/mm^3; platelet count above 75,000 mm^3; serum bilirubin less than 1.2 mg/dl; alanine aminotransferase (ALT) level less than 450 Units; any mucositis must be healing; ascites or pleural effusion must be drained dry; serum creatinine must be normal; creatinine clearance > 60 ml/min; 1 L/M^2 of IV fluid over 6 hours before dosing and 3 L/M^2/day on day of infusion and for 2 days after; alkalinization of urine with sodium bicarbonate; and repeat serum methotrexate and serum creatinine levels at least daily until methotrexate level is below 0.05 micromolar. ▪ Note Drug/lab interactions.

Patient education: Nonhormonal birth control recommended. Continue for at least 3 months after treatment completed. ▪ Avoid alcohol and take only prescribed medications. Reactions can be lethal. ▪ See Appendix D, p. 900.

Maternal/child: Category D: avoid pregnancy. Has caused fetal death and congenital anomalies. ▪ Discontinue breast feeding. ▪ Safety for use in children is limited to chemotherapy.

Elderly: Note Dose adjustments. Diminished hepatic and renal function and increased folate stores may indicate much lower doses. Monitor for early signs of toxicity.

DRUG/LAB INTERACTIONS

The following drugs may enhance methotrexate toxicity when administered concomitantly: alcohol, amiodarone (Cordarone), antibacterials (e.g., tetracycline, chloramphenicol), etretinate (Tegison), acetylated salicylates (e.g., aspirin) nonsteroidal antiinflammatory drugs (NSAIDs) (e.g., indomethacin, ketoprofen, naproxen), penicillins (e.g., amoxicillin, mezlocillin), probenecid, salicylates, any hepatotoxic drug, sulfonamides, para-aminobenzoic acid (PABA), phenylbutazone, phenytoin (Dilantin), pyrimethamine, and trimethoprim (component of trimethoprim-sulfamethoxazole [Bactrim, Septra]); interactions may be life threatening. Monitoring of serum levels and/or reduced doses of methotrexate may be indicated or a longer duration of leucovorin rescue may be required. ■ Omeprazole (Prilosec) increases serum levels of methotrexate. Discontinue several days prior to methotrexate administration. Consider an H_2 antagonist (e.g., ranitidine [Zantac]). ■ Asparaginase antagonizes methotrexate; separate administration by 24 hours. ■ Vitamins with folic acid may alter response to methotrexate. ■ Methotrexate interacts with many drugs such as antidiabetics, charcoal, corticosteroids, other antineoplastics (e.g., procarbazine), thiopurines (e.g., azathioprine [Imuran]), and others to produce potentially serious reactions. ■ Do not administer live vaccines to patients receiving antineoplastic drugs. ■ May decrease phenytoin (Dilantin) serum levels. ■ Procarbazine (Matulane), may increase nephrotoxicity of methotrexate. Allow 72 hours between last dose of procarbazine and first dose of methotreate. ■ Monitor for signs of increased bone marrow suppression with sulfonamides (e.g., sulfisoxazole [Gantrisin], TMP-SMZ [Bactrim]). May also cause TMP-SMZ (Bactrim)-induced megaloblastic anemia. ■ Urinary alkalinizers increase renal excretion and may reduce effectiveness.

SIDE EFFECTS

Toxicity usually dose related. Death can occur from average doses, high doses, drug interactions (e.g., NSAIDs), bone marrow toxicity, and GI toxicity. Acne, alopecia (occasional), chills, cystitis, dehydration, depigmentation, diabetes, diarrhea, edema, enteritis, fever, GI ulceration, gingivitis, hematologic depression, hemorrhage from any site, hepatotoxicity, leukoencephalopathy, menstrual dysfunction, nausea, oral ulceration, pharyngitis, pruritus, pulmonary disease (dry nonproductive cough), rash, septicemia, stomatitis, urticaria, vomiting.

ANTIDOTE

Citrovorum factor, folinic acid (leucovorin) may be given orally, IM, or IV promptly to counteract inadvertent overdose. Citrovorum factor is also indicated as a planned rescue mechanism for large doses of methotrexate required to treat some malignancies. Doses equal to dose of methotrexate are frequently required. Should be given within 1 hour in overdose, 24 hours in rescue. See specific process for overdose and for rescue for high-dose MTX; in leucovorin monograph. Doses up to 150 mg or 100mg/M^2 every 3 hours may be required if serum creatinine is 50% or greater than base line measurement before methotrexate administration. Serum methotrexate must come down to below 0.05 micromolar. Hydration and urinary alkalinization are mandatory to prevent precipitation in renal tubules. Discontinue methotrexate and notify the physician of any side effects. Platelet transfusion may be indicated with thrombocytopenia. Death may occur from the progression of most of these side effects. Symptomatic and supportive therapy is indicated. Charcoal hemoperfusion may be helpful.

METHYLDOPATE HYDROCHLORIDE

Antihypertensive

Aldomet

pH 3.0 to 4.2

USUAL DOSE

250 to 500 mg every 6 hours. Up to 1 Gm every 6 hours is acceptable. Maintain with oral medication in same dosage as soon as practical. Limit the initial dose of methyldopate to 500 mg/day in divided doses if given with antihypertensives other than thiazides; if added to a thiazide regimen, no dose adjustment of the thiazide is necessary.

PEDIATRIC DOSE

5 to 10 mg/kg of body weight every 6 hours. Maximum dose is 65 mg/kg or 3 Gm/24 hr, whichever is less.

DOSE ADJUSTMENTS

Reduced dose may be required in the elderly and with impaired liver and renal function. ■ Note Drug/lab interactions.

DILUTION

Single dose may be diluted in 100 ml of D5W or in sufficient D5W to achieve a final concentration of 10 mg/ml and given as an infusion. *Storage:* Store below 40° C.

INCOMPATIBLE WITH

Alkaline drugs (e.g., barbiturates, sulfonamides), amphotericin B (Fungizone), methohexital (Brevital). Physically compatible with many drugs. Consider specific use and precautions above.

RATE OF ADMINISTRATION

Each dose as an infusion is given over 30 to 60 minutes.

ACTIONS

A moderate antihypertensive drug. Exact mechanism of action is unknown, but is thought to be due to its metabolism to alpha-methyl-norepinephrine which lowers arterial BP through several processes. Reduces both supine and standing BP without affecting cardiac output, glomerular filtration rate, or renal blood flow. Onset of action is 4 to 6 hours and lasts 10 to 16 hours. Extensively metabolized and excreted in urine. Crosses placental barrier and is secreted in breast milk.

INDICATIONS AND USES

Hypertension when parenteral therapy is indicated. ■ Hypertensive crises, especially for patients with renal or coronary insufficiency. Because of delayed onset of action, other agents may be preferred.

CONTRAINDICATIONS

Hypersensitivity to any component, including sulfites; active liver disease (e.g., acute hepatitis or active cirrhosis); coadministration with MAO inhibitors (e.g., selegiline [Eldepryl]); history of previous methydopa therapy being associated with liver disorders.

PRECAUTIONS

More effective combined with diuretics. ■ Use caution in impaired liver and renal function.
Monitor: Check blood pressure every 30 minutes until stabilized at

desired level. Slow response lessens usefulness. ▪ Liver function tests, complete blood cell count, and direct Coombs test indicated. ▪ Observe for adequate urine output. ▪ Note Drug/lab interactions.

Maternal/child: Category B: use in pregnancy and lactation with caution and only if clearly needed.

Elderly: Hypotensive and sedative effects may be increased. ▪ Consider age-related organ impairment.

DRUG/LAB INTERACTIONS

Antihypertensive effects may be reduced by barbiturates, and reduced or reversed by tricyclic antidepressants (e.g., amitriptyline [Elavil]). ▪ Serious elevations in blood pressure may occur with phenothiazines (e.g., promethazine [Phenergan]). ▪ Potentiates oral antidiabetics (e.g., tolbutamide [Orinase]), levodopa, levarterenol (Levophed), and all antihypertensive drugs (e.g., hydralazine [Apresoline]). ▪ May produce adverse mental symptoms with haloperidol. ▪ Capable of paradoxical reactions with cocaine, norepinephrine (Levophed), and phenylephrine (Neo-Synephrine). Severe hypertension can occur. ▪ Concurrent use with MAO inhibitors (e.g., selegiline [Eldepryl]) is contraindicated, may produce hyperexcitability and hypertension. ▪ Lithium toxicity has developed with concurrent use. ▪ Causes false elevated urinary catecholamine response. ▪ May potentiate anesthetics; reduced doses of anesthetics may be required. ▪ Use with nonselective beta blockers (e.g., propranolol [Inderal]) may cause paradoxical hypertension.

SIDE EFFECTS

Anaphylaxis, apprehension, depression, dizziness, dry mouth, edema, elevated alkaline phosphatase, elevated AST (SGOT), fever, hemolytic anemia, nasal congestion, nightmares, paradoxical hypertension, positive Coombs' test, postural hypotension (mild), sedation.

ANTIDOTE

Notify the physician of all side effects. Most can be decreased in severity by reducing dosage. Drug may be discontinued. Dopamine (Intropin) or levarterenol (Levophed) should reverse hypotension of overdose. Hemodialysis may be used in acute overdose.

METHYLENE BLUE

Antidote
Diagnostic agent

Methylthionine chloride

pH 3.0 to 4.5

USUAL DOSE

1% methylene blue, 1 ml equals 10 mg. 1 to 2 mg/kg of body weight is recommended dose. Dose may be repeated in 1 hour if necessary. Do not exceed recommended dose. Continuous infusions may sometimes be indicated (see Rate of Administration).

DILUTION

Usually given undiluted.

Storage: Store below 40° C. Protect from light.

INCOMPATIBLE WITH

Do not mix with any other drug.

RATE OF ADMINISTRATION

IV injection: A single dose should be evenly distributed over 5 minutes. Inject very slowly to prevent toxic effects of local high concentration of the compound.

Continuous infusion: For treatment of methemoglobinemia following an overdose of agents in which there is a prolonged or continuous methemoglobin formation (e.g., dapsone), a continuous infusion may be administered at a rate of 0.1 to 0.15 mg/kg/hr following the initial dose of 1 to 2 mg/kg.

ACTIONS

Low concentrations will convert methemoglobin to hemoglobin (methemoglobin is toxic and gives the blood a chocolate-brown color; it does not carry oxygen). High concentrations convert ferrous iron of hemoglobin to ferric iron, thus forming methemoglobin. Excreted in urine and bile.

INDICATIONS AND USES

Treatment of aquired or idiopathic methemoglobinemia. ▪ Diagnostic dye. ▪ To identify body structures and fistulas. ▪ Has been used for treatment of cyanide poisoning, but sodium nitrate is considered to be safer and more effective.

CONTRAINDICATIONS

Hypersensitivity to methylene blue; intraspinal injection, renal insufficiency.

PRECAUTIONS

May cause cyanosis or cardiac irregularities. ▪ May induce hemolysis in patients deficient in glucose-6-phosphate dehydrogenase.

Monitor: Check hemoglobin; may cause a marked anemia resulting from accelerated destruction of erthrocytes. ▪ Note Precautions.

Patient education: May discolor urine and stool blue-green. Will stain tissue.

Maternal/child: Pregnancy Category C: Safety for use during pregnancy and lactation not established. ▪ Infants under 5 months of age are more susceptible to methemoglobinemia produced by high concentrations of methylene blue.

SIDE EFFECTS

Minor: Nausea, vomiting, bladder irritation, diarrhea, headache.

Major: Abdominal pain, anemia, dizziness, fever, precordial pain, profuse diaphoresis, mental confusion, methemoglobin.

ANTIDOTE

Discontinue the drug upon appearance of any side effect. Remove skin stains with hypochlorite solution.

METHYLERGONOVINE MALEATE

Uterine stimulant (oxytocic)

Methergine

pH 2.7 to 3.5

USUAL DOSE

1 ml (0.2 mg or gr $\frac{1}{320}$); may be repeated every 2 to 4 hours as necessary. A maximum of 5 doses is usually not exceeded.

DILUTION

Check expiration date on vial; methylergonovine deteriorates with age. May be given undiluted. Some clinicians recommend dilution with 5 ml of NS. Do not add to IV solutions. May be given through Y-tube or three-way stopcock of infusion set.

Storage: Store at 15° to 30° C.

INCOMPATIBLE WITH

Limited information available. Do not mix in a syringe with any other drug.

COMPATIBLE WITH

Y-site: Heparin, hydrocortisone sodium succinate (Solu-Cortef).

RATE OF ADMINISTRATION

0.2 mg or fraction thereof over 1 minute. Too-rapid injection may cause severe nausea and vomiting.

ACTIONS

A synthetic oxytocic. It exerts a direct stimulation on the smooth muscle of the uterus. Produces vasoconstriction, increases CVP, elevates BP, and may rarely produce peripheral ischemia. In therapeutic doses the prolonged initial contraction of the uterus is followed by periods of relaxation and contraction. Preferred because it is less likely to cause hypertension. Effective within 1 minute for up to 3 hours. It is probably metabolized in the liver and excreted in feces. Secreted in breast milk.

INDICATIONS AND USES

Routine management after delivery of the placenta. ▪ Postpartum atony. ▪ Hemorrhage. ▪ Subinvolution.

CONTRAINDICATIONS

Hypersensitivity, hypertension, pregnancy before third stage of labor (delivery of the placenta), toxemia.

PRECAUTIONS

Not recommended for use before the delivery of the placenta. Occasionally given after the anterior shoulder is delivered if the obstetrician directs and is present. ▪ IV administration is for emergency use only. IM or oral routes are preferred and should be used after the initial IV dose. ▪ Use caution in presence of sepsis, obliterative vascular disease, and cardiac, hepatic, or renal disease.

Monitor: Monitor blood pressure. ▪ Uterine response may be poor in calcium-deficient patients; calcium replacement may be required for effective response. Avoid or use extreme caution if calcium replacement is needed in patients taking digoxin. ▪ Note Drug/lab interactions.

Maternal/child: Pregnancy Category C: note Contraindications and Precautions. Administration before delivery of the placenta may cause hypoxia and intracranial hemorrhage in the infant, captivation of the placenta, or missed diagnosis of a second infant. ▪ May be given orally during lactation for up to 1 week after delivery.

DRUG/LAB INTERACTIONS

Severe hypertension and cerebrovascular accidents can result with ephedrine, methoxamine (Vasoxyl), and other vasopressors. Chlorpromazine (Thorazine) or hydralazine (Apresoline) IV will reduce this hypertension.

SIDE EFFECTS

Rare in therapeutic doses but may include the following:

Average dose: Allergic phenomena, chest pain (temporary), diaphoresis, dilated pupils, dizziness, dyspnea, headache, hypertension (transient), hypotension, nausea, tinnitus, vomiting, weakness.

Overdose: Abortion, blindness, cerebrovascular accident, convulsions, excitement, gangrene, hypercoagulability, palpitations, severe nausea and vomiting, shock, tachycardia, thirst, tremor, uterine bleeding.

ANTIDOTE

Discontinue the drug immediately at the onset of any side effect and notify the physician. Most side effects are transient unless there is severe toxicity and will be treated symptomatically. Use antiemetics (e.g., prochlorperazine [Compazine], ondansetron [Zofran] for nausea and vomiting. Treat cardiac ischemia with nitroglycerin, seizures with diazepam (Valium) or phenytoin (Dilantin). Treat peripheral ischemia with nitroprusside, tolazoline (Priscoline), or phentolamine (Regitine). Treat hypertension with nitroprusside, chlorpromazine (Thorazine), or hydralazine (Apresoline). Severe poisoning is treated with vasodilator drugs, sedatives, calcium gluconate to relieve muscular pain, and other supportive treatment. Heparin is used to control hypercoagulability.

METHYLPREDNISOLONE SODIUM SUCCINATE

Hormone
(Adrenocorticoid/glucocortoid)
Antiinflammatory

A-MethaPred, Solu-Medrol   pH 7.0 to 8.0

USUAL DOSE

Average dose range is 10 to 250 mg initially. May be repeated every 4 to 6 hours as necessary. IV methylprednisolone is usually given in an emergency situation or when oral dosing is not feasible. Larger doses may be justified by patient condition. Repeat until adequate response, then decrease dose as indicated. Total dose usually does not exceed 1.5 Gm/24 hr. Dose is individualized according to the severity of the disease and the response of the patient and is not necessarily reduced for children. High-dose treatment is utilized until patient condition stabilizes, usually no longer than 48 to 72 hours.

Antiinflammatory: 10 to 40 mg. May be repeated every 4 to 6 hours as necessary.

Life-threatening shock or septic shock (unlabeled and controversial): Highdose "pulse" therapy: Several regimens have been suggested:

30 mg/kg initially. Repeat every 4 to 6 hours or

100 to 250 mg initially. Repeat every 2 to 6 hours or

30 mg/kg as a loading dose, followed by a continuous infusion of 30 mg/kg every 12 hours for 24 to 48 hours.

Acute spinal cord injury high-dose therapy (investigational): Spinal cord injury must be less than 8 hours old and above L-2. The earlier methylprednisolone therapy begins, the better the results.

Loading dose: 30 mg/kg of a specifically diluted solution (See Dilution) evenly distributed over 15 minutes. Maintain IV line with standard IV fluids for 45 minutes, then begin a maintenance dose of 5.4 mg/kg/hr for 23 hours. Discontinue 24 hours after loading dose initiated.

Status asthmaticus: 10 to 250 mg/dose every 4 to 6 hr.

Acute exacerbation of multiple sclerosis: 160 mg as a single dose each day for 7 days. Follow with 64 mg every other day for one month.

Pneumocystis carinii *pneumonia (unlabeled):* Initiate within 24 to 72 hours of initial antibiotic PCP therapy. 30 mg twice daily for 5 days. Follow with 30 mg once daily for 5 days (day 6 through 10). Then reduce to 15 mg once daily for eleven days (day 11 through 21) or until antibiotic regimen is complete.

Severe lupus nephritis (unlabeled): 1 Gm as an infusion over 1 hour for 3 days. Follow with long-term prednisolone oral therapy.

PEDIATRIC DOSE

Antiinflammatory/immunosuppressive: 0.16 to 0.8 mg/kg/24 hr in equally divided doses every 6 to 12 hours. One source suggests that 0.5 mg/kg/day is the minimum dose.

Status asthmaticus: 1 to 2 mg/kg as a loading dose. Maintain with 0.5 to 1 mg/kg every 6 hours.

Severe lupus nephritis (unlabeled): 30 mg/kg every other day for 6 doses. Follow with long-term prednisolone oral therapy.

DOSE ADJUSTMENTS

Reduced dose may be required in the elderly, in patients with renal transplants, and with cyclophosphamide. Note Precautions and Drug/lab interactions.

DILUTION

Available in vials containing 40 mg, 125 mg, 500 mg, 1,000 mg, and 2,000 mg. Each vial has an appropriate amount of diluent. Available in an Act-O-Vial, which is reconstituted by removing the protective cap, turning the rubber stopper a quarter turn, and pressing down, allowing the diluent into the lower chamber. Agitate gently. Using sterile technique, insert a needle through the center of the rubber stopper to withdraw diluted solution. To be diluted only with diluent supplied in Act-O-Vial. May be given direct IV, as an infusion, or further diluted in desired amounts of D5W, D5/NS, or NS. Best if minimally diluted to 0.25 mg/ml; consult pharmacist. Discard unused solutions after 48 hours.

Acute spinal cord injury loading and maintenance doses: Each 1 Gm vial must be diluted to 16 ml with bacteriostatic water to maintain potency and avoid precipitation (62.5 mg/ml). Further dilute in D5W, D5/NS, or

NS with an amount to facilitate dose of 5.4 mg/kg/hr. (Example for a patient weighing 50 kg: [50 kg × 5.4 mg/hr = 270 mg/hr. 270 mg/hr × 23 hours = 6,210 mg total dose.] With a total dose of 6,210 mg at 62.5 mg/ml, you will have 99.36 [100] ml of reconstituted methylprednisolone. Add an additional 100 ml diluent to achieve 31.25 mg/ml. 270 mg/hr is the desired dose for this patient. 270 mg/hr divided by 31.25 mg/ml [strength of solution] equals 8.6. Administer at 8.6 ml/hr to achieve desired dose over 23 hours.)

INCOMPATIBLE WITH

Allopurinol (Zyloprim), aminophylline, calcium gluconate, cephalothin (Keflin), chlorpromazine (Thorazine), ciprofloxacin (Cipro IV), cytarabine (ARA-C), dextrose 5% in 0.45% normal saline, digitoxin (Crystodigin), diltiazem (Cardizem), diphenhydramine (Benadryl), doxapram (Dopram), filgrastim (Neupogen), glycopyrrolate (Robinul), insulin, meperidine (Demerol), metaraminol (Aramine), nafcillin (Unipen), ondansetron (Zofran), paclitaxel (Taxol), penicillin G sodium and potassium, potassium chloride, promethazine (Phenergan), sargramostim (Leukine), thiamylal (Surital), thiopental (Pentothal), tolazoline (Priscoline), vinorelbine tartrate.

RATE OF ADMINISTRATION

Direct IV: Each 500 mg or fraction thereof over 2 to 3 minutes or longer. Direct IV administration is usually route of choice and eliminates possibility of overloading the patient with IV fluids. May be given as an *infusion* in its own diluent over 10 to 20 minutes. At the discretion of the physician, a continuous infusion may be given, properly diluted, over a specified time.

Shock: 30 mg over 15 to 30 min.

Acute spinal cord injury: See Usual dose.

ACTIONS

An adrenocortical steroid with potent metabolic, antiinflammatory actions and innumerable other effects. Has a greater antiinflammatory potency than prednisolone and less tendency to cause excessive potassium and calcium excretion and sodium and water retention. Has four times the potency of hydrocortisone sodium succinate. Has minimal mineralocorticoid activity. Primarily used for antiinflammatory and immunosuppressive effects. May be used in conjunction with other forms of therapy, such as epinephrine for acute allergic reactions or antibiotics in acute infections. Primarily metabolized in the liver and excreted in the urine and feces. 75% excretion occurs within 24 hours, allowing use of very large doses with reasonable safety. Crosses the placental barrier. Secreted in breast milk.

INDICATIONS AND USES

Supplementary therapy for severe allergic reaction (use epinephrine first). ▪ Shock unresponsive to conventional therapy. ▪ Acute exacerbation of multiple sclerosis. ▪ Has numerous other uses when given IM or PO.

Unlabeled uses: High-dose therapy as an adjunct to traditional spinal cord injury management; to improve neurologic recovery in an acute (less than 8 hours old) spinal cord injury above L-2. ▪ Treatment of *Pneumocystis carinii* pneumonia as an adjunct to antibiotics. ▪ Treatment of severe lupus nephritis. ▪ Treatment of septic shock (controversial).

CONTRAINDICATIONS
Absolute contraindications in long-term therapy, except in life-threatening situations: Hypersensitivity to any product component, including sulfites; newborns; systemic fungal infections.

Relative contraindications: Active or latent peptic ulcer, active or healed tuberculosis, acute psychoses, chickenpox, congestive heart failure, diabetes mellitus, diverticulitis, fresh intestinal anastomoses, hypertension, myasthenia gravis, ocular herpes simplex, osteoporosis, pregnancy, psychotic tendencies, renal insufficiency, septic shock, thromboembolic tendencies, vaccinia.

PRECAUTIONS
Not the drug of choice to treat acute adrenocortical insufficiency. ■ To avoid relative adrenocortical insufficiency, do not stop therapy abruptly, taper off. Patient is observed carefully, especially under stress, for up to 2 years; exception is very short-term therapy. ■ Prophylactic antacids may prevent peptic ulcer complications.

Monitor: Monitor electrolytes. May cause sodium retention and potassium and calcium excretion. May cause hypertension secondary to fluid and electrolyte disturbances. ■ May mask signs of infection. ■ May increase insulin needs in diabetics. ■ Administer a single dose before 9AM to reduce suppression of individual's adrenocortical activity. ■ Periodic ophthalmic exams may be necessary with prolonged treatment. ■ Note Drug/lab interactions.

Patient education: Report edema, tarry stools, or weight gain promptly. Anorexia, diarrhea, dizziness, fatigue, low blood sugar, nausea, weakness, weight loss and vomiting; may indicate adrenal insufficiency after dose reduction or discontinuing therapy, report any of these symptoms. ■ May mask signs of infection and/or decrease resistance. ■ Diabetics may have an increased requirement for insulin or oral hypoglycemics. ■ Avoid immunizations with live vaccines. ■ Carry ID stating steroid dependent if receiving prolonged therapy.

Maternal/child: Pregnancy Category C: note Contraindications. ■ Use caution in lactation. Secretion into breast milk less than other glucocorticoids. ■ Observe newborn for hypoadrenalism if mother has received large doses. ■ Monitor growth and development of children receiving prolonged treatment.

Elderly: Reduced muscle mass and plasma volume may require a reduced dose. Monitor blood pressure, blood glucose, and electrolytes carefully. ■ Risk of hypertension and glucocorticoid-induced osteoporosis increased. ■ Avoid aluminum-based antacids (risk of Alzheimer's disease).

DRUG/LAB INTERACTIONS
Aminoglutethimide (Cytadren) and mitotane (Lysodren) suppress adrenal function of corticosteroids; monitor carefully if concurrent use is necessary. ■ Metabolism increased and effects reduced by hepatic enzyme inducing agents (e.g., alcohol, barbiturates [e.g., phenobarbital], hydantoins [e.g., phenytoin (Dilantin), rifampin (Rifadin)]); dose adjustments may be required when adding or deleting from drug profile. ■ Risk of hypokalemia increased with amphotericin B, or potassium-depleting diuretics (e.g., thiazides, furosemide, ethacrynic acid). Monitor potassium levels and cardiac function. Increased risk of digitalis (e.g., digoxin) toxicity secondary to hypokalemia. ■ May

also decrease effectiveness of potassium supplements; monitor serum potassium. ▪ Diuretics decrease sodium and fluid retention effects of corticosteroids; corticosteroids decrease sodium excretion and diuretic effects of diuretics. ▪ Use with cyclosporine in organ transplants is therapeutic but may increase cyclosporine toxicity; use caution. ▪ Clearance decreased and effects increased with estrogens, oral contraceptives, ketoconazole (Nizoral), and macrolide antibiotics (e.g., azithromycin [Zithromax], erythromycin, troleandomycin [TAO]). ▪ May interact with anticoagulants, nondepolarizing muscle relaxants (e.g., doxacurium [Nuromax]), or theophyllines; may inhibit or potentiate action, monitor carefully. ▪ Monitor patients receiving insulin or thyroid hormones carefully; dose adjustments of either or both agents may be required. ▪ Use with ritodrine (Yutopar) has caused pulmonary edema in the mother; discontinue both agents with onset of S/S of pulmonary edema. ▪ May antagonize effects of anticholinesterases (e.g., neostigmine), isoniazid, salicylates, and somatrem; dose adjustments may be required. ▪ Do not vaccinate with attenuatedvirus vaccines (e.g., smallpox) during therapy. ▪ Altered protein-binding capacity will impact effectiveness of this drug. ▪ Note Dose adjustments.

SIDE EFFECTS
Do occur but are usually reversible: Cushing's syndrome; electrolyte and calcium imbalance; euphoria; glycosuria; hyperglycemia; hypersensitivity reactions, including anaphylaxis; hypertension; increased intracranial pressure; menstrual irregularities; peptic ulcer perforation and hemorrhage; protein catabolism; spontaneous fractures; transitory burning or tingling; sweating, headache, or weakness; thromboembolism and many others.

ANTIDOTE
Notify the physician of any side effect. Will probably treat the side effect if necessary. Resuscitate as necessary for anaphylaxis and notify physician. Keep epinephrine immediately available.

METOCLOPRAMIDE HYDROCHLORIDE
GI stimulant
Antiemetic

✤**Maxeran, Octamide PFS, Reglan**
pH 3.0 to 6.5

USUAL DOSE
Radiologic examination of the small bowel: 10 mg (2 ml) as a single dose.
Antiemetic: 2 mg/kg of body weight 30 minutes before giving emetogenic cancer chemotherapy (e.g., cisplatin, dacarbazine). Repeat every 2 hours for 2 doses, then every 3 hours for 3 doses (note Dose adjustments). Another regimen calls for 3 mg/kg 30 minutes before and 90 minutes after emetogenic chemotherapy. Given in combination with dexamethasone and lorazepam or diphenhydramine.
Diabetic gastroparesis: 10 mg immediately before each meal and at bedtime. Use IV for up to 10 days if symptoms are severe. Continue treatment for 2 to 8 weeks orally.

PEDIATRIC DOSE

Radiologic examination of the small bowel: 6 to 14 years: 2.5 to 5 mg.

Under 6 years: 0.1 mg/kg of body weight.

Gastroesophageal reflux or GI dysmotility: 0.2 to 0.4 mg/kg/24 hours in equally divided doses every 6 hours. Maximum dose 0.5 mg/kg/24 hr.

Antiemetic: 1 to 2 mg/kg/dose every 2 to 6 hours. Premedicate with diphenhydramine (Benadryl).

DOSE ADJUSTMENTS

Dose may be reduced to 1 mg/kg if initial doses suppress vomiting. Initial doses may be reduced to 1 mg/kg for less emetogenic regimens. ■ Reduce initial dose by half in the elderly if indicated and in any patient with a creatinine clearance < 40 ml/min. Adjust subsequent doses as indicated. ■ Note Drug/lab interactions.

DILUTION

May be given undiluted if dose does not exceed 10 mg. For doses exceeding 10 mg dilute in at least 50 ml of D5W, NS, D5/½NS, R, or LR, and give as an infusion.

INCOMPATIBLE WITH

Allopurinol, ampicillin, calcium gluconate, cephalothin (Keflin), chloramphenicol (Chloromycetin), cisplatin (Platinol), erythromycin (Erythrocin), furosemide (Lasix), methotrexate (Folex), penicillin G potassium, sodium bicarbonate. Physically compatible with many drugs for up to 48 hours (see literature).

RATE OF ADMINISTRATION

Too-rapid IV injection will cause intense anxiety, restlessness, and then drowsiness.

Direct IV: 10 mg or fraction thereof over 2 minutes.

Infusion: Administer over a minimum of 15 minutes.

ACTIONS

A dopamine antagonist that blocks the stimulation of medullary chemoreceptor trigger zones by dopamine. Inhibits nausea and vomiting. Stimulates tone and amplitude of gastric contractions and increases peristalsis of the duodenum and jejunum increasing gastric emptying. It relaxes the lower esophageal sphincter, pyloric sphincter, and duodenal bulb. Does not stimulate gastric, biliary, or pancreatic secretions. Acts even if vagal innervation not present. Action negated by anticholinergic drugs. Onset of action occurs in 1 to 3 minutes and lasts 1 to 2 hours. Excreted in urine. Secreted in breast milk.

INDICATIONS AND USES

Facilitate small bowel intubation. ■ Stimulate gastric and intestinal emptying of barium to permit radiologic examination of the stomach and small intestine. ■ Prevention of nausea and vomiting associated with emetogenic cancer chemotherapy. ■ Prophylaxis of postoperative nausea and vomiting when nasograstric suction is not indicated. ■ Diabetic gastroparesis.

CONTRAINDICATIONS

Situations in which gastric motility is contraindicated, i.e., gastric hemorrhage, obstruction, or perforation; known hypersensitivity to metoclopramide; patients with epilepsy or patients taking drugs that may also cause extrapyramidal reactions; and pheochromocytoma.

PRECAUTIONS

May produce sedation, extrapyramidal symptoms or Parkinson-like symptoms, similar to those seen with phenothiazines. Use caution in patients with preexisting disease. ■ Tardive dyskinesia (syndrome of potentially irreversible involuntary movements of the tongue, face, mouth, jaw, trunk, or extremities) is usually related to duration of treatment and total cumulative dose. ■ A prolactin-elevating compound; may be carcinogenic. Risk with a single dose almost nonexistent. ■ May cause serious depression and suicidal tendencies; use extreme caution in any patient with a history of depression. ■ May cause methemoglobinemia in premature and full-term neonates at doses exceeding 0.5 mg/kg/24 hr.

Monitor: Monitor vital signs. ■ Pretreatment with diphenhydramine may reduce incidence of extrapyramidal symptoms with larger doses (e.g., antiemetic). ■ Note Precautions and Drug/lab interactions.

Patient education: Use caution performing any task that requires alertness, coordination, or physical dexterity; may produce dizziness and drowsiness. ■ If any involuntary movement of eyes, face, or limbs occurs, notify physician promptly. ■ Avoid alcohol or other CNS depressants (e.g., barbiturates, benzodiazepines [e.g., diazepam (Valium)]).

Maternal/child: Category B. Use caution in pregnancy and lactation. ■ Dose in breast milk is usually within acceptable range for infants. ■ May increase milk production (elevates prolactin). ■ Note Precautions and Side effects.

Elderly: May be more sensitive to therapeutic or adverse effects. ■ Long-term use increases risk of extrapyramidal effects (e.g., parkinsonism, tardive dyskinesia). ■ Note Dose adjustments.

DRUG/LAB INTERACTIONS

Antagonized by anticholinergic drugs (e.g., atropine) and narcotic analgesics (e.g., morphine). ■ Potentiates alcohol, cyclosporine, and succinylcholine. ■ Drugs ingested orally may be absorbed more slowly or more rapidly depending on the absorption site (e.g., inhibits cimetidine, digoxin). ■ Potentiates MAO inhibitors (e.g., selegiline [Eldepryl]); use extreme caution or do not use. ■ Insulin reactions may result from gastric stasis, making diabetic control difficult. Dose or timing of insulin may need adjustment. ■ Extrapyramidal effects may be potentiated with concomitant use of phenothiazines, butyrophenones, and thioxanthines (antipsychotic drugs). ■ Used concurrently, metoclopramide and levodopa have opposite effects on dopamine receptors; metoclopramide is inhibited and levodopa is potentiated.

SIDE EFFECTS

Usually mild, transient, and reversible after metoclopramide discontinued. Occur in 20% to 30% of patients. CNS and GI side effects occur in 81% and 43% respectively of patients treated for cisplatin-induced nausea.

Average dose: Allergic reactions can occur. Anxiety, bowel disturbances, confusion, convulsions, depression (severe, may have suicidal tendencies), dizziness, drowsiness, extrapyramidal reactions, fatigue, hallucinations, headache, insomnia, methemoglobinemia in neonates, nausea, restlessness, tardive dyskinesia. Numerous other side effects may occur.

Overdose: Disorientation, drowsiness, and extrapyramidal reactions.

ANTIDOTE

Notify physician of all side effects. Most will respond to a reduced dose or discontinuation of metoclopramide. Treat overdose or extrapyramidal reactions with diphenhydramine (Benadryl) or benzotropine (Cogentin). Symptoms should disappear within 24 hours. Treat methemoglobinemia with IV methylene blue. Resuscitate as necessary.

METOPROLOL TARTRATE

Beta-adrenergic blocking agent
Antiarrhythmic (Post MI)

Lopressor   pH 7.5

USUAL DOSE

5 mg as an IV bolus dose. Initiate as soon as the patient's hemodynamic condition has stabilized. Repeat at 2-minute intervals for 2 more doses; a total dose of 15 mg (JAMA recommends 5 to 10 mg at 5 minute intervals to a total dose of 15 mg). If IV doses are well tolerated, give 50 mg orally every 6 hours for 48 hours beginning 15 minutes after the last bolus. Follow with an oral maintenance dose of 100 mg twice daily. In patients who do not tolerate the full IV dose start 25 to 50 mg orally within 15 minutes of the last IV dose. Dosage based on degree of intolerance. May have to discontinue metoprolol. Best results achieved if administered within 2 to 4 hours of symptom onset or thrombolytic therapy.

DOSE ADJUSTMENTS

Note Drug/lab interactions. ▪ Not required in impaired renal function.

DILUTION

May be given undiluted.

INCOMPATIBLE WITH

Any other drug in a syringe because of specific use.

COMPATIBLE WITH

Y-site: Meperidine (Demerol), morphine.

RATE OF ADMINISTRATION

A single dose over 1 minute. Monitor ECG, heart rate, and blood pressure and discontinue metoprolol if adverse symptoms occur (bradycardia less than 45 beats/min, heart block greater than first degree, systolic blood pressure less than 100 mm Hg, or moderate to severe cardiac failure).

ACTIONS

Metoprolol is a cardioselective (B_1) adrenergic blocking agent. Its mechanism of action in patients with suspected or definite myocardial infarction is not known. It reduces the incidence of recurrent myocardial infarctions and reduces the size of the infarct and the incidence of fatal arrhythmias. Well distributed throughout the body, it acts within 1 to 2 minutes and lasts about 3 to 4 hours. Metabolized in the liver and throughout the body. Excreted as metabolites in the urine.

INDICATIONS AND USES

To reduce cardiac mortality in hemodynamically stable individuals with suspected or definite myocardial infarction. ▪ Antihypertensive in oral dosage form.

CONTRAINDICATIONS

Heart rate below 45 beats/min, second- or third-degree heart block, significant first-degree heart block (PR interval greater than 0.24 seconds), systolic blood pressure below 100 mm Hg, or moderate to severe cardiac failure.

PRECAUTIONS

Use caution in presence of heart failure controlled by digitalis. Both drugs slow AV conduction. ▪ May mask tachycardia occurring with hypoglycemia in diabetes and tachycardia of hyperthyroidism. ▪ Use with extreme caution in any patient with asthma, bronchospasm, or lung disease. ▪ Discontinuation of beta-blockers prior to OR is controversial (beta-blockade interferes with cardiac response to reflex stimuli); however, some authorities recommend administering throughout perioperative period. May cause arrhythmia, angina, MI, or death if stopped abruptly. ▪ May cause severe bradycardia in patients with Wolff-Parkinson-White syndrome.

Monitor: Continuous ECG, heart rate, and blood pressure monitoring is mandatory during administration of IV metoprolol. ▪ Note Drug/lab interactions.

Patient education: Report any breathing difficulty promptly.

Maternal/child: Category C: safety for use in pregnancy and lactation and in children not established. Has caused some problems during delivery resulting in neonatal bradycardia and low APGAR scores. See literature for guidelines.

Elderly: Use with caution in age-related peripheral vascular disease; risk of hypothermia increased. ▪ May exacerbate mental impairment.

DRUG/LAB INTERACTIONS

Concurrent use with calcium channel blockers (e.g., diltiazem, verapamil) may potentiate both drugs and result in severe depression of myocardium and AV conduction. ▪ Concurrent use with antihypertensive agents may result in excessive hypotension. Dose adjustment may be required. ▪ Effects decreased by cocaine; may result in hypertension, severe bradycardia, or heart block. ▪ Concurrent use within 14 days of MAO inhibitors (selegiline [Eldepryl]) may cause severe hypertension. ▪ Use with sympathomimetic agents (e.g., epinephrine, norepinephrine, phenylephrine) or xanthines (e.g., aminophylline) may negate therapeutic effects of both drugs. ▪ Effects of beta-adrenergic blocking agents may be decreased by ampicillin, antiinflammatory agents, barbiturates, calcium salts, rifampin, salicylates and others. ▪ General anesthetics, cimetidine (Tagamet), furosemide, phenothiazines (e.g., promethazine [Phenergan]), phenytoin (Dilantin), and quinolone antibiotics (e.g., ciprofloxacin) may increase myocardial depressant effects and hypotension. ▪ Potentiates effects of oral antidiabetics, catecholamine-depleting drugs (e.g., reserpine), insulin, lidocaine, narcotics, and skeletal muscle relaxants; monitor carefully, dose adjustment may be required. ▪ Concurrent use with clonidine may precipitate acute hypertension if one or both agents are stopped abruptly. Withdraw metoprolol first. ▪ Effects decreased when hypothyroid patient is converted to a euthyroid state; adjust dose as indicated. ▪ Used concurrently with digitalis or alpha-adrenergic blockers (e.g., phentolamine [Regitine]) as indicated. Use caution; both digitalis and metoprolol slow AV conduction.

SIDE EFFECTS

Bradyarrhythmias, bronchospasm, cardiac failure, confusion, dizziness, dyspnea, first-degree heart block, headache, hypotension, nightmares, pruritus, rash, respiratory distress, second- or third-degree heart block, syncopal attacks, tiredness, vertigo, visual disturbances.

ANTIDOTE

For any side effect, discontinue drug and notify physician immediately. Patients with myocardial infarction may be more hemodynamically unstable; treat with caution. Use atropine for bradycardia; use isoproterenol with caution if atropine not effective. Glucagon 5 to 10 mg IV may be effective if atropine and isoproterenol are not (investigational use). Transvenous cardiac pacing may be needed. Treat hypotension with IV fluids if indicated or vasopressors (dopamine [Intropin] or norepinephrine [Levarterenol]); treat cause of hypotension (e.g., bradycardia). Use all vasopressors with extreme caution; severe hypotension can result. Use digitalis and diuretics at first sign of cardiac failure; dobutamine, isoproterenol, or glucagon may be required. Use aminophylline or isoproterenol (with extreme care) for bronchospasm, glucagon or IV glucose for hypoglycemia. Treat other side effects symptomatically; resuscitate as necessary.

METRONIDAZOLE HYDROCHLORIDE

Antibacterial
Antiprotozoal

**Flagyl IV, Flagyl IV RTU, Metro IV,
Metronidazole Redi-infusion, Metryl IV**

pH 5.0 to 7.0

USUAL DOSE

Anaerobic infections: Begin with an initial loading dose of 15 mg/kg of body weight. Follow with 7.5 mg/kg in 6 hours and every 6 hours thereafter for 7 to 10 days or longer if indicated. Do not exceed 4 Gm in 24 hours.

Complicated intra-adbominal infections: 500 mg every 6 hours given in combination with ciprofloxacin, 400 mg every 12 hours or cefepine 2 Gm every 12 hours.

Prevent postoperative infection in contaminated or potentially contaminated colorectal surgery: 15 mg/kg infused over 30 to 60 minutes and completed 1 hour before surgery. Follow with 7.5 mg/kg in 6 hours and in 12 hours. If *Bacteroides fragilis* is the suspected or confirmed organism, an alternate regimen is to give a 1,500 mg dose at the beginning of surgery to ensure adequate metronidazole levels.

PEDIATRIC DOSE

Safety for use in infants and children not established, but is used for anaerobic infections.

Anaerobic infections: Children and infants over 7 days of age: An initial loading dose of 15 mg/kg. Follow with 7.5 mg/kg every 6 hours. Another source suggests every 8 hours.

Preterm infants: An initial loading dose of 15 mg/kg. 48 hours after loading dose begin 7.5 mg/kg every 12 hours.

Term infants: Same as preterm except begin maintenance dose (7.5 mg/kg) 24 hours after loading dose.

DOSE ADJUSTMENTS

Reduce dose in hepatic disease and in the elderly. Increase intervals in neonates (see Pediatric dose). ▪ Dose adjustment not indicated in anuric patients; accumulated metabolites readily removed by dialysis.

DILUTION

All solutions are prediluted and ready to use (5 mg/ml) except Flagyl IV. Do not use plastic containers in series connections. Risk of air embolism is present. Avoid all contact with aluminum in needles and syringes in all situations. Color change will occur. Flagyl IV requires a specific dilution process; initially add 4.4 ml sterile water or NS for injection (100 mg/ml). Solution must be clear. Will be yellow to yellow-green in color with a pH of 0.5 to 2.0. Must be further diluted to at least 8 mg/ml with NS, D5W, or LR and be neutralized before infusion with 5 mEq of sodium bicarbonate per 500 mg. Mix thoroughly. CO_2 gas will be generated and may require venting.

Storage: Store at room temperature before and after dilution. Discard diluted and neutralized solutions in 24 hours. Do not refrigerate; a precipitate will result. Protect from light when storing.

INCOMPATIBLE WITH

Administer separately per manufacturer's recommendation. Discontinue primary infusion during administration. Aztreonam (Azactam), cefamandole (Mandol), dopamine (Intropin), filgrastim (Neupogen).

RATE OF ADMINISTRATION

Must be given as a slow IV infusion, each single dose over 1 hour. Discontinue primary IV during administration. May be given as a continuous infusion. Rate should be ordered by physician.

ACTIONS

A bactericidal agent with cytotoxic effects, active against specific anaerobic bacteria and protozoa. Widely distributed in therapeutic levels to all body fluids (including abscesses). Levels are directly proportional to dose given. Onset of action is prompt and lasts about 8 hours. Crosses placental and blood-brain barriers. Excreted in urine, some in feces. Secreted in breast milk.

INDICATIONS AND USES

Treatment of serious intraabdominal, skin and skin structure, gynecologic, bone and joint, CNS, and lower respiratory tract infections; bacterial septicemia; and endocarditis caused by susceptible anaerobic bacteria. ■ To provide anaerobic activity when used in combination with ciprofloxacin for the treatment of complicated intra-abdominal infections. ■ Perioperative prophylaxis to reduce infection rates in contaminated or potentially contaminated colorectal surgery. ■ Given orally for antibiotic-related pseudomembranous colitis, amebiasis, and other indications.

Investigational use: As a radiosensitizer to make resistant tumors more susceptible to radiation therapy.

CONTRAINDICATIONS

Hypersensitivity to metronidazole or nitroimidazole derivatives; first trimester of pregnancy.

PRECAUTIONS

A mixed (anaerobic/aerobic) infection will require use of additional appropriate antibiotics. ■ Sensitivity studies indicated to determine susceptibility of the causative organism to metronidazole. ■ Avoid prolonged use of the drug; superinfection caused by overgrowth of nonsusceptible organisms may result. ■ Symptoms of candidiasis may be exacerbated and require treatment. ■ Use caution in patients predisposed to edema and/or taking corticosteroids, in patients with impaired cardiac function (contains 27 to 28 mEq sodium/Gm), CNS disease, or a history of blood dyscrasias. ■ Carcinogenic in rodents; use only when necessary.

Monitor: Rotate IV site frequently to avoid thrombophlebitis. Avoid extravasation. ■ Obtain total and differential leukocyte counts before and after therapy. ■ Monitor serum levels (suggested) and observe for toxicity in patients with hepatic disease receiving reduced doses and in the elderly. ■ Observe patients receiving high doses for extended periods; seizures and peripheral neuropathies may occur; neuropathy may not be reversible. ■ Transfer to oral dosing as soon as practical. ■ Note Drug/lab interactions.

Patient education: Avoid alcohol, alcohol-containing preparations, and disulfiram; toxic reactions will occur.

Maternal/child: Safety for use in pregnancy, lactation, children, and neonates not established. Half-life markedly extended in newborns; adjust intervals (see Pediatric dose). ▪ Note Contraindications.

Elderly: Pharmacokinetics altered in the elderly; monitor serum levels if possible and adjust dose accordingly.

DRUG/LAB INTERACTIONS

Avoid alcohol, alcohol-containing preparations, and disulfiram; toxic reactions will occur. ▪ Barbiturates (e.g., phenobarbital) may inhibit therapeutic action. ▪ May be antagonized by bacteriostatic antibiotics (e.g., chloramphenicol, erythromycin, and tetracyclines); bactericidal action may be negated. ▪ Cimetidine (Tagamet) may increase metronidazole serum levels. ▪ Potentiates hydantoins (e.g., phenytoin [Dilantin]). ▪ Potentiates oral anticoagulants (e.g., warfarin). ▪ May increase lithium levels and cause toxicity. ▪ May cause serious cardiotoxicity with astemizole (Hismanal) or terfenadine; not recommended. ▪ May cause decreased AST (SGOT) levels.

SIDE EFFECTS

Abdominal cramping, anorexia, constipation, cystitis, darkened deep red urine, decreased libido, diarrhea, dizziness, dryness of the mouth, vagina, or vulva; dysuria, epigastric distress, fever, fleeting joint pain, flushing, furry tongue, glossitis, headache, incontinence, metallic taste (expected), nasal congestion, nausea, neutropenia (reversible), painful coitus, pelvic pressure, peripheral neuropathy, polyuria, proctitis, pruritus, pseudomembranous colitis, rash, seizures, stomatitis, syncope, thrombocytopenia (reversible), thrombophlebitis, T-wave flattening, urticaria, vomiting.

ANTIDOTE

Notify physician of all side effects. Treatment will be symptomatic and supportive. Discontinue metronidazole with onset of seizures or signs of peripheral neuropathy (e.g., numbness or paresthesia of an extremity); benefit/risk of therapy must be reconsidered with onset of convulsions or peripheral neuropathy. Rapidly removed by hemodialysis. Treat anaphylaxis and resuscitate as necessary.

MIDAZOLAM HYDROCHLORIDE

Benzodiazepine
Sedative-hypnotic
Anesthetic adjunct
Amnestic

Versed

pH 3.0

USUAL DOSE

Sedation, anxiolysis (anti-anxiety), and/or amnesia for short diagnostic, endoscopic, and therapeutic procedures:

Healthy adults less than 60 years of age: 1 to 2.5 mg immediately before the procedure.

Begin with 1 mg and titrate slowly up to slurred speech or 2.5 mg. Some patients respond adequately to 1 mg. If additional medication is needed wait a full 2 minutes, then titrate additional dosage slowly in small increments (usually no more than 1 mg). Wait a full 2 minutes between each increment. A total dose exceeding 5 mg is rarely necessary. Reduce dose by 30% in the presence of narcotic premedication or other CNS depressants. 25% of the sedating dose can be used for maintenance only when clearly indicated by clinical evaluation.

Patients over 60 years of age or debilitated or chronically ill patients: 1 to 1.5 mg. Begin with 1 mg and titrate slowly up to slurred speech or 1.5 mg. May respond adequately to 1 mg. If additional medication is needed wait a full 2 minutes, then titrate additional dosage in small increments (no more than 1 mg). Wait a full 2 minutes between each increment. A total dose exceeding 3.5 mg is rarely necessary. Reduce dose by 50% in the presence of narcotic premedication or other CNS depressants. 25% of the sedating dose can be used for maintenance only when clearly indicated by clinical evaluation.

Induction of anesthesia before administration of other anesthetic agents and/or maintenance of anesthesia as a component of balanced anesthesia during surgical procedures:

In all patients (unpremedicated and premedicated), allow 2 minutes from initial dose to reach peak effect. If necessary, complete induction with 25% of initial dose or use inhalational anesthesia (e.g., halothane). Doses of any agents used after induction of anesthesia with midazolam may need to be reduced to as little as 25% of the usual initial dose. 25% of the induction dose can be repeated when indicated by lightening of anesthesia.

Unpremedicated patients under 55 years of age: 0.3 to 0.35 mg/kg as an initial dose. A total dose of up to 0.6 mkg/kg has been required; recovery may be prolonged.

Unpremedicated patients over 55 years of age: 0.3 mg/kg as an initial dose.

Unpremedicated debilitated patients or those with severe systemic disease: 0.2 to 0.25 mg/kg as an initial dose. As little as 0.15 mg/kg may be adequate.

Patients premedicated with sedatives or narcotics under 55 years of age: 0.25 mg/kg as an initial dose may be adequate. Range is 0.15 to 0.35 mg/kg of body weight.

Patients premedicated with sedatives or narcotics over 55 years of age (Good risk [ASAI & II]): 0.2 mg/kg as an initial dose may be adequate.

Patients premedicated with sedatives or narcotics who are debilitated or those with severe systemic disease: 0.15 mg/kg as an initial dose may be adequate. Premedication usually includes narcotics (e.g., fentanyl 1.5 to 2 mcg/kg IV 5 minutes before induction, or morphine [up to 0.15 mg/kg IM] or meperidine [up to 1 mg/kg IM]) 1 hour before induction with midazolam. Sedative premedication usually includes hydroxyzine pamoate (Vistaril). 100 mg PO or sodium seconal 200 mg PO 1 hour before induction.

Sedation for anesthesia or treatment in a critical care setting for intubated and mechanically ventilated patients:

Continuous infusion (concentration 0.5 mg/ml). Begin with a *loading dose* of 0.01 to 0.05 mg/kg (0.5 to 4 mg for a typical adult) to rapidly initiate sedation. Infuse over several minutes. May be repeated at 10- to 15- minute intervals until adequate sedation achieved.

For maintenance of sedation: An initial infusion rate of 0.02 to 0.1 mg/kg/hr (1 to 7 mg/hr) may be used. Upper-end doses may be required, but use the lowest recommended doses in patients with residual effects from anesthetic drugs or in those concurrently receiving other sedatives or opiods. Initial infusion rate may be titrated up or down by 25% to 50% to maintain desired level of sedation. Decrease by 10% to 25% every few hours to find the minimum effective infusion rate. The lowest rate that produces the desired level of sedation is recommended. Agitation, hypertension, or tachycardia in response to stimulation in adequately sedated patients may indicate need for an opiod analgesic. Reduced rate of midazolam infusion may be indicated with the addition of an opioid analgesic.

PEDIATRIC DOSE

In all situations dose is based on lean body weight in obese pediatric patients.

Sedation, anxiolysis (antianxiety), and/or amnesia before and during procedures or before anesthesia:

All increments of midazolam are on a mg/kg basis. Total dose will depend on patient response, type and duration of the procedure, and the type and dose of concomitant medications. Titrate dose of midazolam and other concomitant medications slowly to the desired clinical effect. With concomitant medications, dose of midazolam should be reduced (usually by 25% to 30%)). Before beginning a procedure or repeating a dose, wait a full 2 to 3 minutes to fully evaluate the sedative effect. If further sedation is necessary, continue to titrate with small increments at 2- to 3-minute intervals until desired level of sedation achieved. Prolonged sedation and risk of hypoventilation may be associated with higher-end doses.

Non-intubated infants less than 6 months of age: Uncertain when patient transfers from neonatal physiology to pediatric physiology; manufacturer has no specific dosing recommendations. Titrate with very small increments to clinical effect and monitor very carefully for airway obstruction and hypoventilation.

Children 6 months to 5 years of age: Begin with an initial dose of 0.05 to 0.1 mg/kg. Up to 0.6 mg/kg may be required, but a total dose of 6 mg is usually not exceeded.

Children 6 to 12 years of age: Begin with an initial dose of 0.025 to 0.05 mg/kg. Up to 0.4 mg/kg may be required, but a total dose of 10 mg is usually not exceeded.

Children 12 to 16 years of age: See adult dose. May require higher than recommended adult doses, but total dose usually does not exceed 10 mg.

Sedation, anxiolysis, amnesia:

Intubated children in critical care settings: Begin with a loading dose of 0.05 to 0.2 mg/kg. May be allowed to breathe on own through intubation tube but assisted ventilation recommended in children receiving other CNS depressants. In hemodynamically compromised children titrate the loading dose in small increments and monitor for hypotension, respiratory rate, and oxygen saturation. May be followed by a continuous IV infusion at 0.06 to 0.12 mg/kg/hr (1 to 2 mcg/kg/min). Increase or decrease infusion in 25% increments or use supplemental IV injection to maintain desired effect.

Sedation of intubated neonates in critical care settings:

Neonates <32 weeks: A continuous infusion at a rate of 0.03 mg/kg/hr (0.5 mcg/kg/min).

Neonates >32 weeks: A continuous infusion at a rate of 0.06 mg/kg/hr (1 mcg/kg/min).

Do not use loading doses in neonates. Infusion may be run more rapidly for the first several hours to establish therapeutic plasma levels. Reassess rate carefully and frequently to use the lowest possible effective dose and reduce the potential for drug accumulation. Midazolam contains benzyl alcohol and must be used with extreme caution in neonates.

DOSE ADJUSTMENTS

Reduce dose by 30% to 50%, depending on age, in the presence of narcotic premedication or other CNS depressants (See Usual dose) ▪ Reduce dose in congestive heart failure, chronic obstructive pulmonary disease, chronic renal failure, the debilitated, and patients over 55 years of age. Half-life is extended and depressant effects will be potentiated (see Usual dose). ▪ Dose based on lean body weight in obese pediatric patients. ▪ Note Drug/lab interactions.

DILUTION

Read label carefully and confirm mg dose. Available in two strengths, 1 mg/ml and 5 mg/ml.

IV injection: May be diluted with D5W or NS. Dilute in a sufficient amount to permit slow titration, (i.e., 1 mg in 4 ml or 5 mg in 20 ml [0.25 mg/m]). Maximum concentration after dilution should not exceed 0.5 mg/ml.

Infusion: Dilute in either of the above solutions to a maximum concentration of 0.5 mg/ml. 5 ml of a 1 mg/ml (5 mg) in 5 ml of diluent yields 0.5 mg/ml. 5 ml of a 5 mg/ml (25 mg) in 45 ml diluent is usually a 24-hour supply and also yields 0.5 mg/ml. Use a controlled infusion device or at the very least a metriset (60 gtt/ml) to facilitate titration and control flow to prevent overdose.

INCOMPATIBLE WITH

Albumin, ampicillin (Ampicin), bumetanide (Bumex), ceftazidime (Ceptaz), cefuroxime (Zinacef), dexamethasone (Decadron), dimenhydrinate (Dramamine), dobutamine (Dobutrex), foscarnet (Foscavir), furosemide (Lasix), hydrocortisone sodium succinate (Solu-Cortef), imipenem-cilastatin (Primaxin), nafcillin (Unipen), pentobarbital (Nembutal), perphenazine (Trilafon), prochlorperazine (Compazine), ranitidine (Zantac), sodium bicarbonate, sulfamethoxazole-trimethoprim (Bactrim).

RATE OF ADMINISTRATION

IV injection: Sedation: Any single increment of a total dose titrated slowly over at least 2 minutes. Stop at any point that the speech becomes slurred.

Induction of anesthesia: Any single increment of a total dose over 20 to 30 seconds. Rapid injection in any situation may cause respiratory depression or apnea.

Infusion: See Usual dose. The American Academy of Critical Care recommends limiting the use of midazolam in the critical care setting to 24 hours because its metabolites accumulate in peripheral tissue, especially with long-term infusion.

Pediatric rate: Any single increment of a total dose over a minimum of 2 to 3 minutes. Rapid injection or infusion may cause severe hypotension or seizures in infants and neonates; incidence increased with concomitant fentanyl. Note comments under infusion above.

ACTIONS

A short-acting benzodiazepine CNS depressant 3 to 4 times as potent as diazepam. Depressant effects are dependent on dose, route of administration, and the presence or absence of other premedications. Can depress the ventilatory response to CO_2 stimulation. Mechanics of respiration are not adversely affected with usual doses. Mean arterial pressure, cardiac output, stroke volume and systemic vascular resistance may be slightly decreased. May cause heart rates of less than 65/min to rise and more than 85/min to fall. Produces sleepiness and relief of apprehension, and diminishes patient recall very effectively. Onset of action occurs within 3 to 5 minutes. Half-life ranges from 1.8 to 6.4 hours, shorter than that of diazepam (Valium). Metabolized in the liver by cytochrome P_{450} mediation and excreted as metabolites in urine. Crosses the placental barrier. Secreted in breast milk.

INDICATIONS AND USES

To produce sedation, relieve anxiety, and impair memory of perioperative events. ▪ May be used with or without narcotic sedation for conscious sedation before short diagnostic, endoscopic, or therapeutic procedures (e.g., bronchoscopy, gastroscopy, cystoscopy, coronary angiography, cardiac catheterization). ▪ Induction of anesthesia before administration of other anesthetic agents. ▪ As a component in the induction and maintenance of balanced anesthesia in short surgical procedures. ▪ Continuous infusions may be used in intubated and mechanically ventilated patients for sedation as a component of anesthesia or during treatment in a critical care setting.

CONTRAINDICATIONS

Acute narrow-angle glaucoma, known hypersensitivity to midazolam, open-angle glaucoma unless receiving appropriate treatment. Not recommended in pregnancy, childbirth, lactation, shock, coma, acute alcohol intoxication with depression of vital signs.

PRECAUTIONS

Should be used only in a hospital or ambulatory care setting with continuous monitoring of respiratory and cardiac function (e.g., pulse oximetry). Resuscitative drugs (including flumazenil [Romazicon]) and age- and size-appropriate equipment for bag/valve/mask ventilation and intubation must be immediately available. Personnel must be skilled in airway management. ▪ A dedicated individual with no other responsibilities should monitor deeply sedated infants and children throughout any procedure. ▪ A topical anesthetic agent should be used with midazolam during perioral endoscopy, and premedication with a narcotic is recommended in bronchoscopy since increased cough reflex and laryngospasm frequently occur. Premedication with a narcotic is also recommended with balanced anesthesia. ▪ For IV/IM use only. Contains benzyl alcohol. Do not use for intrathecal or epidural administration. ▪ Use caution in neonates. At recommended doses benzyl alcohol is not expected to be toxic, but excessive benzyl alcohol may result in hypotension, metabolic acidosis, and increased incidence of kernicterus, especially in small preterm infants. ▪ Use extreme caution in the elderly, in patients with chronic disease states, decreased pulmonary reserve, and in those with uncompensated acute illness (e.g., severe fluid or electrolyte disturbances); may have increased risks of hypoventilation, airway obstruction, or apnea. Peak effect may take longer. ▪ Note Pediatric dose for additional precautions with infants and children. ▪ Does not protect against increased intracranial pressure or circulatory changes noted with succinylcholine or pancuronium or associated with intubation under light general anesthesia. ▪ Some clinicians prefer midazolam over diazepam because of effectiveness, minimum pain if any on injection, and miscibility with many drugs and solutions.

Monitor: Obtain a careful presedation history (e.g., medical conditions, concomitant meds), and complete a physical exam. Check for airway abnormalities. ▪ Monitor respiratory and cardiac function (e.g., BP, HR, pulse oximetry) continuously. Has caused apnea and cardiac arrest. Monitoring of ECG desirable. Maintain a patent airway and support adequate ventilation. Record assessments using standard assessment charts for scoring, especially in pediatric patients. ▪ Extravasation or arterial administration hazardous. ▪ Bed rest required for a minimum of 3 hours after IV injection. ▪ Note Drug/lab interactions.

Patient education: Do not drive or operate hazardous machinery until the day after surgery or longer. All effects must have subsided. Avoid use of alcohol or other CNS depressants (e.g., antihistamines, barbiturates) for 24 hours after last dose. ▪ May impair memory; request written postop instructions. ▪ Consider birth control options.

Maternal/child: Pregnancy Category D: avoid pregnancy. ▪ Not recommended during pregnancy, labor and delivery, or lactation. ▪ Elimination rate is faster in infants and children. ▪ Neonate has reduced or immature organ function. May be susceptible to profound and/or prolonged respiratory effects. ▪ Note Precautions and Monitor.

Elderly: Note Usual dose and Dose adjustments. Start with a small dose and increase gradually based on response. ▪ More sensitive to therapeutic and adverse effects (e.g., oversedation, ataxia, dizziness). IV injection may be more likely to cause apnea, bradycardia, hypotension, and cardiac arrest. ▪ Note Precautions and Drug/lab interactions.

DRUG/LAB INTERACTIONS

Concurrent use with other CNS depressants (e.g., alcohol, antihistamines, barbiturates, inhalation anesthetics [e.g., halothane], MAO inhibitors [e.g., selegiline (Eldepryl)], narcotics [e.g., morphine, meperidine (Demerol), fentanyl], phenothiazines [e.g., prochlorperazine (Compazine)], thiopental, and tricyclic antidepressants [e.g., imipramine (Tofranil-PM)]) may result in additive effects for up to 48 hours. May produce apnea or prolonged effect, depress ventilatory response to CO_2, or cause hypotension. Reduce doses of midazolam. ▪ Agents that inhibit cytochrome P_{450} activity (e.g., azole antifungals [e.g., ketonconazole (Nizoral), miconazole (Monistat)], cimetidine [Tagamet], diltiazem [Cardizem], verapamil [Isoptin], macrolide antibiotics [e.g., erythromycin], omeprazole [Prilosec], and ranitidine [Zantac]) decrease clearance and increase effects of midazolam resulting in prolonged sedation. ▪ Reduce doses of inhalation anesthetics (e.g., halothane) and/or thiopental when used with midazolam. ▪ Indinavir (Crixivan), nelfinavir (Viracepf), and ritonavir (Norvir) may increase risk of prolonged sedation and respiratory depression. Concurrent use not recommended. Benzodiazepines metabolized by alternate routes may be safer (e.g., lorazepam [Ativan], oxazepam [Serax], temazepam [Restoril]). ▪ May increase serum concentrations of digoxin and phenytoin (Dilantin); monitor digoxin and phenytoin serum levels. ▪ Benzodiazepines decrease clearance and increase toxicity of zidovudine (AZT). ▪ May increase clearance and decrease effectiveness of levodopa. ▪ Hypotensive effects of benzodiazepines may be increased by any agent that induces hypotension (e.g., antihypertensives, bretylium, CNS depressants, diuretics, lidocaine, paclitaxel). Monitor blood pressure during and after use. ▪ Use with rifampin (Rifadin) increases clearance and reduces effects of benzodiazepines. ▪ Theophyllines (Aminophylline) antagonize sedative effects of benzodiazepines. ▪ Clozapine (Leponix) has caused respiratory distress or cardiac arrest in a few patients; use concurrently with extreme caution. ▪ Smoking increases metabolism and clearance of midazolam, decreasing plasma levels and sedative effects.

SIDE EFFECTS

In adults and children, the incidence of cardiorespiratory events is higher in patients undergoing procedures where they are not intubated or are receiving other CNS depressing agents (e.g., fentanyl). Serious cardiorespiratory events may include airway obstruction, apnea, hypotension, oxygen desaturation, respiratory arrest, and/or cardiac arrhythmias or arrest. Inadequate or excessive dosing may cause agitation, combativeness, involuntary movements (e.g., clonic, tonic, muscle tremor), and hyperactivity; may be caused by cerebral hypoxia or be true parodoxical reactions. Other common reactions are coughing, drowsiness, fluctuation in vital signs, headache, hiccups, nausea and vomiting, nystagmus (especially in children), induration, redness, or phlebitis at injection site. Capable of numerous other side effects. Has caused death and hypoxic encephalopathy. Withdrawal may be seen in patients receiving an infusion for extended periods of time.

Overdose: Sedation, somnolence, confusion, impaired coordination, diminished reflexes, coma, and untoward effect on vital signs.

ANTIDOTE

Notify the physician of all side effects. Reduction of dosage may be required or will be treated symptomatically. Discontinue the drug for major side effects or paradoxical reactions. Flumazenil (Romazicon) will reverse all sedative effects of benzodiazepines. A patent airway, artificial ventilation, oxygen therapy and other symptomatic treatment must be instituted promptly. May cause emesis; observe closely. Treat allergic reaction and resuscitate as necessary.

MILRINONE LACTATE

Corotrope, Primacor

Inotropic agent

pH 3.2 to 4.0

USUAL DOSE

50 mcg/kg (0.05 mg/kg) of body weight as the initial loading dose (3.5 mg [3.5 ml] for a 70 kg person).

	Loading dose (ml) using 1 mg/ml Concentration									
	Patient body weight (kg)									
kg	30	40	50	60	70	80	90	100	110	120
ml	1.5	2	2.5	3	3.5	4	4.5	5	5.5	6

Follow with a maintenance infusion of 0.5 mcg/kg/min (35 mcg/min for a 70 kg person). Titrate the infusion dose between 0.375 mcg/kg/min to 0.75 mcg/kg/min (26 mcg/min to 52 mcg/min for a 70 kg person) based on hemodynamic effect. Do not exceed a total dose of 1.13 mg/kg/24 hr, including boluses. Duration of infusion usually does not exceed 48 to 72 hours but has been used for up to 5 days.

DOSE ADJUSTMENTS

Reduced dose required in impaired renal function based on creatinine clearance (see literature).

DILUTION

Loading dose: May be given undiluted, or each 1 mg (1 ml) may be diluted in 1 ml NS or 0.45%S for injection.

Infusion: Dilute with NS, 0.45%S, or D5W. Available prediluted as 200 mcg/ml in 100 ml D5W. Amount of diluent may be increased or decreased based on patient fluid requirements.

Desired infusion Concentration (mcg/ml)	PRIMACOR 1 mg/ml (ml)	Diluent (ml)	Total volume (ml)
100	10	90	100
100	20	180	200
150	10	56.7	66.7
150	20	113	133
200	10	40	50
200	20	80	100

May be given through Y-tube or three-way stopcock of IV infusion set but should never come in contact with furosemide (Lasix) or bumetanide (Bumex). Use only freshly prepared solutions.

Storage: Store at room temperature before dilution; avoid freezing.

INCOMPATIBLE WITH

Bumetanide (Bumex), furosemide (Lasix), procainamide (Pronestyl). Should not be mixed with other drugs until further compatibility data are available.

RATE OF ADMINISTRATION

Loading dose: A single dose over 10 minutes.

Infusion: Use a microdrip (60 gtt/ml) or an infusion pump to deliver milrinone in recommended doses. Manufacturer's dose chart below defines selected dose in mcg/kg/min in infusion rate of ml/hr. Adjust as indicated by physician's orders and progress in patient's condition. Reduce rate or stop infusion for excessive drop in blood pressure.

PRIMACOR infusion rate (ml/hr) using 100 mcg/ml concentration										
Maintenance dose	Patient body weight (kg)									
(mcg/kg/min)	30	40	50	60	70	80	90	100	110	120
0.375	6.8	9	11.3	13.5	15.8	18	20.3	22.5	24.8	27
0.4	7.2	9.6	12	14.4	16.8	19.2	21.6	24	26.4	28.8
0.5	9	12	15	18	21	24	27	30	33	36
0.6	10.8	14.4	18	21.6	25.2	28.8	32.4	36	39.6	43.2
0.7	12.6	16.8	21	25.2	29.4	33.6	37.8	42	46.2	50.4
0.75	13.5	18	22.5	27	31.5	36	40.5	45	49.5	54

PRIMACOR infusion rate (ml/hr) using 150 mcg/ml concentration										
Maintenance dose	Patient body weight (kg)									
(mcg/kg/min)	30	40	50	60	70	80	90	100	110	120
0.375	4.5	6	7.5	9	10.5	12	13.5	15	16.5	18
0.4	4.8	6.4	8	9.6	11.2	12.8	14.4	16	17.6	19.2
0.5	6	8	10	12	14	16	18	20	22	24
0.6	7.2	9.6	12	14.4	16.8	19.2	21.6	24	26.4	28.8
0.7	8.4	11.2	14	16.8	19.6	22.4	25.2	28	30.8	33.6
0.75	9	12	15	18	21	24	27	30	33	36

PRIMACOR infusion rate (ml/hr) using 200 mcg/ml concentration										
Maintenance dose	Patient body weight (kg)									
(mcg/kg/min)	30	40	50	60	70	80	90	100	110	120
0.375	3.4	4.5	5.6	6.8	7.9	9	10.1	11.3	12.4	13.5
0.4	3.6	4.8	6	7.2	8.4	9.6	10.8	12	13.2	14.4
0.5	4.5	6	7.5	9	10.5	12	13.5	15	16.5	18
0.6	5.4	7.2	9	10.8	12.6	14.4	16.2	18	19.8	21.6
0.7	6.3	8.4	10.5	12.6	14.7	16.8	18.9	21	23.1	25.2
0.75	6.8	9	11.3	13.5	15.8	18	20.3	22.5	24.8	27

ACTIONS

A new class of cardiac inotropic agent different in chemical structure and mode of action from digitalis glycosides and catecholemines. Similar to amrinone (Inocor), with fewer side effects. With a loading dose, peak effect occurs within 10 minutes. Continuous administration is required to maintain serum levels. It has positive inotropic action with vasodilator activity. Reduces afterload and preload by direct relaxant effect on vascular smooth muscle. Produces slight enhancement of AV node conduction. Cardiac output is improved without significant increases in heart rate or myocardial oxygen consumption or changes in arteriovenous oxygen difference. Pulmonary capillary wedge pressure, total peripheral resistance, diastolic blood pressure, and mean arterial pressure are decreased. Heart rate generally remains the same. Primary route of excretion is in urine.

INDICATIONS AND USES

Short-term management of congestive heart failure.

CONTRAINDICATIONS

Severe aortic or pulmonary valvular disease in lieu of surgical relief of the obstruction. Hypersensitivity to milrinone or amrinone (Inocor).

PRECAUTIONS

Use caution in impaired renal function; serum levels may increase considerably. ▪ May be given to digitalized patients without causing signs of digitalis toxicity; correct hypokalemia with potassium supplements. ▪ May increase ventricular response in atrial flutter/fibrillation. Consider pretreatment with digitalis. ▪ Additional fluids and electrolytes may be required to facilitate appropriate response in patients who have been vigorously diuresed and may have insufficient cardiac filling pressure. Use caution. ▪ Safety for use in the acute phase of myocardial infarction not established. ▪ May aggravate outflow tract obstruction in hypertrophic subaortic stenosis or severe obstructive aortic or pulmonary valvular disease (see Contraindications).

Monitor: Monitoring of platelets before therapy and at intervals is recommended. ▪ Observe patient continuously; monitoring of ECG, BP, urine output, renal function, fluid and electrolyte changes (especially potassium), and body weight are recommended. ▪ Monitoring of cardiac index, pulmonary capillary wedge pressure, central venous pressure, and plasma concentration is very useful. ▪ Observe for orthopnea, dyspnea, and fatigue. ▪ Reduce rate or stop infusion for excessive drop in blood pressure. ▪ As cardiac output and diuresis improves, a reduction in diuretic dose may be indicated. ▪ Possible risk of arrhythmias. Risk further increased with excessive diuresis and/or hypokalemia. Replace potassium as indicated.

Maternal/child: Pregnancy Category C: safety for use during pregnancy, lactation, and in children not established. Use during pregnancy only if potential benefit justifies potential risk.

Elderly: Consider impaired renal function; may require a reduced dose.

DRUG/LAB INTERACTIONS

Theoretical potential for interaction with calcium channel blockers (e.g., verapamil [Isoptin]); no clinical evidence to date. ▪ May cause additive hypotensive effects with any drug that produces hypotension (e.g., alcohol, benzodiazepines [e.g., diazepam, Versed], lidocaine, paclitaxel). ▪ Note Monitor.

SIDE EFFECTS

Supraventricular and ventricular dysrhythmias including nonsustained ventricular tachycardia do occur. Angina, chest pain, headaches, hypokalemia, hypotension, thrombocytopenia, and tremor have been reported.

ANTIDOTE

Notify the physician of any side effect. Based on degree of severity and condition of the patient, may be treated symptomatically, and dose may remain the same, be decreased, or the milrinone may be discontinued. Reduce rate or discontinue the drug at the first sign of marked hypotension and notify the physician. May be resolved by these measures alone or vasopressors (e.g., dopamine [Intropin]) may be required. Treat dysrhythmias with the appropriate drug. Resuscitate as necessary.

MITOMYCIN   Antineoplastic
                                                        (Antibiotic)

Mitocmycin-C, MTC, Mutamycin   pH 6.0 to 8.0

USUAL DOSE

10 to 20 mg/M^2 as a single dose. May be repeated in 6 to 8 weeks if no bone marrow toxicity occurs. Discontinue drug if no response after two courses of treatment. Total cumulative dose should not exceed 50 mg/M^2. Note Precautions/Monitor.

DOSE ADJUSTMENTS

Subsequent doses based on posttreatment leukocyte and platelet counts. Some sources say to withhold dose for leukocytes below 4,000/mm^3 or platelet count below 100,000/mm^3. Others recommend 70% of the previous dose with leukocytes between 2,000 to 2,999/mm^3 and platelet count between 25,000 to 74,999/mm^3 and 50% of the previous dose with leukocytes below 2,000/mm^3 and platelet count below 25,000/mm^3. ∎ Lower usual dose range is indicated when used with other antineoplastic drugs and radiation.

DILUTION

Specific techniques required; see Precautions. Each 5 mg must be diluted with 10 ml sterile water for injection. Allow to stand at room temperature until completely in solution. May be given through the Y-tube or three-way stopcock of a free-flowing infusion of NS or D5W or further diluted in either of the same solutions or sodium lactate 1/6M and given as an infusion. Stable in D5W for only 3 hours.

Storage: Stable after initial reconstitution at room temperature for 7 days, up to 14 days if refrigerated. When further diluted, stable at room remperature for 3 hours in D5W, 12 hours in NS and 24 hours in lactated Ringer's.

INCOMPATIBLE WITH

Bleomycin (Blenoxane), filgrastim (Neupogen), piperacillin/tazobactam (Zosyn), sargramostim (Leukine), vinorelbine tartrate.

RATE OF ADMINISTRATION

A single dose over 5 to 10 minutes. Infusion rate determined by amount and type of solution. Will maintain potency in 5% dextrose in water for 3 hours.

ACTIONS

A highly toxic antibiotic, antineoplastic agent. Cell cycle phase nonspecific, it is most useful in G and S phases. Interferes with cell division by binding with DNA to slow production of RNA. Rapidly distributed to body tissues and ascitic fluid. Does not cross blood-brain barrier. Metabolized in the spleen, kidneys, and liver. Some excreted in urine.

INDICATIONS AND USES

Treatment of disseminated adenocarcinoma of the stomach or pancreas. Used in combination with other drugs. May be useful in bladder, cervical, breast, bronchogenic, gallbladder, lung, and head and neck carcinoma and malignant melanoma.

CONTRAINDICATIONS

Not recommended as single-agent primary therapy. Known hypersensitivity to mitomycin, thrombocytopenia, coagulation disorders, increased bleeding from other causes, potentially serious infections, serum creatinine above 1.7 mg/100 ml.

PRECAUTIONS

Follow guidelines for handling cytotoxic agents. See Appendix A, p. 893. ▪ Administered by or under the direction of the physician specialist. ▪ Use extreme caution in impaired renal function; see Contraindications.

Monitor: Monitor white blood cells, red blood cells, platelet count, prothrombin time, bleeding time, differential, and hemoglobin before, during, and 7 to 10 weeks after therapy. ▪ Monitor all patients receiving any dose (initial or cumulative) of 60 mg or more for unexplained anemia with fragmented cells on peripheral blood smear, thrombocytopenia, and decreased renal function. ▪ Determine absolute patency of vein; use of an IV catheter is preferred because severe cellulitis and tissue necrosis will result from extravasation. If extravasation occurs, discontinue injection and use another vein. Elevate extremity and apply cold compresses to extravasated area. ▪ May precipitate adult respiratory distress syndrome. Oxygen can be toxic to the lungs; monitor intake carefully and use only enough to provide adequate arterial saturation. ▪ Monitor fluid balance; avoid overhydration. ▪ Be alert for signs of bone marrow depression or infection. ▪ Prophylactic antibiotics may be indicated pending results of C/S in a febrile neutropenic patient. ▪ Prophylactic antiemetics may reduce nausea and vomiting and increase patient comfort.

Patient education: Nonhormonal birth control recommended. ▪ Report IV site burning and stinging promptly. ▪ See Appendix D, p. 900.

Maternal/child: Avoid pregnancy; may produce teratogenic effects on the fetus. ▪ Information on safety in lactation or in children not available; discontinue breast feeding.

Elderly: Consider diminished hepatic function, monitor for early signs of toxicity.

DRUG/LAB INTERACTIONS

Do not administer live vaccines to patients receiving antineoplastic drugs. ▪ May cause shortness of breath, severe bronchospasm, and acute pneumonitis with vinca alkaloids (e.g., vinblastine [Velban]).

SIDE EFFECTS

Alopecia, anaphylaxis, anorexia, bleeding, blurring of vision, cellulitis at injection site, confusion, coughing, diarrhea, drowsiness, dyspnea with nonproductive cough, edema, elevated BUN or serum creatinine, fatigue, fever, headache, hematemesis, hemolytic uremic syndrome (microangiopathic hemolytic anemia [hematocrit less than 25%], irreversible renal failure [serum creatinine greater than 16 mg/dl], and thrombocytopenia [less than 100,000/mm^3]), hemoptysis, hypertension, leukopenia, mouth ulcers, nausea, paresthesias, pneumonia, pruritus, pulmonary edema, purple discoloration of vein, radiographic evidence of pulmonary infiltrates, renal failure, respiratory distress syndrome (adult), skin toxicity, stomatitis, syncope, thrombophlebitis, vomiting.

ANTIDOTE

Most side effects will be treated symptomatically. Keep the physician informed. All are potentially serious and many can be life threatening. Hematopoietic depression requires cessation of therapy until recovery occurs. Discontinue drug if dyspnea, nonproductive cough, or radiographic evidence of pulmonary infiltrates is present. Discontinue drug for any symptoms of hemolytic uremic syndrome. There is no specific antidote. Supportive therapy as indicated will help sustain the patient in toxicity. If extravasation has occurred, L.A. dexamethasone injected into the indurated area with a fine hypodermic needle may be helpful; elevate extremity.

MITOXANTRONE HYDROCHLORIDE

Antineoplastic
(Antibiotic)

Novantrone   pH 3.0 to 4.5

USUAL DOSE

Acute nonlymphocytic leukemia: 10 to 12 mg/M^2/day for 5 days.

Combination initial therapy in acute nonlymphocytic leukemia: 12 mg/M^2/day of mitoxantrone on days 1 through 3 and cytarabine 100 mg/M^2/day as a continuous 24 hour infusion on days 1 through 7. Should a complete remission not be achieved, repeat mitoxantrone, 12 mg/M^2/day for only 2 days, and cytarabine 100 mg/M^2/day for 5 days after all signs or symptoms of severe or life-threatening nonhematologic toxicity have cleared. After full hematologic recovery, some consolidation therapy trials have repeated the second course doses in approximately 6 weeks and again in 4 weeks. Severe myelosuppression occurred in these subsequent courses. Note Precautions/Monitor.

Other malignancies: 12 mg/M^2 once every 3 to 4 weeks.

Prostate cancer: 12 to 14 mg/M^2 as a short IV infusion once every 21 days. Used concurrently with steroids.

DILUTION

Specific techniques required; see Precautions. A single dose must be diluted with at least 50 ml of NS or D5W. May be further diluted in NS, D5W, or D5/NS. Must be given through Y-tube or three-way stopcock of a free-flowing infusion of D5W or NS, or may be diluted in larger amounts of the same solutions and given as a continuous infusion.

Storage: Diluted solution should be used immediately; do not freeze.

INCOMPATIBLE WITH

Heparin, hydrocortisone sodium phosphate in a PVC container (Hydrocortone), paclitaxel (Taxol), piperacillin/tazobactam (Zosyn). Consider toxicity and specific use.

RATE OF ADMINISTRATION

Direct IV: A single dose of properly diluted medication over at least 3 to 5 minutes.

Intermittent infusion: A single dose over 15 to 30 minutes.

Infusion: Sometimes a single dose is given as a continuous infusion over 24 hours. Is combined with cytarabine.

ACTIONS

The first of a new class of synthetic antibiotic antineoplastic agents called anthracenediones. Has achieved complete remissions with a single course of combination therapy. Extensive distribution to tissue occurs rapidly. Has a cytocidal effect on proliferating and nonproliferating cells. Probably not cell cycle specific. Half-life varies from 2.3 to 13 days. Slowly excreted in bile and urine.

INDICATIONS AND USES

Treatment of acute nonlymphocytic leukemia in adults. ▪ Treatment of bone pain in patients with advanced prostate cancer resistant to hormones. Used concurrently with steroids.

Investigational uses: Treatment of solid tumors, including advanced breast cancers, hepatocellular carcinoma, and non-Hodgkin's lymphomas.

CONTRAINDICATIONS

Hypersensitivity to mitoxantrone or other anthracyclines.

PRECAUTIONS

Follow guidelines for handling cytotoxic agents. See Appendix A, p. 893. ▪ Usually administered by or under the direction of the physician specialist. ▪ Will cause severe myelosuppression; use extreme caution in preexisting drug-induced bone marrow suppression. ▪ May cause acute congestive heart failure. ▪ Use caution if liver or renal function impaired. ▪ Urine and sclera may turn bluish in color. ▪ Use of goggles, gloves, and protective gown recommended. Flush skin copiously with warm water should any contact occur. Irrigate eyes immediately in case of contact. Clean spills with 5.5 parts calcium hypochlorite to 13 parts by weight of water for each 1 part of mitoxantrone.

Monitor: Monitoring of white blood cells, red blood cells, platelet count, liver function and kidney function indicated before and during therapy. ▪ Use extreme caution and monitor ECG, chest x-ray, echocardiography, and systolic ejection fraction in patients with preexisting heart disease, previous treatment with daunorubicin (Cerubidine), doxorubicin (Adriamycin), or radiation therapy encompassing the heart. ▪ Because of rapid lysis of cancer cells, initiate hypouricemic therapy with allopurinol or similar agents before beginning treatment. Monitor uric acid levels and maintain hydration. ▪ Observe closely and frequently for all signs of bleeding or infection. ▪ Prophylactic antibiotics may be indicated pending results of C/S in a febrile neutropenic patient. ▪ Has nonvesicant properties but extravasation must be avoided. Should extravasation occur, discontinue injection and use another vein. ▪ Prophylactic antiemetics may reduce nausea and vomiting and increase patient comfort.

Patient education: Nonhormonal birth control recommended. ▪ Report IV site burning or stinging promptly. ▪ See Appendix D, p. 900.

Maternal/child: Category D: avoid pregnancy. May produce teratogenic effects on the fetus. ▪ Discontinue breast feeding. ▪ Safety for use in children not established.

DRUG/LAB INTERACTIONS

Do not administer live vaccines to patients receiving antineoplastic drugs.

SIDE EFFECTS

Abdominal pain, acute congestive heart failure, alopecia (reversible), bleeding, bone marrow suppression (severe with standard doses), cough, decrease in systolic ejection fraction, diarrhea, dyspnea, fever, headache, infections, jaundice, mucositis, nausea, renal failure, seizures, stomatitis, vomiting.

ANTIDOTE

There is no specific antidote. Notify physician of all side effects. Most will be treated symptomatically. Blood and blood products, antibiotics and other adjunctive therapies must be available. Oprelvekin (Numega) has been used to treat thrombocytopenia. Overdose has resulted in death. Peritoneal dialysis or hemodialysis not effective. Supportive therapy as indicated will help sustain the patient in toxicity.

MIVACURIUM CHLORIDE

Neuromuscular blocking agent
(Nondepolarizing)
Anesthesia adjunct

Mivacron   pH 3.5 to 5.0

USUAL DOSE

Must be individualized based on age, weight/degree of obesity, renal, hepatic, and/or other diseases. Clinical duration varies. Use a peripheral nerve stimulator to monitor response to mivacurium, avoid overdose, monitor need for additional relaxant, and monitor adequacy of spontaneous recovery or antagonism. Test dose may be required; (See Dose adjustments).

Adults under balanced anesthesia and to facilitate intubation: 0.15 mg/kg of body weight should provide good conditions for intubation in 2.5 to 3 minutes and provide 15 to 20 minutes of clinical relaxation (time to 25% recovery). Lower doses may result in a longer time for development of satisfactory conditions.

Maintenance dose under balanced anesthesia:

Direct IV: 0.10 mg/kg administered at 25% recovery will extend relaxation another 15 minutes. Determine need for maintenance dose based on beginning symptoms of neuromuscular blockade reversal determined by a peripheral nerve stimulator. Adjust dose based on desired duration. Repeated maintenance doses usually do not produce a cumulative effect.

Infusion: May be used to maintain neuromuscular block. An average of 6 to 7 mcg/kg/min should maintain neuromuscular block at 89% to 99%. *Initiated at time of initial dose:* 4 mcg/kg/min. *After evidence of recovery from initial dose:* 9 to 10 mcg/kg/min. See literature for infusion rate tables.

PEDIATRIC DOSE

Children 2 to 12 years of age under balanced anesthesia: 0.2 mg/kg should provide good conditions for intubation in less than 2 minutes and provide 10 minutes of clinical relaxation. Children require higher doses on a mg/kg basis than adults. Onset and recovery of neuromuscular block occurs more rapidly.

Maintenance dose: Required more frequently. See adult mg/kg maintenance dose for *direct IV* administration.

Infusion to maintain neuromuscular block at 89% to 99% averages 14 mcg/kg/min.

DOSE ADJUSTMENTS

■ If inhalational anesthetics (e.g., isoflurane, enflurane) have been started, reduce dose of mivacurium by 25%. A mivacurium dose may require some reduction with halothane. Reduce maintenance infusion by 35% to 40% or more depending on amount of inhalational anesthetics used. Use with halothane will require a smaller reduction.
■ Reduced dose based on ideal body weight required in obesity (30% or more over ideal body weight). Specific calculation required (males, [106 + (6 × inches in height above 5 feet) ÷ 2.2] = IBW in kg; females, [100 + (5 × inches in height above 5 feet) ÷ 2.2] = IBW in kg). ■ A test dose of 0.015 to 0.020 mg/kg should be used in any patient receiving drugs (see Drug/lab interactions) or with a condition (e.g., cachetic, debilitated, neuromuscular diseases, carcinomatosis) that may potentiate neuromuscular block. Also use a reduced infusion rate for maintenance. ■ A test dose of 0.015 to 0.020 mg/kg should be used in burn patients. Any additional dosing must be regulated by a peripheral nerve stimulator monitor. ■ Length of block is prolonged and maintenance infusion rate must be decreased in the elderly and by as much as 50% based on degree of impairment in liver or renal disease. ■ Reduced doses may be required in clinically significant cardiovascular disease. ■ If used at all for patients with reduced plasma cholinesterase (pseudocholinesterase) activity, do not use an infusion for maintenance in patients homozygous for the atypical plasma cholinesterase gene, and reduce infusion rate in heterozygous patients. ■ Note Drug/lab interactions.

DILUTION

Supplied as 2 mg/ml. May be further diluted in D5W, NS, or other compatible infusion solutions (e.g., D5/NS, LR, D5/LR). Up to 3 ml diluent may be added to each 1 ml mivacurium (yields 0.5 mg/ml, which is the maximum dilution). Also available as a premixed infusion (50 ml of 0.5 mg/ml). See literature for specific instructions on use of flexible plastic containers. Use only if clear and container undamaged.

Storage: Store undiluted product at room temperature (15° to 25° C [59° to 77° F]). Avoid exposure to ultraviolet light; do not freeze. All concentrations for single patient use only. Stable up to 24 hours aseptically diluted and stored in polyvinyl bags at 5° to 25° C (41° to 77° F). Immediate use of diluted product is preferred; discard any unused portion in 24 hours.

INCOMPATIBLE WITH

Alkaline solutions with a pH over 8.5 (e.g., barbiturates). Do not add other drugs to mivacurium. Use of a Y-site and irrigation with NS may be required.

COMPATIBLE WITH

Y-site: D5W, NS, D5/NS, D5/LR, or LR; alfentanil (Alfenta); droperidol (Inapsine); fentanyl (Sublimaze); midazolam (Versed); and sufentanil (Sufenta).

RATE OF ADMINISTRATION

Titrate to desired effect. Use of a peripheral nerve stimulator monitor required.

Direct IV: A single dose over 5 to 15 seconds. Extend administration time to 60 seconds in any patient with a history of clinically significant cardiovascular disease or any patient with a history of histamine sensitivity (release of histamine is related to the dose and speed of injection).

Infusion: Usual dose and pediatric dose includes average rates to maintain neuromuscular block at 89% to 99%. See infusion rate tables. Reduce rate of infusions in specific situations; see Dose adjustments.

Infusion rates for maintenance of neuromuscular block during opioid nitrous oxide/oxygen anesthesia using mivacurium injection (2 mg/ml)									
Drug delivery rate (mcg/kg/min)									
4	5	6	7	8	10	14	16	18	20
Patient weight (kg)	Infusion delivery rate (ml/hr)								
10	1.2	1.5	1.8	2.1	2.4	3	4.2	4.8	5.4	6
15	1.8	2.3	2.7	3.2	3.6	4.5	6.3	7.2	8.1	9
20	2.4	3	3.6	4.2	4.8	6	8.4	9.6	10.8	12
25	3	3.8	4.5	5.3	6	7.5	10.5	12	13.5	15
35	4.2	5.3	6.3	7.4	8.4	10.5	14.7	16.8	18.9	21
50	6	7.5	9	10.5	12	15	21	24	27	30
60	7.2	9	10.8	12.6	14.4	18	25.2	28.8	32.4	36
70	8.4	10.5	12.6	14.7	16.8	21	29.4	33.6	37.8	42
80	9.6	12	14.4	16.8	19.2	24	33.6	38.4	43.2	48
90	10.8	13.5	16.2	18.9	21.6	27	37.8	43.2	48.6	54
100	12	15	18	21	24	30	42	48	54	60

Infusion rates for maintenance of neuromuscular block during opioid nitrous oxide/ oxygen anesthesia using mivacurium premixed infusion (0.5 mg/ml)									
Drug delivery rate (mcg/kg/min)									
4	**5**	**6**	**7**	**8**	**10**	**14**	**16**	**18**	**20**
Patient weight (kg)	Infusion delivery rate (ml/hr)								
10	5	6	7	8	10	12	17	19	22	24
15	7	9	11	13	14	18	25	29	32	36
20	10	12	15	17	19	24	34	38	43	48
25	12	15	18	21	24	30	42	48	54	60
35	17	21	26	29	34	42	59	67	76	84
50	24	30	36	42	48	60	84	96	108	120
60	29	36	43	50	58	72	101	115	130	144
70	34	42	50	59	67	84	118	134	151	168
80	39	48	58	67	77	96	134	154	173	192
90	44	54	65	76	86	108	151	173	194	216
100	48	60	72	84	96	120	168	192	216	240

ACTIONS

A short-acting nondepolarizing neuromuscular blocking agent. Causes skeletal muscle relaxation and paralysis by competing for cholinergic receptors at the motor end-plate. Onset of action is dose dependent. Produces maximal neuromuscular blockade in adults within 2.5 to 5 minutes and adequate blockade lasts from 15 to 20 minutes. In children the onset is faster (1.5 to 3 min) and duration of action shorter (10 min). Length of action extended with numerous disease entities. 95% recovery may take 30 to 40 minutes. At average doses, there is minimal change in mean arterial blood pressure or heart rate. Metabolized by plasma cholinesterases. Excreted mostly as metabolites in bile and urine.

INDICATIONS AND USES

Adjunct to general anesthesia that provides skeletal muscle relaxation during surgery or mechanical ventilation and/or facilitates endotracheal intubation.

CONTRAINDICATIONS

Hypersensitivity to mivacurium or other benzylisoquinolinium agents. Multiple-dose vials contraindicated with a known allergy to benzyl alcohol.

PRECAUTIONS

For IV use only. ■ Administered by or under the direct observation of the anesthesiologist. ■ Neuromuscular diseases (e.g., myasthenia gravis) and other diseases where prolonged block is probable (e.g., carcinomatosis) increase sensitivity to drug. Can cause critical reactions. Test dose required. ■ Resistance may develop in patients with burns, depending on the time elapsed since the initial injury and the size of the area involved. May be offset by reduced plasma cholines-terase activity. Test dose required. ▪ Dehydration and acid-base or serum electrolyte abnormalities may potentiate or antagonize the action. ▪ Bradycardia may be more common because mivacurium has little effect on heart rate and will not counteract bradycardia caused by anesthetic agents or vagal stimulation. ▪ Use caution and reduce maintenance dose in the elderly and in liver or renal dysfunction. Pro-longed duration can occur. ▪ Use extreme caution in patients with clinically significant cardiovascular disease and any patient with a history of allergic reactions; extended rate of administration required. ▪ Use with extreme caution in patients known or suspected to be homozygous for the atypical plasma cholinesterase gene. ▪ No data available on long-term use in patients mechanically ventilated in ICU.

Monitor: This drug produces apnea. Facilities for resuscitation and life support must be available (e.g., intubation equipment, oxygen, controlled artificial ventilation). ▪ Maintain a patent airway and ascertain adequate ventilation at all times. ▪ Neostigmine (Prostigmin) and atropine must be available. ▪ Monitor all vital organ functions until adequate recovery. Maintain adequate hydration. ▪ Use a peripheral nerve stimulator to monitor response and avoid overdose, monitor need for additional relaxant, and monitor adequacy of spontaneous recovery or antagonism. ▪ Patient may be conscious and completely unable to communicate by any means. Has no analgesic properties. ▪ Best if not used until patient is unconscious. ▪ Monitor for early signs of malignant hyperthermia; has not occurred but is a possibility. ▪ Review serum electrolytes and acid-base balance before administration. ▪ Note Drug/lab interactions.

Maternal/child: Pregnancy Category C: use during pregnancy only if benefits justify risks. ▪ Effects on neonate unknown; no studies available. ▪ Safety for use during lactation not established. ▪ Not recommended for infants and children under 2 years of age and benzyl alcohol in multiple dose vials contraindicated in newborns.

Elderly: Duration of block is slightly longer; note Dose adjustments.

DRUG/LAB INTERACTIONS

Observe evidence of recovery from succinylcholine before administra-tion. ▪ Duration of action extended and recovery prolonged by inha-lation anesthetics (e.g., enflurane, isoflurane, halothane). Varying dose reductions required (See Dose adjustments) ▪ Prolongation of neuro-muscular block may occur with many antibiotics (e.g., aminoglyco-sides [e.g., kanamycin (Kantrex), gentamicin (Garamycin)]), bacitracin, clindamycin (Cleocin), colistin (Coly-Mycin S), colistimeth-ate (Coly-Mycin M), clindamycin (Cleocin), polymyxin-B (Aero-sporin), piperacillin, tetracyclines, and with lithium, local anesthetics, diuretics, benzodiazepines (e.g., diazepam [Valium]) and other muscle relaxants, magnesium salts, procainamide (Pronestyl), and quinidine. Test dose and dose reduction required. ▪ Phenytoin (Dilantin) or car-bamazepine (Tegretol) may lengthen time of onset and shorten dura-tion of action; increased dose may be required. ▪ Potentiated by acidosis; inhibited by alkalosis. Electrolyte imbalance (acute [e.g., diarrhea] or chronic [e.g., adrenocortical insufficiency]) and acid-base imbalance are usually mixed; either reaction can occur.

SIDE EFFECTS

Average dose: Flushing is most common (15%). Prolonged action resulting in skeletal muscle weakness to profound and prolonged skeletal muscle paralysis with respiratory insufficiency or apnea is possible. Airway closure caused by relaxation of epiglottis, pharynx, and tongue muscles, bradycardia, bronchospasm, cardiac arrhythmias, dizziness, erythema, fever, injection site reaction, muscle spasms, rash, urticaria, tachycardia, and wheezing occur in less than 1%.

Overdose: Doses over 0.20 mg/kg over 5 to 15 seconds may cause marked hypotension.

ANTIDOTE

All side effects resulting from prolonged action can be medical emergencies. A short-acting drug; a patent airway and controlled continuous ventilation until normal function assured should be adequate. Treat symptomatically and monitor continuously. Neostigmine (Prostigmin [usual dose, 0.03 to 0.06 mg/kg]) or edrophonium (Tensilon [0.5 mg/kg]) are antagonists but should not be given before spontaneous recovery has begun (see specific monograph for complete information). Administer in combination with an anticholinergic agent (e.g., atropine). Identify appropriate time for antagonism, and monitor recovery with peripheral nerve stimulator. Evaluate 5 second head lift and grip strength. Time to recovery is based on level of residual neuromuscular block at time of dosing. The earlier an anticholinesterase is administered, the longer it will be to recovery. Treat marked hypotension with Trendelenburg position, IV fluids, and vasopressors (e.g., dopamine [Intropin]). Resuscitate and treat allergic reactions as indicated.

MORPHINE SULFATE

Narcotic analgesic (agonist)
Adjunct, pulmonary edema

Astramorph PF, Duramorph

pH 2.5 to 7.0

USUAL DOSE

Direct IV: 2.5 to 15 mg/70 kg (gr ¹/₁₆ to ¼). Repeat every 2 to 4 hours as necessary. May be titrated to achieve pain relief with lowest dose (e.g., pain relief in myocardial infarction [1 to 3 mg every 5 min until desired response]). 10 mg (gr ⅙) is adequate for most needs. Dose must be individualized based on response and tolerance. When seeking the required dose to achieve pain relief for an individual patient, increases in increments of at least 25% of the previous ineffective dose are suggested. Lower slightly if pain controlled but patient is too drowsy; or lower dose and increase frequency. Cancer patients suffering with severe chronic pain often require higher doses because of increased tolerance (up to 150 mg/hr has been given). Very high doses (275 to 440 mg/hr) are occasionally used for short periods of time (hours to days) for extreme exacerbations of pain in these drug-tolerant individuals. 1 to 3 mg/kg over 15 to 20 minutes will induce unconsciousness.

Infusion: 1 mg/ml (range is 0.1 to 1 mg/ml) in NS or D5W per controlled infusion device (may be patient activated). Based on a 1 mg/ml dilution an initial loading dose may range from 3 to 5 mg (3 to 5 ml). The continuous background infusion to provide a level of pain relief and maintain patency of the vein may range from 1 to 2.5 mg/hr (1 to 2.5 ml). Additional doses averaging 0.5 to 1.5 mg (0.5 to 1.5 ml) may be activated by the patient at selected intervals every 3 to 60 minutes (averaging 10 to 15 min). Additional boluses (averaging 1 to 2 mg (1 to 2 ml) may be given by health care professionals (e.g., every 30 min prn). In selected cancer patients all of these doses may be considerably higher.

PEDIATRIC DOSE

Usual range is 0.05 to 0.1 mg/kg.

Selected children with severe chronic cancer pain: 0.025 to 2.6 mg/kg/hr (average 0.04 to 0.07 mg/kg/hr).

Selected children with severe pain during sickle cell crisis: 0.03 to 0.15 mg/kg/hr.

Selected children requiring postoperative analgesia: 0.01 to 0.04 mg/kg/hr. Reduce to 0.015 to 0.02 mg/kg/hr in neonates due to reduced elimination and susceptibility to CNS side effects.

DOSE ADJUSTMENTS

Reduced dose and/or extended intervals may be required in impaired renal or hepatic function and in the elderly. ■ Note Drug/lab interactions.

DILUTION

Direct IV: Should be diluted. Use at least 5 ml of sterile water or NS for injection or other IV solutions. May be given through Y-tube or three-way stopcock of infusion set.

Infusion: Each 0.1 to 1 mg is usually diluted in 1 ml NS or D5W and administered via a controlled infusion device that may be patient activated (e.g., a narcotic syringe infuser system). Available in 60 ml amps containing 1 to 2 mg/ml for direct transfer to syringe infuser systems (Astramorph PF and Duramorph are preservative free and expensive; can be used IV, but are the only choice for epidural or intrathecal injection; see drug literature. Infumorph is NOT for IV use). Fluid restriction or high doses may require more concentrated solutions. Concentrations above 5 mg/ml are rarely exceeded. Available in vials containing 25 mg/ml, which must be further diluted before infusion.Is sometimes added to larger amounts (500 ml to 1 L) of IV solution in selected situations and infused via a large volume controlled infusion pump (requires close titration).

INCOMPATIBLE WITH

Acyclovir (Zovirax), aminophylline, amobarbital (Amytal), chlorothiazide (Diuril), furosemide (Lasix), gallium nitrate (Ganite), heparin, meperidine (Demerol), methicillin (Staphcillin), pentobarbital (Nembutal), phenobarbital (Luminal), phenytoin (Dilantin), prochlorperazine (Compazine), promethazine (Phenergan), sargramostim (Leukine), sodium bicarbonate, sodium iodide, thiopental (Pentothal).

RATE OF ADMINISTRATION

Frequently titrated according to symptom relief and respiratory rate. Side effects markedly increased if rate of injection too rapid.

Direct IV: 15 mg or fraction thereof of properly diluted medication over 4 to 5 minutes.

Infusion: Initial loading dose, basal rate (continuous rate of infusion), patient self-administered dose and interval, additional boluses permitted, and total dose for 1 hour should be ordered by physician. Administer initial dose and boluses at rate for direct IV. For continuous infusion and self-administered dose and interval, note range of ml/hr under Usual dose.

ACTIONS

An opium-derivative, narcotic analgesic, which is a descending CNS depressant. It has definite respiratory depressant actions. Pain relief is effected almost immediately and lasts up to 4 to 5 hours (mean is 2 hours). Morphine induces sleep and inhibits perception of pain by binding to opiate receptors, decreasing sodium permeability, and inhibiting transmission of pain impulses. Depresses many other senses or reflexes. Relieves pulmonary congestion, lowers myocardial oxygen requirements, and reduces anxiety. Detoxified in the liver, and excreted in the urine. Crosses the placental barrier. Secreted in breast milk.

INDICATIONS AND USES

Relief of moderate to severe acute and chronic pain (e.g., post-op or cancer pain). ■ Analgesic of choice in pain associated with myocardial infarction. ■ Treatment of acute pulmonary edema associated with left ventricular failure. ■ Pre-op to sedate, decrease anxiety and facilitate induction of anesthesia. ■ Restore uterine tone and contractions in a uterus made hyperactive by oxytocics.

CONTRAINDICATIONS

Acute bronchial asthma, diarrhea caused by poisoning until toxic material eliminated, hypersensitivity to opiates, premature infants or labor and delivery of premature infants, pulmonary edema caused by a chemical respiratory irritant, respiratory depression, upper airway obstruction.

PRECAUTIONS

Use caution in the elderly, in patients with impaired hepatic or renal function, pulmonary disease, and patients on anticoagulation therapy. ▪ Use extreme caution in craniotomy, head injury, and increased intracranial pressure; respiratory depression and intracranial pressure may be further increased. ▪ May cause apnea in asthmatic patients. ▪ Symptoms of acute abdominal conditions may be masked. ▪ May increase ventricular response rate in presence of supraventricular tachycardias. ▪ Cough reflex is suppressed. ▪ Tolerance for the drug gradually increases, but abstinence for 1 to 2 weeks will restore effectiveness. ▪ A marked increase in dose may precipitate seizures in presence of a history of convulsive disorders.

Monitor: Oxygen, controlled respiratory equipment, and naloxone (Narcan) must always be available. ▪ Observe patient frequently to continuously based on amount of dose and monitor vital signs. Keep patient supine; orthostatic hypotension and fainting may occur; less likely with continuous low doses, but observe closely during ambulation. ▪ Uncontrolled pain causes sleep deprivation, decreases pain threshold, and increases pain. When pain is finally controlled, expect the patient to sleep more until recovery from sleep deprivation. ▪ Stool softeners and/or laxatives will be required to avoid constipation and fecal impaction, especially with increased doses and extended use. Maintain adequate hydration. ▪ Note Drug/lab interactions.

Patient education: Avoid alcohol or other CNS depressants (e.g., barbiturates, benzodiazepines [e.g., diazepam (Valium)]). ▪ May cause blurred vision, dizziness, or drowsiness; use caution in tasks that require alertness. ▪ May be habit forming.

Maternal/child: Pregnancy Category C: safety for use in pregnancy or lactation not established. Benefits must outweigh risks. ▪ Note Contraindications.

Elderly: Note Dose adjustments and Precautions. ▪ May be more sensitive to effects (e.g., respiratory depression, constipation, urinary retention). ▪ Analgesia should be effective with lower doses. ▪ Consider age-related organ impairment.

DRUG/LAB INTERACTIONS

Alcohol, hydroxyzine (Atarax), other CNS depressants (e.g., narcotic analgesics, general anesthetics, barbiturates, hypnotics, sedatives) H_2 antagonists (e.g., cimetidine [Tagamet]), and some phenothiazines (e.g., chlorpromazine [Thorazine]) may increase CNS depression, respiratory depression, and hypotension; reduced dose of one or both agents indicated. ▪ Anticholinergics (e.g., atropine) and antidiarrheals may increase risk of constipation or paralytic ileus. ▪ Hypotensive effects will be increased with diuretics (e.g., furosemide [Lasix]), antihypertensive agents (especially ganglionic blockers [e.g., guanethidine (Ismelin)]), or hypotension-producing agents (e.g., antidepressants, benzodiazepines [e.g., diazepam], adrenergic blocking agents [e.g., propranolol], calcium channel blocking agents [e.g., diltiazem], calcium, nitroprusside, nitroglycerin). ▪ Use with buprenorphine (Buprenex) may negate effects. ▪ May antagonize effects of metoclopramide (Reglan). ▪ Markedly reduced doses of MAO inhibitors (e.g., selegiline [Eldepryl]) required with opiates. ▪ Will cause withdrawal symptoms in opiate-dependent patients with naltrexone (Trexan) or buprenorphine (Buprenex). ■ May cause extended respiratory depression or prolonged blockade with neuromuscular blocking agents (e.g., mivacurium [Mivacrom], succinylcholine [Anectine], tubocurarine). ■ Avoid concurrent use with zidovudine (AZT); may increase toxicity of either or both. ■ After several weeks, hepatic metabolism increases and analgesic effect may decrease in smokers.

SIDE EFFECTS

Average dose: Constipation, delayed absorption of oral medications, hypersensitivity reactions, hypothermia, increased intracranial pressure, nausea, neonatal apnea, orthostatic hypotension, respiratory depression (slight), urinary retention, vomiting.

Overdose: Anaphylaxis, Cheyne-Stokes respiration, coma, excitation, hypotension (severe), inverted T wave on ECG, myocardial depression (severe), pinpoint pupils, respiratory depression (severe), tachycardia, death.

ANTIDOTE

With increasing severity of any side effect or onset of symptoms of overdose, discontinue the drug and notify the physician. Naloxone (Narcan) will reverse serious respiratory depression. A patent airway, artificial ventilation, oxygen therapy, and other symptomatic treatment must be instituted promptly. Resuscitate as necessary.

MULTI-VITAMIN INFUSION
Nutritional supplement (vitamin)

Berocca parenteral nutrition, Multivitamin concentrate, M.V.I. -12, M.V.I. Pediatric

USUAL DOSE

One 5 to 10 ml dose every 24 hours.

PEDIATRIC DOSE

MVI Pediatric: Less than 1 kg: 1.5 ml/24 hr

1 to 3 kg: 3.25 ml/24 hr.

Over 3 kg to 11 years of age: 5 ml/24 hr.

DILUTION

Each adult dose must be diluted in at least 500 ml but preferably 1,000 ml of IV fluids. Soluble in commonly used infusion fluids, including dextrose, saline, electrolyte replacement fluids, plasma, and selected protein amino acid products. Do not use if any crystals have formed.

Pediatric dilution: Each dose of *MVI Pediatric* should be added to at least 100 ml of compatible infusion solution.

Storage: Most preparations should be refrigerated. *MVI Pediatric* may be stored at controlled room temperature. Protect from light.

INCOMPATIBLE WITH

Acetazolamide (Diamox), alkaline solutions, amino acids (10% and 5.5% Travasol), bleomycin (Blenoxane), calcium saits, chlorothiazide (Diuril), doxycycline (Vibramycin), erythromycin (Erythrocin), FreAmine III (8.5% amino acid), kanamycin (Kantrex), lincomycin (Lincocin), sodium bicarbonate, streptomycin.

RATE OF ADMINISTRATION

Give at prescribed rate of infusion fluids.

ACTIONS

A multiple vitamin solution containing fat-soluble and water-soluble vitamins in an aqueous solution. Provides B complex and vitamins A, D, and E. It provides daily requirements or corrects an existing deficiency.

INDICATIONS AND USES

Need of optimumal vitamin intake to maintain the body's normal resistance and repair processes, such as after surgery, extensive burns, trauma, severe infectious diseases, and comatose states.

CONTRAINDICATIONS

Known hypersensitivity to thiamine hydrochloride or other components.

PRECAUTIONS

Never used undiluted.

SIDE EFFECTS

Rare when administered as recommended: anaphylaxis, dizziness, fainting.

ANTIDOTE

With onset of any side effect, discontinue administration immediately and notify the physician. Treat anaphylaxis or resuscitate as necessary.

MUROMONAB-CD3

Monoclonal antibody Immunosuppressant

Orthoclone OKT3

pH 6.5 to 7.5

USUAL DOSE

Do not give initial or subsequent doses unless patient temperature is less than 37.8° C (100° F). Administration of IV methylprednisolone sodium succinate 8 mg/kg of body weight 1 to 4 hours before muromonab-CD3 is recommended to reduce side effects of cytokine release syndrome (CRS) associated with the first two to three doses. Acetaminophen and antihistamines may also be used concomitantly. Note Monitor.

Renal allograph rejection: 5 mg/24 hr for 10 to 14 days. Initiate on diagnosis of acute renal rejection.

Cardiac/hepatic allograph rejections: 5 mg/24 hr for 10 to 14 days if rejection has not been reversed by corticosteroid therapy.

PEDIATRIC DOSE

Manufacturer states that it has been used in infants and children at doses less than 5 mg/day. Dose based on immunologic monitoring. Another source recommends 0.1mg/kg/24hr for 10-14 days.

DOSE ADJUSTMENTS

Doses of concomitant immunosuppressive therapy must be reduced to the lowest level compatible with a therapeutic response during muromonab-CD3 therapy. Resume maintenance doses 3 days before completion of muromonab-CD3 therapy.

DILUTION

May be given undiluted. Must be withdrawn from vial through a low protein-binding 0.2 or 0.22 micron filter. Discard filter and attach needle for direct IV administration. Do not shake.

Storage: Keep unopened vials under refrigeration. May have some fine translucent particles. Will not affect potency, and use of filter will clear.

INCOMPATIBLE WITH

Manufacturer states, "Do not give by IV infusion or in conjunction with other drug solutions."

RATE OF ADMINISTRATION

A single dose as an IV bolus in less than 1 minute.

ACTIONS

A murine monoclonal antibody to the T3 (CD3) antigen of human T cells. An immunosuppressive agent that reverses graft rejection by blocking all known T-cell functions. Onset of action is within minutes. CD3 positive cells reappear within several days and reach pretreatment levels in 1 week after daily injections are stopped.

INDICATIONS AND USES

Treatment of acute allograft rejection in renal transplant patients. ■ Treatment of acute rejection in heart and liver transplant patients resistant to standard steroid therapy.

CONTRAINDICATIONS

Hypersensitivity to muromonab-CD3 or any product of murine origin; anti-mouse antibody titer ≥1:1,000; patients in fluid overload as evidenced by chest x-ray or greater than 3% weight gain within the week before treatment; history of seizures or patients who may be predisposed to seizures; pregnancy and lactation.

PRECAUTIONS

Usually administered in the hospital by or under the direction of a physician experienced in immunosuppressive therapy and management of organ transplant patients. Adequate laboratory and supportive medical resources including airway management, emergency drugs and equipment must be available. ■ A protein substance that induces antibodies; use extreme caution if a second course of therapy is needed. ■ May cause lymphomas, skin cancers, or lymphoproliferative disorders. ■ Neuro-psychiatric events including seizures, encephalopathy, cerebral edema, aseptic meningitis and headache have been reported.

Monitor: To reduce incidence of serious side effects, evaluate patients for fluid overload. Must have a clear chest x-ray within 24 hours and have gained no more than 3% above minimal weight present 7 days before injection. ■ Monitor white blood cell count and differential, circulating T cells as CD3 antigen, and 24 hour trough values of muromonab-CD3 (rise rapidly for the first 3 days of treatment and then average 0.9 mcg/ml thereafter during treatment). ■ Monitor renal and hepatic function. ■ Testing for human-mouse antibody titers is strongly recommended (see Contraindications). ■ Observe for fever, chills, dyspnea, and malaise, which frequently occur 30 minutes to 6 hours after a dose. Symptoms of cytokine release syndrome (CRS) may range from flu-like to a life-threatening shock-like reaction. ▪ Anaphylaxis may occur immediately. ▪ May be difficult to distinguish between CRS and anaphylaxis. If hypersensitivity is suspected, do not reexpose patient to muromonab-CD3. ▪ Increased susceptibility to infection; observe closely. Prophylactic antibiotics may be indicated pending results of C/S in a febrile neutropenic patient. ▪ Treat any fever over 37.8° C (100° F) with antipyretics to lower before giving any single dose. ▪ Note Dose adjustments.

Patient education: Side effects from first few doses are expected. Incidence lessens with subsequent doses. ▪ Avoid pregnancy; consider birth control options. ▪ See Appendix D, p. 900. ▪ Review potentially serious symptoms of CRS. ▪ Report difficulty in breathing, swallowing, rapid heart beat, rash or itching immediately. ▪ Use caution performing tasks that require mental alertness.

Maternal/child: Category C: safety for use in pregnancy and men and women capable of conception not established. Use only when absolutely necessary. ▪ Discontinue breast feeding. ▪ Has been used in children over 2 years of age, but safety not established, monitor closely.

DRUG/LAB INTERACTIONS

Do not administer live vaccines to patients receiving immunosuppressive drugs. ▪ Immunosuppressive agents (e.g., azathioprine, cyclophos-phamide, corticosteroids, cyclosporine) increase risk of infection and development of lymphoproliferative disorders. Use reduced doses with caution.

SIDE EFFECTS

Cytokine release syndrome (chills, dyspnea, fever, and malaise) is very common with early doses and can progress to shock; incidence lessens with subsequent doses. Anaphylaxis, chest pain, diarrhea, infections (e.g., cytomegalovirus, Epstein Barr, herpes simplex, *Staphylococcus epidermidis, Pneumocystis carinii, Legionella, Cryptococcus, Serratia*), lymphomas, nausea, serum sickness, severe pulmonary edema, tremors, vomiting, and wheezing have occurred.

ANTIDOTE

Notify the physician of all side effects. Most can be treated symptomatically. Pretreat as indicated in Usual dose to reduce side effects with early doses. Use antipyretics and antihistamines as indicated. Proper patient screening should reduce incidence of pulmonary edema. Shock from CRS may require O_2, IV fluids, corticosteroids, pressoramines (e.g., dopapime [Intropin]), antihistamines (e.g., diphenhydramine [Benadryl]), and intubation. Drug may be decreased or discontinued or other immunosuppressive agents utilized. Resuscitate as necessary.

NAFCILLIN SODIUM
Antibacterial
(Penicillinase-resistant penicillin)

Nafcil, Nallpen, Unipen
pH 6.0 to 8.5

USUAL DOSE
500 mg to 1 Gm every 4 hours.
Endocarditis or osteomyelitis: 1 to 2 Gm every 4 hours.
Meningitis: 100 to 200 mg/kg/24 hours in equally divided doses every 4 to 6 hours.

PEDIATRIC DOSE
Over 1 month of age: 50 to 100 mg/24 hr in equally divided doses every 6 hours in moderate infections. 100 to 200 mg/kg of body weight/24 hr in equally divided doses every 4 to 6 hours has been used in serious infections (e.g., osteomyelitis, pericarditis, endocarditis). IM route preferred; rarely used IV in children.

NEONATAL DOSE
10 to 20 mg/kg every 8 to 12 hours or dosing specific to age and weight.
Over 2,000 Gm; age up to 7 days: 25 mg/kg every 8 hours. 50 mg/kg every 8 hours for meningitis. *Over 7 days of age:* 25 mg/kg every 6 hours. 50 mg/kg every 6 hours for meningitis.
Under 2,000 Gm; age up to 7 days: 25 mg/kg every 12 hours. 50 mg/kg every 12 hours for meningitis. *Over 7 days of age:* 25 mg/kg every 8 hours. 50 mg/kg every 8 hours for meningitis.

DOSE ADJUSTMENTS
May need to decrease dose in patients with severe renal and hepatic impairment.

DILUTION
Each 500 mg vial is diluted with 1.7 ml of sterile water for injection (1 Gm vial with 3.4 ml, 2 Gm vial with 6.8 ml). Each 1 ml equals 250 mg. Further dilute each dose with a minimum of 15 to 30 ml of sterile water, NS, or 0.45%S, or other compatible IV solutions (see literature). Concentration should be 2 to 40 mg/ml. May be given through Y-tube, three-way stopcock, or with additive tubing, or may be added to larger volume of compatible solutions.
Storage: Refrigerate unused medication after initial dilution, and discard after 7 days. Stable in specific solutions at concentrations of 2 to 40 mg/ml for 24 hours at room temperature and 96 hours if refrigerated.

INCOMPATIBLE WITH
Aminoglycosides (e.g., gentamicin, kanamycin), aminophylline, ascorbic acid, aztreonam (Azactam), bleomycin (Blenoxane), cytarbine (ARA-C), diltiazem (Cardizem), fentanyl/droperidol (Innovar), hydrocortisone sodium succinate (Solu-Cortef), insulin, labetalol (Trandate), meperidine (Demerol), methylprednisolone (Solu-Medrol), midazolam (Versed), nalbuphine (Nubain), pentazocine (Talwin), promazine (Sparine), solutions with a pH below 5.0 or over 8.0, verapamil (Isoptin).

RATE OF ADMINISTRATION

Direct IV: Each 500 mg or fraction thereof properly diluted over 5 to 10 minutes.

Intermittent IV: Administration over 30 to 60 minutes may decrease incidence of thrombophlebitis.

Infusion: When diluted in large volumes of infusion fluids, give at rate prescribed.

ACTIONS

A semisynthetic penicillin, used for its bactericidal action against gram-positive organisms, primarily penicillinase-producing staphylococci. Readily distributed into most body fluids and tissues except spinal fluid. Crosses the placental barrier. Primarily excreted through bile; a small amount is excreted in the urine. Secreted in breast milk.

INDICATIONS AND USES

Treatment of infections caused by penicillinase-producing staphylococci.

CONTRAINDICATIONS

Known hypersensitivity to any penicillin or cephalosporin (not absolute).

PRECAUTIONS

Sensitivity studies necessary to determine susceptibility of the causative organism to nafcillin; sometimes difficult to determine accurately. ▪ Avoid prolonged use of the drug; superinfection caused by overgrowth of nonsusceptible organisms may result.

Monitor: Watch for early symptoms of allergic reaction, especially in individuals with a history of allergic problems. ▪ Renal, hepatic, and hematopoietic function should be checked during long-term therapy. ▪ May cause thrombophlebitis, especially in the elderly or with too-rapid injection. Limit IV treatment to 24 to 48 hours when possible. Change to oral therapy as soon as practical. ▪ Electrolyte imbalance and cardiac irregularities from sodium content are possible. Contains 2.9 mEq sodium/Gm. May aggravate CHF. Observe for hypokalemia. ▪ Note Drug/lab interactions.

Patient education: May require alternate birth control.

Maternal/child: Pregnancy Category B: use only if clearly needed. ▪ May cause diarrhea, candidiasis, or allergic response in nursing infants. ▪ Elimination rate markedly reduced in neonates.

Elderly: Note Precautions/Monitor and Dose adjustments.

DRUG/LAB INTERACTIONS

May be antagonized by bacteriostatic antibiotics (e.g., chloramphenicol, erythromycin, tetracyclines), bactericidal action may be negated. ▪ Potentiated by probenecid (Benemid); toxicity may result. ▪ Inhibits aminoglycosides (e.g., gentamicin). Do not mix in same IV container. ▪ Concomitant use with beta-adrenergic blockers (e.g., propranolol [Inderal]) may increase risk of anaphylaxis and inhibit treatment. ▪ Risk of bleeding with anticoagulants (e.g., heparin) is increased. ▪ Inhibits effectiveness of oral contraceptives; breakthrough bleeding or pregnancy could result. ▪ High doses (9 to 12 Gm daily) may decrease serum half-life of warfarin, monitor PT up to 30 days after nafcillin completed. ▪ May decrease clearance and increase toxicity of methotrexate. ▪ May cause false values in common lab tests; see literature.

SIDE EFFECTS

Relatively infrequent except for sensitivity reactions such as anaphylaxis, skin rashes, and urticaria. Bleeding abnormalities, diarrhea, nausea, pruritus, and vomiting have been reported. Hypersensitivity myocarditis (fever, eosinophilia, rash, sinus tachycardia, ST-T changes and cardiomegaly) or pseudomembranous colitis can occur. Higher than normal doses may cause neurologic adverse reactions including convulsions, especially with impaired renal function.

ANTIDOTE

Notify the physician immediately of any adverse symptoms. For severe symptoms discontinue the drug, treat allergic reaction (antihistamines, epinephrine, corticosteroids), and resuscitate as necessary. Hemodialysis or peritoneal dialysis is minimally effective in overdose. Hyaluronidase (Wydase) has been used to treat extravasation.

NALBUPHINE HYDROCHLORIDE

Narcotic analgesic
(Agonist-antagonist)
Anesthesia adjunct

Nubain
pH 3.5

USUAL DOSE

Pain control: 10 mg/70 kg. Repeat every 3 to 6 hours as necessary. Up to 20 mg can be given in a single dose if required. Maximum total daily dose is 160 mg.

Adjunct to balanced anesthesia: A loading dose of 300 mcg (0.3 mg) to 3 mg/kg over 10 to 15 minutes. Maintain desired level of balanced anesthesia with 250 to 500 mcg (0.25 to 0.5 mg)/kg as required. Administered only under the direction of the anesthesiologist.

DOSE ADJUSTMENTS

Reduce dose to one fourth if previous medication a narcotic. Observe for symptoms of withdrawal. Increase to effective dose gradually. ■ Reduced dose may be required in the elderly or debilitated; in impaired liver or renal function; in patients with limited pulmonary reserve; and in the presence of other CNS depressants. ■ Note Drug/lab interactions.

DILUTION

May be given undiluted.

Storage: Prior to use, store at controlled room temperature. Avoid freezing and/or prolonged exposure to light.

INCOMPATIBLE WITH

Allopurinol (Zyloprim), diazepam (Valium), ketorolac (Toradol), nafcillin (Nafcil), pentobarbital (Nembutal), piperacillin/tazobactam (Zosyn), promethazine (Phenergan), sargramostim (Leukine).

RATE OF ADMINISTRATION

Pain control: Each 10 mg or fraction thereof over 3 to 5 minutes. Frequently titrated according to symptom relief and respiratory rate.

Anesthesia adjunct: See Usual dose.

ACTIONS

A synthetic narcotic agonist-antagonist analgesic. It equals morphine in analgesic effect and has one-fourth the antagonist effect of naloxone. Does produce respiratory depression, but this does not increase markedly with increased doses. Pain relief is effected in 2 to 3 minutes and lasts about 3 to 6 hours. Metabolized in the liver. Some excretion in urine. Crosses the placental barrier. Secreted in breast milk.

INDICATIONS AND USES

Relief of moderate to severe pain. ■ Preoperative analgesia. ■ Surgical anesthesia supplement. ■ Obstetric analgesia during labor.

Investigational use: SC administration of 10 mg to reduce pruritus from epidural fentanyl dose.

CONTRAINDICATIONS

Hypersensitivity to nalbuphine or its components (may contain sulfites).

PRECAUTIONS

May precipitate withdrawal symptoms if stopped too quickly after prolonged use or if patient has been on opiates. ■ Use caution in respiratory depression or difficulty from any source, head injury, increased intracranial pressure, biliary surgery, history of drug abuse, the elderly or debilitated, and in impaired liver or kidney function. Reduced doses may be indicated. ■ Use caution in myocardial infarction with nausea and vomiting.

Monitor: Naloxone (Narcan), oxygen, and controlled respiratory equipment must be available. ■ Observe patient frequently and monitor vital signs. ■ Keep patient supine to minimize side effects; orthostatic hypotension and fainting may occur. Observe closely during ambulation. ■ Pain control usually more effective with routinely administered doses. Determine apropriate interval through clinical assessment ■ Note Drug/lab interactions.

Patient education: Avoid use of alcohol or other CNS depressants (e.g., antihistamines, diazepam [Valium]). ■ Request assistance for ambulation. ■ Use caution performing any task that requires alertness; may cause dizziness, euphoria, and sedation. ■ May be habit forming.

Maternal/child: Pregnancy Category C: safety for use in pregnancy or lactation not established. ■ Has been used safely during labor and delivery of term infants, but use caution during labor and delivery of premature infants. ■ Not recommended for children under 18 years.

Elderly: May be more sensitive to effects (e.g., respiratory depression, constipation, dizziness, urinary retention). ■ Analgesia should be effective with lower doses. ■ Consider age-related organ impairment.

DRUG/LAB INTERACTIONS

Potentiated by cimetidine (Tagamet), phenothiazines (e.g., chlorpromazine [Thorazine]), by other CNS depressants such as narcotic analgesics, general anesthetics, alcohol, anticholinergics, antihistamines, barbiturates, hypnotics, neuromuscular blocking agents (e.g., mivacurium [Mivacron]), psychotropic agents, and sedatives. Reduced doses of both drugs may be indicated. ■ May decrease analgesic effects of other narcotics; avoid concurrent use.

SIDE EFFECTS

Anaphylaxis, blurred vision, bradycardia, clammy skin, dizziness, dry mouth, headache, hypertension, hypotension, nausea, respiratory depression, sedation, tachycardia, urinary urgency, vertigo, vomiting.

ANTIDOTE

With increasing severity of any side effect or onset of symptoms of overdose, discontinue the drug and notify the physician. Naloxone hydrochloride (Narcan) will reverse respiratory depression. A patent airway, artificial ventilation, oxygen therapy, and other symptomatic treatment must be instituted promptly.

NALMEFENE HYDROCHLORIDE

Antidote
Narcotic antagonist

Revex

pH 3.9

USUAL DOSE

Manage known or suspected narcotic overdose: nonopioid dependent: (fully reversing dose) 0.5 mg/70 kg. May be followed by 1 mg/70 kg in 2 to 5 minutes if indicated. If no clinical response, additional nalmefene is not indicated.

Suspicion of opioid dependency: Begin with a challenge dose of 0.1 mg/70 kg. If no evidence of withdrawal (e.g., abdominal cramps, anxiety, chills, diaphoresis, gooseflesh, joint pain, myalgia, restlessness, rhinorrhea, vomiting, yawning) in 2 minutes, follow dose recommendations for nonopioid dependent.

Reverse postoperative narcotic depression: (partially reversing dose) 0.25 mcg/kg. Repeat at 2- to 5-minute intervals until ventilation is adequate and the patient is alert without significant pain or discomfort. A total dose above 1 mcg/kg does not provide additional therapeutic effect.

Reversal of Postoperative Opioid Depression	
Body Weight	ml of Nalmefene 100 ug/ml Solution
50 kg	0.125
60 kg	0.15
70 kg	0.175
80 kg	0.2
90 kg	0.225
100 kg	0.25

PEDIATRIC DOSE

Safety for use in children and neonates not established.

DOSE ADJUSTMENTS

Reduce dose to 0.1 mcg/kg if reversing postoperative narcotic depression in a patient known to be at increased cardiovascular risk. Increments should also be reduced to 0.1 mcg/kg. ■ Reduced doses not indicated for single episodes of reversal in impaired hepatic or renal function or in the elderly.

DILUTION

Available in two concentrations. Blue label contains 100 mcg/ml and is primarily used postoperatively. Green label contains 1 mg/ml and is primarily used to manage or reverse known or suspected narcotic overdose. May be given undiluted except in the postoperative patient at increased cardiac risk (1:1 dilution with NS or SW is recommended).

Storage: Store at controlled room temperature.

INCOMPATIBLE WITH

Specific information not available.

RATE OF ADMINISTRATION

Give the initial dose over 15 to 30 seconds. Extend to 60 seconds to prevent dizziness and hypertension in patients with renal failure. Titrate subsequent doses required to desired effect.

ACTIONS

A potent narcotic antagonist similar to naloxone and naltrexone. Prevents or reverses the effects of opioids (e.g., respiratory depression, sedation, hypotension) by competing for opioid receptors. Has no narcotic agonist activity. Onset of action occurs within 2 minutes. Partially reversing doses (1 mcg/kg) have a duration of 30 to 60 minutes. Fully reversing doses (1 mg/70 kg) have an elimination half-life of 10.8 hours (naloxone's is 1.1 hours) so the duration of action is as long as that of most narcotics. It provides protection against renarcotization, sustains reversal of respiratory depression, and reduces the need for repeat doses. Actions are dose proportional. Rapidly distributed. Metabolized in the liver and excreted in urine. Probably crosses the placental barrier. Secreted in breast milk.

INDICATIONS AND USES

Management of known or suspected narcotic overdose. ▪ Complete or partial reversal of narcotic drug effects, including respiratory depression, induced by both natural and synthetic narcotics (including propoxyphene, nalbuphine, pentazocine, and butorphanol).

Unlabeled uses: Reverse the systemic effects of intrathecal opioids.

CONTRAINDICATIONS

Known hypersensitivity to nalmefene.

PRECAUTIONS

Use with caution in patients with opioid dependence; may cause acute withdrawal symptoms. ▪ Use caution in patients at high cardiovascular risk or patients receiving potentially cardiotoxic drugs; arrhythmias (including bradycardia, tachycardia, VT, and VF), hypertension, hypotension, and pulmonary edema have occurred with opioid reversal. ▪ With recommended low doses (incremental doses of 0.25 mcg/kg titrated to desired effect) maintenance of opioid analgesia is maintained. Larger doses or fully reversing doses may produce long-lasting antianalgesic effects; use caution in post-op patients or surgical outpatients. ▪ Withdrawal symptoms may occur in nonopioid dependent patients if high doses of opioids are used during surgery. ▪ Serious adverse cardiovascular or respiratory effects may occur if opioids are used to overcome full blockade in treatment of withdrawal reactions.

Monitor: Before administration, establish a patent airway. Controlled artificial ventilation with oxygen may be indicated. Establish an IV line.

▪ Monitor vital signs and pupil dilation closely; ECG monitoring may be indicated. ▪ Continue to monitor until no reasonable risk of recurrent respiratory depression. ▪ Note Precautions and Drug/lab interactions.

Patient education: Notify physician if pain control medication not adequately effective.

Maternal/child: Pregnancy Category B: use only if clearly needed. ▪ Human studies not available, but was secreted into rat's milk; probably best to postpone breast feeding for 12 to 24 hours. ▪ Safety for use in children and neonates not yet established.

Elderly: No specific recommendations for single episodes of reversal. ▪ Note Precautions.

DRUG/LAB INTERACTIONS

Propoxyphene, methadone, and levo-alpha-acetylmethadol (LAMM) have longer half-lives than nalmefene; observe patient closely. ▪ Reversal of buprenorphine (Buprenex)-induced respiratory depression may be incomplete and require mechanically assisted ventilation. ▪ No adverse interactions to this date with benzodiazepines (e.g., diazepam [Valium], midazolam [Versed]), inhalation anesthetics (e.g., halothane), muscle relaxants (e.g., doxacurium [Nuromax]), and muscle relaxant antagonists (e.g., edrophonium [Enlon], neostigmine [Prostigmin]). ▪ May be an increased risk of seizures with flumazenil (Romazicon).

SIDE EFFECTS

Incidence of side effects is dose related. Many side effects may be caused by abrupt reversal of the effects of the opioid. Hypertension, nausea and vomiting, and tachycardia occur most frequently. Blurred vision, chills, diarrhea, dizziness, drowsiness, fatigue, fever, headache, hypotension, irritability, pain, paranoia, tremor, and vasodilation may occur. Arrhythmias (including bradycardia, tachycardia, VT and VF) and pulmonary edema have occurred.

ANTIDOTE

Notify the physician of any side effect. Treatment will probably be symptomatic. Resuscitate as necessary.

NALOXONE HYDROCHLORIDE

Narcan

Antidote
Narcotic antagonist

pH 3.0 to 4.0

USUAL DOSE

Narcotic overdose: 0.4 to 2 mg. Repeat in 2 to 3 minutes if indicated. The diagnosis of narcotic overdose should be questioned if no response is observed after 10 mg of naloxone. If effective, dosage may be repeated as necessary for recurrence of symptoms.

Postoperative narcotic depression: 0.1 to 0.2 mg at 2- to 3-minute intervals to desired response. Titrate to avoid excessive reduction of narcotic analgesic action.

PEDIATRIC DOSE

Ampoules containing 0.02 mg/ml are available, but larger doses are frequently required. Adult strength is often used to reduce amount of injection and to effect desired response which may require increased or repeat doses. One source states "up to 10 times a dose has been required."

Narcotic overdose: Less than 20 kg: 0.01 to 0.1 mg/kg of body weight initially. Based on estimated degree of overdose and respiratory depression. May repeat every 2 to 3 minutes. May dilute with SW. American Academy of Pediatrics recommends 0.1 mg/kg. Manufacturer recommends 0.01 mg/kg.

Over 20 kg or over 5 years of age: 2 mg. Repeat every 2 to 3 minutes as necessary. A continuous infusion may be used after the initial effective dose. Add 75% to 100% of effective dose to a specific amount of IV fluid and run evenly distributed over 1 hour. For some overdoses (e.g., methadone) weaning in 50% increments may take up to 48 hours. In other situations 6 to 12 hours is adequate. If symptoms recur, rebolus and go back to 100%.

Postoperative narcotic depression: 0.005 to 0.01 mg IV at 2- to 3-minute intervals to desired response.

NEONATAL DOSE

0.01 mg/kg of body weight. Administration into umbilical vein is preferred.

DILUTION

May be given undiluted, diluted with sterile water for injection, or further diluted in NS or D5W and given as an infusion (2 mg in 500 ml equals a concentration of 0.004 mg/ml). Discard infusions after 24 hours.

Storage: Store below 40° C. Protect from light

INCOMPATIBLE WITH

Limited information available. Bisulfites, sulfites, long-chain or high-molecular-weight anions, solutions with an alkaline pH. Confirm physical and chemical stability before mixing with any drug or agent.

RATE OF ADMINISTRATION

Each 0.4 mg or fraction thereof over 15 seconds. Titrate infusion to patient response.

ACTIONS

A potent narcotic antagonist. Overcomes effects of narcotic overdose including respiratory depression, sedation, and hypotension. Unlike other narcotic antagonists, it does not have any narcotic effect itself. Onset of action is within 2 minutes. Duration of action is dependent on dose and route of naloxone administration. Requirement for repeat doses is dependent on amount, type, and route of narcotic administration. Metabolized in the liver and excreted in urine.

INDICATIONS AND USES

Reversal of narcotic depression. ▪ Antidote for natural and synthetic narcotics, (e.g., butorphanol, methadone, nalbuphine, pentazocine, and propoxyphene). ▪ Diagnosis of acute opiate overdose.

Investigational uses: Reversal of alcoholic coma and improvement of circulation in refractory shock.

CONTRAINDICATIONS

Known hypersensitivity to naloxone.

PRECAUTIONS

Does not produce respiratory depression with nonnarcotic drug overdose, a beneficial action. ▪ It is ineffective against respiratory depression caused by barbiturates, anesthetics, other nonnarcotic agents, or pathologic conditions. ▪ Will precipitate acute withdrawal symptoms in narcotic addicts; use caution, especially with newborns of narcotic-dependent mothers. ▪ Use caution in patients with cardiac disease or those receiving cardiotoxic drugs.

Monitor: Symptomatic treatment with oxygen and artificial ventilation as necessary should be continued until naloxone is effective. Observe patient continuously. Duration of narcotic action may exceed that of naloxone.

Maternal/child: Pregnancy Category B: use in pregnancy and lactation only when clearly needed. Safety for use not established. ▪ Note Precautions.

SIDE EFFECTS

Elevated partial thromboplastin time (occasional), hypertension, irritability and increased crying in the newborn, nausea and vomiting, sweating, tachycardia, tremulousness. Overdose postoperatively may result in excitement, hypertension, hypotension, reversal of analgesia, pulmonary edema, ventricular tachycardia and fibrillation.

ANTIDOTE

Notify the physician of any side effect. Treatment will probably be symptomatic. Resuscitate as necessary.

NEOSTIGMINE METHYLSULFATE

Cholinergic
Cholinesterase inhibitor
Antidote
Antimyasthenic

Prostigmin

pH 5.9

USUAL DOSE

Muscle relaxant antagonist: 0.5 to 2 mg. Repeat as required to restore voluntary respiration. 5 mg is the normal maximum total dose. Adminster atropine sulfate, 0.6 to 1.2 mg for each 0.5 to 2 mg of neostigmine. Administer in a separate syringe a few minutes before neostigmine. Use caution and monitor pulse rate. Pulse rate must be at least 80 beats/min. Alternately, glycopyrolate 0.2 mg for each 1 mg of neostigmine can be used and can be mixed in the same syringe as neostigmine.

Treatment of myasthenia gravis: 0.5 mg; titrate carefully; usually given IM.

PEDIATRIC DOSE

Muscle relaxant antagonist: 40 mcg (0.04 mg)/kg of body weight with 20 mcg (0.02 mg)/kg of atropine. An alternate dose regimen is *infants:* 0.025 to 0.1 mg/kg with atropine 0.0125 to 0.05 mg/kg. *Children:* 0.025 to 0.08 mg/kg with atropine 0.0125 to 0.04 mg/kg. Maximum dose is 2.5 mg. Glycopyrolate 0.2 mg for each 1 mg of neostigmine can be used instead of atropine. Note all comments under Usual dose.

Treatment of myasthenia gravis: 0.01 to 0.04 mg/kg. May repeat every 2 to 3 hours. Usually given IM.

DOSE ADJUSTMENTS

Use extreme caution and minimum effective dose in small children, cardiac disease, asthma, epilepsy, hypothyroidism, vagotonia, peptic ulcer, and severely ill patients. Titrate exact dose; evaluate response with a peripheral nerve stimulator device.

DILUTION

Confirm ampoule or vial is for IV use. May be given undiluted. Do not add to IV solutions. May be given through Y-tube or three-way stopcock of infusion set.

Storage: Store below 40° C. Protect from light.

INCOMPATIBLE WITH

Limited information available. Because of specific use and potential toxicity, neostigmine should not be mixed with any other drug.

RATE OF ADMINISTRATION

0.5 mg or fraction thereof over 1 minute.

ACTIONS

An anticholinesterase and antagonist of non-depolarizing neuromuscular blocking agents. Inhibits the enzyme cholinesterase, allowing acetylcholine to accumulate at the myoneural junction. Restores normal transmission of nerve impulses and makes muscle contraction stronger and more prolonged. Onset of action is 4 to 8 minutes. Duration of action is 2 to 4 hours. Hydrolyzed by cholinesterases and metabolized by microsomal enzymes in the liver. Excreted primarily in urine.

INDICATIONS AND USES

Antidote for nondepolarizing muscle relaxants (e.g., doxacurium [Nuromax], mivacurium [Mivacron], tubocurarine [Curare]), atropine, hyoscine. ■ Treatment of myasthenia gravis.

CONTRAINDICATIONS

High concentrations of inhalant anesthesia (e.g., halothane, cyclopropane); known sensitivity to bromides and neostigmine, mechanical intestinal or urinary obstruction, peritonitis.

PRECAUTIONS

A physician should be present when this drug is used IV. ■ Has many additional uses given IM or orally. ■ Edrophonium (Tensilon) can differentiate between myasthenic and cholinergic crisis. ■ Note Dose Adjustments.

Monitor: A peripheral nerve stimulator device should be used to monitor effectiveness. ■ *Caution:* Atropine may mask symptoms of neostigmine overdose. ■ Epinephrine should always be available. ■ Hyperventilate the patient. ■ Note Dose adjustments and Drug/lab interactions.

Maternal/child: Pregnancy Category C: may induce premature labor in pregnancy near term. ■ Transient muscular weakness in swallowing, sucking, and breathing has been observed in neonates of myasthenic mothers. Confirm distinction between cholinergic or myasthenic crisis in neonate with edrophonium test. Treat neonate with IM pyridostigmine 0.05 to 0.15 mg/kg of body weight if indicated. ■ Discontinue breast feeding.

Elderly: Duration of antagonism of neuromuscular blockade prolonged.

DRUG/LAB INTERACTIONS

Potentiates narcotic analgesics (e.g., morphine, codeine, meperidine) and succinylcholine (Anectine). ■ Antagonized by ganglionic blocking agents (e.g., trimethaphan [Arfonad], guanethedine [Ismelin], mecamylamine [Inversine]) and aminoglycoside antibiotics (e.g., gentamycin [Garamycin]). ■ May be inhibited by corticosteroids and magnesium.

SIDE EFFECTS

Usually caused by overdose: abdominal cramps, anorexia, anxiety, bradycardia, cardiac arrhythmias and arrest, cholinergic crises, cold moist skin, convulsion, diaphoresis, diarrhea, hypotension, increased bronchial secretions, increased lacrimation, increased salivation, miosis, muscle cramps, muscle weakness, nausea, pulmonary edema, vomiting.

ANTIDOTE

Atropine sulfate. If side effects occur, discontinue drug and notify the physician. Atropine sulfate in doses of 0.6 mg IV will counteract most side effects and may be repeated every 3 to 10 minutes. Endotracheal intubation or tracheostomy is considered prophylactic in anesthesia or crises. Artificial ventilation, oxygen therapy, cardiac monitoring, adequate suctioning, and treatment of shock or convulsions must be instituted and maintained as necessary. Treat allergic reactions with epinephrine. Pralidoxime chloride (PAM) 2 Gm IV followed by 250 mg every 5 minutes may be required to reactivate cholinesterase and reverse paralysis.

NETILMICIN SULFATE

**Antibacterial
(Aminoglycoside)**

Netromycin

pH 3.5 to 6.0

USUAL DOSE

1.5 to 3.25 mg/kg of body weight every 12 hours. 1.3 to 2.2 mg/kg every 8 hours in serious systemic infections. Dose based on ideal body weight. Adjust according to severity of infection and to peak and trough concentrations. Recent studies suggest that a total daily dose adminstered as a single dose (instead of divided into 2 ro 3 doses) may provide higher peak levels and enhance drug effectiveness while actually reducing or having no adverse effects on risk of toxicity.

PEDIATRIC DOSE

6 weeks to 12 years: 1.8 to 2.7 mg/kg of body weight every 8 hours or 2.7 to 4 mg/kg every 12 hours. Note caution in Dilution.

NEONATAL DOSE

2 to 3.25 mg/kg of body weight every 12 hours. Lower doses may be appropriate because of immature kidney function. Note caution in Dilution.

DOSE ADJUSTMENTS

Reduce daily dose commensurate with amount of renal impairment and/or increase intervals between injections. See manufacturer's specific recommendations. ▪ Reduced dose or extended intervals may be required in the elderly. ▪ Note Monitor and Drug/lab interactions.

DILUTION

Further dilute each single dose in 50 to 200 ml of NS, D5W, D5/NS, or other compatible solutions (see literature).

Pediatric dilution: Pediatric and neonatal concentrations have been discontinued. Use extreme caution to ensure correct dose for neonates and children. Begin with 100 mg/ml concentration for adults, measure with a tuberculin or insulin syringe (e.g., a 3 kg [6½ lb] infant would receive a dose of 6 to 9.75 mg [0.06 to 0.0975 ml] every 12 hours). Decrease volume of diluent for neonates and children based on fluid requirements. Concentrations of 2 to 3 mg/ml acceptable.

Storage: Stable for up to 72 hours.

INCOMPATIBLE WITH

Administer separately. Inactivated in solution with carbenicillin, other penicillins, and most cephalosporins. Allopurinol (Zyloprim), amphotericin B, cefamandole (Mandol), cephalothin (Keflin), dopamine (Intropin), furosemide (Lasix), heparin.

RATE OF ADMINISTRATION

Each single dose over 30 minutes to 2 hours.

ACTIONS

An aminoglycoside antibiotic with neuromuscular blocking action. Bactericidal against specific gram-positive and gram-negative bacilli by interfering with protein synthesis. Well distributed throughout all body fluids. Usual half-life is 2 to 3 hours; half-life prolonged in infants, postpartum females, fever, liver disease and ascites, spinal cord injury, cystic fibrosis, and the elderly; shorter in severe burns. Crosses the placental barrier. Excreted through the kidneys. Secreted in breast milk.

INDICATIONS AND USES

Short-term treatment of serious infections caused by specific organisms. ■ Primarily used when penicillin and other less toxic antibiotics are ineffective or contraindicated. ■ To treat suspected infection in the immuno-suppressed patient. ■ Has been used in patients with previous neurotoxic reactions to aminoglycosides without further toxicity.

CONTRAINDICATIONS

Known netilmicin or aminoglycoside sensitivity, renal failure. Sulfite sensitivity may be a contraindication.

PRECAUTIONS

Use extreme caution if therapy is required over 7 to 10 days; ototoxic and nephrotoxic. ■ Sensitivity studies indicated to determine susceptibility of the causative organism to netilmicin. ■ Superinfection may occur from overgrowth of nonsusceptible organisms. ■ Use caution in infants, children, the elderly, and severely burned patients. ■ Use extreme caution in patients with end-stage renal disease. ■ Contains sulfites and benzyl alcohol. Use caution in patients with asthma. May cause fatal "gasping syndrome" in premature infants.

Monitor: Narrow range between toxic and therapeutic levels. Periodically monitor peak and trough concentrations to avoid peak serum concentrations above 16 mcg/ml and trough concentrations above 4 mcg/ml. Desired range is 6 to 10 and 0.5 to 2 mcg/ml, respectively. ■ Watch for decrease in urine output and rising BUN and serum creatinine. Dose may require decreasing. ■ Routine serum levels and evaluation of hearing are recommended. ■ Maintain good hydration. ■ Monitor serum calcium, magnesium, potassium, and sodium; levels may decline. Depressed levels have caused mental confusion, paresthesia, positive Chvostek and Trousseau signs (provoked spasm of facial and other muscles; occurs in tetany), and tetany in adults; muscle weaknesses and tetany in infants.

■ In extended treatment, monitoring of serum levels, electrolytes, renal, auditory, and vestibular functions daily is recommended. ■ Note Drug/lab interactions.

Patient education: Report promptly dizziness, hearing loss, weakness, or any changes in balance. ■ Consider birth control options.

Maternal/child: Category D: avoid pregnancy. ■ Use during lactation only if absolutely necessary; safety not established. ■ Use with extreme caution in neonates; renal immaturity will prolong half-life. ■ Peak concentrations are generally lower in infants and young children. ■ Note Precautions.

Elderly: Consider less toxic alternatives. ■ Longer intervals between doses may be more important than reduced doses. ■ Monitor renal function and drug levels carefully. Measurement of creatinine clearance more useful than BUN or serum creatinine to assess renal function. ■ Half-life prolonged.

DRUG/LAB INTERACTIONS

Inactivated in solution with penicillins but is synergistic when used in combination with beta-lactam antibiotics (e.g., sulbactam sodium, clavulanate potassium, cephalosporins, penicillins), and vancomycin. Dose adjustment and appropriate spacing required because of physical incompatibilities and interactions. Synergism may be inconsistent; measure aminoglycoside levels. ■ Concurrent use topically or systemically with any other ototoxic or nephrotoxic agents should be avoided. May have dangerous additive effects with anesthetics (e.g., enflurane), other neuromuscular blocking antibiotics (e.g., kanamycin), diuretics (e.g., furosemide [Lasix]), beta-lactam antibiotics (e.g., cephalosporins), vancomycin, and many others. ■ Neuromuscular blocking muscle relaxants (e.g., doxacurium [Nuromax]), succinylcholine [Anectine]) are potentiated by aminoglycosides. ***Apnea can occur.*** ■ Aminoglycosides are also potentiated by anticholinesterases (e.g., edrophonium), antineoplastics (e.g., nitrogen mustard, cisplatin). ■ May be antagonized by bacteriostatic antibiotics (e.g., chloramphenicol, erythromycin, and tetracyclines); bactericidal action may be impacted. ■ Note Side effects.

SIDE EFFECTS

Occur more frequently with impaired renal function, dehydration, higher doses, prolonged administration, in the elderly, and in patients receiving other ototoxic or nephrotoxic drugs.

Minor: Anorexia, burning, dizziness, fever, headache, hypertension, hypotension, itching, lethargy, muscle twitching, nausea, numbness, rash, roaring in ears, tingling sensation, tinnitus, urticaria, vomiting, weight loss.

Major: Blood dyscrasias; convulsions; elevated alkaline phosphatase, bilirubin, BUN, serum creatinine, AST (SGOT), and ALT (SGPT); hearing loss; laryngeal edema; neuromuscular blockade; oliguria; respiratory depression or arrest.

ANTIDOTE

Notify the physician of all side effects. If minor side effects persist or any major symptom appears, discontinue the drug and notify physician. Treatment is symptomatic. In overdose, hemodialysis may be indicated. Monitor fluid balance, creatinine clearance, and plasma levels carefully. Complexation with ticarcillin or carbenicillin (12 to 30 Gm/day) may be as effective as hemodialysis. Consider exchange transfusion in the newborn. Calcium salts or neostigmine may reverse neuromuscular blockade. Resuscitate as necessary.

NICARDIPINE HYDROCHLORIDE

Calcium channel blocker
Antihypertensive

Cardene IV   pH 3.5

USUAL DOSE

Must be individualized based on the severity of hypertension and the response of each patient. Blood pressure decrease is dependent on the rate of infusion and frequency of dose adjustments. Gradual reduction based on clinical situation is best. Avoid too-rapid or excessive drop in blood pressure.

To substitute for oral nicardipine therapy: 5 ml diluted solution/hr (0.5 mg/hr) will achieve similar plasma concentration to an oral dose of 20 mg every 8 hours; 12 ml/hr (1.2 mg/hr) to an oral dose of 30 mg every 8 hours; 22 ml/hr (2.2 mg/hr) to an oral dose of 40 mg every 8 hours.

Gradual reduction of blood pressure in a drug-free patient: Initiate therapy with diluted solution at 50 ml/hr (5.0 mg/hr). May be increased by 25 ml/hr (2.5 mg/hr) every 15 minutes until desired blood pressure reduction is achieved. Do not exceed 150 ml/hr (15 mg/hr).

Rapid reduction of blood pressure in a drug-free patient: Initiate at 50 ml/hr as above, but increases of 25 ml/hr may be given every 5 minutes until desired blood pressure reduction is achieved. Do not exceed 150 ml/hr of diluted solution.

Maintenance: When desired blood pressure is achieved, reduce rate to 30 ml/hr (3 mg/hr). This is the average maintenance rate. Adjust as needed to maintain desired response.

Transfer to an oral antihypertensive agent: The first dose of oral Cardene should be given 1 hour before discontinuing infusion. Initiate any other oral antihypertensive agent on discontinuation of infusion.

DOSE ADJUSTMENTS

Lower doses and slower titration suggested in congestive heart failure and impaired hepatic or renal function.

DILUTION

Each ampoule (25 mg in 10 ml) must be diluted with 240 ml of compatible infusion solution to equal a concentration of 0.1 mg/ml. Compatible in 0.45NS, NS, D5W, D5/0.45NS, D5/NS. Also compatible in D5W with 40 mEq of potassium added.

Storage: Store ampoules in carton, protected from light at controlled room temperature. Has a light yellow color. Diluted solution is stable at room temperature for 24 hours.

INCOMPATIBLE WITH

Lactated Ringer's injection, sodium bicarbonate.

RATE OF ADMINISTRATION

Must be administered as a slow continuous infusion in a concentration of 0.1 mg/ml (25 mg in 250 ml). Adjust as indicated in Usual dose and Dose adjustments.

ACTIONS

The first dihydropyridine calcium channel blocker for IV use. Lowers blood pressure by blocking the entry of calcium ions into the blood vessels. Does not alter serum calcium. Causes coronary and peripheral blood vessels to dilate and relax, reducing systemic vascular resistance. Increases cardiac output, coronary blood flow, and myocardial oxygen supply without increasing cardiac oxygen demand. Reduces blood pressure without significantly affecting cardiac conduction and usually does not depress cardiac function. Begins to reduce blood pressure in minutes; achieves 50% of ultimate decrease in 45 minutes but may not reach final steady state for 24 to 48 hours. When discontinued, can lose 50% of effect within 30 minutes, but gradually decreasing effects persist for up to 50 hours. Effects more prominent in hypertensive than in normotensive volunteers. Extensively metabolized in the liver. Excreted in urine and feces. Crosses placental barrier. Secreted in breast milk.

INDICATIONS AND USES

Short-term treatment of hypertension when oral therapy is not feasible or not desirable. ■ Continuation of hypertensive therapy in chronic hypertensive patients in critical care, surgery, or emergency room.

CONTRAINDICATIONS

Advanced aortic stenosis (reduced diastolic pressure may worsen rather than improve myocardial oxygen balance), hypersensitivity.

PRECAUTIONS

Use caution in patients with coronary artery disease. May cause increase in frequency, duration, or severity of angina. Has improved left ventricle function after beta-blockade. ■ Can lead to worsened failure in congestive heart failure, especially with severe left ventricle dysfunction or use of beta-blockers. ■ Use caution in hypertension of pheochromocytoma; limited experience. ■ May increase hepatic venous pressure; use caution in patients with portal hypertension. ■ Use caution in impaired hepatic or renal function; lower doses indicated. ■ Continue regular dosing on day of surgery and thereafter unless otherwise specified by physician. May cause severe angina or MI if discontinued.

Monitor: Avoid too-rapid or excessive reduction in either systolic or diastolic blood pressure. Monitor blood pressure during and after infusion. ■ If administered via a peripheral vein, change infusion site every 12 hours. ■ Transfer to oral therapy as soon as clinical condition permits. ■ Note Precautions and Drug/lab interactions.

Patient education: Request assistance to change position or ambulate.

Maternal/child: Category C: use during pregnancy only if benefit justifies risk. ■ Discontinue breast feeding. ■ Safety for use in children under 18 not established.

Elderly: Half-life may be prolonged. ■ May cause drug-induced tinnitus.

DRUG/LAB INTERACTIONS

Not a beta-blocker; when used in conjunction with beta-blockers (e.g., atenolol [Tenormin], metoprolol [Lopressor]), beta-blocker withdrawal must be gradual. ■ Cimetidine (Tagamet) increases nicardipine plasma concentrations; monitor carefully. ■ May alter digoxin plasma levels; monitor serum digoxin. ■ May cause hypotension during fentanyl anesthesia if used concomitantly with a beta-blocker; an increased volume of circulating fluids may be required. ■ Will increase plasma levels of cyclosporine (Sandimmune); monitor and decrease cyclosporine dose if indicated. ■ Plasma protein binding of nicardipine not altered with therapeutic concentrations of furosemide (Lasix), propranolol (Inderal), dipyridamole (Persantine), warfarin (Coumadin), quinidine, or naproxen (Naprosyn).

SIDE EFFECTS

Average dose: Generally not serious and are expected consequences of vasodilation; dizziness (1.4%), ECG abnormality including PVCs (1.4%), headache (14.6%), hypotension (5.6%), nausea and vomiting (4.8%), polyuria (1.4%), postural hypotension (1.4%), sweating (1.4%), tachycardia (3.5%). Many other side effects occurred in less than 1% of patients.

Overdose: Bradycardia, confusion, drowsiness, flushing, hypotension (marked), palpitations, slurred speech. Progressive AV block may occur with lethal overdose.

ANTIDOTE

Keep physician informed of all side effects. Headache, hypotension, and tachycardia have required a reduction in dose or discontinuation of nicardipine. When symptoms subside, nicardipine may be restarted at low doses (e.g., 30 to 50 ml/hr) and adjusted to maintain desired blood pressure. In overdose monitor blood pressure, cardiac and respiratory functions; put patients in Trendelenburg position; use vasopressors (e.g., dopamine [Intropin]), for excessive hypotension. IV calcium gluconate may reverse effects of calcium entry blockade.

NITROGLYCERIN IV

Antianginal
Antihypertensive
Vasodilator

Nitro-Bid IV, Nitrostat IV, Tridil   pH 3.0 to 6.5

USUAL DOSE

5 mcg/min initially. Increase by 5 mcg/min increments every 3 to 5 minutes until some blood pressure response is noted. Reduce increments and/or increase time to fine-tune to desired hemodynamic response. If no response at 20 mcg/min, 10 mcg/min increases may be used. Increases of up to 20 mcg/min have been used to achieve desired effect. No fixed optimum dose. Tolerance may develop if administered over 12 to 24 hours.

Unstable angina and congestive heart failure associated with MI: 10 to 20 mcg/min; increase by 5 to 10 mcg/min every 5 to 10 minutes until desired hemodynamic response (current JAMA recommendations).

PEDIATRIC DOSE

0.25 to 0.5 mcg/kg/min initially. May increase by 0.5 to 1 mcg/kg/min increments every 3 to 5 minutes until desired response. Note Maternal/child.

DOSE ADJUSTMENTS

Reduced dose may be required with persistent headache unrelieved by analgesics. Reduce dose gradually when weaning to prevent rebound symptoms.

DILUTION

Available premixed in 250 ml D5W with 25, 50, or 100 mg nitroglycerin or 500 ml with 50, 100, or 200 mg nitroglycerin. All other preparations must be diluted and administered as an infusion. Use only non-PVC plastic or glass infusion bottles and specific (nonpolyvinyl chloride) infusion tubing (provided by manufacturer). Do not use filters. Dilute in a given amount of D5W or NS for infusion. Concentration dependent on initial preparation (0.5 mg/ml or 5 mg/ml) and patient fluid tolerances. 10 ml of 0.5 mg/ml in 250 ml diluent equals 20 mcg/ml (in 1,000 ml, 5 mcg/ml). 10 ml of 5 mg/ml in 250 ml diluent equals 200 mcg/ml (in 1,000 ml, 50 mcg/ml).

See dilution chart, p. 618

Diluent volume (ml)	Quantity of nitroglycerin (5 mg/ml)	Approximate final concentration (mcg/ml)
100	10 mg (2ml)	100
100	20 mg (4 ml)	200
100	40 mg (8 ml)	400
250	25 mg (5 ml)	100
250	50 mg (10 ml)	200
250	100 mg (20 ml)	400
500	50 mg (10 ml)	100
500	100 mg (20 ml)	200
500	200 mg (40 ml)	400

May be used in dilutions from 25 to 500 mcg/ml.

Pediatric dilution: 6 mg nitroglycerin in 100 ml D5W at an infusion rate of 1 ml/hr equals 1 mcg/kg/min.

Storage: Protect vials from light. Solution stable for up to 24 hours.

INCOMPATIBLE WITH

Manufacturer states, "Do not admix with any other drug." Alteplase (tPA), bretylium (Bretylate), hydralazine (Apresoline), phenytoin (Dilantin).

RATE OF ADMINISTRATION

Dependent on patient response and effective dose. Specific adjustments required; see Usual dose. Use extreme caution in patients responsive to initial 5 mcg/min dose. Decrease adjustments and increase time between doses as patient begins to respond. Use of an infusion pump or microdrip (60 gtt/ml) required. Exact and constant delivery mandatory.

Concentration (mcg/ml)	50	100	200	400
Desired dose (mcg/min)	60 microdrops = 1 ml Flow rate (microdrops/min = ml/hr)			
5	6	3	—	—
10	12	6	3	—
15	18	9	—	—
20	24	12	6	3
30	36	18	9	—
40	48	24	12	6
60	72	36	18	9
80	96	48	24	12
120	—	72	36	18
160	—	96	48	24
240	—	—	72	36

Concentration (mcg/ml)	50	100	200	400
Desired dose (mcg/min)	60 microdrops = 1 ml Flow rate (microdrops/min = ml/hr)			
320	—	—	96	48
480	—	—	—	72
640	—	—	—	96

ACTIONS

A vascular smooth-muscle relaxant and vasodilator. Affects arterial and venous beds. Reduces myocardial oxygen consumption, preload, and afterload by reducing systolic, diastolic, and mean arterial blood pressure; central venous and pulmonary capillary wedge pressures; and pulmonary and systemic vascular resistance. Effective coronary perfusion is usually maintained. Low doses (30 to 40 mcg/min) produce venodilation; high doses (150 to 500 mcg/min) produce arteriolar dilation. Widely distributed throughout the body. Onset of action occurs in 1 to 2 minutes and lasts 3 to 5 minutes. Metabolized in the liver and excreted in urine.

INDICATIONS AND USES

Control of blood pressure in perioperative hypertension (especially cardiovascular procedures). ■ Drug of choice in unstable angina or congestive heart failure associated with acute myocardial infarction. May be used in combination with dobutamine (Dobutrex) 2 to 20 mcg/kg/min to produce hemodynamic improvement while reducing risk of ischemic damage. ■ Treatment of angina pectoris if patient unresponsive to therapeutic doses of organic nitrates and/or a beta blocker. ■ Controlled hypotension during surgical procedures.

CONTRAINDICATIONS

Anemia (severe), hypersensitivity to nitrates, hypotension or uncorrected hypovolemia, cerebral hemorrhage, closed-angle glaucoma, head trauma, increased intracranial pressure, pericardial tamponade, constrictive pericarditis.

PRECAUTIONS

Use caution in patients who may be using sildenafil citrate (Viagra). See Drug/lab interactions. ■ Special tubing causes problems with infusion pump control. Patient may still be receiving nitroglycerin even though pump is off or tubing clamped. Low flow rates may actually be higher and not deliver accurate dosage. ■ Plastic (polyvinyl chloride) tubing or containers will absorb up to 80% of diluted nitroglycerin. Use extreme caution and adjust dose if changing tubing, using extension tubings, etc. Absorption greatest with slowest rate. ■ If changing preparations from 0.8 mg/ml to 5.0 mg/ml, use new tubing or clear tubing with a minimum of 15 ml, adjust dose carefully, and observe effects. ■ Use caution in patients with low left ventricular filling pressure or low pulmonary capillary wedge pressure. May have exaggerated response to low dosage. ■ Use caution in hepatic or renal disease, pericarditis, or postural hypotension.

Monitor: Maintain adequate systemic blood pressure and coronary perfusion pressure. Heart rate and blood pressure measurements man-

datory; pulmonary wedge pressure recommended. ▪ Observe for tachycardia, which can decrease diastolic filling time. ▪ Observe for fall in
pulmonary wedge pressure. Precedes arterial hypotension and impending
shock. Reduce or discontinue drug temporarily. ▪ Headache may
improve with analgesics or slightly lower dose; usually improves with
time. ▪ Note Drug/lab interactions.

Maternal/child: Pregnancy Category C: safety for use in pregnancy,
lactation, and in children not established.

Elderly: Hypotensive effects may be increased. ▪ Consider age-related
renal impairment.

DRUG/LAB INTERACTIONS

May cause irreversible hypotension if given within 24 hours of sildenafil
citrate (Viagra). ▪ Potentiated by alcohol (may cause hypotension and
cardiovascular collapse), antihypertensives, aspirin, beta-adrenergic
blockers (e.g., propranolol [Inderal]), other vasodilators, phenothiazines
(e.g., prochlorperazine [Compazine]), and tricyclic antidepressants.
▪ Inhibited by dihydroergotamine and sympathomimetics (e.g., vasopressors [phenylephrine], bronchodilators, decongestants, glaucoma
agents, mydriatics). ▪ Inhibits acetylcholine, histamine, norepinephrine.
▪ Potentiates nondepolarizing muscle relaxants (e.g., tubocurarine
[Curare]); may cause apnea. ▪ May cause marked orthostatic hypotension with calcium channel blockers (e.g., verapamil [Isoptin]). ▪ May
antagonize anticoagulant effects of heparin; monitor. ▪ Concurrent use
with alteplase (tPA); reduces the thrombolytic effects of alteplase.

SIDE EFFECTS

Abdominal pain, allergic reactions (e.g., itching, tracheobronchitis,
wheezing), angina, apprehension, dizziness, headache, hypotension,
methemoglobinemia, muscle twitching, nausea, palpitations, postural
hypotension, restlessness, retrosternal discomfort, tachycardia, vomiting.

Overdose: Bloody diarrhea, colic, confusion, diaphoresis, dyspnea,
flushing, heart block, paralysis, tachycardia, visual disturbances. Severe
hypotension may result in shock, reflex paradoxical bradycardia,
inadequate cerebral circulation, constrictive pericarditis, pericardial
tamponade, decreased organ perfusion, and death.

ANTIDOTE

Notify physician of all side effects. Discontinue if blurred vision or
dry mouth occur. For accidental overdose with severe hypotension and
reflex tachycardia and/or fall in pulmonary wedge pressure, reduce
rate or temporarily discontinue until condition stabilizes. Lower head
of bed (Trendelenburg position). Administer IV fluids. Use O_2 and
assisted ventilation if indicated. An alpha-adrenergic agonist (methoxamine [Vasoxyl] or phenylephrine [Neo-Synephrine]) is rarely
required. Epinephrine and related compounds (dopamine) are contraindicated. Monitor levels and treat methemoglobinemia if indicated with
methylene blue 0.2 ml/kg of body weight (1 to 2 mg/kg) IV and
high-flow oxygen. Treat anaphylaxis and resuscitate as necessary.

NITROPRUSSIDE SODIUM

Antihypertensive
Vasodilator

Nitropress

pH 3.5 to 6.0

USUAL DOSE

Begin with 0.3 mcg/kg of body weight/min. Under continuous blood pressure monitoring, titrate upward very gradually (small increments every 2 to 3 minutes). 3 mcg/kg/min is the average effective dose; range is 0.1 to 5 mcg/kg/min. Small adjustments can lead to major fluctuations in blood pressure. Never exceed 10 mcg/kg/min. If 10 mcg/kg/min does not promote adequate blood pressure reduction in 10 minutes, discontinue administration and use another antihypertensive agent. Cyanide toxicity can occur with as little as 2 mcg/kg/min and could begin to occur after 10 minutes at the maximum dose.

Acute CHF: Titrate as above until one of the following occurs: cardiac output is no longer increasing, perfusion of vital organs would be compromised by further reduction of BP, or maximum infusion rate (10 mcg/kg/min) is reached.

PEDIATRIC DOSE

Begin with 0.3 mcg/kg/min. Adjust slowly to individual response as in Usual dose.

DOSE ADJUSTMENTS

Average effective dose may be as little as 0.5 mcg/kg/min in patients who are receiving other antihypertensive agents by any route.
■ Reduced dose may be required in the elderly.

DILUTION

Each 50 mg must be dissolved with 2 to 3 ml of D5W or sterile water for injection without a preservative. Further dilute this stock solution in a minimum of 250 ml of D5W (manufacturer's recommendation). JAMA suggests NS may be used. Must be administered as an infusion. Larger amounts of solution may be used. 50 mg in 250 ml equals 200 mcg/ml. 50 mg in 500 ml equals 100 mcg/ml. Immediately after mixing, wrap infusion bottle in opaque material (e.g., aluminum foil) to protect from light. Use only freshly prepared solutions; usually discard infusion within 4 hours of mixing. (Literature now states "stable for 24 hours if properly protected.") ■ Solution has a faint brownish tint; discard immediately if highly colored, blue, green, or dark red.

Pediatric dilution: Add 0.6 mg/kg to 100 ml diluent. 1 ml/hr equals 0.1 mcg/kg/min.

INCOMPATIBLE WITH

Haloperidol (Haldol). Manufacturer recommends dilution in D5W only.

COMPATIBLE WITH

Additive: Esmolol in D5W if protected from light.

Y-site: Amrinone (Inocor), atracurium (Tracrium), diltiazem (Cardizem), dobutamine (Dobutrex), dopamine (Intropin), enalaprilat (Vasotec IV), famotidine (Pepcid IV), heparin, indomethacin (Indocin), lidocaine, nitroglycerin, pancuronium (Pavulon), tacrolimus (Prograf), vecuronium (Norcuron). Consult pharmacist to confirm; studies are recent.

RATE OF ADMINISTRATION

Use of an infusion pump (volumetric preferred) required to regulate dose accurately. Increase mcg/kg/min rate as outlined in Usual dose to reduce blood pressure gradually to preset or desired levels. Do not exceed maximum dose. Response should be noted almost immediately. Manufacturer provides an infusion rate chart in ml/hr to achieve initial (0.3 mcg/kg/min) and maximal (10 mcg/kg/min) for 50, 100, and 200 mcg/ml dilutions.

Volume		250 ml		500 ml		1000ml	
sodium nitroprusside		50 mg		50 mg		50 mg	
injection concentration		200 mcg/ml		100 mcg/ml		50 mcg/ml	
pt weight							
kg	lbs	init	max	init	max	init	max
10	22	1	30	2	60	4	120
20	44	2	60	4	120	7	240
30	66	3	90	5	180	11	360
40	88	4	120	7	240	14	480
50	110	5	150	9	300	18	600
60	132	5	180	11	360	22	720
70	154	6	210	13	420	25	840
80	176	7	240	14	480	29	960
90	198	8	270	16	540	32	1080
100	220	9	300	18	600	36	1200

ACTIONS

A potent, rapid-acting antihypertensive agent. Produces peripheral vasodilation through direct action on smooth muscle of the blood vessels. Effective almost immediately. Will lower diastolic blood pressure 30% to 40% or more below pretreatment levels. May increase heart rate and/or cardiac output slightly. Effectiveness ends when IV infusion is stopped. Blood pressure will return to pretreatment levels in 1 to 10 minutes. Rapidly converted to thiocyanate and eventually excreted in the urine.

INDICATIONS AND USES

Drug of choice for hypertensive emergencies. ■ Cardiogenic shock. ■ Controlled hypotension during surgery. ■ Acute congestive heart failure.

Unlabeled: In combination with dopamine to reduce afterload in hypertensive patient with myocardial infarction. ■ Treatment of left ventricular failure in combination with oxygen, morphine, and a loop diuretic.

CONTRAINDICATIONS

Compensatory hypertension, e.g., arteriovenous shunt or coarctation of the aorta; known inadequate cerebral circulation; emergency surgery on moribund patients.

PRECAUTIONS

Use only when adequate personnel and appropriate equipment are available for continuous monitoring. ■ Precipitous decreases in blood pressure can occur quickly. Can lead to irreversible ischemic injuries or death. ■ Cyanide toxicity can occur with doses less than the average effective dose and will begin to occur as the maximum dose of 10 mcg/kg/min is approached. May be rapid, serious, and lethal. ■ Methemoglobinemia may begin to occur within 16 hours if larger doses are required. ■ Use caution in hypothyroidism, increased intracranial pressure, liver or renal impairment, and the elderly. ■ May increase ischemia in myocardial infarction.

Monitor: Determine patency of vein; avoid extravasation. ■ Continuous automatic blood pressure monitoring is mandatory (intra-arterial pressure sensor preferred). Never allow systolic blood pressure to fall below 60 mm Hg. ■ Monitor pulmonary wedge pressure in patients with myocardial infarction or severe congestive heart failure. ■ Oral antihypertensive agents may be given concomitantly to maintain ongoing blood pressure regulation. Reduced nitroprusside dose may be indicated (note Dose adjustments). ■ Measure blood thiocyanate levels daily if dose is 3 mcg/kg/min (1 mcg/kg/min in the anuric patient). Desired level of steady-state thiocyanate is less than 1 mmol/L. Co-administration of sodium thiosulfate in doses 5 to 10 times that of nitroprusside has been used to avoid toxicity with larger doses or necessary long-term therapy; may potentiate hypotensive action; use with extreme caution. ■ In controlled hypotension, monitor blood loss and correct hypovolemia before and during surgery. ■ Persistent hypotension (lasting more than 1 to 10 minutes) after nitroprusside is discontinued is due to another source. ■ Monitor for sodium retention.

Patient education: Report IV site burning or stinging promptly. ■ Request assistance to ambulate.

Maternal/child: Category C: safety for use in pregnancy and in children not yet established. Has caused cyanide toxicity in fetus of ewes, but not in humans. ■ Discontinue breast feeding.

Elderly: Note Dose adjustment and Precautions. ■ Hypotensive effects may be increased. ■ Consider age-related renal impairment.

DRUG/LAB INTERACTIONS

Potentiated by ganglionic blocking agents (e.g., trimethaphan [Arfonad]), volatile liquid anesthesia (e.g., halothane), and circulatory depressants. ■ Will cause profound hypotension with diazoxide (Hyperstat IV.)

SIDE EFFECTS

Usually occur with too-rapid rate of infusion and are reversible: abdominal pain, apprehension, bradycardia, coma, decreased platelet aggregation, diaphoresis, dizziness, ECG changes, flushing, headache, hypotension (profound), ileus, increased intracranial pressure, muscle twitching, nausea, palpitations, rash, restlessness, retching, retrosternal discomfort, venous streaking. With prolonged therapy or overdose, cyanide intoxication (air hunger, bright red venous blood, confusion, elevated cyanide levels, marked clinical deterioration, metabolic acidosis, and death), hypothyroidism, or methemoglobinemia (chocolate brown blood, impaired oxygen delivery even though cardiac output and arterial pO_2 are adequate) can occur.

ANTIDOTE

At first sign of side effects, decrease rate of administration. Never allow systolic blood pressure to fall below 60 mm Hg. If blood pressure begins to rise or side effects persist, notify the physician. Hemodialysis or peritoneal dialysis may be indicated for thiocyanate levels over 10 mg/dl. For massive overdose with signs of cyanide toxicity or tachyphylaxis, discontinue nitroprusside. Cyanide antidote kits contain all needed medications (see sodium nitrite/sodium thiosulfate monograph for complete information). Administer amyl nitrite inhalations for 15 to 30 seconds each minute until 3% sodium nitrite solution can be initiated as an IV infusion or immediately start the infusion (4 to 6 mg/kg) over 2 to 4 minutes. Monitor blood pressure carefully; may cause hypotension which will also require treatment. Next, inject sodium thiosulfate 150 to 200 mg/kg (usually about 12.5 Gm or 50 ml of the 25% solution) in 50 ml of 5% dextrose in water IV over 10 minutes. Observe patient. If signs of overdose reappear, may repeat the above process after 2 hours; but use one-half the original dosage. Sodium nitrite provides a buffer for cyanide by converting HgB into methemoglobin, sodium thiosulfate converts cyanide into thiocyanate which is then excreted in urine. For hypotension, slow or discontinue the IV and put the patient in Trendelenburg position. Should improve in 1 to 10 minutes. Correct hypotension with vasopressors (e.g., dopamine [Intropin]). Treat methemoglobinemia with methylene blue 1 to 2 mg/kg. Use with caution if considerable amounts of cyanide are bound to methemoglobin.

NOREPINEPHRINE   Vasopressor

Levarterenol bitartrate, Levophed   pH 3.0 to 4.5

USUAL DOSE

8 to 12 mcg/min initially (JAMA recommendation is 0.5 to 30 mcg/min), then adjust to maintain desired blood pressure range, usually 2 to 4 mcg/min. Larger doses may be given safely as long as the patient remains hypotensive and blood volume depletion is corrected. 2 mg bitartrate equals 1 mg of norepinephrine. All doses are expressed in terms of norepinephrine.

PEDIATRIC DOSE

1 to 2 mcg/min adjusted to maintain desired blood pressure.

DILUTION

Must be diluted in 250 to 1,000 ml of D5W. D5/NS and given as an IV infusion. 4 mg (4 ml) in 1 L of diluent equals 4 mcg/ml. Final concentration based on fluid volume requirements of the patient. Administration in a dextrose solution reduces loss of potency resulting from oxidation. Normal saline without dextrose is not recommended. Phentolamine (Regitine) 5 to 10 mg and/or heparin sodium to provide 100 to 200 units/hr may be added to the diluent to prevent any sloughing, necrosis, and/or thrombosis from slight leakage along the vein pathway.

INCOMPATIBLE WITH

Aminophyline amobarbital (Amytal), ampicillin (Polycillin), ascorbic acid, cephalothin (Keflin), cephapirin (Cefadyl), chlorpheniramine (Chlor-Trimeton), chlorothiazide (Diuril), diazepam (Valium), heparin, metaraminol (Aramine), methicillin (Staphcillin), oxytocin (Pitocin, Syntocinon), pentobarbital (Nembutal), phenobarbital (Luminal), phenytoin (Dilantin), secobarbital (Seconal), sodium bicarbonate, sodium iodide, streptomycin, tetracycline (Achromycin), thiopental (Pentothal), warfarin (Coumadin), whole blood.

RATE OF ADMINISTRATION

See Usual dose. Use the slowest possible flow rate to correct hypotension gradually and maintain adequate or preset blood pressure. Some response should be noted within 1 to 2 minutes of IV administration. Use of an infusion pump or microdrip (60 gtt/ml) is an aid to correct evaluation of dose. Reduce infusion rate gradually. Avoid sudden discontinuation.

Norepinephrine (Levophed) infusion rate						
Desired dose	4 mg in 1,000 ml D5W or D5/NS 2 mg in 500 ml D5W or D5/NS 4 mcg/ml			8 mg in 1,000 ml D5W or D5/NS 4 mg in 500 ml D5W or D5/NS 8 mcg/ml		
mcg/min	mcg/hr	ml/min	ml/hr	mcg/hr	ml/min	ml/hr
2	120	0.5	30	120	0.25	15
3	180	0.75	45	180	0.375	22.5
4	240	1	60	240	0.5	30
6	360	1.5	90	360	0.75	45
8	480	2	120	480	1	60
9	540	2.25	135	540	1.125	67.5
10	600	2.5	150	600	1.25	75
11	660	2.75	165	660	1.375	82.5
12	720	3	180	720	1.5	90

ACTIONS

Levarterenol is the levo-isomer of norepinephrine. It is a sympathomimetic drug that functions as a peripheral vasoconstrictor (alpha-adrenergic action) and inotropic stimulator of the heart and dilator of coronary arteries (beta-adrenergic action). Dilates the coronary arteries more than twice as much as epinephrine can. It is rapidly inactivated in the body by various enzymes and excreted in changed form in the urine.

INDICATIONS AND USES

All hypotensive states, including those associated with spinal anesthesia, blood reactions, drug reactions, hemorrhage, myocardial infarction, pheochromocytomectomy, septicemia, surgery, sympathectomy, and trauma. ■ Adjunct in treatment of cardiac arrest and profound hypotension.

CONTRAINDICATIONS

Do not use in hypotension from blood loss unless an emergency, in mesenteric or peripheral vascular thrombosis, or with cyclopropane or halothane (inhalant) anesthesia.

PRECAUTIONS

Whole blood or plasma should be given in a separate IV site. May be given through Y-tube connection. ▪ Use caution in the elderly and in those with peripheral vascular disease or ischemic heart disease. ▪ Use caution in previously hypertensive patients. Raise blood pressure no more than 40 mm Hg below preexisting systolic pressure. ▪ Use caution in patients with allergies; some formulations contain sulfites. ▪ Therapy may be continued until the patient can maintain his own blood pressure. Decrease dosage gradually.

Monitor: Check blood pressure every 2 minutes until stabilized at the desired level. Check every 5 minutes thereafter during therapy. Avoid hypertension. ▪ Observe for hypovolemia and replace fluids immediately. In an emergency, norepinephrine can be effective in a hypovolemic state before fluid replacement has been accomplished. ▪ Check flow rate and injection site constantly. ▪ Infusion should be through a large vein, preferably the antecubital vein, to prevent complications of prolonged peripheral vasoconstriction. Avoid veins in the hands, ankles, and legs. Use of the femoral vein may be considered. ▪ Causes severe tissue necrosis, sloughing, and gangrene. Insert a plastic IV catheter or similar intravascular device at least 6 inches long well into the large vein chosen to prevent extravasation into any surrounding tissue. Note Dilution. ▪ Blanching along the vein pathway is a preliminary sign of extravasation. Change the injection site. ▪ Note Drug/lab interactions.

Patient education: Report IV site burning or stinging promptly. ▪ Request assistance to ambulate.

Maternal/child: Pregnancy Category C: use only if clearly needed; benefits must outweigh risks. ▪ Use caution in lactation.

Elderly: Note Precautions.

DRUG/LAB INTERACTIONS

Pressor effects may be potentiated by amphetamines, anesthetics, antihistamines, tricyclic antidepressants (e.g., desipramine [Norpramine]), rauwolfia alkaloids (e.g., reserpine), thyroid preparations, and methylphenidate (Ritalin). ▪ May cause severe hypertension with ergot alkaloids and guanethidine (Ismelin), and severe prolonged hypertension with MAO inhibitors (e.g., selegiline [Eldepryl]). ▪ May cause hypotension and bradycardia with hydantoins (e.g., phenytoin [Dilantin]). ▪ Bretylium and halogenated hydrocarbon anesthetics (e.g., halothane) may cause serious arrhythmias. ▪ Interacts in numerous and sometimes contradictory ways with many drugs.

SIDE EFFECTS

Rare when used as directed; anxiety, arrhythmias (e.g., bradycardia and VT), chest pain, decreased cardiac output, dyspnea, headache, ischemia, necrosis caused by extravasation, pallor, photophobia, seizures, vomiting. Persistent headache may indicate overdose and severe hypertension. Gangrene has been reported.

ANTIDOTE

To prevent sloughing and necrosis in areas where extravasation has occurred, with a fine hypodermic needle inject 5 to 10 mg of phentolamine (Regitine) diluted in 10 to 15 ml of NS liberally throughout the tissue in the extravasated area. Treatment should be started as soon as extravasation is recognized. Atropine may be used to counteract the bradycardia. Notify physician of any side effect. Should a sudden or uncontrolled hypertensive state occur, discontinue levarterenol, notify the physician, and if necessary, treat with an adrenergic blocking agent (e.g., phentolamine [Regitine] or phenoxybenzamine [Dibenzyline]).

OCTREOTIDE ACETATE

Antidiarrheal
Growth hormone suppressant

Sandostatin

pH 3.9 to 4.5

USUAL DOSE

Usually given SC (see Precautions). In most situations begin with a lower dose to allow gradual tolerance to GI side effects. Increase gradually based on patient response and tolerance. Begin SC dosing as soon as practical.

Antidiarrheal (GI tumor): 50 mcg once or twice daily. Increase gradually if indicated.

Antidiarrheal (investigational for AIDS): 100 mcg as an IV bolus over 10 minutes. Follow with a continuous infusion, intermittent infusion, or bolus dose of 10 mcg/hr. Increase gradually to 100 mcg/hr. When adequate control is achieved, decrease to 75 mcg/hr. SC dose range is from 100 mcg up to 3,000 mcg/24 hr.

Carcinoid tumors: 100 to 600 mcg/24 hr in equally divided doses 2 to 4 times daily during first 2 weeks of therapy. Average total daily dose ranges from 300 to 450 mcg, but therapeutic response is obtained with ranges from 50 to 750 mcg. Up to 1,500 mcg/day has been used in selected patients.

Carcinoid crisis (investigational): 100 mcg as an IV bolus. May be given to treat carcinoid crisis during anesthesia or given prior to induction of anesthesia as a prophylactic measure.

Vasoactive intestinal peptide tumors: Average dose range is 200 to 300 mcg/24 hr in equally divided doses 2 to 4 times daily during first 2 weeks of therapy. Average total daily dose ranges from 150 to 750 mcg but therapeutic response usually achieved with doses under 450 mcg/24 hr. Doses of 25 to 50 mcg/hr IV for 2 to 4 days have been used.

Treatment of GI bleeding (investigational): Begin with a loading dose of 50 to 100 mcg. Follow with a continuous infusion of 25 to 50 mcg/hr for 1 to 5 days. Intermittent infusion or bolus doses may be substituted for the continuous infusion.

Growth hormone suppression: 50 mcg every 8 hours is the initial dose. Increase dose gradually as indicated by IGF-1 levels (see Monitor). Another study suggests an initial dose of 100 mcg equally distributed over 24 hours as a continuous infusion. Increase by 100 mcg each 24-hour period. Acromegaly has been suppressed at doses of 300 to 500 mcg/24 hr. May be maintained at home with infusions through an implantable IV or SC pump or SC dosing of 50 to 100 mcg every 8 hours.

Antihypoglycemic: Life-threatening hypoglycemia secondary to insulinoma (investigational): 100 mcg as an IV bolus.

Reduce output from GI or pancreatic fistulas (investigational): 50 to 200 mcg every 8 hours. In one study, 250 mcg/hr was given as a continuous infusion for 48 hours, followed with SC dosing. Fistula became dry within 72 hours and eventually closed.

PEDIATRIC DOSE

Experience is limited, but seems to be well tolerated in infants and young children.

1 to 10 mcg/kg of body weight/24 hours has been effective in various conditions (e.g., as an antidiarrheal).

Nesidioblastosis (pancreatic tumors [investigational]): 1 mcg/kg/hr as an IV infusion until vasoactive intestinal peptide (VIP) levels fall and fluid absorption is normal. Follow with SC dosing.

DOSE ADJUSTMENTS

In all situations dose adjustment may be required on a daily basis to maintain symptomatic control. After initial 2 weeks of therapy, gradually decrease dose to achieve therapeutically effective maintenance dose. ▪ Reduce dose in the elderly; half-life extended and clearance decreased. ▪ Half-life markedly extended in severe renal failure requiring dialysis. Reduction of maintenance dose indicated. ▪ Note Drug/Lab interactions.

DILUTION

May be given undiluted or may be diluted with 50 to 200 ml of NS or D5W and given as an intermittent infusion or further diluted and given as a continuous infusion.

Storage: Prior to use store in refrigerator (2° to 8° C [36° to 46° F]) and protect from light. May store at room temperature on day of use. Diluted solution stable for 24 hours.

INCOMPATIBLE WITH

Total parenteral nutrition solutions, insulin, and IV fat emulsion 10%. Octreotide is added to TPN in actual practice, but is not recommended by the manufacturer; consult pharmacist. If used as an additive with insulin, octreotide markedly increases adsorption of insulin and reduces availability.

RATE OF ADMINISTRATION

Direct IV: A single dose over 3 minutes.

Intermittent infusion: A single dose over 15 to 30 minutes.

Continuous infusion: Give at a rate consistent with the required hourly dose in an amount of fluid appropriate for the specific patient.

ACTIONS

A long-acting octapeptide. Mimics the actions of the natural hormone somatostatin, suppressing secretion of serotonin, gastroenteropancreatic peptides (e.g., gastrin, vasoactive intestinal peptide, insulin, glucagon, secretin, motilin, pancreatic polypeptide), and growth hormone. Decreases splanchnic blood flow. Stimulates fluid and electrolyte absorption from GI tract and prolongs GI transit time. Readily absorbed from subcutaneous injection site, and about 65% bound to plasma protein. Half-life longer than the natural hormone (1.5 hours compared to 1 to 3 minutes). Action may extend to 12 hours. Some excreted unchanged in urine.

INDICATIONS AND USES

To suppress or inhibit the severe diarrhea and flushing episodes associated with carcinoid tumors. ▪ Treatment of profuse watery diarrhea associated with vasoactive intestinal peptide tumors (VIPomas). ▪ Treatment of acromegaly to suppress growth hormone and achieve normalization of growth hormone and IGF-1 levels.

Investigational uses: Treatment of severe diarrhea in patients with AIDS. Carcinoid crisis during anesthesia, adjunct to treatment of life-threatening hypoglycemia, treatment of GI bleeding. Adjunct to pancreatectomy and treatment of GI or pancreatic fistulas.

CONTRAINDICATIONS

Sensitivity to octreotide acetate or any of its components.

PRECAUTIONS

▪ IV use is limited to emergency situations. SC injection with rotation of injection sites is preferred route of administration. ▪ May decrease size of tumors and slow rate of growth and metastases. Data not definitive. ▪ Use caution in patients with diabetes; requirements for insulin, sulfonylureas, and diazoxide may be altered.

Monitor: Observe for transient hyper- or hypoglycemia during induction and dose changes because of changes in balance of hormones (e.g., insulin, glucagon, and growth hormone). ▪ Monitor fluids and electrolytes carefully. ▪ 5-HIAA, plasma serotonin, and plasma substance P may be useful lab studies to evaluate patient response with carcinoid tumor. Measurement of plasma vasoactive intestinal peptide will be helpful in VIPoma. ▪ In acromegaly, initial response may be monitored with growth hormone levels at 1- to 4-hour intervals for 8 to 12 hours after a dose. IGF-1 levels every 2 weeks and/or multiple growth hormone levels taken 0 to 8 hours after administration may be used to make dose adjustments. ▪ Can alter fat absorption and decrease gallbladder motility; observe for gallbladder disease. Baseline and periodic ultrasound of gallbladder and bile ducts indicated in long-term SC therapy. Periodic fecal fat and carotene studies also indicated. ▪ Monitor base line and periodic thyroid function tests, especially in long-term SC therapy. ▪ Note Dose adjustments and Drug/Lab interactions.

Patient education: Instruct patient and/or family in appropriate skills if self-administration indicated. To avoid or lessen incidence of GI side effects, schedule injections between meals and at bedtime.

Maternal/child: Category B: although studies do not indicate harm to the fetus, use in pregnancy and lactation only if clearly needed. ▪ Has been used without adverse effects in infants over 1 month and children, but safety and efficacy is not established.

Elderly: Note Dose adjustments. ▪ May be more sensitive to side effects, observe carefully.

DRUG/LAB INTERACTIONS

Use caution in patients receiving concomitant beta-blockers (e.g., atenolol [Tenormin], propranolol [Inderal] calcium channel blockers (e.g., diltiazem [Cardizem], verapamil [Calan]) or any agents used for fluid and electrolyte balance. Will require adjustment in these therapies as symptoms are controlled by octreotide. ▪ May inhibit effectiveness of cyclosporine and may result in transplant rejection. ▪ Markedly increases adsorption of insulin and reduces availability. ▪ Concurrent use with oral antidiabetic agents, glucagon, growth hormone, or insulin may cause hypo- or hyperglycemia. Monitor patient carefully and adjunct dose of these agents as indicated.

SIDE EFFECTS

Most side effects are of mild to moderate severity and of short duration. Abdominal pain/discomfort, abnormal stools, anorexia, anxiety, biliary sludge, cholelithiasis, constipation, convulsions, depression, diarrhea, dizziness, drowsiness, fatigue, fat malabsorption, flatulence, fluttering sensation, GI bleeding, headache, heartburn, hepatitis, hyperesthesia, hyperglycemia, hypoglycemia, increase in liver enzymes, insomnia, irritability, jaundice, nausea, pounding in the head, rectal spasm, swollen stomach, vomiting. Many other side effects occur in less than 1% of patients.

ANTIDOTE

Keep physician informed of all side effects. A dose adjustment of either octreotide or other concomitant therapies may be required. Symptomatic and supportive treatment may be indicated. Overdose will cause hyperglycemia or hypoglycemia depending on tumor involved and endocrine status of patient. Discontinue osctreotide temporarily, notify the physician, and monitor the patient carefully. Symptomatic treatment should be sufficient.

OFLOXACIN

Antibacterial (Fluoroquinolone)

Floxin I.V.   pH 3.5 to 5.8

USUAL DOSE

200 to 400 mg every 12 hours. Dose and duration of treatment are based on mild to moderate infection and specific diagnosis. Normal renal function required. Dose and serum levels similar by oral or IV route. Transfer to oral dose as soon as practical. IV administration should not be used for more than 10 days (no studies available on longer use).

Exacerbation of chronic bronchitis, community-acquired pneumonia, and uncomplicated skin and skin structure infections: 400 mg every 12 hours for 10 days.

Acute uncomplicated gonorrhea: A single dose of 400 mg.

Chlamydial infections (cervicitis/urethritis): 300 mg every 12 hours for 7 days.

Pelvic inflammatory disease: 400 mg every 12 hours for 10 to 14 days.

Cystitis: 200 mg every 12 hours for 3 to 7 days depending on causative organism (see literature).

Complicated urinary tract infections: 200 mg every 12 hours for 10 days.

Prostatitis due to E. coli: 300 mg every 12 hours for up to 6 weeks.

DOSE ADJUSTMENTS

Increase interval between doses to 24 hours if creatinine clearance is between 10 and 50 ml/min. Reduce dose by one-half and increase interval to 24 hours if creatinine clearance is less than 10 ml/min. See literature for additional information. ■ Note Drug/lab interactions.

DILUTION

Available premixed and ready for use in infusion bottles (400 mg in 100 ml 5% dextrose) and in plastic infusion containers (200 mg in 50 ml and 400 mg in 100 ml 5% dextrose). All contain 4 mg/ml. Do not hang plastic containers in a series; may cause air embolism; see packaging for specific preparation and administration directions. Also available in 10 ml vials (40 mg/ml) and 20 ml vials (20 mg/ml). Vials must be diluted to a final maximum concentration of 4 mg/ml. May be further diluted to concentrations as low as 0.4 mg/ml. To yield 4 mg/ml, dilute 200 mg dose (5 ml of 40 mg/ml or 10 ml of 20 mg/ml) with 50 ml diluent; 300 mg dose (7.5 ml of 40 mg/ml or 15 ml of 20 mg/ml) with 75 ml diluent; and 400 mg dose (10 ml of 40 mg/ml or 20 ml of 20 mg/ml) with 100 ml diluent. Compatible diluents are NS, D5W, D5/0.45%S, D5NS, LR, or Plasma-Lyte 56; 5% dextrose in half-normal saline with 0.15% potassium chloride; 5% sodium bicarbonate; sodium lactate (⅙ molar lactate); and water for injection.

Storage: A clear, colorless to slightly yellow solution. Vials stable to expiration date at room temperature before opening. Contains no preservative; all preparations are intended for single use only. If using a vial that will yield more than one dose, dilute all at one time. Diluted solutions stable at controlled room temperature for 3 days, up to 14 days if refrigerated. May be frozen for up to 6 months. Do not force thaw (e.g., microwave or water bath) and do not refreeze. Discard any unused portion of premixed solutions and/or opened vials.

INCOMPATIBLE WITH

Manufacturer recommends ofloxacin be administered separately. Never administer in the same IV or through the same tubing with any solution containing metal ions (e.g., calcium, copper, iron, magnesium, zinc); may chelate with these ions. Always flush line before and after administration of any other drug through the same IV line.

RATE OF ADMINISTRATION

A single dose must be equally distributed over 60 minutes as an infusion. Too-rapid administration may cause hypotension, increase incidence of anaphylaxis, local site inflammation, or other side effects. May be given through a Y-tube or three-way stopcock of infusion set. Temporarily discontinue other solutions infusing at the same site and flush tubing before and after ofloxacin.

ACTIONS

A synthetic broad-spectrum antimicrobial agent, a fluoroquinolone. Bactericidal to a wide range of aerobic and anaerobic gram-negative and gram-positive organisms through interference with an enzyme needed for synthesis of bacterial DNA. Onset of action is prompt, and serum levels are dose related. Steady state is achieved after 4 doses. Half-life averages 4 to 6 hours. Readily distributed to body fluids and tissue. Therapeutic levels found in blister fluid, cervix, lung tissue, ovary, prostatic fluid and tissue, skin, and sputum. Well absorbed in patients with cystic fibrosis. Activity not affected by beta-lactamase production. Resistant chlamydia strains may emerge. Minimal metabolism occurs in the liver (less than other quinolones). Excreted as unchanged drug in the urine. Small amounts found in bile and feces. Crosses placental barrier. Secreted in breast milk.

INDICATIONS AND USES

Treatment of mild to moderate lower respiratory, skin and skin structure, urinary tract and prostate infections, pelvic inflammatory disease, and sexually transmitted diseases. Effective against specific organism (see literature). ■ Used in multi-drug-resistant organism infections when other antiinfectives are ineffective or cannot be used. ■ Additional appropriate therapy required if anaerobic organisms are suspected of contributing to the infection. ■ Not effective in the treatment of syphilis.

CONTRAINDICATIONS

Known hypersensitivity to ofloxacin or any other quinolone antimicrobial agent (e.g., norfloxacin [Noroxin], ciprofloxacin [Cipro]).

PRECAUTIONS

For IV use only. ▪ Safety and effectiveness in severe infections not established. ▪ Culture and sensitivity studies indicated to determine susceptibility of the causative organism to ofloxacin. ▪ *Pseudomonas aeruginosa* may develop resistance during treatment. Ongoing culture and sensitivity studies indicated. ▪ Prolonged use may cause superinfection because of overgrowth of nonsusceptible organisms. ▪ Use with caution in patients with known CNS disorders that predispose to seizures (e.g., epilepsy, severe cerebral arteriosclerosis, concomitant drug therapy). ▪ May cause ophthalmologic abnormalities (e.g., cataracts). Incidence increases with length of treatment.

Monitor: May cause anaphylaxis with the first or succeeding doses, even in patients without known hypersensitivity. Emergency equipment must always be available. ▪ Maintain adequate hydration to prevent concentrated urine throughout treatment. May form crystals in alkaline urine. ▪ Test all patients with gonorrhea for syphilis at time of diagnosis and in 3 months. Requires additional treatment. ▪ Monitor hematopoietic, hepatic, and renal systems during prolonged treatment. ▪ Use of larger veins will help to reduce incidence of allergic reactions with incidence of local irritation. Symptoms of local irritation do not preclude further administration of ofloxacin unless they recur or worsen. Generally resolve when infusion complete. ▪ Note Drug/lab interaction.

Patient education: Consider birth control options. ▪ Report skin rash or any other hypersensitivity reaction promptly. ▪ Avoid excessive sunlight or artificial ultraviolet light. Potential for photosensitivity may cause severe sunburn. Wear dark glasses outdoors. ▪ Dizziness or lightheadedness may interfere with ambulation and motor coordination. ▪ Effects of caffeine or theophylline preparations may be increased. Limit or eliminate concurrent use. Monitor if use necessary. ▪ Note Precautions/Monitor and Drug/lab interactions.

Maternal/ child: Pregnancy Category C: not recommended. Benefits must outweigh risks. High doses have caused maternal and fetal toxicity. ▪ Discontinue breast feeding. ▪ Safety for use in children under 18 years of age not established. Has caused arthropathy and osteochondrosis in juvenile animals.

Elderly: Percent of side effects similar to younger adults. Half-life extended to 7 or 8 hours with normal renal function.

DRUG/LAB INTERACTIONS

Other quinolones have caused serious or fatal reactions with theophylline (e.g., cardiac arrhythmia or arrest, respiratory failure, seizures, status epilepticus). If must be used concomitantly, monitor serum levels of theophylline and decrease dose as appropriate. No problems have occurred, but observe closely with caffeine. ▪ Serum levels may be increased with cimetidine (Tagamet). ▪ Serum levels may be decreased with antineoplastics agents (e.g., cisplatin, doxorubicin [Adriamycin]). ▪ Cyclosporine serum levels and nephrotoxic effects may be increased with concomitant use. ▪ Administration with febufen (a NSAID that is not approved for use in the U.S.) may increase CNS toxicity. ▪ May potentiate oral anticoagulants (e.g., warfarin [Coumadin]); monitor prothrombin times. ▪ Probably potentiated by probenicid; may require dose adjustment based on ofloxacin serum levels. ▪ Concurrent administration with procainamide may decrease procainamide levels. ■ Note Side effects.

SIDE EFFECTS

Average: Abdominal pain and cramps, altered sense of taste, chest pain (1% to 3%), decreased appetite, diarrhea (4%), dizziness (5%), dry mouth, external genital pruritus in women (6%), fatigue, flatulence, GI distress, headache (9%), insomnia (7%), local site reactions (e.g., erythema, phlebitis, swelling), nausea (10%), nervousness, pharyngitis, phototoxicity, pruritus, pseudomembranous colitis, pyrexia, rash, somnolence, taste disturbances, trunk pain, vaginal discharge (3%), vaginitis (5%), visual disturbances, and vomiting. Capable of numerous other reactions in less than 1% of patients. Allergic reactions (anaphylaxis, cardiovascular collapse, death, dyspnea, edema [facial, laryngeal, or pharyngeal], eosinophilia, fever, hepatic necrosis, itching, jaundice, loss of consciousness, rash, urticaria); cardiac arrest; CNS stimulation (confusion, hallucinations, light-headedness, restlessness, seizures, tingling, toxic psychosis, tremors) can occur.

Overdose: Disorientation, dizziness, drowsiness, facial swelling and numbness, hot and cold flushes, nausea, slurring of speech.

ANTIDOTE

Keep physician informed of all side effects. Many will require symptomatic treatment; monitor closely. Discontinue ofloxacin at the first appearance of a skin rash or any other sign of hypersensitivity or at the onset of any CNS symptom, pseudomembranous colitis, or phototoxicity. Treat allergic reactions with epinephrine (Adrenalin), airway management, oxygen, IV fluids, antihistamines (e.g., diphenhydramine [Benadryl]), corticosteroids (e.g., Solu-Cortef), and pressor amines (e.g., dopamine [Intropin]) as indicated. Treat CNS symptoms as indicated. May require diazepam (Valium) for seizures. Mild cases of colitis may respond to discontinuation of oflaxacin. Oral vancomycin (Vancocin) or metronidazole (Flagyl) is the treatment of choice for antibiotic-related pseudomembranous colitis. Adequate hydration and supplementation of electrolytes and proteins usually indicated. Maintain hydration in overdose. No specific antidote; not removed by hemodialysis or peritoneal dialysis. Maintain patient until drug is excreted.

ONDANSETRON HYDROCHLORIDE

Zofran

Antiemetic
5HT$_3$ receptor antagonist

pH 3.3 to 4.0

USUAL DOSE

A single 32 mg dose or 0.15 mg/kg of body weight (first in a sequence of three doses) 30 minutes before giving emetogenic cancer chemotherapy (e.g., cisplatin, methotrexate). Given as an intermittent infusion. Repeat 0.15 mg/kg dose at 4 and 8 hours after the first dose. Alternate *investigational regimens* are 10 to 15 mg every 3 hours as an intermittent infusion; or a continuous infusion of 30 mg over 12 hours, or 60 mg over 24 hours. In selected situations doses are used every 3 hours to supplement the continuous infusion; based on symptoms, response, and tolerance of individual patient. These doses exceed present FDA approvals.

Postoperative nausea: Adults and children weighing ≥ *40 kg:* 4 mg before anesthesia induction or immediately after surgery. Although repeat doses have not been studied, they are commonly given at 3- to 4-hour intervals.

PEDIATRIC DOSE

Children 4 to 18 years of age: 0.15 mg/kg of body weight 30 minutes before giving emetogenic cancer chemotherapy. Given as an intermittent infusion. Repeat 0.15 mg/kg/dose at 4 and 8 hours after the first dose.

Postoperative nausea: Children 2 to 12 years of age weighing ≤ *40 kg:* 0.1 mg/kg before anesthesia induction or immediately after surgery. Note comments under Adult dose.

DOSE ADJUSTMENTS

No dose adjustment required for the elderly or in renal or hepatic disease.

DILUTION

Direct IV: 4 mg dose may be given undiluted.

Intermittent IV: A single dose should be diluted in 50 ml of NS, D5W, D5/0.45%S, D5/NS. Now available as 32 mg in 50 ml D5W.

Infusion: May be further diluted in larger amounts of the above solutions. Also compatible in 10% mannitol and Ringer's injection. A precipitate will form in alkaline solutions.

Storage: Store unopened vials at CRT or refrigerate. Stable at CRT for 48 hours after dilution.

INCOMPATIBLE WITH

Acyclovir (Zovirax), allopurinol (Zyloprim), aminophylline, amphotericin B (Fungizone), ampicillin, ampicillin and sulbactam (Unasyn), cefoperazone (Cefobid), fluorouracil (5-FU), furosemide (Lasix), ganciclovir (Cytovene), lorazepam (Ativan), methylprednisolone (Solu-Medrol), mezlocillin (Mezlin), piperacillin (Pipracil), sargramostim (Leukine). Precipitate will form in alkaline solutions (e.g., sodium bicarbonate, barbiturates).

COMPATIBLE WITH

Y-site: Up to 4 hours with aztreonam (Azactam), cefazolan (Kefzol), ceftazidime (Ceptaz), fluconazole (Diflucan), and ranitidine (Zantac) 0.5 or 2 mg/ml (with ondansetron 0.03, 0.1, or 0.3 mg/ml),

RATE OF ADMINISTRATION

Direct IV: (Postop N/V) A single dose over at least 30 seconds, 2 to 5 minutes preferred.

Intermittent IV adults and children: A single dose equally distributed over 15 minutes.

Infusion: Evenly distributed over 12 to 24 hours.

ACTIONS

A selective antagonist of serotonin receptors. Chemotherapeutic agents such as cisplatin increase the release of serotonin from specific cells in the GI tract, causing emesis. By antagonizing these receptors, chemotherapy-induced nausea and vomiting are prevented. Lacks the activity at dopamine receptors of metoclopramide (Reglan), so it does not cause sedation. No correlation between plasma levels and antiemetic activity. Metabolized by specific hepatic enzymes; onset of action is prompt and lasts about 4 hours. May last only 2 to 3 hours in children under 15 years of age. Excreted in feces and urine. May be secreted in breast milk.

INDICATIONS AND USES

Prevention of nausea and vomiting associated with initial and repeat courses of emetogenic cancer chemotherapy, including high-dose cisplatin, nonplatinum agents, and radiation therapy. Has been shown to be effective with cyclophosphamide (Cytoxan), doxorubicin (Adriamycin), etoposide (VePesid), fluorouracil (Adrucil), ifosfamide (Ifex), methotrexate (Folex), mitoxantrone (Novantrone), and vincristine (Oncovin). ■ Prevention or treatment of postoperative nausea. ■ Used orally for prevention of nausea and vomiting, including N/V associated with radiotherapy. Recently approved for IM injection as an alternative to IV in the prevention of post-op nausea and vomiting.
Investigational use: Treatment of panic disorder.

CONTRAINDICATIONS

Hypersensitivity to ondansetron.

PRECAUTIONS

Sterile technique imperative in withdrawing a single dose from the multidose vial. Available as a single-dose vial and in 4- and 8-mg tablets. ■ Not indicated instead of gastric suction or intestinal peristalsis. Use in abdominal surgery or in patients with chemotherapy induced nausea and vomiting may mask a progressive ileus or gastric distension.
Monitor: Observe closely. Ambulate slowly to avoid orthostatic hypotension. ■ Stool softeners or laxatives may be required to prevent constipation.
Patient education: May cause dizziness or fainting; request assistance to ambulate. ■ Report promptly difficulty breathing, tightness in the chest, or wheezing.
Maternal/child: Category B: no evidence of impaired fertility or harm to fetus. Use in pregnancy only if potential benefit justifies potential risk. ■ Use caution if required during lactation. ■ Safety for use in children under 3 years of age not established.
Elderly: Note Dose adjustments.

DRUG/LAB INTERACTIONS

Even though metabolized in the liver and changes in clearance rates do occur, no specific drug interactions requiring dose adjustments have been identified.

SIDE EFFECTS

Abdominal pain or discomfort, constipation, cramps, dizziness, faintness, headache, lightheadedness, transient elevation of AST (SGOT) or ALT (SGPT). Other side effects have occurred (e.g., bronchospasm, extrapyramidal reaction, rash) in fewer than 1% of patients. Overdose caused sudden blindness in one patient.

ANTIDOTE

Most side effects will be treated symptomatically. Keep physician informed as indicated. Overdose of 10 times the usual dose has not caused significant problems. Treat anaphylaxis and resuscitate as necessary.

ORPHENADRINE CITRATE

Skeletal muscle relaxant
(Central acting)

Banflex, Flexoject, Flexon,
Myolin, Norflex, Orphenate

pH 5.0 to 6.0

USUAL DOSE
60 mg (2 ml) every 12 hours.

DILUTION
May be given undiluted, or a single dose may be diluted in 5 to 10 ml of sterile water for injection.

Storage: Store at CRT.

INCOMPATIBLE WITH
No specific information available. Note Precautions and Contraindications.

RATE OF ADMINISTRATION
60 mg or fraction thereof over 5 minutes.

ACTIONS
A diphenhydramine derivative with anticholinergic effects. Exact mechanism of action is unknown, but may be related to its analgesic properties. Does not directly relax tense skeletal muscles. Onset of action is immediate. Half-life of parent compound is 14 hours. Metabolized in the liver. Excreted in feces and urine.

INDICATIONS AND USES
Acute spasm of voluntary muscle, especially posttraumatic, discogenic, and tension spasms. ■ Treatment of nicotine-induced convulsions.

CONTRAINDICATIONS
Achalasia, bladder neck obstruction, cardiospasm, glaucoma, hypersensitivity to orphenadrine citrate or its components (contains bisulfites), myasthenia gravis, prostatic hypertrophy, pyloric or duodenal obstruction, stenosing peptic ulcer.

PRECAUTIONS
Equal effectiveness produced by IM or oral route. Use IV only when necessary for rapid onset of action. ■ Use caution in tachycardia, cardiac arrhythmias, cardiac decompensation, coronary insufficiency, pregnancy, and lactation. ■ Norflex contains sulfites; use caution to prevent allergic response.

Monitor: Keep patient in recumbent position for at least 15 minutes to avoid postural hypotension.

Patient education: Avoid alcohol and other CNS depressants. ■ May cause dizziness, drowsiness, and visual disturbances. ■ Request assistance for ambulation. ■ Use caution in any task requiring alertness.

Maternal/child: Safety for use in pregnancy and lactation not established; benefits must outweigh risks. ■ Not recommended for children.

Elderly: May cause confusion. ■ Sensitivity to anticholinergic effects (dry mouth, urinary retention). ■ Consider age-related renal impairment; may preclude use.

DRUG/LAB INTERACTIONS
Absorption of many oral drugs inhibited or potentiated due to decreased GI motility. ■ Not recommended for concomitant use with propoxyphene (Darvon) or perphenazine (Trilafon). ■ Potentiates anticholinergic drugs and thiazide diuretics. ■ Inhibits haloperidol and phenothiazines (e.g., prochlorperazine [Compazine]).

SIDE EFFECTS
Usually associated with higher doses or too-rapid administration: blurred vision, dizziness, drowsiness, dry mouth, excitation, headache, lightheadedness, nausea, palpitations, pupil dilation, tachycardia, urinary retention, urticaria, vomiting, weakness. Anaphylactic reactions can occur (rare).

Overdose: Deep coma, cardiac arrhythmias, tonic and clonic seizures, shock, respiratory arrest, death.

ANTIDOTE
Notify the physician of any side effects. Reduction of dosage will probably relieve them. For symptoms of hypersensitivity, discontinue the drug, notify the physician, and treat symptomatically. Treat overdose promptly. Resuscitate as necessary.

OXACILLIN SODIUM
Antibacterial
(Penicillinase-resistant penicillin)

Bactocil, Prostaphlin   pH 6.0 to 8.5

USUAL DOSE
Over 40 kg (88 lb): 250 mg to 1 Gm or more every 4 to 6 hours. Maximum dose is 20 Gm/24 hr.

PEDIATRIC DOSE
Under 40 kg: 50 to 100 mg/kg of body weight/24 hr in equally divided doses every 4 to 6 hours. Maximum dose is 100 to 300 mg/kg/24 hr.

INFANT DOSE
Under 2,000 Gm; age up to 14 days: 25 mg/kg every 12 hr. *15 to 30 days of age:* 25 mg/kg every 8 hr.

Over 2,000 Gm; age up to 14 days: 25 mg/kg every 12 hr. *15 to 30 days of age:* 25 mg/kg every 6 hr.

DOSE ADJUSTMENTS
Decreased dose may be required in severe renal impairment.

DILUTION
Each 500 mg or fraction thereof should be diluted in 5 ml of sterile water or NS for injection. May be further diluted for intermittent or continuous infusion in 50 to 1,000 ml of D5W, D5/NS, NS, LR, or other compatible IV solutions to a final concentration of 0.5 to 40 mg/ml (see literature).

Storage: Diluted solution stable for at least 6 hours. See literature.

INCOMPATIBLE WITH
Acidic solutions, amikacin (Amikin), cytarabine (ARA-C), levarterenol (Levophed), metaraminol (Aramine), verapamil (Isoptin).

RATE OF ADMINISTRATION

Too-rapid rate may cause seizures.

Direct IV: 1 Gm (10 ml) or fraction thereof slowly over 10 minutes.

Intermittent IV: A single dose over 10 to 30 minutes.

Infusion: May be administered in specific IV solutions (check literature) over up to a 6-hour period.

ACTIONS

A semisynthetic penicillin with bactericidal effect against penicillinase-producing organisms. Easily distributed into most body fluids, including trace amounts in spinal fluid. Crosses the placental barrier. Excreted primarily in the urine. Secreted in breast milk.

INDICATIONS AND USES

Infection caused by penicillinase-producing staphylococci.

CONTRAINDICATIONS

Known sensitivity to any penicillin or cephalosporin (not absolute).

PRECAUTIONS

Sensitivity studies necessary to determine susceptibility of the causative organism to oxacillin. ■ Superinfection caused by overgrowth of nonsusceptible organisms is a possibility. ■ Change to oral therapy as soon as practical.

Monitor: Periodic liver, kidney, and hematopoietic studies are advised. ■ Electrolyte imbalance and cardiac irregularities from sodium content are possible. Contains 2.8 mEq sodium/Gm. May aggravate CHF. Observe for hypokalemia. ■ Note Drug/lab interactions.

Patient education: May require alternate birth control.

Maternal/child: Pregnancy Category B: use only if clearly needed. ■ May cause diarrhea, candidiasis, or allergic response in nursing infants. ■ Limited experience in use on premature infants and neonates. Use with caution. Elimination rate markedly reduced in neonates.

Elderly: Note Precautions/ Monitor and Dose Adjustments.

DRUG/LAB INTERACTIONS

May be used concurrently with aminoglycosides (e.g., gentamicin [Garamycin]) but must be administered in separate infusions; inactivates aminoglycosides. ■ May be antagonized by bacteriostatic antibiotics (e.g., chloramphenicol, erythromycin, tetracyclines); bactericidal action may be negated. ■ Potentiated by probenecid (Benemid); toxicity may result. ■ May potentiate heparin. ■ Concomitant use with beta-adrenergic blockers (e.g., propranolol [Inderal]) may increase risk of anaphylaxis and inhibit treatment. ■ May decrease clearance and increase toxicity of methotrexate. ■ May inhibit effectiveness of oral contraceptives; breakthrough bleeding or pregnancy could result. ■ May cause false values in common lab tests, see literature.

SIDE EFFECTS

Relatively infrequent: diarrhea, elevated AST (SGOT), hepatic dysfunction, hypersensitivity with anaphylaxis, nausea, pruritus, skin rash, thrombophlebitis, transient hematuria in newborns, urticaria, vomiting. Hypersensitivity myocarditis (fever, eosinophilia, rash, sinus tachycardia, ST-T changes and cardiomegaly) and pseudomembranous colitis can occur. Higher than normal doses may cause neurologic adverse reactions including convulsions; especially with impaired renal function.

ANTIDOTE

Notify the physician of any adverse symptoms. For severe symptoms, discontinue the drug, treat allergic reaction (antihistamines, epinephrine, corticosteroids), and resuscitate as necessary. Hemodialysis or peritoneal dialysis are minimally effective in overdose.

OXYMORPHONE HYDROCHLORIDE

Narcotic analgesic (agonist)

Numorphan

pH 2.7 to 4.5

USUAL DOSE

0.5 mg initially. May repeat every 2 to 4 hours. Up to 1.5 mg may be required.

When seeking the required dose to achieve pain relief for an individual patient, increases in increments of at least 25% of the previous dose are suggested. Lower slightly if pain controlled but patient is too drowsy, or lower dose and increase frequency.

DOSE ADJUSTMENTS

Reduced dose or extended intervals may be required in the elderly, in hepatic or renal disease, and in emphysema. ■ Note Drug/lab interactions.

DILUTION

Each dose should be diluted with 5 ml of sterile water or NS. May give through Y-tube or three-way stopcock of infusion set.

Storage: Store below 40° C. Protect from light.

INCOMPATIBLE WITH

Specific information not available (consider similarity to morphine).

RATE OF ADMINISTRATION

A single dose properly diluted over 2 to 5 minutes. Usually titrated according to symptom relief and respiratory rate.

ACTIONS

An opium derivative and CNS depressant closely related to morphine. Ten times more potent than morphine milligram for milligram. Onset of action is prompt and lasts 3 to 4 hours. Detoxified in the liver and excreted in the urine. Crosses placental barrier. Secreted in breast milk.

INDICATIONS AND USES

Relief of moderate to severe pain. ■ Support of anesthesia. ■ Obstetric analgesia. ■ Relief of anxiety in dyspnea of acute left ventricular failure and pulmonary edema.

CONTRAINDICATIONS

Acute bronchial asthma, children under 12 years of age, diarrhea caused by poisoning until toxic material eliminated, known hypersensitivity to opiates, premature infants and labor and delivery of premature infants, pulmonary edema caused by chemical respiratory irritant, upper airway obstruction.

PRECAUTIONS

Use caution in the elderly and in patients with impaired hepatic or renal function and pulmonary disease. ▪ Use extreme caution in craniotomy, head injury, and increased intracranial pressure; respiratory depression and intracranial pressure may be further increased. ▪ May cause apnea in the asthmatic. ▪ Symptoms of acute abdominal conditions may be masked. ▪ May increase ventricular response rate in presence of supraventricular tachycardias. ▪ Cough reflex is suppressed. ▪ Tolerance to oxymorphone gradually increases. A marked increase in dose may precipitate seizures in presence of a history of convulsive disorders.

Monitor: Oxygen, controlled respiratory equipment, and naloxone (Narcan) must be available. ▪ Observe patient frequently and monitor vital signs. Keep patient supine; orthostatic hypotension and fainting may occur. Uncontrolled pain causes sleep deprivation, decreases pain threshold, and increases pain; when pain is finally controlled, expect the patient to sleep more until recovery from sleep deprivation.

Patient education: Avoid alcohol or other CNS depressants (e.g., barbiturates, benzodiazepines [e.g., diazepam (Valium)]). ▪ May cause blurred vision, dizziness, or drowsiness; use caution in tasks that require alertness. ▪ May be habit forming.

Maternal/child: Safety for use in pregnancy or lactation not established (note Contraindications).

Elderly: Note Dose adjustments and Precautions. ▪ May be more sensitive to effects (e.g., respiratory depression, constipation, urinary retention). ▪ Analgesia should be effective with lower doses. ▪ Consider age-related organ impairment.

DRUG/LAB INTERACTIONS

Potentiated by phenothiazines and other CNS depressants such as narcotic analgesics, alcohol, antihistamines, barbiturates, cimetidine (Tagamet), hypnotics, sedatives, MAO inhibitors (e.g., selegiline [Eldepryl]), neuromuscular blocking agents (e.g., tubocurarine), and psychotropic agents. Reduced dosages of both drugs may be indicated.

SIDE EFFECTS

At equianalgesic doses, may cause more nausea, vomiting, and euphoria than morphine.

Minor: Anorexia, constipation, dizziness, skin rash, urinary retention, urticaria.

Major: Anaphylaxis, hypotension, respiratory depression, somnolence.

ANTIDOTE

Notify the physician of any side effect. If minor side effects progress or any major side effect occurs, discontinue the drug and notify the physician. Treat anaphylaxis as indicated or resuscitate as necessary. Naloxone hydrochloride (Narcan) will reverse serious respiratory depression.

OXYTOCIN INJECTION

Oxytocic
Antihemorrhagic

Pitocin

pH 2.5 to 4.5

USUAL DOSE

Determined by uterine response and intended use, dilution, and rate of administration. Oxytocins must be administered by only one route at a time. For instance, do not combine oral and IV routes. Piggyback oxytocin into a normal saline IV without oxytocins, see Precautions.

Induction of labor: Begin with 0.5 to 2 milliunits/min (mU/min). See Dilution and Rate of administration.

Control of postpartum bleeding: 10 units at 10 to 40 mU/min, following delivery of the infant(s) and preferably the placenta(s). See Dilution and Rate of administration.

Incomplete or inevitable abortion: 10 Units at 10 to 20 mU/min, a second source says 10 to 40 mU/min. See Dilution and Rate of administration.

Postabortion hemorrhage (unlabeled): 10 Units at 20 to 100 mU/min. See Dilution and Rate of administration.

Oxytocin challenge test (investigational): Infuse properly diluted oxytocin (10 mU/ml) at an initial rate of 0.5 mU/min. Gradually increase rate until contractions are every 3 to 4 minutes. Monitor fetal heart rate concurrently. Observe signs of fetal distress with contractions. Distress indicates inadequate placental reserve. Stop infusion.

DILUTION

In all situations rotate gently to distribute medication through solution.

Induction of labor: Dilute 1 ml (10 units) in 1 liter of NS, D5W, LR, or D5/NS for infusion (10 mU/ml). This dilution is also used for the *oxytocin challenge test.*

Control of postpartum bleeding: Dilute 1 to 4 ml (10 to 40 units) in 1 liter of above infusion fluids (10 to 40 mU/ml).

Incomplete or inevitable abortion/postabortion hemorrhage: Dilute 1 ml (10 units) in 500 ml of above infusion fluids (20 mU/ml).

Storage: Store at CRT or under refrigeration, depending on manufacturer.

INCOMPATIBLE WITH

Levarterenol (Levophed), prochlorperazine (Compazine), sodium bisulfites, warfarin (Coumadin).

RATE OF ADMINISTRATION

Given only as an IV infusion. Use of an infusion pump or other accurate control device is required. In all situations, use the minimum effective rate and monitor strength, frequency, and duration of contractions; resting uterine tone, fetal heart rate (in induction of labor), and maternal blood pressure at least every 15 minutes or more often if indicated.

Induction of labor: Begin with 0.5 to 2 mU/min (0.05 to 0.2 ml), increase in increments of 1 to 2 mU/min at 30- to 60-minute intervals until contractions simulate normal labor. Maximum dose rarely exceeds 9 to 10 mU/min at term, average is 2 to 5 mU/min. Reduce by similar increments when desired frequency of contractions is reached and labor has progressed to 5 to 6 cm. 6 mU/min provides oxytocin levels similar

to spontaneous labor. Pre-term inductions may require somewhat higher doses (one source suggests a maximum of 20 mU/min), use caution.
Control of postpartum bleeding: Rate of infusion must control uterine atony. Begin with 10 to 40 mU/min. Increase or decrease rate as indicated. Proceed quickly but with caution because of strength of solution.
Incomplete or inevitable abortion: 10 to 40 mU/min.
Postabortion hemorrhage: 20 to 100 mU/min.

ACTIONS

A synthetic posterior pituitary hormone that will produce rhythmic contraction of uterine smooth muscle. Its effectiveness depends on the level of uterine excitability, which usually increases as a pregnancy progresses. Very rapid acting, it has a shorter duration of action than ergot derivatives (half-life of 1 to 6 minutes). Duration of action is approximately 1 hour. Is the drug of choice for induction of delivery. Probably detoxified in the liver and through enzymatic processes and excreted in the urine. Has a weak antidiuretic effect.

INDICATIONS AND USES

After selective patient evaluation by the physician, it is used to induce or stimulate labor at term or before. ■ To control postpartum bleeding. ■ To treat incomplete or inevitable abortion. ■ Treatment of postabortion hemorrhage.
Investigational use: Oxytocin challenge test.

CONTRAINDICATIONS

Cephalopelvic disproportion, fetal malpresentation, hypersensitivity, hypertonic uterine contractions, lack of satisfactory progress with adequate uterine activity, obstetrical emergencies (e.g., abruptio placentae), prolonged use in uterine inertia, serious medical or obstetric conditions (past or present), toxemia (severe), vaginal delivery contraindicated (e.g., active herpes genitalis, cord presentation or prolapse, invasive cervical carcinoma, total placenta previa and vasa previa). Note precautions.

PRECAUTIONS

A normal saline IV without oxytocins must be hung, connected by Y-tube or three-way stopcock, and ready for use in adverse reactions. ■ Should be administered only in the hospital; the physician must be immediately available. ■ Use in fetal distress, hydramnios, partial placenta previa, prematurity, borderline cephalopelvic disproportion, and any condition that may cause uterine rupture (e.g., cesarean section (previous), uterine surgery, uterine overdistention, past history of uterine sepsis) is not recommended except in unusual circumstances. ■ Oxytocin challenge test is an antepartum test of uteroplacental insufficiency in high-risk pregnancy. Test done only by a qualified physician.
Monitor: Monitor blood pressure, fetal heart tones, strength and timing of contractions, and resting uterine tone at least every 15 minutes or more often if indicated. Continuous observation of patient required. ■ Monitor oral fluid intake and observe for signs of fluid retention. Water intoxication has caused maternal death. ■ Note Precautions and Drug/lab interactions.
Maternal/child: Has no use before induction of labor; note Contraindications. ■ May be found in breast milk; consider postponing nursing for 24 hours after discontinued.

DRUG/LAB INTERACTIONS

Severe hypertension can result in the presence of local anesthesia, regional anesthesia (caudal or spinal), and with dopamine (Intropin), ephedrine, epinephrine, methoxamine (Vasoxyl), and other vasopressors. Chlorpromazine (Thorazine) IV will reduce this hypertension.

SIDE EFFECTS

Maternal: Anaphylaxis, cardiac arrhythmias, fatal afibrinogenemia, fluid retention leading to water intoxication and coma, convulsion, and death; hypertension, increased blood loss, nausea, pelvic hematoma, PVCs, postpartum hemorrhage, severe uterine hypertonicity, spasm or contraction; subarachnoid hemorrhage, uterine rupture, vomiting.

Fetal: Bradycardia, brain damage, CNS damage, death, low Apgar scores, neonatal jaundice, retinal hemorrhage.

ANTIDOTE

Nausea and vomiting are tolerable and can be treated symptomatically. Immediately call the physician's attention to any side effect noted or suspected; many can be fatal. Discontinue the drug immediately for any signs of fetal distress, uterine hyperactivity, tetanic contractions, uterine resting tone exceeding 15 to 20 mm H_2O, or water intoxication. Use of a Y-connection or three-way stopcock, allowing the oxytocin drip to be discontinued while the vein is kept open, is required. Turn mother on side (prevent fetal anoxia) and administer oxygen. Restriction of fluids, diuresis, hypertonic saline solutions IV, correction of electrolyte imbalance, control of convulsions with cautious use of barbiturates, or the use of magnesium sulfate may be required. These side effects can occur during labor and delivery and into the postpartum period. Careful evaluation and selection of patients eliminate many hazards, but be prepared for an emergency.

PACLITAXEL

Antineoplastic (Miscellaneous)

Taxol

pH 4.4 to 5.6

USUAL DOSE

Premedication: Must be premedicated before each dose to prevent severe hypersensitivity reactions. Usual regimen includes oral dexamethasone (Decadron) 20 mg 12 and 6 hours before; IV diphenhydramine (Benadryl) 50 mg 30 to 60 minutes before; and IV cimetidine (Tagamet) 300 mg or ranitidine (Zantac) 50 mg 30 to 60 minutes before dosing with paclitaxel. When premedicating patients with AIDS-related Kaposi's sarcoma, reduce the dose of oral dexamethasone to 10 mg at 12 and 6 hours before the doses of IV diphehydramine and IV cimetidine or ranitidine remain as above.

Metastatic ovarian cancer: 135 or 175 mg/M^2 as an infusion. Repeat every 3 weeks. Premedication, specific parameters, and specific equipment required before or during administration; see Premedication, Dose adjustments and Precautions/Monitor. Larger doses, with or without filgrastim (G-CSF, Neupogen), have produced similar responses. Note rate of administration.

First-line treatment of ovarian cancer: 135 mg/M^2 as an infusion over 3 hours. Follow with cisplatin 75 mg/M^2 as an infusion over 24 hours. Repeat every 3 weeks. Note comments in metastatic ovarian cancer section.

Breast cancer: 175 mg/M^2 as an infusion. Repeat every 3 weeks. Note all comments under ovarian cancer above. Administer filgrastim (G-CSF) 5 mcg/kg/dose on days 3 through 10. Doses of paclitaxel up to 250 mg/M^2 were used in initial studies. Most effective dose not yet established.

AIDS-related Kaposi's sarcoma: 135 mg/M^2 as an infusion. Repeat every 3 weeks or 100 mg/M^2 repeated every 2 weeks. Note all comments under Premedication and ovarian cancer above and Dose adjustments below.

DOSE ADJUSTMENTS

Reduce dose by 20% for subsequent courses in patients who experience severe peripheral neuropathy or severe neutropenia (neutrophils < 250 to 500 cells/ mm^3) for 1 week or longer. ▪ Withhold therapy if neutrophils below 1,500/mm^3 or platelets below 100,000/mm^3. ▪ Dose reduction may be considered in impaired hepatic function, at this time, it is not considered in impaired renal function. ▪ In AIDS related Kaposi's sarcoma the parameters are slightly different. Initiate or repeat paclitaxel only if neutrophil count (≥1,000/mm^3; reduce dose by 20% in patients who experience severe neutropenia (neutrophils < 500/mm^3 for a week or longer); use concomitant filgrastim (G-CSF) as clinically indicated.

DILUTION

Specific techniques required; see Precautions. Must be diluted and given as an infusion. May leach the toxic plasticizer DEHP from PVC infusion bags or sets; prepare and store in bottles (glass, polypropylene) or plastic bags (polypropylene, polyolefin) and administer through polyethylene-lined administration sets. Compatible with NS, D5W, D5/NS, or D5/R. Final concentration of 0.3 to 1.2 mg/ml required. For a 135 mg/M^2 dose, a large adult (body surface about 2 M^2) will receive 270 mg (45 ml of paclitaxel at 6 mg/ml). Will require dilution in an additional 180 ml to make a 1.2 mg/ml concentration or 855 ml to make a 0.3 mg/ml concentration. Solution may appear hazy.

Storage: May be stored at controlled room temperature or refrigerated prior to dilution. Diluted for infusion, it is stable at room temperature for up to 27 hours.

INCOMPATIBLE WITH

Consider toxicity and specific use. Amphotericin B (Fungizone), chlorpromazine (Thorazine), hydroxyzine (Vistaril), methylprednisolone sodium succinate (Solu-Medrol), mitoxantrone (Novantrone).

RATE OF ADMINISTRATION

A single dose properly diluted must be equally distributed over 3 hours. Use of an in-line filter not greater than 0.22 microns required. Use of a metriset (60 gtt/ml) or an infusion pump appropriate to control flow. More dilute concentrations (0.6 to 0.3 mg/ml) are being administered over 3 to 6 hours by some oncologists.

ACTIONS

An antineoplastic. A novel antimicrotubule agent. Paclitaxel derived from the bark of pacific yew has now been replaced by paclitaxel produced semisynthetically from a renewable source (needles and twigs of the Himalayan yew). Both are chemically identical. Through specific processes it stabilizes microtubules, thus preventing depolymerization.

This action inhibits the normal dynamic reorganization of the microtuble network essential for vital interphase and mitotic cellular functions. Also induces abnormal bundles of microtubules throughout the cell cycle and multiple asters of microtubules during mitosis. More active in patients who have not received previous chemotherapy. Distribution and/or tissue (protein) binding is extensive. Evidence suggests metabolism in the liver; high concentrations occur and are probably excreted through bile. Minimal excretion of unchanged drug occurs in urine.

INDICATIONS AND USES

Treatment of metastatic carcinoma of the ovary after failure of first-line or subsequent chemotherapy. ■ First-line treatment for ovarian cancer. ■ Metastatic breast cancer. Refractory to initial chemotherapy or for a relapse within 6 months. ■ Second-line treatment of AIDS-related Kaposi's sarcoma. Prior therapy should have included an anthracycline (e.g., doxorubicin, idarubicin) unless contraindicated.

Investigational uses: First-line treatment for metastic breast cancer. ■ Adencarcinoma of the upper GI tract. ■ Advanced head and neck cancer. ■ Advanced non-small-cell lung cancer. ■ Hormone-refractory prostate cancer. ■ Leukemias. ■ Previously untreated extensive-stage small-cell lung cancer.

CONTRAINDICATIONS

Baseline neutropenia <1,500 cells/mm^3, history of prior severe hypersensitivity reactions to paclitaxel or other drugs formulated in polyoxyethylated castor oil (Cremophor EL [e.g., cyclosporine, teniposide]).

PRECAUTIONS

Follow guidelines for handling cytotoxic agents. See Appendix A, p. 893. ■ Usually administered by or under the direction of the physician specialist. ■ Adequate diagnostic and treatment facilities must be readily available. ■ Use caution in patients with cardiac conduction abnormalities, CHF, MI within previous 6 months, and severe hepatic impairment. ■ Myelosuppression may be more frequent and more severe in patients who have received prior radiation therapy. ■ Preexisting neuropathies resulting from prior therapies are not a contraindication for paclitaxel therapy. ■ Various studies show that incidence and severity of neurotoxocity and hematologic toxicity increase with dose, especially above 190 mg/M^2.

Monitor: Use caution to prevent bone marrow depression. Dose dependent and is the dose-limiting toxicity. Obtain base line CBC with differential. Monitor frequently during therapy and before each dose. Note Dose adjustments. ■ Obtain base line ECG; arrhythmias occur frequently. Continuous cardiac monitoring required for all patients with an abnormal base line ECG or those who experienced conduction arrhythmias during administration of a previous dose. ■ Most severe hypersensitivity reactions occur in the first hour; monitor all vital signs including blood pressure frequently. Incidence seems to decrease with subsequent doses. ■ Observe closely for signs of infection. Prophylactic antibiotics may be indicated pending results of C/S in a febrile neutropenic patient. ■ Use prophylactic antiemetics to reduce nausea and vomiting and increase patient comfort.

Patient education: Avoid pregnancy; nonhormonal birth control recommended. ■ Review of monitoring requirements and adverse events before therapy imperative. ■ Report any unusual or unexpected symptoms, side effects, or signs of infection (e.g, chills, fever, night sweats) as soon as possible. ■ See Appendix D, p. 900. ■ Obtain name and telephone number of a contact person for emergencies, questions, or problems. ■ Seek resources for counseling or supportive therapy.

Maternal/child: Pregnancy Category D: avoid pregnancy. May cause fetal harm. ■ Discontinue breast feeding. ■ Safety for use in children not established.

DRUG/LAB INTERACTIONS

Dexamethasone, diphenhydramine, cimetidine, and ranitidine do not affect protein binding of paclitaxel. ■ To reduce potential for profound myelosuppression when using paclitaxel and cisplatin concurrently, give paclitaxel first, then cisplatin. ■ Ketoconazole (Nizoral) concomitantly may inhibit metabolism and increase toxicity. ■ Other inhibitors of cytochrome P_{450} iso enzyme CYP2C8 (e.g., cyclosporine [Sandimmune], dexamethasone [Decadron], diazepam [Valium], etoposide, quinidine, teniposide [Vumon], testosterone, verapamil [Calan]) may also inhibit metabolism of paclitaxel and increase toxicity. ■ Neurotoxicity and symptomatic motor dysfunction occurring with higher doses (> 250 mg/M^2) may be potentiated by cisplatin and filgrastim (G-CSF). ■ May cause additive effects with bone marrow–depressing agents or agents that cause blood dyscrasias (e.g., amphotericin B, antithyroid agents, azathioprine, chloramphenicol, ganciclovir, interferon, plicamycin, zidovudine) and radiation therapy. Reduced doses may be required. ■ Do not administer chloroquine or live virus vaccines to patients receiving antineoplastic agents.

SIDE EFFECTS

Dose dependent and generally reversible, but may be fatal. All patients were premedicated to prevent hypersensitivity. Abnormal ECG (all patients [30%]), abnormal ECG with normal baseline (19%), alopecia (82%), anemia <11 Gm/dl (90%) <8 Gm/dl (24%), arthralgia/myalgia (55%), bleeding (19%), bradycardia (10%), diarrhea (43%), elevated bilirubin (8%), elevated alkaline phosphatase (23%), elevated AST (SGOT) (16%), fever (19%), hypersensitivity reactions (moderate, e.g., dyspnea, flushing, rash [39%]; severe, e.g., chest pain, dyspnea, hypotension [2%]), hypotension (23%), infections (chills, fever, nightsweats [35%]), leukopenia <4,000/mm^3 (93%) <1,000 mm^3 (26%), mucositis (39%), nausea and vomiting (59%), neutropenia <2,000/mm^3 (92%) <500/mm^3 (67%), peripheral neuropathy (any [62%], severe [4%]), thrombocytopenia <100,000/mm^3 (27%) <50,000/mm^3 (10%). A grand mal seizure occurred in one patient.

ANTIDOTE

Keep physician informed of all side effects. Most will be treated symptomatically as indicated. Most hypersensitivity reactions will subside with temporary discontinuation of paclitaxel, and incidence seems to decrease with subsequent doses. Severe reactions may require epinephrine (Adrenalin), antihistamines (e.g., diphenhydramine [Benadryl]), corticosteroids (e.g., dexamethasone [Decadron]), or bronchodilators (e.g., albuterol (Ventolin), theophylline [aminophylline]). Most should not be rechallenged, but some patients tolerated subsequent doses. Neutropenia can be profound, and the nadir usually occurs about day 11. Recovery is generally rapid and spontaneous but may be treated with filgrastim (G-CSF, Neupogen). Severe thrombocytopenia (nadir day 8 or 9) may require platelet transfusions, has been treated with oprelvekin (Numega). Severe anemia (<8 Gm/dl) may require packed cell transfusions, moderate anemia (<11 Gm/dl) may be treated with epoetin alfa (Epogen). Hypotension and bradycardia do not usually occur at the same time except in hypersensitivity. Treat only if symptomatic. Some arrhythmias (e.g., nonspecific repolarization abnormalities, sinus tachycardia, and PVCs) are common and may not require intervention. Treat any serious or symptomatic arrhythmia (e.g. conduction abnormalities, ventricular tachycardia) promptly and monitor continuously during subsequent doses. Neurologic symptoms tend to worsen with each course; note Dose adjustments. Usually improve within several months. Severe peripheral neuropathies or seizure may necessitate discontinuation of paclitaxel. There is no specific antidote for overdose. Supportive therapy will help sustain the patient in toxicity. Resuscitate if indicated.

PAMIDRONATE DISODIUM
Antihypercalcemic
(Bisphosphonate)

APD, Aredia   pH 6.0 to 7.4

USUAL DOSE

Moderate hypercalcemia (corrected serum calcium of 12 to 13.5 mg/dl): One dose of 60 to 90 mg as an infusion.

Severe hypercalcemia (corrected serum calcium greater than 13.5 mg/dl): One dose of 90 mg as an infusion. Serum calcium levels should fall into the normal range (8.5 to 10.5 mg/100 ml [1 dl], corrected for serum albumin).

Experience is limited, but retreatment with the same dose may be considered if hypercalcemia recurs; wait at least 7 days from completion of first infusion to allow full response. Always used in conjunction with adequate hydration and appropriate testing. Note Precautions/Monitor.

Paget's disease: 30 mg/day as an infusion for 3 consecutive days. Selected patients have been retreated with the same dose when indicated. Experience limited; see note above.

Osteolytic bone lesions of multiple myeloma: 90 mg as an infusion once every 30 days. Optimal duration of therapy not known.

Osteolytic bone metastases of breast cancer: 90 mg as an infusion every 3 to 4 weeks.

DOSE ADJUSTMENTS

Lower-dose regimen may be appropriate in impaired renal or hepatic function. No experience with creatinine above 5.0 mg/100 ml (1 dl).

■ Note Precautions.

DILUTION

Reconstitute each 30, 60, or 90 mg vial with 10 ml sterile water for injection. Dissolve completely (3, 6, or 9 mg/ml).

Hypercalcemia of malignancy: Further dilute a single daily dose in 1,000 ml NS (preferred), 0.45 NS, or D5W. A minimum of 500 ml diluent may be used if absolutely necessary in patients with compromised cardiovascular status.

Paget's disease: Further dilute a single daily dose in 500 ml of the above solutions.

Osteolytic bone lesions of multiple myeloma: Further dilute each 90 mg dose in 500 ml of above solutions.

Osteolytic bone metastases of breast cancer: Further dilute each 90 mg dose in 250 ml of above solutions.

Storage: Before reconstitution, store at controlled room temperature. After reconstitution, may be refrigerated for up to 24 hours. Stable after dilution for 24 hours at room temperature.

INCOMPATIBLE WITH

Calcium-containing solutions (e.g., Ringer's solutions). Manufacturer states, "should be given in a single intravenous solution and line separate from all other drugs."

RATE OF ADMINISTRATION

Use of a microdrip (60 gtt/ml) or an infusion pump recommended for even distribution. Too-rapid infusion rate may lead to overdose, elevated BUN and creatinine levels, and renal tubular necrosis. Rate recommendations vary considerably. They are based on specific clinical trials for each diagnosis. In some trials a rate of up to 1 mg/min has been used with caution.

Hypercalcemia of malignancy: A 60 mg dose equally distributed over 4 hours and a 90 mg dose equally distributed over 24 hours.

Paget's disease: A single dose over 4 hours.

Osteolytic bone lesions of multiple myeloma: A single dose over 4 hours.

Osteolytic bone metastases of breast cancer: A single dose over 2 hours.

ACTIONS

A bisphosphonate hypocalcemic agent. Reduces serum calcium concentrations by inhibiting accelerated bone resorption. Binds to preformed bone surfaces and may block bone mineral dissolution. Effectively inhibits the accelerated bone resorption resulting from osteoclast hyperactivity induced by various tumors. Does not inhibit bone formation and mineralization. Plasma levels achieve some reduction in calcium levels in 24 to 48 hours, and maximal response in 4 to 7 days. In two studies a single dose normalized serum calcium by day 7 in 61% to 70% of patients treated with 60 mg and 100% of those treated with 90 mg. Maintains duration of normocalcemia/hypocalcemia longer than etidronate (Didronel). Rapidly adsorbed by bone with some transit through the liver. Slowly excreted in urine.

INDICATIONS AND USES

Treatment of moderate to severe hypercalcemia of malignancy in patients with or without bone metastasis, in conjunction with adequate hydration. Symptoms of hypercalcemia may include anorexia, bone pain, confusion, constipation, dehydration, depression, fatigue, lethargy, muscle weakness, nausea and vomiting, and polyuria. Severe dehydration may lead to renal insufficiency. With high levels of serum calcium, cardiac manifestations (e.g., bradycardia, cardiac arrest, ventricular arrhythmias), and neurologic symptoms (e.g., coma, seizures, and death) may occur. ■ Treatment of Paget's disease. ■ Adjunct in treatment of osteolytic lesions of multiple myeloma and osteolytic bone metastases of breast cancer.

CONTRAINDICATIONS

Hypersensitivity to pamidronate or other bisphosphonates (e.g., etidronate [Didronel], alendronate [Fossmax]).

PRECAUTIONS

Calcium is bound to serum protein; concentration fluctuates with changes in blood volume. Changes in serum calcium (especially during rehydration) may not reflect true plasma levels. Measurement with ionized calcium levels is preferred. If unavailable, all calcium measurement should be corrected for albumin to establish a basis for treatment and evaluation of treatment. ■ Mild or asymptomatic hypercalcemia will be treated with conservative measures (e.g., saline hydration, with or without diuretics [after correcting hypovolemia]). Consider patient's cardiovascular status. Corticosteroids may be indicated if the underlying cancer is sensitive (e.g., hematologic cancers). ■ Use in the treatment of hypercalcemia associated with hyperparathyroidism or with other non-tumor-related conditions has not been adequately studied. ■ May be used adjunctively with chemotherapy, radiation, or surgery. ■ *Osteolytic bone lesions of multiple myeloma:* Limited information available on use in multiple myeloma patients with a serum creatinine greater than 3 mg/dl. *Monitor:* Obtain base line measurements of serum calcium (corrected for serum albumin), electrolytes, phosphate, magnesium, and creatinine and CBC with differential and hematocrit/hemoglobin. Monitor all closely as indicated by baseline results (may be daily). Serum phosphate levels will decrease and usually require treatment. ■ Monitor serum alkaline phosphatase during therapy for Paget's disease. ■ Patients with cancer-related hypercalcemia are frequently dehydrated. Must be adequately hydrated orally and/or IV before treatment is initiated. Hydration with saline is preferred to facilitate renal excretion of calcium and correct dehydration. A pretreatment urine output of 2 L/day is recommended. Maintain adequate hydration and urine output throughout treatment. ■ Avoid overhydration in patients with compromised cardiovascular status. Observe frequently for signs of fluid overload. Correct hypovolemia before using diuretics. ■ Monitor patients with preexisting anemia, leukopenia, or thrombocytopenia very carefully during treatment and the first 2 weeks following treatment. ■ *Osteolytic bone lesions of multiple myeloma:* Adequately hydrate patients with marked Bence-Jones proteinuria and dehydration before pamidronate infusion.

Patient education: Regular visits and assessment of lab tests imperative. ■ Dietary restriction of calcium and vitamin D may be required. ■ Take only prescribed meds. ■ Report abdominal cramps, chills, confusion, fever, muscle spasms, sore throat and/or any new medical problems promptly.

Maternal/child: Category C: use in pregnancy has not been studied; use only if clearly needed. ■ Safety for use during lactation not established. ■ Safety for use in children not established.

Elderly: Monitor fluid and electrolyte status carefully to avoid overhydration. Use of lower fluid volume (see Dilution) may be required.

DRUG/LAB INTERACTIONS

Use with furosemide (Lasix) does not affect calcium-lowering action. ■ Does not interfere with any known primary cancer therapy. ■ Effects may be antagonized by calcium-containing preparations or vitamin D; avoid use.

SIDE EFFECTS

Average dose: Abdominal pain, anemia, anorexia, bone pain, constipation, fever (mild and transient), generalized pain, hypertension, hypocalcemia (abdominal cramps, confusion, muscle spasms), infusion site reaction (e.g., induration and pain on palpation, redness, swelling), urinary tract infections, vomiting. Fluid overload, hypokalemia, hypomagnesemia, and hypophosphatemia occur frequently with use of concurrent fluid and diuretics.

Overdose: Occurs less frequently with lower dose range (30 to 60 mg). Fever (high), hypocalcemia, hypotension, leukopenia or lymphopenia (fever, chills, sore throat), transient taste perversion. Elevated BUN and creatinine clearance levels and renal tubular necrosis may occur with excessive dose or rate of administration.

ANTIDOTE

Keep physician informed of side effects. Some may respond to symptomatic treatment. Magnesium, phosphorus, and potassium may require replacement if depletion too severe. If mild, all will probably return toward normal in 7 to 10 days. For asymptomatic or mild to moderate hypocalcemia (6.5 to 8.0 mg/100 ml [1 dL] corrected for serum albumin), short-term calcium therapy (e.g., calcium gluconate) may be indicated. Discontinue drug for any symptoms of overdose. Monitor serum calcium and use vigorous IV hydration, with or without diuretics for 2 to 3 days. Monitor intake and output to ensure adequacy and balance. Use short-term IV calcium therapy if indicated. High fever may respond to steroids. Red blood cell transfusions may be required in anemia. Treat anaphylaxis and resuscitate as indicated.

PANCURONIUM BROMIDE

Neuromuscular blocking agent
(Nondepolarizing)
Anesthesia adjunct

Pavulon   pH 4.0

USUAL DOSE

Adults and children: Must be individualized, depending on previous drugs administered and degree and length of muscle relaxation required. Succinylcholine must show signs of wearing off before pancuronium is given. 0.04 to 0.1 mg/kg of body weight initially. 0.01 mg/kg in increments as required to maintain muscle relaxation; usually 25 to 60 minute intervals.

Endotracheal intubation: 0.06 to 0.1 mg/kg.

NEONATAL DOSE

Extreme sensitivity to pancuronium exists during the first month of life. Begin with a test dose of 0.02 mg/kg and assess responsiveness.

DOSE ADJUSTMENTS

Note Drug/lab interactions; marked reduction of pancuronium dose may be required. ■ A higher total dose may be required in biliary or hepatic disease, but onset is slower and neuromuscular block is prolonged.

DILUTION

May be given undiluted.

Storage: Best if stored in refrigerator. Will maintain potency at room temperature for up to 6 months.

INCOMPATIBLE WITH

Diazepam (Valium),

RATE OF ADMINISTRATION

A single dose over 60 to 90 seconds.

ACTIONS

A skeletal muscle relaxant five times as potent as tubocurarine chloride (curare). Causes paralysis by interfering with neural transmission at the myoneural junction. Onset of action is dose dependent. Peak effect occurs in 3 to 4 minutes and lasts 30 to 45 minutes. It may take another 30 minutes or up to several hours before complete recovery occurs. Excreted in the urine.

INDICATIONS AND USES

Adjunctive to general anesthesia to facilitate endotracheal intubation and to relax skeletal muscles during surgery or mechanical ventilation.
■ Paralytic agent when no other drug has controlled severe agitation, inhibiting specific treatments in intensive care units.

CONTRAINDICATIONS

Known hypersensitivity to pancuronium or bromides; first trimester of pregnancy.

PRECAUTIONS

Usually administered by or under the direct observation of the anesthesiologist. ■ Repeated doses may produce a cumulative effect. ■ Impaired pulmonary function or respiratory deficiencies can cause critical reactions. ■ Use caution in impaired liver or kidney function, in patients with tachycardia, and in any patient who might develop adverse effects from an increase in heart rate. ■ Myasthenia gravis increases sensitivity to drug. ■ Long-term use (i.e., intensive care) may result in prolonged paralysis or skeletal muscle weakness.

Monitor: This drug produces apnea. Controlled artificial ventilation with oxygen must be continuous and under direct observation at all times. Maintain a patent airway. ■ Use a peripheral nerve stimulator to monitor response to pancuronium and avoid overdose. ■ Patient may be conscious and completely unable to communicate by any means. Pancuronium has no analgesic properties. ■ Action is altered by dehydration, electrolyte imbalance, body temperatures, and acid base imbalance. ■ Hyperkalemia may cause cardiac dysrhythmias and increased paralysis. ■ Note Precautions and Drug/lab interactions.

Maternal/child: Pregnancy Category C: unknown potential hazards to fetus; benefits must outweigh risks. Not recommended in first trimester.
■ Has caused rare severe skeletal muscle weakness in neonates undergoing mechanical ventilation.

Elderly: Delay in onset time may be caused by slower circulation time in cardiovascular disease, old age, or edematous states; allow more time for drug to achieve maximum effect.

DRUG/LAB INTERACTIONS

May cause severe arrhythmias with inhalant anesthetics (e.g., enflurane, halothane), and in patients on chronic tricyclic antidepressant therapy (e.g., amitriptyline [Elavil]). ■ Potentiated by hypokalemia, some carcinomas, many antibiotics (e.g., aminoglycosides [kanamycin (Kantrex), gentamicin (Garamycin)], bacitracin, colistin [Coly-Mycin S], colistimethate [Coly-Mycin M], polymyxin-B [Aerosporin], tetracyclines, piperacillin), calcium salts, CO_2, diuretics, diazepam (Valium) and other muscle relaxants, digitalis, magnesium sulfate, quinidine, morphine, lidocaine, meperidine, propranolol (Inderal), succinylcholine, and others. May need to reduce dose of pancuronium; use with caution. ■ Recurrent paralysis may occur with quinidine. ■ Antagonized by acetylcholine, anticholinesterases, aminophylline, azathioprine, carbamazepine, and potassium. ■ Succinylcholine must show signs of wearing off before pancuronium is given. Use caution.

SIDE EFFECTS

Prolonged action resulting in respiratory insufficiency or apnea and tachycardia. Airway closure caused by relaxation of epiglottis, pharynx, and tongue muscles. Hypersensitivity reactions are possible. Anaphylaxis, histamine release, hypotension, and shock may occur.

ANTIDOTE

All side effects are medical emergencies. Treat symptomatically. Controlled artificial ventilation must be continuous. Pyridostigmine (Mestinon) or neostigmine (Prostigmin) given with atropine will probably reverse the muscle relaxation. Not effective in all situations; may aggravate severe overdose. Resuscitate as necessary.

PAPAVERINE HYDROCHLORIDE

Vasodilator
(Peripheral)

pH 3.0 to 4.5

USUAL DOSE

1 to 4 ml (30 to 120 mg) every 3 hours as indicated. Second dose may be given in 10 minutes only when treating extrasystoles.

PEDIATRIC DOSE

1.5 mg/kg of body weight every 6 hours.

DOSE ADJUSTMENTS

Note Drug/lab interactions.

DILUTION

May be given undiluted or may be diluted in an equal amount of sterile water for injection. Usually not added to IV solutions. May be given through Y-tube or three-way stopcock of infusion set.

INCOMPATIBLE WITH

Alkaline solutions, aminophylline, bromides, diatrizoate meglumine, iodides, ioxaglate meglumine, lactated Ringer's injection.

RATE OF ADMINISTRATION

1 ml (30 mg) or fraction thereof over 2 minutes. Rapid IV injection may cause death.

ACTIONS

A nonnarcotic opium alkaloid, it is a direct smooth muscle relaxant and antispasmodic. Relaxation is noted in vascular system and bronchial musculature and in GI, biliary, and urinary tracts. More effective on muscle in spasm, it has an affinity for the smooth muscle of blood vessels. Affects cardiac muscle to depress conduction and increase refractory period. Improved circulation and muscle relaxation decrease pain. Metabolized in the liver and excreted in the urine.

INDICATIONS AND USES
Vascular spasm associated with an acute myocardial infarction. ▪ Peripheral or pulmonary embolism. ▪ Peripheral vascular disease and cerebral angiospastic states. ▪ Visceral spasm of ureteral, biliary, or GI colic. ▪ Angina pectoris.

CONTRAINDICATIONS
Complete AV heart block.

PRECAUTIONS
Rarely used; active therapeutic value is questioned. ▪ Rapid IV injection may cause death. ▪ IM injection is preferred. ▪ Use with caution in glaucoma and impaired liver function. ▪ Large doses can depress AV and intraventricular conduction, resulting in arrythmias.
Monitor: Observe patient continuously, monitor vital signs. ▪ Note Drug/lab interactions.
Patient education: Avoid alcohol and other CNS depressants. ▪ May cause dizziness and drowsiness; request assistance for ambulation. ▪ Use caution in any task requiring alertness.
Maternal/child: Category C: safety for use in pregnancy and lactation and in children not established.
Elderly: Risk of hypothermia may be increased.

DRUG/LAB INTERACTIONS
May be used with narcotics if the relaxant effect is not adequate to relieve discomfort. Narcotic dosage should be reduced. ▪ Antagonizes effects of levodopa.

SIDE EFFECTS
Minor: Blurred or double vision, diaphoresis, discomfort (generalized), flushing, hypertension (slight), hypotension, respiratory depth increase, scleral jaundice, sedation, tachycardia.
Major: Respiratory depression, seizures, ventricular ectopic rhythms, sudden death.

ANTIDOTE
Notify the physician of any minor side effects. If minor symptoms progress or any major side effect appears, discontinue the drug immediately and notify the physician. Treatment of toxicity will be symptomatic and supportive. Consider diazepam (Valium) or phenytoin (Dilantin) for convulsions. Anesthesia with thiopental and paralysis with a neuromuscular blocking agent (e.g., tubocurarine [curare]) may be required. Use dopamine (Intropin) for hypotension. Calcium gluconate may reduce toxic cardiovascular effects. Monitor ECG. Resuscitate as necessary.

PEGASPARGASE

Antineoplastic
(Miscellaneous)

Oncaspar, PEG-L-asparaginase

pH 7.3

USUAL DOSE

2,500 international units (IU)/M^2 every 14 days as an infusion. Most frequently used as a component of a multiple agent protocol. Infrequently used in the same dose as a single agent. Note Precautions.

PEDIATRIC DOSE

Over 1 year of age with body surface area less than 0.6 M^2: 82.5 IU/kg of body weight every 14 days.

Body surface area greater than 0.6 M^2: Same as adult dose.

DOSE ADJUSTMENTS

Adjust dose based on patient response and toxicity.

DILUTION

Specific techniques required; see Precautions. Available preservative free in 5 ml vials containing 750 IU/ml. Must be further diluted with 100 ml of NS or D5W and administered through the Y-tube or three-way stopcock of a free-flowing infusion of similar solutions. Do not shake; mix gently. Use only clear solutions.

Storage: Appearance the same but activity is destroyed if accidentally frozen. *Do not administer!* Refrigerate before dilution. For single-dose use only, do not reenter vial, discard unused portions. Discard any time solution is cloudy or after 48 hours at room temperature.

INCOMPATIBLE WITH

Specific information not available. Consider incompatible in syringe or solution because of toxicity and specific use.

RATE OF ADMINISTRATION

A single dose evenly distributed over 1 to 2 hours. Slow rate of infusion as indicated by side effects.

ACTIONS

An oncolytic agent. A modified version of L-asparaginase (native asparaginase derived from *Escherichia coli*) that rapidly depletes asparagine from cells. Some malignant cells have a metabolic defect that makes them unable to synthesize asparagine as normal cells do. They are dependent on exogenous asparagine for survival. Plasma half-life does not appear to be influenced by dose levels, nor does it correlate with age, sex, surface area, renal or hepatic function, diagnosis, or extent of disease. Measurable for up to 15 days. Cannot be detected in urine.

INDICATIONS AND USES

Treatment of acute lymphoblastic leukemia in patients who require L-asparaginase but have developed hypersensitivity to its native form. Primarily used as part of a multiple agent protocol with other chemotherapeutic agents (e.g., cytarabine, daunorubicin, doxorubicin, methotrexate, vincristine). Should be used as a single agent only when multiagent chemotherapy is considered inappropriate. Safety and effectiveness have been established in patients between 1 and 21 years of age with known previous hypersensitivity to native L-asparaginase.

Investigational use: Treatment of acute lymphocytic leukemia.

CONTRAINDICATIONS

Pancreatitis, past history of pancreatitis, significant hemorrhagic events associated with prior L-asparaginase therapy, and patients who have had previous serious allergic reactions (e.g., bronchospasm, generalized urticaria, hypotension, laryngeal edema, hypotension) or other unacceptable adverse reactions to pegaspargase (Oncaspar).

PRECAUTIONS

Follow guidelines for handling cytotoxic agents. See Appendix A, p. 893. ▪ Must be administered by or under the direction of the physician specialist (e.g., medical oncologist). ▪ Freezing destroys activity; see Storage. ▪ Intramuscular is the preferred route of administration; incidence of allergic reactions, hepatotoxicity, coagulopathy, and gastrointestinal and renal disorders are lower. ▪ May cause severe hepatic and central nervous system toxicity; use caution. ▪ May be at increased risk for bleeding or thrombosis. ▪ Note Drug/lab interactions.

Monitor: Observe patient carefully during and for at least 1 hour after infusion. ▪ Appropriate treatment for resuscitation and/or anaphylaxis must always be available. Risk may be increased if patient has had reactions to native asparaginase or is over 21 years of age. ▪ Frequent monitoring of blood counts, bone marrow evaluation, serum amylase, blood sugar, uric acid, and liver and kidney function are necessary. ▪ Monitoring of fibrinogen, PT, and PTT may be indicated to determine effects on plasma proteins. ▪ Allopurinol, increased fluid intake, and alkalinization of the urine may be required to reduce uric acid levels. ▪ Nausea and vomiting can be severe. Prophylactic administration of antiemetics recommended to increase patient comfort. ▪ Predisposition to infection probable. ▪ Prophylactic antibiotics may be indicated pending results of C/S in febrile neutorpenic patient.

Patient education: Report all symptoms promptly, incidence of allergic reaction is significant and risk of bleeding is increased. ▪ All meds including nonprescription drugs must be evaluated. Contact physician before changing any meds. ▪ Verbalize all questions. ▪ Assess birth control requirements. ▪ See Appendix D, p. 900.

Maternal/child: Category C: effect on fetus unknown. Evaluation of benefit versus risk is necessary for anyone who is pregnant or may become pregnant. ▪ Discontinue breast feeding.

Elderly: Consider age-related organ toxicity.

DRUG/LAB INTERACTIONS

Potential for increased risk of bleeding or thrombosis; may be exacerbated with concurrent administration of drugs with anticoagulant effects (e.g., heparin, coumadin, dipyridamole [Persantine], aspirin, or NSAIDs [e.g., indomethacin]). ▪ Use extreme caution with hepatotoxic agents (e.g., other chemotherapeutic agents, alcohol, NSAIDs, phenytoin [Dilantin]) especially in the presence of liver dysfunction. May cause severe hepatic and CNS toxicity. ▪ May inhibit action of drugs dependent on protein synthesis or cell replication (e.g., methotrexate). ▪ May interfere with the enzymatic detoxification of other drugs; particularly in the liver. ▪ Depletes serum protein; may increase the toxicity of protein bound drugs.

SIDE EFFECTS

May be more toxic in adults than in children. Allergic reactions occur more frequently in patients hypersensitive to native asparaginase (60%

versus 12% in nonsensitized patients) and may be dose limiting. Allergic reactions (e.g., bronchospasm, chills, dyspnea, edema, erythema, fever, pain, rash, urticaria), coagulopathy, fever, hepatotoxicity, increased ALT (SGPT), malaise, nausea and vomiting (over 5%), hyperglycemia requiring insulin therapy (3%), pancreatitis (clinical) (1%), thrombosis (4%). Has caused fatal fulminating pancreatitis. Capable of causing numerous other side effects in 1% to 5% of all patients.

ANTIDOTE

Notify physician of all side effects. Reduced rate of administration may be helpful. Pegaspargase may have to be discontinued until recovery or permanently discontinued. Symptomatic and supportive treatment is indicated. Treat allergic reactions promptly with epinephrine, corticosteroids, oxygen, and antihistamines. There is no specific antidote.

PENICILLIN G AQUEOUS

Antibacterial
(Penicillin)

Penicillin G potassium, Penicillin G sodium,
Pfizerpen

pH 6.0 to 8.5

USUAL DOSE

1 to 20 million units/24 hr equally distributed over 24 hours as a continuous infusion or equally divided in 4 to 6 intermittent infusions. Doses up to 80 million units/24 hr have been given in life-threatening infections. (400,000 units equals approximately 250 mg.)

PEDIATRIC DOSE

100,000 to 400,000 units/kg of body weight/24 hr in equally divided doses every 4 to 6 hours. Dosage can vary greatly and must be adjusted according to the severity of the infection. Treat congenital syphilis for 10 to 14 days. Maximum dose is 24,000,000 units.

NEONATAL DOSE

Under 1,200 Gm: 25,000 units/kg of body weight every 12 hours (meningitis 50,000 units).

Under 2,000 Gm; Age 0 to 7 days: 25,000 units/kg every 12 hours (meningitis, 50,000 units). *Over 7 days:* 25,000 units/kg every 8 hours (meningitis, 75,000 units).

Over 2,000 Gm; age 0 to 7 days: 25,000 units/kg every 8 hours (meningitis, 50,000 units). *Over 7 days:* 25,000 units/kg every 6 hours (meningitis, 56,250 units).

Congenital syphilis: Treat for 10 to 14 days.

Age 0 to 7 days: 50,000 units/kg every 12 hours.

Age 7 to 28 days: 50,000 units/kg every 8 hours.

Over 28 days of age: 50,000 units/kg every 6 hours.

DOSE ADJUSTMENTS

Reduce dose in impaired renal function. ■ Note Drug/lab interactions.

DILUTION

Initial dilution must be with sterile water for injection. Direct flow of water against sides of the vial while gently rotating vial. Shake vigorously. Directions on vial should be followed to provide desired number of units per milliliter. Available with 1, 5, 10, and 20 million units per vial. May be added to NS or dextrose solutions for infusion.

INCOMPATIBLE WITH

To preserve bactericidal action, do not mix other agents with penicillin in the infusion solution. Acid media, alcohol 5% in dextrose, alkaline media, amikacin (Amikin), aminophylline, amphotericin B (Fungizone), ascorbic acid, cephalothin (Keflin), chlorpromazine (Thorazine), dextran, dopamine (Intropin), heparin, hydroxyzine (Vistaril), IV fat emulsion 10%, lincomycin (Lincocin), metaraminol (Aramine), metoclopramide (Reglan), pentobarbital (Nembutal), phenytoin (Dilantin), prochlorperazine (Compazine), promazine (Sparine), promethazine (Phenergan), sodium bicarbonate, thiopental (Pentothal), trifluoperazine (Stelazine), vancomycin. For penicillin sodium add: bleomycin (Blenoxane) (Vancocin), cytarabine (ARA-C), hydroxyzine (Vistaril), methylprodnisolone (Solu-medrol), potassium chloride (KCl).

RATE OF ADMINISTRATION

Penicillin is not given by direct IV route. Administer as ordered as continuous IV drip; for example, 5 million units in 1,000 ml of D5W over 12 hours. Is sometimes given by intermittent infusion (1/6 or 1/4 of a daily dose in 100 ml over 1 to 2 hours every 4 to 6 hours). Dosage level must be maintained to provide therapeutic serum levels. Too-rapid administration or excessive doses may cause electrolyte imbalance and/or seizures. Stable at room temperature for at least 24 hours.

ACTIONS

Bactericidal against penicillin-sensitive microorganisms during the stage of active multiplication. Distributed into most body fluids. Distribution into spinal fluid is minimal unless inflammation is present. Crosses the placental barrier. Excreted in the urine. Secreted in breast milk. Available in a potassium salt containing 1.7 mEq of potassium and 0.3 mEq sodium in 1 million units or a sodium salt containing 2 mEq sodium in 1 million units.

INDICATIONS AND USES

Severe infections caused by penicillin G-sensitive gram-positive, gram-negative, and anaerobic microorganisms (e.g., streptococcal, pneumococcal, Vincent's gingivitis, spirochetal infections, meningitis, endocarditis). ■ Prophylaxis against bacterial endocarditis in specific situations.

CONTRAINDICATIONS

Known sensitivity to any penicillin or cephalosporin (not absolute).

PRECAUTIONS

Sensitivity studies necessary to determine susceptibility of the causative organism to penicillin. ■ Avoid prolonged use of drug, superinfection caused by overgrowth of nonsusceptible organisms may result. ■ Allergic reactions are most likely to occur in patients with a history of sensitivity to multiple allergens. ■ Potassium penicillin most frequently used. Doses over 10,000,000 units may cause fatal hyperkalemia; especially in patients with renal insufficiency.

Monitor: Periodic evaluation of renal and hematopoietic systems is recommended in prolonged therapy. ▪ Electrolyte imbalance from potassium or sodium content is very possible. Monitor closely. ▪ Observe for thrombophlebitis. ▪ Note Drug/lab interactions.

Patient education: May require alternate birth control.

Maternal/child: Pregnancy Category B: use only if clearly needed. ▪ May cause diarrhea, candidiasis, or allergic response in nursing infants. ▪ Elimination rate markedly reduced in neonates.

DRUG/LAB INTERACTIONS

Inactivated by acids, alkalies, oxidizing agents, and carbohydrate solutions with an alkaline pH. Optimum pH range 6.0 to 7.0. ▪ May be antagonized by bacteriostatic antibiotics (e.g., chloramphenicol, erythromycin, tetracyclines), bactericidal action may be negated. ▪ Risk of bleeding with anticoagulants (e.g., heparin) is increased. ▪ Inactivates aminoglycosides (gentamicin e.g., [Garamycin]); administer in separate infusions. ▪ Probenecid decreases elimination of penicillin resulting in prolonged blood levels. May be desirable or may cause toxicity. ▪ May decrease effectiveness of oral contraceptives; breakthrough bleeding or pregnancy could result. ▪ Concomitant use with potassium supplements or potassium-sparing diuretics (e.g., spironolactone [Aldactone]) may increase risk of hyperkalemia. ▪ May decrease clearance and increase toxicity of methotrexate. ▪ May cause false values in common lab tests; see literature.

SIDE EFFECTS

Minor: Arthralgia, chills, edema, fever, prostration, skin rash, urticaria.

Major: Acute interstitial nephritis, anaphylaxis, convulsions, hemolytic anemia, hyperreflexia, neurotoxicity, potassium poisoning with coma, sodium-induced congestive heart failure. Hypersensitivity myocarditis (fever, eosinophilia, rash, sinus tachycardia, ST-T changes and cardiomegaly) and pseudomembranous colitis can occur. Higher than normal doses may cause neurologic adverse effects including convulsions, especially with impaired renal function.

ANTIDOTE

For all side effects, discontinue the drug, treat the allergic reaction or resuscitate as necessary, and notify the physician. Treat minor side effects symptomatically according to physician's order. Removed by hemodialysis.

PENTAMIDINE ISETHIONATE

Antiprotozoal

♣Pentacarinat, Pentam 300

pH 4.09 to 5.4

USUAL DOSE

Treatment of pneumocystis carinii: 4 mg/kg of body weight once daily for 14 days. Note Precautions/Monitor. Has been used up to 21 days, benefits not defined.

Pneumocystis prophylaxis: 4 mg/kg once each month. May be given every 2 weeks if indicated.

Leishmania, visceral (investigational): 2 to 4 mg/kg once daily for up to 15 days.

Leishmania, cutaneous (investigational): 2 to 4 mg/kg once or twice a week until lesions heal.

Trypanosoma gambiense (investigational): 4 mg/kg once daily for 10 days.

PEDIATRIC DOSE

Pneumocystis carinii: 4 mg/kg once daily for 12 to 14 days.

Pneumocystis prophylaxis: See adult dose.

Leishmania donovani: 2 to 4 mg/kg once daily for 15 days. Up to 21 days have been suggested but risks with therapy over 14 days may be increased.

Trypanosoma gambiense: See adult dose.

DOSE ADJUSTMENTS

Reduced dose in renal failure may be indicated.

DILUTION

Initially dilute each 300 mg or fraction thereof in 3 to 5 ml sterile water or D5W. Dilute 200 mg vial of ♣Pentacarinat with 2 ml. A single dose must be further diluted in 50 to 250 ml of D5W (♣Pentacarinat 200 or 300 mg in 500 ml) and given as an infusion.

Storage: Stable at room temperature for 24 hours. Discard unused portion. Protect dry product and reconstituted solution from light.

INCOMPATIBLE WITH

Aldesleukin (Proleukin), cefazolin (Kefzol), cefoperazone (Cefobid), cefotaxime (Claforan), cefoxitin (Mefoxin), ceftizidime (Ceptaz), ceftriaxone (Rocephin), fluconazole (Diflucan), foscarnet (Foscavir). Consider incompatible in syringe or solution because of specific use and frequent side effects.

RATE OF ADMINISTRATION

A single dose should be evenly distributed over 60 minutes.

Leishmania, visceral and cutaneous: A single dose evenly distributed over 1 to 2 hours.

ACTIONS

An antiprotozoal agent. Specifically active against *Pneumocystis carinii*. It is thought to interfere with nuclear metabolism and inhibit the synthesis of DNA, RNA, phospholipids, and proteins. Route of metabolism is unknown. Excreted partially in urine. May accumulate in renal failure.

INDICATIONS AND USES
Treatment and prophylaxis of *Pneumocystis carinii* pneumonia (PCP).
Investigational use: Treatment of trypanosomiasis and visceral and cutaneous leishmaniasis. Aerosol used prophylactically to prevent PCP in high-risk patients.

CONTRAINDICATIONS
None if the diagnosis of *Pneumocystis carinii* pneumonia is confirmed.

PRECAUTIONS
Specific use only; establish correct diagnosis. ▪ Trimethoprim/sulfamethoxazole is the drug of choice for treatment of *Pneumocystis* pneumonia. Pentamidine causes numerous and serious side effects and is indicated only if the patient does not respond to or tolerate TMP/SMX. ▪ Use extreme caution in patients with hypertension, hypotension, hypoglycemia, hyperglycemia, hypocalcemia, leukopenia, thrombocytopenia, anemia, hepatic or renal dysfunction, ventricular tachycardia, pancreatitis, and Stevens-Johnson syndrome.
Monitor: Before, during, and after therapy obtain a BUN and serum creatinine (daily), CBC, platelet count, alkaline phosphatase, bilirubin, AST (SGOT), ALT (SGPT), serum calcium, and ECG. ▪ Has caused fatalities resulting from severe hypotension, hypoglycemia, and cardiac arrhythmias even with the administration of the first dose. Keep patient supine, observe continuously for any sign of adverse reaction, and monitor blood pressure continuously during infusion and afterward until stable. ▪ Emergency equipment for resuscitation must be immediately available. ▪ Monitor blood glucose levels daily during therapy and several times after therapy is complete. Pancreatic necrosis and very high plasma insulin levels have occurred. May also cause hyperglycemia and diabetes mellitus.
Patient education: May cause severe hypotension; remain lying down until blood pressure is stable. ▪ Report any unusual bleeding or bruising.
Maternal/child: Pregnancy Category C: use only when clearly needed during pregnancy and lactation. Hazards to fetus or infant are unknown. ▪ Discontinue breast feeding.

SIDE EFFECTS
Occur in more than 50% of patients and may be life threatening. Some side effects occur after the course of treatment is completed. Acute renal failure, anemia, anorexia, bad taste in mouth, cardiac arrhythmias including ventricular tachycardia, confusion, dizziness, elevated serum creatinine and liver function tests, fever, hallucinations, hyperglycemia, hyperkalemia, hypocalcemia, hypoglycemia, hypotension, leukopenia, nausea, neuralgia, phlebitis, rash, thrombocytopenia.

ANTIDOTE
Discontinue the drug and resuscitate as necessary for any life-threatening side effects. Notify physician of all side effects. Symptomatic treatment is indicated.

PENTAZOCINE (LACTATE)

Talwin

Narcotic analgesic
(Agonist-antagonist)

pH 4.0 to 5.0

USUAL DOSE

5 to 30 mg. May repeat every 3 to 4 hours or decrease to 5 to 15 mg and repeat every 2 hours. 360 mg equals maximum dose in 24 hours.

DOSE ADJUSTMENTS

Reduced dose may be required in the elderly or debilitated; in impaired liver or renal function; in patients with limited pulmonary reserve, and in the presence of other CNS depressants; use caution. ■ Increased dose may be required in smokers. ■ Note Precautions and Drug/lab interactions.

DILUTION

May be given undiluted. It is preferable to dilute each 5 mg with at least 1 ml of sterile water for injection.

Storage: Prior to use, store at controlled room temperature. Avoid freezing.

INCOMPATIBLE WITH

All barbiturates, aminophylline, glycopyrrolate (Robinul), heparin, nafcillin (Nafcil), sodium bicarbonate.

RATE OF ADMINISTRATION

Each 5 mg or fraction thereof over 1 minute.

ACTIONS

A synthetic narcotic agonist-antagonist with a potent analgesic action, pentazocine is somewhat less effective than morphine and meperidine in equivalent doses. Onset of action is prompt, 2 to 3 minutes, and lasts about 2 hours. Metabolized in the liver. Excreted in urine. Crosses the placental barrier. Secreted in breast milk.

INDICATIONS AND USES

Relief of moderate to severe pain. ■ Preoperative medication. ■ Support of anesthesia. ■ Obstetric analgesia.

CONTRAINDICATIONS

Hypersensitivity to pentazocine or its components (contains sulfites); pathologic brain conditions.

PRECAUTIONS

Use with caution in bronchial asthma, relief of biliary pain, history of drug abuse, myocardial infarction (especially if nausea and vomiting are present; increases cardiac workload), decreased renal or hepatic function, respiratory depression from any cause, a history of seizures and in patients with head injury or increased intracranial pressure. ■ Mild narcotic antagonist. May precipitate withdrawal symptoms in patients accustomed to narcotics. ■ May provide less effective analgesia in heavy smokers.

Monitor: Naloxone (Narcan), oxygen, and controlled respiratory equipment must always be available. ■ Observe patient continuously during injection and frequently thereafter. Monitor vital signs. Keep patient supine to minimize side effects, orthostatic hypotension and fainting may occur. Observe closely during ambulation. ■ Pain control usually more effective with routinely administered doses. Determine appropriate interval through clinical assessment. ■ Note Drug/lab interactions.

Patient education: Avoid use of alcohol or other CNS depressants (e.g., antihistamines, diazepam [Valium]). ■ Request assistance for ambulation. ■ May be habit forming.

Maternal/child: Pregnancy Category C: safety for use in pregnancy, lactation, and children under 12 years not established. ■ Use extreme caution if necessary during delivery of premature infants.

Elderly: May be more sensitive to effects (e.g., respiratory depression, constipation, dizziness, urinary retention). ■ Analgesia should be effective with lower doses. ■ Consider age-related organ impairment.

DRUG/LAB INTERACTIONS

Potentiated by cimetidine (Tagamet), and other CNS depressants such as narcotic analgesics, general anesthetics, alcohol, anticholinergics, antihistamines, barbiturates, hypnotics, sedatives, psychotropic agents, MAO inhibitors, and neuromuscular blocking agents (e.g., mivacurium [Mivacron]). Reduced doses of both drugs may be indicated. ■ May decrease analgesic effects of other narcotics; avoid concurrent use. ■ Metabolism and clearance increased in smokers, analgesic effects may be decreased.

SIDE EFFECTS

Allergic reactions, apprehension, blurred vision, circulatory depression, confusion, constipation, cramps, depression, diarrhea, disorientation, double vision, dreams, drug dependence, dry mouth, dyspnea, facial edema, floating feeling, flushing, hallucinations, headache, hypertension, insomnia, muscle tremor, neonatal apnea, nervousness, nystagmus, paresthesias, perspiration, pruritus, respiratory depression, sedation, seizures, shock, tachycardia, taste alteration, urinary retention, uterine contraction depression.

ANTIDOTE

For any side effect, discontinue the drug and notify the physician. Treat side effects symptomatically. For overdose or respiratory depression, naloxone hydrochloride (Narcan) is the antidote of choice. If naloxone is not available, methylphenidate (Ritalin) may be of value in respiratory depression (only available in oral form).

PENTOBARBITAL SODIUM

Nembutal sodium

Barbiturate
Sedative-hypnotic
Anticonvulsant

pH 9.0 to 10.5

USUAL DOSE

100 mg initially. Wait 1 full minute between each dose to determine drug effect. Additional doses in increments of 25 to 50 mg may be given as indicated. Maximum dosage ranges from 200 to 500 mg.

Barbiturate coma: Loading dose: 3 to 10 mg/kg over 30 minutes to 3 hours. **Maintenance dose:** 1.5 to 2 mg/kg every 1 to 2 hours or an infusion of 0.5 to 3 mg/kg/hr. Adjust to maintain pentobarbital blood level between 110 and 177 mM/L (25 to 40 mg/dl) or ICP below 25 Torr.

PEDIATRIC DOSE

1 to 3 mg/kg slowly until asleep. Maximum dose 100 mg/24 hr.

Barbiturate coma: See adult dose: An alternate source suggests **Loading dose:** 10 to 15 mg/kg over 1 to 2 hours. **Maintenance dose:** Begin with 1 mg/kg/hr; increase to 2 to 3 mg/kg/hr to maintain EEG burst suppression.

DOSE ADJUSTMENTS

Reduce dose in impaired renal or hepatic function, usually required in the debilitated or elderly. ■ Note Drug/lab interactions.

DILUTION

May be given undiluted or, preferably, may be further diluted in sterile water, NS, or Ringer's injection. Any desired amount of diluent may be used. 9 ml of diluent with 1 ml of pentobarbital (50 mg) equals 5 mg/ml. Use only absolutely clear solutions.

INCOMPATIBLE WITH

Atropine, benzquinamide (Emete-Con), brompheniramine (Dimetane-Ten), butorphanol (Stadol), cefazolin (Kefzol), chlordiazepoxide (Librium), chlorpheniramine (Chlor-Trimeton), chlorpromazine (Thorazine), cimetidine (Tagamet), clindamycin (Cleocin), codeine, diphenhydramine (Benadryl), droperidol (Inapsine), dymenhydrinate (Dramamine), ephedrine, erythromycin (Ilotycin), fentanyl, fructose solutions, glycopyrrolate (Robinul), hydrocortisone sodium succinate (Solu-Cortef), hydroxyzine (Vistaril), insulin (aqueous), kanamycin (Kantrex), levorphanol (Levo-Dromoran), meperidine (Demerol), methadone, methyldopa (Aldomet), midazolam (Versed), morphine, nalbuphine (Nubain), norepinephrine (Levophed), opium alkaloids, pancuronium (Pavulon), penicillins, pentazocine (Talwin), phenytoin (Dilantin), prochlorperazine (Compazine), promazine (Sparine), promethazine (Phenergan), ranitidine (Zantac), sodium bicarbonate, streptomycin, succinylcholine (Anectine), thiamine (Betalin-S), triflu-promazine (Vesprin), vancomycin (Vancocin).

RATE OF ADMINISTRATION

50 mg or fraction thereof over 1 minute. Titrate slowly to desired effect. Rapid injection rate may cause symptoms of overdose (e.g., serious respiratory depression).

Barbiturate coma: See specific dose recommendations.

ACTIONS

A sedative, hypnotic barbiturate of short duration with anticonvulsant effects. Pentobarbital is a CNS depressant. Onset of action is prompt by the IV route and lasts about 3 to 4 hours. Will effectively depress the motor cortex if adequate doses are administered. Pain perception is unimpaired. Reportedly reduces cerebral blood flow and thus reduces cerebral edema and intracranial pressure. Detoxified in the liver and excreted fairly quickly in the urine in changed form. Crosses the placental barrier. Secreted in breast milk.

INDICATIONS AND USES

Preanesthetic sedation. ▪ Dental and minor surgical sedation. ▪ Control of convulsions caused by disease and drug poisoning. ▪ Short-term hypnotic. ▪ Sedation in psychotic states.

Investigational uses: High doses have been used to induce coma in the management of cerebral ischemia and increased intracranial pressure. Has been most effective in patients under 35 years of age or in closed head injuries.

CONTRAINDICATIONS

Acute or chronic pain, delivery (when maximum drug effect would be at the time of delivery), history of porphyria, known hypersensitivity to barbiturates, severely impaired liver function especially with any signs of hepatic coma, severe respiratory disease or depression.

PRECAUTIONS

IV route usually reserved for critical situations. ▪ Use caution in status asthmaticus, shock, severe renal or liver disease, depressive states after convulsions, shock and in the elderly. ▪ Use caution in acute or chronic pain. ▪ Status epilepticus can occur from too-rapid withdrawal. ▪ May be habit forming. Use caution in the presence of fever, diabetes, hyperthyroidism, or severe anemia; may increase side effects. ▪ Benzodiazepines (diazepam [Valium], midazolam [Versed]) generally preferred for sedation.

Monitor: Record blood pressure, pulse, and respiration every 3 to 5 minutes. Keep patient under constant observation. ▪ Maintain a patent airway. ▪ Treat the cause of a convulsion. ▪ Highly alkaline; determine absolute patency of vein; use of large veins preferred to prevent thrombosis. Avoid extravasation. Intraarterial injection will cause gangrene. ▪ Monitor phenytoin and barbiturate levels when both drugs are used concurrently. ▪ Monitor hematopoietic, renal, and hepatic systems in extended therapy. ▪ Note Drug/lab interactions.

Patient education: Avoid alcohol and other CNS depressants (e.g., antihistamines, diazepam [Valium]) ▪ May be habit forming. ▪ May require alternate birth control.

Maternal/child: Category D: avoid pregnancy; will cause birth defects. ▪ May cause drowsiness in the nursing infant. ▪ Note Contraindications. ▪ May cause paradoxical excitement in children.

Elderly: Often have increased sensitivity to barbiturates; may cause marked excitement, depression, confusion, and increased risk of barbiturate-induced hypothermia. ▪ Note Dose adjustments and Precautions. ▪ Consider age-related hepatic or renal impairment.

DRUG/LAB INTERACTIONS

Use extreme caution if any other CNS depressants have been given, such as alcohol, narcotic analgesics, anesthetics, antidepressants, antihistamines, hypnotics, MAO inhibitors, phenothiazines, sedatives, aminoglycoside antibiotics, or tranquilizers; potentiation with respiratory depression may occur. ■ Inhibits effectiveness of propranolol (Inderal), corticosteroids, doxycycline (Vibramycin), oral anticoagulants, oral contraceptives, quinidine, and theophylline. Capable of innumerable interactions with many drugs. ■ May increase orthostatic hypotension with furosemide (Lasix). ■ Monitor phenytoin and barbiturate levels when both drugs are used concurrently. ■ May inhibit vitamin D metabolism with extended use.

SIDE EFFECTS

Average dose: Depression, dermatitis, facial edema, fever, hypotension, neonatal apnea, pain at or below injection site, respiratory depression (hypoventilation), thrombocytopenic purpura.

Overdose: Apnea, coma, cough reflex depression, flat EEG (reversible unless hypoxic damage has occurred), hypotension, laryngospasm, lowered body temperature, pulmonary edema, renal shutdown, respiratory depression, sluggish or absent reflexes.

ANTIDOTE

Discontinue drug immediately for pain at or below injection site. Notify the physician of any side effects. Symptomatic and supportive treatment are most important in overdose. Maintain an adequate airway with artificial ventilation if indicated. Keep the patient warm. IV volume expanders (dextran) and IV fluids will help maintain adequate circulation. Diuretics or hemodialysis will promote the elimination of the drug. Vasopressors (dopamine [Intropin]) will maintain blood pressure.

PENTOSTATIN   Antineoplastic (Antibiotic)

DCF, 2-deoxycoformycin, Nipent   pH 7.0 to 8.5

USUAL DOSE

4 mg/M^2 every other week. Evaluation and prehydration is required before administration; see Precautions/Monitor. If there is no major toxicity and improvement is continuous, treat until a complete response is achieved; then administer two additional doses. Do not treat beyond 12 months.

DOSE ADJUSTMENTS

Reduced dose and benefit-versus-risk assessment may be required with impaired renal function (creatinine clearance below 60 ml/min); insufficient data available. ■ Withhold dose if serum creatinine elevated; obtain creatinine clearance. ■ Withhold dose if the absolute neutrophil count falls from a base line of greater than 500 cells/mm^3 before therapy to less than 200 cells/mm^3 during treatment. Resume treatment when count returns to predose levels.

DILUTION

Specific techniques required; see Precautions. Diluent (5 ml sterile water) provided; dissolve completely; will yield 2 mg/ml. May be given direct IV or further diluted in 25 to 50 ml NS or D5W; 25 ml yields 0.33

mg/ml, 50 ml yields 0.18 mg/ml. Treat spills or waste with a 5% sodium hypochlorite solution before disposal.

Storage: Refrigerate before initial reconstitution. Store at room temperature and use within 8 hours after initial reconstitution or dilution for infusion.

INCOMPATIBLE WITH

Specific information not available. May decompose more readily in acidic solutions. Should be considered incompatible in syringe or solution with any other drug because of toxicity and specific use.

RATE OF ADMINISTRATION

Direct IV: A single dose over 1 minute.

Infusion: A single dose over 20 to 30 minutes. In either situation follow with an additional 500 ml of prehydration infusion fluids.

ACTIONS

Mechanism of action is not known, but it is cytotoxic as a result of its potent inhibition of the enzyme adenosine deaminase (ADA). Blocks DNA and RNA synthesis and causes DNA damage. Average terminal half-life of 6 hours is extended to 18 hours in patients with impaired renal function (creatinine clearance less than 50 ml/min). Inhibits ADA for up to 1 week; actual response may not occur for months. Crosses blood-brain barrier. Primarily excreted in urine.

INDICATIONS AND USES

Treatment of hairy cell leukemia (HCL).

Investigational uses: May be used in combination or sequentially with SC interferon-alpha-2b (Intron A). Treatment of non-hodgkins lymphoma, mycosis fungoides, adult t-cell lymphoma, chronic lymphocytic leukemia, rheumatoid arthritis.

CONTRAINDICATIONS

Hypersensitivity to pentostatin.

PRECAUTIONS

Follow guidelines for handling cytotoxic agents. See Appendix A, p. 893. ■ Assess drug profile before administration. ■ Myelosuppression, especially neutropenia, is most severe during the first few courses of treatment. ■ Must consider risk/benefit in patients with some bone marrow depression, the possibility of chickenpox or herpes zoster, a history of gout or urate renal stones, renal function impairment, or previous cytotoxic drug or radiation therapy. Use extreme caution. ■ After 6 months of treatment, assess for response; if partial or complete response is not evident, discontinue treatment. If partial response is evident, reevaluate as indicated but do not treat beyond 12 months.

Monitor: Monitor complete blood count and serum creatinine before each dose and as indicated. Blood chemistries including serum uric acid, and a creatinine clearance assay are required before and during treatment. ■ Prehydration with 500 to 1,000 ml 5% dextrose in half-normal saline or an equivalent is required. An additional 500 ml is required post administration. ■ Treatment of patients with infection may exacerbate symptoms and cause death. Control infection before treatment initiated. Withhold treatment if an active infection occurs; resume when infection is controlled. ■ Prophylactic antiemetics recommended (e.g., prochlorperazine [Compazine], ondansetron [Zofran]); continue for 48 to 72 hours. ■ Observe closely for severe rashes, nervous system toxicity, and myelosuppression (especially after initial cycles); pentostatin may have to be withheld or discontinued. ▪ For severe neutropenia beyond the initial cycles, evaluate for disease status, including a bone marrow examination. ▪ Assess response to treatment with periodic monitoring of peripheral blood for hairy cells. Bone marrow aspirates and biopsies may be required at 2 to 3 month intervals.

Patient education: Consider birth control options; nonhormonal birth control recommended. ▪ Report rashes, symptoms of infection or bruising and bleeding immediately. ▪ See Appendix D, p. 900.

Maternal/child: Category D: avoid pregnancy; can cause fetal harm. ▪ Discontinue breast feeding. ▪ Safety for use in children and adolescents under 18 not established.

Elderly: Consider decreased renal function.

DRUG/LAB INTERACTIONS

Assess drug profile before administration. ▪ Do not use with fludarabine (Fludara); may increase risk of fatal pulmonary toxicity. ▪ May cause skin rash with allopurinol. ▪ Elevates liver function tests; usually reversible. ▪ Do not administer live vaccines to patients receiving antineoplastic drugs. ▪ Uric acid levels may increase, increased dose of gout agents (e.g., colchicine, probenicid, sulfinpyrazone [Anturane]) may be indicated. ▪ Leukopenia and thrombocytopenia increased by agents causing blood dyscrasias (e.g., anticonvulsants [phenytoin (Dilantin)], penicillins, phenothiazines, and many others).

SIDE EFFECTS

Allergic reactions, anemia, anorexia, chills, cough, diarrhea, fatigue, fever, GU disorders, headache, hepatic disorders/elevated liver function tests, infection, leukopenia, lung disorders, myalgia, nausea, neurologic disorders/CNS, pain, rashes, skin disorders, thrombocytopenia, upper respiratory infections, and vomiting occur in 10% of patients and may require discontinuation of treatment. Abdominal pain, abnormal thinking, abnormal vision, abnormal ECG, anxiety, arthralgia, asthenia, back pain, bronchitis, cardiac arrhythmias, chest pain, confusion, conjunctivitis, constipation, depression, dizziness, dry skin, dyspnea, dysuria, ear pain, ecchymosis, eczema; elevated BUN, creatinine, and LDH; epistaxis, eye pain, flatulence, flu syndrome, hematuria, hemorrhage, herpes simplex, herpes zoster, insomnia, lung edema, lymphadenopathy, maculopapular rash, malaise, neoplasm, nervousness, paresthesia, peripheral edema, petechia, pharyngitis, pneumonia, pruritus, rhinitis, seborrhea, sinusitis, skin discoloration, somnolence, stomatitis, sweating, thrombophlebitis, vesiculobullous rash, weight loss, and death have occurred in 3% to 10% of patients.

ANTIDOTE

Keep physician informed of all side effects; most will be treated symptomatically if indicated. Withhold dose and notify physician for elevated serum creatinine, absolute neutrophil count below 200 cells/mm^3, myelosuppression, infection, CNS toxicity, or severe rash. Overdose may cause death due to severe renal, hepatic, pulmonary, or CNS toxicity. There is no specific antidote. Supportive therapy as indicated will help sustain the patient.

PERPHENAZINE

Trilafon

USUAL DOSE

1 mg, repeat as necessary, allowing 2 to 3 minutes between doses, only until symptoms are controlled. Do not exceed 5 mg.

DOSE ADJUSTMENTS

Reduced dose (one-third to one-half) may be indicated in the elderly.
- Note Drug/lab interactions.

DILUTION

Check label on ampoule. Only single-dose, 5 mg ampoules may be given IV. Handle carefully; may cause contact dermatitis. Each 5 mg (1 ml) must be diluted with 9 ml of NS. Shake well. 1 ml will equal 0.5 mg. May be further diluted and given as an infusion under observation of anesthesiologist (use an infusion pump or a microdrip, 60 gtt/ml). Sensitive to light.

Storage: Store at CRT. Slightly yellow color does not affect potency. Discard if markedly discolored.

INCOMPATIBLE WITH

Aminophylline, cefoperazone (Cefobid), midazolam (Versed), opium alkaloids, oxytocin, pentobarbital (Nembutal), secobarbital (Seconal), thiopental (Pentothal).

RATE OF ADMINISTRATION

0.5 mg or fraction thereof over 1 minute.

ACTIONS

A phenothiazine derivative said to be approximately ten times more potent than chlorpromazine (Thorazine) with effects on the central, autonomic, and peripheral nervous systems. Has weak to moderate sedative effects, moderate anticholinergic effects, and strong antiemetic and entrapyramidal effects. Onset of action is prompt and lasting. Metabolized by the liver and excreted in urine and feces.

INDICATIONS AND USES

Control of severe nausea and vomiting, intractable hiccups, or acute symptoms such as violent retching during surgery.

CONTRAINDICATIONS

Comatose or severely depressed states; hypersensitivity to phenothiazines or its components (contains bisulfites) in the presence of existing blood dyscrasias, bone marrow depression or liver disease, or in patients receiving large doses of other CNS depressants (e.g, antihistamines, barbiturates, or narcotics).

PRECAUTIONS

Use IV only when absolutely necessary. ■ May mask diagnosis of brain tumor, drug intoxication, and intestinal obstruction. ■ Use caution in coronary disease, respiratory disease, severe hypertension or hypotension, glaucoma and epilepsy. ■ Anticholinergic and cardiac effects may be troublesome during anesthesia. For patients receiving phenothiazines, discontinue preoperatively if they will not be continued after surgery.

Monitor: Keep patient in supine position and monitor blood pressure and pulse between doses. ▪ Temperature without etiology indicates drug intolerance.

Patient education: Request assistance for ambulation; may cause dizziness or fainting. ▪ Possible skin and eye sensitivity; avoid unprotected exposure to sun. ▪ Avoid use of alcohol or other CNS depressants (e.g., antihistamines, barbiturates. ▪ Use caution performing tasks requiring alertness.

Maternal/child: Safety for use in pregnancy and lactation not established. ▪ May cause paradoxical excitement in children. ▪ Not recommended for use in children under 12 years.

Elderly: Note Dose adjustments and Precautions. ▪ May cause paradoxical excitement. ▪ May have increased sensitivity to postural hypotension, anticholinergic, and sedative effects. ▪ Increased risk of extrapyramidal side effects (e.g., tardive dyskinesia, parkinsonism).

DRUG/LAB INTERACTIONS

Increased CNS, respiratory depression and hypotensive effects with CNS depressants (e.g., narcotics, barbiturates, alcohol, anesthetics). Reduced dose of these agents usually indicated, may have less potentiating effect than other phenothiazines. ▪ Additive effects with MAO inhibitors (e.g., selegiline [Eldepryl]), anticholinergics, antihistamines, antihypertensives, hypnotics, muscle relaxants, rauwolfia alkaloids, and thiazide diuretics, dose adjustment may be necessary. ▪ Risk of cardiotoxicity increased with pimozide (Orap) and sparfloxacin (Zagam); concurrent use not recommended. ▪ May increase cardiac depressant effects of quinidine, concurrent use should be avoided. ▪ Use of epinephrine not recommended; may cause preciptious hypotension. ▪ Use caution during anesthesia with barbiturates (e.g., methohexital, thiopental); may increase frequency and severity of hypotension and neuromuscular excitation. ▪ Capable of innumerable other interactions.

SIDE EFFECTS

Usually transient if drug is discontinued, but may require treatment if severe: anaphylaxis, blurring of vision, cardiac arrest, dermatitis, dizziness, dryness of mouth, dysphagia, extrapyramidal symptoms (e.g., abnormal positioning, extreme restlessness, pseudoparkinsonism, weakness of extremities), elevated blood pressure, excitement, hypersensitivity reactions, hypotension, slurred speech, spastic movements (especially about the face), tachycardia, temperature without etiology, tightness of the throat, tongue discoloration, tongue protrusion, and many others. Overdose can cause convulsions, hallucinations, and death.

ANTIDOTE

Discontinue the drug at onset of any side effect and notify the physician. Counteract hypotension with IV fluids, or norepinephrine (Levophed) or phenylephrine (Neo-synephrine) and extrapyramidal symptoms with benztropine mesylate (Cogentin) or diphenhydramine (Benadryl). Epinephrine is contraindicated for hypotension; further hypotension will occur. Use diazepam (Valium) or phenobarbital for convulsions or hyperactivity. Phenytoin may be helpful in ventricular arrhythmias. In treating respiratory depression and unconsciousness, avoid analeptics such as doxapram (Dopram); they may cause convulsions. Resuscitate as necessary.

PHENOBARBITAL SODIUM

Barbiturate
Sedative-hypnotic
Anticonvulsant

Luminal sodium

pH 8.5 to 10.5

USUAL DOSE

Use only enough medication to achieve the desired effect. May take up to 15 minutes to reach peak levels in the brain; guard against overdose and excessive respiratory depression.

Hypnotic: 100 to 325 mg.

Sedative: 30 to 120 mg/day in 2 or 3 divided doses.

Anticonvulsant: 200 to 320 mg. May be repeated if necessary. Maximum dose usually does not exceed 600 mg.

Status epilepticus: Loading dose: 10 to 20 mg in single or divided doses. May give an additional 5 mg/kg every 15 to 30 minutes up to a maximum dose of 30 mg/kg. *Maintenance dose:* 1 to 3 mg/kg/24 hr or 0.5 to 1.5 mg/kg every 12 hours.

PEDIATRIC DOSE

Preop sedation: 1 to 3 mg/kg of body weight 60 to 90 minutes before procedure.

Status epilepticus: Loading dose: 15 to 18 mg/kg as a single dose or in divided doses. May give an additional 5 mg/kg every 15 to 30 minutes up to a maximum dose of 30 mg/kg.

Maintenance dose: Infants: 2.5 to 3 mg/kg every 12 hours.

Ages 1 to 5: 3 to 4 mg/kg every 12 hours.

Ages 6 to 12: 2 to 3 mg/kg every 12 hours.

Over 12 years of age: 0.5 to 1.5 mg/kg every 12 hours. Up to 12 mg/kg/24 hours has been used in maintenance doses. Note instructions in Usual dose.

NEONATAL DOSE

Status epilepticus: Loading dose: 15 to 20 mg/kg as a single dose or in divided doses.

Maintenance dose: 1.5 to 2 mg/kg every 12 hours; may be increased to 2.5 mg/kg every 12 hours if needed. Note instructions in Usual dose.

DOSE ADJUSTMENTS

Reduce dose in impaired renal or hepatic function, usually required in the debilitated or elderly. ■ Note Drug/lab interactions.

DILUTION

Sterile powder must be slowly diluted with sterile water for injection. Use a minimum of 3 ml of diluent. Also available in sterile vials and tubexes. Best if further diluted up to 10 ml with sterile water for injection. Solutions from powder form must be freshly prepared. Use only absolutely clear solutions. Discard powder or solution exposed to air for 30 minutes.

INCOMPATIBLE WITH

Acidic solutions, alcohol 5% in dextrose, aminophylline, atracurium (Tracrium), benzquinamide (Emete-Con), calcium chloride, cephalothin (Keflin), chlorpromazine (Thorazine), cimetidine (Tagamet), clindamycin (Cleocin), codeine, dimenhydrinate (Dramanate), diphenhydramine (Benadryl), droperidol (Inapsine), ephedrine, erythromycin (Ilotycin), hydralazine (Apresoline), hydrocortisone sodium succinate (Solu-Cortef), hydromorphone (Dilaudid), hydroxyzine (Vistaril), isoproterenol (Isuprol), insulin (aqueous), kanamycin (Kantrex), levorphanol (Levo-Dromoran), magnesium sulfate, meperidine (Demerol), metaraminol (Aramine), methadone, methyldopa (Aldomet), morphine, norepinephrine (Levophed), pancuronium bromide (Pavulon), parabens, penicillin G potassium, pentazocine (Talwin), phenytoin (Dilantin), phytonadione (Aquamephyton), polymixin-B (Aerosporin), procaine (Novocain), prochlorperazine (Compazine), promazine (Sparine), promethazine (Phenergan), propiomazine (Largon), ranitidine (Zantac), sodium bicarbonate, streptomycin, succinylcholine (Anectine), thiamine, trifluoperazine (Stelazine), tripelennamine (Pyribenzamine), vancomycin (Vancocin), warfarin (Coumadin).

RATE OF ADMINISTRATION

60 mg (gr 1) or fraction thereof over 1 minute. Titrate slowly to desired effect. Rapid injection rate may cause symptoms of overdose (e.g., serious respiratory depression).

Status epilepticus: A single loading dose over 10 to 15 minutes.

ACTIONS

A sedative, hypnotic barbiturate of long duration with potent anticonvulsant effects. Phenobarbital is a CNS depressant. Onset of action is prompt by the IV route and becomes rapidly more intense. Effects last from 6 to 10 hours. Will effectively depress the motor cortex with small doses. Pain perception is unimpaired. Rapidly absorbed by all body tissues and excreted in changed form in the urine. Excreted more readily in alkaline urine. Crosses the placental barrier. Secreted in breast milk.

INDICATIONS AND USES

Prolonged sedation (medical and psychiatric). ▪ Anticonvulsant.

CONTRAINDICATIONS

History of porphyria, impaired renal function, impaired hepatic function especially with any signs of hepatic coma, known hypersensitivity to barbiturates, previous addiction, severe respiratory depression including dyspnea, obstruction, or cor pulmonale.

PRECAUTIONS

IV route usually reserved for critical situations. ▪ Use caution in elderly and debilitated patients and those with asthma, pulmonary disease, shock, and impaired renal or hepatic function. ▪ Status epilepticus can occur from too-rapid withdrawal. ▪ May be habit forming. Use caution in acute or chronic pain. ▪ Benzodiazepines (diazepam [Valium], midazolam [Versed]) generally preferred for sedation.

Monitor: Keep patient under constant observation. Record vital signs every hour, or more often if indicated. ▪ Maintain a patent airway. ▪ Monitor hematopoietic, renal and hepatic systems in any extended therapy. ▪ Treat the cause of a convulsion. ▪ Keep equipment for artificial ventilation available. ■ Highly alkaline, determine absolute patency of vein; use of large veins preferred to prevent thrombosis. Avoid extravasation. Intraarterial injection will cause gangrene. ■ Monitor phenytoin and barbiturate levels when both drugs are used concurrently. ■ Note Drug/lab interactions.

Patient education: Avoid alcohol or other CNS depressants (e.g., antihistamines, diazepam [Valium]). May be habit forming. ■ May require alternate birth control.

Maternal/child: Category D: avoid pregnancy: will cause birth defects. ■ May cause drowsiness in the nursing infant. ■ Note Precautions.

Elderly: Note Dose Adjustments and Precautions. ■ Often have increased sensitivity to barbiturates; may cause marked excitement, depression, confusion and increased risk of barbiturate induced hypothermia. ■ Consider age-related hepatic or renal impairment.

DRUG/LAB INTERACTIONS
Use extreme caution if any other CNS depressants have been given, such as alcohol, narcotic analgesics, anesthetics, antidepressants, antihistamines, hypnotics, MAO inhibitors, phenothiazines, sedatives, aminoglycoside antibiotics, tranquilizers. Potentiation with respiratory depression may occur. ■ Inhibits effectiveness of propranolol (Inderal), corticosteroids, doxycycline (Vibramycin), oral anticoagulants, oral contraceptives, quinidine, and theophylline. Capable of innumerable interactions with many drugs. ■ May increase orthostatic hypotension with furosemide (Lasix). ■ Monitor phenytoin (Dilantin), felbamate (Felbatol), and barbiturate levels when any combination of these drugs is used concurrently. ■ May inhibit vitamin D metabolism with extended use.

SIDE EFFECTS
Rarely occur with slow injection of average doses.

Average dose: Depression, dermatitis, facial edema, fever, headache, hypotension, nausea, neonatal apnea, respiratory depression (hypoventilation), thrombocytopenic purpura, vertigo.

Overdose: Apnea, coma, cough reflex depression, delirium, flat EEG (reversible unless hypoxic damage has occurred), hypotension, laryngospasm, lowered body temperature, pulmonary edema, renal shutdown, respiratory depression, sluggish or absent reflexes, stupor.

ANTIDOTE
Notify the physician of any side effects. Symptomatic and supportive treatment is most important in overdose. Maintain an adequate airway with artificial ventilation if indicated. Keep the patient warm. IV volume expanders (dextran) and other IV fluids will help maintain adequate circulation. Diuretics may promote the elimination of the drug. Vasopressors (e.g., dopamine [Intropin]) will maintain blood pressure.

PHENTOLAMINE MESYLATE

Alpha-adrenergic blocking agent
Antihypertensive
Vasodilator

Regitine

pH 4.5 to 6.5

USUAL DOSE

Phentolamine is available on an allocation basis from the manufacturer (Novartis). Hospitals are allowed to keep 2 boxes on hand, otherwise request must be faxed to manufacturer aft (973) 503-5695 (24 hours). Include a copy of the prescription (Doctor's order), a written request for the required supply, and the name and address of a wholesaler for billing purposes. Telephone (888) 669-6682.

Preoperative: 5 mg 1 to 2 hours before surgery. May be repeated. During surgery the same doses are used as indicated to control epinephrine intoxication.

Prevent necrosis caused by norepinephrine (Levophed): Add 10 mg to each 1,000 ml of IV solution containing norepinephrine or dopamine.

Test dose for diagnosis of pheochromocytoma: 2.5 to 5 mg.

Treatment of Congestive heart failure (investigational): 5 to 10 mg in 500 ml of D5W given at a rate of 0.17 to 0.4 mg/min.

PEDIATRIC DOSE

Preoperative: 1 mg, 0.1 mg/kg of body weight, or 3 mg/M^2 1 to 2 hours before surgery. Repeat as indicated (see adult dose).

Prevent necrosis caused by norepinephrine (Levophed): Add 0.1 to 0.2 mg/kg up to a maximum of 10 mg to each 1,000 ml of IV solution containing norepinephrine.

Test dose for diagnosis of pheochromocytoma: 1 mg.

DILUTION

Each 5 mg should be diluted with 1 ml of sterile water for injection. May be further diluted with 5 to 10 ml of sterile water for injection. Use only freshly prepared solutions.

Storage: Store below 40° C.

INCOMPATIBLE WITH

Iron salts.

RATE OF ADMINISTRATION

Each 5 mg or fraction thereof over 1 minute. Inject test dose rapidly after pressor response to venipuncture has subsided.

ACTIONS

An alpha-blocking agent that competitively antagonizes endogenous and exogenous alpha agents (e.g., epinephrine and norepinephrine). Has positive chronotropic and inotropic effects on cardiac muscle as well as vasodilator effects on vascular smooth muscle. Onset of action is prompt. Half-life is approximately 19 minutes. Metabolic fate is undetermined.

INDICATIONS AND USES

Prevention and treatment of hypertensive episodes of pheochromocytoma preoperatively and during surgery. ■ Prevention and treatment of necrosis and sloughing occurring with dopamine (Intropin) and norepinephrine (Levophed). ▪ Definitive diagnosis of pheochromocytoma.

Investigational uses: Treatment of congestive heart failure, hypertensive crisis due to MAO inhibitor/sympathomimetic amine interactions and rebound hypertension after discontinuation of clonidine, propranolol, or other hypertensive agents.

CONTRAINDICATIONS

Coronary artery disease, coronary insufficiency, hypersensitivity to phentolamine, myocardial infarction (previous or present).

PRECAUTIONS

Use caution in gastritis or peptic ulcer disease. ▪ Use care in the presence of any arrhythmia. It is preferable to have a normal sinus rhythm. ▪ MI, cerebrovascular spasm and cerebrovascular occlusion have occurred following administration, usually in association with marked hypotensive episodes. ▪ For diagnosis of pheochromocytoma, urinary tests such as vanillymandelic acid (VMA) are safer and more accurate. Phentolamine is used only when absolutely necessary. Specific procedure must be followed. Consult with physician and pharmacist.

Monitor: Monitor vital signs every 2 minutes.

Maternal/child: Category C, safety for use during pregnancy and lactation not established. Use with extreme caution and only when clearly indicated.

Elderly: Risk of phentolamine-induced hypothermia may be increased.

DRUG/LAB INTERACTIONS

Antagonizes effects of epinephrine and ephedrine.

SIDE EFFECTS

Minor: Abdominal pain, diarrhea, dizziness, hypotension, nasal stuffiness, nausea, tachycardia, tingling of skin, weakness, vomiting.

Major: Cardiac arrhythmias, cerebrovascular occlusion, cerebrovascular spasm, hypotension (severe), myocardial infarction, shock, tachycardia, vomiting under anesthesia.

ANTIDOTE

For minor side effects, notify the physician. If symptoms progress or any major side effect occurs, discontinue drug and notify the physician immediately. Elevation of legs, volume expanders (e.g., albumin, hetastarch) and administration of norepinephrine are recommended for treatment of hypotension. Do not use epinephrine. Maintain the patient as indicated. If tachycardia or cardiac arrhythmias occur, defer use of digitalis derivatives if possible until rhythm returns to normal.

PHENYLEPHRINE HYDROCHLORIDE

Neo-Synephrine

Vasopressor

pH 3.0 to 6.5

USUAL DOSE

Mild to moderate hypotension or hypotensive emergencies during spinal anesthesia: 0.2 mg. From 0.1 to 0.5 mg may be used initially. May be repeated every 10 to 15 minutes. Never exceed 0.5 mg in a single dose. Highly individualized. Start with a small dose, giving only as much of the drug as required to alleviate undesirable symptoms.

Severe hypotension and shock- or drug-related hypotension: Begin infusion at 100 to 180 mcg/min until blood pressure stabilized at a low normal for specific individual. Maintain with 40 to 60 mcg/min. Titrate to desired effect.

Paroxysmal supraventricular tachycardia: 0.25 to 0.5 mg has been given as a rapid IV bolus. If additional doses are required to achieve adequate response, increase in increments of 0.1 to 0.2 mg and never exceed a total single dose of 1 mg. Adenosine may be the drug of choice.

PEDIATRIC DOSE

Mild to moderate hypotension: 5 to 20 mcg/kg of body weight per dose. May be repeated every 10 to 15 minutes. Do not exceed adult dose.

Severe hypotension and shock- or drug-related hypotension: Begin an infusion at 0.1 to 0.5 mcg/kg/min. Titrate to desired effect. Do not exceed a maximum total dose of 5 mg.

Paroxysmal supraventricular tachycardia: 5 to 10 mcg/kg/dose as a rapid IV bolus. May repeat dose or double a dose and repeat every 5 minutes until desired systolic blood pressure reached.

DOSE ADJUSTMENTS

Hypotension of powerful peripheral adrenergic blocking agents, chlorpromazine, or pheochromocytomectomy may require carefully calculated increased dose therapy.

DILUTION

Direct IV: Dilute 1 ml of a 10 mg/ml solution with 9 ml of sterile water for injection to prepare a final concentration of 1 mg/ml.

Infusion: Dilute 10 mg in 500 ml of NS or D5W to provide a 1:50,000 solution (20 mcg/ml). May increase to 20 or 30 mg in 500 ml if necessary (40 to 60 mcg/ml).

Pediatric infusion: Add 0.6 mg/kg to 100 ml diluent. 1 ml/hr equals 0.1 mcg/kg/min.

Storage: Protect from light.

INCOMPATIBLE WITH

Alkaline solutions, iron salts, phenytoin (Dilantin).

RATE OF ADMINISTRATION

Direct IV: Single dose over 20 to 30 seconds to treat paroxysmal supraventricular tachycardia; over 1 minute in other situations.

Infusion: Regulate drip rate to provide and maintain individual's low normal blood pressure. Use an infusion pump or microdrip (60 gtt/ml) to administer.

ACTIONS

A sympathomimetic, similar to epinephrine. Acts primarily on alpha adrenergic receptors. A potent long-lasting vasoconstrictor. Unique in that it slows the heart rate, increases stroke volume, and does not induce any change in rhythm of the pulse. Renal vessel constriction will occur. Repeated injections produce comparable results. Effective within seconds and lasts about 15 minutes. Metabolic fate and route of excretion have not been determined. Uptake of drug into tissue and some metabolism by the liver have been documented.

INDICATIONS AND USES

Maintain adequate blood pressure in inhalation and spinal anesthesia, shocklike states, drug-induced hypotension, and hypersensitivity reactions. ▪ Treat paroxysmal supraventricular tachycardia. ▪ Prolong anesthesia.

Unlabeled use: Specific antidote for hypotension produced by chlorpromazine hydrochloride (Thorazine).

CONTRAINDICATIONS

Hypertension, ventricular tachycardia and hypersensitivity to phenylephrine.

PRECAUTIONS

Blood volume depletion should be corrected. May be administered concurrently with blood volume replacement. ▪ Use extreme caution in the elderly, hyperthyroidism, bradycardia, partial heart block, myocardial disease, or severe arteriosclerosis. ▪ Contains bisulfites; use caution in allergic individuals.

Monitor: Check blood pressure every 2 minutes until stabilized at the desired level. ▪ Discontinue IV administration if vein infiltrates or is thrombosed; can cause tissue necrosis and sloughing. ▪ Note Precautions, Drug/lab interactions.

Maternal/child: Pregnancy Category C: safety for use in pregnancy or lactation not established.

Elderly: Note Precautions, may have increased sensitivity to effects.

DRUG/LAB INTERACTIONS

Potentiated by tricyclic antidepressants (e.g., desipramine [Norpramin]), guanethidine, MAO inhibitors (e.g., selegiline [Eldepryl]), other vasopressors (epinephrine [Adrenalin]); ergot alkaloids or oxytocic agents (e.g, ergonovine, oxytocin); hypertensive crisis and death can result. ▪ Use caution with digitalis, bretylium, or halogenated hydrocarbon anesthetics (e.g., halothane, isoflurane); arrhythmias may occur.

SIDE EFFECTS

Bradycardia, fullness of head, headache, hypertension, tingling of extremities, tremulousness, ventricular extrasystoles, ventricular tachycardia (short paroxysms), vertigo.

ANTIDOTE

To prevent sloughing and necrosis in areas where extravasation has occurred, with a fine hypodermic needle inject 5 to 10 mg of phentolamine (Regitine) diluted in 10 to 15 ml of normal saline liberally throughout the tissue in the extravasated area. Treatment should be started as soon as extravasation is recognized. Notify the physician of all side effects. IM injection may be preferable. Treat hypertension with phentolamine (Regitine). Treat cardiac arrhythmias as indicated. Treat bradycardia with atropine. Resuscitate as necessary.

PHENYTOIN SODIUM

Hydantoin
Anticonvulsant
Antiarrhythmic

Dilantin, Dilantin sodium   pH 12.0

USUAL DOSE

In all situations, transfer to oral therapy 12 to 24 hours after a loading dose or as soon as practical. Note Precautions.

Status epilepticus, anticonvulsant: A *loading dose* of 10 to 20 mg/kg. Follow with *maintenance doses* of 100 mg every 6 to 8 hours. Do not exceed a total dose of 1.5 Gm. Lethal dose estimated at 2 to 5 Gm. If seizure not terminated, consider other anticonvulsants, barbiturates, or anesthesia. IV diazepam may be the drug of choice for initial treatment. Concurrent administration of phenytoin in the lesser doses is suggested by clinicians to maintain control.

Antiarrhythmic: 50 to 100 mg at 5 to 15 minute intervals until the arrhythmia is abolished or side effects occur. Do not exceed a total dose of 15 mg/kg or 1 Gm.

PEDIATRIC DOSE

Status epilepticus, anticonvulsant: 250 mg/M^2 followed by maintenance doses of 4 to 8 mg/kg/24 hr in divided doses every 8 to 12 hours. An alternate regimen for children of all ages is a loading dose of 15 to 20 mg/kg. Follow with a maintenance dose for age (listed below):

Neonates: Begin with 5 mg/kg/24 hr in equally divided doses every 8 to 12 hours. Range is 5 to 8 mg/kg/24 hours.

Infants and children: Begin with 5 mg/kg/24 hr in equally divided doses every 8 to 12 hours. Range varies according to age: *6 months to 3 years:* 8 to 10 mg/kg/24 hr. *4 to 6 years:* 7.5 to 9 mg/kg/24 hr. *7 to 9 years:* 7 to 8 mg/kg/24 hr. *10 to 16 years:* 6 to 7 mg/kg/24 hr. Maintenance dose should not exceed 20 mg/kg/24 hr. Loading dose not included in this total. Note comments in Usual dose.

Antiarrhythmic: 1.25 mg/kg every 5 minutes until arrhythmia abolished or side effects occur. Do not exceed a total dose of 15 mg/kg. Maintenance dose is 2.5 to 5 mg every 12 hours.

DOSE ADJUSTMENTS

Use caution, lower dose, and slower rate of administration in the seriously ill, elderly, cachetic patients, and in impaired liver or renal function. ▪ In obesity calculate dose on ideal body weight plus 1.33 of excess over ideal; phenytoin preferentially distributes into fat. ▪ Dose adjustment may be required based on serum albumin levels. ▪ Note Drug/lab interactions.

DILUTION

Available as 100 or 250 mg ampoules, syringes, or vials. Usually not added to IV solutions. May be injected through Y-tube or three-way stopcock of infusion set of a compatible solution. Use solution only when completely dissolved and clear; discard if hazy or if a precipitate forms. May be light yellow in color. Recent studies have utilized infusion solutions (NS) prepared immediately before use in suitable concentrations (less than 6.7 mg/ml) to facilitate required rate and fluid limitations or requirements. Method not recommended by manufacturer but is in common use (see Incompatible with). According to most studies, a 0.22 micron in-line filter is required.

Storage: Store between 15° and 30° C.

INCOMPATIBLE WITH

Any other drug in syringe or solution. Will precipitate if pH is altered. Clear tubing with NS if possible before and after administration through Y-tube or three-way stopcock.

RATE OF ADMINISTRATION

Very alkaline; follow each injection with sterile NS to reduce local venous irritation. Best to flush before and after with NS.

Anticonvulsant: 25 to 50 mg or fraction thereof over 1 minute. A rate of 0.5 to 3 mg/kg/min (not to exceed 25 mg/min) has been suggested for neonates and pediatric patients. Another source suggests 1 mg/min. Limit rate to 25 mg/min in the elderly.

Antiarrhythmic: 25 mg or fraction thereof over 2 to 3 minutes.

Infusion: Should be completed within 1 hour. Do not exceed direct IV rate. Best if infusion is piggybacked to a compatible primary IV so phenytoin can be discontinued if side effects occur but IV can be kept open.

ACTIONS

A synthetic anticonvulsant, chemically related to barbiturates. Selectively stabilizes seizure threshold and depresses seizure activity in the motor cortex. Effective control in emergency treatment of seizures may take 15 to 20 minutes because of rate of injection required. Also exerts a depressant effect on the myocardium by selectively elevating the excitability threshold of the cell, reducing the cell's response to stimuli. Readily absorbed, phenytoin is metabolized in the liver and excreted in changed form in the urine. Crosses placental barrier. Secreted in breast milk.

INDICATIONS AND USES

Control of grand mal and psychomotor seizures. ■ Treatment of status epilepticus (grand mal seizures).

Unlabeled use: Treatment of supraventricular and ventricular arrhythmias including those caused by digitalis intoxication. Especially useful for patients who are unable to tolerate quinidine or procainamide.

CONTRAINDICATIONS

Bradycardia, sinoatrial, second- or third-degree heart block, Stokes-Adams syndrome; known sensitivity to hydantoin derivatives.

PRECAUTIONS

Because of benefits provided by fosphenytoin (Cerebyx)—e.g., solubility in IV solutions, improved infusion site tolerance, more rapid rate of administration, and well-tolerated IM option—Parke-Davis wants to discontinue injectable phenytoin (Dilantin). Generic products will still be available. ■ Status epilepticus can occur from abrupt withdrawal of hydantoins. ■ Not effective for petit mal seizures; com bined therapy required if both conditions present. ▪ Use caution in hypotension and severe myocardial insufficiency. ▪ Use caution with low serum albumin level, and adjust dose as indicated. Phenytoin is 90% bound to serum protein and a reduced albumin causes an increase in free drug availability. ▪ Lymphadenopathy has been reported. Monitoring and change in anticonvulsant therapy may be indicated. ▪ Discontinue phenytoin if skin rash appears. ▪ Hyperglycemia and blood dyscrasias have been reported.

Monitor: Narrow margin of error between therapeutic and toxic dose. Plasma levels above 10 mcg/ml usually control seizure activity. The acceptable range is 5 to 20 mcg/ml. Toxicity begins with nystagmus and may be seen at levels less than 20 mcg/ml. ▪ Periodic monitoring of CBC, platelets, albumin, urinalysis, hepatic and renal function is recommended. ▪ Monitor ECG and blood pressure continuously. ▪ Observation of patient symptoms and effectiveness of all medications is imperative. ▪ Determine absolute patency of vein. Avoid extravasation. Very alkaline; follow each injection with sterile NS to reduce local venous irritation. ▪ Patients maintained with phenytoin should be given a dose the morning of surgery to maintain adequate serum levels. ▪ Note Drug/lab interactions.

Maternal/child: Capable of numerous interactions in pregnant women. May cause birth defects (see literature). ▪ Alterations in phenytoin kinetics in pregnant women may necessitate periodic monitoring of serum levels. ▪ Discontinue nursing.

Elderly: Note Dose adjustments and Rate of administration. ▪ May have elevated serum concentrations because of slow metabolism. ▪ Low serum albumin causing a decrease in protein binding may result in increased sensitivity to phenytoin.

DRUG/LAB INTERACTIONS

Capable of innumerable catastrophic drug interactions; review of drug profile by pharmacist imperative. Serum levels may be increased by alcohol (acute ingestion), anticoagulants, antidepressants, antifungal agents (e.g., fluconazole, miconazole, ketoconazole), antihistamines, benzodiazepines (e.g., diazepam [Valium]), chloramphenicol, cimetidine (Tagamet), disulfiram (Antabuse), estrogens, fluoxetine (Prozac), metronidazole, myocardial depressants, paroxetine (Paxil), phenothiazines, sulfonamides, valproic acid, and others. Toxicity and fatality may result. ▪ Serum levels may be decreased by chronic alcohol ingestion, antineoplastics, antituberculosis drugs, barbiturates, carbamazepine (Tegretol), folic acid, leucovorin, rifampin, theophylline, and others resulting in reduced phenytoin effect. ▪ May increase serum levels of CNS depressants, folic acid antagonists, and muscle relaxants. ▪ Inhibits corticosteroids, digitalis, diuretics, itraconazole (Sporanox), levodopa, quinidine, ranitidine (Zantac), and others. ▪ Severe hypotension and bradycardia result with concomitant administration with dopamine (Intropin) and all other sympathomimetic antihypertensive drugs. ▪ In one case report, a patient stabilized on phenytoin and valproic acid experienced seizures and a reduction in antiepileptic drug serum concentration when acyclovir was added to the regimen. ▪ Alters some clinical laboratory tests.

SIDE EFFECTS

Minor: Ataxia, confusion, dizziness, drowsiness, fever, hyperplasia of gums, nervousness, nystagmus, skin eruptions, tremors, visual disturbances.

Major: Bradycardia, cardiac arrest, heart block, hypotension, respiratory arrest, tonic seizures, ventricular fibrillation.

ANTIDOTE

Notify the physician of any side effects. If minor symptoms progress or any major side effect occurs, discontinue the drug and notify the physician. Maintain a patent airway and resuscitate as necessary. Symptoms of heart block or bradycardia may be reversed with IV atropine. Epinephrine may also be useful. Hemodialysis may be required in overdose.

PHOSPHATE

Electrolyte replenisher
Antihypophosphatemic

Potassium phosphate, Sodium phosphate

pH 5.0 to 7.8

USUAL DOSE

Dependent on individual needs of the patient. In total parenteral nutrition (TPN), 10 to 15 mM (310 to 465 mg) of phosphorus/liter of TPN solution should maintain normal serum phosphate. Larger amounts may be required. 1 mM equals 31 mg.

Acute hypophosphatemia: Adults and children: 0.16 to 0.32 mM/kg (5 to 10 mg/kg) of body weight as a **loading dose** equally distributed over 6 hours. Maintain **children** with 0.5 to 1.5 mM/kg/24 hr (15 to 45 mg/kg/24 hr). Maintain **adults** with 48.4 to 64.5 mM/24 hr (1.5 to 2 Gm/24 hr).

INFANT DOSE

Infants receiving TPN: 1.5 to 2 mM/kg (46.5 to 62 mg) of body weight/day.

DILUTION

Must be diluted in a larger volume of suitable IV solution and given as an infusion. Soluble in all commonly used IV solutions except protein hydrolysate. Mix thoroughly.

INCOMPATIBLE WITH

Calcium salts, dextrose in Ringer's, dobutamine (Dobutrex), Ionosol solutions (specific), magnesium, Ringer's lactate. Mix thoroughly after each addition of supposedly compatible drugs or solutions. TPN solutions requiring the addition of phosphates and calcium salts must be mixed by the pharmacist to avoid a precipitate of calcium phosphate. Specific amounts, calculations, order, and temperature (precipitate forms more readily at room temperature) are required. Two deaths have been reported.

RATE OF ADMINISTRATION

0.2 mM of phosphate/kg/hr is the maximum infusion rate. Potassium phosphate will be further limited by the maximum rate for potassium. Consider sodium/potassium content. Infuse slowly. Rapid infusion may cause phosphate or potassium intoxication. Serum calcium may be reduced rapidly causing hypocalcemic tetany.

ACTIONS

Involved in bone deposition. Helps to maintain calcium levels, has a buffering effect on acid-base equilibrium, and influences renal excretion of the hydrogen ion. Normal levels in adults, 3.0 to 4.5 mg/dl of serum; in children, 4.0 to 7.0 mg/dl. Excreted in urine.

INDICATIONS AND USES

To prevent or correct hypophosphatemia in patients with restricted or no oral intake.

CONTRAINDICATIONS

Any disease with high phosphate or low calcium levels, hyperkalemia (potassium phosphate), hypernatremia (sodium phosphate).

PRECAUTIONS

Rapid infusion may cause phosphate, sodium, or potassium intoxication. Serum calcium may be reduced rapidly causing hypocalcemic tetany. ■ Use sodium phosphate with caution in renal impairment, cirrhosis, cardiac failure, or any edematous, sodium-retaining state. ■ Use potassium phosphate with caution in cardiac disease, renal disease, and digitalized patients. ■ Note Incompatible with.

Monitor: Monitor serum calcium, potassium, phosphate, chlorides, and sodium. Discontinue when serum phosphate exceeds 2 mg/dl. ■ Note Drug/lab interactions.

Maternal/child: Category C: safety for use in pregnancy not established.

DRUG/LAB INTERACTIONS

May cause hyperkalemia with potassium-sparing diuretics (e.g., amiloride) or angiotensin-converting enzyme inhibitors (e.g., enalapril [Vasotec]).

SIDE EFFECTS

Elevated phosphates; reduced calcium levels and hypocalcemic tetany; elevated potassium levels causing cardiac arrhythmias; flaccid paralysis; heaviness of the legs; hypotension; listlessness; mental confusion; paresthesia of the extremities.

ANTIDOTE

For any side effect, discontinue the drug and notify the physician. Restore serum calcium with calcium gluconate or chloride. Shift potassium from serum to cells with 150 ml of ⅙ molar sodium lactate or 10% to 20% dextrose with 10 units regular insulin for each 20 Gm dextrose at 300 to 500 ml/hr. Correct acidosis with sodium bicarbonate. Reduce sodium by restriction, diuretics, or hemodialysis. Resuscitate as necessary.

PHYSOSTIGMINE SALICYLATE

Cholinergic
Cholinesterase inhibitor
Antidote

Antilirium

pH 5.8

USUAL DOSE

Anticholinergic toxicity: 0.5 to 2 mg initially. 1 to 4 mg may be repeated as necessary as life-threatening signs recur (arrhythmias, convulsions, deep coma). Maximum dose is 4 mg in 30 minutes.

Postanesthesia: 0.5 to 1 mg initially. Repeat at 10 to 30 minute intervals until desired results obtained.

PEDIATRIC DOSE

To be used in life-threatening situations only. 0.02 mg/kg/dose. May be repeated at 5 to 10 minute intervals only if toxic effects persist and there is no sign of cholinergic effects. Maximum total dose is 2 mg.

DILUTION

May be given undiluted. Do not add to IV solutions. May be given through Y-tube or three-way stopcock of infusion set.

INCOMPATIBLE WITH

No specific information available. Because of potential toxicity, should not be mixed with any other drug.

RATE OF ADMINISTRATION

Rapid IV administration may cause bradycardia, hypersalivation, respiratory distress, and convulsions. 1 mg or fraction thereof over 1 to 3 minutes.

Pediatric rate: 0.5 mg or fraction thereof over at least 1 minute.

ACTIONS

An extract of *Physostigma venenosum* seeds. It inhibits the destructive action of acetylcholinesterase and prolongs and exaggerates the effects of acetylcholine. Stimulates parasympathetic nerve stimulation (pupil contraction, increased intestinal musculature tonus, bronchial constriction, salivary and sweat gland stimulation). Does enter the CNS. Onset of action occurs in 5 minutes and lasts about 1 hour. Rapidly hydrolyzed by cholinesterases.

INDICATIONS AND USES

To reverse CNS toxic effects caused by drugs capable of producing anticholinergic poisoning (e.g., atropine, scopolamine), other anticholinergic/antispasmodic agents (e.g., phenothiazines, antihistamines) and anticholinergic antiparkinson agents (e.g., benztropine [Cogentin], trihexyphenidyl [Artane]).

Investigational uses: Treatment of delirium tremens and Alzheimer's disease.

CONTRAINDICATIONS

Asthma, cardiovascular disease, diabetes, gangrene, mechanical obstruction of the intestines or urogenital tract, vagotonic states, patients receiving choline esters, depolarizing neuromuscular blocking agents (succinylcholine), or tricyclic antidepressants (e.g., amitriptyline [Elavil]).

PRECAUTIONS

Rapid IV administration may cause bradycardia, hypersalivation, respiratory distress, and convulsions. ▪ Contains bisulfites; use caution in allergic individuals.

Monitor: Atropine must always be available. ▪ Monitor vital signs. ▪ Note Drug/lab interactions.

Maternal/child: Safety for use in pregnancy and lactation not established. ▪ Has caused muscular weakness in neonates of mothers treated with other cholinesterase inhibitors for myasthenia gravis. ▪ May contain benzyl alcohol; do not use in neonates.

DRUG/LAB INTERACTIONS

Potentiates succinylcholine (Anectine) and other choline esters (e.g., bethanecol). ▪ May antagonize CNS depressant effects of diazepam (Valium). ▪ May cause serious complications, including death, with tricyclic antidepressants (e.g., amitriptyline [Elavil]).

SIDE EFFECTS

Anxiety, bradycardia, cholinergic crisis (overdose), coma, convulsions, defecation, delirium, disorientation, emesis, hallucinations, hyperactivity, hypersalivation, hypersensitivity, nausea, respiratory distress, salivation, seizures, sweating, urination.

ANTIDOTE

Keep physician informed of side effects. For excessive nausea or sweating, reduce dose. Discontinue drug for bradycardia, convulsions, excessive defecation, emesis, salivation, or urination, or respiratory distress. Treat cholinergic side effects (e.g., arrhythmias, bronchoconstriction) or hypersensitivity with the specific antagonist atropine sulfate in doses of 0.6 mg IV. May be repeated every 3 to 10 minutes. Endotracheal intubation or tracheostomy are considered prophylactic in anesthesia or crisis. Artificial ventilation, oxygen therapy, cardiac monitoring, adequate suctioning, and treatment of shock or convulsions must be instituted and maintained as necessary.

PHYTONADIONE

Vitamin (prothrombogenic)
Antidote
Antihemorrhagic

Aquamephyton, vitamin K₁

pH 5.0 to 7.0

USUAL DOSE

IV not route of choice; has caused death. Note Precautions. A single dose is preferred, but it may be repeated if clinically indicated. Use the smallest dose that achieves effective results to prevent clotting hazards.

Anticoagulant-induced (warfarin or dicumerol) hypoprothrombinemia: 2.5 to 10 mg. Doses up to 25 mg, and rarely, 50 mg, may be needed. May repeat in 6 to 8 hours if initial response is not adequate.

Hypoprothrombinemia from other causes: 2 to 25 mg (rarely 50 mg), depending on the severity of the deficiency and the response obtained.

PEDIATRIC DOSE

Anticoagulant-induced (warfarin or dicumerol) hypoprothrombinemia in infants and children: 1 to 2 mg/dose.

Hypoprothrombinemia from other causes in infants and children: A single dose of 1 to 2 mg.

NEWBORN DOSE

Neonatal hemorrhagic diseases (prophylaxis or treatment): 0.5 to 1.0 mg IM or SC. Rarely given IV.

DOSE ADJUSTMENTS

Note Drug/lab interactions.

DILUTION

May be diluted only with NS, D5/NS, or D5W. Dilution with at least 10 ml of diluent is recommended to facilitate prescribed rate of administration. Photosensitive; protect from light in all dilutions. Discard after single use.

INCOMPATIBLE WITH

Acid pH barbiturates, ascorbic acid, cyanocobalamin (vitamin B_{12}), dextran, dobutamine (Dobutrex), pentobarbital (Nembutal), phenobarbital (Luminal), phenytoin (Dilantin), ranitidine (Zantac), vancomycin (Vancocin), warfarin (Coumadin).

RATE OF ADMINISTRATION

Each 1 mg or fraction thereof over 1 minute or longer.

ACTIONS

Vitamin K, a fat-soluble vitamin, is essential for the hepatic production of four blood coagulation factors including prothrombin. These factors are required for normal blood clotting. Results should be detectable in 1 to 2 hours. Usually controls hemorrhage in 3 to 6 hours, and normal prothrombin levels should be obtained in 12 to 14 hours. Metabolized completely by the body.

INDICATIONS AND USES

Anticoagulant-induced prothrombin deficiency (warfarin or dicumarol). ■ Hemorrhagic disease of the newborn. ■ Hypoprothrombinemia resulting from antibacterial therapy and salicylates. ■ Hypoprothrombinemia resulting from obstructive jaundice, biliary fistula, sprue, ulcerative colitis, celiac disease, intestinal resection, cystic fibrosis of the pancreas, and regional enteritis—these diseases limit the absorption and synthesis of vitamin K.

CONTRAINDICATIONS

Hypersensitivity to components.

PRECAUTIONS

IV is not route of choice; used only when IM or SC routes cannot be used. Use extreme caution; has caused death with the first injection. ■ Supplement with whole blood transfusion if indicated. ■ Now the only vitamin K product for IV use. ■ Do not use to counteract anticoagulant effects of heparin, not effective; protamine sulfate is indicated. ■ When phytonadione is used in a patient for whom anticoagulant therapy is indicated, the same clotting hazards that existed prior to beginning anticoagulant therapy will recur. Use the smallest dose of phytonadione possible and monitor PT.

Monitor: Note Drug/lab interactions. ■ Dose and effect determined by prothrombin times. Keep the physician informed. ■ Pain and swelling at injection site can occur.

Maternal/child: Pregnancy Category C: safety for use not established. ▪ Use caution during lactation. ▪ Use extreme caution in premature infants and neonates. Excessive doses may cause increased bilirubinemia. Severe hemolytic anemia, hemoglobinuria, kernicterus, brain damage and death may occur.

DRUG/LAB INTERACTIONS

Discontinue drugs adversely affecting the coagulation mechanism if possible (e.g., salicylates, antibiotics). ▪ May cause temporary resistance to prothrombin-depressing oral anticoagulants by increasing amount of phytonadione in the liver and blood. Anticoagulation will require larger doses of same or use of heparin sodium.

SIDE EFFECTS

Cyanosis, diaphoresis, dizziness, dyspnea, hypotension, peculiar taste sensations, tachycardia, transient flushing sensation. Anaphylaxis, shock, and death have occurred with IV injection.

ANTIDOTE

Should not be necessary if dosage is accurately calculated before administration. Action can be reversed by warfarin or heparin if indicated. Discontinue the drug and notify the physician of any side effects. For most side effects the physician will probably choose to continue the drug at a decreased rate of administration. Treat allergic reactions as necessary.

PIPECURONIUM BROMIDE

Neuromuscular blocking agent
(Nondepolarizing)
Anesthesia adjunct

Arduan

pH 6.0

USUAL DOSE

Must be individualized based on age, sex, weight/degree of obesity, renal, hepatic, and/or other diseases. Clinical duration varies greatly. Always based on ideal body weight because pipecuronium is poorly soluble in fat. Normal renal function required.

Endotracheal intubation: 0.07 to 0.085 mg/kg of ideal body weight (70 to 85 mcg/kg) to provide 1 to 2 hours of clinical relaxation (time to 25% recovery).

Following succinylcholine and after recovery from succinylcholine paralysis: 0.05 mg/kg (50 mcg/kg) to provide approximately 45 minutes of clinical relaxation. Doses up to 70 to 85 mcg will provide longer periods of relaxation.

Maintenance dose: 0.010 to 0.015 mg/kg (10 to 15 mcg/kg) administered at 25% recovery will extend relaxation another 50 minutes to 1 hour. Determine need for maintenance dose based on beginning symptoms of neuromuscular blockade reversal determined by a peripheral nerve stimulator.

PEDIATRIC DOSE

Children 1 to 14 years: 0.057 mg/kg (57 mcg/kg) to provide 18 to 52 minutes of clinical relaxation. May be less sensitive than adults. No data on maintenance doses available for children.

INFANT DOSE

3 months to 1 year: 0.04 mg/kg (40 mcg/kg) to provide 10 to 44 minutes of clinical relaxation. Sensitivity similar to adults. No data on maintenance doses available for infants. Do not use in newborns.

DOSE ADJUSTMENTS

Reduced dose and specific calculation required in impaired renal function (see literature). ■ Reduced dose based on ideal body weight required in obesity. ■ Reduced dose may be required in impaired hepatic function, the elderly, and patients with edema or cardiovascular disease. ■ Reduce dose in presence of inhalational anesthetics (e.g., isoflurane, enflurane) and with other drugs that prolong neuromuscular blockade. ■ Note Drug/lab interactions. ■ Use of any dose lower than 70 mcg/kg to reduce clinical duration requires extra care during intubation.

DILUTION

Must be reconstituted before administration. Available as 10 mg/vial (yields 1 mg/ml diluted with 10 ml). Compatible with NS, D5W, D5/NS, D5LR, and sterile water for injection. Bacteriostatic water when supplied contains 0.9% benzyl alcohol; do not use in newborns.

Storage: Protect from light. Refrigerate and use within 24 hours if reconstituted with sterile water for injection or any IV solution. If reconstituted with bacteriostatic water (contains benzyl alcohol), it is stable at room temperature or refrigerated for 5 days. Discard unused portion.

INCOMPATIBLE WITH

Specific information not available.

RATE OF ADMINISTRATION

A single dose over 5 to 15 seconds. Titrate to desired effect. Use a peripheral nerve stimulator to monitor response, avoid overdose, monitor need for additional relaxant, and monitor adequacy of spontaneous recovery or antagonism.

ACTIONS

A long-acting nondepolarizing neuromuscular blocking agent. Causes skeletal muscle relaxation and paralysis by competing for cholinergic receptors at the motor end-plate. Onset of action is dose dependent. Produces maximum neuromuscular blockade within 3 to 5 minutes and lasts from 1 to 2 hours. Length of action extended based on degree of renal impairment. It may take another 30 minutes or up to several hours before complete recovery occurs. Does not cause cardiovascular effects associated with other neuromuscular blocking agents (e.g., pancuronium [Pavulon]). Excreted mostly as unchanged drug in urine.

INDICATIONS AND USES

Only recommended in procedures lasting 90 minutes or longer. Adjunct to general anesthesia, to provide skeletal muscle relaxation during surgery. ■ Facilitate endotracheal intubation.

CONTRAINDICATIONS

None known. Not recommended for use in obstetrics (C-section), prior to or following other nondepolarizing neuromuscular blocking agents (e.g., atracurium [Tracrium], pancuronium [Pavulon]), or during prolonged mechanical ventilation in the ICU.

PRECAUTIONS

For IV use only. ■ Administered only by or under the direct observation of the anesthesiologist. ■ Myasthenia gravis and other neuromuscular diseases increase sensitivity to drug. Can cause critical reactions. Shorter-acting muscle relaxants (atracurium [Tracrium]) preferred. ▪ Bradycardia may be more common because pipecuronium has little effect on heart rate, and will not counteract bradycardia caused by opioid anesthetic agents or vagal stimulation. ▪ Use extreme caution in renal dysfunction; shorter-acting drugs (e.g., atracurium [Tracrium], vecuronium [Norcuron]) have a more predictable duration of action.

Monitor: This drug produces apnea. Controlled artificial ventilation with oxygen must be continuous and under direct observation at all times. Maintain a patent airway. Neostigmine (Prostigmin) and atropine must be available. ▪ Monitor all vital organ functions until adequate recovery. ▪ Use a peripheral nerve stimulator to monitor response to pipecuronium, avoid overdose, monitor need for additional relaxant, and monitor adequacy of spontaneous recovery or antagonism. ▪ Patient may be conscious and completely unable to communicate by any means. Has no analgesic properties. ▪ Monitor for early signs of malignant hyperthermia; has not occurred but is a possibility. ▪ Note Drug/lab interactions.

Maternal/child: Pregnancy Category C: use during pregnancy only if benefits justify risks. ▪ Effects on neonate unknown, no studies available, duration of action exceeds duration of cesarean section. ▪ Safety for use during lactation not established. ▪ Not recommended for infants less than 3 months of age. ▪ No data on maintenance dosing in infants or children.

Elderly: Note Dose adjustments. ▪ Delay in onset time may be caused by slower circulation time in cardiovascular disease, old age, or edematous states; allow more time for drug to achieve maximum effect.

DRUG/LAB INTERACTIONS

Do not use before succinylcholine (Anectine) to reduce side effects. ▪ Duration of action extended and recovery prolonged by inhalation anesthetics (e.g., enflurane, isoflurane, halothane). ▪ Prolongation of neuromuscular block may occur with many antibiotics (e.g., aminoglycosides [e.g., kanamycin (Kantrex), gentamicin (Garamycin)]), bacitracin, colistin [Coly-Mycin S], colistimethate [Coly-Mycin M], polymixin-B [Aerosporin], tetracyclines). ▪ Recurrent paralysis may occur with quinidine. ▪ Potentiated by acidosis; inhibited by alkalosis. Electrolyte imbalance (acute [e.g., diarrhea] or chronic [e.g., adrenocortical insufficiency]) and acid-base imbalance are usually mixed; either reaction can occur. ▪ Potentiated by magnesium salts.

SIDE EFFECTS

Bradycardia, hypertension, and hypotension are most common. Prolonged action resulting in skeletal muscle weakness to profound and prolonged skeletal muscle paralysis with respiratory insufficiency or apnea is possible. Airway closure caused by relaxation of epiglottis, pharynx, and tongue muscles, anuria, cardiac arrhythmias, hyperkalemia, hypersensitivity reactions, and hypoglycemia can occur.

ANTIDOTE

All side effects resulting from prolonged action can be medical emergencies. Controlled ventilation must be continuous. Treat symptomatically and monitor continuously. Neostigmine (Prostigmin [usual dose, 0.04 mg/kg]) is an antagonist but should not be given before spontaneous recovery has begun. Administer atropine before neostigmine. Identify appropriate time for antagonism and monitor recovery with peripheral nerve stimulator. Evaluate 5 second head lift and grip strength. Time to recovery is based on level of residual neuromuscular block at time of dosing. The earlier an anticholinesterase is administered, the longer it will be to recovery. Action of antagonist may wear off before pipecuronium.

PIPERACILLIN SODIUM

Antibacterial
(Extended-spectrum penicillin)

Pipracil   **pH 5.5 to 7.5**

USUAL DOSE

3 to 4 Gm every 4, 6, 8, or 12 hours depending on severity of infection. Maximum dose usually 24 Gm/24 hr. Usual duration of therapy is 10 to 14 days. Continue at least 2 days after symptoms of infection disappear.

Perioperative prophylaxis: 2 to 4 Gm 30 minutes to 1 hour before incision. Repeat every 4 to 6 hours for up to 24 hours if indicated. Specific doses for specific procedures (see literature).

PEDIATRIC DOSE

200 to 300 mg/kg/24 hr in equally divided doses every 4 to 6 hours.

Cystic fibrosis in children under 12 years of age: 300 to 600 mg/kg/24 hr in equally divided doses every 4 to 6 hours.

NEONATAL DOSE

100 mg/kg every 12 hours.

DOSE ADJUSTMENTS

Reduce dose only in severe renal impairment with creatinine clearance temporarily below 40 ml/min. May be given to patients undergoing hemodialysis and peritoneal dialysis (see literature for dose).

DILUTION

Each 1 Gm or fraction thereof should be reconstituted with at least 5 ml of SW or NS. Shake vigorously to dissolve. May be further diluted to desired volume (50 to 100 ml) with D5W, NS, or other compatible infusion solutions (see literature or compatibility chart on back cover) and given as an intermittent infusion. Also available in ADD-vantage vials for use with ADD-vantage diluent containers. See manufacturer's directions for preparation, dilution, and administration.

Storage: Stable at room temperature for 24 hours.

INCOMPATIBLE WITH

Aminoglycosides (e.g., amikacin, colistimethate, gentamicin, kanamycin, streptomycin, tobramycin), amphotericin B (Fungizone), chloramphenicol, filgrastim (Neupogen), fluconazole (Diflucan), lincomycin, ondansetron (Zofran), polymyxin B, promethazine (Phenergan), sargramostin (Leukine), vinorelbine tartrate.

RATE OF ADMINISTRATION

Too-rapid injection may cause seizures.

Direct IV: A single dose over 3 to 5 minutes.

Intermittent infusion: A single dose properly diluted over 30 minutes.

Discontinue primary IV infusion during administration. Slow infusion rate for pain along venipuncture site.

ACTIONS

An extended-spectrum penicillin. Bactericidal against a variety of gram-negative and gram-positive bacteria including aerobic and anaerobic strains. Especially effective against *Klebsiella* and *Pseudomonas*. Well distributed in all body fluids, tissue, and bone and through inflamed meninges. Onset of action is prompt. Excreted in bile and urine. Crosses the placental barrier. Secreted in breast milk.

INDICATIONS AND USES

Treatment of serious lower respiratory tract, intraabdominal, urinary tract, gynecologic, skin and skin structure, bone and joint, and gonococcal infections and septicemia caused by susceptible organisms. May be used in either liver or renal impairment since excretion occurs in bile and urine. Frequently used to initiate therapy in serious infections because of broad spectrum. ▪ Perioperative prophylaxis.

CONTRAINDICATIONS

History of allergic reaction to any penicillin or cephalosporin (not absolute).

PRECAUTIONS

Sensitivity studies indicated to determine susceptibility of the causative organism to piperacillin. ▪ Avoid prolonged use of drug; superinfection caused by overgrowth of nonsusceptible organisms may result. ▪ Incidence of side effects increased in patients with cystic fibrosis.

Monitor: Watch for early symptoms of allergic reaction. ▪ Periodic evaluation of renal, hepatic, and hematopoietic systems and serum potassium is recommended in prolonged therapy. Observe for hypokalemia and increased bleeding tendencies. ▪ Observe for electrolyte imbalance and cardiac irregularities. Contains 1.85 mEq sodium/Gm. May aggravate CHF. ▪ Confirm patency of vein; avoid extravasation or intraarterial injection. ▪ Note Drug/lab interactions.

Patient education: May require alternate birth control.

Maternal/child: Pregnancy Category B: use only if absolutely necessary in pregnancy and lactation. ▪ May cause diarrhea, candidiasis, or allergic response in nursing infants. ▪ Safety for use in children under 12 years not established but is used.

Elderly: No problems documented. Age-related decrease in renal function may require decreased dose.

DRUG/LAB INTERACTIONS

Frequently used concurrently with aminoglycosides (e.g., tobramycin [Nebcin]), but must be administered in separate infusions; inactivates aminoglycosides. ▪ Concomitant use with beta-adrenergic blockers (e.g., propranolol [Inderal]) may increase risk of anaphylaxis and inhibit treatment. ▪ Risk of bleeding may be increased with anticoagulants (e.g., heparin); monitoring of coagulation tests may be indicated. Use caution. ▪ May be antagonized by bacteriostatic antibiotics (e.g., chloramphenicol, erythromycin, tetracyclines); bactericidal action may be negated. ▪ May inhibit effectiveness of oral contraceptives; could result in breakthrough bleeding or pregnancy. ▪ Probenecid decreases rate of piperacillin elimination resulting in higher and more prolonged blood levels. May be desirable or may cause toxicity. ■ May prolong neuromuscular blockade with vecuronium (Norcuron). ■ May decrease clearance and increase toxicity of methotrexate. ■ May cause false urine protein reactions with various tests; see Side effects and/or literature.

SIDE EFFECTS

Anaphylaxis, convulsions, diarrhea, dizziness, elevated serum creatinine, BUN, alkaline phosphatase, LDH, serum bilirubin, AST (SGOT), and ALT (SGPT); fatigue, headache, hypokalemia, increased creatinine or BUN, leukopenia, muscle relaxation (prolonged), nausea, neutropenia, pruritus, pseudomembranous colitis, thrombocytopenia, thrombophlebitis, skin rash, vomiting. Hypersensitivity myocarditis can occur (fever, eosinophilia, rash, sinus tachycardia, ST-T changes and cardiomegaly). Higher than normal doses may cause neurologic adverse reactions including convulsions; especially with impaired renal function.

ANTIDOTE

Notify the physician immediately of any adverse symptoms. For severe symptoms, discontinue the drug, treat allergic reaction (antihistamines, epinephrine, corticosteroids), and resuscitate as necessary. Hemodialysis is effective in overdose.

PIPERACILLIN SODIUM AND TAZOBACTAM SODIUM

Antibacterial
(Extended-spectrum penicillin and beta-lactamase inhibitor)

Zosyn

USUAL DOSE

Measurement of both drugs is included in the total dose; for every 1 Gm of piperacillin there is 0.125 Gm of tazobactam (8:1 ratio). 12 Gm piperacillin/1.5 Gm tazobactam/24 hours given as 3.375 (3 Gm piperacillin/0.375 Gm taxobactam) every 6 hours. Doses up to 4.5 Gm every 4 to 8 hours have been used. Usual duration of therapy is 7 to 10 days, based on severity of infection and patient progress.

Nosocomial pneumonia: 3.375 Gm every 4 hours. Use an aminoglycoside also. Continue aminoglycoside if *P. aeruginosa* is isolated, discontinue if it is not isolated.

DOSE ADJUSTMENTS

Reduce dose in renal impairment with a creatinine clearance between 20 to 40 ml/min to 2.25 Gm every 6 hours; below 20 ml/min to 2.25 Gm every 8 hours. May be given to patients undergoing hemodialysis and peritoneal dialysis. Dose in hemodialysis is 2.25 Gm every 8 hours with a single dose of 0.75 Gm following each dialysis period. Supplemental doses not required in peritoneal dialysis. Measure serum levels to further adjust dose as needed. ■ No dose adjustment needed in impaired liver function. ■ Dose reduction may be required in the elderly.

DILUTION

Each 1 Gm of piperacillin content should be reconstituted with a least 5 ml of suitable diluent (e.g., SW or NS with or without preservatives, D5W, 6% Dextran in saline). May be further diluted to desired volume (50 to 100 ml) with the compatible infusion solutions above and given as an intermittent infusion. Also available in ADD-vantage vials for use with ADD-vantage diluent containers. See manufacturer's directions for preparation, dilution, and administration.

Storage: Use single-dose vials immediately after reconstitution; discard any unused portion after 24 hours at room temperature or 48 hours if refrigerated. Stable for up to 7 days after dilution if refrigerated, 3 months if frozen.

INCOMPATIBLE WITH

Manufacturer recommends temporarily discontinuing other solutions infusing at the same site to avoid compatibility problems. Acyclovir (Zovirax), aminoglycosides (e.g., amikacin gentamicin kanamycin streptomycin tobramycin) amphotericin B (Fungizone), chloramphenicol chlorpromazine (Thorazine), cisplatin (Platinol), colistimethate dacarbazine (DTIC), daunorubicin (Cerubidine), dobutamine (Dobutrex), doxorubicin (Adriamycin), doxycycline (Vibramycin), droperidol (Inapsine), famotidine (Pepcid IV), ganciclovir (Cytovene), haloperidol (Haldol), hydroxyzine (Vistaril), idarubicin (Idamycin), lactated Ringer's solution, lincomycin, miconazole (Monistat IV), minocycline (Minocin), mitomycin (Mutamycin), mitoxantrone (Novantrone), nalbuphine (Nubain), ondansetron (Zofran), polymyxin B (Aerosporin), prochlorperazine (Compazine), promethazine (Phenergan), streptozocin (Zanosar), vancomycin (Vancocin), vinorelbine (Navelbine).

COMPATIBLE WITH

Appropriate amounts of potassium chloride as an additive.

RATE OF ADMINISTRATION

A single dose over 30 minutes as an intermittent infusion. Slow infusion rate for pain along venipuncture site. See Incompatible with.

ACTIONS

An antimicrobial agent that combines the extended-spectrum penicillin piperacillin with the potent beta-lactamase inhibitor tazobactam. May be used in suspected polymicrobial infections due to its broad spectrum of activity; spectrum is superior to many other agents. Bactericidal against all three classes of bacterial pathogens; gram-positive and gram-negative aerobes, anaerobes, and enterococci that may be resistant to other antibiotics. Well distributed in all body fluids and tissues. Mean tissue concentrations are 50% to 100% of plasma concentrations. Peak levels are achieved immediately at the completion of an infusion. Plasma half-life ranges from 0.7 to 1.2 hours. Extended two-fold (piperacillin) to four-fold (tazobactam) if creatinine clearance under 40 mcg/ml. Primarily excreted rapidly in urine. Crosses the placental barrier. Secreted in breast milk.

INDICATIONS AND USES

Treatment of infections caused by piperacillin-resistant beta-lactamase—producing strains of specific microorganisms in the following conditions: intraabdominal (e.g., appendicitis complicated by rupture or abscess and peritonitis), gynecologic (e.g., postpartum endometritis and pelvic inflammatory disease), skin and skin structure (complicated and uncomplicated, e.g., cellulitis, cutaneous abscesses, and ischemic/ diabetic foot infection), and pneumonia. ■ Used in combination with aminoglycosides for infections in neutropenic patients or nosocomial pneumonia.

Unlabeled use: Treatment of septicemia.

CONTRAINDICATIONS

History of allergic reaction to any penicillin, cephalosporin, or beta-lactamase inhibitors (not absolute).

PRECAUTIONS

Sensitivity studies indicated to determine susceptibility of the causative organism to piperacillin. ■ Avoid prolonged use of drug; super-infection caused by overgrowth of nonsusceptible organisms may result. ■ Use caution in patients with CHF or those with a history of bleeding disorders or GI disease (e.g., colitis). ■ Incidence of side effects may be increased in patients with cystic fibrosis. ■ Continue at least 2 days after symptoms of infection disappear.

Monitor: Watch for early symptoms of allergic reaction. ■ Periodic evaluation of renal, hepatic, and hematopoietic systems and serum potassium is recommended in prolonged therapy. May cause hypokalemia; observe closely. ■ Contains 2.35 MEq of sodium/Gm. Observe for electrolyte imbalance and cardiac irregularities. May aggravate CHF. ■ Confirm patency of vein; avoid extravasation or intraarterial injection. ■ Observe for increased bleeding tendencies in all patients but especially those with impaired renal function. ■ Note Drug/lab interactions.

Patient education: Report promptly: fever, rash, sore throat, unusual bleeding or bruising, severe stomach cramps, and/or diarrhea, seizures. ■ May require alternate birth control.

Maternal/child: Category B: Use during pregnancy only if clearly needed. ■ May cause diarrhea, candidiasis, or allergic response in nursing infants. ■ Safety for use in children under 12 years not established.

Elderly: No problems documented. Consider age-related impaired renal function.

DRUG/LAB INTERACTIONS

Frequently used concurrently with aminoglycosides (e.g., tobramycin [Nebcin]) but must be administered in separate infusions; inactivates aminoglycosides. ■ Does not affect pharmacokinetics of vancomycin; may be given without dose adjustment. ■ Concomitant administration with probenecid decreases rate of elimination resulting in higher and more prolonged blood levels. May be desirable or may cause toxicity. ■ Use caution with anticoagulants (e.g., heparin), thrombolytic agents (e.g., alteplase [tPA], anistreplase [Eminase]), platelet aggregation inhibitors (e.g., aspirin, NSAIDs, dextran, dipyridamole, plicamycin). Risk of bleeding is increased. Monitoring of coagulation tests may be indicated. Concurrent use with thrombolytic agents is not recommended; may increase risk of severe hemorrhage. ■ May be antagonized by bacteriostatic antibiotics (e.g., chloramphenicol, erythromycin, and tetracyclines); bactericidal action may be negated ■ May decrease clearance and increase toxicity of methotrexate. ■ May inhibit effectiveness of oral contraceptives; could result in breakthrough bleeding or pregnancy. ■ May prolong neuromuscular blockade with vecuronium (Norcuron). ■ May cause false urine protein reactions with various tests and false-positive glucose with Clinitest. ■ Note Side effects.

SIDE EFFECTS

Hypokalemia, increased PTT, and prolonged prothrombin time. Most other side effects are usually mild to moderate and transient. Abdominal pain (1.3%), agitation (2.1%), anxiety (1.2%), chest pain (1.3%), constipation (7.7%), diarrhea (11.3%), dizziness (1.4%), dyspnea (1.1%), dyspepsia (3.3%), edema (1.2%), elevated liver function tests, fever (2.4%), headache (7.7%), hypertension (1.6%), insomnia (6.6%), moniliasis (1.6%), nausea (6.9%), pain (1.7%), positive Coombs' test, pruritus (3.1%), rash (e.g., bullous, eczematoid, maculopapular, urticarial [4.2%]), rhinitis (1.2%), vomiting (3.3%). Anaphylaxis can occur. Transient leukopenia and eosinophilia can occur with prolonged therapy. Higher than normal doses may cause neurologic adverse reactions including convulsions.

ANTIDOTE

Notify the physician immediately of any adverse symptoms. For severe symptoms, discontinue the drug, treat allergic reaction (antihistamines, epinephrine, corticosteroids, airway management, oxygen), and resuscitate as necessary. Use anticonvulsants (e.g., diazepam [Valium]) or barbiturates (e.g., phenobarbital) for seizures. Hemodialysis is effective in overdose.

PLASMA PROTEIN FRACTION
Plasma volume expander

Plasmanate, Plasma-Plex, Plasmatein, Protenate
pH 6.7 to 7.3

USUAL DOSE

Variable, depending on indication for use, condition of patient, and response to therapy. Range is from 250 to 1,500 ml/24 hr. Each 500 ml bottle yields 25 Gm of plasma protein. Suggested initial doses are as follows:

Shock: 250 to 500 ml.

Burns: 500 to 1,000 ml.

Hypoproteinemia, 1,000 to 1,500 ml/24 hr.

PEDIATRIC DOSE

Treatment of acute shock: 6.6 to 30 ml/kg of body weight.

DILUTION

Available as a 5% solution buffered with saline in 250 and 500 ml bottles with injection sets. Plasmanate also available in a 50 ml size. No further dilution is required. Do not use if solution turbid or a sediment visible. Use immediately after opening and discard any unused portion. Contains no preservatives.

Storage: Store at CRT.

INCOMPATIBLE WITH

Alcohol, norepinephrine (Levophed), protein hydrolysate (amino acid products).

RATE OF ADMINISTRATION

Variable, depending on indication, present blood volume, and patient response. Adjust or slow rate according to clinical response and rising blood pressure. Averages are:

Normal blood volume: 1 ml/min.

Treatment of shock and burns in adult: 5 to 8 ml/min. Higher rates may be tolerated if necessary. Rapid infusion (over 10 ml/min) may cause hypotension. Decrease flow rate as patient improves.

Treatment of shock in infants and children: 5 to 10 ml/min. Do not exceed 10 ml/min in children.

Treatment of hypoproteinemia: Single 500 ml dose over 1 hour. For larger amounts the maximum rate is 100 ml/hr.

ACTIONS

A sterile natural plasma protein substance containing at least 83% albumin, no more than 17% alpha and beta globulins, and no more than 1% gamma globulin. Contains 130 to 160 mEq sodium/liter. It expands intravascular volume, prevents marked hemoconcentration, and maintains appropriate electrolyte balance in burns.

INDICATIONS AND USES

Emergency treatment of hypovolemic shock caused by burns, infections, surgery, or trauma (may also be due to dehydration in infants and children). ■ Temporary treatment of hemorrhage when whole blood unavailable. ■ Hypoproteinemia until cause determined and corrected. ■ Prevention of hemoconcentration and maintenance of electrolyte balance in burn patients.

CONTRAINDICATIONS

Cardiac failure, cardiopulmonary bypass, history of allergic reactions to albumin, normal or increased intravascular volume, severe anemia.

PRECAUTIONS

May be given without regard to blood group or type. ■ Not effective for coagulation mechanism defects. ■ Added protein, fluid, and sodium load requires caution in hepatic or renal impairment. ■ If continuous protein loss occurs or edema is present, normal serum albumin (25%) may be the preferred product.

Monitor: Monitor vital signs (including central venous pressure if possible) and urine output every 5 to 15 minutes for 1 hour and hourly thereafter depending on condition. ■ For treatment of shock, observe carefully for bleeding points that may not have been evident at lower pressures. ■ Whole blood may be indicated for considerable red blood cell loss or anemia caused by administration of large amounts of plasma protein fraction. ■ Additional fluids are required for dehydrated patients. Tissue dehydration caused by osmotic action of plasma proteins can be acute. ■ May cause vascular overload, monitor for signs of pulmonary edema or heart failure (e.g., dyspnea, fluid in the lungs, abnormal increases in BP or CVP). ■ Hemoglobin, hematocrit, electrolyte, and serum protein evaluations are necessary during therapy.

Maternal/child: Category C: safety for use in pregnancy not established.

DRUG/LAB INTERACTIONS

May cause an elevated alkaline phosphatase level.

SIDE EFFECTS

Allergic and/or pyrogenic reactions can occur. Incidence of toxicity is low when administered with appropriate caution. Slight nausea can occur. Hypotension can be sudden if administered too rapidly.

ANTIDOTE

Notify the physician of all symptoms and side effects. Discontinue infusion for sudden hypotension. Decrease flow rate if indicated and treat symptomatically. Resuscitate as necessary.

PLICAMYCIN

Antineoplastic
(Antibiotic)
Antihypercalcemic

Mithracin, Mithramycin

pH 7.0

USUAL DOSE

Testicular tumors: 25 to 30 mcg/kg of body weight/24 hr. Repeat daily for 8 to 10 days unless significant side effects or toxicity occur. Repeat at monthly intervals if indicated.

Hypercalcemia and hypercalciuria: 25 mcg/kg of body weight/24 hr for 3 or 4 days. Repeat weekly as required to maintain normal calcium levels.

PEDIATRIC DOSE

Hypercalcemia with malignancies: 25 mcg/kg/dose as an infusion daily for 1 to 4 days. Repeat at weekly intervals as needed or maintain with 1 to 3 doses weekly.

DOSE ADJUSTMENTS

Dose based on average weight in presence of edema or ascites.

DILUTION

Specific techniques required; see Precautions. Each 2.5 mg vial must be initially diluted with 4.9 ml of sterile water for injection (1 ml equals 500 mcg). A single daily dose must be further diluted in 1,000 ml of D5W or D5/NS and given as an infusion. Do not use a filter smaller than 5 microns. Loss of potency will occur. Prepare fresh daily and discard any unused portion.

Pediatric dilution: Same as for adults.

Storage: Store in refrigerator before dilution.

INCOMPATIBLE WITH

Cellulose, ester fibers, iron, trace element solutions. Consider toxicity and specific use.

RATE OF ADMINISTRATION

A single dose every 24 hours over 4 to 6 hours. Extend to 4 to 8 hours in children.

ACTIONS

A potent antibiotic, antineoplastic agent. Interferes with cell division by binding with DNA to inhibit and slow production of RNA. Exact mechanism unknown. Well distributed to kidney, liver, bone, and cerebrospinal fluid. Cytotoxic to HeLa cell tissue culture and some animal tumors. Also acts to lower serum calcium in patients with cancer. Metabolized in the liver. Some excretion in urine.

INDICATIONS AND USES

Testicular tumors not treatable with surgery and/or radiation.
■ Hypercalcemia and hypercalciuria associated with many advanced neoplasms.

CONTRAINDICATIONS

Thrombocytopenia, thrombocytopathy, coagulation disorders or any susceptibility to bleeding, impairment of bone marrow function, lack of hospital and laboratory facilities.

PRECAUTIONS

■ Follow guidelines for handling cytotoxic agents. See Appendix A, p. 893. ■ Administered by or under the direction of the physician specialist. ■ Use extreme caution in impaired renal or hepatic function.
Monitor: Determine absolute patency of vein; cellulitis and tissue necrosis may result from extravasation. Discontinue injection, use another vein. Elevate extremity and apply warm moist heat to the extravasated area.
■ Severe sudden onset of hemorrhage and even death can result from use. ■ Maintain hydration and correct any electrolyte imbalance before treatment. ■ Monitor renal and hepatic function and electrolytes (especially calcium, potassium, and phosphorus.) ■ Monitor platelet count, prothrombin time, and bleeding time during and after therapy.
■ Observe closely for all signs of infection. ■ Prophylactic antibiotics may be indicated pending results of C/S in a febrile neutropenic patient.
■ Prophylactic antiemetics may reduce nausea and vomiting and increase patient comfort.
Patient education: Consider birth control options; nonhormonal birth control recommended. ■ Report IV site burning or stinging promptly.
■ Calcium and vitamin D supplementation or restriction may be necessary depending on indication. ■ Report unusual bleeding or bruising, bloody nose, chills, dark urine, fever, rashes, sore throat, tarry stools, or yellowing of eyes or skin. ■ Do not lie down after eating.
■ See Appendix D, p. 900.
Maternal/child: Category X: avoid pregnancy. ■ Discontinue breast feeding.
Elderly: Monitor fluid and electrolyte status carefully to avoid overhydration. ■ Monitor for early signs of toxicity. ■ Consider age-related organ impairment.

DRUG/LAB INTERACTIONS

Risk of bleeding increased with anticoagulants (e.g., heparin, warfarin [Coumadin]), thrombolytic agents (e.g., alteplase [tPA]), NSAIDs (e.g., indomethacin [Indocin], ibuprofen [Advil]), aspirin, dextran, dipyridamole (Persantine), sulfinpyrazone (Anturane), or valproic acid. Concurrent use not recommended. ■ Potential for toxicity increased with bone marrow depressants (e.g., antineoplastics [e.g., cisplatin], colchicine, eflornithine [Orindyl]), hepatotoxic agents (e.g., alcohol, estrogens), or nephrotoxic agents (e.g., acyclovir, aminoglycosides [e.g., tobramycin], amphotericin B). May be antagonized by calcium or vitamin D preparations. ■ Do not administer live virus vaccines to patients receiving antineoplastic drugs.

SIDE EFFECTS

Minor: Anorexia, depression, diarrhea, drowsiness, fever, flushing, headache, nausea, skin rash, stomatitis, vomiting.
Major: Abnormal clot retraction, abnormal liver function tests, abnormal

renal function tests, elevation of bleeding and clotting time, epistaxis (severe), hematemesis, hemoglobin depression, leukopenia (unusual), platelet count depression, prothrombin content depression, serum calcium, phosphorus, and potassium depression.

ANTIDOTE

Minor side effects will be treated symptomatically. Discontinue the drug and notify the physician immediately of any major side effects. Plateletrich plasma may help to elevate platelet count. Provide immediate treatment or supportive therapy as indicated; bleeding episodes can be fatal. If extravasation has occurred, long-acting dexamethasone injected into the indurated area with a fine hypodermic needle may be helpful. Apply moderate heat.

PORFIMER SODIUM

Photofrin

Photosensitizing agent
Antineoplastic

pH 7.0 to 8.0

USUAL DOSE

A course is a two-stage process requiring administration of both drug and light.

A single IV injection of 2 mg/kg of porfimer sodium is the *first stage*. No further injection of porfimer sodium should be given in any one course of therapy.

Illumination with nonthermal laser light at 40 to 50 hours postinjection is the *second stage*. Standard endoscopic techniques are used for light administration and débridement. The laser system must be approved for delivery of a stable power output at a wavelength of 630± nm. Light is delivered to the tumor by cylindrical OPTIGUIDE™ fiber optic diffusers passed through the operating channel of an endoscope/bronchoscope. The choice of diffuser tip length depends on the length of the tumor. Diffuser length should be sized to avoid exposure of nonmalignant tissue to light and to prevent overlapping of previously treated malignant tissue. A second laser light application may be given 96 to 120 hours after injection. Before providing a second laser light treatment, the residual tumor should be gently débrided. Vigorous débridement may cause esophageal tumor bleeding.

Espohageal cancer: 2 mg/kg of porfimer sodium as an IV injection. A light dose of 300 joules/cm of tumor length should be delivered by the specific process outlined above. Light exposure time is set to 12 minutes and 30 seconds.

Endobronchial cancer: 2 mg/kg of porfimer sodium as an IV injection. A light dose of 200 joules/cm of tumor length should be delivered by the specific process outlined above. Light exposure time is set to 8 minutes and 20 seconds.

Up to three courses may be given, but each must be separated by at least 30 days. Evaluate patients with esophageal cancer for the presence of a tracheoesophageal or bronchoesophageal fistula before each course. Evaluate all patients for possible erosion of the tumor into a major blood vessel.

PEDIATRIC DOSE

Safety and effectiveness for use in children not established.

DOSE ADJUSTMENTS

No adjustments required.

DILUTION

Specific techniques required; see Precautions. Prepare immediately before use. Each vial of porfimer sodium must be reconstituted with 31.8 ml of D5W or NS. Concentration will be 2.5 mg/ml. Shake well until dissolved. An opaque solution; detection of particulate matter by visual inspection is difficult. Withdraw desired dose. Must be protected from bright light and used immediatley.

Storage: Store unopened vials at controlled room temperature in carton to protect from light.

INCOMPATIBLE WITH

Manufacturer states, "Do not mix Photofrin® with other drugs in the same solution."

RATE OF ADMINISTRATION

A single dose equally distributed over 3 to 5 minutes.

ACTIONS

The first light-activated drug (photosensitizing agent) for use in photodynamic therapy (PDT) to be approved in the United States. After IV infusion it is allowed to circulate. It accumulates and is retained in tumors, skin, and organs of the reticuloendothelial system (e.g., liver, spleen) while largely clearing from other tissues. Has no apparent effect on tumors until it is activated by selective delivery of light (usually 40 to 50 hours postinfusion). Light activation induces a photochemical, not a thermal, effect, that produces an active form of oxygen and releases thromboxane A_2. This process causes vasoconstriction, activation and aggregation of platelets, and increased clotting that contribute to ischemic necrosis leading to tissue and tumor death. In patients with esophageal cancer, ability to swallow is improved, as is quality of life. Elimination half-life is very prolonged, up to several weeks. Highly protein bound.

INDICATIONS AND USES

Palliative treatment of patients with completely obstructing esophageal cancer or partially obstructing esophageal cancers that are unsuitable for treatment with thermal laser therapy. ▪ Treatment of microinvasive endobronchial non-small cell lung cancer in patients for whom surgery and radiotherapy are not indicated.

Investigational uses: Treatment of bladder cancer (approved for use in Canada). Studies are in progress on other tumors accessible by scope and fiberoptics to deliver light (e.g., colon).

CONTRAINDICATIONS

Known allergies to porphyrins, an existing tracheoesophageal or bronchoesophageal fistula, porphyria, or tumors eroding into a major blood vessel.

PRECAUTIONS

Use rubber gloves and eye protection during preparation and administration. Avoid any skin or eye contact since that area will become photosensitive. Wipe up spills with a damp cloth. Dispose of all contaminated materials in a polyethylene bag to avoid accidental contact by others. Protection from light will be necessary if accidental exposure or overexposure occurs. Note process in Patient education. ■ Administered by or under the direction of the physician specialist with appropriate knowledge of the selected laser system. Facilities for monitoring the patient and responding to any medical emergency must be availble. ■ Requires laser systems and a fiber-optic diffuser to activate. The FDA has approved several photodynamic lasers and the Optiguide® fiber-optic diffuser for use with porfimer sodium. ■ Avoid exposure of skin and eyes to direct sunlight or bright indoor light (See Patient education) ■ In the original studies for esophageal tumors, some experienced investigators indicated that natural sloughing action in the esophagus might be sufficient and débridement could needlessly traumatize the area. However, débridement is now recommended after each light activation to minimize the potential for obstruction caused by necrotic debris. ■ A minimum of 4 weeks after radiation therapy is complete is recommended before treatment with PDT (photodynamic therapy). This allows the acute inflammation produced by radiotherapy to subside. ■ 2 to 4 weeks should be allowed after PDT is complete before beginning any radiotherapy.

Esophageal tumors: Not recommended if the esophageal tumor is eroding into the trachea or bronchial tree; tracheoesophageal or bronchoesophageal fistula may result from treatment. ■ Use extreme caution in patients with esophageal varices. Light should not be given directly to the variceal area because of the high risk of bleeding.

Endobronchial cancer: Interstitial fiber placement is preferred to intraluminal activation in noncircumferential endobronchial tumors that are soft enough to penetrate. Results in less exposure of the normal bronchial mucosa to light. ■ Patients with obstructing lung cancer who have received prior radiation therapy have a higher incidence of fatal hemoptysis. ■ An endobronchial tumor that invades deeply into the bronchial wall may create a fistula as the tumor resolves. ■ Use with extreme caution in endobronchial tumors located where treatment-induced inflammation could obstruct the airway (e.g., long or circumferential tumors of the trachea, tumors of the carina that involve both mainstem bronchi circumferentially, or circumferential tumors in the mainstem bronchus in patients with prior pneumonectomy).

Monitor: Obtain baseline CBC and monitor for anemia due to tumor bleeding. ■ Prevent extravasation at the injection site. Should extravasation occur, area must be protected from light. ■ Opiates may be required to control pain. ■ Observe patients carefully; most are critically ill, and many complications could occur. ■ Monitor patients with *endobronchial tumors* closely between the laser light therapy and the mandatory débridement bronchoscopy for any evidence of respiratory distress, inflammation, mucositis, or necrotic debris that may cause obstruction of the airway. Immediate bronchoscopy may be required to remove secretions and debris to open the airway. ■ Monitor for hemoptysis; may be a sign of progressive disease, or may result from resolution of a tumor that has eroded into a pulmonary artery. ■ Photosensitivity not tranferable through skin to caregivers. ■ Note Precautions, Patient education, and Drug/lab interactions.

Patient education: Must observe precautions to avoid exposure of skin and eyes to direct sunlight or bright indoor light for 30 days. Photosensitivity is due to residual drug, which is present in all parts of the skin. Ambient indoor light is beneficial as it gradually inactivates the remaining drug through a photobleaching reaction. Do not remain in a darkened room. Do expose skin to ambient indoor light. Avoid bright indoor light from examination lamps, dental lamps, operating room lamps, and unshaded light bulbs. Limit time outdoors to necessary excursions and completely cover body with clothing and shade your face before going out. Ultraviolet sunscreens are of no value because photoactivation is caused by visible light, not UV rays. Eyes will be sensitive to sun, bright lights, and car headlights; wear dark sunglasses with an average white light transmittance of < 4%. After several weeks and before exposing any area of skin to direct sunlight or bright indoor light, test a small area of skin (not the face) for residual photosensitivity. Expose the small area of skin for 10 minutes. If no photosensitivity reaction (redness, swelling, or blistering) occurs within 24 hours, gradually resume normal outdoor activities. Exercise caution and increase skin exposure gradually. If some photosensitivity reaction occurs, continue precautions for 2 more weeks and then retest. Retest level of photosensitivity if travelling to a different geographic area with greater sunshine. ■ Report chest pain (caused by inflammatory response within the area of treatment); may require prescription pain medication. ■ Effective contraception necessary for women of childbearing age.

Maternal/child: Category C: use during pregnancy only if benefits justify potential risk to fetus. Effective contraception necessary for women of childbearing age. Has caused maternal and fetal toxicity in rats and rabbits (increased resorptions, decreased litter size, and reduced fetal body weight). ■ Discontinue breast feeding; not known if it is secreted in breast milk, but serious reactions could occur in the infant. ■ Safety and effectiveness in children not established.

Elderly: Dose modification based on age is not required.

DRUG/LAB INTERACTIONS

No specific studies have been completed, but the following interactions are likely to occur.

Use with other photosensitizing agents (e.g., griseofulvin, phenothiazines [e.g., prochlorperazine (Compazine)], sulfonamides [sulfisoxazole (Gantrisin), ophthalmic solutions (AK-Sulf)], sulfonylurea hypoglycemic agents [tolbutamide (Orinase)], tetracyclines [doxycycline (Vibramycin)], thiazide diuretics [chlorothiazide (Diuril)]) could increase the photosensitivity reaction. ■ Antitumor activity may be decreased by dimethyl sulfoxide, beta-carotene, ethanol, formate, mannitol. ■ Antitumor activity may also be decreased by allopurinol (Zyloprim), calcium channel blockers (e.g., diltiazem [Cardizem]), prostaglandin synthesis inhibitors (NSAIDs [e.g., ibuprofen (Motrin)]), and tissue ischemia. ■ Effectiveness may be reduced by drugs that decrease clotting (e.g., heparin, alteplase [tPA]), vasoconstriction (e.g., nicardipine [Cardene]), or platelet aggregation (e.g., dipyradamole [Persantine], ticlopidine [Ticlid]). ■ Glucocorticoid hormones (e.g., dexamethasone [Decadron]) given before or with PDT may reduce the effectiveness of porfimer by inhibiting the production of thromboxane A_2.

SIDE EFFECTS

Photosensitivity can be severe. May cause constipation. ■ Most toxicities are local effects in the region of illumination and occasionally in surrounding tissues. Usually an inflammatory response induced by the photodynamic effects.

Esophageal tumors: Bronchoesophageal or tracheoesophageal fistula can occur as a result of the disease or treatment, including débridement. Abdominal pain, anemia (more prevalent if tumor is located in the lower third of the esophagus), anorexia, arrhythmias (atrial fibrillation [more prevalent if tumor is located in the middle third of the esophagus], tachycardia), candidiasis, chest pain, coughing, dyspepsia, dysphagia, dyspnea, edema, eructation, esophageal edema (more prevalent if tumor is located in the upper third of the esophagus), esophageal tumor bleeding, esophageal stricture, esophagitis, fever, hematemesis, hypertension, hypotension, insomnia, nausea, pleural effusion, and vomiting may occur, as well as numerous others.

Endobronchial tumors: Coughing, dyspnea (may be life-threatening), mucositis reaction (e.g., edema, exudate, and mucous plug obstruction), stricture, ulceration. Fatal hemoptysis has occurred (higher incidence in patients who have received radiation therapy).

ANTIDOTE

If an overdose of porfimer sodium is given, do not give the laser light treatment. Porfimer sodium is not dialyzable. Increased side effects and damage to normal tissue can be expected if an overdose of light is given. Keep physician informed of all side effects; most will be treated symptomatically. Some may be life-threatening. Respiratory obstruction may require immediate bronchoscopy and removal of the obstruction with suction or forceps. Stent placement may be required in endobronchial stricture. Chest pain may require the use of opiates.

POTASSIUM ACETATE AND POTASSIUM CHLORIDE

Electrolyte replenisher
Antihypokalemic

pH 4.0 to 8.0

USUAL DOSE

Starting dose based on losses, desired replacement, or maintenance. 20 to 60 mEq/24 hr. 200 mEq/24 hr is usually not exceeded. Up to 400 mEq/24 hr has been given in selected situations (e.g., serum potassium less that 2 mEq/L) with extreme caution.

PEDIATRIC DOSE

1 to 4 mEq/kg of body weight/24 hr. Do not exceed 40 mEq/day.

DOSE ADJUSTMENTS

Reduce dose in impaired renal function.

DILUTION

Each individual dose must be diluted in a larger volume of suitable IV solution and given as an infusion. Soluble in commonly used IV solutions. 40 mEq/liter is the preferred dilution. 80 mEq/liter is the usual maximum concentration and must be administered with caution.

In replacement therapy more concentrated doses may be used and must be administered with extreme caution. 40 mEq/100 ml is commonly used and must be controlled by an infusion pump. *Up to 100 mEq/100 ml has been administered through a central line (to avoid phlebitis); must be controlled by an infusion pump.* Direct injection of any concentrated solution can be instantly fatal. Avoid layering of potassium by thoroughly agitating the prepared IV solution. Do not add potassium to an IV bottle in the hanging position; remove from hanger to guarantee dispersion throughout solution. In severe hypokalemia, solutions without dextrose are preferred (dextrose might decrease serum potassium level). Use only clear solutions.

INCOMPATIBLE WITH

Amikacin (Amikin), amphotericin B (Fungizone), blood or blood products, diazepam [Valium], dobutamine (Dobutrex), ergotamine (Ergotrate), fat emulsion 10%, mannitol, methylprednisolone (Solu-Medrol), penicillin G sodium, phenytoin (Dilantin), promethazine (Phenergan). Consult with pharmacist if mixing required.

RATE OF ADMINISTRATION

A maximum of 10 mEq/hr of potassium chloride in any given amount of infusion fluid should not be exceeded. With serious potassium depletion (under 2 mEq/liter serum), 20 to 40 mEq/hr has been given with extreme caution. Use of an infusion pump is recommended in all situations, required with any dose exceeding 60 mEq/24 hr.

Pediatric rate: 0.5 to 1 mEq/kg/hr. Do not exceed 10 mEq/hr.

ACTIONS

Helps to maintain osmotic pressure and ion balance. Flow of potassium into the cell (serum deficiency) increases membrane resting potential and decreases membrane permeability. Flow of potassium out of the cell (serum excess) decreases resting membrane potential and increases membrane permeability. Essential for intracellular tonicity, nerve impulse transmission, cardiac, skeletal, and smooth muscle contraction, normal renal function, metabolism of carbohydrates and proteins, and enzyme reactions. Excreted in urine.

INDICATIONS AND USES

Prophylaxis or treatment of potassium deficiency (e.g., hypokalemia due to diuretic therapy, digitalis intoxication, low dietary potassium intake, vomiting and diarrhea, diabetic acidosis, metabolic alkalosis, corticosteroid therapy, increased renal excretion resulting from acidosis, hemodialysis).

CONTRAINDICATIONS

Any disease or condition in which high potassium levels may occur through potassium retention or other processes (e.g., acute dehydration, adrenocortical insufficiency [untreated Addison's disease]), adynamica episodica hereditaria [periodic loss of strength or weakness], anuria, azotemia, crush syndrome, heat cramps, hyperkalemia from any cause, oliguria, patients on digitalis with severe or complete heart block, postoperative oliguria (early [except during GI drainage]), renal failure, severe hemolytic reactions.

PRECAUTIONS

Impaired renal function or adrenal insufficiency can cause potassium intoxication, which can develop rapidly and without symptoms.

- Loss of chloride usually accompanies potassium depletion and may cause hypochloremic alkalosis. Treat cause of potassium depletion in addition to giving potassium. ▪ Potassium phosphate is preferred for specific intracellular deficiency not caused by alkalosis, since phosphate is the usual ion attached to potassium in the body. Not used in the presence of kidney failure. ▪ Alkalyzing potassiums (e.g., acetate, citrate) are preferred for potassium deficiency patients with renal tubular acidosis. Metabolic acidosis and hyperchloremia are most likely present. ▪ Use potassium acetate with caution in patients with metabolic or respiratory alkalosis.

Monitor: Routine serum potassium, calcium, and sodium levels, pH, ECGs, adequate hydration, and evaluation of adequate urine output are mandatory. Only extracellular potassium can be measured; intracellular potassium equals 98% of total body potassium. Entire clinical picture must be considered. ▪ Normal daily requirements; *newborn,* 2 to 6 mEq/kg/24 hr; *children,* 2 to 3 mEq/kg/24 hr; *adults,* 40 to 80 mEq/24 hr. ▪ Continuous cardiac monitoring is preferable for infusion of over 10 mEq of potassium in 1 hour. ▪ Confirm absolute patency of vein. Extravasation will cause necrosis. Local pain and phlebitis may occur with concentrations greater than 40 mEq/liter. ▪ Note Drug/lab interactions.

Patient education: Report burning or stinging at IV site promptly.

Maternal/child: Pregnancy Category C: effect unknown; use caution and only if clearly needed in pregnancy and lactation.

Elderly: Assessment of renal function and appropriate dose adjustments indicated. ▪ Increased risk of hyperkalemia.

DRUG/LAB INTERACTIONS

Potentiated by angiotensin-converting enzyme inhibitors (e.g., captopril (Capoten), enalaprilat (Vasotec), lisinopril (Prinivil, Zestril). ▪ Digitalis intoxication may occur with hypokalemia. Use caution if discontinuing potassium after stabilization in patients taking digitalis. ▪ Potassium-sparing diuretics (e.g., spironolactone [Aldactone], triamterene [Dyrenium, and a component of Dyazide and Maxzide]) may cause hyperkalemia.

SIDE EFFECTS

Abdominal pain, bradycardia, cardiac arrest, confusion, diarrhea, dysphagia, ECG changes (including increased amplitude of T wave, decreased amplitude of R wave, below base line depression of S wave, disappearing P wave, PR prolongation), hyperkalemia, nausea, respiratory distress, weakness, ventricular fibrillation, voluntary muscle paralysis, vomiting. Progression of side effects may cause death.

ANTIDOTE

For any side effect, discontinue the drug and notify the physician. Death may result from potassium levels of 8 mEq/liter. For severe hyperkalemia (over 6.5 mEq/liter plasma); use IV sodium bicarbonate 40 to 160 mEq over 5 minutes to correct acidosis. Repeat in 10 to 15 minutes if ECG still abnormal. Initially, one ampoule of 50% dextrose may be given into a large vein. Follow with IV dextrose, 10% to 20%, with 1 unit of regular insulin for every 3 Gm of dextrose (or 5 to 10 units insulin for each 20 Gm of dextrose) and infuse at 300 to 500 ml over 1 hour. 150 ml of ⅙ molar sodium lactate is rarely used as a substitute. Eliminate potassium-containing foods and medicines.

Monitor ECG continuously. If P waves are absent, give calcium gluconate or chloride 0.5 to 1 Gm over 2 minutes (exceeds usual rate of administration). Do not use if patient receiving digitalis. All of these measures cause a shift of potassium into the cells and may be used simultaneously. Sodium polystyrene sulfonate (Kayexalate) orally or as retention enemas is used to actually remove potassium from the body. Hemodialysis or peritoneal dialysis may be useful. Use caution in the digitalized patient; too-rapid removal of potassium may cause digitalis toxicity. Resuscitate as necessary. For extravasation, inject area with 1% procaine and hyaluronidase (Wydase). Use a 27- or 25-gauge needle. Apply warm moist compresses.

PRALIDOXIME CHLORIDE

Protopam chloride

Antidote
(Anticholinesterase antagonist)

pH 3.5 to 4.5

USUAL DOSE

Organophosphate pesticide poisoning: 1 to 2 Gm initially. Repeat in 1 hour if indicated. If muscle weakness continues, additional doses can be given with extreme caution; usually every 8 to 12 hours (has been given more frequently). Atropine must be given before pralidoxime but after adequate ventilation has been established. Give atropine, 2 to 4 mg IV, after cyanosis disappears, then give initial dose of pralidoxime. Repeat atropine every 10 minutes until atropine toxicity (delirium, dilated pupils, dry mouth, muscle twitching, pulse 140 beats/min). Ventricular fibrillation can occur if oxygenation is inadequate. Maintain atropinization for at least 48 hours.

Organophosphate chemical poisoning: Usually administered IM by an autoinjector system (survival technology). Atropine must be given first. After the effects of atropine are apparent (e.g., dry mouth), give pralidoxime 600 mg. Repeat both drugs at 15 minute intervals times 2 if indicated. If muscle weakness persists, seek medical help; IV doses as above may be required.

Anticholinesterase overdose (e.g., neostigmine, pyridostigmine): 1 to 2 Gm followed by 250 mg every 5 minutes.

PEDIATRIC DOSE

Organophosphate pesticide or chemical poisoning. Give atropine 0.05 to 0.1 mg/kg. Refer to adult dose for order of administration and specific criteria. Dose of pralidoxime is 20 to 50 mg/kg of body weight initially. Repeat in 1 hour and then at 8- to 12-hour intervals if muscle weakness persists (has been given more frequently).

DOSE ADJUSTMENTS

Reduce dose in renal impairment.

DILUTION

Each 1 Gm of sterile powder is diluted with 20 ml of sterile water for injection. Should be further diluted in 100 ml of NS and given as an IV infusion.

Storage: Use promptly after reconstitution and discard any remaining solution.

INCOMPATIBLE WITH

Any other drug in syringe or solution because of specific use.

RATE OF ADMINISTRATION

Too-rapid injection may cause laryngospasm, muscle rigidity, or tachycardia. Do not exceed a rate of 200 mg/minute.

Direct IV: Each 1 Gm or fraction thereof over 5 minutes. Used only if pulmonary edema present or infusion not practical.

Infusion (preferred): A single dose over 15 to 30 minutes.

ACTIONS

An anticholinesterase antagonist that reactivates cholinesterase inhibited by phosphate esters. It reverses nicotinic effects (e.g., muscle weakness, respiratory depression, and CNS effects caused by organophosphate poisoning) while atropine reverses muscarinic effects (e.g., bradycardia, bronchoconstriction, excessive secretions). Rapidly dispersed throughout body fluids. Onset of action is within 10 to 40 minutes; half-life is short (about 1.2 hours), requiring repeated doses as more poison is absorbed into the GI tract. Partially metabolized by the liver. Most of a single dose is excreted within 6 hours in the urine.

INDICATIONS AND USES

An antidote (treatment adjunct) in organophosphate pesticide or chemical poisoning. Primarily useful for many phosphate ester insecticide poisons with anticholinesterase activity (e.g., diazinon, malathion) or chemicals with anticholinesterase activity (e.g., nerve gas).

■ Control of overdose of anticholinesterase drugs used to treat myasthenia gravis. Confirm diagnosis with edrophonium (Tensilon).

CONTRAINDICATIONS

Hypersensitivity to any component of the product. Not recommended in carbamate poisoning (increases toxicity of Sevin [carbamate insecticide]).

PRECAUTIONS

In poisoning: May be ineffective if more than 24 to 48 hours has passed since exposure; some response may be obtained in severe poisoning. Caregivers must protect themselves from contamination. Wear gowns and gloves. ■ Remove contaminated clothing and cleanse contaminated skin surfaces, hair, and fingernails with water, baking soda solution, and alcohol. ■ Gently flush eyes with water for at least 15 minutes. ■ Diazepam (Valium) may be required to stop convulsions. ■ Use caution in myasthenia gravis; may cause a myasthenic crisis.

Monitor: Before any medication is given, establish and maintain an adequate airway and controlled respiration as indicated. Suction of secretions and oxygen usually required. Draw blood samples for baseline RBC acetylcholinesterase and pseudocholinesterase concentrations. ■ In suspected poisoning, initiate treatment without waiting for lab confirmation of diagnosis. Combined with a history of possible poisoning, a RBC cholinesterase concentration less than 50% of normal is indicative of organophosphate ester poisoning. ■ Gastric lavage and activated charocoal are indicated if organophosphates are ingested; most effective if started within 30 minutes of ingestion. Avoid emesis as patient may lose consciousness and aspirate. ■ Monitor vital signs and ECG continuously. ■ Maintain adequate urine output. ■ Toxicity may recur as poison is absorbed from bowel. ■ Note Drug/lab interactions.

Maternal/child: Pregnancy Category C: effects not known, use only if clearly needed. ▪ Safety for lactation and children not established.

DRUG/LAB INTERACTIONS

Potentiates barbiturates increasing CNS depression. ▪ CNS depressants (e.g., anticonvulsants, antihistamines, muscle relaxants, narcotics, reserpine compounds, phenothiazines) and xanthines (e.g., aminophylline, caffeine) will intensify the effects of organophosphate poisoning and defeat effectiveness of treatment. ▪ Succinylcholine may cause prolonged respiratory paralysis. ▪ Thiamine delays excretion of pralidoxime.

SIDE EFFECTS

Blurred vision, diplopia, dizziness, drowsiness, headache, hyperventilation, impaired accommodation, increased diastolic and systolic BP, laryngospasm, muscle rigidity, muscular weakness, nausea, pharyngeal pain, tachycardia, transient elevated AST, ALT, and CPK. Excitement and manic behavior may occur (atropinization) if pralidoxime is delayed after atropine has been given.

ANTIDOTE

Has not been needed. Patient should be observed for atropine intoxication. Maintain vital signs by any means necessary.

PREDNISOLONE SODIUM PHOSPHATE

Hormone
(Adrenocorticoid/glucocorticoid)
Antiinflammatory
Immunosuppressant

Hydeltrasol, Key-Pred SP, Predicort-RP,
Prednisolone phosphate

pH 7.0 to 8.0

USUAL DOSE

4 to 60 mg/24 hr initially. 10 to 20 mg every 4 to 8 hours may be given. Total dose usually does not exceed 400 mg every 24 hours. Dosage individualized according to the oral dose it is replacing, the severity of the disease, and the response of the patient. In adrenocortical insufficiency, additional use of a concomitant mineralocorticoid (e.g., fludrocortisone [Florinef]) may be indicated.

PEDIATRIC DOSE

Adrenocortical insufficiency: 0.14 mg/kg/day in 3 equally divided doses. Given every third day. Another reference suggests 0.04 to 0.25 mg/kg or 1.5 to 7.5 mg/M^2 IM or IV one or two times daily. Often given orally. Note comment on mineralocorticoid in Usual dose.

DOSE ADJUSTMENTS

Reduced dose may be required in the elderly. Note Drug/lab interactions.

DILUTION

May be given without mixing or dilution. Always use a separate syringe for Hydeltrasol. May be added to NS or D5W and given by

IV infusion. Use solution within 24 hours of dilution. Sensitive to heat.

INCOMPATIBLE WITH

Calcium gluceptate, calcium gluconate, dimenhydrinate (Dramamine), metaraminol (Aramine), methotrexate, polymyxin B (Aerosporin), prochlorperazine (Compazine), promazine (Sparine), promethazine (Phenergan). Not generally mixed with any other drug in a solution.

RATE OF ADMINISTRATION

10 mg or fraction thereof over 1 minute. Decrease rate of injection if any complaints of burning or tingling along injection site.

ACTIONS

Rapidly absorbed synthetic adrenocortical steroid with potent metabolic and antiinflammatory actions. It is three to four times more potent than hydrocortisone. Has minimal mineralocorticoid activity. Metabolized by the liver and excreted in the urine. Crosses the placental barrier. Secreted in breast milk.

INDICATIONS AND USES

To replace oral corticosteroid therapy (e.g., prednisone) when oral dosing is not feasible. ▪ Adrenocortical insufficiency: total, relative, and operative. Use of a concomitant mineralocorticoid (e.g., hydrocortisone IV or fludrocortisone [oral]) may be required. ▪ Acute exacerbations of disease for patients on steroid therapy. ▪ Has numerous other uses by other routes of administration (e.g., IM, intraarticular, intralesional, soft-tissue injection.).

CONTRAINDICATIONS

Absolute contraindications, except in life-threatening situations: Hypersensitivity to any product component including sulfites; systemic fungal infections.

Relative contraindications: Active or latent peptic ulcer, active or healed tuberculosis, acute psychoses, chickenpox, diabetes mellitus, diverticulitis, fresh intestinal anastomoses, hypertension, myasthenia gravis, ocular herpes simplex, osteoporosis, pregnancy, psychotic tendencies, renal insufficiency, thromboembolic tendencies, vaccinia.

PRECAUTIONS

To avoid adrenocortical insufficiency, do not stop therapy abruptly; taper off. Patient is observed carefully, especially if under stress, for up to 2 years. ▪ Prophylactic antacids may prevent peptic ulcer complications. ▪ Periodic ophthalmic exams may be necessary with prolonged treatment. ▪ Note Drub/lab interactions.

Monitor: May increase insulin needs in diabetes. ▪ Monitor electrolytes periodically. May cause sodium retention and potassium and calcium excretion. May cause hypertension secondary to fluid and electrolyte disturbances. ▪ Administer a single dose before 9 AM to reduce suppression of individual's own adrenocortical activity. ▪ May mask signs of infection. ▪ Periodic ophthalmic exams may be necessary with prolonged treatment. ▪ Note Drug/lab interactions.

Patient education: Report edema, tarry stool, or weight gain promptly. ▪ Anorexia, diarrhea, dizziness, fatigue, low blood sugar, nausea, weakness, weight loss, and vomiting may indicate adrenal insufficiency after dose reduction or discontinuing therapy; report any of these symptoms. ▪ Consider birth control options with high dose or prolonged therapy. ▪ May mask signs of infection and/or decrease resistance.

■ Diabetics may have an increased requirement for insulin or oral hypoglycemics. ■ Avoid immunization with live vaccines. ■ Carry ID stating steroid dependent if receiving prolonged therapy.

Maternal/child: Pregnancy Category C: note Contraindications. ■ Use caution in lactation. Secretion into breast milk less than some other glucocorticoids. ■ Observe newborn for hypoadrenalism if mother has received large doses. ■ Monitor growth and development of children receiving prolonged treatment.

Elderly: Reduced muscle mass and plasma volume may require a reduced dose. Monitor blood pressure, blood glucose, and electrolytes carefully. ■ Higher risk of glucocorticoid-induced osteoporosis. ■ Avoid aluminum-based antacids (risk of Alzheimer's disease).

DRUG/LAB INTERACTIONS

Aminoglutethimide (Cytadren) and mitotane (Lysodren) suppress adrenal function of corticosteroids. Monitor carefully if concurrent use is necessary. ■ Metabolism increased and effects reduced by hepatic enzyme inducing agents (e.g., alcohol, barbiturates [e.g., phenobarbital], hydantoins [e.g., phenytoin (Dilantin), rifampin (Rifadin)]); dose adjustment may be required when adding or deleting from drug profile. ■ Risk of hypokalemia increased with amphotericin B, or potassium-depleting diuretics (e.g., thiazides, furosemide, ethacrynic acid). Monitor potassium levels and cardiac function. Increased risk of digitalis toxicity (e.g., digoxin) secondary to hypokalemia. ■ May also decrease effectiveness of potassium supplements; monitor serum potassium. ■ Diuretics decrease sodium and fluid retention effects of corticosteroids; corticosteroids decrease sodium excretion and diuretic effects of diuretics. ■ May antagonize effects of anticholinesterases (e.g., neostigmine), isoniazid, salicylates, and somatrem. Dose adjustments may be required. ■ Use with cyclosporine in organ transplants is therapeutic but may increase cyclosporine toxicity. ■ Clearance decreased and effects increased with estrogens, oral contraceptives, and ketoconazole (Nizoral). ■ May interact with anticoagulants, nondepolarizing muscle relaxants (e.g., doxacurium [Nuromax]) or theophyllines to inhibit or potentiate action; monitor carefully. ■ Monitor patients receiving insulin or thyroid hormones carefully; dose adjustments of either or both agents may be required. ■ Use with ritodrine (Yutopar) has caused pulmonary edema in the mother; discontinue both agents with onset of S/S of pulmonary edema. ■ Do not vaccinate with attenuated-virus vaccines (e.g., smallpox) during therapy. ■ Altered protein-binding capacity will impact effectiveness of this drug. ■ Note Dose adjustments.

SIDE EFFECTS

Do occur, but are usually reversible: anaphylaxis, Cushing's syndrome (moon face, fat pads, etc.), decrease in spermatozoa, euphoria, fat emboli, fluid and electrolyte imbalance with edema, increased intracranial pressure, menstrual irregularities, peptic ulcer with perforation and hemorrhage, protein catabolism with negative nitrogen balance, relative adrenocortical insufficiency, spontaneous fractures, suppression of growth, transitory burning or tingling, and many others.

ANTIDOTE

Notify the physician of any side effect. Will probably treat the side effect. Resuscitate as necessary for anaphylaxis and notify the physician. Keep epinephrine immediately available.

PROCAINAMIDE HYDROCHLORIDE

Pronestyl

Antiarrhythmic

pH 4.0 to 6.0

USUAL DOSE

Loading dose: 0.2 to 1 Gm (100 mg/ml). 100 mg every 5 minutes or 20 mg every 1 minute may be given as an infusion until arrhythmia suppressed or 500 mg is administered. Wait 10 minutes to allow adequate distribution, then resume dosing until arrhythmia suppressed or maximum initial dose (1 Gm or 17 mg/kg) is reached, or side effects appear (e.g., hypotension, QRS complex widening by 50%).

Maintenance dose: After arrhythmia suppressed or maximum dose reached, follow initial dose with an infusion of 1 to 4 mg/min (may require up to 6 mg/min). Titrate to control arrhythmias. Maintain with oral procainamide as soon as possible but at least 4 hours after last IV dose.

PEDIATRIC DOSE

2 to 5 mg/kg of body weight. Do not exceed 100 mg/dose. Repeat as indicated every 10 to 30 minutes. Maximum dose in 24 hours is 30 mg/kg or 2 Gm. An alternate dose regimen is 2 to 6 mg/kg as a loading dose given over 5 minutes; follow with a maintenance infusion of 20 to 80 mcg/kg/min to control arrhythmias.

DOSE ADJUSTMENTS

Maintenance dose may be reduced in impaired or reduced renal function and in individuals over age 50. ■ Note Drug/lab interactions.

DILUTION

Direct IV: Dilute each 100 mg with 5 to 10 ml of D5W.

Infusion: Add 1 Gm of procainamide to 50, 250, or 500 ml of D5W. Yields 20 mg/ml, 4 mg/ml, or 2 mg/ml respectively. 20 mg/ml should only be used as a loading dose. 2 and 4 mg/ml dilutions may be used for loading or maintenance based on fluid restrictions. Solution should be clear; may be light yellow. Discard if darker than light amber.

Pediatric infusion: Loading dose: Add a calculated loading dose (2 to 5 mg/kg) to a minimum of 10 ml D5W for each 100 mg or fraction thereof. More diluent may be used based on size of child and fluid restriction. *Maintenance infusion:* See chart under Pediatric rate of administration.

Storage: Photosensitive; protect from light. Store at controlled room temperature.

INCOMPATIBLE WITH

Amrinone (Inocor), bretylium (Bretylate), esmolol (Brevibloc), ethacrynic sodium (Edecrin), milrinone (Primacor), phenytoin (Dilantin). Physically compatible with many drugs. However, combination is not practical because of individualized rate adjustments necessary to achieve desired effects.

RATE OF ADMINISTRATION

20 mg or fraction thereof over 1 minute. Use an infusion pump or a microdrip (60 gtt/ml) for infusion to deliver a constant rate. Up to 50 mg may be given direct IV over 1 minute with extreme caution. After

stabilized with loading dose, follow with a maintenance infusion at 1 to 6 mg/min.

Procainamide infusion rate (Adults)						
Desired dose	1 gm in 500 ml D5W 2mg/ml			1 gm in 250 ml D5W 4 mg/ml		
mg/min	mg/hr	ml/min	ml/hr	mg/hr	ml/min	ml/hr
1	60	0.5	30	60	0.25	15
2	120	1	60	120	0.5	30
3	180	1.5	90	180	0.75	45
4	240	2	120	240	1	60
5	300	2.5	150	300	1.25	75
6	360	3	180	360	1.5	90

Procainamide infusion rate (Pediatric)		
Desired dose	200 mg in 500 ml D5W 400 mcg/ml	200 mg in 125 ml D5W 1600 mcg/ml
mcg/ kg/min	ml/min × kg = ml/kg/min	ml/min × kg = ml/kg/min
20	0.05 ml × wt in kg	0.0125 ml × wt in kg
30	0.075 × wt in kg	0.01875 × wt in kg
40	0.1 ml × wt in kg	0.025 × wt in kg
50	0.125 × wt in kg	0.03125 × wt in kg
60	0.15 × wt in kg	0.0375 × wt in kg
70	0.175 × wt in kg	0.04375 × wt in kg
80	0.2 × wt in kg	0.05 × wt in kg

Example: To deliver 30 mcg/min to a child weighing 20 kg, multiply 0.075 (ml/min) × 20 (wt in kg) = an infusion rate of 1.5 ml/min.

ACTIONS

A procaine derivative. Exerts a depressing antiarrhythmic action on the heart, slowing the rate, slowing conduction, reducing myocardial irritability, and prolonging the refractory period. Decreases membrane permeability of the cell and prevents loss of sodium and potassium ions. Onset of action should occur in 2 to 3 minutes. Half-life is 3 to 4 hours. Crosses the placental barrier. Plasma levels decrease slowly; partially metabolized to the active metabolite NAPA; remaining drug excreted in the urine.

INDICATIONS AND USES

Suppress PVCs and recurrent ventricular tachycardia when lidocaine is contraindicated or has not suppressed ventricular arrhythmias. ■ Treat wide-complex tachycardias difficult to distinguish from VT (lidocaine preferred). ■ Rarely used in atrial fibrillation, paroxysmal atrial tachycardia, or arrhythmias caused by anesthesia. Safer drugs (e.g., verapamil, diltiazem) are readily available.

CONTRAINDICATIONS

Complete atrioventricular heart block, second- and third-degree AV block unless an electrical pacemaker is operative, preexisting QT prolongation, torsades de pointes, known sensitivity to procainamide or any other local anesthetic of the ester type, myasthenia gravis, systemic lupus erythematosus.

PRECAUTIONS

Oral or IM administration is the route of choice; IV route for emergencies only. ▪ Use extreme caution in first- or second-degree blocks, ventricular tachycardia after a myocardial infarction, digitalis intoxication, CHF, any structural heart disease, and impaired liver or reduced kidney function. ▪ Predigitalize or cardiovert patients with atrial flutter or fibrillation to reduce incidence of sudden increase in ventricular rate as atrial rate is slowed. ▪ Some clinicians recommend giving a dose the night before surgery and then discontinuing until after surgery. If an arrhythmia occurs, use lidocaine for ventricular arrhythmias and calcium channel blockers (e.g., diltiazem, verapamil) or beta-blockers (e.g., atenolol, propranolol) for supraventricular arrhythmias. Resume dosing post-op and utilize oral dosing as soon as possible.

Monitor: Monitor the patient's ECG and blood pressure continuously. Keep patient in a supine position. Avoid a hypotensive response. ▪ Discontinue IV use when the cardiac arrhythmia is interrupted or when the ventricular rate slows without regular atrioventricular conduction. ▪ Small emboli may be dislodged when atrial fibrillation is corrected. ▪ Monitor blood levels of procainamide and NAPA (active metabolite) in patients with renal impairment and in any patient receiving a constant infusion over 3 mg/min for more than 24 hours. ▪ Monitor CBC, including WBC, differential, and platelets with continued use; fatal blood dyscrasis have occurred with usual doses. ▪ Note Drug/lab interactions.

Maternal/child: Pregnancy Category C: safety for use in pregnancy and lactation and in children not established. Consider quinidine as an alternate for use during pregnancy.

Elderly: Half-life prolonged; renal excretion reduced about 25% at age 50 and 50% at age 75. ▪ Increased risk of hypotension.

DRUG/LAB INTERACTIONS

Potentiates or is potentiated by neuromuscular blocking antibiotics (e.g., kanamycin [Kantrex]), anticholinergics (e.g., atropine), thiazide diuretics, antihypertensive agents, muscle relaxants, succinylcholine (Anectine), cimetidine (Tagamet), and others. ▪ May cause serious arrhythmias with other antiarrhythmic agents (e.g., digitalis, disopyramide [Norpace], lidocaine [Xylocaine], quinidine). Lower doses of both drugs may be required. ▪ Antagonizes anticholinesterases (e.g., neostigmine). ▪ Alcohol may increase hepatic metabolism. ▪ Concurrent use with ofloxacin (Floxin) may decrease procainamide serum levels. ▪ May elevate AST (SGOT) levels.

SIDE EFFECTS

Anorexia, bleeding, bruising, chills, dizziness, fever, flushing, giddiness, hallucinations, joint swelling or pain, mental confusion, nausea, skin rash, tremor, vomiting, weakness. May indicate onset of more serious side effects.

Major: Blood dyscrasias (e.g., agranulocytosis, bone marrow depression, hypoplastic anemia, neutropenia, thrombocytopenia); hypotension with a blood pressure drop over 15 mm Hg, lupus erythematosus-like symptoms, PR interval prolongation, QRS complex widening, QT interval prolongation, ventricular asystole, ventricular fibrillation, ventricular tachycardia.

ANTIDOTE

Notify the physician of any side effect. If minor symptoms progress or any major side effect appears, discontinue the drug immediately and notify the physician. Use dopamine (Intropin) or phenylephrine hydrochloride (Neo-Synephrine) to correct hypotension. Treatment of toxicity is symptomatic and supportive. Infusion of ⅙ molar sodium lactate injection may reduce cardiotoxic effects. Hemodialysis may be indicated or urinary acidifiers may increase renal clearance. Resuscitate as necessary. Depending on arrhythmia, quinidine or lidocaine is an effective alternate. Consider insertion of a ventricular pacing electrode as a precautionary measure in case serious AV block develops.

PROCHLORPERAZINE EDISYLATE

Phenothiazine
Antiemetic
Antipsychotic

Compazine, ✽Stemetil

pH 4.2 to 6.2

USUAL DOSE

A single IV dose should not exceed 10 mg. The maximum daily IV dose should not exceed 40 mg.

Control of severe nausea and vomiting: 2.5 to 10 mg, may be repeated one time in 1 to 2 hours if indicated.

Control of severe nausea and vomiting in adult surgical patients: 5 to 10 mg 15 to 30 minutes prior to induction of anesthesia or to control symptoms during or after surgery. Repeat once if necessary.

Management of nausea and vomiting in emetic-inducing chemotherapy (investigational): One source suggests 10 to 20 mg 30 minutes before and 3 hours after treatment. Another source suggests 30 to 40 mg 30 minutes before and 3 hours after treatment. A third source suggests 0.8 mg/kg 30 minutes before and 3 hours after treatment and cites precipitous hypotension with larger doses; but another source suggests 2 mg/kg for highly emetogenic agents (e.g., cisplatin, dacarbazine) and 1 mg/kg for less emetogenic agents. Begin 30 minutes before chemotherapy, repeat every 2 hours for 2 doses, then every 3 hours for 3 doses. Treat extrapyridmal symptoms with diphenhydramine (Benadryl) IM. These doses have not been recommended by the manufacturer and exceed the recommended maximum daily IV dose of 40 mg/24 hr. In addition recommended doses of newer agents (e.g., ondanestron [Zofran]) may be more effective.

Control of severe vascular and tension headaches (investigational): 10 mg given as an injection over 2 minutes. Sometimes given concurrently with dihydroergotamine 1 mg as an infusion over 30 minutes. Another regimen administers 3.5 mg of prochlorperazine over 5 minutes followed by dexamethasone 20 mg over 10 minutes.

PEDIATRIC DOSE

IV route not recommended for children, safety has not been established (see Contraindications, Precautions, Maternal/child).

DOSE ADJUSTMENTS

Reduced dose may be indicated in the elderly. ■ Note Drug/lab interactions.

DILUTION

May be given undiluted or each 5 mg (1 ml) may be diluted with 9 ml of NS (preferred). 1 ml will equal 0.5 mg. Larger amounts of NS may be used. May add doses over 10 mg to 50 ml to 1 liter of commonly used IV solution (e.g., D5W, NS, D5/0.45NS, Ringer's or LR), and give as an intermittent or prolonged infusion. Handle carefully; may cause contact dermatitis. Sensitive to light. Slightly yellow color does not affect potency. Discard if markedly discolored.

Storage: Store below 40° C and protect from light.

INCOMPATIBLE WITH

Aldesleukin (Proleukin), allopurinol (Zyloprim), amitostine (Ethyol), aminophylline, amobarbital (Amytal), amphotericin B, ampicillin, calcium gluceptate, calcium gluconate, chloramphenicol (Chloromycetin), chlorothiazide (Diuril), dexamethasone (Decadron), dimenhydrinate (Dramamine), epinephrine (Adrenalin), erythromycin (Ilotycin), filgrastim (Neupogen), fludarabine (Fludara), foscarnet (Foscavir), furosemide (Lasix), gallium nitrate (Ganite), heparin, hydrocortisone sodium succinate (Solu-Cortef), hydromorphone (Dilaudid), kanamycin (Kantrex), ketorolac (Toradol), levallorphan (Lorfan), methicillin (Staphcillin), methohexital (Brevital), midazolam (Versed), morphine, oxytocin, paraldehyde, penicillin G potassium and sodium, pentobarbital (Nembutal), phenobarbital (Luminal), phenytoin (Dilantin), piperacillin/tazobactam (Zozyn), prednisolone (Hydeltrasol), secobarbital (Seconal), sulfisoxazole (Gantrisin), thiopental (Pentothal), vancomycin (Vancocin). *Should be considered incompatible in syringe with any other drug.*

RATE OF ADMINISTRATION

Direct IV: Each 5 mg or fraction thereof over 1 minute.

Infusion: May be given at ordered rate, or rate may be increased or decreased as symptoms indicate. Use an infusion pump or a microdrip (60 gtt/ml) for infusion.

Management of nausea and vomiting associated with emetic-inducing chemotherapy: A single dose over 15 to 20 minutes as an ***Intermittent IV.***

ACTIONS

A phenothiazine derivative approximately six times more potent than chlorpromazine (Thorazine), with effects on the central, autonomic, and peripheral nervous systems. Has weak anticholinergic effects, moderate sedative effects and strong extrapyramidal effects. A potent antiemetic, acting both centrally at the chemorecptor trigger zone and peripherally by blocking the vagus nerve in the GI tract. Onset of action is prompt and lasting. Metabolized in the liver and excreted in urine and feces.

INDICATIONS AND USES

Control of severe nausea and vomiting. ▪ Antipsychotic drug (other routes of administration usually utilized).

Investigational uses: Use of higher doses to control nausea and vomiting associated with emetic-inducing chemotherapy. ▪ Treatment of severe vascular and tension headaches.

CONTRAINDICATIONS

Children under 2 years or 10 kg (22 lb), comatose or severely depressed states, hypersensitivity to phenothiazines, lactation and pregnancy, except labor and delivery; do not use in pediatric surgery.

PRECAUTIONS

Use IV only when absolutely necessary. IV not recommended for children. ▪ May mask diagnosis of other conditions including Reyes syndrome, brain tumor, drug intoxication, and intestinal obstruction. ▪ Use caution in coronary disease, epilepsy, glaucoma and severe hypertension or hypotension. ▪ Neuroleptic malignant syndrome, characterized by hyperpyrexia, muscle rigidity, autonomic instability and altered mental status has been reported with phenothiazine use. ▪ Anticholinergic and cardiac effects may be troublesome during anesthesia. For patients receiving phenothiazines, taper and discontinue preoperatively if they will not be continued after surgery. ■ May discolor urine pink to reddish brown. ■ Photosensitivity of skin is possible. ■ May cause paradoxical excitation in children and the elderly. ■ May contain sulfites; use caution in patients with allergies.

Monitor: Keep patient in supine position and monitor blood pressure and pulse before administration and between doses. ■ Note Drug/lab interactions.

Patient education: Avoid use of alcohol or other CNS depressants (e.g., antihistamines, barbiturates). ■ Request assistance for ambulation; may cause dizziness or fainting. ■ Use caution performing tasks that require alertness. ■ May cause skin and eye photosensitivity. Avoid unprotected exposure to sun.

Maternal/child: Safety for use in pregnancy, lactation and children not established. Note Contraindications. ■ Incidence of extrapyramidal reactions is relatively high in children, especially in the presence of acute illness (e.g., measles, chicken pox, gastroenteritis) .

Elderly: Note Dose adjustments and Precautions. ■ May have increased sensitivity to postural hypotension, anticholinergic and sedative effects. ■ Increased risk of extrapyramidal side effects (e.g., tardive dyskinesia, parkinsonism).

DRUG/LAB INTERACTIONS

Use with epinephrine not recommended; may cause precipitous hypotension. ■ Increased CNS respiratory depression, and hypotensive effects with narcotics, alcohol, anesthetics, barbiturates, reduced doses of these agents usually indicated. ■ Additive effects with MAO inhibitors (e.g., selegiline [Eldepryl]), anticholinergics, antihistamines, antihypertensives, hypnotics, muscle relaxants, phenytoin (Dilantin), propranolol (Inderal), rauwolfia alkaloids, and thiazide diuretics, dose adjustment may be necessary. ■ Risk of cardiotoxicity increased with pimozide (Orap) and sparfloxacin (Zagam); concurrent use not recommended. ■ May diminish effects of oral anticoagulants. ■ May lower seizure threshold. Dose adjustment of anticonvulsants may be necessary. ■ Use caution during anesthesia with barbiturates (e.g., methohexital, thiopental); may increase frequency and severity of hypotension and neuromuscular excitation. ■ Capable of innumerable other interactions.

SIDE EFFECTS

Usually transient if drug discontinued but may require treatment if severe: anaphylaxis, blurring of vision, cardiac arrest, dermatitis, dizziness, dryness of mouth, dysphagia, elevated blood pressure, extrapyramidal symptoms (e.g., abnormal positioning, extreme restlessness, pseudoparkinsonism, weakness of extremities), excitement, fever without etiology, hypersensitivity reactions, hypotension, slurred speech, spastic movements (especially about the face), tachycardia, tightness of the throat, tongue discoloration, tongue protrusion, and many others. Overdose can cause convulsions, hallucinations, and death.

ANTIDOTE

Discontinue the drug at onset of any side effect and notify the physician. Counteract hypotension with IV fluids and norepinephrine (Levophed) or phenylephrine (Neo-synephrine) and extrapyramidal symptoms with benztropine mesylate (Cogentin) or diphenhydramine

(Benadryl). Epinephrine is contraindicated for hypotension. Further hypotension will occur. Use diazepam (Valium) or phenobarbital for convulsions or hyperactivity. Phenytoin may be helpful in ventricular arrhythmias. In treating respiratory depression and unconsciousness, avoid analeptics such as doxapram (Dopram); they may cause convulsions. Resuscitate as necessary.

PROMAZINE HYDROCHLORIDE

Phenothiazine
Antiemetic
Sedative/hypnotic
Antipsychotic

Prozine, Sparine

pH 4.0 to 5.5

USUAL DOSE

50 to 150 mg. If not effective within 30 minutes, additional doses up to a total of 300 mg may be administered (note Actions and Precautions).

DOSE ADJUSTMENTS

Reduced dose may be indicated in the elderly. ▪ Note Drug/lab interactions.

DILUTION

May be given undiluted, or may dilute with NS. Concentration should not exceed 25 mg/ml. 1 ml (25 to 50 mg) diluted with 9 ml of NS equals 2.5 to 5 mg/ml. Handle carefully; may cause contact dermatitis.

Storage: Store below 40° C. Protect from light.

INCOMPATIBLE WITH

Aminophylline, amobarbital (Amytal), ampicillin (Polycillin), atropine, chloramphenicol (Chloromycetin), chlorothiazide (Diuril), dimenhydrinate (Dramamine), epinephrine (Adrenalin), heparin, hydrocortisone phosphate, hydrocortisone sodium succinate (Solu-Cortef), methicillin (Staphcillin), methohexital (Brevital), nafcillin (Unipen), NS (may have minimal potency loss), penicillin G potassium and sodium, pentobarbital (Nembutal), phenobarbital (Luminal), phenytoin (Dilantin), prednisolone (Hydeltrasol), sodium bicarbonate, thiopental (Pentothal), warfarin (Coumadin).

RATE OF ADMINISTRATION

25 mg or fraction thereof over 1 minute, titrate to effect.

ACTIONS

A phenothiazine derivative with effects on the central, autonomic, and peripheral nervous systems. Has strong anticholinergic and sedative effects, moderate extrapyramidal and antiemetic effects, and weak antipsychotic effects. Onset of action is prompt and lasting. Metabolized in the liver and excreted in urine and feces. Rarely used, other more effective agents (e.g., haloperidol) are more commonly used.

INDICATIONS AND USES

Management of psychiatric disorders.

Unlabeled uses: Preoperative sedation, antiemetic.

CONTRAINDICATIONS

Bone marrow depression, children under 12 years, comatose or severely depressed states, hypersensitivity to phenothiazines, lactation and pregnancy, except labor and delivery.

PRECAUTIONS

IV administration is not recommended. ▪ Use IV only when absolutely necessary. Reserve for acutely agitated, hospitalized patients. Rarely used, other more effective agents (e.g., haloperidol) are more commonly used. ▪ Use with caution in the presence of cerebral arteriosclerosis, coronary heart disease, severe hypertension or hypotension, epilepsy, heat exhaustion, glaucoma, liver disease, and respiratory problems. ▪ May mask diagnosis of brain tumor, drug intoxication, and intestinal obstruction. ▪ In large doses, extrapyramidal and antiemetic, effects are moderate. Hypotensive effects are very prominent. ▪ Neuroleptic malignant syndrome, characterized by hyperpyrexia, muscle rigidity, autonomic instability and altered mental status has been reported with phenothiazine use. ▪ Anticholinergic and cardiac effects may be troublesome during anesthesia. For patients receiving phenothiazines, taper and discontinue preoperatively if they will not be continued after surgery. ▪ May discolor urine pink to reddish brown. ▪ Photosensitivity of skin is possible. ▪ May contain sulfites; use caution in patients with allergies.

Monitor: Establish unquestionable patency of vein. Avoid extravasation. ▪ Intraarterial injection will cause gangrene. ▪ Monitor blood pressure and pulse before administration and between doses. Keep patient in supine position. ▪ Note Drug/lab interactions.

Patient education: Request assistance for ambulation; may cause dizziness or fainting. ▪ Possible skin and eye sensitivity; avoid unprotected exposure to sun. ▪ Avoid use of alcohol or other CNS depressants (e.g., antihistamines, barbiturates) ▪ Use caution in tasks requiring alertness.

Maternal/child: Safety for use in pregnancy, lactation, and children not established. Note Contraindications.

Elderly: Note Dose adjustments. ▪ May have increased sensitivity to postural hypotension, anticholinergic, and sedative effects. ▪ Increased risk of extrapyramidal side effects (e.g., tardive dyskinesia, parkinsonism).

DRUG/LAB INTERACTIONS

Increased CNS, respiratory depression, and hypotensive effects with narcotics, alcohol, anesthetics, barbiturates; reduced doses of these agents usually indicated. ▪ Additive effects with MAO inhibitors (e.g., pargyline [Eutonyl]), anticholinergics, antihistamines, antihypertensives, hypnotics, muscle relaxants, phenytoin (Dilantin), propranolol (Inderal), rauwolfia alkaloids, and thiazide diuretics; dose adjustment may be necessary. ▪ May lower seizure threshold; dose adjustment of anticonvulsants may be necessary. ▪ Use with epinephrine not recommended; may cause precipitous hypotension. ▪ Risk of cardiotoxicity increased with pimozide (Orap) and sparfloxacin (Zagam), concurrent use not recommended. ▪ Use caution during anesthesia with barbiturates (e.g., methohexital, thiopental); may increase frequency and severity of hypotension and neuromuscular excitation. ▪ Capable of innumerable other interactions.

SIDE EFFECTS

Usually transient if drug is discontinued but may require treatment if severe; considered less toxic than prochlorperazine. Anaphylaxis, blurring of vision, cardiac arrest, cerebral edema, convulsions, dermatitis, dizziness, dryness of mouth, dysphagia, extrapyramidal symptoms (e.g., abnormal positioning, extreme restlessness, pseudoparkinsonism, weakness of extremities), elevated blood pressure, excitement, hypersensitivity reactions, hypotension, slurred speech, spastic movements (especially about the face), tachycardia, temperature without etiology, tightness of the throat, tongue discoloration, tongue protrusion, and many others.

ANTIDOTE

Discontinue drug at onset of any side effect and notify physician. Counteract hypotension with norepinephrine (Levophed) or phenylephrine (Neo-synephrine) and IV fluids; extrapyramidal symptoms with benztropine mesylate (Cogentin) or diphenhydramine (Benadryl). Epinephrine is contraindicated for hypotension. Further hypotension will occur. Use diazepam (Valium) or phenobarbital for convulsions or hyperactivity. Phenytoin may be helpful in ventricular arrhythmias. In treating respiratory depression and unconsciousness, avoid analeptics such as doxapram (Dopram); may cause convulsions. Resuscitate as necessary.

PROMETHAZINE HYDROCHLORIDE

Phenothiazine
Antiemetic
Sedative-hypnotic

Anergan 25, Phenazine 25, Phenergan, Prometh-25, Prorex, Prothazine, V-Gan 25

pH 4.0 to 5.5

USUAL DOSE

Nausea and vomiting: 12.5 to 25 mg every 4 to 6 hours as needed.

Allergic conditions: 25 mg. May repeat in 2 hours if necessary. Change to oral therapy as soon as possible.

Sedation; Nighttime: 25 to 50 mg.

Sedation; Perioperative: 25 to 50 mg. May combine with a reduced dose of narcotic analgesic and an anticholinergic drug (e.g., atropine)

Sedation; Labor and delivery: 50 mg during early stage of labor. When labor fully established, may administer 25 to 75 mg with a reduced dose of a narcotic analgesic. May repeat every 4 hours to a maximum dose of 100 mg.

PEDIATRIC DOSE

Nausea and vomiting: 0.25 to 0.5 mg/kg of body weight every 4 to 6 hours. IV rarely used. Do not exceed one half of adult dose.

Preoperative sedation: 1.1 mg/kg. May be combined with a narcotic analgesic and an anticholinergic drug (e.g., atropine).

DOSE ADJUSTMENTS

Reduced dose may be indicated in the elderly. Note Drug/lab interactions.

DILUTION

May be given undiluted or may dilute with NS. Concentration should not exceed 25 mg/ml. 1 ml (25 to 50 mg) diluted with 9 ml of NS equals 2.5 to 5 mg/ml. Slightly yellow color does not alter potency. Discard if greatly discolored. Administer through Y-tube or three-way stopcock of a free-flowing IV.

Storage: Store at CRT. Protect from light.

INCOMPATIBLE WITH

Aldesleukin (Proleukin), allopurinol (Zyloprim), aminophylline, calcium gluconate, carbenicillin (Geopen), cefoperazone (Cefobid), chloramphenicol (Chloromycetin), chlordiazepoxide (Librium), chlorothiazide (Diuril), codeine, dextran, diatrizoate sodium and meglumine, dimenhydrinate (Dramamine), foscarnet (Foscavir), furosemide (Lasix), heparin, hydrocortisone sodium succinate (Solu-Cortef), iodipamide sodium and meglumine, iothalamate meglumine (60%), iothalamate sodium (80%), ketoralac (Toradol), methicillin (Staphcillin), methohexital (Brevital), methylprednisolone (Solu-Medrol), morphine, nalbuphine (Nubain), penicillin G potassium and sodium, pentobarbital (Nembutal), phenobarbital (Luminal), phenytoin (Dilantin), piperacillin/tazobactam (Zosyn), Potassium chloride (Kcl), Prednisolone sodium phosphate (Hydeltrasol), secobarbital (Seconal), thiopental (Pentothal).

RATE OF ADMINISTRATION

Each 25 mg or fraction thereof over 1 minute.

ACTIONS

A phenothiazine derivative with effects on the central, autonomic, and peripheral nervous systems. It has antihistaminic, antiemetic, anticholinergic and sedative effects. As an antihistamine, it competitively blocks the H_1 histamine receptor, antagonizing most of the effects of histamine to at least some degree. Potentiates respiratory depression, sedative, and hypotensive effects of narcotics and other CNS depressants. Has no analgesic effects and does not potentiate analgesic effects of narcotics. Onset of action is prompt. Duration of action is 4 to 6 hours. Primarily metabolized in the liver and excreted in the urine.

INDICATIONS AND USES

Prophylaxis or treatment of minor transfusion reactions. ■ Treatment of hypersensitivity reactions. ■ Treatment of acute nausea, vomiting, and motion sickness. ■ Sedation to meet surgical and obstetric needs. ■ Adjunct to analgesics for control of postoperative pain.

CONTRAINDICATIONS

Bone marrow depression, comatose or severely depressed states, hypersensitivity to phenothiazines, jaundice, lactation, pregnancy. Never inject into an artery or SC.

PRECAUTIONS

Ampoule must state "for IV use". Use with extreme caution in children and the elderly; note Maternal/child and Elderly under Precautions. ■ May cause paradoxical excitation in children and the elderly. ■ Use phenothiazines with extreme caution in children with a history of sleep apnea, a family history of sudden infant death syndrome, or in the presence of Reye's syndrome. ■ Use with caution in patients with asthma, bladder neck obstruction, bone marrow depression, cardiovascular disease, glaucoma, liver dysfunction, prostatic hypertrophy, or stenosing peptic ulcer disease. ■ May mask diagnosis of other conditions including Reye's syndrome, brain tumor, drug intoxication, and intestinal obstruction. ■ May lower seizure threshold; use extreme caution in patients with known seizure disorders and with narcotics or local anesthetics that also lower seizure threshold. ■ May contain sulfites; use caution in patients with allergies. ■ Anticholinergic and cardiac effects may be troublesome during anesthesia. For patients receiving phenothiazines, taper and discontinue preoperatively if they will not be continued after surgery.

Monitor: Determine absolute patency of vein; extravasation will cause necrosis. ■ Keep patient in supine position. Monitor blood pressure and pulse before administration and between doses. ■ Sedative effect may require ambulation to be monitored. ■ Note Drug/lab interactions.

Patient education: Avoid use of alcohol or other CNS depressants (e.g., antihistamines, barbiturates). ■ Request assistance for ambulation; may cause dizziness or fainting. ■ Use caution performing tasks that require alertness. ■ May cause skin and eye photosensitivity. Avoid unprotected exposure to sun. ■ Report stinging or burning at IV site promptly.

Maternal/child: Category C: Safety for use in pregnancy, lactation, and children not established. ■ Do not use in premature infants or neonates. ■ Do not use for vomiting of unknown etiology in children. ■ Excessively large doses of antihistamines in children have caused hallucination, convulsions, and death. ■ Incidence of extrapyramidal reactions is relatively high in children, especially in the presence of acute illness (e.g., measles, chicken pox, gastroenteritis). ■ Note Precautions and Contraindications.

Elderly: Note Dose adjustments and Precautions. ■ May cause confusion, dizziness, hyperexcitability, hypotension and/or sedation. ■ Increased sensitivity to anticholinergic effects (e.g., dry mouth, urinary retention). ■ Increased risk of extrapyramidal side effects (e.g., tardive dyskinesia, parkinsonism).

DRUG/LAB INTERACTIONS

Increased CNS respiratory depression and hypotensive effects with narcotics, alcohol, anesthetics, and barbiturates; reduced doses of these agents usually indicated. ■ Additive effects with MAO inhibitors (e.g., selegiline [Eldepryl]), anticholinergics, antihistamines, antihypertensives, hypnotics, muscle relaxants, phenytoin (Dilantin), propranolol (Inderal), rauwolfia alkaloids, and thiazide diuretics; dose adjustment may be necessary. ■ Use with epinephrine not recommended; may cause precipitous hypotension. ■ Risk of cardiotoxicity increased with pimozide (Orap) and sparfloxacin (Zagam), concurrent use not recommended. ■ May lower seizure threshold. Dose adjustment of anticonvulsants may be necessary. ■ Does not potentiate analgesic effects of narcotics. ■ May produce apnea with neuromuscular blocking antibiotics (e.g., gentamicin). ■ Contraindicated with quinidine, epinephrine, and thiazide diuretics. ■ Use caution during anesthesia with barbiturates (e.g., methohexital, thiopental), may increase frequency and severity of hypotension and neuromuscular excitation. ■ Capable of innumerable other interactions.

SIDE EFFECTS

Average dose: Blurring of vision, dizziness, dryness of mouth, hyperexcitability, hypersensitivity reactions, hypertension (rare), hypotension (mild), nightmares, spastic movements of upper extremities.

Overdose: Anaphylaxis, cardiac arrest, coma, convulsions, deep sedation, respiratory depression. All side effects of phenothiazines are possible, but rarely occur. See prochlorperazine (Compazine).

ANTIDOTE

Discontinue the drug at onset of any side effect and notify the physician. Counteract hypotension with norepinephrine (Levophed) or phenylephrine (Neo-synephrine) and IV fluids; extrapyramidal symptoms with benztropine mesylate (Cogentin) or diphenhydramine (Benadryl). Epinephrine is contraindicated for hypotension. Further hypotension will occur. Use diazepam (Valium) or phenobarbital for convulsions or hyperactivity. Phenytoin may be helpful in ventricular arrhythmias. In treating respiratory depression and unconsciousness, avoid analeptics such as doxapram (Dopram); they may cause convulsions. Resuscitate as necessary.

PROPOFOL INJECTION

General anesthetic
Anesthesia adjunct
Sedative-hypnotic

Diprivan   pH 7.0 to 8.5

USUAL DOSE

Induction of anesthesia: Must be individualized and titrated to desired response.

Healthy adults less than 55 years of age: 40 mg every 10 seconds until induction onset (approximately 2 to 2.5 mg/kg).

Adults over 55 years of age, debilitated or ASA III, or IV risk patients: 20 mg every 10 seconds until induction onset (approximately 1 to 1.5 mg/kg).

Neurosurgical patients: 20 mg every 10 seconds until induction onset (approximately 1 to 2 mg/kg). Infusion of slow injection (20 mg over 10 sec) is used to avoid significant hypotension and decrease in cerebral perfusion pressure.

Maintenance of anesthesia: Must be titrated to desired clinical effect.

Adults less than 55 years of age: Immediately follow induction with an infusion of 100 to 200 mcg/kg/min (6 to 12 mg/kg/hr) or an intermittent bolus in increments of 25 to 50 mg as needed.

Adults over 55 years of age, debilitated or ASA III, or IV risk patients: Immediately follow induction with an infusion of 50 to 100 mcg/kg/min (3 to 6 mg/kg/hr). Do NOT use a rapid intermittent bolus in these patients.

Neurosurgical patients: Immediately follow induction with an infusion of 100 to 200 mcg/kg/min (6 to 12 mg/kg/hr). Do NOT use a rapid intermittent bolus in these patients.

Initiation of MAC sedation: MAC sedation rates are approximately 25% of those used for anesthesia. Must be individualized.

Healthy adults less than 55 years of age: An infusion of 100 to 150 mcg/kg/min (6 to 9 mg/kg/hr) or a slow injection of 0.5 mg/kg over 3 to 5 minutes. Slow infusion or slow injection techniques are preferable to rapid bolus administration.

Adults over 55 years of age, debilitated or ASA III, or IV risk patients: Most patients require doses similar to healthy adults. Must be given as a slow infusion (preferred) or as a slow injection over 3 to 5 minutes. Do NOT give as a rapid bolus.

Maintenance of MAC sedation:

Healthy adults less than 55 years of age: Maintain with an infusion (preferred) of 25 to 75 mcg/kg/min (1.5 to 4.5 mg/kg/hr) or incremental bolus doses of 10 to 20 mg.

Adults over 55 years of age, debilitated or ASA III, or IV risk patients: Most patients require 20% reduction of the adult dose; an infusion of 20 to 60 mcg/kg/min (1.2 to 3.6 mg/kg/hr). Do not use bolus doses.

Sedation of intubated mechanically ventilated or respiratory controlled ICU patients: Given as a continuous infusion. Begin with an initial dose of 5 mcg/kg/min (0.3 mg/kg/hr) over 5 minutes. Allow at least 5 minutes between adjustments to reach peak drug effect and to avoid hypotension. Increase slowly over 5 to 10 minutes by 5 to 10 mcg/kg/min (0.3 to 0.6 mg/kg/hr) to desired level of sedation. Individualize to patient condition, response, blood lipid profile, and vital signs. Some clinicians recommend reducing dose by approximately ½ for elderly (over 55 years) and debilitated.

Maintenance of sedation in mechanically ventilated or respiratory-controlled ICU patients: 5 to 50 mcg/kg/min as a continuous infusion slowly titrated to desired level of sedation. Temporarily reduce dose once each day to assess neurologic and respiratory function. Average maintenance dose **under 55 years** is 38 mcg/kg/min; **over 55 years,** 20 mcg/kg/min. Average maintenance dose for **post-coronary artery bypass graft (CABG) patients** is usually low (median of 11 mcg/kg/min) because of high intraoperative opiates.

Relief of cholestatic pruritus (investigational): 1 to 1.5 mg/kg/hr as a continuous infusion for 3 days.

PEDIATRIC DOSE

Induction of anesthesia in children 3 years or older: Must be individualized and titrated to disired response. 2.5 to 3.5 mg/kg adminstered over 20 to 30 seconds.

Maintenance of anesthesia in children 3 years or older: Must be titrated to desired clinical effect. Immediatley follow induction with an infusion of 125 to 300 mcg/kg/min (7.5 to 18 mg/kg/hr).

DOSE ADJUSTMENTS

All situations: See Usual dose for specific reduced doses required for adults over 55 years of age, debilitated or ASA III, or IV risk patients.
■ Reduced dose required in presence of other CNS depressants. (See Drug/lab interactions). ■ No dose adjustment required for gender, chronic hepatic cirrhosis, or chronic renal failure.

ICU sedation: Adjust infusion to maintain a light level of sedation through the wake-up assessment or weaning process.

DILUTION

Supplied in ready-to-use vented vials containing 10 mg/ml. Shake well before use. May be further diluted only with D5W. Do not dilute to a concentration less than 2 mg/ml (4 ml diluent to 1 ml propofol yields 2 mg/ml). More stable in glass than in plastic. Strict aseptic technique imperative; emulsion supports rapid growth of microorganisms. Do not use with evidence of emulsion separation. Prepare immediately before each use. Flush IV line at end of every 6 hours in extended procedures to remove residual propofol.

Storage: Protect from light and store below 22° C (72° F) but do not refrigerate. Discard infusion and tubing every 12 hours.

INCOMPATIBLE WITH

Do not coadminister through same IV catheter with blood, plasma, or serum. Do not mix with any other agent prior to administration.

COMPATIBLE WITH

Y-site: D5W, 0.2% or 0.45% NS, LR, or D5/LR.

RATE OF ADMINISTRATION

Use of a syringe pump or volumetric pump recommended to provide controlled infusion rates. See Usual dose for specific rates for specific age and/or indication. Extend rate based on age, debilitation, or calculated risk. Must be individualized and titrated to desired level of sedation and changes in vital signs. Monitor respiratory function continuously. Continuous administration preferable to intermittent to avoid periods of undersedation or oversedation. Too-rapid administration (bolus dosing, too-rapid increase in infusion rate, overdose) can cause severe cardiorespiratory complications, especially in adults over 55 years, debilitated or ASA III, or IV risk patients. In all anesthesia, higher rates are generally required for the first 15 minutes, then appropriate responses can usually be maintained with a decrease of 30% to 50%. Always titrate rates downward until there is a mild response to surgical stimulation. This avoids administration at rates higher than clinically necessary. Control increased response to surgical stimulation or lightening of anesthesia (increased pulse rate, blood pressure, sweating and/or tearing) with bolus injections of 25 to 50 mg (adults under 55 years of age only); slow injection of reduced doses or by increasing the infusion rate (adults under or over 55 years of age). If control not effective within 5 minutes, consider use of an opioid, barbiturate, vasodilator, or inhalation agent.

ACTIONS

A potent emulsified IV sedative hypnotic agent. Action is dose and rate dependent. Can provide conscious (verbal contact maintained) or unconscious sedation, depending on dose. Produces hypnosis rapidly and smoothly with minimal excitation, usually within 40 seconds. Depth of sedation easily and rapidly controlled by adjusting rate of infusion. Rapid onset of action facilitates accurate titration and minimizes oversedation. Due to extensive redistribution from the central nervous system to other tissues and high metabolic clearance, recovery from anesthesia or sedation is rapid. Most patients are awake and responsive to verbal commands and oriented in 8 minutes. Metabolized in the liver and excreted as metabolites in urine. Has minimal impact on cardiac output, but changes may occur because of assisted or controlled ventilation, additional opioids or other CNS depressants, intubation, or surgical stimulation. Crosses placental barrier. Secreted in breast milk.

INDICATIONS AND USES

Induce and/or maintain anesthesia as part of a balanced anesthetic technique for inpatient and outpatient surgery. ■ Initiate and maintain monitored anesthesia care (MAC) during diagnostic procedures (e.g., colonoscopy, dental procedures) and in conjunction with local/regional anesthesia during surgical procedures. ■ Continuous sedation and control of stress responses in intubated or respiratory controlled ICU patients (e.g., post-CABG, postsurgical, neuro/head trauma, ARDS, COPD, asthma, status epilepticus, tetanus). Continuous infusions of low doses allows controlled recovery of consciousness when required and for assessment.

Investigational uses: Subhypnotic doses used to treat morphine-induced (cholestatic) pruritus. ■ Treatment of status epilepticus refractory to standard anticonvulsant therapy.

CONTRAINDICATIONS

Known hypersensitivity to propofol or its components (e.g., soybean oil, glycerol, egg lecithin, sodium hydroxide) or any time general anesthesia or sedation is contraindicated.

PRECAUTIONS

All situations: For IV use only. Administered by or under the direct observation of the anesthesiologist. Must have responsibility only for anesthesia during surgery and/or procedures. ■ Staff must be skilled in medical management of critically ill patients, cardiovascular resuscitation, and airway management. ■ Use caution in patients with compromised myocardial function, intravascular volume depletion, or abnormally low vascular tone (e.g., sepsis); may be more susceptible to hypotension. ■ An emulsion; use caution in patients with lipid metabolism disorders (e.g., diabetic hyperlipidemia, pancreatitis, and primary hyperlipoproteinemia). ■ May cause convulsions during recovery phase in patients with epilepsy. ■ Use caution in patients with increased intracranial pressure or impaired cerebral circulation. Decrease in mean arterial pressure may cause decreases in cerebral perfusion. ■ Has no analgesic properties. Provide pain relief or local anesthetic as indicated. Has been used successfully with midazolam (Versed), 1 to 3 mg, for initial induction. Midazolam provides better amnesia and causes less pain on injection, whereas propofol sustains sedation and allows more rapid recovery.

ICU sedation: Monitor tryglcerides with long-term use (ICU sedation). Adjust if fat inadequately cleared from body and reduce other lipid administration.

Monitor: All situations: Correct fluid volume deficiencies before administration. ■ Will cause transient local pain during IV injection; minimize by using larger veins and lidocaine previous to injection. Use with midazolam reduces awareness of this pain. ■ Apnea may occur during induction and last for more than 60 seconds. Intubation equipment, controlled ventilation equipment, oxygen, and facilities for resuscitation and life support must be available. Maintain a patent airway and ascertain adequate ventilation at all times. ■ All vital signs must be monitored continuously. Use of a respiratory monitor required. ■ Hypotension common during first 60 minutes, monitor closely. Significant hypotension or cardiovascular depression can be profound. ■ To prevent profound bradycardia, anticholinergic agents (e.g., atropine, glycopyrrolate [Robinul]) may be required to modify increases in vagal tone due to concomitant agents (e.g., succinylcholine [Anectine]) or surgical stimulation. ▪ Bed rest required for a minimum of 3 hours after IV injection or satisfy specific hospital rules for discharge. ▪ Note Drug/lab interactions.

ICU sedation: Observe for signs and symptoms of pain, may indicate need for opioids for analgesia not an increase in propofol dose. ▪ Benzodiazepines (e.g., diazepam [Valium]) and/or neuromuscular blocking agents (e.g., mivacurium [Mivacron], succinylcholine [Anestine]) may also be used. ▪ Dose may be reduced carefully to allow patient to awaken to a lighter level of sedation allowing neurologic and respiratory assessment daily. Avoid rapid awakening; will cause anxiety, agitation, and resistance to mechanical ventilation. ▪ Discontinue opioids and paralytic agents and optimize respiratory function prior to weaning from mechanical ventilation. ▪ Maintain light sedation until 15 minutes before extubation.

Patient education: Avoid alcohol or other CNS depressants (e.g., antihistamines, benzodiazepines) for 24 hours following anesthesia. ▪ Do not perform tasks requiring mental alertness (e.g., driving, operating hazardous machinery, or sign legal documents) until the day after surgery or longer. All effects must have subsided.

Maternal/child: Category B: use during pregnancy only if clearly needed. ▪ Not recommended for use in obstetric procedures, including cesarean section; no assurance of safety for fetus. ▪ Not recommended for use during lactation. ▪ Has been approved for pediatric anesthesia. Not recommended for use in children under 3 years of age. Serious adverse effects, including fatalities occurred during ICU sedation in children with respiratory infections and/or with doses in excess of recommendations for adults.

Elderly: Dose requirements decrease after age 55 due to reduced clearance and higher blood levels. Minimize undesirable cardiorespiratory depression (hypotension, apnea, airway obstruction, and/or oxygen desaturation) by using reduced doses and rates of administration. Note Usual dose and Dose adjustments.

DRUG/LAB INTERACTIONS

Potentiated by inhalational anesthetics (e.g., enflurane, halothane, isoflurane, nitrous oxide), narcotics (e.g., morphine, meperidine [Demerol], fentanyl [Sublimaze]), sedatives (e.g., barbiturates, benzodiazepines [e.g., diazepam (Valium), midazolam (Versed)], chloral hydrate, droperidol [Inapsine]). Anesthetic and sedative effects increased; systolic, diastolic, mean arterial pressure, and cardiac output are decreased. Reduce dose of propofol to maintain desired level of anesthesia or sedation. ▪ No significant adverse interactions noted to date with neuromuscular blocking agents (e.g., succinylcholine [Anectine], pipecuronium [Arduan], tubocurarine [Curare]). ▪ Neuroexcitatory effects of propofol may cause seizures in patients receiving chlordiazepoxide (Librium) or antidepressants (e.g., fluoxetine [Prozac], maprotilene [Ludiomil]).

SIDE EFFECTS

More likely to occur during loading boluses, with supplemental boluses or higher rate of administration. Apnea; bradycardia (profound); cough; dyspnea; headache; hypotension; hypoventilation; injection site burning, pain, stinging; nausea, and upper airway obstruction are most common. Urine may be green. Abdominal cramping, anaphylaxis (including bronchospasm, erythema, and hypotension), bucking/jerking/thrashing, clonic/myclonic movement (rarely including convulsions and opisthotonus), dizziness, fever, flushing, hiccough, hypertension, tingling/numbness/coldness at injection site, twitching, and vomiting may occur.

Overdose: Cardiorespiratory depression (hypotension, apnea, airway obstruction, and/or oxygen desaturation).

ANTIDOTE

Keep physician informed of all side effects. Reduction of dose may be required or will be treated symptomatically. Discontinue the drug for major side effects, paradoxical reactions, or accidental overdose. A short-acting drug, a patent airway, and continuous controlled ventilation with oxygen until normal function assured should be adequate. Treat bradycardia and/or hypotension with increased rate of IV fluids, Trendelenburg position, vasopressors (e.g., dopamine [Intropin]). Anticholinergic agents (e.g., atropine or glycopyrrolate [Robinul]) may be required. Treat allergic reaction and resuscitate as necessary.

PROPRANOLOL HYDROCHLORIDE

Beta-adrenergic blocking agent
Antiarrhythmic

Inderal   pH 2.8 to 3.5

USUAL DOSE

0.5 to 3 mg given 1 mg at a time. If there is no change in rhythm for at least 2 minutes after the initial dose, cycle may be repeated one time. (JAMA recommends 0.1 mg/kg divided into 3 equal doses and given at 2 to 3 minute intervals.) *No further propranolol may be given by any route for at least 4 hours.* Best results achieved if administered within 2 to 4 hours of symptom onset or thrombolytic therapy.

PEDIATRIC DOSE (UNLABELED)

0.01 to 0.1 mg/kg. Maximum dose is 1 mg. Repeat at 6- to 8-hour intervals if needed.

Tetralogy spells: 0.15 to 0.25 mg/kg/dose may be given slowly. May repeat once in 15 minutes.

DOSE ADJUSTMENTS

Note Drug/lab interactions. ■ Reduce dose gradually to avoid rebound angina, myocardial infarction, or ventricular arrhythmias. ■ Note Drug/lab interactions.

DILUTION

Each 1 mg can be diluted in 10 ml of D5W or may be given undiluted. May be diluted in 50 ml of NS for infusion.

INCOMPATIBLE WITH

Any other drug in a syringe or solution because of toxicity. Note Precautions and Contraindications. *Y-site:* Diazoxide (Hyperstat IV). *Compatible at Y-site* with alteplase (tPA).

RATE OF ADMINISTRATION

Each 1 mg or fraction thereof must be given over 1 minute to avoid excessive hypotension and/or cardiac standstill. Give a single dose as an infusion over 10 to 15 minutes. Allow adequate time for distribution. Observe monitor and discontinue propranolol as soon as rhythm change occurs. Extend rate of administration in pediatric patients.

ACTIONS

Propranolol is a beta-adrenergic blocker with antiarrhythmic effects. Cardiac response to sympathetic nerve stimulation is inhibited, slowing the heart rate (especially ventricular rate) by inhibiting atrioventricular conduction, decreasing the force of cardiac contractility, and decreasing arterial pressure and cardiac output. Well distributed throughout the body, the onset of action occurs within 1 to 2 minutes and lasts about 4 hours. Metabolized in the liver. Some excreted in the urine.

INDICATIONS AND USES

Management of cardiac arrhythmias such as paroxysmal atrial tachycardia, sinus tachycardia, atrial or ventricular extrasystoles, and atrial flutter and fibrillation; and tachyarrhythmia caused by digitalis intoxication, anesthesia (other than chloroform and ether, etc.), thyrotoxicosis, and catecholamines (epinephrine, norepinephrine). Reserve IV use for life-threatening situations. ▪ Ventricular tachycardia and arrhythmias caused by tumor manipulation during excision of pheochromocytoma after treatment with an alpha-adrenergic blocking agent. ▪ Reduce cardiac mortality, recurrent MI, and incidence of ventricular fibrillation in hemodynamically stable individuals with suspected or definite myocardial infarction. ▪ Reduce blood pressure in systolic hypertension caused by hyperdynamic beta-adrenergic circulatory state that occurs in younger persons.

CONTRAINDICATIONS

Allergic rhinitis, bronchial asthma, bronchospasm, cardiogenic shock, complete heart block, congestive heart failure (unless caused by tachycardia), chronic obstructive pulmonary disease, hypersensitivity to beta-adrenergic blocking agents, right ventricular failure caused by pulmonary hypertension, second-degree heart block, sinus bradycardia.

PRECAUTIONS

Oral administration is preferred. Use IV administration only when necessary. ▪ Not considered the drug of choice for arrhythmias in myocardial infarction. ▪ Used concurrently with digitalis or alpha-adrenergic blockers as indicated. ▪ Use with extreme caution in asthmatics, patients with lung disease or bronchospasm, diabetics, or patients with a history of hypoglycemia. May cause hypoglycemia and mask the symptoms. ▪ Discontinuation of beta-blockers prior to OR is controversial (beta blockade interferes with cardiac response to reflex stimuli); however, some authorities recommend administering throughout the perioperative period. May cause arrhythmia, angina, MI, or death if stopped abruptly. ▪ IV dose used during surgery to replace an oral dose should be $\frac{1}{10}$ of the oral dose. ▪ May cause severe bradycardia in patients with Wolff-Parkinson-White syndrome.

Monitor: Continuous ECG and blood pressure monitoring is mandatory during administration of IV propranolol. Monitoring of pulmonary wedge pressure or central venous pressure is recommended. Discontinue the drug when a rhythm change is noted and wait to note full effect before giving additional medication if indicated. ■ Note Precautions and Drug/lab interactions.

Patient education: Report any breathing difficulty promptly.

Maternal/child: Pregnancy Category C: safety for use in pregnancy and lactation and in children not established. Use only when clearly indicated.

Elderly: Use with caution in age-related peripheral vascular disease; risk of hypothermia increased. ■ May exacerbate mental impairment.

DRUG/LAB INTERACTIONS

Effects of both drugs may be reduced with xanthines (e.g., aminophylline) or theophylline levels may increase; monitor carefully. ■ Cimetidine (Tagamet), haloperidol (Haldol), propafenone (Rythmol), and quinolone antibiotics (e.g., ciprofloxacin [Cipro IV]) inhibit propranolol metabolism; reduced dose may be required. Hypotension and bradycardia may be life-threatening with haloperidol. ■ Potentiates benzodiazepines (e.g., diazepam [Valium]) by inhibiting their metabolism; consider use of atenolol (Tenormin). ■ Potentiates ergot alkaloids (e.g., dihydroergotamine [D.H.E. 45]); monitor for peripheral ischemia; reduce ergot dose or discontinue beta-blocker. ■ May be synergistic, additive, or toxic with other cardiac agents (e.g., calcium channel blockers [e.g., verapamil (Isoptin), diltiazem (Cardizem)], digitalis, lidocaine, phenytoin [Dilantin], procainamide [Pronestyl], quinidine). Arrhythmias and/or severe depression of the myocardium and AV conduction can result. Monitor cardiac function; decrease dose of both drugs as indicated. ■ Added hypotensive effect with disopyramide (Persantine), diuretics (e.g., furosemide), other antihypertensive agents (e.g., enalaprilat, nitroglycerin), some phenothiazines (e.g., chlorpromazine [Thorazine]), and reserpine. Reduced dose of one or both drugs may be indicated or consider use of atenolol. ■ Will cause severe bradycardia with MAO inhibitors (e.g., selegiline [Eldepryl]). ■ Use with clonidine may precipitate acute hypertension or aggravate rebound hypertension if clonidine stopped abruptly; discontinue propranolol several days before gradual withdrawal of clonidine. ■ Antihypertensive effects inhibited by NSAIDs (e.g., ibuprofen [Motrin], indomethacin [Indocin]); avoid combination. ■ Effects antagonized by atropine (counteract bradycardia) and somewhat by tricyclic antidepressants (e.g., amitryptyline [Elavil]) or nefazodone (Serzone). ■ Large doses of isoproterenol (Isuprel) may be required to overcome effects of propranolol; use extreme caution, glucagon safer. ■ Use extreme caution with sympathomimetics (e.g., epinephrine), alpha receptor stimulation may be unopposed. Severe hypertension, bradycardia, and heart block can result from concurrent use (will require use of chlorpromazine, hydralazine, aminophylline, and/or atropine to treat). May be indicated in overdose of propranolol. ■ May increase postural hypotension with prazosin (Minipress). ■ May prolong or counteract effects of nondepolarizing muscle relaxants (e.g., pancuronium (Pavulon). ■ May increase anticoagulant effects of warfarin. ■ May mask symptoms of hypoglycemia with insulin and sulfonylureas and result in prolonged hypoglycemia. ■ Reduce dose of propranolol when patients on thioamines (e.g., propylthiouracil [PTU], methimazole [Tapazole]) become euthyroid. ■ Some authorities recommend that beta-adrenergic blockers be discontinued 48 hours before major surgery (beta blockade interferes with cardiac response to reflex stimuli). If continued, use caution administering general anesthetics that depress the myocardium (e.g., cyclopropane, trichlorethylene). ■ BUN may be elevated in patients with imparied renal function. ■ May increase triglycerides. ■ Can interfere with numerous diagnostic and physiologic tests. Consult literature. ■ Metabolism and release of catecholamines increased in smokers; increased doses may be required. May also interfere with therapeutic effects in treatment of angina.

SIDE EFFECTS

AV conduction delays, bradyarrhythmias, bronchospasm, cardiac failure, cardiac standstill, erythematous rash, hallucination, hypotension, laryngospasm, paresthesia of the hands, respiratory distress, syncopal attacks, vertigo, visual disturbances.

ANTIDOTE

For any side effect, discontinue the drug and notify the physician immediately. Effects can be reversed by dopamine, isoproterenol, or levarterenol, but protracted severe hypotension may result. Unresponsive hypotension and bradycardia may be reversed by glucagon 5 to 10 mg over 30 seconds followed by a continuous infusion of 5 mg/hr (see glucagon monograph). Use atropine for bradycardia, digitalis and diuretics for cardiac failure, epinephrine for hypotension, aminophylline and isoproterenol (with extreme care) for bronchospasm, and glucagon for hypoglycemia. Treat other side effects symptomatically and resuscitate as necessary.

PROTAMINE SULFATE
Antidote
(Heparin antagonist)

pH 6.0 to 7.0

USUAL DOSE

1 mg for approximately every 100 USP units of heparin. May be repeated if needed in 10 to 15 minutes. Never exceed 50 mg in any 10-minute period or 100 mg in 2 hours. Dose adjusted as indicated by coagulation studies. Any dose over 100 mg in 2 hours should be justified by coagulation studies (has its own anticoagulant effect). The dose of protamine required decreases rapidly with the time elapsed after heparin injection. (30 minutes after IV heparin, 0.5 mg of protamine will neutralize 100 USP units of heparin).

DOSE ADJUSTMENTS

Because heparin disappears rapidly from the system, reduce dose of protamine based on length of time elapsed since heparin dose (up to one-half if 30 minutes has elapsed). ■ Prompt administration of protamine sulfate may also decrease dose requirements.

DILUTION

Most preparations are prediluted and ready for use. Each 50 mg of powder is diluted with 5 ml sterile water or bacteriostatic water for injection. Shake vigorously. May be further diluted with at least an equal volume of NS or D5W. May be given as an infusion by diluting in a given amount of the same infusion solutions.

Storage: Refrigerate before dilution. Use immediately after dilution. Discard remaining medication. Some literature states, "Stable for 72 hr diluted with bacteriostatic water if refrigerated."

INCOMPATIBLE WITH

Cephalosporins, diatrizoate meglumine 52%; diatrizoate sodium 8% and 60%, ioxaglate meglumine 39.3%, ioxaglate sodium 19.6%, penicillins. Should be considered incompatible in syringe or solution with any other drug because of individualized rate adjustment necessary to produce desired effects.

RATE OF ADMINISTRATION

50 mg (5 ml) or fraction thereof over 10 minutes. Do not exceed 50 mg in 10 minutes. As an infusion, may be given over 2 to 3 hours with dosage titrated according to coagulation studies. Use infusion pump or microdrip (60 gtt/ml) to administer. Too-rapid administration can cause anaphylaxis, bradycardia, dyspnea, flushing, sensation of warmth, or severe hypotension. Hypertension has also occurred.

ACTIONS

An anticoagulant if administered alone. In the presence of heparin, protamine forms a stable salt, neutralizing the anticoagulant effect of both drugs. Each 1 mg of protamine can neutralize approximately 100 USP units of heparin. Onset of action is within 0.5 to 1 minute. Duration of action is about 2 hours.

INDICATIONS AND USES

To neutralize the anticoagulant activity of heparin in severe heparin overdosage. ■ Neutralization of heparin administered during extracorporeal circulation in arterial and cardiac surgery or dialysis procedures.

CONTRAINDICATIONS

None when used as indicated.

PRECAUTIONS

Potential for hypersensitivity increased in patients with allergies to fish, previous exposure to protamine (e.g., protamine insulin), and in infertile or vasectomized men (may have antiprotamine antibodies). ■ Pulmonary edema and/or circulatory collapse may occur in patients undergoing cardiac bypass surgery; etiology unknown.

Monitor: Facilities to treat shock must be available. ■ After cardiac surgery, even with adequate neutralization, further bleeding may occur any time within 24 hours (heparin "rebound"). Observe the patient continuously. Additional protamine sulfate may be indicated.

Maternal/child: Pregnancy Category C: safety for use in pregnancy, lactation, or children not established.

SIDE EFFECTS

Occur more frequently with too-rapid injection; anaphylaxis, back pain, bradycardia, dyspnea, feeling of warmth, flushing, lethargy, nausea, severe hypertension or hypotension, vomiting. Acute pulmonary hypertension, capillary leak and noncardiogenic pulmonary edema, circulatory collapse, or pulmonary edema may occur.

ANTIDOTE

Discontinue the drug and notify the physician, who may recommend a decrease in rate of administration or, if side effects are severe, symptomatic treatment such as administration of whole blood, vasopressors (e.g., dopamine [Intropin]) for hypotension, atropine for bradycardia, and oxygen for dyspnea. Resuscitate as necessary.

PROTEIN (AMINO ACID) PRODUCTS   Nutritional therapy

Aminess 5.2%; Aminosyn 3.5%, 3.5% M, 5%, 7%, 10%; Aminosyn 7% and 8.5% with electrolytes; Aminosyn (pH 6) 10%; Aminosyn HBC 7%; Aminosyn II 3.5%, 3.5% M, 5%, 7%, 8.5%, and 10%; Aminosyn II 7%, 8.5%, and 10% with electrolytes; Aminosyn II 3.5% in 5% or 25% dextrose; Aminosyn II 5% in 25% dextrose; Aminosyn II 4.25% in 10%, 20%, and 25% dextrose; Aminosyn PF 7% and 10%; Aminosyn RF 5.2%; 4% Branch Amin; Clinimix 2.75% in 5% dextrose; Clinimix 4.25% in 5%, 10%, 20%, and 25% dextrose; Clinimix 5% in 15%, 20%, and 25% dextrose; Clinimix E 2.75% in 5% and 10% dextrose with electrolytes and calcium; Clinimix E 4.25% in 5%, 10%, and 25% dextrose with electrolytes and calcium; Clinimix E 5% in 15%, 20%, and 25% dextrose with electrolytes and calcium; crystalline amino acid infusions; FreAmine HBC 6.9%; FreAmine III 8.5%, 10%, and 3% and 8.5% with electrolytes; HepaAmine; hyperalimentation; Nephramine 5.4%; Novamine; Novamine 15%; ProcalAmine; protein hydrolysates; RenAmin; total parenteral nutrition; Travasol 2.75% in 5%, 10%, and 25% dextrose; Travasol 4.25% in 5%, 10%, and 25% dextrose; Travasol 5.5%, 8.5%, and 10% without electrolytes; Travasol 3.5% M, 5.5% and 8.5% with electrolytes; TrophAmine 6% and 10%   pH 5.0 to 7.0

USUAL DOSE

0.5 to 2 gm/kg of body weight/24 hrs. Actual dose will depend on several factors including protein requirements, disease state, physical condition, and weight. Protein amino acid products are available in general, renal failure, hepatic failure/encephalopathy, and metabolic stress formulations. Note Precautions/Monitor.

PEDIATRIC INFANT DOSE

1.5 to 3 gm/kg of body weight/24 hrs. Actual dose will depend on several factors including age, protein requirements, disease state, physical condition, and weight. Infants and children require different percentages of all components. Another source suggests an average TPN maintenance dose of 2.5 Gm amino acids/kg/day. Dextrose kcal (nutritional calories) must be added (range is from 100 to 300 kcal/kg/day). Another source recommends specific total non-protein calories by weight; less than 10 kg, 100 cal/kg; 10 to 20 kg, 1,000 calories plus 50 cal/kg for each kg over 10; greater than 20 kg, 1,500 calories plus 20 cal/kg for each kg over 20. Total may include IV fat calories.

DILUTION

Dilute under strict aseptic techniques according to manufacturer's specific instructions. Most commonly mixed with dextrose (nonprotein calorie source), electrolytes, vitamins, and trace elements to provide total parenteral nutrition (TPN) or peripheral parenteral nutrition (PPN). Intravenous lipids, providing a second nonprotein calorie source and a source of essential fatty acids, may be mixed with the dextrose/amino acid solution or run simultaneously. Use promptly after mixing; laminar flow hood preferred; refrigerate briefly if necessary, and discard any unused portion. Use only clear solutions, observe against adequate light for particulate matter or evidence of container damage.

Storage: Manufacturer recommends refrigeration after any additives (e.g., IV lipids, electrolytes, minerals) are added. When prepared for home use, has been refrigerated for up to 14 days (dextrose and amino acids) or up to 7 days with lipids added. Leave vitamins (e.g., MVI) out until time of adminstration.

INCOMPATIBLE WITH

Amicacin (Amikin), amobarbital (Amytal), amphotericin B (Fungizone), ampicillin (Polycill-N), cefoperazone (Cefobid), cephalothin (Keflin), cephradine (Velosef), chlorothiazide (Diuril), ganciclovir (Cytovene), gentamicin (Garamycin), imipenem-cilastatin (Primaxin), indomethacin (Indocin), methyldopa (Aldomet), iron dextran (Imferon), IV fat emulsion 10%, kanamycin (Kantrex), metronidazole (Flagyl IV), mezlocillin (Mezlin), midazolam (Versed), multivitamins (M.V.I. -12), penicillins, piperacillin (Pipracil), ranitidine (Zantac), sodium bicarbonate, thiopental (Pentothal), many other drugs, and whole blood. Most incompatibilities relate to the preparation (chloride as opposed to phosphate), amount of medication added, other additives present, and thoroughness of mixing. Consult with the pharmacist before mixing any drugs in protein (amino acid) products. Many TPN solutions contain some phosphate. The addition of calcium salts may cause a precipitate. These additives must be mixed by the pharmacist. Specific amounts, calculations, temperature (precipitate forms more readily at room temperature), and order of dilution are required. Manufacturers suggest that only required nutritional products should be added, but H_2 receptors (e.g., cimetidine, ranitidine), insulin, and heparin are frequently added. Many other drugs are compatible for at least 12 hours.

RATE OF ADMINISTRATION

Begin parenteral nutrition at 1 to 2 ml/min and increase gradually as tolerated until the target rate is reached. With the correct parenteral nutrition formulation; fluid, protein, and calorie requirements should be met at the target rate. *Total daily dose should be evenly distributed over the 24-hour period. Maintain a constant drip rate.* Use of infusion pump and microfilter (0.22 micron for dextrose and amino acids, 1.2 micron for solutions with lipids [3 in 1]) recommended. Precipitate very difficult to detect in solutions that contain lipids. There are specific situations (e.g., cyclic TPN primarily used in home care patients) where a daily dose is given over less than 24 hours. Range is from 10 to 14 hours. Usually administered overnight allowing individuals requiring prolonged TPN to maintain their daytime activities.

Pediatric rate: Usually begin with a one half strength nutritional solution at 60 to 70 ml/kg/day. May be gradually increased over 48 hours until full strength and increased to 125 to 150 ml/kg/day. Note all comments under adult Rate of administration.

ACTIONS

Supplies essential and nonessential amino acids and calories with the intent of promoting protein production (anabolism) and preventing protein breakdown (catabolism), promotes wound healing, and acts as a buffer in intracellular and extracellular body fluids. Various brands supply additional calories with alcohol, fructose, or glucose. These additional calories permit available protein to be used for repair of tissue in addition to meeting basic caloric needs.

INDICATIONS AND USES

To prevent nitrogen loss or to reverse negative nitrogen balance in severe illness when oral alimentation is not practical for prolonged periods or normal GI absorption is impaired.

CONTRAINDICATIONS

Hypersensitivity to any component, acidosis, anuria, azotemia, decreased circulating blood volume, severe liver disease, metabolic disorders with impaired amino acid metabolization.

PRECAUTIONS

Catheter insertion for administration of central parenteral nutrition is a sterile surgical procedure (must be a large vein [subclavian or superior vena cava preferred]; 50% glucose is a sclerosing solution). ■ Peripheral veins are suitable for specific products (peripheral parenteral nutrition), when amino acid products are diluted with 2.5%, 5%, or 10% dextrose. ■ Amino acids given without carbohydrates may cause ketone accumulation. ■ Use caution in impaired hepatic function; may cause serum amino acid imbalances, metabolic alkalosis, prerenal azotemia, hyperammonemia, stupor, and coma. ■ Use caution in impaired renal function; may further increase BUN. ■ Fatty infiltration of the liver, acute respiratory failure, and difficulty in weaning hypermetabolic patients from the respirator may be caused by excessive carbohydrate calories.

Monitor: Specific base line studies are required before administration: CBC, platelet count, prothrombin time, BUN, serum creatinine, electrolytes, glucose, triglycerides, cholesterol, albumin, bilirubin, liver function tests (e.g., AST, ALT, LDH), weight, body length and head circumference (in infants), and immunocompetence. Repeat lab tests as indicated during therapy. ■ Monitor intake and output, weight, and during stabilization (3 to 5 days), measure urine glucose, and ketones every shift. After stabilization, measurement of urine glucose and ketones every 8 hours is suggested. ■ Follow a strict, regular aseptic routine to care for insertion site. ■ Single-port central venous catheters to be used only for the nutritional regime. Do not draw blood samples, transfuse blood, or administer other medications. Pseudoagglutination and thrombosis can occur, risk of contamination is great, and validity of results is compromised. Multiple-port central venous catheters may be used for these additional procedures. Observe specific protocols. ■ Monitor BUN frequently. Discontinue infusion if BUN exceeds normal postprandial limits and continues to rise. ■ Blood ammonia levels important especially in infants. ■ Check frequently for any signs of extravasation. ■ Observe for any signs of infection. ■ Additional insulin coverage may be required, especially when dosage is increased too rapidly or with maximum doses. ■ To prevent rebound hypoglycemia, decrease rate gradually over at least 24 hours to discontinue administration. Follow with use of fluids containing 5% to 10% dextrose for several days. ■ Discard any single bottle after 24 hours. Replace administration set every 24 to 48 hours.

Maternal/child: Use hypertonic dextrose (component of parenteral nutrition) with extreme caution in low-birth-weight or septic infants. May cause severe hyperglycemia. ■ Hyperammonemia is of particular significance in infants. Can cause mental retardation; measure blood ammonia frequently.

DRUG/LAB INTERACTIONS
Tetracycline may reduce protein-sparing effects.

SIDE EFFECTS
Abdominal pains, anaphylaxis, bone demineralization, changes in levels of consciousness, convulsions, dehydration, edema at the site of injection, electrolyte imbalances, glycosuria, hyperammonemia, hyperglycemia, hyperpyrexia, hypertension, metabolic acidosis and/or alkalosis, osmotic dehydration, phlebitis and thrombosis, pulmonary edema, rebound hypoglycemia, septicemia, vasodilation, vomiting, weakness.

ANTIDOTE
Notify the physician of all side effects. An alternate brand may cause fewer problems, or amounts of glucose or additives may be adjusted to correct the problem. Many of the side effects listed will respond to a reduced rate. Some will require catheter insertion at a new site. Treat symptomatically and resuscitate as necessary. Stop infusion immediately for any signs of acute respiratory distress. May represent pulmonary embolus or intestitial pneumonitis, which may be caused by a precipitate of electrolytes (e.g., calcium and phosphates) in the solution.

PROTIRELIN
Thypinone, Thyrel-TRH

Diagnostic agent

pH 6.5

USUAL DOSE
200 to 500 mcg. 500 mcg is optimum dose. Specific procedure required (see Precautions).

PEDIATRIC DOSE
Ages 6 to 16 years: 7 mcg/kg of body weight up to 500 mcg. Experience is limited in infants and children under 6 years of age, but the same dose has been used.

DILUTION
May be given undiluted.

Storage: Store below 40° C.

INCOMPATIBLE WITH
Specific information not available. Consider specific use.

RATE OF ADMINISTRATION
A single dose over 15 to 30 seconds.

ACTIONS
This synthetic hormone is similar to natural thyrotropin-releasing hormone produced by the hypothalamus. It increases release of

thyroid-stimulating hormone (TSH) from the anterior pituitary. TSH levels peak in 20 to 30 minutes and return to baseline in about 3 hours. Protirelin half-life is about 5 minutes. Eliminated renally.

INDICATIONS AND USES
An adjunct in: diagnostic assessment of thyroid function. ▪ Diagnostic procedures in pituitary or hypothalamic dysfunction. ▪ Evaluation of the effectiveness of thyrotropin suppression with T_4 in patients with nodular or diffuse goiter. ▪ Primary hypothyroidism to facilitate adjustment of thyroid hormone dosage.

CONTRAINDICATIONS
Known hypersensitivity to protirelin or its components.

PRECAUTIONS
▪ Assay methods and thus results vary with each laboratory performing this test. Test should be interpreted by a physician familiar with hypothalmic-pituitary-thyroid physiology. ▪ Discontinue liothyronine (T_3) 7 days before test and medications containing levothyroxine (T_4) 14 days before test except when testing effectiveness of thyroid suppression with T_4 or for adjustment of thyroid dose. ▪ Adrenocortical drugs used in maintenance therapy of hypopituitarism may be continued. Only large doses will reduce the TSH response. ▪ TSH response is reduced by repeated administration of protirelin. If repeat testing is necessary, wait at least 7 days. ▪ Will not differentiate primary hypothyroidism from normal. Do not administer to patients in whom marked, rapid changes in blood pressure would be dangerous unless potential benefit outweighs potential risk.

Monitor: Patient should remain supine throughout the test. Moderate transient hypertension is frequent; monitor BP before protirelin administration and frequently thereafter until it returns to pretreatment baseline. ▪ Draw one blood sample for TSH assay just before injection, and another 30 minutes after injection. ▪ Note Drug/lab interactions.

Maternal/child: Category C. Safety for use during pregnancy not established.

DRUG/LAB INTERACTIONS
Response may be inhibited by aspirin and levodopa. ▪ Elevated serum lipids may interfere with TSH assay. Fasting for 6 hours or eating a low fat meal prior to the test is recommended (except in patients with hypopituitarism).

SIDE EFFECTS
Occur frequently; are usually minor and subside quickly. Abdominal discomfort, bad taste, breast enlargement and leakage in lactating women, dry mouth, flushed sensation, headache, hypertension, hypotension, lightheadedness, nausea, urge to urinate. Anxiety, convulsions in patients with epilepsy or brain damage, drowsiness, pressure in the chest, sweating, tightness in the throat, tingling sensation, and transient amaurosis in patients with pituitary tumors may occur.

ANTIDOTE
Notify physician and manage side effects as indicated by severity. Treat allergic reactions and resuscitate as necessary.

PYRIDOSTIGMINE BROMIDE

Cholinergic
(Cholinesterase inhibitor)
Antidote
Antimyasthenic

Mestinon, Regonol   pH 5.0

USUAL DOSE

Myasthenia gravis: One-thirtieth of the oral dose or about 2 mg. Highly individualized. Observe for cholinergic crisis.

Muscle relaxant antagonist: 0.1 to 0.25 mg/kg of body weight (usually 10 to 20 mg) as a single dose. Give atropine first (See Precautions) and maintain ventilation.

PEDIATRIC DOSE

Myasthenia gravis or muscle relaxant antagonist: 0.05 to 0.15 mg/kg/dose every 4 to 6 hr. Maximum single dose 10 mg. Note instructions in adult doses.

DILUTION

May be given undiluted. Do not add to IV solutions. May be given through Y-tube or three-way stopcock of infusion set.

INCOMPATIBLE WITH

Unstable in alkaline solutions. Because of potential toxicity, pyridostigmine should not be mixed with any other drug.

RATE OF ADMINISTRATION

Myasthenia gravis: 0.5 mg or fraction thereof over 1 minute.

Muscle relaxant antagonist: 5 mg or fraction thereof over 1 minute.

ACTIONS

An anticholinesterase muscle stimulant and antagonist of skeletal muscle relaxants. Inhibits the enzyme cholinesterase, allowing acetylcholine to accumulate at the myoneural junction. Restores normal transmission of nerve impulses and makes muscle contraction stronger and more prolonged. Has fewer side effects and longer duration of action than neostigmine (Prostigmin).

INDICATIONS AND USES

Treatment of myasthenia gravis during physically stressful situations when oral dosing is not practical (labor, postpartum, surgery). ■ Antagonist to nondepolarizing muscle relaxants (e.g., gallamine [Flaxedil], tubocurarine [curare]).

CONTRAINDICATIONS

Known sensitivity to anticholinesterase agents or bromides, mechanical intestinal or urinary obstruction, urinary tract infections, patients taking mecamylamine.

PRECAUTIONS

A physician should be present when this drug is used. IM route preferred. ■ Edrophonium (Tensilon) can differentiate between increased symptoms of myasthenia and cholinergic crisis. ■ Use caution in bronchial asthma, cardiac arrhythmias, and patients receiving anticholinesterase drugs.

Monitor: Used as a curariform antagonist; administer atropine sulfate, 0.6 to 1.2 mg IV, immediately before pyridostigmine. *Caution:* atropine may mask symptoms of pyridostigmine overdose. Cholinergic crisis may result. ■ Maintain a patent airway and use artificial ventilation as indicated. ■ Epinephrine and atropine should always be available. ■ A peripheral nerve stimulator device can monitor effectiveness.

Maternal/child: Safety for use in pregnancy not established. ■ Discontinue breast feeding. ■ May induce premature labor in pregnancy near term. Transient muscular weakness in swallowing, sucking, and breathing has been observed in neonates of myasthenic mothers. Confirm distinction between cholinergic and myasthenic crisis in neonate with edrophonium test. Treat neonate with IM pyridostigmine 0.05 to 0.15 mg/kg if indicated.

Elderly: Duration of antagonism of neuromuscular blockade prolonged.

DRUG/LAB INTERACTIONS

Potentiates narcotic analgesics (e.g., morphine, meperidine) and succinylcholine (Anectine). ■ Antagonizes anesthetics (ether), ganglionic blocking agents (e.g., trimethaphan [Arfonad]), and aminoglycoside antibiotics (e.g., kanamycin [Kantrex]); neuromuscular block may be accentuated. ■ May be inhibited by corticosteroids and magnesium.

SIDE EFFECTS

Usually caused by overdose: abdominal cramps, anorexia, anxiety, bradycardia, cardiac arrhythmias and arrest, cholinergic crisis, cold moist skin, convulsions, diaphoresis, diarrhea, hypotension, increased bronchial secretions, increased lacrimation, increased salivation, miosis, muscle cramps, muscle weakness, nausea, pulmonary edema, respiratory paralysis with apnea, skin rash (bromide), thrombophlebitis, vomiting.

ANTIDOTE

Atropine sulfate. If side effects occur, discontinue the drug and notify the physician. Atropine sulfate in doses of 0.6 mg IV will counteract most side effects and may be repeated every 3 to 10 minutes. Endotracheal intubation or tracheostomy is considered prophylactic in anesthesia or crisis. Artificial ventilation, oxygen therapy, cardiac monitoring, adequate suctioning, and treatment of shock or convulsions must be instituted and maintained as necessary. Treat allergic reactions with epinephrine. Pralidoxime chloride 1 to 2 Gm IV followed by 250 mg every 5 minutes may be required to reactivate cholinesterase and reverse paralysis.

PYRIDOXINE HYDROCHLORIDE

Nutritional supplement (vitamin)
Antidote

Hexa-Betalin, Vitamin B$_6$ pH 2.0 to 3.8

USUAL DOSE

Pyridoxine dependency syndrome: 30 to 600 mg/day.

Drug-induced pyridoxine deficiency: 50 to 200 mg/day for 3 weeks. Follow with 25 to 100 mg/day as needed.

Prophylaxis or treatment of pyridoxine deficiency in patients receiving parenteral nutrition: May be added to parenteral nutrition; dose will depend on patient condition.

INH poisoning (>10gm): (unlabeled use): 4 gm IV followed by 1 gm IM every 30 minutes. Total pyridoxine dose should equal ingested INH dose.

Cycloserine poisoning (unlabeled use): 300 mg/day. Higher doses may be required.

Hydrazine poisoning (unlabeled use): 25 mg/kg. Give one-third of dose IM and remainder as a 3 hour infusion.

Gyrometra mushroom poisoning (unlabeled use): 25 mg/kg over 15 to 30 minutes. Repeat as needed.

PEDIATRIC DOSE

Pyridoxine-dependent seizures: 10 to 100 mg.

DOSE ADJUSTMENTS

Removed by hemodialysis. Dialysis patients may require higher doses.

DILUTION

May be given by direct IV administration undiluted or added to most IV solutions and given as an infusion.

Storage: Store below 40° C unless otherwise stated by manufacturer. Deteriorates in excessive heat; protect from heat and light.

INCOMPATIBLE WITH

Sufficient information not available; alkaline solutions, iron salts, oxidizing solutions.

RATE OF ADMINISTRATION

50 mg or fraction thereof over 1 minute if given undiluted.

ACTIONS

Vitamin B_6 is water soluble. It is a coenzyme necessary for the metabolism of proteins, carbohydrates, and lipids. Involved in many reactions including the conversion of tryptophan to nicotinamide and serontin, breakdown to glucose-1-phosphate, synthesis of gamma aminobutyric acid (GABA) in the CNS (energy transformation in brain and nerve cells), and synthesis of heme. Metabolized by the liver, and excreted in the urine.

INDICATIONS AND USES

Prophylaxis and treatment of pyridoxine deficiency. Deficiency may be due to inadequate diet, inborn error of metabolism or concomitant drug use.

Unlabeled uses: Treatment of INH, hydrazine, and cycloserine poisoning. Treatment of neurological effects of Gyrometra mushroom poisoning. Nausea and vomiting associated with pregnancy.

CONTRAINDICATIONS

Known sensitivity to pyridoxine.

PRECAUTIONS

Used IV only when oral dosage not acceptable. ■ Deficiency can cause abnormal EEG. ■ Need for pyridoxine increases with amount of protein in diet. ■ Chronic administration of large doses may cause adverse neurological effects.

Maternal/child: Pregnancy Category A: requirements are increased in pregnancy and lactation. Do not exceed RDA. ■ Large doses in utero can cause pyridoxine-dependency syndrome in newborn. ■ May inhibit lactation. ■ Safety for use in children not established.

DRUG/LAB INTERACTIONS

An antagonist to levodopa. Does not antagonize carbidopa/levodopa combination (Sinemet). ■ Isoniazid is a vitamin B_6 antagonist and will cause deficiency disease. Cycloserine, penicillamine, hydralazine, oral contraceptives may increase pyridoxine requirements. ■ May decrease phenobarbital and phenytoin (Dilantin) levels. ■ Excessive doses may elevate AST.

SIDE EFFECTS

Almost nonexistent; some slight flushing or feeling of warmth may occur. With larger doses, ataxia, low folic acid levels, paresthesias, somnolence, and withdrawal seizures in infants with high maternal doses may occur.

ANTIDOTE

No antidote is known or has been needed. Symptomatic treatment of side effects may be indicated.

QUINIDINE GLUCONATE INJECTION

Antiarrhythmic

pH 5.5 to 7.0

USUAL DOSE

Antiarrhythmic: 200 mg. Repeat as indicated to control arrhythmia. 330 mg or less effective in most patients. Up to 1 Gm has been required. A test dose of 200 mg IM for idiosyncrasy is desired if time permits. Maintain with an oral quinidine preparation. Do not exceed 5 Gm total dose in 24 hours.

Plasmodium falciparum *malaria:* A loading dose of 15 mg/kg in 250 ml NS as an infusion over 4 hours. 24 hours from initial dose begin 7.5 mg/kg in 125 to 250 ml NS over 4 hours. Repeat every 8 hours for 7 days or transfer to oral therapy. An alternate regimen is a loading dose of 10 mg/kg in 250 ml NS as an infusion over 1 to 2 hours. Follow immediately with 0.02 mg/kg/min for up to 72 hours, until parasitemia less than 1% or transferred to oral therapy.

PEDIATRIC DOSE

2 to 10 mg/kg every 3 to 6 hours. Use IV only when other routes not possible.

DOSE ADJUSTMENTS

Note Drug/lab interactions.

DILUTION

800 mg (10 ml) must be diluted in at least 40 ml of D5W. 1 ml of properly diluted solution equals 16 mg quinidine. Use only clear colorless solutions.

INCOMPATIBLE WITH

Alkalies and iodides, amiodarone (Cordarone), atracurium (Tracrium), furosemide (Lasix), heparin. Most other drugs in syringe or solution. Combination impractical because of possible side effects and need to determine effectiveness. Has been shown to be compatible with brety-lium cimetidine, and verapamil, through Y-tube connection.

RATE OF ADMINISTRATION

1 ml (16 mg) or fraction thereof of properly diluted solution over 1 minute. Use an infusion pump or microdrip (60 gtt/ml). Too-rapid administration may cause a marked decrease in arterial pressure.

ACTIONS

A dextro-isomer of quinine. Exerts a depressing antiarrhythmic action on the heart, slowing the rate, slowing conduction, reducing myocardial contractility, and prolonging the refractory period. Increases potassium levels within the cells while it decreases sodium levels. Can have a vasodilating effect. Onset of action occurs when an effective blood concentration has been reached (15 to 30 minutes usually) and lasts 4 to 6 hours. Metabolized in the liver, most of the drug is excreted in the urine. Crosses placental barrier. Secreted in breast milk.

INDICATIONS AND USES

Cardiac arrhythmias, including atrial fibrillation, atrial flutter, premature asystoles, supraventricular tachycardia, ventricular tachycardia, and paroxysmal rhythms. ▪ Treatment of life-threatening *Plasmodium falciparum* malaria.

CONTRAINDICATIONS

Partial AV or complete heart block, any severe intraventricular conduction defects (including digitalis toxicity), aberrant impulses and abnormal rhythms due to escape mechanism, history of drug-induced torsades de pointes, history of long QT syndrome, known hypersensitivity to quinidine or cinchona, (e.g., febrile reactions, skin eruption, thrombocytopenia), myasthenia gravis, history of thrombocytopenic purpura with quinidine administration.

PRECAUTIONS

Oral or IM administration is route of choice. ▪ Use extreme caution in first- or second-degree blocks, extensive myocardial damage, digitalis intoxication, and impaired liver or kidney function. ▪ Use caution in atrial flutter or fibrillation; may require pretreatment with digitalis to prevent progressive reduction of AV block and an extremely rapid ventricular rate. ▪ Any other antiarrhythmic agent may cause new, increased, or more severe arrhythmias (e.g., more frequent PVCs, ventricular tachycardia or fibrillation, torsades de pointes). ▪ Lidocaine or procainamide is generally used in preference to quinidine. ▪ Doses used for *P. falciparum* malaria may cause hypotension, increased QRS and QT intervals, and cinchonism (e.g., dizziness, ringing in ears). ▪ Some clinicians recommend giving a dose the night before surgery and then discontinuing until after surgery. If arrhythmia occurs, use lidocaine for ventricular arrhymias and calcium channel blockers (e.g., verapamil) or beta-blockers (e.g., atenolol, propranolol) for supraventricular arrhythmias. Resume dosing postop and utilize oral dosing as soon as possible. ▪ Note Drug/lab interactions.

Monitor: Monitor patient's ECG and blood pressure continuously (plus parasitemia in malaria). Too-rapid administration may cause a marked decrease in arterial pressure. ▪ Keep patient in supine position. ▪ Discontinue IV use when the normal sinus rhythm returns, the heart rate falls to 120 beats/min, or any signs of cardiac toxicity occur (increased PR and QT intervals, over a 50% prolongation of QRS complex, or P waves disappear). ▪ Monitor serum levels if quinidine is used over 48 hours. ▪ Note Drug/lab interactions.

Patient education: Report breathing difficulty, dizziness, headache, nausea, ringing in the ears, skin rash, or visual disturbances promptly.

Maternal/child: Category C: safety for use in pregnancy not established, but no congenital defects have been reported in years of use. ■ Safety for use in lactation and in children not established.

Elderly: Half-life prolonged; frequency and severity of side effects may be increased.

DRUG/LAB INTERACTIONS

Potentiates or is potentiated by other antiarrhythmics (e.g., amiodarone [Cordarone]), anticholinergics (e.g., atropine), anticoagulants, antihypertensive agents, cimetidine (Tagamet), nondepolarizing neuromuscular blockers (e.g., tubocurarine, mivacurium), neuromuscular blocking antibiotics (e.g., kanamycin [Kantrex]), phenothiazines (e.g., prochlorperazine [Compazine]), reserpine, ritonavir (Norvir), succinylcholine (Anectine), thiazide diuretics, tricyclic antidepressants (e.g., amitriptyline [Elavil]), urinary alkalinizers, and others. May produce fatal cardiac arrhythmias, prolonged neuromuscular block, and other serious side effects. ■ Use caution with digitalis, procainamide, metoprolol, and propranolol. Lower doses of both drugs may be required.
■ Inhibited by barbiturates (e.g., phenobarbital), cholinergic agents (e.g., edrophonium, neostigmine), nifedipine, phenytoin (Dilantin), and rifampin; adjust dose. ■ May cause severe hypotension with verapamil, especially in patients with hypertrophic cardiomyopathy.
■ Increased levels of disopyramide (Norpace) and decreased levels of quinidine occur when used together. ■ May decrease analgesic activity of codeine. ■ A case report suggests concurrent use with erythromycin may increase serum levels of quinidine. ■ May cause increased serum skeletal muscle creatine phosphokinase. ■ Triamterene (Dyrenium) interferes with fluorescent measurement of serum levels.

SIDE EFFECTS

Minor: Apprehension, cramps, deafness (transitory), diaphoresis, fever, headache, nausea, rash, tinnitus, urge to defecate, urge to void, vertigo, visual disturbances, vomiting.

Major: Potentially fatal arrhythmias including atrioventricular heart block, cardiac standstill, prolonged PR or QT intervals, or 50% widening of QRS complex, tachycardia, ventricular fibrillation, acidosis, arthralgia, coma, confusion, hypokalemia, hypotension (acute), lethargy, myalgia, paresthesia, respiratory depression or arrest, thrombocytopenia purpura, seizures, urticaria.

ANTIDOTE

Notify the physician of any side effects. If minor symptoms progress or any major side effect appears, discontinue the drug immediately and notify the physician. Use fluid replacement and dopamine (Intropin), metaraminol (Aramine), or norepinephrine (Levophed) to correct hypotension and 1/6 molar sodium lactate to block effects of quinidine on the myocardium. Use phenytoin (Dilantin) or lidocaine for tachyarrhythmias. In overdose, monitoring of blood gases, electrolytes, and acidification of urine (avoid alkalinization) are indicated; cardiac pacing may be required. Treatment of toxicity is symptomatic and supportive. Hemodialysis may be indicated. Do not administer CNS depressants in overdose. Resuscitate as necessary. Depending on original arrhythmia, procainamide or lidocaine is effective alternate.

RANITIDINE

H₂ antagonist
Antiulcer agent
Gastric acid inhibitor

Zantac

pH 6.7 to 7.3

USUAL DOSE

Direct IV or intermittent infusion: 50 mg (2 ml) every 6 to 8 hours. Increase frequency of dose, not amount, if necessary for pain relief. 50 mg every 8 to 12 hours may be used short term to replace an oral dose of 150 mg every 12 hours in patients unable to take oral meds. Do not exceed 400 mg/day.

Continuous infusion: 150 mg may be given as a continuous infusion equally distributed over 24 hours. To maintain intergastric acid secretion rates at 10 mEq/hr or less, dose range may be higher in patients with pathologic hypersecretory syndrome (Zollinger-Ellison). Literature suggests an initial dose of 1 mg/kg/hr. Measure gastric acid output in 4 hours. If above 10 mEq/hr or symptoms recur, adjust dose upward in 0.5 mg/kg/hr increments. Up to 2.5 mg/kg/hr has been used.

Additive for total parental nutrition (TPN): 70% to 100% of an average 24 hour dose has been used equally distributed over 24 hours as a continuous infusion. May be supplemented with intermittent doses as needed.

Prevention of pulmonary aspiration during anesthesia: 50 mg 60 to 90 minutes before anesthesia.

Control of acute upper GI bleeding: 150 mg over 24 hours.

Prevention of stress ulcers: 0.125 to 0.25 mg/kg/hr.

PEDIATRIC DOSE

1 to 2 mg/kg/24 hr in equally divided doses every 6 to 8 hours.

DOSE ADJUSTMENTS

Increase intervals between injections to achieve pain relief with least frequent dosage in impaired renal function. If the creatinine clearance is less than 50 ml/min, reduce dose to 50 mg/24 hrs. Gradually increase to 50 mg/18, 12, or 6 hours with caution if indicated. Adjust schedule to be given after dialysis.

DILUTION

Direct IV: Each 50 mg must be diluted with 20 ml of NS or other compatible infusion solution for injection (D5W, D10W, LR, 5% sodium bicarbonate). Concentration of solution must be no greater than 2.5 mg/ml. Additional diluent may be used.

Intermittent infusion: Available premixed as a 0.5 mg/ml solution in 100 ml or each 50 mg may be diluted in 100 ml (0.5 mg/ml) of D5W or other compatible infusion solution and given piggyback. Concentration of solution should be no greater than 0.5 mg/ml. Manufacturer recommends discontinuing primary IV during intermittent infusion to avoid incompatibilities. Do not use premixed plastic containers in series connections; may cause air embolism.

Continuous infusion: Total daily dose may be diluted in 250 ml of D5W or other compatible infusion solution. For Zollinger-Ellison patients, concentration of solution must be no greater than 2.5 mg/ml.

In all situations, avoid any contact with aluminum during administration (e.g., needles). Inspect for color and clarity. Slight darkening of solution does not affect potency. Compatible in selected TPN solutions for 24 hours (consult pharmacist).

Storage: Stable at room temperature for 48 hours after dilution.

INCOMPATIBLE WITH

Amphotericin B (Fungizone), atracurium (Tracrium), cefamandole (Mandol), cefazolin (Ketzol), cefoxitin (Mefoxin), ceftazidime (Tazicef), cefuroxime (Kefurox), cephalothin (Keflin), chlorpromazine (Thorazine), clindamycin (Cleocin), diazepam (Valium), ethacrynic acid (Edecrin), hetastarch (Hespan), hydroxyzine (Vistaril), metaraminol (Aramine), midazolam (Versed), opium alkaloids, pentobarbital (Nembutal), phenobarbital (Luminal), phytonadione. Do not add any other drugs to premixed ranitidine (Aquamephyton) in plastic containers.

RATE OF ADMINISTRATION

Too-rapid administration has precipitated rare instances of bradycardia, tachycardia, and PVCs.

Direct IV: Each 50 mg or fraction thereof at a rate not to exceed 4 ml/min diluted solution (20 ml over 5 min).

Intermittent infusion: Each 50 mg dose over 15 to 20 minutes. Should not exceed a rate of 5 to 7 ml/min.

Continuous infusion: Total daily dose equally distributed over 24 hours. Should not exceed a rate of 6.25 mg/hr (10.7 ml/hr if 150 mg [6 ml ranitidine] is diluted in 250 ml). Use of infusion pump preferred to avoid complications of overdose or too-rapid administration.

ACTIONS

A histamine H_2 antagonist, it inhibits both daytime and nocturnal basal gastric acid secretion. It also inhibits gastric acid secretion stimulated by food, histamine, bentazole, and pentagastrin. Not an anticholinergic agent. Does not lower calcium levels in hypercalcemia. Onset of action is prompt and effective for 6 to 8 hours. 5 to 12 times more potent than cimetidine. Metabolized in the liver. Excreted in the urine. Crosses placental barrier. Secreted in breast milk.

INDICATIONS AND USES

Short-term treatment of intractable duodenal ulcers and pathologic hypersecretory conditions in the hospitalized patient. ■ Treatment of active benign gastric ulcers in those patients unable to take oral medication. ■ Treatment of erosive gastroesophageal reflux disease (GERD) and erosive esophagitis diagnosed by endoscopy. ■ Additive to TPN to simplify fluid and electrolyte management (decreases the volume and chloride content of gastric secretions).

Investigational use: Preoperatively to prevent pulmonary aspiration of acid during anesthesia. ■ Control of acute upper GI bleeding. ■ Prevention of stress ulcers.

CONTRAINDICATIONS

Known hypersensitivity to ranitidine or its components.

PRECAUTIONS

Use antacids concomitantly to relieve pain. ■ Gastric malignancy may be present even though patient is asymptomatic. ■ Use caution in patients with impaired hepatic function. ■ Gastric pain and ulceration may recur after medication stopped. ▪ Effects maintained with oral dosage. Total treatment usually discontinued after 6 weeks.

Monitor: Observe frequently; monitor vital signs and pain levels. ▪ Monitor ALT (SGPT) if therapy exceeds 400 mg for over 5 days. ▪ Change to oral dose when appropriate. ▪ Note Drug/lab interactions.

Patient education: Stop smoking or at least avoid smoking after the last dose of the day. ▪ May increase blood alcohol levels.

Maternal/child: Pregnancy Category B: use during pregnancy or lactation only when clearly needed. ▪ Safety for use in children not established.

Elderly: Safety and effectiveness consistent with younger ages; consider reduced renal function.

DRUG/LAB INTERACTIONS

May potentiate warfarin-type anticoagulants; monitor prothrombin times. ▪ Potentiates effects of alcohol, procainamide (Pronestyl), sulfonylureas (Glipizide). ▪ May potentiate theophyllines (e.g., aminophylline). ▪ May inhibit gastric absorption of ketoconazole (Nizoral). ▪ Clinical effect (inhibition of nocturnal gastric secretions) may be reversed by cigarette smoking. ▪ Elevated ALT (SGOT), slight elevation in serum creatinine, and a false-positive for urine protein with Multistix may occur.

SIDE EFFECTS

Abdominal discomfort, burning and itching at IV site, constipation, diarrhea, headache (severe), and nausea and vomiting are the most common side effects. Allergic reactions (bronchospasm, fever, rash, eosinophilia) can occur. Agitation, arthralgias, bradycardia, confusion, depression, dizziness, elevated SGPT, hallucinations, hepatitis (reversible), impotence, insomnia, malaise, muscular pain, PVCs, somnolence, tachycardia, and vertigo occur rarely. Note Drug/lab interactions.

ANTIDOTE

Notify physician of all side effects. May be treated symptomatically or may respond to decrease in frequency of dosage. Resuscitate as necessary for overdose. Hemodialysis or peritoneal dialysis may be indicated in overdose.

REMIFENTANIL HYDROCHLORIDE

Narcotic analgesic (agonist)
Anesthesia adjunct

Ultiva

pH 2.5 to 3.5

USUAL DOSE

General anesthesia and continuing as an analgesic into the immediate postoperative period: Not recommended as the sole anesthetic agent because it may not cause loss of consciousness and it has a high incidence of apnea, muscle rigidity, and tachycardia. Given concomitantly with reduced doses of other anesthetics (e.g., isoflurane, midazolam [Versed], propofol [Diprivan], and/or thiopental [Pentothal]); see Dose adjustments and Drug/lab interactions. Individualize based on patient response. May be premedicated with benzodiazepines (e.g., diazepam [Valium], midazolam [Versed]). *If intubation is to occur less than 8 minutes after the start of a remifentanil infusion, an initial dose of 1 mcg/kg may be administered over 30 to 60 seconds. See table below:

Phase	Continuous IV infusion (mcg/kg/min)	Infusion dose range (mcg/kg/min)	Supplemental IV bolus dose (mcg/kg)
Induction of anesthesia (through intubation)	0.5-1*		
Maintenance of anesthesia with:			
Nitrous oxide (66%)	0.4	0.1-2	1
Isoflurane (0.4 to 1.5 MAC)	0.25	0.05-2	1
Propofol (100 to 200 mcg/kg/min)	0.25	0.05-2	1
Continuation as an analgesic into the immediate post-operative period	0.1	0.025-0.2	not recommended

Monitored anesthesia care:

Method	Timing	Remifentanil alone	Remifentanil + 2 mg midazolam
Single IV dose	Given 90 seconds before local anesthetic	1 mcg/kg over 30 to 60 seconds	0.5 mcg/kg over 30 to 60 seconds
Continuous IV infusion	Beginning 5 minutes before local anesthetic	0.1 mcg/kg/min	0.05 mcg/kg/min
	After local anesthetic	0.05 mcg/kg/min (Range:0.025-0.2 mcg/kg/min)	0.025 mcg/kg/min (Range: 0.025-0.2 mcg/kg/min)

PEDIATRIC DOSE

Children 2 to 12 years of age: Same mcg/kg dose as adults; note all comments. 25 mcg/ml dilution recommended.

DOSE ADJUSTMENTS

Reduce starting dose by 50% in the elderly (over 65 years of age), then cautiously titrate to effect. ■ Base starting dose on ideal body weight in obese patients (>30% over their IBW). ■ No dose adjustment required in patients with atypical cholinesterase or in chronic or severe renal or hepatic dysfunction. ■ Dose may be reduced up to 75% with other anesthetic agents; see Drug/lab interactions. ■ See Precautions.

DILUTION

To reconstitute add 1 ml of diluent for each mg of remifentanil (1 mg/ml). Compatible with SW, D5W, D5/NS, NS, 0.45 NS, D5/LR, and LR (has reduced stability). Shake well. Must be further diluted to a final concentration of 25, 50, or 250 mcg/ml with additional amounts of the above solutions (see table below):

Amount of reconstituted remifentanil in each vial	Amount of diluent	Final volume after reconstitution and dilution	Final concentration
1 mg	39 ml	40 ml	
2 mg	78 ml	80 ml	25 mcg/ml
5 mg	195 ml	200 ml	
1 mg	19 ml	20 ml	
2 mg	38 ml	40 ml	50 mcg/ml
5 mg	95 ml	100 ml	
5 mg	15 ml	20ml	250 mcg/ml

Pediatric dilution: 25 mcg/ml dilution recommended.
Storage: Store between 2° to 25° C. Stable for 24 hours at room temperature after reconstituted and diluted with above solutions. Stability reduced to 4 hours with lactated Ringer's injection.

INCOMPATIBLE WITH

Limited information available. Do not administer into the same IV tubing as blood or blood products.

COMPATIBLE WITH

Y-site: Propofol (Diprivan).

RATE OF ADMINISTRATION

Use of an infusion device required. Injection site should be close to the venous cannula, and all IV tubing should be flushed when the infusion is discontinued to prevent delayed effects. Rapid elimination and lack of accumulation permits titration of infusion rate without concern for prolonged duration. Every 0.1 mcg/kg/min change in the infusion rate will lead to a 2.5 ng/ml change in blood concentration within 5 to 10 minutes (note Precautions). Skeletal muscle rigidity is related to the dose and speed of administration. In any situation infusion rates greater than 0.2 mcg/kg/min may cause respiratory depression.

Anesthesia induction: If intubation is to occur less than 8 minutes after the start of a remifentanil infusion, an initial dose of 1 mcg/kg over 30 to 60 seconds may be given.

Anesthesia maintenance: Titrate upward in 25% to 100% increments or downward in 25% to 50% increments every 2 to 5 minutes to attain desired level of opioid effect. Supplemental bolus doses of 1 mcg/kg may be given every 2 to 5 minutes in response to light anesthesia or episodes of intense surgical stress. If infusion rates >1 mcg/kg/min are required, consider increasing concomitant anesthetic agents to increase the depth of anesthesia.

Continuation as an analgesic during the immediate postoperative period: Adjust rate in 0.025 mcg/kg/min increments every 5 minutes to balance level of analgesia and respiratory rate. Administer alternate analgesics to control postoperative pain before discontinuing remifentanil.

Monitored anesthesia care (MAC): See table in Usual dose. Titrate to patient comfort, analgesia, and adequate respiration; do not use sedation as a criteria for titration, may cause muscle rigidity and respiratory depression. Note Contraindications and Precautions.

After placement of a local or regional block with MAC: To reduce risk of hypoventilation, decrease infusion rate to 0.05 mcg/kg/min; thereafter titrate in increments of 0.025 mcg/kg/min at 5-minute intervals to balance level of analgesia and respiratory rate.

IV infusion rates of remifentanil (ml/h) for a 25-mcg/ml solution

Infusion rate (mcg/kg/min)	Patient weight (kg)									
	10	20	30	40	50	60	70	80	90	100
0.0125	0.3	0.6	0.9	1.2	1.5	1.8	2.1	2.4	2.7	3
0.025	0.6	1.2	1.8	2.4	3	3.6	4.2	4.8	5.4	6
0.05	1.2	2.4	3.6	4.8	6	7.2	8.4	9.6	10.8	12
0.075	1.8	3.6	5.4	7.2	9	10.8	12.6	14.4	16.2	18
0.1	2.4	4.8	7.2	9.6	12	14.4	16.8	19.2	21.6	24
0.15	3.6	7.2	10.8	14.4	18	21.6	25.2	28.8	32.4	36
0.2	4.8	9.6	14.4	19.2	24	28.8	33.6	38.4	43.2	48

IV infusion rates of remifentanil (ml/h) for a 50-mcg/ml solution

Infusion rate (mcg/kg/min)	Patient weight (kg)							
	30	40	50	60	70	80	90	100
0.025					2.1	2.4	2.7	3
0.05		2.4	3	3.6	4.2	4.8	5.4	6
0.075	2.7	3.6	4.5	5.4	6.3	7.2	8.1	9
0.1	3.6	4.8	6	7.2	8.4	9.6	10.8	12
0.15	5.4	7.2	9	10.8	12.6	14.4	16.2	18
0.2	7.2	9.6	12	14.4	16.8	19.2	21.6	24
0.25	9	12	15	18	21	24	27	30
0.5	18	24	30	36	42	48	54	60
0.75	27	36	45	54	63	72	81	90
1	36	48	60	72	84	96	108	120
1.25	45	60	75	90	105	120	135	150
1.5	54	72	90	108	126	144	162	180
1.75	63	84	105	126	147	168	189	210
2	72	96	120	144	168	192	216	240

IV infusion rates of remifentanil (ml/h) for a 250-mcg/ml solution

Infusion rate (mcg/kg/min)	Patient weight (kg)							
	30	40	50	60	70	80	90	100
0.1	0.72	0.96	1.2	1.44	1.68	1.92	2.16	2.4
0.15	1.08	1.44	1.8	2.16	2.52	2.88	3.24	3.6
0.2	1.44	1.92	2.4	2.88	3.36	3.84	4.32	4.8
0.25	1.8	2.4	3	3.6	4.2	4.8	5.4	6
0.5	3.6	4.8	6	7.2	8.4	9.6	10.8	12
0.75	5.4	7.2	9	10.8	12.6	14.4	16.2	18
1	7.2	9.6	12	14.4	16.8	19.2	21.6	24
1.25	9	12	15	18	21	24	27	30
1.5	10.8	14.4	18	21.6	25.2	28.8	32.4	36
1.75	12.6	16.8	21	25.2	29.4	33.6	37.8	42
2	14.4	19.2	24	28.8	33.6	38.4	43.2	48

ACTIONS

An opioid agonist analgesic with rapid onset (1 minute) and peak effect (3 to 5 minutes) and short duration of action (5 to 10 minutes). Effects and side effects are dose dependent. There is direct correlation between dose, blood levels, and response. Blood concentration decreases 50% in 3 to 6 minutes after a 1-minute infusion or after prolonged continuous infusion due to rapid distribution and elimination and is independent of duration of drug administration. Recovery from effects occurs within 5 to 10 minutes. New steady state concentrations occur within 5 to 10 minutes after changes in infusion rates. Serum concentrations, volume of distribution, clearance, and half-life in children 2 to 12 years were similar to adults. Rapidly metabolized by specific blood and tissue esterases.

INDICATIONS AND USES

An analgesic agent for use during induction and maintenance of general anesthesia for inpatient and outpatient procedures and for continuation as an analgesic in a postoperative anesthesia care unit or intensive care setting. ▪ Analgesic component of monitored anesthesia care.

CONTRAINDICATIONS

Known hypersensitivity to remifentanil or other fentanyl analogs (e.g., alfentanil, fentanyl, sulfentanil). ▪ Contains glycine; do not use for epidural or intrathecal administration. ▪ **IV bolus doses should be used only during the maintenance of general anesthesia. Administration of bolus doses simultaneously with a continuous infusion to spontaneously breathing patients is not recommended.**

PRECAUTIONS

For IV use only. ▪ Intended for use by or under the direct supervision of the anesthesiologist. Must have responsibility only for anesthesia during surgery and/or procedures. Staff must be skilled in medical management of critically ill patients, cardiovascular resuscitation, and airway management. ▪ Analgesia usually achieved with minimal decrease in respiratory rate with infusions of 0.05 to 0.1 mcg/kg/min producing blood concentrations of 1 to 3 ng/ml. Supplemental doses of 0.5 to 1 mcg/kg, incremental increases in infusion rate >0.05 mcg/kg/min, and blood concentrations exceeding 5 ng/ml (typically produced by infusions of 0.2 mcg/kg/min) have caused transient and reversible respiratory depression, apnea, and muscle rigidity. ▪ May cause chest wall rigidity (inability to ventilate) after single doses of >1 mcg/kg administered over 30 to 60 seconds or infusion rates >0.1 mcg/kg/min; peripheral muscle rigidity may occur at lower doses. May also cause chest wall rigidity with doses <1 mcg/kg when given concurrently with a continuous infusion of remifentanil. May be prevented or lessened by prior or concurrent administration of a hypnotic (propofol or thiopental) or a neuromuscular blocking agent (e.g., atracurium). ▪ With a 1-minute infusion of <2 mcg/kg, remifentanil will cause dose-dependent hypotension and bradycardia in premedicated patients undergoing anesthesia. Additional doses >2 mcg/kg do not produce further decreases. ▪ Respiratory depression is dose related, but due to a lack of drug accumulation; recovery of respiratory drive is more rapid and less variable than other similar agents. Rate of respiratory recovery will vary depending on concurrent anesthetics (e.g., N_2O, propofol, isoflurane). ▪ Use caution in very obese patients; may have increased potential for cardiovascular or respiratory problems. ▪ Increased risk of respiratory depression in patients with impaired respiratory function; use caution. ▪ Use caution in patients with bradycardia; HR may decrease further. ▪ Intraoperative awareness has been reported. ▪ Has not been used for longer than 16 hours in ICU patients.

Monitor: Oxygen, intubation equipment, controlled ventilation equipment, naloxone (Narcan), neuromuscular blocking agents (e.g., mivacurium [Mivacron]), and facilities for resuscitation and life support must always be available. Maintain a patent airway and ascertain adequate ventilation at all times. A conscious patient will appear to be asleep and may forget to breathe unless commanded to do so. ▪ Can cause rigidity of respiratory muscles; may require a muscle relaxant (benzodiazepine) or neuromuscular blocking agent to relax muscles and permit artificial ventilation. ▪ All vital signs must be monitored continuously. Use of a respiratory monitor and monitoring of oxygen saturation required. Supplemental oxygen always required for general anesthesia; strongly recommended for MAC. ▪ Keep patient supine; orthostatic hypotension and fainting may occur. ▪ Flush IV line before discontinuing an infusion of remifentanil. ▪ Establish adequate postoperative analgesia before discontinuing an infusion of remifentanil. ▪ Note Precautions. ▪ Monitor for 30 to 60 minutes after anesthesia complete. Effect of remifentanil will be offset within 5 to 10 minutes, but respiratory depression may still occur from concomitant anesthetics.

Patient education: Avoid alcohol or other CNS depressants (e.g., antihistamines, diazepam [Valium]). ▪ Blurred vision, dizziness, drowsiness, or lightheadedness may occur; use caution. ▪ Do not perform tasks requiring mental alertness (e.g., driving, operating hazardous machinery, or signing legal documents) until the day after surgery or longer.

Maternal/child: Pregnancy Category C: Use only when clearly needed; benefit must justify risk to fetus. ▪ May cause respiratory depression and other opioid effects in the newborn if used before or during labor and delivery; safety not demonstrated. ▪ Other fentanyl analogs are secreted in breast milk; remifentanil not yet studied, use caution during lactation. ▪ Safety for use in infants and children under 2 years of age not established.

Elderly: Note Dose adjustments. Increased sensitivity to effects and clearance reduced by 25%, but blood concentrations fall as rapidly after remifentanil is discontinued. Incidence of hypotension may be increased; nausea and vomiting may be decreased.

DRUG/LAB INTERACTIONS

Respiratory depression increased and prolonged with other concurrent anesthetics (e.g., N_2O, propofol, isofluane). ▪ Nonspecific esterases in blood products may inactivate remifentanil. ▪ Clearance is not altered by concomitant use of thiopental, isoflurane, propofol, or temazepam (Restoril) during anesthesia; is synergistic with hypnotics (e.g., propofol, thiopental), inhaled anesthetics (e.g., isoflurane), and benzodiazepines (e.g., midazolam). Risk of hypotension and respiratory depression increased. Doses of these agents have been reduced by up to 75%. ▪ No drug interactions to date with atracurium (Tracium), mivacurium (Mivacron), esmolol (Brevibloc), antiglaucoma agents (echothiophate), neostigmine (Prostigmin), or physostigmine (Antilirium). ▪ During monitored anesthesia care concurrent administration with midazolam 4 to 8 mg increased the rate of respiratory depression even when the dose of remifentanil was reduced by 50%. ▪ Does not prolong the duration of muscle paralysis from succinylcholine in animals. ▪ Hypothermic cardiopulmonary bypass may reduce clearance by 20%, increasing effects.

SIDE EFFECTS

Minor: Chills, dizziness, fever, flushing, headache, nausea, pain at IV site, postoperative pain, pruritus, shivering, sweating, vomiting, warm sensation.

Major: Apnea, bradycardia, hypertension, hypotension, respiratory depression, skeletal muscle rigidity, tachycardia. Many other serious side effects can occur, including other arrhythmias.

Overdose: Apnea, bradycardia, chest wall rigidity, hypoxemia, hypotension, seizures.

ANTIDOTE

Keep physician informed of all side effects. Minor side effects will be tolerated or treated symptomatically. Major side effects or overdose may be life threatening and must be treated immediately. Antagonized by opioid antagonists; short-acting opioid antagonists should be adequate (e.g., naloxone [Narcan]). Reversal of opioid effects may lead to acute pain and sympathetic hyperactivity. Maintain a patent airway, with oxygen, and artificial ventilation as needed. Respiratory depression in spontaneously breathing patients is usually managed by decreasing the rate of infusion by 50% or temporarily discontinuing remifentanil. Bradycardia and hypotension can be reversed by reducing the rate of infusion or the dose of concurrent anesthetics. Bradycardia may require atropine or glycopyrrolate. Hypotension may require IV fluids or catecholamines (e.g., ephedrine, epinephrine, norepinephrine). Treat excessive muscle rigidity during induction of anesthesia by administering a neuromuscular blocking agent (e.g., succinylcholine) and concurrent induction medications (e.g., thiopental). Treat excessive muscle rigidity in spontaneously breathing patients by decreasing the rate, discontinuing remifentanil, or administering a neuromuscular blocking agent or naloxone. Hypertension may require antihypertensives (e.g., nitroglycerin). Treatment of seizures may require benzodiazepines (e.g., diazepam [Valium]).

RESPIRATORY SYNCYTIAL VIRUS IMMUNE GLOBULIN INTRAVENOUS

Immunizing agent (passive)

RespiGam, RSV-IGIV

PEDIATRIC DOSE

750 mg/kg as a single dose IV infusion. Administer the first dose prior to the respiratory syncytial virus (RSV) season (early November through April in the northern hemisphere). Repeat monthly throughout the season.

DILUTION

No dilution required; ready to infuse in a 50 mg/ml solution. Should be clear and colorless. Do not shake vial; avoid foaming. Remove the tab portion of the vial cap and clean with 70% alcohol before puncturing with infusion set. Note Incompatible with.

Storage: Refrigerate unopened vials. Begin infusion within 6 hours and complete within 12 hours after single-use vial is entered.

INCOMPATIBLE WITH

Should be administered through a separate IV line. If piggy-backing is necessary, the preexisting line must contain only 2½%, 5%, 10%, or 20% dextrose in water or NS. Dilution must not exceed 1 part RSV-IGIV to 2 parts dextrose solution at the Y-connection.

RATE OF ADMINISTRATION

An infusion pump is required to deliver a constant rate; an in-line filter larger than 15 microns may be used. Slow rate of infusion at onset of patient discomfort or for any adverse reactions (e.g., anxiety, dizziness, hypotension, pruritus). Begin with 1.5 ml/kg/hr for the first 15 minutes. If no discomfort or adverse effects, may be increased to 3 ml/kg/hr from 15 to 30 minutes and to 6 ml/kg/hr from 30 minutes to the end of the infusion. Monitor closely during and after each rate change. Slower rates of infusion may be indicated in ill children. Never exceed 6 ml/kg/hr.

ACTIONS

A specialty immunoglobulin (IgG) containing neutralizing and protecting antibodies to RSV. Capable of neutralizing each of 62 different RSV clinical isolates of subgroups A and B. Pooled from adult human plasma selected for high titers of neutralizing antibody against RSV. RSV antibody content is 5 to 10 times that of standard Intravenous Immune Globulin. Purified and standardized by several specific methods (e.g., solvent-detergent viral inactivation process to decrease the possibility of transmission of bloodborne pathogens [e.g., HIV, hepatitis]). Mean half-life of a single dose is 22 to 28 days.

INDICATIONS AND USES

Prevention of serious lower respiratory tract infection caused by RSV in children under 24 months of age with bronchopulmonary dysplasia (BPD) or a history of premature birth (≤ 35 weeks gestation). Has reduced the incidence and duration of RSV hospitalization and severity of RSV illness in these high-risk infants. ■ Has not been shown to be effective for the treatment of RSV infection.

CONTRAINDICATIONS

History of a prior severe hypersensitivity reaction to RSV-IGIV or other immunoglobulin preparations, patients with isolated IgA deficiency or preexisting anti-IgA antibodies.

PRECAUTIONS

Use caution; infants with underlying pulmonary disease may be more susceptible to fluid overload; may respond to rate reduction or require loop diuretics (e.g., bumetanide [Bumex] or furosemide [Lasix]). ■ Not recommended for use in children with clinically apparent fluid overload. ■ Aseptic meningitis syndrome (AMS) has been reported in a few patients. Symptoms (e.g., drowsiness, fever, headache, [severe], muscle rigidity, nausea and vomiting, painful eye movements) may occur within a few hours or up to 2 days following infusion. Other causes of meningitis must be ruled out. Seems to occur with higher doses (2 Gm/kg) and subsides with discontinuation of IGIV.

Monitor: Assess vital signs and cardiopulmonary status. At a minimum, must be done prior to infusion, before each rate increase, and thereafter at 30-minute intervals until 30 minutes after the infusion is complete. Observe for symptoms of fluid overload (e.g., increases in heart rate, respiratory rate, retractions, and rales). ▪ Loop diuretics, epinephrine, and diphenhydramine must be readily available. Note Antidote.

Maternal/child: Pregnancy Category C: use only if clearly indicated. ▪ Safety for use in infants with congenital heart disease (CHD) has not been established. A somewhat larger number of life-threatening adverse events occurred during trial in infants with CHD with right-to-left shunts who underwent surgery.

DRUG/LAB INTERACTIONS

May interfere with immune response to live-virus vaccines (e.g., measles, mumps, rubella). Reimmunization is recommended at least 10 months after RSV-IGIV is discontinued, if appropriate. The American Association of Pediatrics (AAP) recommends deferring primary immunization with these agents until 9 months after the last dose of RSV-IGIV. ▪ Effect on antibody responses to DPT, haemophilus influenza type b (Hib), and oral polio virus is unknown; booster doses may be indicated 3 to 4 months after RSV-IGIV is discontinued. The AAP states "current data do not support the need for supplemental doses of these vaccines in infants receiving RSV-IGIV."

SIDE EFFECTS

Abdominal cramps, anxiety, arthralgia, chest tightness, dizziness, dyspnea, flushing, hypotension, myalgia, palpitations, pruritus may occur and may be related to the rate of infusion. Mild fluid overload and/or mild decreases in oxygen saturation may occur. Full range of allergic symptoms including anaphylaxis may occur. Is made from human plasma; process attempts to eliminate risk of hepatitis or HIV infection.

Overdose: Fluid overload.

ANTIDOTE

Reduce rate immediately for patient discomfort, mild hypotension, S/S of fluid overload, or other signs of adverse reaction. Keep physician informed. Treat fluid overload with loop diuretics (e.g., bumetanide, furosemide) if indicated. Discontinue immediately for precipitous hypotension, anaphylaxis, or severe allergic reaction, and treat acute allergic symptoms with epinephrine and diphenhydramine (Benadryl). Hypotension should resolve quickly; may require dopamine (Intropin).

RETEPLASE RECOMBINANT

Thrombolytic agent
(Recombinant)

Retavase, r-PA

pH 7.0 to 7.4

USUAL DOSE

Administered concomitantly with heparin. Give a 5,000 Unit IV bolus of heparin prior to the initial injection of reteplase, then give 10 Units (10 ml) of reteplase as an IV injection. Follow with a 1,000 Unit/hr continuous IV infusion of heparin for at least 24 hours. Give a second 10 Unit bolus of reteplase 30 minutes after the first. Note Dilution, Incompatible with, and Rate of administration. Aspirin is also used either during or following heparin treatment; an initial dose of 160 to 350 mg is followed by doses of 75 to 350 mg.

DOSE ADJUSTMENTS

The second bolus should not be given if serious bleeding in a critical location (e.g., intracranial, gastrointestinal, retroperitoneal, pericardial) occurs before it is due to be given.

DILUTION

Supplied in a kit with all components for reconstitution. Each kit contains a package insert, and two of each of the following: single-use reteplase vials (10.8 Units each), single-use diluent vials of SW (10 ml each), sterile 10-ml syringes with 20-gauge needles attached, sterile dispensing pins, sterile 20-gauge needles for administration, and alcohol swabs. Withdraw diluent with 20-gauge needle. Discard needle and put dispensing pin on syringe of diluent. Transfer diluent to vial of reteplase. Pin and syringe should remain in place while vial is swirled to dissolve reteplase. *Do not shake.* When completely dissolved, withdraw 10 ml reconstituted solution into the syringe (vials are 0.7 ml overfilled). Remove dispensing pin and replace with a 20-gauge needle for administration.

Storage: Kit should remain sealed to protect contents from light. Store at 2° to 25° C (36° to 77° F). Do not use beyond expiration date. Contains no preservatives; should be reconstituted immediately before use, but may be stored at room temperature if used within 4 hours. Discard all unused solution and supplies.

INCOMPATIBLE WITH

Manufacturer states, "should be given via an IV line in which no other medication is being simultaneously injected or infused. No other medication should be added to the injection solution containing reteplase." Incompatible with heparin; do not administer heparin in the same IV line unless the line is flushed with a minimum of 30 to 50 ml NS or D5W before and after reteplase.

RATE OF ADMINISTRATION

Heparin: First 1,000 Units over 1 minute. After this test dose, the balance of 4,000 Units may be given over 1 minute. Follow with an infusion of 1,000 Units/hr.

Reteplase: A single dose evenly distributed over 2 minutes. To avoid incompatibilities and ensure delivery of both doses, be sure to flush line with a minimum of 30 to 50 ml NS or D5W before and after each injection.

ACTIONS

A recombinant plasminogen activator. Exerts its thrombolytic action by generating plasmin from plasminogen through a specific process. Plasmin then degrades the fibrin matrix of the thrombus. Potency is expressed in units, which are specific to reteplase. With therapeutic doses, a decrease in circulating fibrinogen makes the patient susceptible to bleeding. Onset of action is prompt, effecting patency of the vessel within 90 minutes in most patients. The FDA has allowed the manufacturer to claim superiority over alteplase at achieving patency within 90 minutes. Prompt opening of arteries increases probability of improved cardiac function. Half-life is 13 to 16 minutes. Cleared from the plasma by the liver and kidneys. Mean fibrinogen level should return to baseline value within 48 hours.

INDICATIONS AND USES

Management of acute myocardial infarction (AMI) in adults for the improvement of ventricular function following AMI, the reduction of the incidence of congestive failure, and the reduction of mortality associated with AMI. Treatment should begin as soon as possible after the onset of symptoms of AMI. ■ Current AHA and JAMA recommendations identify thrombolytic agents as Class 1 therapy in patients younger than 70 years with recent onset of chest pain (within 6 hours) consistent with AMI and at least 0.1 mV of ST segment elevation in at least two ECG leads. Use in all other patients based on age, accurate diagnosis, and time from onset of chest pain.

CONTRAINDICATIONS

Active internal bleeding, arteriovenous malformation or aneurysm, bleeding diathesis, history of cerebral vascular accident, intracranial or intraspinal surgery or trauma within 2 months, intracranial neoplasm, severe uncontrolled hypertension.

PRECAUTIONS

Administered under the direction of a physician knowledgeable in its use and with appropriate diagnostic and laboratory facilities available. ■ Reperfusion arrhythmias occur frequently (e.g., sinus bradycardia, accelerated idioventricular rhythm, PVCs, ventricular tachycardia); have antiarrhythmic meds available at bedside. ■ A greater alteration of hemostatic status than with heparin. Strict bed rest indicated to reduce risk of bleeding. Use extreme care with the patient; avoid any excessive or rough handling or pressure (including too-frequent BPs); avoid invasive procedures (e.g., arterial puncture, venipuncture, IM injection). If these procedures are absolutely necessary, use extreme precautionary methods (use radial artery instead of femoral; small-gauge catheters and needles, and sites that are easily observed and compressible where bleeding can be controlled; avoid handling of catheter sites, and use extended pressure application of up to 30 minutes). Minor bleeding occurs often at catheter insertion sites. Avoid use of razors and toothbrushes. ■ Use extreme caution and weigh risks against anticipated benefits in the following situation: recent major surgery (e.g., coronary artery bypass graft, obstetrical delivery, organ biopsy), previous puncture of noncompressible vessels (e.g., jugular, subclavian), cerebrovascular disease, recent GI or GU bleeding, recent trauma, hypertension (e.g., systolic BP ≥180 mm Hg and/or diastolic BP ≥110 mm Hg), high likelihood of left heart thrombus, (e.g., mitral stenosis with atrial fibrillation), acute pericarditis, subacute bacterial endocarditis, hemostatic defects including those secondary to severe hepatic or renal disease, severe hepatic or renal dysfunction, pregnancy, diabetic hemorrhagic retinopathy or other hemorrhagic ophthalmic conditions, septic thrombophletitis or occluded AV cannula at a seriously infected site, advanced age, patients currently receiving oral anticoagulants (e.g., warfarin [Coumadin]), any other condition in which bleeding constitutes a significant hazard or would be particularly difficult to manage because of its location. ▪ Simultaneous therapy with continuous infusion of heparin is used to reduce the risk of rethrombosis. Markedly increases risk of bleeding. ▪ Standard treatment for myocardial infarction continues simultaneously with reteplase therapy except if temporarily contraindicated (e.g., arterial blood gases unless absolutely necessary. ▪ No experience with patients receiving repeat courses of reteplase. ▪ Cholesterol embolization has been reported and may be fatal.

Monitor: Best to establish separate IV lines for reteplase and heparin. If not appropriate be sure to flush the IV line before and after each injection of reteplase. ▪ Baseline ECG, CPK, and clotting studies (TT, PTT, CBC, fibrinogen level, platelets) and baseline assessment (patient condition, pain, hematomas, petechiae, or recent wounds) should be completed before administration. Type and cross-match may also be ordered. ▪ Monitor ECG continuously, and record strips with greatest ST segment elevation initially and every 15 minutes for at least 4 hours. A 12-lead ECG is indicated when therapy is complete. ▪ Maintain strict bed rest; monitor the patient carefully and frequently for anginal pain and signs of bleeding; observe catheter sites at least every 15 minutes and apply pressure dressings to any recently invaded site; watch for hematuria, hematemesis, bloody stool, petechiae, hematoma, flank pain, muscle weakness; do neuro checks every hour. Continue until normal clotting function returns. ▪ Watch for extravasation. ▪ Note Precautions and Drug/lab interactions.

Patient education: Compliance with all measures to minimize bleeding (e.g., strict bed rest) is very important. ▪ Avoid use of razors, toothbrushes, and other sharp items. ▪ Use caution while moving to avoid excessive bumping. ▪ Report all episodes of bleeding and apply local pressure if indicated. Expect oozing from IV sites.

Maternal/child: Pregnancy Category C. Has resulted in hemorrhage leading to spontaneous abortions in rabbits. Safety for use in pregnancy, lactation, and children not established.

Elderly: Note Indications and Precautions. ▪ May have poorer prognosis following AMI and pre-existing conditions that may increase risk of intracranial bleeding. Select patients carefully to maximize benefits.

DRUG/LAB INTERACTIONS

Interaction of reteplase with other cardioactive drugs has not been studied. ▪ Use caution with drugs that may alter platelet function (e.g., abciximab [ReoPro], aspirin, dipyridamole [Persantine], NSAIDs [e.g., indomethacin], phenylbutazone [Butazolidin]). Risk of bleeding will be increased if used concomitantly. ▪ Risk of bleeding with concomitant use of heparin and vitamin K antagonists (e.g., warfarin

[Coumadin]) is markedly increased. ■ Coagulation tests will be unreliable; specific procedures can be used; notify the lab of reteplase use.

SIDE EFFECTS

Bleeding is most common: internal (GI tract, GU tract, intracranial, respiratory, or retroperitoneal sites), epistaxis, gingival, and superficial or surface bleeding (venous cutdowns, arterial punctures, sites of recent surgical intervention). Reperfusion arrhythmias are common; other serious arrhythmias may occur. A few allergic reactions, as well as fever, hypotension, nausea, and vomiting, have occurred. Cholesterol embolism has been reported and may be fatal. Clinical S/S may include acute renal failure, gangrenous digits, hypertension, infarctions (e.g., bowel, cerebral, myocardial, or spinal cord), pancreatitis, "purple toe" syndrome, renal artery occlusion.

ANTIDOTE

Notify physician of all side effects. Note even the minutest bleeding tendency. Oozing at IV sites is expected. Control minor bleeding by local pressure. For severe bleeding in a critical location, discontinue second dose of reteplase if it has not been given and any heparin therapy immediately. Whole blood, packed red blood cells, cryoprecipitate, fresh-frozen plasma, platelets, desmopressin, tranexamic acid, and aminocaproic acid may all be indicated. Topical preparations of aminocaproic acid may stop minor bleeding. Consider protamine if heparin has been used. Treat bradycarcia with atropine, reperfusion arrhythmias with lidocaine or procainamide; VT or VF may require cardioversion. Treat minor allergic reactions symptomatically. Discontinue drug and treat anaphylaxis as indicated; resuscitate as necessary. Discontinue therapy if any symptoms of cholesterol embolism occur.

RH$_O$ (D) IMMUNE GLOBULIN INTRAVENOUS (HUMAN)

Immunizing agent (passive)
Platelet count stimulator

Rh$_o$ (D)-IGIV, WinRho SD

pH 6.5 to 7.6

USUAL DOSE

Treatment of immune thrombocytopenic purpura (ITP): Adults and children: 250 IU (50 mcg)/kg of body weight as the initial dose. May be given as a single dose or divided in two and given on two consecutive days. A maintenance dose of 125 to 300 IU (25 to 60 mcg)/kg may be given. Dose and frequency based on patients clinical response (e.g., RBC, hemoglobin, reticulocyte levels, and platelet counts). Note Dose adjustments.

Pregnancy, pre-delivery: 1,500 IU (300 mcg) at 28 weeks gestation. If administered early in the pregnancy, it should be repeated at 12-week intervals to maintain an adequate level of passively acquired anti-Rh.

Pregnancy, post-delivery: 600 IU (120 mcg) as soon as possible after delivery of a confirmed Rh$_o$ (D) positive baby. Usually given no later than 72 hours post-delivery. If the Rh status of the infant is unknown at 72 hours, administer to the mother at that time. Should be given as soon as possible up to 28 days after delivery.

Post-abortion, amniocentesis (after 34 weeks' gestation), or any other manipulation late in pregnancy (after 34 weeks' gestation): 600 IU (120 mcg) immediately after abortion or procedure associated with increased risk of Rh isoimmunization. Must be given within 72 hours.

Post-amniocentesis before 34 weeks' gestation or after chorionic villus sampling: 1,500 IU (300 mcg) immediately after the procedure. Repeat every 12 weeks during the pregnancy.

Threatened abortion: 1,500 IU (300 mcg) as soon as possible.

Transfusion: Administer within 72 hours after exposure for treatment of incompatible blood transfusions or massive fetal hemorrhage. Give up to 3,000 mcg every 8 hours until the total dose is administered. Total dose for Rh+ blood is 45 IU (9 mcg)/ml of blood administered. Total dose for Rh+ red cells is 90 IU (18 mcg)/ml of red cells administered.

PEDIATRIC DOSE
Treatment of ITP: See Usual dose and Dose adjustments.

DOSE ADJUSTMENTS
Treatment of ITP: Adults and children: If the hemoglobin level is less than 10 Gm/dl, reduce the initial dose to 125 to 200 IU (25 to 40 mcg)/kg to minimize the risk of increasing the severity of anemia in the patient.

Suppression of Rh isoimmunization: A large fetomaternal hemorrhage may cause an incorrect evaluation by standard tests of the amount of Rh_o(D)-IGIV required. Assess the amount of hemorrhage and adjust dose accordingly.

DILUTION
Each vial must be reconstituted with 2.5 ml of NS, provided by manufacturer. Use as many vials as are required to achieve desired dose. Available in 600 IU and 1,500 IU vials. After reconstitution 600 IU vial delivers 240 IU (48 mcg)/ml and 1,500 IU vial delivers 600 IU (120 mcg)/ml. 5 IU equals 1 mcg.

Storage: Store unopened vials in refrigerator. Note expiration date. Do not freeze. Reconstituted vials can be stored in the refrigerator but must be used within 4 hours of reconstitution.

INCOMPATIBLE WITH
Specific information not available. Manufacturer states, "should not be administered with other products." Dilute only with NS.

RATE OF ADMINISTRATION
A single dose as an IV injection over 3 to 5 minutes.

ACTIONS
A specialty immunoglobulin containing human plasma protein fraction, consisting primarily of IgG. A 1,500 IU vial contains 300 mcg of anti-Rh_o(D), which can effectively suppress the immunizing potential of approximately 17 ml of Rh_o(D)-positive blood cells, and, in addition, contains 25 to 40 mg of nonspecific gammaglobulin. Pooled from source plasma selected for high titers of Rh_o(D) antibody. Purified and standardized by several specific methods (e.g., solvent-detergent viral inactivation process to decrease the possibility of transmission of bloodborne pathogens [e.g., HIV, hepatitis]). Similar to native IgG that normally circulates in human plasma and has a similar half-life. Crosses the blood-brain barrier.

INDICATIONS AND USES

To increase platelet count and prevent excessive hemorrhage in non-splenectomized Rh$_o$(D)-positive children with acute or chronic immune thrombocytopenic purpura (ITP), adults with chronic ITP, or children and adults with ITP secondary to HIV infection. ■ Suppression of Rh isoimmunization in nonsensitized Rh$_o$(D)-negative women during the normal course of pregnancy, within 72 hours after spontaneous or induced abortions, amniocentesis, chorionic villus sampling, ruptured tubal pregnancy, abdominal trauma or transplacental hemorrhage, unless the blood type of the fetus or father is known to be Rh$_o$(D)-negative. ■ Suppression of Rh isoimmunization in Rh$_o$(D)-negative female children and female adults in their childbearing years transfused with Rh$_o$(D)-positive red blood cells or blood components containing Rh$_o$(D)-positive red blood cells.

CONTRAINDICATIONS

All uses: History of a prior severe hypersensitivity reaction to human immune globulin preparations; patient with isolated IgA deficiency or preexisting IgA antibodies.

Treatment of ITP: Not recommended for use in Rh$_o$(D)-negative or splenectomized individuals.

Suppression of Rh isoimmunization: ■ For suppression of Rh isoimmunization in the mother. *DO NOT ADMINISTER TO THE INFANT.* Not recommended for use in Rh$_o$(D)-negative individuals shown to be Rh immunized by standard screening tests.

PRECAUTIONS

Confirm vial label—must state for IV or IV/IM use; several similar products are for IM use only (e.g., RhoGam). ■ IV route required for ITP. ■ If the hemoglobin level is less than 8 Gm/dl, use with extreme caution; may increase severity of anemia. ■ If a large fetomaternal hemorrhage occurs late in pregnancy or after delivery Rh$_o$(D) IGIV should be administered in sufficient doses if there is any doubt about the mother's blood type.

Monitor: Treatment of ITP: Obtain baseline RBC, hemoglobin, reticulocyte levels, and platelet counts. Monitor during therapy to determine clinical response. Given to Rh$_o$ (D)-positive patients, in this situation, interaction with RBC usually cause some degree of RBC hemolysis; observe carefully. *Pregnancy:* Maintain accurate records of Rh factor and Rh$_o$ (D)-IGIV. ■ Obtain CBC and other appropriate lab work based on procedure or situation. ■ Monitor vitals signs if indicated. *All Uses:* Note Precautions.

Patient education: ITP: May cause a considerable drop in hemoglobin; follow-up testing important. ■ Report feelings of dizziness, tiredness, weakness.

Maternal/child: Pregnancy Category C: use only if clearly needed. ■ Specific information not available on safety during lactation. ■ For the suppression of Rh isoimmunization in the mother; do not administer to the infant.

Elderly: No specific information available.

DRUG/LAB INTERACTIONS

Interaction with other drugs has not been evaluated.

SIDE EFFECTS
ITP: Destruction of $Rh_o(D)$ red cells resulting in decreased hemoglobin (range was 0.4 to 6.1 Gm/dl).

Prophylaxis in pregnancy: Only 26 out of 9,905 women had treatment failures resulting in development of $Rh_o(D)$ antibodies. *All uses:* Chills, discomfort at the injection site, fever, and headache occur most frequently.

ANTIDOTE
Keep physician informed of side effects; may require symptomatic treatment. *ITP:* Treatment may have to be discontinued if drop in hemoglobin too severe. Transfusion may be required.

RIFAMPIN

**Antibacterial
(Antituberculosis)**

Rifadin

pH 7.8 to 8.8

USUAL DOSE
Tuberculosis: 600 mg daily as a single dose. Prescribed concurrently with at least one other antituberculin drug (e.g., ethambutol [Myambutol], isoniazid, pyrazinamide, or streptomycin).

Meningococcal carriers: 600 mg daily as a single dose for 4 days or 600 mg every 12 hours for 2 days. In all situations use oral dose form as soon as practical.

PEDIATRIC DOSE
Tuberculosis: 10 to 20 mg/kg of body weight daily as a single dose. Do not exceed 600 mg. See information in adult dose.

NEONATAL DOSE
Meningococcal carriers: Under 1 month of age: 5 mg/kg every 12 hr for 2 days.

Over 1 month of age: 10 mg/kg every 12 hr for 2 days.

DOSE ADJUSTMENTS
Dose reduction to 10 mg/kg/day may be required in the debilitated or elderly. ■ Reduced dose required in impaired hepatic function. ■ No dose adjustment is necessary in impaired renal function; serum concentrations do not change. ■ Note Drug/lab interactions.

DILUTION
Each 600 mg vial must be initially diluted in 10 ml of sterile water for injection (60 mg/ml). Swirl gently to dissolve. Withdraw desired dose and further dilute in 500 ml (preferred) or 100 ml of D5W. If dextrose is contraindicated, NS may be used but will slightly decrease the stability of the solution. 100 ml dilution used only in selected situations.

Storage: Use solution diluted in D5W within 4 hours; solution diluted in NS stable for 24 hours. Protect from light prior to dilution.

INCOMPATIBLE WITH
Diltiazem (Cardizem), minocycline (Minocin), sodium lactate.

RATE OF ADMINISTRATION

A single dose equally distributed as an infusion over 3 hours. In selected situations a single dose diluted in 100 ml may be administered over 30 minutes.

ACTIONS

A semisynthetic antituberculosis antibiotic. Has a bactericidal or bacteriostatic action that is effective in susceptible cells during cell division or at the resting stage. Onset of peak plasma levels is prompt, and average levels are maintained for 8 to 12 hours based on dose. Rapidly absorbed throughout the body and present in many organs and body fluids including CSF. Metabolized in the liver and excreted in bile. Crosses the placental barrier. Secreted in breast milk.

INDICATIONS AND USES

Treatment or retreatment of tuberculosis when the drug cannot be taken by mouth. ■ Treatment of asymptomatic carriers of *Neisseria* meningitis. Not indicated for treatment of meningococcal infection because of rapid emergence of resistant meningococci.

CONTRAINDICATIONS

Hypersensitivity to any rifamycins; individuals with liver disease are at higher risk for complications.

PRECAUTIONS

For IV use only. Do not administer IM or SC. ■ Risk of liver damage is markedly increased if impaired liver function is present. Hepatotoxicity, hepatic encephalopathy, and death associated with jaundice have occurred in patients with liver disease and when rifampin is given with other hepatotoxic agents (e.g., isoniazid, halothane). Discontinue one or both drugs for signs of hepatocellular damage. ■ Susceptibility tests required before use as treatment for asymptomatic carriers of *Neisseria* meningitis and if positive cultures persist after use. ■ May exacerbate porphyria. ■ Urine, feces, saliva, sputum, sweat, and tears may be colored red-orange. Soft contact lenses may be permanently stained. CSF may be light yellow. ■ Reduced biliary excretion of contrast media for gallbladder studies may occur.

Monitor: Obtain a complete blood count, bilirubin level, and transaminase level prior to initiating rifampin. Draw a blood sample for base line chemistries. ■ Monitor ALT (SGPT) and AST (SGOT) prior to therapy and every 2 to 3 weeks during therapy. ■ Notify physician immediately if flu-like symptoms develop; may be due to hepatotoxicity. ■ Thrombocytopenia has occurred. Reversible if rifampin is discontinued as soon as purpura occurs. Cerebral hemorrhage has occurred when rifampin has been continued or resumed after the appearance of purpura. Contact physician immediately if purpura occurs. ■ Confirm patency of IV; avoid extravasation. Restart IV at a new site for any signs of inflammation or irritation. ■ Do all lab tests and affected radiology studies before daily dose of medication. ■ Note Drug/lab interactions.

Patient education: Use of nonhormonal contraceptives recommended. ■ Avoid use of alcohol or other hepatotoxic agents (e.g., acetamenaphen [Anacin-3, Tylenol], NSAIDs [ibuprofen (Motrin)], phenothiazines [e.g., promethazine (Phenergan)], some antineoplastic agents, sulfonamides). ■ May cause reddish orange discoloration of feces, saliva, sputum, sweat, urine, and tears. ■ May discolor soft contact lenses.

Maternal/child: Has teratogenic potential. Safety for use during pregnancy not established. Benefit must outweigh risk. See literature for best combinations with least known risk. ■ Administration during the last few weeks of pregnancy may cause postnatal hemorrhages in mother and infant; treatment with vitamin K may be required. ■ Closely monitor neonates of rifampin-treated mothers for adverse effects. ■ Discontinue breast feeding if mother requires treatment.

Elderly: Risk of hepatitis increased after age 50. ■ Note Dose adjustments.

DRUG/LAB INTERACTIONS

Hepatotoxicity, hepatic encephalopathy, and death associated with jaundice have occurred when rifampin is given with other hepatotoxic agents (e.g., isoniazid, halothane). Discontinue one or both drugs for signs of hepatocellular damage. ■ Inhibits activity and decreases plasma levels of acetaminophen (Tylenol), analgesics (e.g., narcotics), barbiturates (e.g., phenobarbital), benzodiazepines (e.g., diazepam [Valium]), beta-blockers (e.g., propranolol [Inderal]), chloramphenicol, clofibrate (Atromid-S), corticosteroids (e.g., prednisone), cyclosporine (Sandimmune), dapsone, digoxin and digitoxin, disopyramide (Norpace), estrogens, haloperidol (Haldol), hydantoins (e.g., phenytoin [Dilantin]), methadone, mexiletine (Mexitil), oral antidiabetics (tolbutamide), oral anticoagulants (warfarin [Coumadin]), oral contraceptives, quinidine, tacrolimus (Prograf), theophyllines (e.g., aminophylline), tocainide (Tonocard), verapamil (Isoptin). Increased doses of these drugs may be required. Monitor carefully; obtain prothrombin daily when used with oral anticoagulants (e.g., warfarin); use of nonhormonal contraceptives recommended during rifampin therapy; and diabetes may be more difficult to control. ■ Treatment failure of ketoconazole (Nizoral) or rifampin may occur when given concomitantly. ■ May reduce effectiveness of zidovudine (AZT). Rifampin increases clearance and reduces serum levels of zidovudine. ■ Inhibited by clofazimine (Lamprene). Decreases rate of absorption and delays peak plasma levels of rifampin. ■ Potentiated by probenecid. ■ May cause hypertension with enalapril (Vasotec). ■ Para-aminosalicylic acid (PAS) will decrease serum levels of rifampin. Drugs should be taken at least 8 hours apart. ■ Pyrazinamide may also reduce rifampin serum levels. ■ May cause an early rise in bilirubin during initial days of treatment; should subside. Throughout treatment transient abnormalities in liver function tests will occur. ■ Therapeutic levels inhibit assays of serum folate and vitamin B_{12}.

SIDE EFFECTS

Average dose: Anaphylaxis may occur even with repeat doses. Abnormal liver function tests, anorexia, ataxia, behavioral changes, conjunctivitis (exudative), cramps, diarrhea, dizziness, edema of face and extremities, epigastric distress, eosinophilia, fatigue, flushing, flu-like symptoms (e.g., chills, fever, headache, malaise, muscle and bone pain), gas, heartburn, hematuria, hemolytic anemia, hepatic reactions, hepatitis, hypotension, leukopenia, menstrual disturbances, mental confusion, myopathy (rare), muscle weakness, nausea, numbness (generalized), pain in extremities, purpura, pruritus, rash, renal failure (acute), shortness of breath, sore mouth and tongue, thrombocytopenia, urticaria, visual disturbances, vomiting, wheezing.

Overdose: Bilirubin levels increase rapidly; brown-red discoloration of feces, skin, sweat, tears, and urine is proportional to amount of overdose; lethargy, nausea, and vomiting are immediate; liver enlargement and tenderness; unconsciousness.

ANTIDOTE

With increasing severity of any side effect, alterations in liver function tests, flu-like symptoms, purpura, thrombocytopenia, or symptoms of overdose, discontinue the drug and notify the physician immediately. Forced diuresis will promote excretion. Bile drainage may be indicated in the presence of seriously impaired hepatic function lasting more than 24 to 48 hours. Hemodialysis may be useful. Treat anaphylaxis and resuscitate as necessary.

RITODRINE HYDROCHLORIDE

Uterine relaxant
(Tocolytic)

Yutopar

pH 4.8 to 5.5

USUAL DOSE

Begin with 0.05 mg/min (0.17 ml/min or 10 gtt/min). Gradually increase by 0.05 mg/min (0.17 ml/min or 10 gtt/min) every 10 minutes until desired result obtained or until maternal heart rate reaches 130 beats per minute. Usual effective dose is 0.15 to 0.35 mg/min. Continue infusion for at least 12 hours after contractions cease, then begin oral ritodrine. Administer first oral dose 30 minutes before IV is discontinued. IV dosing may be repeated if preterm labor recurs. Note Precautions/Monitor.

DOSE ADJUSTMENTS

Note Drug/lab interactions.

DILUTION

Each 150 mg must be diluted in 500 ml of D5W. NS, Ringer's solution, or Hartmann's solution may increase the risk of pulmonary edema and should be used only when dextrose is not appropriate (e.g., diabetes mellitus). Concentration will be 0.33 mg/ml. A more concentrated solution may be prepared if fluid restriction is required. Do not use if solution discolored or contains particulate matter or precipitate.

Storage: Store below 40° C. Discard solution after 48 hours.

INCOMPATIBLE WITH

Should be considered incompatible in solution with any other drug because of specific use, accurate rate calculation, and potential for additive toxicity.

RATE OF ADMINISTRATION

Specific instructions included under Usual dose. Usually effective between 0.15 and 0.35 mg/min (0.50 to 1.17 ml/min or 30 to 70 gtt/min). Use of a microdrip chamber (60 gtt/ml) required; infusion pump preferred. Estimates based on suggested dilution. Adjust if more or less diluent is used. Highly individualized based on patient's response and side effects.

ACTIONS

A beta-adrenergic receptor agonist (primarily B_2) that acts to inhibit contractility of uterine smooth muscle. May cause an increase in heart rate, blood glucose, insulin, and free fatty acids and a widening of the pulse pressure. Onset of action is prompt and lasts about 2 hours. Crosses the placental barrier. Metabolized in the liver and excreted in the urine.

INDICATIONS AND USES
To arrest preterm labor in suitable patients.

CONTRAINDICATIONS
Before the twentieth week of pregnancy; conditions during pregnancy that are hazardous to the mother or infant (e.g., antepartum hemorrhage, cardiac disease [maternal], chorioamnionitis, diabetes mellitus [uncontrolled], eclampsia [or severe preeclampsia]), hypersensitivity to ritodrine or its components, hyperthyroidism (maternal), intrauterine fetal death, pulmonary hypertension, preexisting maternal medical conditions adversely affected by beta-mimetic drugs (bronchial asthma treated with beta-mimetics or steroids, cardiac arrhythmias with tachycardia or digitalis intoxication, hypovolemia, hypertension [uncontrolled], and pheochromocytoma).

PRECAUTIONS
Most effective if begun as soon as diagnosis of preterm labor established and contraindications are ruled out. ■ Use extreme caution if indicated in a mother with mild to moderate preeclampsia, hypertension, or diabetes. ■ May contain bisulfites; use caution in patients with allergies.
Monitor: Obtain maternal base line ECG to rule out heart disease. ■ Monitor uterine contractions, maternal heart rate, blood pressure, and fetal heart rate every 5 minutes until stable, every 15 to 30 minutes thereafter until infusion discontinued. ■ Maintain adequate hydration, but avoid fluid overload and observe for signs of pulmonary edema (may unmask unknown cardiac disease). Respiratory rate above 20 or pulse rate sustained at 140 or above may indicate onset of pulmonary edema. ■ Maintain patient in left lateral position during infusion to minimize hypotension. ■ Evaluate fetal maturity (sonography). ■ Maternal hyperglycemia must be monitored and treated if indicated. May precipitate reactive hypoglycemia in the infant. ■ Monitor insulin, glucose, and electrolyte levels in selected patients or long-term therapy. Normal levels will be altered. ■ Note Drug/lab interactions.

DRUG/LAB INTERACTIONS
Corticosteroids concomitantly may precipitate pulmonary edema. ■ Inhibited by beta-adrenergic blockers (e.g., propranolol [Inderal]). ■ Potentiated by other sympathomimetic amines (e.g., epinephrine [Adrenalin], dopamine [Intropin]). Effects may be additive. Do not administer concurrently; allow adequate time intervals before initiating therapy with any sympathomimetic drug. ■ Cardiovascular effects (cardiac arrhythmias, hypotension) potentiated by diazoxide (Hyperstat IV), magnesium sulfate, meperidine (Demerol), and general anesthetics. ■ Increased hypertension may occur with atropine.

SIDE EFFECTS
Anaphylaxis, anxiety, cardiac arrhythmias, chest pain, constipation, decreased diastolic pressure, diarrhea, epigastric distress, elevated systolic pressure, erythema, glycosuria, headache, hemolytic icterus, hyperventilation, ileus, jitteriness, lactic acidosis, malaise, nausea, nervousness, palpitations, pulmonary edema, pulse pressure widened, restlessness, tachycardia, tightness of the chest, tremor, vomiting.

ANTIDOTE

Keep physician informed of all side effects. Most side effects are expected and will be tolerated or treated symptomatically (note Drug/lab interactions). Marked hypotension, tachycardia, cardiac arrhythmias, and other signs of beta-adrenergic stimulation will require discontinuation of the drug. Uterine relaxation may persist for several hours, and oral therapy may be considered. A beta-blocker (propranolol [Inderal]) may be required. Discontinue drug and treat anaphylaxis as indicated. At first signs of fluid overload or pulmonary edema, notify physician immediately and treat as indicated.

RITUXIMAB

Recombinant monoclonal antibody
Antineoplastic

Rituxan   pH 6.5

USUAL DOSE

Premedication: Acetaminophen (Tylenol) and diphenhydramine (Benadryl) should be considered as premedication before each dose to prevent or attenuate severe hypersensitivity reactions.

CD20 positive, B-cell non-Hodgkin's lymphoma: 375 mg/M^2 as an IV infusion once each week for four doses (days 1, 8, 15, and 22). Note Drug/lab interactions.

PEDIATRIC DOSE

Safety and effectiveness for use in children not established.

DOSE ADJUSTMENTS

No dose adjustments recommended. Note Rate of administration.

DILUTION

Each single dose must be further diluted to a final concentration of 1 to 4 mg/ml with NS or D5W. 500 mg (50 ml) in 450 ml will yield 1mg/ml; 500 mg (50 ml) in 75 ml will yield 4 mg/ml. Gently invert to mix solution. Discard any unused portion left in vial. No incompatibilities with polyvinylchloride or polyethylene bags have been observed.

Storage: Refrigerate vials at 2° to 8° C (36° to 46° F) and protect from light. Do not use beyond expiration date. Diluted solutions may be refrigerated for 24 hours and are stable at room temperature for an additional 12 hours.

INCOMPATIBLE WITH

Manufacturer states "rituximab should not be mixed or diluted with other drugs."

RATE OF ADMINISTRATION

Must be given as an infusion. *Do not administer as an IV push or bolus.* Hypersensitivity reactions are a a common occurrence and may be prevented or lessened with premedication and a reduced rate of infusion.

First infusion: Begin with an initial rate of 50 mg/hr (at this rate a 500 mg dose would be infused over 10 hours). If no discomfort or adverse effects occur, may be gradually increased by 50 mg/hr increments at 30 minute intervals to a maximum rate of 400 mg/hr. At any time that discomfort or adverse effects occur, reduce the rate of infusion. Discontinue the infusion for severe reactions and treat as indicated (see Antidote). When symptoms have completely resolved, the infusion can be restarted at half the previous rate.

Subsequent infusions: If no discomfort or adverse effects occurred with the first infusion, subsequent infusions may begin with an initial rate of 100 mg/hr and increased by 100 mg/hr increments at 30 minute intervals to a maximum rate of 400 mg/hr. Note all precautionary measures under first infusion.

ACTIONS

An antineoplastic agent. A chimeric murine/humanized $(Ig)G_1$ monoclonal antibody produced by recombinant DNA technology. Designed to bind to the CD20 antigen found on the surface of normal and malignant B lymphocytes. Results in a rapid and sustained depletion (cytotoxity) of circulating and tissue-based B cells. Depletion was sustained for 6 to 9 months posttreatment in 83% of patients. B-cell recovery begins at appoximately 6 months, and most levels return to normal by 12 months following completion of treatment. May sensitize drug-resistant human B-cell lymphoma cell lines to cytotoxic chemotherapy. Detected in serum for 3 to 6 months after completion of therapy. Average serum half-life was 59.8 hours (range 11.1 to 104.6) after the first infusion and 174 hours (range 26 to 442 hours) after the fourth infusion. Wide range may reflect variable tumor burdens and decreasing numbers of CD20 positive B-cells with repeated infusions. Peak and trough serum levels were inversely correlated with baseline values for the number of circulating CD20 positive B-cells and measures of disease burden. IgG, antibodies may cross the placental barrier and may be secreted in breast milk.

INDICATIONS AND USES

Treatment of patients with relapsed or refractory low-grade or follicular CD20 positive B-cell non-Hodgkin's lymphoma.

CONTRAINDICATIONS

Known hypersensitivity or anaphylactic reactions to murine proteins, rituximab, or any of its components.

PRECAUTIONS

May be given on an outpatient basis. ■ Hypersensitivity reactions (e.g., hypotension, bronchospasm, and angioedema) have occurred, especially with the first infusion. May respond to a decrease in rate of infusion, but emergency equipment, oxygen, and drugs (including epinephrine, antihistamines, and corticosteroids) must be available for immediate use. ■ Use caution in patients who either have or develop HAMA/HACA titers; may have allergic reactions when treated with rituximab or other murine or chimeric monoclonal antibodies. ■ Safety of immunization with vaccines, particularly live viral vaccines, and the ability of the patient to respond to vaccines following rituximab therapy has not been studied. ■ Experience with patients who have received more than one course of rituxmab is limited. Reporting of adverse events were similar. ■ Note Rate of administration and Drug/lab interactions.

Monitor: Obtain baseline CBC and platelet count and repeat at regular intervals. Repeat more frequently in patients who develop cytopenias (e.g., leukopenia, neutropenia, thrombocytopenia). ▪ Observe patient continuously for symptoms of allergic reactions; more frequent during the first infusion, but can occur at any time. ▪ Monitor HR and BP frequently. ▪ ECG monitoring required during and in the immediate posttreatment period in patients with preexisting cardiac conditions and in any patient who develops or has previously developed a clinically significant arrhythmia during treatment. ▪ Observe closely for signs of infection. Prophylactic antibiotics may be indicated pending results of C/S in a febrile neutropenic patient. ▪ Use prophylactic antimetics to reduce nausea and vomiting and increase patient comfort. ▪ Note Premedication in Usual dose, Rate of administration, and Drug/lab interactions.

Patient education: Avoid pregnancy; nonhormonal birth control recommended. ▪ Review monitoring requirements and potential side effects before therapy. ▪ Report any unusual or unexpected symptoms or side effects promptly. ▪ See Appendix D, p. 900.

Maternal/child: Category C: Avoid pregnancy; could potentially cause fetal B-cell depletion. Use only if clearly needed. ▪ Discontinue nursing until circulating drug levels are no longer detectable. ▪ Safety and effectiveness in children not established.

Elderly: Specific information not available. Use caution and observe closely.

DRUG/LAB INTERACTIONS

Transient hyoptension may occur during rituximab infusion; consider withholding antihypertensive medications 12 hours before rituximab infusion. ▪ No specific drug interaction studies have been done to this date. ▪ Pharmacokinetics of rituximab remained similar to rituximab alone when given in combination with CHOP chemotherapy (cyclophosphamide, doxorubicin, vincristine, prednisone).

SIDE EFFECTS

Hypersensitivity or infusion-related side effects generally occur within 30 minutes to 2 hours of beginning of first infusion. Fever and chills are most common. Other frequent symptoms include: abdominal pain, angioedema (sensation of tongue or throat swelling), asthenia, bronchospasm, dizziness, dyspnea, fatigue, flushing, headache, hypotension, myalgia, nausea, pain at disease sites, pruritus, rash, rhinitis, throat irritation, urticaria, and vomiting. Cardiac arrhythmias (e.g., supraventricular and ventricular tachycardia), anemia, leukopenia, neutropenia, and thrombocytopenia have occurred in some patients. In addition to the above, anorexia, depression, night sweats, peripheral edema, respiratory symptoms, and tachycardia were reported in patients who had been retreated.

ANTIDOTE

Keep physician informed of all side effects. Most will be treated symptomatically as indicated. Hypersensitivity or infusion-related side effects generally resolve with slowing or interruption of the rituximab infusion and with supportive care (IV saline, diphenhydramine, and acetaminophen). Most patients who have had non–life-threatening reactions have been able to complete the full course of therapy. Discontinue the infusion immediately for any life-threatening side effect (e.g., bronchospasm, severe cardiac arrhythmias, severe hypotension). Treat anaphylaxis with oxygen, antihistamines (diphenhydramine), epinephrine, and corticosteroids. Maintain a patent airway. Treat arrhythmias if indicated and monitor ECG until recovery and with subsequent doses. Treat hypotension with IV fluids, Trendelenburg position, and, if necessary, vasopressors (e.g., norepinephrine [Levophed], dopamine [Intropin]). Resuscitate if indicated.

ROCURONIUM BROMIDE

Neuromuscular blocking agent
(Nondepolarizing)
Anesthesia adjunct

Zemuron   pH 4.0

USUAL DOSE

Must be individualized, depending on previous drugs administered and degree and length of muscle relaxation required. Should be used with adequate anesthesia and after unconsciousness induced. A peripheral nerve stimulator should be used to measure neuromuscular function during administration in order to monitor drug effect, determine the need for additional doses, and confirm recovery from neuromuscular block. See Precautions and Drug/lab interactions.

Rapid sequence intubation: 0.6 to 1.2 mg/kg of body weight as an initial dose. Patient should be appropriately premedicated and adequately anesthetized. Should provide excellent or good intubating conditions within 2 minutes.

Tracheal intubation: 0.6 mg/kg regardless of anesthetic technique as an initial dose. Neuromuscular block sufficient for intubation usually achieved in 2 minutes (range 0.4 to 6 minutes), maximum blockade within 3 minutes, and provides 15 to 85 minutes (average 31) of clinical relaxation. A 0.45 mg/kg dose may be used. Intubation usually achieved in 2 minutes (adequate block range 0.8 to 6.2 minutes), maximum blockade within 4 minutes, and provides 12 to 31 minutes (average 22) of clinical relaxation. With this lower dose, expect a more rapid time to 25% recovery (12 to 15 minutes). Larger bolus doses of 0.9 mg/kg or 1.2 mg/kg may be used in selected patients without adverse effects to the cardiovascular system. Maximum blockade occurs within 3 minutes, and provides 27 to 111 or 38 to 160 minutes of clinical relaxation (average 58 or 67 minutes).

Maintenance dose: 0.1, 0.15, and 0.2 mg/kg administered at 25% recovery will extend relaxation another 12 (range 2 to 31), 17 (range 6 to 50), and 24 (range 7 to 69) minutes. Should not be administered until recovery of neuromuscular function is evident. Repetitive dosing may produce a clinically insignificant cumulative effect. Usually given as a bolus, may be given as an infusion (see Rate of administration).

PEDIATRIC DOSE

0.6 mg/kg in children under halothane anesthesia as an initial dose. Intubation usually achieved in one minute, maximum blockade within 1 minute (range 0.5 to 3.3 minutes). Provides 24 to 68 minutes (average 41) of clinical relaxation in *infants 3 months to 1 year of age* and 17 to 41 minutes (average 27) of clinical relaxation in *children 1 to 12 years of age.*

Maintenance dose: 0.075 to 0.125 mg/kg administered at 25% recovery will extend relaxation for 7 to 10 minutes. Alternately, 0.012 mg/kg/min may be given as an infusion when twitch response returns to 10% of control. Adjust rate based on twitch response to peripheral nerve stimulation. Spontaneous recovery similar to adults in infants 3 months to 1 year, but more rapid in children 1 to 12 years.

DOSE ADJUSTMENTS

Initial dose (0.6 mg/kg) should be based on actual body weight in obese patients. ■ Reduced initial and maintenance doses may be required in presence of some inhalation anesthetics (e.g., isoflurane, enflurane) and with other drugs that prolong neuromuscular blockade (See Drug/lab interactions). ■ Reduced dose (especially maintenance) may be required in impaired renal or hepatic function. ■ Rapid sequence induction in patients with ascites requires up to 0.6 mg/kg; duration will be prolonged. ■ Reduced dose indicated in cachectic or debilitated patients, and those with neuromuscular diseases (e.g., myasthenia gravis) or carcinomatosis. ■ Patients with burns, cerebral palsy, disuse atrophy, denervation, or direct muscle trauma, may be resistant and require increased doses. ■ Chronic use of anticonvulsants may require increased doses. ■ Dose reduction not indicated in patients with reduced plasma cholinesterase activity. ■ Note Drug/lab interactions.

DILUTION

Direct IV: May be given undiluted or diluted in sterile water for injection.
Infusion: May be further diluted in NS, D5W, D5/NS, D5/LR. Diluting each 1 mg (0.1 ml) with 1 to 10 ml of solution yields 1 to 0.1 mg/ml.
Storage: Refrigerate vials (preferred); do not freeze. Vials stable at room temperature for up to 30 days. Use diluted solutions within 24 hours. Discard unused solution.

INCOMPATIBLE WITH

Alkaline solutions (e.g., barbiturates, phenytoin [Dilantin], sodium bicarbonate). Do not administer through the same needle.

RATE OF ADMINISTRATION

Peripheral nerve stimulator required; see Usual dose.
Direct IV: A single dose over 5 to 15 seconds as the initial or maintenance dose. Titrate to desired effect.
Infusion: 0.01 to 0.012 mg/kg/min as a maintenance dose after early evidence of spontaneous recovery from intubating dose. Because of rapid redistribution, if begun after more than 10% of recovery additional boluses may be required. Must be individualized. When desired level of neuromuscular block is achieved, usual rate is 0.004 to 0.016 mg/kg/min.
Pediatric infusion rate: 0.012 mg/kg/min. Note comments under adult infusion.

ACTIONS

A nondepolarizing neuromuscular blocking agent with a rapid to intermediate onset of action depending on dose. Causes skeletal muscle relaxation and paralysis by competing for cholinergic receptors at the motor end-plate. Action is antagonized by acetylcholinesterase inhibitors (e.g., neostigmine and edrophonium). Excellent to good intubating conditions are dose dependent and more rapid than with other similar agents. Rapid distribution half-life is 1 to 2 minutes and slower distribution half-life is 14 to 18 minutes. Elimination half-life is 1.4 hrs. Somewhat bound to plasma protein (30%). Has minimal impact on the cardiovascular system, although cases of tachycardia have been reported. May cause some histamine release, usually not clinically significant. Metabolized in the liver and excreted in bile and urine. Crosses placental barrier.

INDICATIONS AND USES

Adjunct to general anesthesia to facilitate rapid sequence and routine tracheal intubation and to provide skeletal muscle relaxation during surgery or mechanical ventilation.

CONTRAINDICATIONS

Known hypersensitivity to rocuronium. Not recommended for rapid-sequence induction in cesarean section.

PRECAUTIONS

For IV use only. ■ Administered only by or under the direct observation of the anesthesiologist. ■ Time of onset is similar but duration of action is variable in impaired renal function and prolonged 1.5 times in impaired hepatic function; use with caution. ■ May cause increased pulmonary vascular resistance; use caution in patients with pulmonary hypertension or valvular heart disease. ■ Use caution and allow time for drug to achieve onset of effects in altered circulation time (e.g., cardiovascular disease, advanced age). ■ Myasthenia gravis and other neuromuscular diseases increase sensitivity to drug. May cause critical reactions; test dose may be indicated. ■ Has not been studied for long-term use in the ICU. Tolerance to rocuronium may develop. Continuous use of a peripheral nerve stimulator mandatory if employed in this situation. Note Usual dose and Dose adjustments. May cause prolonged paralysis or skeletal muscle weakness during weaning. ■ Flush eyes with water for at least 10 minutes for accidental contact.

Monitor: This drug produces apnea. Controlled artificial ventilation with oxygen must be continuous and under direct observation at all times. Maintain a patent airway. Neostigmine (Prostigmin) or edrophonium (Enlon, Tensilon) and atropine must be available. ■ Monitor all vital organ functions until adequate recovery. ■ Use a peripheral nerve stimulator to monitor response to recuronium, avoid overdose, monitor need for additional relaxant, and monitor adequacy of spontaneous recovery or antagonism. ■ Patient may be conscious and completely unsable to communicate by any means. Must be used with adequate anesthesia or sedation, has no analgesic properties. ■ Action may be altered by dehydration, electrolyte imbalance, body temperatures, and acid-base imbalance; monitor closely. ■ Monitor for early signs of malignant hyperthermia; has not occurred but is a possibility. ■ Note Drug/lab interactions. ■ If extravasation occurs, discontinue infusion and use another vein.

Maternal/child: Pregnancy Category B: benefits must justify potential risk to fetus. No teratogenic effects noted in rats. ■ (See Contraindications). ■ Safety for use during lactation and in infants under 3 months of age not established. ■ May cause a transient increase in heart rate after intubation in children who do not receive atropine before induction.

Elderly: Effects not significantly different from other adults. Slightly prolonged clinical duration may occur. Consider slower circulation time in cardiovascular disease, advanced age, edematous states, and impaired liver function.

DRUG/LAB INTERACTIONS

Duration of action extended and recovery prolonged by inhalation anesthetics (e.g., enflurane, isoflurane, halothane). Effects less if rocuronium administered first, but reduced dose (especially maintenance doses) still required. ▪ Patients receiving chronic anticonvulsants (e.g., carbamazapine [Tegretol], phenytoin [Dilantin]), theophyllines (e.g., aminophylline), or phenyelphrine (Neo-Synephrine) may be resistant to nondepolarizing muscle relaxants and require higher doses. ▪ Prolongation of neuromuscular block may occur with many antibiotics (e.g., aminoglycosides [e.g., gentamicin (Garamycin), tobramycin (Nebcin)]), bacitracin, colistin [Coly Mycin S], colistimethate [Coly Mycin M], polymixin-B [Aerosporin], tetracycline, vancomycin); magnesium salts, lithium, procainamide, quinidine, and other nondepolarizing muscle relaxants. Reduced doses of rocuronium may be required. ▪ May cause recurrent paralysis with quinidine. ▪ Succinycholine (Anectine) must show signs of wearing off before rocuronium is given. Use before succinycholine to reduce side effects has not been studied.

SIDE EFFECTS

Occurred in less than 1% of patients. Abnormal electrocardiogram, arrhythmia (e.g., tachycardia) bronchospasm, hiccup, hyper- or hypotension (transient), injection site edema, nausea, pruritus, rash, rhonchi, wheezing.

Overdose: Prolonged action resulting in skeletal muscle weakness to prolonged skeletal muscle paralysis with respiratory insufficiency or apnea is possible. Airway closure caused by relaxation of epiglottis, pharynx, and tongue muscles can occur.

ANTIDOTE

All side effects resulting from overdose or prolonged action can be medical emergencies. Controlled ventilation and oxygen must be continuous. Treat symptomatically and monitor continuously. Once spontaneous recovery has reached 25%, the neuromuscular block produced by rocuronium is readily reversed by neostigmine (Prostigmin [usual dose, 0.04 mg/kg (range 0.01 to 0.09)]) or edrophonium (Enlon, Tensilon [usual dose 0.5 mg/kg (range 0.3 to 1)]). Administer atropine before neostigmine or edrophonium. Reversal to 75% recovery usually occurs within 15 minutes. Rarely, additional antagonists may be required.

SAMARIUM SM 153 LEXIDRONAM INJECTION

Radiopharmaceutical
Bisphosphonate

Quadramet, SM 153

pH 7.0 to 8.5

USUAL DOSE

Measured by a suitable radioactivity calibration system (e.g., radioisotope dose calibrator) immediately before use by the radiation oncologist. Significant radioactivity; verify dose and patient.

1 mCi/kg. Should be given undiluted through a secure in-dwelling catheter and followed with a saline flush. Flushing of IV line before injection appropriate (see Incompatibilities).

DOSE ADJUSTMENTS

Use caution in calculating dose in very thin or very obese patients; dose adjustments in patients at the extremes of weight have not been studied. ■ Dose adjustment not required based on gender, in the elderly, or in impaired hepatic function. ■ Patients with renal insufficiency have not been studied.

DILUTION

Special techniques required; see Precautions. Available frozen in 2 ml (100 mCi) and 3 ml (150 mCi) vials in a lead shield package. Thaw at room temperature and use within 8 hours of thawing. Given undiluted (see Usual dose).

Storage: Store frozen at −10° to −20° C in a lead shielded container until use. Drug product expires 48 hours after the time of calibration noted on the label, or 8 hours after thawing, whichever is earlier.

INCOMPATIBLE WITH

Manufacturer states, "Samarium SM 153 should not be diluted or mixed with other solutions." Contains calcium and may be incompatible with solutions that contain molecules that can complex with and form calcium precipitates (e.g., phosphates, intravenous fat emulsion).

RATE OF ADMINISTRATION

Total desired dose over 1 minute. Flushing of IV line before injection appropriate, flushing following injection recommended.

ACTIONS

An injectable radioisotope and therapeutic agent. Consists of radioactive samarium and a tetraphosphonate chelator (ethylenediaminetetramethylenephosphonic acid [EDTMP]). Has an affinity for bone and concentrates in areas of bone turnover. The greater the number of metastatic lesions, the more skeletal uptake of SM 153 radioactivity. Accumulates in osteoblastic lesions more than in normal bone (ratio of 5 to 1). Emits beta rays that palliate metastatic bone pain, and emits gamma rays permitting imaging on conventional gamma cameras. Specific mechanism of action unknown. Half-life is 46.3 hours (1.93 days). Nearly 85% of radioactivity cleared from plasma within 30 minutes, 99% in 5 hours. Excreted intact primarily in urine (19% to 50% [mean 35%] within 6 hours, balance within 12 hours). The greater the number of metastatic lesions, the less radioactivity is excreted. Pain remission has lasted an average of 4 months (range 1 to 11 months). Retreatment after relapse has been effective.

INDICATIONS AND USES

Relief of pain in patients with confirmed osteoblastic metastatic bone lesions that enhance on radionuclide bone scan.

Investigational uses: Treatment of rheumatoid arthritis, Paget's disease of bone, and ankylosing spondylitis.

CONTRAINDICATIONS

Known hypersensitivity to EDTMP or similar bisphosphonate compounds (pamidronate [Aredia], etidronate [Didronel]).

PRECAUTIONS

Follow specific guidelines for handling radioactive agents to ensure minimum radiation exposure to patients and occupational workers consistent with appropriate patient management. Contact radiation safety officer. ▪ Radiopharmaceuticals usually administered by or under the direction of the physician specialist whose experience and training have been approved by the appropriate government agency. ▪ Confirm presence of bone metastases before therapy. ▪ Will cause moderate bone marrow depression; evaluate current clinical and hematologic status and bone marrow response history to treatment with myelotoxic agents. ▪ Not recommended for use in patients with evidence of compromised bone marrow reserve from previous therapy or disease involvement. Benefits must outweigh risks. ▪ Use caution in cancers (e.g., metastatic prostate cancer) that may be associated with disseminated intravascular coagulation (DIC). ▪ Use caution in patients whose platelet counts are falling or who have other clinical or laboratory findings suggesting DIC. ▪ Use caution in patients at risk for developing hypocalcemia. EDTMP is a chelating agent; ECG changes or arrhythmias may occur with or without the presence of hypocalcemia (has not been studied in humans). ▪ Because of hydration requirements, use with caution in patients with CHF or renal insufficiency. ▪ Does not prevent the development of spinal cord compression and is *not indicated* for the treatment of spinal cord compression. ▪ Note Monitor and Drug/lab interactions. ▪ Do not release patients until their radioactivity levels and exposure comply with federal and local regulations.

Monitor: Obtain baseline CBC platelets, and serum electrolytes. Beginning 2 weeks after admininstration, monitor CBC and platelets weekly for at least 8 weeks or until recovery of adequate bone marrow function. Repeat serum electrolytes at intervals. ▪ Adequate oral or IV hydration important to promote urinary excretion; a minimum of 500 ml before injection is recommended. ▪ ECG monitoring and serum calcium levels indicated in patients at risk for developing hypocalcemia or arrhythmias with or without the presence of hypocalcemia (see Precautions). ▪ Encourage frequent voiding to minimize radiation exposure to the bladder. ▪ Catheterize incontinent patients to minimize risk of radioactive contamination of clothing, bed linen, and the patient's environment. ▪ Samarium SM153 is not indicated for treatment of spinal cord compression. It does not prevent the development of spinal cord compression due to underlying disease. If S/S of spinal cord compression occur (e.g., pain, paresthesias, sensory loss, muscular weakness, spasticity, wasting, loss of sphincter control), diagnostic and therapeutic measures must be taken immediately to avoid permanent disability. ▪ A 40% to 50% decrease in WBCs and platelets is expected; nadir usually occurs between 3 and 5 weeks, returns to baseline within 8 weeks. ▪ Observe for S/S of infection. Use of prophylactic antibiotics may be indicated pending results of C/S in a febrile neutropenic patient. ▪ Use analgesics and antiemetics as indicated for patient comfort. ▪ Note Patient education.

Patient education: Avoid pregnancy; birth control recommended for men and women. See Maternal/child. ▪ See Appendix D, p. 900. ▪ Pain may be slightly increased for up to 2 to 3 days after injection (flare reaction), usually mild and self-limiting; use pain medication as needed. ▪ During the first 12 hours following administration the following precautions are necessary: Patient must inform any health professional caring for them that they have received SM 153. Radioactivity will be present in excreted urine and feces; use of a toilet instead of a urinal is preferred. Flush toilet several times after each use. Any spilled urine must be wiped up completely, and hands should be washed thoroughly. If blood or urine gets onto clothing, the clothing should be washed separately or stored for 1 to 2 weeks to allow for decay of the SM 153. ▪ Pain relief may begin to occur in 4 to 7 days; all patients in studies reported pain relief within 14 days. Maximum decrease in pain is expected in 3 to 4 weeks. As pain is decreased, need for pain med should also decrease. Effects may last for a few or many months (range is 1 to 11 months). ▪ Regular monitoring of blood count is imperative. ▪ Follow usual diet and activity patterns. As pain improves, patients may be able to do more than previously; do not overdo.

Maternal/child: Category D: Avoid pregnancy, can cause fetal harm. Women of childbearing age should have a negative pregnancy test before administration of SM 153. Both men and women should use an effective method of contraception after the administration of SM 153. ▪ Discontinue breast feeding. ▪ Safety and effectiveness for use in children under 16 years of age not established.

Elderly: Consider decreased renal function. Possibility of delayed excretion and need for extended precautions.

DRUG/LAB INTERACTIONS

Drug-drug interactions have not been studied. ▪ Potential for additive effects on bone marrow with chemotherapy or external beam radiation are unknown. Do not administer SM 153 concurrently unless benefits outweigh risks. Not recommended until bone marrow recovery is adequate.

SIDE EFFECTS

Primary side effects are transient increase in bone pain after injection (flare reaction) and bone marrow depression (leukopenia, thrombocytopenia). Numerous other side effects, including anemia, arrhythmias, DIC, hypertension, or hypotension, may occur. May be caused by SM 153 or by the underlying disease (see literature).

ANTIDOTE

Keep physician informed of patient status and results of blood studies. Appropriate transfusions or blood modifiers (e.g., epoetin-alfa [Epogen, Procrit], filgrastim [Neupogen], sargramostim [Leukine], oprelvekin [Numega]) may be indicated to treat bone marrow toxicity. Treat transient increase in bone pain with analgesics. Treat other side effects (e.g., arrhythmias, hypotension) as indicated.

SARGRAMOSTIM

Colony-stimulating factor
Antineutropenic

GM-CSF, human granulocyte-macrophage
colony-stimulating factor, Leukine

pH 7.1 to 7.7

USUAL DOSE

Myeloid reconstitution after allogenic or autologous bone marrow transplantation: 250 mcg/M^2/day as a 2-hour infusion daily for 21 days. Initial infusion must begin 2 to 4 hours after bone marrow infusion and not less than 24 hours after the last dose of chemotherapy and 12 hours after the last dose of radiation. Post—marrow infusion absolute neutrophil count (ANC) should be less than 500 cells/mm^3.

Engraftment delay or failure of bone marrow transplantation: 250 mcg/M^2/day as a 2-hour infusion daily for 14 days. Wait for 7 days; if engraftment has not occurred, repeat 14 day course of 250 mcg/M^2. Wait an additional 7 days; if engraftment has still not occurred, give a 14 day course of 500 mcg/M^2. If engraftment does not occur, further courses or dose increases are not indicated. Note time restrictions on chemotherapy and radiation above and in Drug/lab interactions.

Neutrophil recovery following chemotherapy in acute myelogenous leukemia (AML) in adults 55 years of age or older: 250 mcg/M^2/day as an infusion over 4 hours. Begin on day 11 or 4 days after induction chemotherapy is complete. Day 10 bone marrow should be hypoplastic with fewer than 5% blasts. Repeat sargramostim daily until absolute neutrophil count (ANC) is greater than 1,500/mm^3 for three consecutive days or a maximum of 42 days. Use same criteria if a second cycle of induction chemotherapy is indicated.

Mobilization of peripheral blood progenitor cells: 250 mcg/M^2/day as a 24-hour continuous infusion (or give SC once daily). Continue at the same dose until adequate numbers of progenitor stem cells are collected. Collection of progenitor cells (apheresis) usually begins about day 5 and is repeated daily. All cells are stored until predetermined targets are achieved. After immunosuppression with selected antineoplastic bone marrow depressant agents to neutralize remaining tumor cells or ineffective leukocytes, the collected progenitor stem cells are reinfused into the patient by IV infusion. This process has been used primarily in patients who were not candidates for bone marrow transplant; however, it is increasingly being used instead of bone marrow transplant.

Post-peripheral blood progenitor cell transplantation: 250 mcg/M^2/day as a 24-hour continuous infusion (or give SC once daily). Begin immediately following infusion of harvested progenitor cells and continue until an ANC is greater than 1,500/mm^3 for three consecutive days. Neutrophil recovery occurs somewhat sooner in patients receiving sargramostim stimulation. Results in a shorter time to platelet and RBC transfusion independence.

DOSE ADJUSTMENTS

May require reduced dose in impaired renal or hepatic function. Based on individual patient response. ■ For an ANC above 20,000 cells/mm^3, WBC above 50,000 cells/mm^3, or a platelet count above 500,000/mm^3, reduce dose by one half or temporarily discontinue. ■ Note Antidote.

DILUTION

Now available in liquid form (reconstituted) or each 250 or 500 mcg vial of the dry product must be reconstituted with 1 ml sterile water for injection with or without preservative. Confirm expiration date to ensure valid product. Direct diluent to the side of the vial and swirl gently. Avoid foaming or vigorous agitation. Do not shake. Either product must be further diluted in NS for infusion. If the final concentration of sargramostim will be below 10 mcg/ml, albumin (human) must be added to the NS before addition of the sargramostim (1 ml of 5% albumin to each 50 ml NS). This will prevent adsorption of the drug into the components of the IV delivery system. Liquefied product contains benzyl alcohol. Use sterile technique; enter vial only to dilute and/or to withdraw a single dose. Discard any unused portion. Should be clear and colorless.

Storage: Must be refrigerated in all forms; do not freeze or shake. Reconstituted with SW without preservatives or any diluted solution should be used within 6 hours. Reconstituted with bacteriostatic SW (benzyl alcohol preservative) or the new liquid preparation can be refrigerated for up to 20 days.

INCOMPATIBLE WITH

Manufacturer recommends that no medication other than albumin be added to the infusion solution.

Y-site incompatibility: Sargramostim concentration is 10 mcg/ml. Acyclovir (Zovirax), amphotericin B (Fungizone), ampicillin (Polycillin-N), ampicillin sulbactam (Unasyn), cefonicid (Monocid), cefoperazone (Cefobid), ceftazidime (Fortaz), chlorpromazine (Thorazine), ganciclovir (Cytovene), haloperidol (Haldol), hydrocortisone sodium phosphate, hydrocortisone sodium succinate (Solu-Cortef), hydromorphone (Dilaudid), hydroxyzine (Vistaril), imipenem-cilastatin (Primaxin), lorazepam (Ativan), methylprednisolone sodium succinate (Solu-Medrol), mitomycin (Mutamycin), morphine, nalbuphine (Nubain), ondansetron (Zofran), piperacillin (Pipracil), sodium bicarbonate, tobramycin (Nebcin), vancomycin (Lyphocin).

COMPATIBLE WITH

Y-site if sargramostim at 10 mcg/ml concentration: Amikacin (Amikin), aminophylline, aztreonam (Azactam), bleomycin (Blenoxane), butorphanol (Stadol), calcium gluconate, carboplatin (Paraplatin), carmustine (BCNU), cefazolin (Kefzol), cefotaxime (Claforan), cefotetan (Cefotan), ceftizoxime (Cefizox), ceftriaxone (Rocephin), cefuroxime (Zinacef), cimetidine (Tagamet), cisplatin (Platinol), clindamycin (Cleocin), cyclophosphamide (Cytoxan), cyclosporine (Sandimmune), cytarabine (ARA-C), dacarbazine (DTIC), dactinomycin (Cosmegen), dexamethasone (Decadron), diphenhydramine (Benadryl), dopamine (Intropin), doxorubicin (Adriamycin), doxycycline (Vibramycin), droperidol (Inapsine), etoposide (VePesid), famotidine (Pepcid), fentanyl (Sublimaze), fluconazole (Diflucan), fluorouracil (5 FU), furosemide (Lasix), gentamicin (Garamycin), heparin, idarubicin (Idamycin), ifosfamide (Ifex), immune globulin IV (Polygam), magnesium sulfate, mannitol (Osmitrol), mechlorethamine (nitrogen mustard), meperidine (Demerol), mesna, methotraxate (Folex), metoclopramide (Reglan), metronidazole (Flagyl), mezlocillin (Mezlin), miconazole (Monistat), minocycline (Minocin), mitoxantrone (Novantrone), netilmicin (Netromycin), pentostatin

(Nipent), piperacillin/tazobactam (Zozyn), potassium chloride, prochlorperazine (Compazine), promethazine (Phenergan), ranitidine (Zantac), teniposide (Vumon), ticarcillin (Ticar), ticarcillin/clavulanate (Timentin), trimethoprim-sulfamethoxazole (Bactrim), vinblastine (Velban), vincristine (Oncovin), zidovudine (AZT).

RATE OF ADMINISTRATION

See Usual dose. Each single dose must be evenly distributed over 2, 4, or 24 hours. Do not use an in-line membrane filter. Reduce rate or temporarily discontinue for onset of any side effects that cause concern (e.g., allergic reaction).

ACTIONS

Colony-stimulating factors are glycoproteins that bind to specific hematopoietic cell surface receptors and stimulate proliferation, differentiation commitment, and some end-cell functional activation. Utilizing recombinant DNA technology, sargramostim is produced in a yeast *(Saccharomyces cerevisiae)*. It differs slightly from endogenous GM-CSF. It induces partially committed progenitor cells to divide and differentiate in the granulocyte-macrophage pathways. Can also activate mature granulocytes and macrophages. It is a multilineage factor and has dose-dependent effects. It increases the cytotoxicity of monocytes toward certain neoplastic cell lines and activates polymorphonuclear neutrophils to inhibit the growth of tumor cells. It significantly improves the time to neutrophil recovery (engraftment), decreases length of hospitalization, shortens the duration of infectious episodes, and decreases antibiotic usage. Patients with fewer impaired organs have the best opportunity for improvement in survival. Detected in the serum in 5 minutes; peak levels are reached 2 hours after injection and last at least 6 hours.

INDICATIONS AND USES

Acceleration of hematopoietic recovery (myeloid engraftment) in patients undergoing allogenic or autologous bone marrow transplantation. ■ Bone marrow transplantation failure or engraftment delay. ■ Neutrophil recovery following chemotherapy in acute myelogenous leukemia (AML); safety for use in adults under 55 years not established. ■ Mobilzation of peripheral blood progenitor cells. ■ Stimulate neutrophil recovery post peripheral blood progenitor cell transplantation.

Unlabeled uses: Increase WBC in myelodysplastic syndromes and in AIDS patients receiving zidovudine. ■ Correct neutropenia in aplastic anemia. ■ Decrease transplantation-associated organ system damage, especially in kidney and liver transplants.

CONTRAINDICATIONS

Hypersensitivity to any components of sargramostim or yeast products; patients with leukemic myeloid blasts in the bone marrow or peripheral blood equal to 10% or more.

PRECAUTIONS

Should be administered under the direction of a physician knowledgeable about appropriate use. ■ Use caution if considered for use in any malignancy with myeloid characteristics. Can act as a growth factor for any tumor type, particularly myeloid malignancies. ■ Can be effective in patients receiving purged bone marrow if the purging process preserves a sufficient number of progenitors. ■ Effects may be limited in patients previously exposed to intensive chemotherapy or radiation therapy. ■ Neutralizing antibodies may form after receiving sargramostim and may inhibit therapeutic effect.

Monitor: Obtain a complete blood count with differential before administration and twice weekly thereafter to monitor for excessive leukocytosis (WBC greater than 50,000 cells/mm^3; or an absolute neutrophil count [ANC] greater than 20,000 cells/mm^3). ■ If blast cells appear or disease progression occurs, treatment should be discontinued. ■ Anemia, leukocytopenia, and thrombocytopenia occur as side effects of various procedures; monitor carefully. ■ Observe for fluid retention; may cause peripheral edema, pleural effusion, and/or pericardial effusion. May occur more frequently in individuals with preexisting lung disease or cardiac disease, including a history of arrhythmias. Use with caution. ■ Use with caution in patients with preexisting renal or hepatic dysfunction; an increased serum creatinine or increased bilirubin and hepatic enzymes may occur. Reversible if drug discontinued. Monitor renal and hepatic function biweekly. ■ Flushing, hypotension, and syncope may occur, especially with the initial dose. Reduce rate or stop temporarily.

Patient education: Promptly report any symptoms of infection (e.g., fever) or allergic reaction (e.g., itching, swelling, redness at the injection site).

Maternal/child: Has been used in more than 100 children from 4 months of age to 18 years with similar experience to the adult population, even though literature says safety not established. ■ Pregnancy Category C: safety for use in pregnancy and lactation not established; use only if clearly needed. ■ Liquefied product contains benzyl alcohol; do not use in premature infants.

DRUG/LAB INTERACTIONS

Do not administer within 24 hours preceding or following chemotherapy or within 12 hours preceding or following radiotherapy. Rapidly dividing cells and the success of the treatment would be adversely affected by chemotherapy and radiation. ■ Myeloproliferative effects may be potentiated by lithium or corticosteroids; use with caution.

SIDE EFFECTS

Asthenia, diarrhea, malaise, peripheral edema, rash, and urinary tract disorders are most common. Allergic reactions, including anaphylaxis, are possible; arthralgia, capillary leak syndrome, dyspnea, fever, headache, hypoxia, local injection site reactions, myalgia, pericardial effusion, peripheral edema, pleural effusion, and supraventricular arrhythmias have been reported.

ANTIDOTE

Discontinue sargramostim for anaphylaxis, if blast cells appear, or there is progression of underlying disease. A maximum dose limit has not been determined; for accidental overdose, discontinue and monitor for WBC increase and respiratory symptoms. For an ANC above 20,000 cells/mm^3, WBC above 50,000 cells/mm^3, or a platelet count above 500,000/mm^3, reduce dose by one half or temporarily discontinue. Blood count should return to base line level in 3 to 7 days. For any side effect that causes concern, reduce dose or temporarily discontinue. Keep physician informed. Treat anaphylaxis and resuscitate as necessary.

SCOPOLAMINE HYDROBROMIDE

Hyoscine hydrobromide

Anticholinergic

pH 3.5 to 6.5

USUAL DOSE

Anticholinergic: 0.3 to 0.6 mg (300 to 600 mcg or gr $\frac{1}{200}$ to $\frac{1}{100}$).

Antiemetic: 0.3 to 0.6 mg. One source suggests a single dose, another repeat in 6 to 8 hours as needed. Up to 1 mg has been used.

Anesthesia adjunct: 0.6 mg 3 to 4 times a day as a sedative-hypnotic, 0.32 to 0.65 mg to promote amnesia.

PEDIATRIC DOSE

Anticholinergic or Antiemetic: 6 mcg (0.006 mg)/kg of body weight or 200 mcg/M^2 as a single dose. Maximum dose is 0.3 mg.

DOSE ADJUSTMENTS

Note Drug/lab interactions. Reduced dose may be required in the elderly, debilitated, or patients with chronic lung disease.

DILUTION

Dilute desired dose in at least 10 ml of sterile water for injection.

Storage: Store below 40° C. Protect from light.

INCOMPATIBLE WITH

Alkalies. Physically compatible with many drugs.

RATE OF ADMINISTRATION

0.6 mg or fraction thereof over 1 minute.

ACTIONS

Anticholinergic agent that inhibits the muscarinic actions of acetylcholine. It dilates the pupils, decreases glandular secretions, relaxes smooth muscle tissue, temporarily increases heartrate, has a calming, sedative action that produces a partial amnesia, and produces less tenacious sputum postoperatively. It is widely distributed throughout the body. Onset of action is 30 minutes. Duration of action is 4 hours. Metabolized by the liver and excreted in urine. Crosses the placental barrier. May be secreted in breast milk.

INDICATIONS AND USES

Alone or with sedatives for preanesthetic medication. ■ Biliary tract disorders. ■ Gastric hypermotility. ■ Antiemetic. ■ Motion sickness. ■ Combined with analgesic or hypnotics in obstetrics. ■ Available as a transdermal patch to prevent nausea and vomiting of anesthetics or opiate analgesia.

CONTRAINDICATIONS

Known sensitivity to hyoscine, narrow-angle glaucoma, acute hemorrhage with unstable cardiovascular status, asthma, hepatic disease, intestinal atony of the elderly or debilitated, myasthenia gravis, myocardial ischemia, obstructive disease of the GI or GU tracts, paralytic ileus, renal disease, pyloric stenosis, prostatic hypertrophy, severe ulcerative colitis, tachycardia, toxic megacolon.

PRECAUTIONS

Most frequently used SC or IM. Rarely given IV. ■ Use with caution in asthma, hepatic disease, prostatic hypertrophy, in the elderly, in infants and small children, and in debilitated patients with chronic lung disease. ■ Note Maternal/child.

Monitor: Note Precautions, Maternal/child, Elderly and Drug/lab interactions.

Patient education: Report difficulty urinating. ■ Use caution in any task requiring alertness.

Maternal/child: Crosses the placenta, but adverse effects to the fetus have not been reported; however, one source has suggested that it may cause respiratory depression and hemorrhage in the neonate ■ Use in obstetrics is limited; use caution. ■ May inhibit lactation. Toxicity to nursing infants possible. ■ Note Precautions.

Elderly: Note Dose adjustments, Precautions/Monitor, and Contraindications. ■ May cause agitation, confusion, drowsiness, or excitement. ■ Observe for constipation and/or urinary retention.

DRUG/LAB INTERACTIONS

Potentiated by amantadine, antidepressants (e.g., amitriptyline [Elavil]), antihistamines, antiparkinson agents, benzodiazepines (e.g., diazepam [Valium]), buclizine, isoniazid, MAO inhibitors (e.g., selegiline [Eldepryl]), meperidine (Demerol), nitrates, orphenadrine, phenothiazines (e.g., chlorpromazine [Thorazine]), procainamide (Pronestyl), and quinidine. Reduced dose of either or both drugs may be indicated. ■ Antagonized by guanethidine, histamine, reserpine, and others. Hyoscine does interact with many drugs and potentiates the effects of both. Sometimes this is a desired interaction, as with morphine. ■ Use caution with cholinergics, digitalis, digoxin, diphenhydramine (Benadryl), levodopa, and neostigmine. May cause adverse effects. ■ Potentiates atenolol (Tenormin), sympathomimetics (e.g., terbutaline), nitrofurantoin, and thiazide diuretics. ■ Use with methotrimeprazine (Levoprome) may cause a drop in blood pressure and tachycardia. ■ May decrease effectiveness of ketoconazole (Nizoral).

SIDE EFFECTS

Mild in therapeutic doses, aggravated with overdose; anticholinergic psychosis, delirium, dry mouth, excitement, fever (heat loss by evaporation is inhibited), flushing, hallucination, hypertension, restlessness, slow reaction of pupils to light, tachycardia, thirst, urinary retention.

Overdose: Coma, respiratory failure, and unconsciousness.

ANTIDOTE

Wide margin of safety between therapeutic and lethal dosage. Notify physician of aggravated side effects. Neostigmine methylsulfate, 0.5 to 1 mg IV, may be used for symptomatic treatment, as may sedatives and barbiturates.

SECOBARBITAL SODIUM

Barbiturate
Sedative-hypnotic
Anticonvulsant

Seconal sodium   pH 9.7 to 10.5

USUAL DOSE (FOR ADULTS AND CHILDREN):
Moderate sedation: 1 to 1.5 mg/kg of body weight.
Prior to nerve block in dentistry: 100 to 150 mg.

Hypnotic: 2 mg/kg (50 to 250 mg).

Convulsions due to tetanus: 5.5 mg/kg.

Any dose may be repeated in 3 to 4 hours as indicated. 250 mg is usual maximum single dose, but 500 mg is never exceeded. Use only enough medication to achieve desired effect.

PEDIATRIC DOSE

Anticonvulsant in tetanus: 3 to 5 mg/kg or 125 mg/M^2/dose.

Status epilepticus: 15 to 20 mg/kg over 15 minutes.

DOSE ADJUSTMENTS

Reduced dose indicated in impaired renal or hepatic function, usually required in the debilitated or the elderly. ■ Note Drug/lab interactions.

DILUTION

Dilute with sterile water for injection. Any desired amount of diluent may be used. 9 ml of diluent with 1 ml of secobarbital (50 mg) equals 5 mg/ml. Use only absolutely clear solutions.

Storage: Store in refrigerator; protect from light.

INCOMPATIBLE WITH

Atracurium (Tracrium), benzquinamide (Emete-Con), chlordiazepoxide (Librium), chlorpromazine (Thorazine), cimetidine (Tagamet), clinda-mycin (Cleocin), codeine, diphenhydramine (Benadryl), droperidol (Inapsine), ephedrine, erythromycin (Ilotycin), glycopyrrolate (Robinul), hydrocortisone sodium succinate (Solu-Cortef), insulin (aqueous), isoproterenol (Isuprel), levorphanol (Levo-Dromoran), meperidine (Demerol), metaraminol (Aramine), methadone, methyldo-pate (Aldomet), norepinephrine (Levophed), pancuronium bromide (Pavulon), penicillin G potassium, pentazocine (Talwin), phenytoin (Dilantin), phytonadione (Aquamephyton), procaine (Novocain), prochlorperazine (Compazine), promethazine (Phenergan), propiom-azine (Largon), sodium bicarbonate, streptomycin, succinycholine (Anectine), thiamine (Betalin-S), vancomycin (Vancocin).

RATE OF ADMINISTRATION

50 mg or fraction thereof over 1 minute. Never exceed a rate of 50 mg or fraction thereof over 15 seconds. Titrate slowly to desired effect. Rapid injection rate may cause symptoms of overdose (e.g., serious respiratory depression).

ACTIONS

A sedative, hypnotic barbiturate of short duration with anticonvulsant effects. Secobarbital is a CNS depressant. Onset of action is prompt by IV route and lasts about 3 or 4 hours. Will effectively depress motor cortex if adequate doses are administered. Pain perception is unimpaired. Rapidly absorbed by all body tissues and excreted fairly quickly in the urine in changed form. Crosses placental barrier. Secreted in breast milk.

INDICATIONS AND USES

Preanesthetic sedation. ■ Dental and minor surgical sedation. ■ Control of convulsions caused by tetanus. ■ Sedation in psychotic states.

CONTRAINDICATIONS

Delivery (when maximum drug effect would be achieved at the time of delivery), history of porphyria, severely impaired liver function especially with any signs of hepatic coma, known hypersensitivity to barbiturates, premature delivery, severe respiratory depression.

PRECAUTIONS

IV route usually reserved for critical situations. ■ Use caution in asthma, pulmonary and cardiovascular diseases, toxemia of pregnancy, history of bleeding, impaired renal or hepatic function, shock, uremia, and depressive states after a convulsion. ■ Use caution in the presence of fever, diabetes, hyperthyroidism, or severe anemia; untoward reactions may occur. ■ Status epilepticus can occur from too-rapid withdrawal. ■ May be habit forming; use caution in acute or chronic pain. ■ Benzodiazepines (diazepam [Valium], midazolam [Versed]) generally preferred for sedation.

Monitor: Highly alkaline; determine absolute patency of vein; use of large veins preferred to prevent thrombosis. Avoid extravasation. Intraarterial injection will cause gangrene. ■ Record blood pressure, pulse, and respiration every 3 to 5 minutes. Keep patient under constant observation. ■ Monitor hematopoietic, renal, and hepatic systems in extended therapy. ■ Maintain a patent airway. Keep equipment for artificial ventilation available. ■ Treat the cause of a convulsion. ■ Note Drug/lab interactions.

Patient education: May not drive or perform other tasks requiring alertness if given on an outpatient basis. ■ Avoid alcohol or other CNS depressants (e.g., antihistamines, diazepam [Valium]) ■ May be habit forming. ■ May require alternate birth control.

Maternal/child: Category D: avoid pregnancy: will cause birth defects. ■ Note Contraindications. ■ May cause drowsiness in the nursing infant. ■ May cause paradoxical excitement in children.

Elderly: Note Dose adjustments. ■ May have increased sensitivity to barbiturates, may cause marked excitement, depression, confusion, and increased risk of barbiturate induced hypothermia. ■ Consider reduced renal or hepatic function.

DRUG/LAB INTERACTIONS

Use extreme caution if any other CNS depressants have been given such as alcohol, narcotic analgesics, anesthetics, antidepressants, antihistamines, hypnotics, MAO inhibitors, phenothiazines, sedatives, neuromuscular blocking antibiotics, or tranquilizers. Potentiation with respiratory depression may occur. ■ Inhibits effectiveness of propranolol (Inderal), corticosteroids, doxycycline (Vibramycin), oral anticoagulants, oral contraceptives, quinidine, and theophylline. Capable of innumerable interactions with many drugs. ■ May increase orthostatic hypotension with furosemide (Lasix). ■ Monitor phenytoin and barbiturate levels when both drugs are used concurrently. ■ May inhibit vitamin D metabolism with extended use.

SIDE EFFECTS

Average dose: Depression, dermatitis, facial edema, fever, hypotension, neonatal apnea, respiratory depression (hypoventilation), thrombocytopenic purpura.

Overdose: Apnea, coma, cough reflex depression, flat EEG (reversible unless hypoxic damage has occurred), hypotension, laryngospasm, lowered body temperature, pulmonary edema, sluggish or absent reflexes, renal shutdown, respiratory depression.

ANTIDOTE

Notify the physician of any side effects. Symptomatic and supportive treatment is most important in overdose. Maintain an adequate airway with artificial ventilation if indicated. Keep the patient warm. IV volume expanders (dextran) and IV fluids will help maintain adequate circulation. Diuretics or hemodialysis will promote the elimination of the drug. Vasopressors (e.g., dopamine [Intropin]) will maintain blood pressure.

SECRETIN
Secretin-Boots, Secretin-Ferring

Diagnostic agent

pH 2.5 to 5.0

USUAL DOSE

IV test dose: 0.1 to 1 clinical unit (CU). If no reaction in one minute, administer diagnostic dose.

Pancreatic function testing and procedure for obtaining desquamated pancreatic cells for cytopathology: 1 CU/kg of body weight as a single dose.

Diagnosis of gastrinoma (Zollinger-Ellison syndrome): 2 CU/kg as a single dose.

DILUTION

Check expiration date. Dilute vial containing 75 CU with 7.5 ml of NS to provide a solution of 10 CU/ml. Avoid vigorous shaking. Use diluted solution immediately and discard unused portion.

Storage: Store at -20° C. May store at or below 25° C for up to 3 weeks.

INCOMPATIBLE WITH

Specific information not available. Should be considered incompatible with any drug in the syringe because of specific use.

RATE OF ADMINISTRATION

A single dose evenly distributed over 1 minute.

ACTIONS

A gastrointestinal peptide hormone. It acts to increase the bicarbonate content and volume of pancreatic secretions. Peak output occurs in 30 minutes and may continue for 2 hours. Failure to achieve a predetermined level of bicarbonate or volume of secretions after secretin administration is indicative of pancreatic dysfunction. Also acts to stimulate gastrin release in patients with gastrinoma, whereas little or no change in gastrin levels is seen in normal subjects. Secretin is degraded in the liver and by enzymes in the blood and has a serum half-life of 18 minutes.

INDICATIONS AND USES

Diagnosis of pancreatic exocrine disease. ▪ Diagnosis of gastrinoma (Zollinger-Ellison syndrome). ▪ May aid in the diagnosis of some hepatobiliary diseases by providing cells for cytopathologic examination.

CONTRAINDICATIONS

Known hypersensitivity to secretin, acute pancreatitis until attack subsided.

PRECAUTIONS

Use with extreme caution in pancreatitis; note Contraindications. ▪ Patients who have undergone a vagotomy or who have inflammatory bowel disease may be hyporesponsive to secretin test. ▪ A greater than normal volume response to secretin stimulation, which can mask coexisting pancreatic disease, may be seen in some patients with alcoholic or other liver diseases.

Monitor: Pancreatic dysfunction diagnosis is accomplished by inserting a specific double-lumen gastric tube after a 12-hour fast. Correct positioning under fluoroscopic guidance is required. Aspirate gastric contents continuously to prevent passage into the duodenum. Collect duodenal contents for 10 to 20 minutes until a clear, bile-stained, uncontaminated fluid with a pH greater than or equal to 6.0 is obtained. Obtain two uncontaminated baseline samples of duodenal fluids 10 minutes apart. Administer secretin (usually done by physician). Collect four duodenal samples in separate sterile specimen containers (one sample at 10 minutes, one at 20 minutes, one at 40 minutes, and the last at 1 hour after administration of secretin). Sometimes the samples are collected at four 20-minute intervals. ■ Gastrinoma diagnosis begins with a 12-hour fast. Draw two blood samples for fasting (baseline) serum gastrin levels. Administer secretin. Collect blood samples at 1, 2, 5, 10, and 30 minutes for serum gastrin concentrations.

Maternal/child: Defer use in pregnancy if possible; safety not established and fluoroscopy required. ■ Use caution in lactation. ■ Safety for use in children not established.

DRUG/LAB INTERACTIONS

Inhibited by anticholinergics (e.g., atropine).

SIDE EFFECTS

Allergic reactions from impure preparations and/or repeat injections do occur. Thrombophlebitis can occur.

ANTIDOTE

Discontinue the drug immediately for any signs of allergic reaction. Treat anaphylaxis with epinephrine, antihistamines (e.g., diphenhydramine [Benadryl]), vasopressors (e.g., dopamine [Intropin]), aminophylline, and corticosteroids as indicated. Maintain a patent airway and resuscitate as necessary.

SERMORELIN ACETATE

Geref

Hormone
Diagnostic agent

pH 5.5

USUAL DOSE

1 mcg/kg of body weight as a single test dose. Schedule in the morning following an overnight fast. Specific procedure required. Draw venous blood samples for growth hormone determinations 15 minutes before, immediately prior to administration, and every 15 minutes times four after administration. Use a 3 ml NS flush immediately after injection of sermorelin.

DILUTION

Each 50 mcg ampoule must be diluted with a minimum of 0.5 ml of the 2 ml NS provided. Solution must be clear and used immediately after reconstitution. Do not use if cloudy or discolored. Discard any unused material.

Storage: Dry powder stable for 1 year from date of manufacture if stored in refrigerator.

INCOMPATIBLE WITH

Specific information not available. Consider incompatible in syringe or solution due to specific use.

RATE OF ADMINISTRATION

A single dose as a bolus injection followed by a 3 ml NS flush.

ACTIONS

A sterile lyophilized white powder, this synthetic hormone is identical in amino acid composition to endogenous natural growth hormone-releasing factor (GHRF, GRF). Increases plasma growth hormone concentrations by direct stimulation of the somatotroph cells of the anterior pituitary gland to release growth hormone. Does not have stimulatory effects on the secretion of other pituitary hormones (e.g., prolactin, TSH, FSH, LH, or ACTH). An increase in peak levels begins within 5 minutes, and maximum levels occur 30 to 60 minutes after injection. Plasma half-life is 6 to 8 minutes. Rapidly distributed and then degraded to an inactive fragment.

INDICATIONS AND USES

Evaluation of the ability of the somatotroph of the pituitary gland to secrete growth hormone (GH). ■ Used SC for treatment of idiopathic growth hormone deficiency in children with growth failure and as an adjunct to gonadotropin therapy in ovulation induction for infertility (orphan designation).

CONTRAINDICATIONS

Hypersensitivity to sermorelin acetate or any of its components (e.g., mannitol, albumin).

PRECAUTIONS

A normal plasma GH response (28 +/- 15 ng/ml within 30 minutes) to sermorelin acetate demonstrates that the somatotroph is intact. 50% of patients who do not respond to standard testing will show a normal response to sermorelin. GH deficiency may still be the result of hypothalamic dysfunction in the presence of an intact somatotroph. ■ Test is most easily interpreted when there is a subnormal response to conventional provocative testing and a normal response to sermorelin. The site of dysfunction cannot be determined if both conventional and sermorelin testing result in subnormal GH responses. ■ Not useful in the diagnosis of acromegaly. ■ Discontinue exogenous growth hormone therapy at least 1 week before testing. ■ Response may be inhibited by obesity, hyperglycemia, and elevated plasma fatty acids.

Monitor: Note Precautions and Drug/lab interactions.

Maternal/child: Safety for use in pregnancy and lactation not established. Has been shown to produce minor variations in fetuses of rats and rabbits. Use during pregnancy or lactation only if benefits outweigh risk.

DRUG/LAB INTERACTIONS

Do not test in the presence of drugs that directly affect the pituitary secretion of somatotropin (e.g., insulin, glucocorticoids [e.g., dexamethasone, cortisone, prednisone], cyclooxygenase inhibitors [e.g., aspirin or indomethacin]). ■ Transiently elevated somatotropin levels can occur with clonidine, levodopa, and insulin-induced hypoglycemia. ▪ Response inhibited by muscarinic antagonists (e.g., atropine), antithyroids (e.g., propylthiouracil), and in hypothyroid patients.

SIDE EFFECTS

Average dose: Allergic reactions (e.g., redness, swelling, and urticaria at the injection site [25% of patients develop antibodies]); flushing of the face; headache; nausea; pain at the injection site; paleness; strange taste in the mouth; tightness in the chest; transient warmth; vomiting.

Overdose: Blood pressure and heart rate changes have been reported with doses over 10 mcg/kg. Cardiovascular collapse is conceivable but has not happened.

ANTIDOTE

Notify physician of all side effects; may be transient or may require symptomatic treatment. Treat allergic reactions with diphenhydramine (Benadryl) or epinephrine. Resuscitate as necessary.

SINCALIDE   Diagnostic agent
Kinevac   pH 5.5 to 6.5

USUAL DOSE

Contraction of the gallbladder: 0.02 mcg/kg of body weight (1.4 mcg/70 kg [154 lb]). May give a second dose of 0.04 mcg/kg in 15 minutes if satisfactory contraction of the gallbladder does not occur. After the injection, take x-rays at 5-minute intervals to visualize the gallbladder and 1-minute intervals during the first 5 minutes to visualize the cystic duct.

Secretin-sincalide test of pancreatic function: Initiate a 60 minute infusion of secretin 0.25 units/kg. IV test dose required; refer to secretin. Follow in 30 minutes through a separate IV site with a 30 minute infusion of sincalide 0.02 mcg/kg.

DILUTION

Each 5 mcg vial must be initially diluted with 5 ml of sterile water for injection. Use diluted solution immediately and discard unused portion.

Contraction of the gallbladder: May be given without additional dilution.

Secretin-sincalide test of pancreatic function: Further dilute the calculated dose (1.4 mcg/70 kg [1.4 ml]) in 30 ml NS for injection. Further dilute the calculated dose of secretin in 60 ml NS for injection.

Storage: Store at room temperature before dilution.

INCOMPATIBLE WITH

Specific information not available. Should be considered incompatible with any drug in the syringe or solution because of specific use.

RATE OF ADMINISTRATION

Contraction of the gallbladder: A single dose evenly distributed over 30 to 60 seconds.

Secretin-sincalide test of pancreatic function: Evenly distribute secretin over 60 minutes (approximately 1 ml/min). Evenly distribute sincalide over 30 minutes (approximately 1 ml/min).

ACTIONS

Causes the gallbladder to contract and evacuate bile in a manner similar to endogenous cholecystokinin. Maximum effect is achieved in 5 to 15 minutes. Causes delayed gastric emptying and increased intestinal motility. When given in conjunction with secretin, both the volume of pancreatic secretion and the output of bicarbonate and protein enzymes are increased. By analyzing and measuring the duodenal aspirate, pancreatic function (volume of the secretion, bicarbonate concentration, amylase content) can be assessed.

INDICATIONS AND USES

To provide a sample of gallbladder bile for analysis of its composition (aspirated from the duodenum). ■ To stimulate pancreatic secretion for analysis of its composition and examination of cytology. Used in conjunction with secretin. Specimen aspirated from the duodenum. ■ Postevacuation cholecystography when indicated and intake of a fatty meal is not desired.

CONTRAINDICATIONS

Known hypersensitivity to sincalide.

PRECAUTIONS

Small gallbladder stones may be evacuated from the gallbladder. They could lodge in the cystic duct or common bile duct. Not highly probable because contraction of the gallbladder is not complete.

Maternal/child: Safety for use during pregnancy not established; use only when benefits outweigh risk to fetus. ■ Safety for use in children not established.

SIDE EFFECTS

Abdominal discomfort, abdominal pain, and urge to defecate usually occur because of delayed gastric emptying and increased intestinal motility. Dizziness, flushing, and nausea may occur.

ANTIDOTE

Keep physician informed of side effects. Assist patient with comfort measures. Resuscitate as necessary.

SODIUM ACETATE

Electrolyte replenisher
Antihyponatremic
Alkalizing agent

pH 6.0 to 7.0

USUAL DOSE

Determined by nutritional needs, evaluation of electrolytes, and degree of hyponatremia. Available in 2 mEq and 4 mEq/ml concentrations. Each ml provides 2 or 4 mEq each of sodium and acetate.

DILUTION

Must be added to larger volumes of IV infusion solutions including total parenteral nutrition. Use only clear solutions.

Storage: Store at room temperature. Discard unused portion.

INCOMPATIBLE WITH

None when used as indicated.

RATE OF ADMINISTRATION

Administer at prescribed rate for infusion solutions. Rapid or excessive administration may produce sodium overload, water retention, alkalosis, or hypokalemia.

ACTIONS

An alkalizing agent and sodium salt. Sodium is the predominant cation of extracellular fluid. It controls water distribution throughout the body. Hypothalamus osmoreceptors, sensitive to osmolarity changes in the blood, control serum sodium concentration (142 mEq/L). Body fluid is lost when sodium content decreases and retained when sodium content increases. The acetate ion is metabolized to bicarbonate, thus providing a source of bicarbonate. It also acts as a hydrogen ion receptor.

INDICATIONS AND USES

To prevent or correct hyponatremia in patients with restricted intake, especially in individualized IV formulations when basic needs are not met by standard solutions. ■ Treatment of mild to moderate acidotic states. ■ Source of sodium ions in hemodialysis and peritoneal dialysis.

CONTRAINDICATIONS

Patients with hypernatremia or water retention.

PRECAUTIONS

Use with caution in impaired renal function, congestive heart failure, hypertension, peripheral or pulmonary edema, any condition resulting in salt retention, and in patients receiving corticosteroids. ■ Use acetate-containing solutions with extreme caution in patients with metabolic or respiratory alkalosis and/or impaired hepatic function. ■ Temporary therapy in acidosis. Treatment of primary condition must be instituted. ■ Sodium bicarbonate is the drug of choice for use in severe acidosis that requires immediate correction.

Monitor: Evaluate electrolytes frequently during treatment. ■ Evaluate fluid balance. ■ Rapid or excessive administration may produce alkalosis or hypokalemia. Cardiac arrhythmias may result from an intracellular shift of potassium. Many other complications may arise from electrolyte imbalance.

Maternal/child: Pregnancy Category C: safety not established, use only if clearly needed.

SIDE EFFECTS

Hypernatremia, sodium level over 147 mEq/L, is most common (congestive heart failure, delirium, dizziness, edema, fever, flushing, headache, hypotension, oliguria, pulmonary edema, reduced salivation and lacrimation, respiratory arrest, restlessness, swollen tongue, tachycardia, thirst, weakness). Alkalosis and fluid or solute overload can occur.

ANTIDOTE

Notify the physician of any side effect. Reduce rate and notify physician at first sign of congestion or fluid overload. May be treated by sodium restriction and/or use of diuretics (e.g., furosemide [Lasix]) or dialysis. Resuscitate as necessary.

SODIUM BICARBONATE

Electrolyte replenisher
Alkalizing agent

pH 7.0 to 8.5

USUAL DOSE

Adjusted according to pH, Paco$_2$, calculated base deficit, clinical response, and fluid limitations of the patient. In the presence of a low CO_2 content, adjust gradually to avoid unrecognized alkalosis. Correction to a CO_2 of 20 mEq/L within 24 hours will most likely result in a normal pH if the cause of acidosis is controlled and normal kidney function is present. Average dose for most indications is 2 to 5 mEq/kg/24 hr in adults and children.

Cardiac arrest: 1 mEq/kg of body weight, only when appropriate (see Precautions; evidence supports little benefit and use may be detrimental). Repeat half dose in 10 minutes if indicated by blood pH and PaCO$_2$.

PEDIATRIC DOSE

For neonates and children up to 2 years of age, dose must never exceed 8 mEq/kg/24 hr of a 4.2% or more dilute solution. (See Usual dose.)

DILUTION

Available as:

4.2% sodium bicarbonate solution: 5 mEq/10 ml (0.5 mEq/ml).

5% sodium bicarbonate solution: 297.5 mEq/500 ml (0.595 mEq/ml).

7.5% sodium bicarbonate solution: 44.6 mEq/50 ml or 8.9 mEq/10 ml (0.892 mEq/ml).

8.4% sodium bicarbonate solution: 50 mEq/50 ml or 10 mEq/10 ml (1 mEq/ml).

neut (4% sodium bicarbonate solution): 2.4 mEq/5 ml (0.48 mEq/ml). Use limited to a buffering solution. Will raise pH of IV fluids and medications. Never used as a systemic alkalinizer.

May be given in prepared solutions. 7.5% and 8.4% solutions should be diluted with equal amount of water for injection, or dilute with compatible IV solutions, depending on desired dosage and desired rate of administration. 4.2% or a more dilute solution is preferred for infants and children. Use only clear solutions.

INCOMPATIBLE WITH

5% alcohol with 5% dextrose, amino acids, amiodarone (Cordarone), ascorbic acid, atropine, calcium chloride, calcium gluconate, carboplatin (Paraplatin), carmustine (BiCNU), cefotaxime (Claforan), chlorpromazine (Thorazine), ciprofloxacin (Cipro IV), cisplatin (Platinol), codeine, corticotropin (ACTH), dobutamine (Dobutrex), dopamine (Intropin), epinephrine (Adrenalin), fat emulsion 10%, glycopyrrolate (Robinul), hydromorphone (Dilaudid), idarubicin (Idamycin), imipenem-cilastatin (Primaxin), insulin (aqueous), Ionosol solutions, isoproterenol (Isuprel), labetalol (Normodyne), lactated Ringer's injection, levorphanol (Levo-Dromoran), lincomycin (Lincocin), magnesium sulfate, meperidine (Demerol), methadone, methicillin (Staphcillin), metoclopramide (Reglan), midazolam (Versed), morphine, norepinephrine (Levophed), penicillin G potassium, pentobarbital (Nembutal), pentazocine (Talwin), phenobarbital (Luminal), procaine (Novocain), promazine (Sparine), Ringer's injection, secobarbital (Seconal), sodium lactate injection ($\frac{1}{6}$ molar), streptomycin, succinycholine (Anectine), thiopental (Pentothal), ticarcillin/clavulanate (Timentin), tubocurarine (Curare), vancomycin (Vancocin), vinorelbine.

RATE OF ADMINISTRATION

Flush IV line thoroughly before and after administration. Usual rate of administration of any solution is 2 to 5 mEq/kg over 4 to 8 hours. Do not exceed 50 mEq/hr. Decrease rate for children. Note Pediatric dose. Rapid or excessive administration may produce alkalosis, hypernatremia, hypokalemia, and hypocalcemia. Cardiac arrhythmias may result from an intracellular shift of potassium. Will also produce pain and irritation along injection site.

Cardiac arrest: Up to 1 mEq/kg of body weight properly diluted over 1 to 3 minutes.

ACTIONS

An alkalizing agent and sodium salt. Helps to maintain osmotic pressure and ion balance. It is the buffering agent in blood. Bicarbonate ion elevates blood pH promptly. 99% reabsorbed with normal kidney function. Only 1% is excreted in the urine.

INDICATIONS AND USES

Metabolic acidosis (blood pH below 7.2 or plasma bicarbonate of 8mEq/L or less) caused by circulatory insufficiency resulting from shock or severe dehydration, extracorporeal circulation of blood, severe renal disease, cardiac arrest (note Precautions), uncontrolled diabetes with ketoacidosis (low-dose insulin preferred), and primary lactic acidosis. ■ Hyperkalemia. ■ Hemolytic reactions requiring alkalinization of urine to reduce nephrotoxicity. ■ Severe diarrhea. ■ Barbiturate, methyl alcohol, or salicylate intoxication. ■ Buffering solution to raise pH of IV fluids and medications.

CONTRAINDICATIONS

Diuretics known to produce hypochloremic alkalosis (e.g., thiazides), edema, hypertension, hypocalcemia, (alkalosis may produce CHF, convulsions, hypertension, and tetany), hypochloremia (from vomiting, GI suction, or diuretics), impaired renal function, metabolic alkalosis, respiratory alkalosis or acidosis, and any situation in which the administration of sodium could be clinically detrimental.

PRECAUTIONS

Temporary therapy in metabolic acidosis. Treatment of primary condition must be instituted. Best to partially correct acidosis and allow compensatory mechanisms to complete the correction. ■ Use with caution in cardiac, liver, or renal disease; CHF, fluid/solute overload, elderly and postoperative patients with renal or cardiovascular insufficiency, and in patients receiving corticosteroids. ■ Use in cardiac arrest only after difibrillation, cardiac compression, intubation, ventilation, and more than one trial of epinephrine have been used. ■ Adequate alveolar ventilation should control acid-base balance in most arrest situations except prolonged cardiac arrest, arrested patients with preexisting metabolic acidosis, hyperkalemia, or tricyclic or barbiturate overdose.

Monitor: Confirm absolute patency of vein. Extravasation may cause chemical cellulitis, necrosis, ulceration, or sloughing. ■ Flush IV line throughly before and after administration; many incompatabilities. ■ Determine blood pH, Po_2, Pco_2, and electrolytes several times daily during intensive treatment and daily in most other situations. Determine base excess or deficit in infants and children (dose = $0.3 \times$ kg $\times$ base deficit). Notify physician of all results. ■ Rapid or excessive administration may produce alkalosis, hypokalemia, and hypocalcemia. Cardiac arrhythmias may result from an intracellular shift of potassium. Many other complications may arise from electrolyte imbalance. ■ Use only 50 ml ampoules in cardiac arrest to prevent accidental overdose. Recent practice indicates smaller doses may be appropriate when indicated in cardiac arrest and may prevent secondary alkalosis. Adequate alveolar ventilation is imperative. Evaluate patient response and blood gases.

Maternal/child: Category C: safety for use in pregnancy not established; use only if clearly needed. ■ Use caution in lactation. ■ Doses in excess of 8 mEq/kg/24 hr and/or given too rapidly (10 ml/min) may cause intracranial hemorrhage, hypernatremia, and decrease in cerebrospinal fluid pressure in neonates and children under 2 years.

Elderly: Contains sodium; use caution in the elderly with renal or cardiovascular insufficiency with or without CHF (note Precautions).

DRUG/LAB INTERACTIONS

Inhibits tetracyclines, chlorpropamide, lithium carbonate, methotrexate, and salicylates. ■ Potentiates anorexiants (e.g., amphetamines), sympathomimetics (e.g., ephedrine, dopamine [Intropin]), flecainide, mecamylamine, and quinidine.

SIDE EFFECTS

Rare when used with caution: alkalosis, (hyperirritability and tetany), hypernatremia (edema, CHF), hypokalemia, local site pain with venous irritation.

ANTIDOTE

Discontinue the drug and notify the physician of any side effect. Hypokalemia usually occurs with alkalosis. Sodium and potassium chloride must be supplemented as indicated for correction. Treatment of alkalosis often results in more alkalosis. Rebreathing expired air from a paper bag may help to control beginning symptoms of alkalosis. Calcium gluonate may help in severe alkalosis. Administration of a balanced hypotonic electrolyte solution (Isolyte H, Normosol-M, Plasma-lyte 56) with sodium and potassium chloride added may help to excrete the bicarbonate ion in the urine. Ammonium chloride may be indicated. Treat tetany as indicated (calcium gluconate). Treat extravasation with injection of lidocaine or hyaluronidase (Wydase). Use a 27- or 25-gauge needle. Elevate the extremity and apply warm moist compresses. Resuscitate as necessary.

SODIUM CHLORIDE

Electrolyte replenisher
Antihyponatremic

pH 4.8

USUAL DOSE

Highly individualized and related to specific condition, concentration of salts in the plasma, and/or loss of body fluids.

Hypotonic: (0.45% [one-half normal saline], 4.5 Gm of sodium chloride/L or 77 mEq of sodium and 77 mEq of chloride [≈155 mOsm/L]) 2 to 4 L/24 hr.

Isotonic: (0.9% [normal saline], 9 Gm of sodium chloride/L or 154 mEq of sodium and 154 mEq of chloride [≈310 mOsm/L]), 1.5 to 3 L/24 hr. *Bacteriostatic isotonic normal saline* contains benzyl alcohol as a preservative. It is used in small amounts (usually 1 to 2 ml) as a diluent for injectable drugs (IV, IM, SC) or to flush peripheral lines. Do not exceed 30 ml/24 hr in adults. Never used in neonates.

Hypertonic: Calculate sodium deficit. Total body water [TBW] is 45% to 50% in females and 50% to 60% in males.

Na deficit in mEq = TBW [desired - observed plasma Na]

Hypertonic contains (3% 30 Gm of sodium chloride/L or 513 mEq of sodium and 513 mEq of chloride [≈1,030 mOsm/L] or 5%, 50 Gm of sodium chloride/L or 855 mEq of sodium and 855 mEq of chloride [≈1,710 mOsm/L]), 200 to 400 ml/24 hr. Continue until serum sodium is 130 mEq/L or neurologic symptoms improve. Occasionally may have to be repeated within the 24-hour period. See Precautions.

Concentrated: To be used only as an additive in parenteral fluid therapy (14.6% contains 2.5 mEq of sodium and chloride/ml; 23.4% contains 4 mEq of sodium and chloride/ml).

DILUTION

Available as **Hypotonic** 25 ml, 50 ml, 150 ml, 250 ml, 500 ml, 1L; **isotonic** (2 ml, 3 ml, 5 ml, 10 ml, 20 ml, 25 ml, 30 ml, 50 ml, 100 ml, 150 ml, 250 ml, 500 ml, 1 liter); or **hypertonic** (500 ml) solution in vials and/or bottles for injection or infusion and ready for use. Isotonic and hypotonic sodium chloride are frequently combined with D5W or D10W. **Concentrated** must be diluted before use. Used only as an additive in parenteral fluids. Permits specific mEq for mEq replacement of sodium and chloride without contributing to fluid overload. Available in 14.6% strength in 20 ml, 40 ml, and 200 ml; 23.4% strength in 30 ml, 50 ml, 100 ml, and 200 ml.

Bacteriostatic isotonic available in 2 ml, 10 ml, and 30 ml vials ready for use as a diluent. Never use in neonates.

Storage: Store at controlled room termperature. Do not freeze.

INCOMPATIBLE WITH

Amphotericin B (Fungizone), fat emulsion 10%, mannitol norepinephrine (Levophed).

RATE OF ADMINISTRATION

Isotonic and hypotonic: A single daily dose equally distributed over 24 hours. Rate is dependent on age, weight, and clinical condition of the patient.

Hypertonic: One-half the calculated dose over at least 8 hours. Do not exceed 100 ml over 1 hour. Too-rapid infusion may cause local pain and venous irritation; reduce rate for tolerance.

Concentrated: Properly diluted in parenteral fluids and equally distributed over 24 hours. Never exceed hypertonic rate (see above) based on actual mEq of sodium chloride.

ACTIONS

Sodium is the predominant cation of extracellular fluid. It controls water distribution throughout the body. Hypothalamus osmoreceptors, sensitive to osmolarity changes in the blood, control serum sodium concentration (142 mEq/L). Body fluid is lost when sodium content decreases and retained when sodium content increases. Readily absorbed in kidney tubules. Frequently exchanged for hydrogen and potassium ions. Excess excreted in urine.

INDICATIONS AND USES

Replace lost sodium and chloride ions in the body (e.g., hyponatremia or low salt syndrome). ▪ Maintain electrolyte balance.

Hypotonic: Water replacement without increase of osmotic pressure or serum sodium levels; treatment of hyperosmolar diabetes requiring considerable fluid without excess sodium.

Isotonic: To replace sodium and chloride lost from vomiting because of obstructions and/or aspiration of GI fluids; treatment of metabolic alkalosis with fluid loss and sodium depletion. ▪ Diluent in parenteral preparations. ▪ To initiate and terminate blood transfusions without hemolyzing red blood cells. ▪ Maintain patency and perform routine irrigations of many types of intravascular devices (e.g., catheters, implanted ports). ▪ Antidote for drug-induced hypercalcemia. Given concurrently with furosemide (Lasix). ▪ Priming solution in hemodialysis procedures.

Hypertonic: Used only when high sodium and/or chloride content without large amounts of fluid is required (e.g., electrolyte and fluid loss replaced with sodium-free fluids, excessive water intake resulting in drastic dilution of body water, emergency treatment of severe salt depletion, addisonian crisis, diabetic coma).

Concentrated: Used to meet the specific requirements of patients with unusual fluid and electrolyte needs (e.g., special problems of sodium electrolyte intake or excretion).

CONTRAINDICATIONS

Hypernatremia; fluid retention; situations where sodium or chloride could be detrimental. 3% and 5% sodium chloride solutions are contraindicated with elevated, normal, or slightly decreased serum sodium and chloride levels. Bacteriostatic sodium chloride is contraindicated in newborns.

PRECAUTIONS

Use caution in circulatory insufficiency, congestive heart failure, edema with sodium retention, kidney dysfunction, hepatic disease, hypoproteinemia, in the elderly or debilitated individuals, and in patients receiving corticosteroids. ▪ Use with caution in surgical patients (note Monitor). ▪ More than 1 liter of normal saline may cause hypernatremia, which can result in loss of bicarbonate ions and acidosis. ▪ Change IV tubing at least every 48 hours. ▪ All uses require preservative-free solutions except the limited use of bacteriostatic NS as a diluent or flushing agent. ▪ Inadvertent direct injection or absorption of concentrated sodium chloride may cause sudden hypernatremia, cardiovascular shock, CNS disorders, extensive hemolysis, cortical necrosis of the kidneys and severe local tissue necrosis with extravasation. Use extreme caution.

Monitor: Maintain accurate intake and output; monitor electrolytes and acid-base balance, especially in prolonged therapy. ▪ Monitor vital signs as indicated. ▪ Monitor for signs of hyponatremia (sodium <135 mEq/L [e.g., disorientation, headache, lethargy, nausea, weakness]). May progress to coma and seizures. ▪ NS can cause sodium retention resulting in fluid retention, edema, and circulatory overload during or immediately after surgery. Observe closely. Rarely used unless salt depletion factors are present. ▪ Excessive administration of potassium-free solutions may cause hypokalemia. ▪ Before and during use of hypertonic or concentrated sodium chloride, determine osmolar concentrations and chloride and bicarbonate content of the serum. Observe patient continuously to prevent pulmonary edema. ▪ With hypertonic or concentrated solutions, use a small needle and a large vein to reduce venous irritation and avoid extravasation (note Precautions).

Maternal/child: Category C: safety for use during pregnancy not established; use only if clearly needed. ▪ Use caution in lactation. ▪ Benzyl alcohol preservative in bacteriostatic sodium chloride has caused toxicity in newborns. Do not use. ▪ Safety for use in children not established.

Elderly: Incidence of adverse reactions may be increased; monitor carefully, especially with renal or cardiac insufficiency with or without CHF. ▪ Note Precautions.

SIDE EFFECTS

Due to sodium excess: aggravation of existing acidosis, anorexia, cellular dehydration, deep respiration, disorientation, distention, edema, hydrogen loss, hyperchloremic acidosis, hypertension, increased BUN, nausea, oliguria, potassium loss, pulmonary edema, water retention, weakness. Excessive excretion of crystalloids to maintain normal osmotic pressure will increase excretion of potassium and bicarbonate and further increase acidosis. Other salts (e.g., iodide and bromide) used for therapy will also be excreted rapidly.

ANTIDOTE

Discontinue or decrease the rate of infusion and notify the physician of side effects. Sodium excess can be treated by sodium restriction and/or use of diuretics or hemodialysis to remove excessive amounts. Observe the patient carefully and treat symptomatically. Save balance of fluid for examination.

SODIUM NITRITE AND SODIUM THIOSULFATE

Antidote

pH 7.0 to 9.0/pH 6.0 to 9.5

USUAL DOSE

Cyanide poisoning and treatment of nitroprusside-induced cyanide toxicity:
Following administration of amyl nitrite inhalant or immediately if an IV line is in place, give 300 mg (10 ml) 3% sodium nitrite IV followed by sodium thiosulfate 12.5 Gm IV (125 ml 10% solution or 50 ml 25%). 150 to 200 mg/kg is an alternate dosing schedule for sodium thiosulfate. One half of the initial dose of both drugs may be repeated in 2 hours if signs of toxicity persist.

Prophylaxis against nitroprusside induced cyanide toxicity (Sodium thiosulfate only): Coadministration of sodium thiosulfate in doses 5 to 10 times that of nitroprusside has been used to avoid toxicity with larger doses or necessary long-term therapy. May potentiate hypotensive action, use with caution.

Arsenic poisoning (Sodium thiosulfate only [unlabeled use]): 100 mg (1 ml 10% solution, 0.4 ml 25%) on the first day. Increase dose by 100 mg each day until 500 mg dose is reached. Thereafter, give 500 mg every other day as needed.

Prophylaxis against cisplatin induced nephrotoxicity (Sodium thiosulfate only [unlabeled use]): A standard dose has not been established. A common recommendation is a bolus dose of 4 gm/M^2 (range is 3 to 7.5 gm/M^2) prior to cisplatin administration followed by an infusion of 2 gm/M^2/hr for 5 to 12 hours as cisplatin is being instilled.

PEDIATRIC DOSE

Cyanide poisoning or treatment of nitroprusside-induced cyanide toxicity:
Following administration of amyl nitrite inhalant, or immediately if an IV line is in place, give 180 to 240 mg (6 to 8 ml) of 3% sodium nitrite/M^2 (or 4 to 6 mg/kg [0.2 ml/kg]) followed by sodium thiosulfate 7 Gm/M^2 (70 ml of 10% solution/M^2 or 28 ml of 25% solution/M^2). Do not exceed adult doses.

DILUTION

Both may be given undiluted.

Storage: Ampoule must be airtight for storage. Store at CRT.

INCOMPATIBLE WITH

Acids, oxidizing agents, salts of heavy metals.

RATE OF ADMINISTRATION

Cyanide poisoning: Sodium nitrite at 2.5 ml/min; sodium thiosulfate, a single dose equally distributed over 10 minutes or longer.

Arsenic poisoning: Each 100 mg or fraction thereof equally distributed over at least 2 minutes.

ACTIONS

Sodium nitrite produces methemoglobinemia that combines with the cyanide ion to make cyanmethemoglobin. It dissociates to make free cyanide, which is then converted to thiocyanate by sodium thiosulfate. The end product is excreted in urine.

INDICATIONS AND USES

A cyanide antidote kit containing sodium thiosulfate, sodium nitrate and amyl nitrite is used to facilitate the removal of cyanide in intoxication and in nitroprusside-induced cyanide toxicity. ▪ Sodium thiosulfate is also used for prophylaxis against nitroprusside-induced cyanide toxicity and as an injection into tissue infiltrated by extravasation of mechlorethamine.

Unlabeled use: Sodium thiosulfate may be used in the treatment of arsenic poisoning and for prophylaxis against cisplatin-induced nephrotoxicity in the intraperitoneal treatment of ovarian cancer.

CONTRAINDICATIONS

None when used for specific indication.

PRECAUTIONS

Read instructions supplied in kit thoroughly. ▪ Dimercaprol (BAL) IM is more commonly used as an antidote for arsenic poisoning. ▪ If there is reasonable suspicion of cyanide toxicity, initiate treatment immediately (usually before lab results are known).

Monitor: Monitor the patient very carefully, maintain a patent airway, and provide oxygen. ▪ Control BP with IV fluids and vasopressors (e.g., dopamine [Intropin]), and correct acidosis if indicated (may not appear until more than 1 hour after dangerous cyanide levels occur). Measurement of cyanide levels and arterial blood gases to determine venous hyperoxemia and acidosis may be indicated. Measurment of methemoglobin concentrations may be indicated.

Maternal/child: Pregnancy Category C: use only when clearly needed.

SIDE EFFECTS

Abdominal pain, angina, apprehension, dizziness, headache (severe), hypotension, involuntary passing of urine and feces, nausea and vomiting, paradoxical bradycardia, restlessness, tachycardia, weakness, vertigo.

ANTIDOTE

Keep physician informed of all side effects; will be treated symptomatically. Rapid infusion of sodium nitrite may cause excessive vasodilation and hypotension. A decrease in rate of administration may be necessary. Resuscitate as indicated.

SODIUM PHOSPHATE P$_{32}$

Antineoplastic
(Radiopharmaceutical)

pH 5.0 to 6.0

USUAL DOSE

Measured by appropriate radioactivity calibration system immediately before administration by the radiation oncologist. See literature for specific calibrations.

Polycythemia vera: Leukocyte count should be 5,000/mm^3 or more, and platelet count should be above 150,000/mm^3. 2.3 millicuries (mCi)/M^2 as an initial dose. Average is 3 to 5 mCi; range is 1 to 8 mCi depending on stage of disease and patient size. Must be individualized. May repeat

in 12 weeks if necessary. Should be used with adjunctive phlebotomy.
Chronic leukemia: Leukocyte count should be 20,000/mm³ or more. One source says 1 to 3 mCi, another 6 to 15 mCi.
Skeletal metastases: Leukocyte count should be 5,000/mm³ or more and platelet count should be above 100,000/mm³. 10 to 21 mCi given in divided doses over a 3 to 4 week schedule. See literature for sample schedule.

DOSE ADJUSTMENTS
Reduced doses or extended intervals may be required in the elderly.

DILUTION
Specific techniques required; see Precautions. May be given undiluted. May be given direct IV or through Y-tube or three-way stopcock of a free-flowing IV infusion. May be further diluted in 50 to 100 ml NS, D5W, or D5/NS and given as an infusion. Use only clear, colorless solutions. Do not use chromic sodium phosphate P₃₂; it is for intracavitary therapy and is green and cloudy.
Storage: Stored at room temperature in special containers in specific areas.

INCOMPATIBLE WITH
Specific information not available. Consider incompatible with any other drug in syringe or solution because of radioactivity and specific use.

RATE OF ADMINISTRATION
Direct IV: Total desired dose over 2 to 3 minutes.
IV infusion: Total dose over 30 minutes.

ACTIONS
Phosphorus is required in the metabolic and proliferative activity of cells. Radioactive phosphorus concentrates in rapidly proliferating tissue (e.g., bone marrow, spleen, liver). Beneficial only when in direct contact with malignancy or absorbed into bone. Half-life is 14.3 days. Decays by beta emission.

INDICATIONS AND USES
Treatment of polycythemia vera, chronic myelocytic leukemia, and chronic lymphocytic leukemia. ■ Palliative treatment of selected patients with multiple areas of skeletal metastases.
Unlabeled use: Treatment of essential thrombocytothemia.

CONTRAINDICATIONS
Sequential treatment with a chemotherapeutic agent. See Usual dose for specific limitations based on leukocyte and platelet counts.

PRECAUTIONS
Rarely used. Follow specific guidelines for handling radioactive agents to ensure minimum radiation exposure to patients and occupational workers consistent with appropriate patient management. Contact radiation safety officer. ■ Radiopharmaceuticals usually administered in the hospital by or under the direction of the physician specialist whose experience and training have been approved by the appropriate government agency. ■ Oral administration in a fasting patient may be as effective as IV administration. ■ Not usually effective in retinoblastomas. ■ Use radiopharmaceuticals when indicated within 10 days of onset of menses in women of childbearing age. Bone pain may be temporarily increased in patients pretreated with testosterone.
Monitor: Monitor CBC and platelet count at regular intervals. ■ Prepare

IV set-up and prime IV tubing in advance. Ensure there will be no dripping or spills of radioactive material. ■ Maintain adequate hydration. ■ Use of prophylactic antibiotics may be indicated pending results of C/S in a febrile neutropenic patient.

Patient education: Avoid pregnancy. Nonhormonal birth control recommended. ■ See Appendix D, p. 900.

Maternal/child: Category C: safety for use in pregnancy not established. Use only when clearly indicated and benefits exceed hazards to fetus. ■ Discontinue breast feeding. ■ Safety for use in children not established. ■ Note Precautions.

Elderly: May be more sensitive to effects of radiation. ■ Note Dose adjustments.

DRUG/LAB INTERACTIONS

Concurrent use with bone marrow depressants (e.g., antineoplastics [carboplatin, daunorubicin], chloramphenicol) may increase bone marrow toxicity.

SIDE EFFECTS

Anemia, leukopenia, and thrombocytopenia may occur with larger therapeutic doses. 15% of patients with polycythemia may develop acute leukemia.

ANTIDOTE

Keep physician informed of patient status and results of blood and bone marrow studies. Appropriate transfusions or blood modifiers (e.g., epoetin-alfa [Epogen, Procrit], filgrastin [Neupogen], sargramostim [Leukine], oprelvekin [Numega]) may be indicated to treat bone marrow toxicity.

STREPTOKINASE
Kabikinase, Streptase

Thrombolytic agent

pH 6.0 to 8.0

USUAL DOSE

Coronary artery thrombi: 1.5 million IU direct IV within 6 hours of onset of symptoms of acute transmural myocardial infarction. An alternative is 20,000 IU given directly into coronary artery within 6 hours of onset of symptoms of acute transmural myocardial infarction. Follow with 2,000 IU/min for 1 hour. Total dose equals 140,000 IU. Other protocols are in use. Recent studies suggest that alteplase (tPA) is the drug of choice.

Deep vein thrombosis, pulmonary or arterial embolism, arterial thrombosis:
Loading dose: 250,000 IU.

Maintenance dose: 100,000 IU/hour for 24 to 72 hours depending on diagnosis. May be increased based on thrombin time evaluations.

Arteriovenous cannula occlusion: 250,000 IU into each occluded limb of cannula.

DILUTION

All uses except cannula occlusion: Each vial (250,000, 600,000, 750,000, or 1,500,000 IU) must be diluted with 5 ml of NS (preferred) or D5W. Add diluent slowly, direct to sides of vial, roll and tilt gently. Do not shake. Further slowly dilute each vial to a total volume of 45 ml (preferred). May be diluted to a maximum of 500 ml in 45 ml increments (preferred). Discard solution with large amounts of flocculation or any solution remaining after 24 hours. Can be infused through a 0.8 micron or larger pore filter.

Arteriovenous cannula occlusion: Each vial (250,000 IU) must be diluted with 2 ml sodium chloride for injection. Use care in dilution as above.

Storage: Refrigerate after initial dilution. Discard after 24 hours.

INCOMPATIBLE WITH

Most references and manufacturer state, "Do not add any medications to solution or to Y-site." Another source suggests *Y-site compatibility* with dobutamine (Dobutrex), dopamine (Intropin), heparin, lidocaine, nitroglyerin. Consult pharmacist.

RATE OF ADMINISTRATION

Volumetric or syringe infusion pump required. Reconstituted streptokinase will alter drop size and impact correct dosage with drop size mechanisms.

Direct IV use for coronary artery thrombi: 1.5 million IU dose evenly distributed over 60 minutes.

Coronary artery thrombi: Bolus dose over 15 to 30 seconds via coronary catheter placed by Judkins or Sones technique directly to thrombosed site verified by selective coronary angiography. Follow with 2,000 IU/min for 60 minutes.

Deep vein thrombosis, pulmonary arterial embolism, arterial thrombi: Loading dose: a single dose equally distributed over 25 to 30 minutes.

Maintenance dose: 100,000 IU or more as ordered equally distributed every hour for 24 to 72 hours. Dissolution of arterial thrombi may occur in 24 hours or less; deep vein thrombi may take up to 72 hours.

Arteriovenous cannula occlusion: A single dose slowly (do not force) into each occluded limb of cannula. Clamp for 2 hours, then aspirate contents, flush with saline, and reconnect.

ACTIONS

An enzyme prepared from filtrates of beta-hemolytic streptococci. It combines with plasminogen and converts it to plasmin, which degrades fibrin clots, fibrinogen, and other plasma proteins. This activation takes place within a thrombus as well as on the surface. Onset of action is prompt and may last up to 12 to 24 hours. End products of this activity possess an anticoagulant effect. Bleeding may be very difficult to control.

INDICATIONS AND USES

Lysis of coronary artery thrombi. JAMA standards identify thrombolytic agents as Class I therapy in patients younger than 70 years with chest pain consistent with acute MI and at least 0.1 mV of ST segment elevation in at least two ECG leads. Use in all other patients based on age, accurate diagnosis, and time from onset of chest pain. ■ Lysis of acute massive pulmonary emboli if one or more lobes are involved or if hemodynamics are unstable. ■ Lysis of an equivalent amount of thrombi in other vessels (deep veins). ■ Lysis of acute arterial thrombi and arterial emboli. ■ Clearing of occluded arteriovenous cannulae as an alternative to surgical revision.

CONTRAINDICATIONS

Active internal bleeding, cerebral vascular accident within 2 months, intracranial or intraspinal surgery, intracranial neoplasm, hypersensitivity to streptokinase.

PRECAUTIONS

Administered only in the hospital under the direction of a physician knowledgeable in its use and with appropriate diagnostic and laboratory facilities available. ▪ For coronary catheter procedure, diagnosis of acute myocardial infarction must be confirmed and the site of the coronary thrombosis confirmed with selective angiography. Concurrent heparin therapy may be required in this situation. ▪ Diagnosis of pulmonary or other emboli should be confirmed. Best results obtained if started within 5 to 7 days of onset of pulmonary emboli; 3 to 4 days of onset of DVT, and 3 days of onset of arterial thrombi. Discontinue streptokinase if thrombin time or other lysis parameters are not above 1½ times normal in 4 hours. Excessive resistance may be present. ▪ Use extreme caution in presence of atrial fibrillation or mitral stenosis with atrial fibrillation; very high risk of stroke from dislodged emboli. ▪ Prior sensitization to streptokinase increases risk of allergic reaction in subsequent courses of treatment. ▪ Use extreme caution in the following situations: any surgical procedure, biopsy, lumbar puncture, thoracentesis, paracentesis, multiple cutdowns, or intraarterial diagnostic procedures within 10 days; ulcerative wounds; recent trauma with possible internal injury; visceral malignancy; pregnancy and first 10 days postpartum; any lesion of GI or GU tract with a potential for bleeding (e.g., diverticulitis, ulcerative colitis); severe hypertension; acute or chronic hepatic or renal insufficiency; uncontrolled hypocoagulable state; chronic lung disease with cavitation; rheumatic valvular disease; subacute bacterial endocarditis; and any condition where bleeding might be hazardous or difficult to manage because of location.

Monitor: Establish a separate IV line for streptokinase. ▪ Observe patient continuously. Obtain hematocrit, platelet count, activated PTT, thrombin time, prothrombin time, and CPK before therapy. ▪ Diphenhydramine (Benadryl) 50 mg IV prophylactically is recommended. ▪ In 4 hours and during therapy thrombin time or prothrombin time changes are monitored and will reflect effectiveness of treatment. Keep physician continuously informed. Request specific parameters for notifying physician after initial supervised injection. ▪ Coronary thrombi may lyse in 1 hour; continue treatment to ensure complete lysis. ▪ Monitor ECG and record strips with greatest ST segment elevation initially and every 15 minutes for at least 4 hours. ▪ Monitor blood pressure frequently. ▪ When thrombin time is less than twice the normal control value, initiate heparin infusion to keep PTT at 60 seconds. Prompt, easy treatment of direct IV a distinct advantage over catheter procedure. ▪ Maintain strict bed rest and apply pressure dressings to any recently invaded site. ▪ A greater alteration of hemostatic status than with heparin; use care in handling patient; avoid arterial puncture, venipuncture, and IM injection. Use extreme precautionary methods (use of radial artery, not femoral; extended pressure application of up to 30 minutes) if above procedures absolutely necessary. Minor bleeding occurs often at streptokinase insertion sites. Do not reduce or stop streptokinase as lytic activity will be increased and cause more bleeding. ▪ Monitor for hypotension and arrhythmias during therapy; atrial and ventricular arrhythmias can occur. ▪ Intensive follow-up therapy with continuous infusion of heparin (without a loading dose) is indicated in all situations to prevent recurrent thrombosis. Begin in about 3 to 4 hours of completion of streptokinase, when the thrombin time or aPTT is reduced to less than twice the normal control value. ■ Do not take blood pressure in lower extremities; thrombi may be dislodged. ■ Attempt to clear arteriovenous cannulae occlusions with good syringe technique and heparinized saline before using streptokinase. Allow effect of heparin to diminish. Instruct patient to exhale and hold his breath any time the catheter is not connected to the IV tubing or a syringe to prevent air from entering the open catheter and thus the circulatory system.

Patient education: Report any signs of allergic reaction promptly (e.g., itching, rash, shortness of breath). ■ Compliance with all measures to minimize bleeding (e.g., strict bed rest) is very important. ■ Avoid use of razors, toothbrushes, and other sharp items. ■ Use caution while moving to avoid excessive bumping. ■ Report all episodes of bleeding and apply local pressure if indicated.

Maternal/child: Pregnancy Category C: use only if clearly needed. Safety for use in pregnancy, lactation, or children not established.

Elderly: Note Indications and Precautions. ■ May have poorer prognosis following MI and pre-existing conditions that may increase risk of intracranial bleeding. Select patients carefully to maximize benefits.

DRUG/LAB INTERACTIONS

Simultaneous use of anticoagulants not recommended except for coronary artery thrombi. Do not use either drug until the effects of the previous drug are diminished. ■ Avoid use of drugs that may alter platelet function (e.g., aspirin, indomethacin, phenylbutazone).

SIDE EFFECTS

Allergic reactions, including anaphylaxis, are not uncommon with streptokinase. Arrhythmias, hypotension. Fever increase of 1° to 2° F is common. Bleeding can be life threatening.

ANTIDOTE

Notify physician of all side effects. Note even the minutest bleeding tendency. Therapy may have to be discontinued with serious blood loss and bleeding not controlled by local pressure. Whole blood, packed red blood cells, cryoprecipitate, fresh-frozen plasma, platelets, desmopressin, tranexamic acid, and aminocaproic acid may all be indicated. Do not use dextran. Topical preparations of aminocaproic acid may stop minor bleeding. Consider protamine if heparin has been used. Treat bradycardia with atropine, reperfusion arrhythmias with lidocaine or procainamide; VT or VF may require cardioversion. If hypotension occurs, reduce rate promptly. If not resolved, vasopressors (e.g., dopamine [Intropin]), Trendelenburg position, and suitable plasma expanders (e.g., albumin, plasma protein fraction [Plasmanate], or hetastarch) may be indicated. Treat minor allergic reactions symptomatically. Discontinue drug and treat anaphylaxis as indicated; resuscitate as necessary.

STREPTOMYCIN SULFATE

Antibacterial
(Aminoglycoside)
Antituberculosis

pH 5.0 to 8.0

USUAL DOSE

Mycobacterium *tuberculosis:* 12 to 15 mg/kg daily. Calculation is be based on ideal body weight not actual weight. 12 to 27 mg/kg has been used safely. Doses over 20 mg/kg are usually given every other day. Used in combination with isoniazid (INH), rifampin (Rifadin), and pyrazinamide. Maximum suggested total cumulative dose over the course of therapy is 120 Gm.

Mycobacterium avium *complex:* 11 to 13 mg/kg daily. Part of a multiple drug regimen of three to five agents.

DOSE ADJUSTMENTS

Reduced dose required in renal impairment and/or nitrogen retention. ■ Reduce dose in patients over 60 years based on age, renal function, and eighth nerve impairment. ■ Elevated peak drug concentrations require a reduced dose. ■ Note Drug/lab interactions.

DILUTION

Prepared solution equals 400 mg/ml. Further dilute total daily dose to a volume of 100 ml with D5W or D5/NS.

Storage: Refrigerate undiluted ampoules. Diluted solution is stable for 24 hours at room temperature. According to the National Jewish Center guidelines, the current formulation from Pfizer is stable for up to 30 days after dilution if refrigerated.

INCOMPATIBLE WITH

Amobarbital (Amytal), amphotericin B (Fungizone), ampicillin, chlorothiazide (Diuril), erythromycin gluceptate, heparin, methicillin, methohexital (Brevital), norepinephrine (Levophed), pentobarbital (Nembutal), phenobarbital (Luminal), phenytoin (Dilantin), secobarbital (Seconal), sodium bicarbonate.

RATE OF ADMINISTRATION

Total daily dose, properly diluted, as an infusion over 30 minutes. Slow rate to 60 minutes if any tingling or dizziness occurs during administration or if elevated peak drug concentrations occur.

ACTIONS

An aminoglycoside antibiotic with potential neuromuscular blocking action. Inhibits protein synthesis in bacterial cells. Bactericidal against specific gram-negative organisms and bacilli. Well distributed through all organ tissues except the brain (unless meninges inflamed). Peak serum levels of 25 to 50 mcg/ml occur promptly and gradually decrease to 12.5 to 25 mcg/ml over 5 to 6 hours. Usual half-life is 2.5 hours. Half-life is prolonged in infants, postpartum females, liver disease and ascites, spinal cord injury, cystic fibrosis, and the elderly. May be prolonged up to 100 hours in end-stage renal disease. Half-life is shorter in anemia, severe burns, and fever. Crosses the placental barrier. 30% to 90% excreted in urine with 24 hours.

INDICATIONS AND USES

Treatment of *Mycobacterium* tuberculosis when one or more of the following drugs (ethambutol [Myambutol], isoniazid [INH], rifampin [Rifadin], or pyrazinamide) is contraindicated because of toxicity, intolerance, or drug resistance. Increased rates of drug resistance and/or concomitant HIV infection are more common than in previous times. Usual four drug regimen is either ethambutol or streptomycin with isoniazid, rifampin, and pyrazinamide. IV administration is especially useful in cachectic patients or those needing prolonged streptomycin therapy.

Investigational uses: *Mycobacterium avium* complex, a common infection in AIDS patients. ■ Prophylactically after coronary artery bypass surgery.

CONTRAINDICATIONS

Known streptomycin sensitivity. Known aminoglycoside sensitivity may be a contraindication due to cross sensitivity.

PRECAUTIONS

Labeled for IM use only; probably due to impurities in early preparations. New formulations are being given safely IV; check your hospital's policy in case an informed consent or release is required. ■ Handle with care, may cause skin sensitivity reactions. ■ Used only when other less hazardous agents are ineffective or contraindicated. ■ Adequate laboratory and audiometic testing facilities must be available. ■ Sensitivity studies necessary to determine susceptibility of causative organism to streptomycin. ■ Superinfection may occur from overgrowth of nonsusceptible organisms. ■ May contain sulfites; use caution in patients with asthma. ■ For additional questions, consultations may be obtained from the Division of Infectious Disease at National Jewish Center (800-423-8891, ext. 1279).

Monitor: Monitor serum BUN, creatinine, calcium, magnesium, potassium, and sodium before therapy and weekly. ■ Calcium, magnesium, potassium, and sodium levels may decline and require replacement. ■ Observe for any adverse effects including at the infusion site. ■ High serum levels increase risk of ototoxicity and neurotoxicity. Assess adequacy of dose and clearance of drug with serum streptomycin concentrations (2 to 6 hours after a timed dose) initially and every 2 to 4 weeks. Peak therapeutic levels are between 20 and 30 mcg/ml. Serum levels over 50 mcg/ml may be toxic. ■ Watch for decrease in urine output, rising BUN and serum creatinine, and declining creatinine clearance levels. Dose may require decreasing, serum levels should not exceed 25 mcg/ml if any kidney damage is present. ■ Assess vestibular function toxicity weekly (Romberg test, past point, heel to toe, and lateral nystagmus). ■ Assess ototoxicity with audiograms every 2 to 4 weeks. ■ All of the above monitoring may be done more frequently if indicated. Permanently implanted central venous catheters allow treatment on an outpatient basis. Blood work may be done every 2 weeks and all other tests every 4 weeks when stable enough to be treated as an outpatient. ■ Maintain good hydration. Dehydration may increase risk of nephrotoxicity, monitor closely if vomiting, diarrhea, or other events which may cause dehydration occur. ■ National Jewish Center uses chromatographic assay to determine streptomycin serum levels; concomitantly administered antibiotics do not have to be withheld when collecting samples for analysis. ■ Usual length of treatment for tuberculosis is 1 year. Discontinue streptomycin therapy whenever toxic symptoms appear, impending toxicity is feared, organisms become resistant, or full therapeutic effect is achieved. ■ In long-term therapy, alkalinization of urine may minimize renal irritation. ■ Note Drug/lab interactions.

Patient education: Report promptly any changes in balance, dizziness, hearing loss or weakness. ■ Consider birth control options.

Maternal/child: Category D: avoid pregnancy; has caused total irreversible bilateral deafness in infants whose mothers received streptomycin during pregnancy. ■ Discontinue breast feeding. ■ Has caused CNS depression including stupor, flaccidity, coma, and deep respiratory depression in very young infants.

Elderly: Risk of toxicity increased; note Dose adjustments.

DRUG/LAB INTERACTIONS

Inactivated in solution with penicillins but is synergistic when used in combination with beta-lactam antibiotics (e.g., cephalosporins, penicillins) and vancomycin. Dose adjustment and appropriate spacing required because of physical incompatibilities and interactions. Synergism may be inconsistent; measure aminoglycoside levels. ■ Concurrent use with any other neutotoxic, ototoxic, or nephrotoxic agents should be avoided. May have dangerous additive effects with other aminoglycosides (e.g., gentamicin, neosporin), diuretics (e.g., furosemide [Lasix], mannitol), beta-lactam antibiotics (e.g., cephalosporins), colistin (Coly-Mycin-S), polymixin-B (Aerosporin), vancomycin, cyclosporine, and many others. ■ May be antagonized by bacteriostatic antibiotics (e.g., chloramphenicol, erythromycin, and tetracycline); bactericidal action may be impacted. ■ Anesthetics (e.g., enflurane) and neuromuscular blocking muscle relaxants (e.g., doxacurium [Nuromax], succinylcholine [Anectine]) are potentiated by aminoglycosides. Respiratory paralysis and *apnea can occur.* ■ Aminoglycosides are potentiated by anticholinesterases (e.g., edrophonium), antineoplastics (e.g., nitrogen mustard, cisplatin). ■ Note Side effects.

SIDE EFFECTS

Occur more frequently with impaired renal function, higher doses, prolonged administration, dehydration, in the elderly, and in patients receiving other ototoxic or nephrotoxic drugs. Allergic reactions (e.g., angioneurotic edema, anaphylaxis, itching, rash, urticaria), apnea, azotemia, cochlear ototoxicity (hearing loss and deafness), eosinophilia, exfoliative dermatitis, hemolytic anemia, facial parasthesias, fever, leukopenia, muscular weakness, neuromuscular blockade, pancytopenia, roaring in the ears, thrombocytopenia, tinnitus, vestibular ototoxicity (nausea and vomiting, vertigo). Least nephrotic of the aminoglycosides but nephrotoxicity does occur. Has caused severe chilling (rigors) with penicillins if spacing is not adequate.

ANTIDOTE

Notify the physician of all side effects. Discontinue streptomycin with any evidence of renal impairment, ototoxicity, or vestibular toxicity. Tinnitus, roaring noises, or a sense of fullness in the ears indicate a need for audiometric examination. Auditory changes are usually irreversible and bilateral and may be partial or total. Vestibular symptoms are reversible if detected early. A reduction in dose may be required or an alternate drug used. In overdose hemodialysis may be indicated. Monitor fluid balance, creatinine clearance, and plasma levels carefully. Complexation with ticarcillin (12 to 30 Gm/day) may be as effective as hemodialysis. Calcium salts or neostigmine may reverse neuromuscular blockade. Resuscitate as necessary.

STREPTOZOCIN

Antineoplastic (Alkylating agent/nitrosurea)

Zanosar

pH 3.5 to 4.5

USUAL DOSE

500 mg/M^2 for 5 consecutive days. Repeat every 6 weeks until maximum benefit or treatment-limiting toxicity observed. May also give 1,000 mg/M^2 weekly for 2 doses. May then increase up to 1,500 mg/M^2 to achieve therapeutic response if significant toxicity not observed. Overall cumulative dose to onset of response is 2,000 mg/M^2. Maximum response is usually achieved with 4,000 mg/M^2 total cumulative dose.

DOSE ADJUSTMENTS

Reduce dose in impaired renal function, note Precautions/Monitor. ■ Reduce dose or discontinue drug if mild proteinuria occurs. ■ Can be used with other antineoplastic drugs in reduced doses to achieve tumor remission.

DILUTION

Specific techniques required; see Precautions. Each 1 Gm vial must be diluted with 9.5 ml NS or D5W (100 mg/ml). Usually further diluted in larger amounts (50 to 250 ml) of the same solutions.

Storage: Store in refrigerator before and after dilution. Discard within 12 hours of dilution. Contains no preservatives. Protect from light.

INCOMPATIBLE WITH

Consider toxicity and specific use. Allopurinol (Zyloprim), penicillin/tazobactam (Zosyn).

RATE OF ADMINISTRATION

A single dose in minimum diluent may be given over 5 to 15 minutes. Increase injection time if additional diluent used or if indicated for patient comfort. Has been given as a continuous infusion over 5 days. Reduced some side effects but increased some CNS side effects.

ACTIONS

An alkylating agent of the nitrosurea group with antitumor activity, cell cycle phase nonspecific. Has a diabetogenic (hyperglycemic) effect resulting from selective uptake into and toxicity to pancreatic islet beta cells. Disappears from the blood serum rapidly. Concentrates in the liver and kidneys. Excreted primarily in urine.

INDICATIONS AND USES

Suppress or retard neoplastic growth in metastatic pancreatic islet cell carcinoma. Use limited by renal toxicity to those with symptomatic or progressive metastatic disease.

Investigational uses: Treatment of adrenocortical and colon cancers and Hodgkin's lymphoma.

CONTRAINDICATIONS

Hypersensitivity to streptozocin. Severely impaired liver or renal function may be a contraindication.

PRECAUTIONS

Follow guidelines for handling cytotoxic agents. See Appendix A, p. 893. ▪ Administered by or under the direction of the physician specialist. ▪ Marked decrease in leukocyte and platelet counts has occurred and may be fatal.

Monitor: Renal toxicity is dose related, cumulative, and can be fatal. Monitor renal function before, weekly, and for 4 weeks after each course of therapy (serial urinalysis, BUN, plasma creatinine, serum electrolytes, creatinine clearance). Reduce dose or discontinue drug if mild proteinuria occurs. Further deterioration of renal function may occur. ▪ Determine absolute patency and quality of vein and adequate circulation of extremity. Severe cellulitis may result from extravasation. If extravasation occurs, discontinue injection; use another vein. ▪ Have IV dextrose available especially with the first dose. Sudden release of insulin may precipitate hypoglycemia. Monitor serum glucose at periodic intervals. ▪ Monitor CBC and liver function tests weekly. ▪ Nausea and vomiting have occurred in all patients and can be severe. Prophylactic administration of antiemetics recommended. ▪ Observe for any signs of infection. Use of prophylactic antibiotics may be indicated pending results of C/S in a febrile neutropenic patient. ▪ Maintain hydration. ▪ Note Drug/lab interactions.

Patient education: Avoid pregnancy, nonhormonal birth control recommended. ▪ Report IV site burning or stinging promptly. ▪ See Appendix D, p. 900.

Maternal/child: Category C: No studies in pregnant women, benefits must outweigh risks. Produces teratogenic effects in rats. Has mutagenic potential. ▪ Discontinue breast feeding.

DRUG/LAB INTERACTIONS

Do not administer live vaccines to patients receiving antineoplastic drugs. ▪ Concurrent use with hepatotoxic or nephrotoxic medications and radiation therapy may increase toxicity and could be fatal. ▪ Phenytoin (Dilantin) may decrease therapeutic effects.

SIDE EFFECTS

Anemia, decreased platelet count (precipitous), diarrhea, elevated AST (SGOT) and LDH, hepatic toxicity (usually reversible), hypoalbuminemia, hypoglycemia, insulin shock, leukopenia (precipitous), nausea and vomiting (severe), proteinuria, thrombocytopenia. Two cases of diabetes insipidus have been reported.

ANTIDOTE

Notify physician of all side effects. Nausea and vomiting, hematologic changes, and renal toxicity (proteinuria) may require dose reduction or discontinuation of the drug. There is no specific antidote. Supportive therapy as indicated will help sustain the patient in toxicity. For extravasation, elevate extremity, consider injection of long-acting dexamethasone (Decadron LA) or hyaluronidase (Wydase) throughout extravasated tissue. Use a 27- or 25-gauge needle. Apply warm moist compresses.

STRONTIUM-89 CHLORIDE INJECTION

Radiopharmaceutical

Metastron

pH 4.0 to 7.5

USUAL DOSE

Measured by a suitable radioactivity calibration system immediately prior to use by the radiation oncologist. Significant radioactivity, verify dose and patient. See literature for specific calibrations.

148 MBq, 4 mCi. An alternate dose is 1.5 to 2.2 MBq/kg, 40 to 60 mcCi/kg of body weight may be used. Any repeat dose should be based on individual response to therapy, current symptoms, and hematologic status. Not recommended at intervals of less than 90 days.

DILUTION

Special techniques required; see Precautions. Available as a 10 ml vial containing 148 MBq, 4 mCi (average single dose). May be given undiluted direct IV.

Storage: Keep inside its transportation shield whenever possible. Store at controlled room temperature.

INCOMPATIBLE WITH

Specific information not available. Consider incompatible with any other drug in syringe or solution because of radioactivity and specific use.

RATE OF ADMINISTRATION

Total desired dose over 1 to 2 minutes. A flushing sensation may occur with too rapid administration.

ACTIONS

An injectable radioisotope. Selectively irradiates sites of primary and metastatic bone with minimal irradiation of soft tissue (maximum range is 8 mm). Uptake by bone is increased at sites of metastatic bone disease as compared to normal bone, concentrating the radiation dose to these lesions. Relieves bone pain and reduces painful progression of new sites even when other therapies have not been effective. Retained in normal bone for 14 days, retained in metastatic bone lesions much longer. Half-life is 50.5 days. Decays by beta emission. Rapidly cleared from plasma. Primarily excreted in urine. 33% excreted in feces. Crosses the placental barrier.

INDICATIONS AND USES

Relief of bone pain in patients with painful skeletal metastases.

CONTRAINDICATIONS

None known.

PRECAUTIONS

Radiopharmaceuticals usually administered by or under the direction of the physician specialist whose experience and training have been approved by the appropriate government agency. ■ Confirm presence of bone metastases prior to therapy. ■ Not indicated for use in patients with cancer not involving bone. ■ Onset of pain relief is delayed (7 to 20 days post injection), not recommended if life expectancy is very short. ■ Use with caution in patients with platelet

counts below 60,000/mm^3 and white cell counts below 2,400/mm^3.
■ Benefits must outweigh risks if used in patients with evidence of seriously compromised bone marrow from previous therapy or disease infiltration or in patients with impaired renal function.

Monitor: Follow specific guidelines for handling radioactive agents to ensure minimum radiation exposure to patients and occupational workers consistent with appropriate patient management. Contact radiation safety officer. ■ Monitor complete blood counts including platelets before treatment and at least every other week. A 30% platelet depression is normal; nadir usually occurs between 12 and 16 weeks. Recovery is very slow, up to 6 months. ■ Catheterize incontinent patients to minimize risk of radioactive contamination of clothing, bed linen, and the patient's environment. ■ Use of prophylactic antibiotics may be indicated pending results of C/S in a febrile neutropenic patient.

Patient education: Avoid pregnancy; nonhormonal birth control recommended. ■ See Appendix D, p. 900. ■ Pain may be slightly increased after a few days; may last for 2 to 3 days; use pain medication as needed. ■ As pain is decreased need for pain meds should also decrease. Effects usually last for several months (average is 6 months). ■ Regular monitoring of blood count imperative. ■ During the first week after injection the following precautions are necessary: patient must inform any health professional caring for them that they have received strontium-89. Use of a toilet instead of a urinal is preferred, flush twice. Wipe up any spilled urine with a tissue and flush it away. Patient must wash hands after using the toilet. Immediately wash any linen or clothes that becomed stained with urine, feces, or blood. Wash separately from other clothes and rinse thoroughly. Ask for instructions if urine collection device is used. Wash away any spilled blood from cuts. ■ Follow usual diet and activity patterns. As pain improves, patient may be able to do more than previously; don't overdo. ■ Manufacturer provides a patient information sheet.

Maternal/child: Category D: avoid pregnancy. May cause fetal harm. ■ Discontinue breast feeding. ■ Safety for use in children under 18 years not established.

Elderly: Consider decreased renal function. Possibility of delayed excretion and need for extended precautions.

DRUG/LAB INTERACTIONS
Specific information not available.

SIDE EFFECTS
Bone marrow toxicity is expected. Transient increase in bone pain at 36 to 72 hours after injection.

ANTIDOTE
Keep physician informed of patient status and results of blood studies. Appropriate transfusions or blood modifiers may be indicated to treat bone marrow toxicity. Treat transient increase in bone pain with analgesics.

SUCCINYLCHOLINE CHLORIDE

Neuromuscular blocking agent
(Depolarizing)
Anesthesia adjunct

Anectine, Quelicin, Sucostrin

pH 3.0 to 4.5

USUAL DOSE

0.3 to 1.1 mg/kg of body weight initially for short-term muscle relaxation (average is 0.6 mg/kg). Should be administered after unconsciousness induced to reduce patient discomfort. If muscle relaxation must be sustained over a long period of time, maintain with intermittent IV injections of 0.04 to 0.07 mg/kg at appropriate intervals or with a continuous infusion of 0.5 to 10 mg/min (average is 2.5 to 4.3 mg/min). Monitoring with a peripheral nerve stimulator advisable to avoid overdose, especially with a continuous infusion. Highly individualized, depending on response and degree of relaxation required. 1 mg/kg of body weight is sufficient to cause respiratory paralysis. Never exceed 150 mg total dose. A test dose of 0.1 mg is sometimes used to test patient sensitivity and recovery time.

Electroshock therapy: 10 to 30 mg 1 minute prior to shock.

PEDIATRIC DOSE

Infants and small children: 1 to 2 mg/kg (most sources say 2 mg/kg).

Older children and adolescents: 1 mg/kg. To sustain muscle relaxation in all pediatric patients maintain with intermittent injections of 0.3 to 0.6 mg/kg/dose at 5 to 10 minute intervals. Monitoring with a peripheral nerve stimulator advisable. Continuous infusion not recommended; increased risk of malignant hyperpyrexia.

DOSE ADJUSTMENTS

Minimal doses with extreme care are required in patients with low plasma pseudocholinesterase (e.g., abnormal body temperatures, anemia, burns, cancer, collagen diseases, dehydration, exposure to neurotoxic insecticides, malnutrition, myxedema, patients with a recessive hereditary trait, pregnancy, severe liver disease or cirrhosis, and patients receiving antimalarials, antineoplastics, chlorpromazine [Thorazine], echothiophate iodide [Phospholine], irradiation, MAO inhibitors [e.g., selegiline (Eldepryl)], neostigmine, oral contraceptives, or pancuronium). Use a test dose of 5 to 10 mg or cautiously administer a 0.1% infusion.

DILUTION

May be given undiluted if short-term muscle relaxation is desired. For intermittent or continuous infusion during anesthesia add 1 Gm of succinylcholine to 500 ml or 1 liter of D5W, D5/NS, or NS. 1 ml of diluted solution delivers 2 mg (1 mg) of succinylcholine. For all other uses, 100 mg in 1 liter delivers 0.1 mg succinylcholine. Use only freshly prepared solutions.

Storage: Store in refrigerator after dilution. Multidose vials stable at room temperature for up to 14 days. Powder for infusion may be stored at room temperature before preparation.

INCOMPATIBLE WITH

Alkaline solutions, barbiturates (e.g., amobarbital [Amytal], methohexital [Brevital], pentobarbital [Nembutal], phenobarbital, secobarbital [Seconal], thiopental [Pentothal]), chlorpromazine (Thorazine), nafcillin (Unipen).

RATE OF ADMINISTRATION

Too-rapid rate may cause profound bradycardia and rarely asystole. Incidence of bradycardia higher with a second dose.

Direct IV: Single initial dose over 30 seconds.

Intermittent or continuous infusion: Variable, depending on individual response and muscle relaxation required. Use an infusion pump or microdrip (60 gtt/ml) for accuracy. Never exceed 10 mg/min.

ACTIONS

An ultra-short-acting depolarizing skeletal muscle relaxant. Causes paralysis by interfering with neural transmission at the myoneural junction. Onset of action is within 0.5 to 1 minute. Duration of peak effect is 4 to 10 minutes. Metabolized to succinic acid and choline. Only a small amount is excreted by the kidneys. Crosses placental barrier in small amounts.

INDICATIONS AND USES

Skeletal muscle relaxation during operative and manipulative procedures. ▪ Facilitate management of patients undergoing mechanical ventilation. ▪ Termination or prevention of convulsive episodes resulting from drug toxicity or electroshock therapy.

CONTRAINDICATIONS

Hypersensitivity to succinylcholine, family history of malignant hyperthermia, genetic disorders of plasma pseudocholinesterase, myopathies associated with elevated CPK values, acute narrow-angle glaucoma, penetrating eye injuries.

PRECAUTIONS

Primarily used by or under the direct observation of the anesthesiologist. ▪ Small doses of nondepolarizing muscle relaxants (e.g., tubocurarine) will reduce severity of muscle fasciculations and incidence of myoglobinuria (occurs more frequently in children) but may cause a prolonged mixed block. ▪ Incidence of bradycardia increased with repeat dosing. ▪ May cause prolonged blockade with hypocalemia, hypokalemia, and cardiovascular, hepatic, or pulmonary disorders. ▪ May cause serious cardiac arrhythmias, including cardiac arrest in patients who are digitalized or on quinidine, as well as those with electrolyte imbalance, hyperkalemia, or severe trauma. Use extreme caution. ▪ Patients with pre-existing hyperkalemia, or those with spinal cord injuries, paralysis, or degenerative or dystrophic neuromuscular disease may become severely hyperkalemic with succinylcholine; use caution. ▪ Prolonged respiratory paralysis may occur in patients with low plasma pseudocholinesterase (see Dose Adjustments; decreased plasma cholinesterase activity potentiates this drug). ▪ Muscle fasciculation may cause additional trauma in patients with fractures or muscle spasm. ▪ May cause cardiac arrest in children with undiagnosed Duchenne's muscular dystrophy; note Monitor. ▪ Patients with myasthenia gravis may be resistant to succinylcholine. ▪ May increase intraocular pressure. ▪ May convert to a nondepolarizing block during repeated or prolonged administration. Respiratory depression and apnea are common. Use a peripheral nerve stimulator to confirm diagnosis before treating with anticholinergic agents and atropine (See Antidote)

Monitor: This drug may produce apnea. Controlled artificial ventilation must be available and under direct observation at all times. ■ Observe for early signs of malignant hyperthermic crisis (jaw muscle spasm, lack of laryngeal relaxation, rigidity, and unresponsive tachycardia). ■ Continuous ECG monitoring recommended. Observe for peaked T-waves; may be an early sign of Duchenne's muscular dystrophy. Occurs more often in males under 8 years. ■ Monitor for increased intragastric pressure; avoid regurgitation and possible aspiration. ■ Note Precautions and Drug/lab interactions.

Maternal/child: Category C: use extreme caution in pregnancy. There is greater potential for prolonged apnea because of increased sensitivity to succinylcholine in pregnant women. If used during cesarean section; apnea and flaccidity may occur in the neonate depending on mother's dose. ■ Use caution in lactation. ■ A few occurrences of hyperkalemiainduced cardiac arrest have been noted in male pediatric patients.

Elderly: Delay in onset time may be caused by slower circulation time in cardiovascular disease, old age, or edematous states; allow more time for drug to achieve maximum effect.

DRUG/LAB INTERACTIONS

May cause a prolonged mixed block with nondepolarizing muscle relaxants (e.g., atracurium, tubocurarine). ■ May cause cardiac arrhythmias in digitalized patients resulting from a sudden loss of potassium from muscle cells. ■ Potentiated by neuromuscular blocking antibiotics (e.g., aminoglycosides [e.g., kanamycin, neomycin]), selected non-penicillin antibiotics (e.g., bacitracin, colistimethate, polymyxins, tetracyclines, vancomycin), beta-adrenergic blocking agents (e.g., propranolol [Inderal]), furosemide (Lasix), procainamide (Pronestyl), organic phosphate compounds (insecticides), anticholinesterase drugs (e.g., neostigmine, edrophonium), cimetidine (Tagamet), cyclophosphamide (Cytoxan), isoflurane, lidocaine, lithium carbonate, quinine, quinidine, and magnesium salts. ■ Increased neuromuscular blockade and prolonged respiratory depression may occur for several days after cyclophosphamide therapy is stopped. ■ Potentiated by amphotericin B and thiazide diuretics in patients with electrolyte imbalance (e.g., hypocalcemia, hypokalemia); reduced dose indicated. ■ Incidence of cardiac arrhythmias and/or malignant hyperthermia may be increased with inhalation anesthetics (e.g., cyclopropane, halothane). ■ Incidence of cardiac arrhythmias may be increased by narcotic analgesics. ■ May cause muscle paralysis and respiratory collapse with vancomycin. ■ Capable of innumerable other drug interactions. ■ Inhibited by previous administration of diazepam (Valium).

SIDE EFFECTS

Minor: Bradycardia, or other cardiac arrhythmias, histamine release, hyperkalemia, muscular twitching, myoglobinemia, myoglobinuria, rash, respiratory depression, salivation (excessive).

Major: Cardiac arrhythmias, hyperthermia, malignant hyperthermic crisis, prolonged apnea with progression to a phase II block (usually results from repeated or prolonged administration).

ANTIDOTE

Discontinue drug with onset of any major side effect. An anesthesiologist should be present. Controlled artificial ventilation must be continuous. Endotracheal intubation or tracheostomy is considered prophylactic if necessary for adequate respiratory exchange. Confirm diagnosis of phase II block by using a peripheral nerve stimulator; presence of muscle twitch must also have returned for at least 20 minutes. Both of these are necessary before reversal with anticholinesterase drugs (e.g., neostigmine) is attempted. Whole blood transfusion may restore absent cholinesterase activity and stimulate voluntary respiration in unresponsive cases. Atropine should help to control bradycardia. Treat malignant hyperthermic crisis symptomatically with cooling measures, restoration of electrolyte balance, IV fluids, and maintenance of urinary output. Sodium bicarbonate may be indicated. Dantrolene may be indicated. IV calcium, bicarbonate, and glucose with insulin concurrent with hyperventilation have been used to resuscitate children with Duchenne's muscular dystrophy. Resuscitate as necessary.

SULFAMETHOXAZOLE-TRIMETHOPRIM

Antibacterial
Antiprotozoal

Bactrim, Co-trimoxazole, Septra, SMZ-TMP, TMP-SMZ   pH 10.0

USUAL DOSE

Doses listed are based on the trimethoprim component of the drug.

Severe urinary tract infections and shigellosis in adults and children over 2 months of age: 8 to 10 mg/kg of body weight in equally divided doses every 6, 8, or 12 hours for 14 days (urinary tract infections) or 5 days (shigellosis).

Pneumocystis carinii *pneumonitis in adults and children over 2 months of age:* 15 to 20 mg/kg in equally divided doses every 6 or 8 hours for up to 14 days.

DOSE ADJUSTMENTS

Reduce dose by one-half for creatinine clearance between 15 and 30 ml/min; note Contraindications. ■ Reduced dose may be indicated in the elderly. ■ Note Monitor and Drug/lab interactions.

DILUTION

Each 5 ml ampoule must be diluted in 125 ml D5W and given as an infusion. Reduce diluent to 75 ml for each ampoule only if fluid restriction required. Standard dilution must be used within 6 hours; fluid restriction dilution must be used within 2 hours. Available in 5, 10, 20, and 30 ml vials. Concentration per ml same as 5 ml ampoule. Discard if cloudiness or crystallization is present.

Storage: Store at room temperature; do not refrigerate.

INCOMPATIBLE WITH

Do not mix in syringe or solution with any other drug (manufacturer's directive). Fluconazole (Diflucan), foscarnet (Foscavir), midazolam (Versed), NS, vinorelbine (Navelbine).

RATE OF ADMINISTRATION

A single dose must be infused over 60 to 90 minutes. When administered by an infusion device, thoroughly flush all lines used to remove any residual sulfamethoxazole-trimethoprim. Avoid rapid infusion or bolus injection.

ACTIONS

A broad-spectrum antibacterial and antiprotozoal combination agent with bacteriocidal action effective against gram-positive and gram-negative organisms. Blocks sequential steps in the folic acid pathway, preventing the synthesis of nucleic acids and proteins essential to many bacteria. Combination contains 400 mg sulfamethoxazole and 80 mg trimethoprim per each 5 ml. Widely distributed in all body fluids and tissues, including cerebrospinal fluid, sputum, and bile. Onset of action is prompt and serum levels are maintained up to 10 hours. Metabolized in the liver and up to 60% is excreted in urine in 24 hours. Crosses placental barrier. Secreted in breast milk. Partially removed by hemodialysis.

INDICATIONS AND USES

Severe urinary tract infections. ▪ *Pneumocystis carinii* pneumonia. ▪ Shigellosis. ▪ Prophylaxis in neutropenic patients. ▪ Used orally in HIV and other immunocompromised patients to prevent pneumonia.
Investigational use: Treatment of cholera and salmonella type infections.

CONTRAINDICATIONS

Creatinine clearance below 15 ml/min, hypersensitivity to trimethoprim or sulfonamides, megaloblastic anemia resulting from folate deficiency, nursing mothers, pregnancy at term and infants less than 2 months of age (may cause hemolytic anemia, jaundice and kernicterus), streptococcal pharyngitis.

PRECAUTIONS

Sensitivity studies indicated to determine susceptibility of the causative organism to sulfamethoxazole-trimethoprim. ▪ Not for IM use. ▪ Use caution in impaired liver or renal function, possible folate deficiency, allergic individuals, bronchial asthma, porphyria, glucose 6-phosphate dehydrogenase (G-6PD) deficiency, and in the elderly. ▪ A sulfonamide drug; allergic reactions can occur. Use caution in patients with a history of hypersensitivity to furosemide (Lasix), thiazide diuretics (e.g., chlorothiazide), sulfonylureas (e.g., tolbutamide), or carbonic anhydrase inhibitors (e.g., acetazolamide). ▪ Some products contain bisulfites; use caution in patients with allergies. ▪ Incidence of side effects markedly increased in AIDS patients. May not tolerate or respond to this drug.
Monitor: Maintain adequate hydration to prevent crystalluria and stone formation. ▪ CBC required before and during therapy. Discontinue for any significant reduction in a blood-forming element. Urinalysis and renal function tests also indicated. ▪ If extravasation occurs, discontinue and restart at a new site. May cause phlebitis. ▪ Monitor closely if any signs of rash appear or have appeared in previous infusions. Several cases of life-threatening reactions have occurred. ▪ Note Precautions and Drug/lab interactions.
Patient education: Maintain adequate hydration. ▪ Report bruising or bleeding, fever, rash, or sore throat promptly. ▪ Possible skin photosensitivity. Avoid unprotected exposure to sunlight.

Maternal/child: Pregnancy Category C: no adequate studies. May interfere with folic acid metabolism in mother and fetus. Benefits must outweigh risks. ■ May contain benzyl alcohol. ■ Note Contraindications. ■ Discontinue breast feeding. ■ Two infants who developed a rash had life-threatening reactions when SMZ/TMP was restarted:
Elderly: Note Dose adjustments. ■ Increased risk of severe side effects (e.g., bone marrow depression, decrease in platelets with or without purpura, skin reactions) especially in impaired renal or liver function or with other drugs (e.g., diuretics).

DRUG/LAB INTERACTIONS
May be potentiated by probenecid. ■ May inhibit cyclosporine (Sandimmune) and increase nephrotoxicity. ■ May potentiate warfarin (Coumadin), phenytoin (Dilantin), oral hypoglycemics, dapsone, and zidovudine (Retrovir, AZT). ■ May displace methotrexate from its binding sites, increasing free fraction of methotrexate and its potential for toxicity. ■ May interfere with serum methotrexate assay and Jaffe assay for creatinine. ■ Note Precautions.

SIDE EFFECTS
All side effects of sulfonamides including allergic reaction are possible. Nausea, vomiting, and rash occur most frequently. Ataxia, convulsions, tremors, and respiratory depression are symptoms of major toxicity. With high doses or administration over an extended period of time, bone marrow depression (leukopenia, megaloblastic anemia, thrombocytopenia) may occur.

ANTIDOTE
Notify the physician of any side effect. Discontinue the drug at any sign of major toxicity or bone marrow depression. Some sources recommend leucovorin 5 to 15 mg daily for treatment of bone marrow depression. Peritoneal dialysis is not effective in toxicity; hemodialysis may be moderately effective in reducing serum levels. Acidification of urine may increase excretion. Treat anaphylaxis with epinephrine, corticosteroids, antihistamines, and vasopressors as indicated.

TACROLIMUS   Immunosuppressant
FK 506, Prograf

USUAL DOSE
Note Precautions. IV route used for patients unable to take oral medications; risk of anaphylaxis increased with IV administration.
Prophylaxis of organ rejection in kidney or liver transplant: Adults and children: 0.03 to 0.05 mg/kg/day as a continuous infusion is the recommended starting dose. (Dose recommendations have been lowered by the manufacturer [were 0.05 to 0.1] and dose regimens vary among transplant centers and approved or investigational use [range 0.01 to

0.05].) Begin no sooner than 6 hours after transplantation. Adults usually receive doses at the lower end of the range. Children usually require doses at the upper end of the range. Individualized adjustment based on clinical assessment of rejection (e.g., trough blood concentrations) or patients' tolerance is imperative and may be required on a daily basis. Adjunctive adrenal corticosteroid therapy early post transplant is recommended. Initiate oral tacrolimus therapy as soon as feasible. Oral doses vary with specific organ transplant and in adults and children (see literature). Total dose in mg/kg/day is given in equally divided doses every 12 hours. Begin 8 to 12 hours after IV tacrolimus is discontinued.

Treatment of organ rejection in kidney or liver transplants and prophylaxis or treatment of other solid organ transplants (investigational): 0.01 to 0.05 mg/kg/day. Note all comments and protocol above.

Prophylaxis of graft-versus-host disease (investigational): 0.04 mg/kg/day as a continuous infusion started the day prior to bone marrow transplant. Note all comments and protocol above.

Treatment of graft-versus-host disease (investigational): 0.1 mg/kg/day as an infusion in equally divided doses every 12 hours. Administer each infusion over 4 hours. Note all comments and protocol above.

DOSE ADJUSTMENTS
Use lowest dosing range initially for paitents with impaired renal or hepatic function; (pre or post transplant). Nephrotoxicity may be increased and further reductions may be required; should be based on tacrolimus trough levels in blood. ■ Delay tacrolimus therapy up to 48 hours in patients with post operative oliguria. ■ Lower doses may be appropriate for maintenance. ■ Note Monitor and Drug/lab interactions.

DILUTION
A 24-hour dose must be diluted with an appropriate amount of NS or D5W. Desired concentration is between 4 and 20 mcg/ml. May leach phthalate from polyvinylchloride containers; use diluents in glass or polyethylene infusion bottles. Chart provides some dose and dilution examples.

Desired dose (mg/kg)	Wt (kg)	Total dose	Amount of diluent (ml)	mcg/ml
0.08	20	1.6 mg/24 hr	250	6.4
			100	16
0.05	60	3 mg/24 hr	500	6
			250	12
0.04	100	4 mg/24 hr	1,000	4

Storage: Store at controlled room temperature prior to dilution. Discard diluted solution in 24 hours.

INCOMPATIBLE WITH
Limited information available. Should not be mixed with solutions of pH 9 or greater (e.g., acyclovir [Zovirax], ganciclovir [Cytovene]). May be compatible at Y-site with many drugs; consult pharmacist.

RATE OF ADMINISTRATION

A single dose properly diluted and equally distributed over 24 hours as a continuous infusion. Use of a metriset (60 gtt/min) or infusion pump suggested.

ACTIONS

A potent immunosuppressive agent. Prolongs survival of allogeneic kidney and liver transplants. Suppresses some humoral immunity (within the body fluids) but suppresses cell-mediated reactions to a greater extent (e.g., allograft rejection, delayed type hypersensitivity, collagen-induced arthritis, experimental allergic encephalomyelitis, graft-versus-host disease). Inhibition of T lymphocyte activation results in immunosuppression. Highly protein bound. Metabolized primarily by the P_{450} enzyme system to up to 10 metabolites. Minimal excretion in urine. Crosses the placental barrier. Secreted in breast milk.

INDICATIONS AND USES

Prophylaxis of organ rejection in allogeneic kidney and liver transplants in conjunction with adrenal corticosteroids. Studies show a reduction in rejection episodes as compared to other immunosuppressants and a reduced use of steroids and antilymphocytes (e.g., antilymphocyte globulin, antithymocyte globulin) to reduce rejection and retain some resistance to infection.

Investigational uses: Treatment of organ rejection in kidney or liver transplants. Prophylaxis and treatment of organ rejection in bone marrow, heart, pancreas, pancreatic island cell, and small bowel transplants. ■ Treatment of autoimmune diseases and severe recalcitrant psoriasis.

CONTRAINDICATIONS

Hypersensitivity to tacrolimus or polyoxyl 60 hydrogenated castor oil.

PRECAUTIONS

For IV use only. Oral dosing preferred; begin as soon as feasible. ■ Usually administered in the hospital by or under the direction of a physician experienced in immunosuppressive therapy and management of organ transplant patients. ■ Adequate laboratory and supportive medical resources must be available. ■ Risk of anaphylaxis increased by IV route versus oral route; use caution. ■ Use caution in impaired renal function; increases in serum creatinine may require dose reduction or use of an alternate immunosuppressant. ■ May cause lymphomas and other malignancies (especially of skin), and has been associated with a lymphoproliferative disorder (LPD) related to Epstein-Barr virus. ■ Antiviral prophylaxis (e.g., acyclovir, ganciclovir, immune globulin) may be advisable in some patients.

Monitor: Obtain baseline CBC, differential, platelets, electrolytes, BUN, and serum creatinine. Monitor regularly during therapy. ■ Contains a castor oil derivative and alcohol; observe continuously for signs of an allergic reaction for the first 30 minutes of the infusion and frequently thereafter. A source of oxygen and epinephrine must always be available. ■ Monitor urine output and serum creatinine carefully. Overt nephrotoxicity occurs more frequently early after transplant resulting in increased serum creatinine and decreased urine output. ■ Monitor tacrolimus blood levels to evaluate rejection, toxicity, need for dose reduction, and patient compliance. Whole blood median trough concentrations (measured by ELISA) may vary considerably during the first week but then stabilize; rejection is minimized with median ranges from 9.8 ng/ml to 19.4 ng/ml; but target ranges will depend on indication and protocol. ■ Monitor all parameters to evaluate possibility of organ rejection. ■ Monitor blood pressure; antihypertensives may be indicated. ■ Monitor serum potassium and magnesium levels. May cause hyperkalemia or hypomagnesemia. ■ May cause hyperglycemia, monitor carefully; treatment may be required. ■ Observe for signs of infection (e.g., fever, sore throat, tiredness) or unusual bleeding or bruising. ■ Use of prophylactic antibiotics may be indicated pending results of C/S in a febrile neutropenic patient. ■ Note Precautions and Drug/lab interactions.

Patient education: Nonhormonal birth control preferred to oral contraceptives to reduce complications of drug interactions. ■ Emphasize need for frequent routine lab work, compliance imperative. ■ Interacts with many medications. Discuss any changes in drug regimen (prescription or non-prescription) with doctor or pharmacist. ■ Inform of increased risk of neoplasia. ■ See Appendix D, p. 900.

Maternal/child: Pregnancy Category C: use only if necessary; benefits must outweigh risk to fetus. Has been associated with hyperkalemia and renal dysfunction in the fetus. ■ Discontinue breast feeding. ■ Is used in children but safety and efficacy not established. ■ Appears to be an increased risk for LPD and primary Epstein-Barr virus infection in immunosuppressed children.

Elderly: Consider age-related organ impairment.

DRUG/LAB INTERACTIONS

May be used concurrently only with adrenocorticosteroids. Do not use simultaneously with cyclosporine (Sandimmune). If a change of immunosuppressants is indicated (tacrolimus to cyclosporine or cyclosporine to tacrolimus), avoid additive nephrotoxicity by waiting for at least 24 hours before starting the alternate drug. If elevated blood concentrations are present, further extend the interval between the two drugs. ■ Use extreme caution with other nephrotoxic agents (e.g., aminoglycosides [gentamicin, tobramycin], amphotericin B [Fungizone], cisplatin [Platinol]). ■ Do not use potassium-sparing diuretics (e.g., spironolactone [Aldactone]); increases risk of hyperkalemia. ■ Calcium channel blockers (e.g., diltiazem [Cardizem], nicardipine [Cardene], verapamil [Isoptin]), antifungal agents (e.g., clotrimazole [Mycelex], fluconazole [Diflucan], itraconazole [Sporanox], ketoconazole [Nizoral]), bromocriptine (Parlodel), cimetidine (Tagamet), clarithromycin (Biaxin), cyclosporine (Sandimmune), danazol (Cyclomen), erythromycin, methylprednisone (Medrol), metoclopramide (Reglan) may inhibit the P_{450} enzyme system and increase tacrolimus blood levels, increasing toxicity potential. ■ Anticonvulsants (e.g., carbamazepine [Tegretol], phenobarbital, phenytoin [Dilantin]), and rifamycins (e.g., rifabutin [Mycobutin], rifampin [Rifadin]), may induce the P_{450} enzyme system, decreasing effectiveness and leading to decreased tacrolimus blood levels and organ rejection. ■ Avoid vaccinations and do not use live vaccines in patients receiving tacrolimus.

SIDE EFFECTS

Occur in a majority of patients and are more pronounced at higher doses. May improve somewhat over time. Nephrotoxicity (abnormal renal function with increased serum creatinine and BUN, oliguria), and neurotoxicity (delirium, headache, insomnia, paresthesia, tremor, seizures) may be dose limiting. Abdominal pain, abnormal liver function tests, anemia, anorexia, ascites, asthenia, atelectasis, back pain, blood dyscrasias, coma, constipation, diarrhea, dyspnea, fever, hyperglycemia, hyper- or hypokalemia, hypertension, hypomagnesemia, leukocytosis, nausea, peripheral edema, pleural effusion, pruritus, rash, seizures, thrombocytopenia, urinary tract infections, vomiting. Many other side effects have occurred in less than 3% of patients.

ANTIDOTE

Notify the physician of all side effects. Most will be treated symptomatically. Tacrolimus may be decreased or disconttinued or alternate immunosuppressive agents substituted. Nephrotoxicity, neurotoxicity, or hematopoietic depression may require temporary reduction of dose or discontinuation of therapy. Dialysis is not effective in overdose. Discontinue immediately if anaphylaxis occurs and treat with oxygen, epinephrine, corticosteroids, and/or antihistamines (e.g., diphenhydramine [Benadryl]). Resuscitate as necessary.

TENIPOSIDE

Antineoplastic
(Mitotic inhibitor)

VM-26, Vumon   pH 4.0 to 6.5

USUAL DOSE

Acute lymphocytic leukemia (ALL): 165 mg/M^2 in combination with cytarabine 300 mg/M^2 twice weekly for 8 to 9 doses. An alternate regimen includes 250 mg/M^2 in combination with vincristine 1.5 mg/M^2 once each week for 4 to 8 weeks plus predisone 40 mg/M^2 orally for 28 days.

Neuroblastoma (investigational): 130 to 180 mg/M^2 once each week as a single agent. In combination with other antineoplastic agents, 100 mg/M^2 once every 21 days.

Non-Hodgkin's lymphoma (investigational): 30 mg/M^2/day for 10 days, 30 mg/M^2/day every 5 days, or 50 to 100 mg/M^2 once each week as a single agent. In combination with other antineoplastic agents, 60 to 70 mg/M^2 once each week.

Small cell lung cancer (investigational): 80 to 90 mg/M^2 daily for 5 days.

DOSE ADJUSTMENTS

Reduce dose by one half in patients with Down syndrome and leukemia (increased sensitivity to myelosuppressive chemotherapy). Higher doses may be used in subsequent courses based on degree of myelosuppression and mucositis. Must be individualized. ■ Reduced dose may be necessary in severe renal or hepatic impairment. ■ Reduced dose may be indicated in combination therapy. ■ Withhold dose if platelets less than 50,000/mm^3 or absolute neutrophil count less than 500/mm^3. Do not restart until adequate recovery.

DILUTION

Specific techniques required; see Precautions. Must be diluted and given as an infusion. May leach the toxic plasticizer DEHP from PVC infusion bags or sets; prepare and store in bottles (glass, polypropylene) or plastic bags (polypropylene, polyolefin) and administer through polyethylene-lined administration sets (e.g., lipid administration sets or low DEHP-containing nitroglycerin sets). Undiluted tenoposide has caused acrylic or ABS plastic devices to crack and leak; handle carefully during dilution process. Compatible with NS or D5W. Final concentration of 0.1, 0.2, 0.4, or 1 mg/ml desired. Contains 10 mg/ml. 100 mg (10 ml) in 990 ml yields 0.1 mg/ml, in 490 ml yields 0.2 mg/ml, in 240 ml yields 0.4 mg/mg, in 90 ml yields 1 mg/ml. Precipitation may occur at recommended concentrations, especially with excessive agitation. Avoid contact of diluted solution with any other drugs or fluids; flush IV line with D5W or NS before and after administration.

Storage: Refrigerate unopened ampoules in original packaging. Do not refrigerate diluted solutions; 1 mg/ml should be administered within 4 hours; all other dilutions are stable at controlled room temperature for up to 24 hours.

INCOMPATIBLE WITH

Heparin. Because of potential for precipitation, compatibility with any drug, infusion fluid, infusion material, or IV pump cannot be assured. Note rate of administration and Precautions/Monitor.

RATE OF ADMINISTRATION

Total desired dose, properly diluted and evenly distributed over at least 30 to 60 minutes. Infusion time may be extended. Flush IV line with D5W or NS before and after administration to avoid precipitation of teniposide in IV catheter. Rapid infusion may cause marked hypotension or increased nausea and vomiting.

ACTIONS

An antineoplastic agent. A semisynthetic derivative of podophyllotoxin related to etoposide. Cell cycle specific for the late S or early G_2 phase. Cytotoxic effects are related to the relative number of single- and doublestrand DNA breaks produced in cells. Active against certain murine leukemias with acquired resistance to cisplatin, doxorubicin, amsacrine, daunorubicin, mitoxantrone, or vincristine. Highly protein bound; limits distribution within the body (a beneficial effect). Plasma levels increase with dose. Distribution half-life is approximately 1 hour, terminal half-life 5 hours. Method of metabolism is not known. Only about 10% excreted as unchanged drug in urine.

INDICATIONS AND USES

Induction therapy in refractory childhood acute lymphoblastic leukemia. Used in combination with other antineoplastic agents.

Investigational uses: A second-line single agent or combination therapy in neuroblastoma in patients who have not responded or who have relapsed on other regimens. ■ A second-line single agent or combination therapy in non-Hodgkin's lymphoma in patients who are refractory to other regimens. ■ Small cell lung cancer.

CONTRAINDICATIONS

Hypersensitivity to teniposide, etoposide, (no cross-sensitivity to date), or a history of prior severe hypersensitivity reactions to other drugs formulated in Cremophor EL (e.g., cyclosporine, paclitaxel).

PRECAUTIONS

Follow guidelines for handling cytotoxic agents. See Appendix A, p. 893. ■ Usually administered by or under the direction of the physician specialist. ▪ Adequate diagnostic and treatment facilities must be readily available. ▪ Use caution in patients with impaired hepatic or renal function; may reduce plasma clearance and increase toxicity. ▪ Incidence of hypersensitivity may be increased in patients with brain tumors or neuroblastoma. ▪ Acute CNS depression and hypotension occurred in patients receiving high-dose teniposide pretreated with antiemetic drugs; use caution. ▪ Children with ALL in remission on teniposide maintenance therapy have shown an increased risk of developing secondary acute nonlymphocytic leukemia (ANLL). ▪ Plasma drug levels decline following IV infusion in children; in adults levels increase with dose. No cumulative toxicity has been reported.

Monitor: Use caution to prevent bone marrow depression; occurs early with indicated doses and can be profound. Obtain base line hemoglobin, white blood cell count with differential, and platelet count. Monitor frequently during therapy, before each dose, and after therapy. Note Dose adjustments. ▪ Severe hypersensitivity reactions can occur with the first dose of teniposide and may be life-threatening. Epinephrine, oxygen, and other emergency supplies must be at the bedside. Monitor patient continuously and take vital signs very frequently during the first hour and at intervals thereafter. ▪ Monitor renal and hepatic function tests before and during therapy. ▪ Determine absolute patency and quality of vein and adequate circulation of extremity. Avoid extravasation; can cause local tissue necrosis and thrombophlebitis. ▪ Precipitation sufficient to occlude central venous access catheters has occurred; monitor infusion closely, and flush thoroughly before and after administration. ▪ Use prophylactic antiemetics to increase patient comfort. ▪ Steady-state volume of distribution increases with a decrease in plasma albumin levels; monitor children with hypoalbuminemia carefully. ▪ If severe myelosuppression occurs, bone marrow examination should be repeated before a decision to continue therapy is made. ▪ Observe closely for signs of infection. Prophylactic antibiotics may be indicated pending results of C/S in a febrile neutropenic patient.

Patient education: Report IV site burning or stinging promptly. ▪ Avoid pregnancy, nonhormonal birth control recommended. ▪ Report any signs of hypersensitivity promptly (e.g., chills, difficult breathing, fever, flushing, rapid heartbeat, rash). ▪ Secondary acute nonlymphocytic leukemia (ANLL) has been reported (see Precautions). ▪ Interacts with many medications. Discuss all drugs (prescription or non-prescription) with doctor or pharmacist. ▪ See Appendix D, p. 900.

Maternal/child: Pregnancy Category D: avoid pregnancy. May cause fetal harm. ▪ Potential for serious adverse reactions in nursing infants; discontinue breast feeding. ▪ Contains benzyl alcohol; not recommended for use in premature infants. ▪ Intended for use in children, but note Precautions/Monitor.

Elderly: Monitor renal, hepatic, and hematologic function closely.

DRUG/LAB INTERACTIONS

Sodium salicylate, sulfamethizole, and tolbutamide displace teniposide from protein-binding sites. Can cause substantial increases in free drug levels and increase toxicity of teniposide. ▪ May result in clinically significant drug interactions with other drugs highly bound to protein (e.g., buprenorphine, calcium channel blocking agents [e.g., diltiazem, verapamil], phenothiazines [e.g., prochlorperazine (Compazine)]). ■ May increase plasma clearance and increase intracellular levels of methotrexate. ■ Phenobarbital and phenytoin (Dilantin) increase clearance of tenoposide; may reduce effectiveness. ■ Depressant and hypotensive effects of antiemetics may be additive with alcohol in teniposide.

SIDE EFFECTS

Most are reversible if detected early. Hypersensitivity reactions (e.g., bronchospasm, chills, dyspnea, facial flushing, fever, hypertension, hypotension, tachycardia, urticaria) have occurred in 5% of patients, and can be fatal if not treated promptly. Myelosuppression (anemia [88%], leukopenia [89%], neutropenia [95%], thrombocytopenia [85%]) occurs early, can be profound, and recovery can be delayed. Alopecia (9%), bleeding (5%), diarrhea (33%), fever (3%), hypotension/cardiovascular (2%), infection (12%), mucositis (76%), nausea and vomiting (29%), rash (3%), thrombophlebitis. Hepatic dysfunctions, metabolic abnormalities, neurotoxicity, and renal dysfunction have occurred in less than 1% of patients.

ANTIDOTE

Keep physician informed of all side effects. Symptomatic treatment is often indicated. Discontinue tenoposide and treat hypersensitivity reactions immediately (epinephrine [Adrenalin], antihistamines [e.g., diphenhydramine (Benadryl)], cimetidine [Tagamet], corticosteroids [e.g., dexamethasone (Decadron)], bronchodilators [e.g., theophylline (Aminophylline)], IV fluids). Consider risk/benefit before rechallenging any patient who has had a severe hypersensitivity reaction. Pretreatment with corticosteroids and antihistamines and constant observation are imperative. For other severe side effects (e.g., myelosupression), drug dose may be reduced or it may be discontinued. Consider filgrastim (G-CSF, Neupogen) for neutropenia, platelet transfusion for thrombocytopenia, packed cell transfusions or epoetin alfa (Epogen) for anemia. Consider diazepam (Valium) or phenytoin (Dilantin) for seizures. Hypotension is usually due to a rapid infusion rate; discontinue temporarily. Trendelenburg position and IV fluids should reverse the hypotension; vasopressors (e.g., dopamine [Intropin]) may be required. In addition to antiemetics (e.g., ondansetron [Zofran]), rate reduction may reduce nausea and vomiting. For extravasation, discontinue the drug immediately and administer into another site. Consider injection of long-acting dexamethasone (Decadron LA) throughout extravasated tissue. Use a 27- or 25-gauge needle. Elevate extremity; moist heat may be helpful. Resuscitate as necessary.

TERBUTALINE SULFATE

Brethine, Bricanyl

Uterine relaxant
(Sympathomimetic)

pH 3.0 to 5.0

USUAL DOSE

All IV doses are investigational. Literature recommends hydrating the patient with IV fluids (5% dextrose in lactated Ringer's or 0.45% saline) for 30 minutes. If no adverse effects, try oral terbutaline 2.5 mg. If contractions remain strong and regular after 30 minutes, begin IV dosing at 10 mcg/min initially (120 gtt/min if 60 gtt = 1 ml, 30 gtt/min if 15 gtt = 1 ml). Gradually increase by 5 mcg/min at 10 to 20 minute intervals until desired result obtained or a maximum dose of 25 mcg/min is reached (some literature states 80 mcg/min). Continue infusion for 30 to 60 minutes after contractions cease. Reduce infusion by 5 mcg/min at 30 minute intervals, until the lowest effective maintenance dose is reached. Maintain this dose for at least 8 hours after uterine contractions have ceased. Immediately follow with SC therapy at 250 mcg every 6 hours for 3 days followed by oral terbutaline 5 mg 3 times daily (some follow immediately with oral dosing eliminating SC).

DILUTION

Each 5 mg (five 1 mg ampoules) must be diluted in 1,000 ml of D5W for infusion. Use NS only when dextrose is not appropriate (e.g., diabetes mellitus). Concentration will be 5 mcg/ml. Use only clear, colorless solutions. Discard solution after 48 hours.

Storage: Store ampoules at room temperature; protect from light.

INCOMPATIBLE WITH

Bleomycin (Blenoxane). Should be considered incompatible in solution with any other drug because of specific use, accurate rate calculation, and potential for additive toxicity.

COMPATIBLE WITH

Y-site: Insulin; consult pharmacist.

RATE OF ADMINISTRATION

Specific instructions included under usual dose. Use of a microdrip (60 gtt/ml) required; infusion pump preferred. Estimates based on suggested dilution. Adjust if more or less diluent is used. Highly individualized based on patient's response and side effects.

ACTIONS

A beta-adrenergic stimulator. Primary actions are bronchodilation and inhibition of uterine smooth muscle contractility. Increases pulse rate and widens pulse pressure moderately. Onset of action is prompt and lasts about 2 hours. Metabolized in the liver. Crosses the placental barrier. Primary excretion in the urine. Secreted in breast milk.

INDICATIONS AND USES

All IV uses are investigational. To arrest preterm labor. ■ Temporarily prevent labor during preparation for operative delivery. ■ Prevent fetal distress during transportation to a hospital.

CONTRAINDICATIONS

Before the twentieth week of pregnancy; conditions during pregnancy that are hazardous to the mother or infant (e.g., antepartum hemorrhage, cardiac disease [maternal], chorioamnionitis, diabetes mellitus [uncontrolled], eclampsia [or severe preeclampsia], hypersensitivity to terbutaline or its components, hyperthyroidism [maternal], intrauterine fetal death, pulmonary hypertension, preexisting maternal medical conditions adversely affected by beta-mimetic drugs [bronchial asthma treated with beta-mimetics or steroids], cardiac arrhythmias with tachycardia or digitalis intoxication); hypovolemia; hypertension (uncontrolled); and pheochromocytoma. *Probable contraindications* may include infection; placenta abruptio; placenta previa; premature rupture of the membranes; severe Rh disease, including erythroblastosis fetalis.

PRECAUTIONS

Not FDA-approved for IV use. Both manufacturers state their product is for SC use only and state "not for IV use." Is being used IV throughout the United States and in other countries. Considered by many to be as effective as ritodrine (Yutopar), to have fewer serious side effects, and to be more economical. ■ Generally used in patients with preterm labor with regular uterine contractions at less than 10 minute intervals. A complete evaluation of the mother must be made (e.g., history, physical, prenatal record, reports from previous ultrasound, routine lab including urine culture and sensitivity). *This is an experimental drug. Although it has been used for this purpose for many years, your hospital may require a documented informed consent.* ■ Most effective if begun as soon as diagnosis of preterm labor established. ■ Use extreme caution if indicated in maternal mild to moderate preeclampsia, hypertension, or diabetes.

Monitor: Obtain maternal baseline ECG to rule out heart disease. Monitor frequency and duration of uterine contractions, maternal pulse rate, blood pressure, and fetal heart rate every 5 minutes until stable, every 15 minutes thereafter until infusion discontinued. ■ Maintain adequate hydration, but avoid fluid overload and observe for signs of pulmonary edema. Respiratory rate above 20 or pulse rate sustained at 150 or above may indicate onset of pulmonary edema. Infusion time exceeding 24 hours, sodium-containing solution, and multiple pregnancy may precipitate pulmonary edema. ■ Evaluate fetal maturity (sonography). ■ Maternal hyperglycemia must be monitored and treated if indicated. May precipitate reactive hypoglycemia in the infant. Monitor insulin, glucose, and electrolyte levels in selected patients or long-term therapy. Normal levels will be altered. ■ Note Drug/lab interactions.

Maternal/child: Category B: safety for use in pregnancy not established (note Contraindications). ■ Delay breast feeding until drug has cleared maternal system. ■ Not for use in children.

DRUG/LAB INTERACTIONS

Inhibited by beta-adrenergic blockers (e.g., propranolol [Inderal]). ■ Potentiated by other sympathomimetic amines (e.g., epinephrine [Adrenalin], dopamine [Intropin]). Effects, including cardiovascular effects, may be additive. Do not administer concurrently; allow adequate time intervals before initiating therapy with any sympathomimetic drug. ■ MAO inhibitors (e.g., selegiline [Eldepryl]) or tricyclic antidepressants (e.g., amitriptyline [Elavil]) will potentiate effects on the vascular system.

SIDE EFFECTS

Maternal: Allergic reactions including anaphylaxis; cardiac dysrhythmias; chest pain; chest discomfort or burning sensation; decreased diastolic pressure; diaphoresis; dizziness; drowsiness; dyspnea; elevated systolic pressure; flushing; headache; hyperglycemia; hyperinsulinemia; hyperlactacidemia; hypocalcemic nausea; hypokalemia; myocardial ischemia; nervousness; pain at injection site; palpitations; pulmonary edema; pulse pressure widening; sweating; tachycardia; tremors; vomiting; weakness.
Fetal: Tachycardia, neonatal hypoglycemia.

ANTIDOTE

Keep physician informed of all side effects. Notify immediately if contractions persist (terbutaline ineffective) or if any signs of maternal or fetal stress occur. Some side effects are expected and will be tolerated or treated symptomatically (note Drug/lab interactions). Marked hypotension, tachycardia, cardiac arrhythmias, and other signs of beta-adrenergic stimulation will require discontinuation of the drug. Uterine relaxation may persist for several hours, and SC and oral therapy instead of IV may be considered. Discontinue drug and treat anaphylaxis as indicated. At first signs of fluid overload or pulmonary edema, notify physician immediately and treat as indicated. Additional reasons for discontinuing terbutaline are: evidence of overt amnionitis; fetal distress; fetal heart rate above 200/min, maternal heart rate above 150/min, or respiratory rate less than 10/min; persistent maternal arrhythmia; progressive cervical dilatation to greater than 7 cm.

TERIPARATIDE ACETATE   Diagnostic agent
Parathar

USUAL DOSE

200 units. Specific procedure required (see Precautions and manufacturer's literature).

PEDIATRIC DOSE

Children over 3 years of age: 3 units/kg of body weight. Do not exceed 200 units.

DILUTION

Diluent provided; 10 ml equals 200 units. Must be used within 4 hours. Discard any unused reconstituted solution.

INCOMPATIBLE WITH

Specific information not available. Consider specific use.

RATE OF ADMINISTRATION

A single dose equally distributed over 10 minutes.

ACTIONS

A synthetic polypeptide hormone containing the active fragment of human parathyroid hormone. Two effects of this hormone are to stimulate the release of cyclic adenosine monophosphate (cAMP) in the urine and to increase urinary excretion of phosphate. These effects make it useful as a diagnostic agent.

INDICATIONS AND USES

To distinguish between hypoparathyroidism and pseudohypoparathyroidism in patients with clinical laboratory evidence of hypocalcemia, which may be caused by either condition.

CONTRAINDICATIONS

Hypersensitivity to teriparatide or any component of this preparation.

PRECAUTIONS

Use caution in borderline hypercalcemic patients (10.5 mg/dl); a single dose can cause hypercalcemia. ▪ Not intended for recurrent or chronic use.

Monitor: To differentiate between hypoparathyroidisms (modified Ellsworth-Howard test) the patient must drink 200 ml of water/hr beginning two hours before the study begins and every hour until it is complete. This ensures adequate urine output. Collect a baseline urine specimen in the 60 minute period immediately before administration of teriparatide. Collect urine specimens from 0 to 30 minutes, 30 to 60 minutes, and 60 to 120 minutes. All specimens must be in separate containers and labeled appropriately. Measurement of urinary cAMP and phosphate must be corrected for creatinine excretion. Change in urinary cAMP excretion in the 0- to 30-minute period is the most sensitive indicator for separation of hypoparathyroidisms. ▪ Patients with hypothyroidism show a greater increase in cAMP and a greater urinary excretion of phosphate (see manufacturer's literature). ▪ Allergic reactions may be caused by peptide content. Have epinephrine available.

Maternal/child: Pregnancy Category C: safety for use in pregnancy and lactation not established; use only when clearly indicated. ▪ Limited date available on children over 3 years of age.

SIDE EFFECTS

Allergic reactions including anaphylaxis; cramps, diarrhea, hypercalcemia, hypocalcemia, metallic taste, nausea, pain at injection site, tingling of extremities. Hypertensive crisis occurred in one patient with a history of hypertension.

ANTIDOTE

Notify physician and manage side effects as indicated by severity. Treat allergic reactions with epinephrine. If hypercalcemia occurs, discontinue drug immediately and ensure adequate hydration. Treat hypocalcemia with calcium if indicated. Resuscitate as necessary.

THIAMINE HYDROCHLORIDE

Betalin S, vitamin B₁

Nutritional supplement (vitamin)

pH 2.5 to 4.5

USUAL DOSE

Wet beriberi with myocardial failure: 5 to 30 mg 3 times daily. Intradermal test dose (¹⁄₁₀₀ of actual dose) recommended in suspected sensitivity. Observe for 30 minutes.

Wernicke's encephalopathy: 100 mg daily for 3 days. Up to 500 mg may be required in the first 24 hours with extreme caution.

PEDIATRIC DOSE

Infantile beriberi with myocardial failure: 10 to 25 mg/24 hr.

DILUTION

May be given by direct IV administration or added to most IV solutions and given as an infusion.

Storage: Can be refrigerated; protect from freezing and from light.

INCOMPATIBLE WITH

Erythromycin (Erythrocin), kanamycin (Kantrex), streptomycin. Solutions with neutral or alkaline pH such as barbiturates (e.g., amobarbital [Amytal], phenobarbital [Luminal]), carbonates, citrates, acetates, sulfites.

RATE OF ADMINISTRATION

100 mg or fraction thereof over 5 minutes. For 100 mg or larger doses, equal distribution over an extended time as an infusion is preferred.

ACTIONS

A water-soluble vitamin, thiamine is necessary to most metabolic processes in humans, especially carbohydrate metabolism. Widely distributed in all body tissues, metabolized in the liver, and excreted in urine.

INDICATIONS AND USES

Prophylaxis or treatment of thiamine deficiency syndromes including beriberi (wet or dry), Wernicke's encephalopathy, or peripheral neuritis.

CONTRAINDICATIONS

Known hypersensitivity to thiamine hydrochloride.

PRECAUTIONS

Not commonly administered IV; PO or IM is preferred. ▪ Rarely used alone, it is more often administered as a multiple B vitamin. ▪ In thiamine deficiency, administer thiamine before giving any glucose load to prevent the sudden onset of Wernicke's encephalopathy or add 100 mg to each of the first few liters of IV fluid to avoid precipitating heart failure. ▪ Requirements may be increased in certain conditions (e.g, alcoholism, burns, GI disease or malabsorption). ▪ Supplementation is necessary in patients receiving total parenteral nutrition (usually administered as a multivitamin).

Patient education: Dietary consultation indicated to prevent relapse.

Maternal/child: Pregnancy Category A: use only if clearly needed. ■ Use caution in lactation.

SIDE EFFECTS

Anaphylaxis and death caused by sensitivity reaction can occur with IV administration. Recent studies have shown that allergic reactions can occur with equal frequency by any route. Incidence after IV administration is less than 0.1%. May increase in frequency with repeat injections. Other reactions include feeling of warmth, nausea, pruritus, pain, sweating, urticaria, and weakness.

ANTIDOTE

Discontinue the drug, treat allergic reaction or resuscitate as necessary, and notify the physician.

THIOPENTAL SODIUM

Barbiturate
General anesthetic
Anticonvulsant

Pentothal Sodium

pH 10.0 to 11.0

USUAL DOSE

Administer a test dose of 25 to 75 mg. Wait at least 1 minute and assess patient reaction and sensitivity.

Convulsions: 75 to 125 mg. Up to 250 mg may be required. Use only enough medication to achieve desired effect.

Increased intracranial pressure in neurosurgical patients: 1.5 to 5 mg/kg intermittently as needed to reduce ICP.

Narcoanalysis: 100 mg/min with patient counting backward from 100. Discontinue when counting confused and before sleep.

DOSE ADJUSTMENTS

Reduce dosage and use caution in the elderly, in cardiovascular disease, hypotension, shock, medication potentiation, impaired renal or liver function, Addison's disease, myxedema, elevated blood urea, elevated intracranial pressure, asthma, severe anemia, and myasthenia gravis. ■ Note Drug/lab interactions.

DILUTION

Each 500 mg of sterile thiopental powder must be reconstituted with at least 20 ml of SW for injection (supplied) to make a 2.5% solution. Each 1 ml equals 25 mg. The 20 ml of 2.5% solution may be further diluted to 125 to 250 ml in NS or D5W to provide a 0.2% to 0.4% solution for infusion. Solutions stronger than a 2.5% concentration will cause hemolysis. Prepared solutions also available. Use only freshly prepared clear solutions. Discard unused portion after 24 hours.

INCOMPATIBLE WITH

Acid solutions, amikacin (Amikin), aminophylline, arginine, atracurium (Tracrium), benzquinamide (Emete-Con), calcium salts, cephalothin (Keflin), cephapirin (Cefadyl), cimetidine (Tagamet), clindamycin (Cleocin), chlorpromazine (Thorazine), codeine, dimenhydrinate (Dramamine), diphenhydramine (Benadryl), doxapram

(Dopram), droperidol (Inapsine), ephedrine, fentanyl (sublimaze), glyco-pyrrolate (Robinul), hydromorphone (Dilaudid), insulin (aqueous), levorphanol (Levo-Dromoran), magnesium sulfate, meperidine (De-merol), metaraminol (Aramine), methadone, methyldopate (Aldomet), methylprednisolone (Solu-Medrol), morphine, norepinephrine (Lev-ophed), para-aminobenzoic acid (PABA), penicillins, procaine (No-vocain), prochlorperazine (Compazine), promazine (Sparine), prometh-azine (Phenergan), Ringer's solutions, sodium bicarbonate, solutions with more than 5% sugar, succinylcholine (Anectine), trimethaphan (Ar-fonad), tubocurarine (curare).

RATE OF ADMINISTRATION
Each 25 mg or fraction thereof over 1 minute. Titrate slowly to desired effect. Rapid injection rate may cause symptoms of overdose (e.g., serious respiratory depression).

ACTIONS
An ultra-short-acting barbiturate and CNS depressant that produces hypnosis and anesthesia without analgesia. Has potent anticonvulsant effects. Onset of action is prompt and lasts about 15 to 30 minutes. Rapidly distributes into all body tissues. Some is retained in fatty tissue, causing sustained or delayed effect. Excreted in changed form in the urine. Crosses the placental barrier. Secreted in breast milk.

INDICATIONS AND USES
Administration generally limited to the anesthesiologist. ■ Control of convulsive states during or after anesthesia. ■ Decrease intracranial pressure in neurosurgical patients (adequate ventilation required). ■ Narcoanalysis or narcosynthesis.

CONTRAINDICATIONS
History of porphyria, known hypersensitivity to barbiturates, status asthmaticus, suitable veins not available.

PRECAUTIONS
Usually administered by or under direct observation of a physician. 1-time use is most common (e.g., anesthesia). ■ Note Dose adjust-ments.
Monitor: Record vital signs every 3 to 5 minutes. Keep patient under constant observation. ■ Treat the cause of the convulsion. ■ Maintain a patent airway and have equipment for artificial ventilation available. ■ Highly alkaline, determine absolute patency of vein. Extravasation will cause necrosis and sloughing; intraarterial injection can cause gangrene. ■ Note Drug/lab interactions.
Patient education: Avoid alcohol or other CNS depressants (e.g., antihis-tamines, diazepam [Valium]) for 24 hours. ■ Possibility of psychomotor impairment for 24 hours. Use caution in any task requiring alertness.
Maternal/child: Category C: Safety for use in pregnancy not established. Benefits must outweigh risks. ■ Only small amounts appear in breast milk, delay breast feeding. ■ May cause paradoxical excitement in children.
Elderly: Note Dose adjustments. ■ May have increased sensitivity to barbiturates; may cause marked excitement, depression, confusion and increased risk of barbiturate induced hypothermia. ■ Recovery of cognitive and psychomotor functions may be slower. ■ Consider reduced hepatic function.

DRUG/LAB INTERACTIONS

Use with extreme caution if any other CNS depressants have been given, such as alcohol, narcotic analgesics, anesthetics, antidepressants, antihistamines, hypnotics, MAO inhibitors, phenothiazines, sedatives, neuromuscular blocking antibiotics, or tranquilizers. Potentiation with respiratory depression and/or increased excitability may occur. ■ Anesthesia extended with probenicid, reduced dose may be indicated. ■ Anesthetic effects may be increased with sulfisoxazole. ■ Monitor phenytoin and barbiturate levels when both drugs are used concurrently. ■ A single dose may affect BSP and liver function studies.

SIDE EFFECTS

Average dose: Depression, dermatitis, facial edema, fever, hypotension, neonatal apnea, respiratory depression (hypoventilation), thrombocytopenic purpura. Anaphylactic reactions can occur.

Overdose: Apnea, cardiac arrhythmias, coma, cough reflex depression, flat EEG (reversible unless hypoxic damage has occurred), hypotension, hypothermia, laryngospasm, pulmonary edema, renal shutdown, respiratory depression, sluggish or absent reflexes.

ANTIDOTE

Call any side effect to the physician's attention. Symptomatic and supportive treatment is most important in overdosage. Keep the patient warm. IV volume expanders (dextran) and IV fluids will help maintain adequate circulation. Diuretics and ventilation will promote the elimination of the drug. Vasopressors (e.g., dopamine [Intropin]) will maintain blood pressure. For extravasation, local injection of 1% procaine will relieve pain and promote vasodilation. Local heat application may be helpful.

THIOTEPA

Antineoplastic
(Alkylating agent/nitrosurea)

Tespa, Thioplex, TSPA

pH 7.6

USUAL DOSE

0.3 to 0.4 mg/kg of body weight as initial dose. Maintenance dose and frequency adjusted according to blood cell counts before and after treatment. Usually given at 1 to 4 week intervals. Dose based on average weight in presence of ascites or edema.

DOSE ADJUSTMENTS

Reduce dose or discontinue if WBC or platelet count falls rapidly. ■ Usually contraindicated but can be used with extreme caution and in low doses in patients with existing hepatic, renal, or bone marrow damage if benefits outweigh risks.

DILUTION

Specific techniques required; see Precautions. Each 15 mg of drug is diluted with 1.5 ml of sterile water for injection (10 mg/ml). Shake solution gently and allow to stand until clear. A hypotonic solution, it should be filtered through a 0.22-micron filter and further diluted with NS before administration. May then be given through Y-tube or three-way stopcock of a free-flowing IV infusion. Final solution should be clear; do not use if hazy, opaque, or a precipitate is present. Thioplex is a new formulation with a longer shelf-life and will gradually replace Tespa.

Storage: Must be refrigerated before and after reconstitution. Protect from light at all times. Use reconstituted solution within 8 hours. Use diluted solution immediately.

INCOMPATIBLE WITH

Cisplatin (Platinol), filgrastim (Neupogen), minocycline (Minocin), vinorelbine (Navelbine).

COMPATIBLE WITH

Y-site: Allopurinol (Zyloprim), melphalan (Alkeran), piperacillin/ tazobactam (Zosyn); consult pharmacist.

RATE OF ADMINISTRATION

60 mg or fraction thereof over 1 minute direct IV.

ACTIONS

An alkylating agent of the nitrosurea group with antitumor activity. Cell cycle phase nonspecific. Thought to have a radiomimetic action, which releases ethylenimine radicals that disrupt DNA bonds and destroy actively dividing cells. Well distributed, it is metabolized in the liver and excreted as metabolites in the urine.

INDICATIONS AND USES

To suppress or retard neoplastic growth in adenocarcinomas of the breast and ovary. ■ Also used intracavitary to treat some bladder cancers and to control intracavitary effusion secondary to neoplastic disease (toxicity still occurs from systemic absorption).

CONTRAINDICATIONS

Hepatic, renal, or bone marrow damage unless need is greater than the risk; known hypersensitivity to thiotepa.

PRECAUTIONS

Follow guidelines for handling cytotoxic agents. See Appendix A, p. 893. ■ Administered by or under the direction of the physician specialist. ■ Use caution in leukopenia, thrombocytopenia, recent radiation therapy, and infection. ■ Note Dose adjustments and Side effects.

Monitor: Daily blood cell and platelet counts are necessary during initial treatment and weekly thereafter until 3 weeks after therapy is discontinued. Very toxic to hematopoietic system. ■ Be alert for signs of bone marrow depression or infection. Use of prophylactic antibiotics may be indicated pending results of C/S in a febrile neutropenic patient. ■ Allopurinol may prevent formation of uric acid crystals. ■ Prophylactic antiemetics may increase patient comfort. ■ Note Drug/lab interactions.

Patient education: Nonhormonal birth control recommended for patient and partner. ■ See Appendix D, p. 900.

Maternal/child: Category D: avoid pregnancy. Will produce teratogenic effects on the fetus. Has a mutagenic potential. ■ Discontinue breast feeding. ■ Safety for use in children not established.

Elderly: Consider possibility of impaired organ function.

DRUG/LAB INTERACTIONS

May cause irreversible bone marrow damage with other antineoplastic drugs, radiation therapy, or any drugs that cause bone marrow depression. Allow complete recovery verified by white blood cell count before using a second agent. ■ Potentiates neuromuscular blocking agents (e.g., pancuronium [Pavulon], succinylcholine [Anectine]). May cause prolonged apnea, especially with concurrent use of other antineoplastic agents. ■ Do not administer live virus vaccines to patients receiving antineoplastic drugs.

SIDE EFFECTS

Minor: Amenorrhea, anorexia, dizziness, fever, headache, hives, hyperuricemia, nausea, pain at injection site, skin rash, throat tightness, vomiting.

Major: Anaphylaxis, bone marrow depression, hemorrhage, intestinal perforation, septicemia. Hematopoietic toxicity (anemia, leukopenia, thrombocytopenia) may be life threatening, is dose related, and does occur with usual doses.

ANTIDOTE

Minor side effects will be treated symptomatically if necessary. Discontinue the drug and notify the physician of major side effects. If platelet count below 150,000/mm^3 or white blood cells below 3,000/mm^3, discontinue use and notify physician. Administration of whole blood, platelets, or leukocytes may be required. Blood modifiers (e.g., epoetin-alfa [Epogen, Procrit], filgrastin [Neupogen], sargramostin [Leukine], oprelvekin [Numega]) may be indicated to treat bone marrow toxicity. Treat allergic reaction as indicated.

TICARCILLIN DISODIUM

Antibacterial (Extended-spectrum penicillin)

Ticar

pH 6.0 to 8.0

USUAL DOSE

150 to 300 mg/kg of body weight/24 hr in divided doses every 3, 4, or 6 hours. All doses vary depending on the severity of the infection. Maximum dose is 24 Gm/24 hr.

PEDIATRIC DOSE

Under 40 kg (88 lb): 50 to 300 mg/kg of body weight/24 hr in divided doses every 4, 6, or 8 hours. Do not exceed adult dose.

NEONATAL DOSE

Under 1,200 Gm; age up to 4 weeks: 75 mg/kg of body weight every 12 hours.

Under 2,000 Gm; age up to 7 days: 75 mg/kg every 12 hours. *Over 7 days of age:* 75 mg/kg every 8 hours.

Over 2,000 Gm; age up to 7 days: 75 mg/kg every 8 hours. *Over 7 days of age:* 75 mg/kg every 6 hours.

DOSE ADJUSTMENTS

Reduce daily dose commensurate with amount of renal or hepatic impairment. Intervals between injections should also be increased.

DILUTION

Each 1 Gm or fraction thereof is diluted with 4 ml of sterile water for injection. Further dilution of each gram with an additional 20 to 50 ml or more of sterile water for injection, D5W, NS, or sodium lactate ⅙ M is required for direct IV administration or intermittent piggyback infusion to decrease vein irritation. May be added to larger volumes and given as a continuous infusion. Also available in a 3 gm ADD-Vantage vial for use with ADD-Vantage diluent containers. Stable at room temperature for at least 48 hours.

INCOMPATIBLE WITH

All aminoglycosides (e.g., amikacin [Amikin], gentamicin [Garamycin], kanamycin [Kantrex], netilmicin [Netromycin], tobramycin [Nebcin]), colistimethate (Coly-Mycin M), doxapram (Dopram), fluconazole (Diflucan), vancomycin (Vancocin).

RATE OF ADMINISTRATION

Too-rapid injection may cause seizures. Slow infusion rate for pain along venipuncture site.

Direct IV: 1 Gm or fraction thereof over 5 minutes or more to reduce vein irritation.

Intermittent infusion: A single dose over 30 minutes to 2 hours. In neonate give over 10 to 20 minutes.

Continuous infusion: At specified rate not to exceed rate and concentration of intermittent infusion.

ACTIONS

An extended-spectrum penicillin. Bactericidal for many gram-negative, gram-positive, and anaerobic organisms. Large doses with high blood levels are well tolerated. Distributes into cerebrospinal fluid only if inflammation is present. Crosses the placental barrier. Excreted in the urine. Secreted in breast milk.

INDICATIONS AND USES

Bacterial septicemia, acute and chronic infections of the respiratory tract, skin and soft tissue, intraabdominal area, female pelvis, genital tract, and urinary tract. ▪ Useful in infections complicated by impaired renal functions or in patients receiving immunosuppressive or oncolytic drugs.

CONTRAINDICATIONS

Known penicillin or cephalosporin sensitivity (not absolute).

PRECAUTIONS

Sensitivity studies indicated to determine susceptibility of the causative organism to ticarcillin. ▪ Superinfection caused by overgrowth of nonsusceptible organisms can occur. ▪ Incidence of side effects increased in patients with cystic fibrosis. ▪ Continue for at least 2 days after symptons of infection have disappeared.

Monitor: Periodic evaluation of renal, hepatic, hematopoietic systems and serum potassium is recommended in prolonged therapy. Observe for hypokalemia and increased bleeding tendencies. ▪ Observe for electrolyte imbalance and cardiac irregularities. Contains 4.7 to 5 mEq sodium/Gm. May aggravate CHF. ▪ Note Drug/lab interactions.

Patient education: May require alternate birth control.

Maternal/child: Pregnancy Category B: use only if clearly needed. ▪ May cause diarrhea, candidiasis, or allergic response in nursing infants. ▪ Elimination rate markedly reduced in neonates.

Elderly: No problems documented. Age-related decrease in renal or hepatic function may require decrease in dose.

DRUG/LAB INTERACTIONS

Probenecid decreases rate of ticarcillin elimination resulting in higher and more prolonged blood levels. May be desirable or may cause toxicity. ■ Gentamicin and tobramycin used concurrently in severe infection but must be administered in separate infusions; penicillins inactivate aminoglycosides. ■ May be antagonized by bacteriostatic antibiotics (e.g., chloramphenicol, erythromycin, and tetracyclines); bactericidal action may be negated. ■ Concomitant use with beta-adrenergic blockers (e.g., propranolol [Inderal]) may increase risk of anaphylaxis and inhibit treatment. ■ May increase risk of bleeding; monitoring of coagulation tests may be indicated. Use caution with anticoagulants (e.g., heparin). ■ May inhibit effectiveness or oral contraceptives; break-through bleeding or pregnancy could result. ■ Monitoring of serum lithium indicated with concurrent use. Sodium may alter renal excretion. ■ May decrease clearance and increase toxicity of methotrexate. ■ May cause false urine protein reactions with various tests. See Side effects and/or literature.

SIDE EFFECTS

Abnormal clotting time or prothrombin time, anaphylaxis, anemia, convulsions, elevated serum creatinine, alkaline phosphatase, LDH, serum bilirubin, AST (SGOT) and ALT (SGPT), eosinophilia, fever, hypokalemia, leukopenia, nausea, neutropenia, phlebitis, pruritus, pseudomembranous colitis, skin rash, thrombocytopenia, urticaria, vomiting. Hypersensitivity myocarditis can occur (fever, eosinophilia, rash, sinus tachycardia, ST-T changes and cardiomegaly). Higher than normal doses may cause neurologic adverse reactions including convulsions; especially with impaired renal function.

ANTIDOTE

Notify the physician immediately of any adverse symptoms. For severe symptoms, discontinue the drug, treat allergic reaction (epinephrine, antihistamines, corticosteroids), and resuscitate as necessary. Hemodialysis is effective in overdose.

TICARCILLIN DISODIUM AND CLAVULANATE POTASSIUM

Antibacterial
(Extended-spectrum penicillin and
beta-lactamase inhibitor)

Timentin

pH 5.5 to 7.5

USUAL DOSE

3.1 Gm of preparation available contains 3 Gm ticarcillin to 0.1 Gm clavulanate.

Over 60 kg (130 lb): 3.1 Gm every 4 to 6 hours.

Under 60 kg: 200 to 300 mg/kg of body weight/24 hr in equally divided doses every 4 to 6 hours. Doses vary depending on the severity of the infection, susceptibility of the organism, and condition of the patient. Treatment usually continued for 10 to 14 days; may be extended if required.

Surgical prophylaxis (unlabeled): 3.1 Gm 30 to 60 minutes before start of surgery or as soon as the umbilical cord is clamped in cesarean section. Repeat at 4 hour intervals for 3 doses.

PEDIATRIC DOSE

Infants and children 3 months to 16 years of age and < 60 kg: 50 mg/kg every 6 hours. Base dose on the ticarcillin component. In serious infections, increase to 50 mg/kg every 4 hours. Note Contraindications.

Children with cystic fibrosis: 350 to 400 mg ticarcillin and 11.7 to 17 mg clavulanate/kg/24 hr. Give in equally divided doses every 4 to 6 hours.

NEONATAL DOSE

Safety for use in infants under 3 months of age not established but has been used. Base dose on ticarcillin component. Note Contraindications.

Under 1,200 Gm; age up to 4 weeks: 75 mg/kg of body weight every 12 hours.

Under 2,000 Gm; age up to 7 days: 75 mg/kg every 12 hours. *Over 7 days of age:* 75 mg/kg every 8 hours.

Over 2,000 Gm; age up to 7 days: 75 mg/kg every 8 hours. *Over 7 days of age:* 75 mg/kg every 6 hours.

DOSE ADJUSTMENTS

Reduce total daily dose if renal function impaired. Calculated according to degree of impairment (see literature). ▪ Reduce dose in impaired hepatic function. ▪ Reduced dose may be indicated in the elderly.

DILUTION

Each 3.1 Gm or fraction thereof is diluted with 13 ml of sterile water or NS (200 mg/ml). Shake well. A single dose must be further diluted in 50 to 100 ml or more of D5W, NS, or LR's and given as an intermittent infusion. Also available in ADD-Vantage vials for use with ADD-Vantage diluent containers.

Storage: Stable at room temperature for at least 6 hours or for 72 hours under refrigeration. Stability extended after further dilution (see literature).

INCOMPATIBLE WITH

All aminoglycosides (e.g., amikacin [Amikin], gentamicin [Garamycin], kanamycin [Kantrex], tobramycin [Nebcin]), colistimethate (Coly-Mycin), sodium bicarbonate.

RATE OF ADMINISTRATION

Intermittent infusion: A single dose over 30 minutes. May be given through Y-tube or three-way stopcock of infusion set. Discontinue primary IV during administration. Too-rapid injection may cause seizures. Slow infusion rate for pain along venipuncture site.

ACTIONS

An extended-spectrum penicillin. Bactericidal for many gram-negative, gram-positive, and anaerobic organisms. This specific formulation extends activity by protecting ticarcillin from degradation by B-lactamase enzymes. Large doses with high blood levels are well tolerated. Widely distributed in all body fluids and tissues. Distributes into cerebrospinal fluid only if inflammation is present. Peak serum levels achieved by end of infusion. Crosses the placental barrier. Excreted in the urine. Secreted in breast milk.

INDICATIONS AND USES

Bacterial septicemia, acute and chronic infections of the respiratory tract, skin and skin structure, bone and joint, endometrium, and urinary tract caused by beta-lactamase-producing organisms. Useful in infections complicated by impaired renal functions or in patients receiving immunosuppressive or oncolytic drugs.
Unlabeled use: Surgical prophylaxis.

CONTRAINDICATIONS

Known sensitivity to penicillins, cephalosporins, or beta-lactamase inhibitors (not absolute). ▪ Not recommended in infants and children under 16 years of age for the treatment of septicemia or infections where the suspected or proven pathogen is *haemophilus influenza* type B.

PRECAUTIONS

Specific process sensitivity studies indicated to determine susceptibility of the causative organism to ticarcillin and clavulanate. ▪ Superinfection caused by overgrowth of nonsusceptible organisms can occur. ▪ Use caution in patients with CHF or those with a history of bleeding disorders or GI disease (e.g., colitis). ▪ Incidence of side effects increased in patients with cystic fibrosis. ▪ Continue for at least 2 days after signs and symptoms of infection have disappeared.
Monitor: Periodic evaluation of renal, hepatic, and hematopoietic systems and serum potassium is recommended in prolonged therapy. Observe for electrolyte imbalance and cardiac irregularities. Observe for hypokalemia. Contains 4.75 mEq sodium/Gm. May aggravate CHF. ▪ Observe for increased bleeding tendencies in all patients but especially those with impaired renal function. ▪ Note Drug/lab interactions.
Patient education: Report promptly: fever, rash, sore throat, unusual bleeding or bruising, severe stomach cramps and/or diarrhea, seizures. ▪ May require alternate birth control.
Maternal/child: Pregnancy Category B: use only if clearly needed. Studies in rats have not shown adverse effects on the fetus. ▪ May cause diarrhea, candidiasis, or allergic response in nursing infants. ▪ Is used in

infants over under 3 months of age but safety for use not established. *Elderly:* No problems documented; age-related decrease in renal or hepatic function may require decreased dose.

DRUG/LAB INTERACTIONS

Probenecid decreases rate of ticarcillin elimination, resulting in higher and more prolonged blood levels of ticarcillin; will not affect clavulanate levels. May be desirable or may cause toxicity. ▪ Aminoglycosides (e.g., gentamicin, tobramycin) used concurrently in severe infection but must be administered in separate infusions at least 1 hour apart; inactivates aminoglycosides. ▪ May be antagonized by bacteriostatic antibiotics (e.g., chloramphenicol, erythromycin, tetracyclines), bactericidal action may be negated. ▪ Concomitant use with beta-adrenergic blockers (e.g., propranolol [Inderal]) may increase risk of anaphylaxis and inhibit treatment. ▪ Use caution with anticoagulants (e.g., heparin), thrombolytic agents (e.g., [tPA], anistreplase [Eminase]), platelet aggregation inhibitors (e.g., aspirin, NSAIDs, dextran, dipyridamole, plicamycin). Risk of bleeding may be increased. Monitoring of coagulation tests may be indicated. Concurrent use with thrombolytic agents is not recommended; may increase risk of severe hemorrhage. ▪ May inhibit effectiveness of oral contraceptives; breakthrough bleeding or pregnancy could result. ▪ Monitoring of serum lithium indicated with concurrent use; increased sodium may alter renal excretion. ▪ May decrease clearance and increase toxicity of methotrexate. ▪ Clavulanic acid may cause a false-positive Coombs' test. ▪ May cause false urine protein reactions with various tests; see Side effects and/or literature.

SIDE EFFECTS

Anaphylaxis; anemia; arthralgia; chest discomfort; chills; convulsions; diarrhea; disturbances of taste and smell; elevated alkaline phosphatase, BUN, LDH, serum bilirubin, AST (SGOT), and ALT (SGPT); eosinophilia; fever; flatulence; epigastric pain; headache; hypernatremia; hypokalemia; increased bleeding time; leukopenia; myalgia; nausea; neutropenia; phlebitis; prolonged clotting time or prothrombin time; pruritus; pseudomembranous colitis; skin rash; stomatitis; thrombocytopenia; urticaria; vomiting. Hypersensitivity myocarditis can occur (fever, eosinophilia, rash, sinus tachycardia, ST-T changes and cardiomegaly). Higher than normal doses may cause neurologic adverse reactions including convulsions; especially with impaired renal function.

ANTIDOTE

Notify the physician immediately of any adverse symptoms. For severe symptoms, discontinue the drug; treat allergic reaction (epinephrine, antihistamines, corticosteroids), and resuscitate as necessary. Hemodialysis may be indicated in overdose.

TOBRAMYCIN SULFATE

Antibacterial
(Aminoglycoside)

Nebcin

pH 3.0 to 6.5

USUAL DOSE

3 mg/kg of body weight/24 hr equally divided into 3 doses and given every 8 hours. Up to 5 mg/kg equally divided into 3 or 4 doses may be given if indicated. Reduce to usual dose as soon as feasible. Dose based on lean body weight plus 40% for obese patients.

Recent studies suggest that a total daily dose administered as a single dose (instead of divided into 2 to 3 doses) may provide higher peak levels and enhance drug effectiveness while actually reducing or having no adverse effects on risk of toxicity.

Patients with cystic fibrosis: 5 to 7.5 mg/kg/24 hr equally divided into 3 doses and given every 8 hours.

PEDIATRIC DOSE

Same as adult dose. Another source suggests 6 to 7.5 mg/kg of body weight/24 hr in 3 or 4 equally divided doses.

NEWBORN DOSE

1 week of age or less: 4 mg/kg of body weight/24 hr in two equal doses every 12 hours. Lower doses may be safer because of immature kidney function. 2.5 mg/kg every 18 hours or 3 mg/kg every 24 hours may provide acceptable peak and trough levels in neonates weighing less than 2,000 Gm.

DOSE ADJUSTMENTS

Reduce daily dose commensurate with amount of renal impairment and/or increase intervals between injections. Measurement of serum concentrations following a loading dose of 1 mg/kg is suggested. Adjust dose accordingly. ■ Reduced doses or extended intervals may be required in the elderly. ■ Note Drug/lab interactions.

DILUTION

Prepared solutions equal 10 or 40 mg/ml. Further dilute each single dose in 50 to 100 ml of NS or D5W and administer through an additive tubing. Also available in ADD-Vantage vials for use with ADD-Vantage diluent containers. Reduce volume of diluent proportionately for children.

INCOMPATIBLE WITH

Allopurinol (Zyloprim), cefamandole (Mandol), clindamycin (Cleocin), heparin, hetastarch (Hespan), indomethacin (Indocin), sargramostim (Leukine), any calcium or magnesium ions. Administer separately; inactivated in solution with penicillins and most cephalosporins. Note Precautions and Drug/lab interactions.

RATE OF ADMINISTRATION

Each single dose, properly diluted, over a minimum of 20 and a maximum of 60 minutes.

ACTIONS

An aminoglycoside antibiotic with potential neuromuscular blocking action. Inhibits protein synthesis in bacterial cells. Bactericidal against specific gram-negative and bacilli, including *Escherichia coli, Kleb-*

siella, Proteus, and *Pseudomonas*. Well distributed through all body fluids. Usual half-life is 2 to 2.5 hours. Half-life is prolonged in infants, post-partum females, fever, liver disease and ascites, spinal cord injury, cystic fibrosis, and the elderly; shorter in severe burns. Crosses the placental barrier. Excreted in the kidneys.

INDICATIONS AND USES

Short-term treatment of serious infections caused by susceptible organisms, (e.g., septicemia, meningitis [concentration low, combine with intrathecal], peritonitis). ▪ Primarily used when penicillin and other less toxic antibiotics ineffective or contraindicated. ▪ Concurrent therapy with a penicillin or cephalosporin sometimes indicated.

CONTRAINDICATIONS

Known tobramycin or aminoglycoside sensitivity. Sulfite sensitivity may be a contraindication.

PRECAUTIONS

Use extreme caution if therapy is required over 7 to 10 days. ▪ Sensitivity studies necessary to determine susceptibility of causative organism to tobramycin. ▪ Superinfection may occur from overgrowth of nonsusceptible organisms. ▪ Use caution in infants, children, and the elderly. ▪ May contain sulfites; use caution in patients with asthma.

Monitor: Watch for decrease in urine output, rising BUN and serum creatinine, and declining creatinine clearance levels. Dose may require decreasing. ▪ Routine evaluation of hearing is recommended. ▪ Narrow range between toxic and therapeutic levels. Periodically monitor peak and trough concentrations to avoid peak serum concentrations above 12 mcg/ml and trough concentrations above 2 mcg/ml. Therapeutic levels are between 4 and 8 mcg/ml. ▪ Maintain good hydration. ▪ Monitor serum calcium, magnesium, potassium, and sodium; levels may decline. ▪ In extended treatment, monitoring of serum levels, electrolytes, renal, auditory and vestibular functions daily is recommended. ▪ Note Drug/lab interactions.

Patient education: Report promptly dizziness, hearing loss, weakness, or any changes in balance. ▪ Consider birth control options.

Maternal/child: Category D: avoid pregnancy; use during pregnancy and lactation only when absolutely necessary. Potential hazard to fetus. ▪ Peak concentrations are generally lower in infants and young children. ▪ Use extreme caution in premature infants and neonates; immature kidney function will result in prolonged half-life. ▪ Note Precautions.

Elderly: Consider less toxic alternatives. ▪ Monitor renal function and drug levels carefully. Measurement of creatinine clearance more useful than BUN or serum creatinine to assess renal function. ▪ Half-life prolonged;longer intervals between doses may be more important than reduced doses. ▪ Note Precautions, Dose adjustments, and Side effects.

DRUG/LAB INTERACTIONS

Inactivated in solution with penicillins but is synergistic when used in combination with beta-lactam antibiotics (e.g., sulbactam sodium, clavulanate potassium, cephalosporins, penicillins) and vancomycin. Dose adjustment and appropriate spacing required because of physical incompatibilities and interactions. Synergism may be inconsistent; measure aminoglycoside levels. ▪ Concurrent use topically or systemically with any other ototoxic or nephrotoxic agents should be avoided. May have dangerous additive effects with anesthetics (e.g., enflurane), other neuromuscular blocking antibiotics (e.g., kanamycin), diuretics (e.g., furosemide [Lasix]), beta-lactam antibiotics (e.g., cephalosporins), vancomycin, and many others. ■ Neuromuscular blocking muscle relaxants (e.g., doxacurium [Nuromax], succinylcholine [Anectine]) are potentiated by aminoglycosides. *Apnea can occur.* ■ May be antagonized by bacteriostatic antibiotics (e.g., chloramphenicol, erythromicin, and tetracycline); bactericidal action may be impacted. ■ Aminoglycosides are potentiated by anticholinesterases (e.g., edrophonium), antineoplastics (e.g., nitrogen mustard, cisplatin). ■ Note Side effects.

SIDE EFFECTS

Occur more frequently with impaired renal function, higher doses, prolonged administration, dehydration, in the elderly, and in patients receiving other ototoxic or nephrotoxic drugs.

Minor: Dizziness; fever; headache; increased AST (SGOT), ALT (SGPT), and serum bilirubin; itching; lethargy; rash; roaring in the ears; urticaria; vomiting.

Major: Apnea; blood dyscrasias; cylindruria; elevated BUN, nonprotein nitrogen (NPN), and creatinine; hearing loss; leukocytosis, neuromuscular blockade; oliguria; proteinuria; seizures (large doses); tinnitus; vertigo.

ANTIDOTE

Notify the physician of all side effects. If minor side effects persist or any major symptom appears, discontinue the drug and notify the physician. Treatment is symptomatic or a reduction in dose may be required. In overdose hemodialysis may be indicated. Monitor fluid balance, creatinine clearance, and plasma levels carefully. Complexation with ticarcillin or carbenicillin (12 to 30 Gm/day) may be as effective as hemodialysis. Consider exchange transfusion in the newborn. Calcium salts or neostigmine may reverse neuromuscular blockade. Resuscitate as necessary.

TOLAZOLINE HYDROCHLORIDE

Priscoline

Pulmonary antihypertensive

pH 3.0 to 4.0

NEONATAL DOSE

1 to 2 mg/kg of body weight as an initial loading dose. Follow with an infusion of 1 to 2 mg/kg/hr. Usually discontinued within 36 to 48 hours.

DILUTION

May be given undiluted. May be given through Y-tube or three-way stopcock of infusion set. May be further diluted to be given as an infusion. Compatible with many commonly used solutions (e.g., Dextran 6% in dextrose or saline, dextrose in water or saline, fructose in water or saline, invert sugar in water or saline, Ionosol products, lactated Ringer's injection, normal or half-normal saline, Protein hydrolysate 5%, Ringer's injection, sodium lactate ⅙ molar). Amount of diluent based on total dose and fluid needs of infant. May be given through Y-tube or three-way stopcock of infusion set.

INCOMPATIBLE WITH

Ethacrynic acid (Edecrin), hydrocortisone sodium succinate (Solu-Cortef), indomethacin (Indocin), methylprednisolone sodium succinate (Solu-Medrol).

RATE OF ADMINISTRATION

Loading dose: Administer over 10 minutes directly into scalp or upper extremity vein (to maximize delivery to pulmonary artery). See Neonatal dose for maintenance infusion.

ACTIONS

An alpha adrenergic blocking agent. Decreases peripheral resistance and increases venous capacitance. Usually reduces pulmonary arterial pressure and vascular resistance. Additional actions include sympatho-mimetic activity (e.g, cardiac stimulation), parasympathomimetic activity (e.g, GI tract stimulation), and histamine stimulation. Onset of action is within 30 minutes; half-life in neonates is from 3 to 10 hours. Excreted in the urine.

INDICATIONS AND USES

Treatment of persistent pulmonary hypertension of the newborn (when systemic arterial oxygenation cannot be adequately sustained by usual supportive care of oxygen and mechanical ventilation).

CONTRAINDICATIONS

Hypersensitivity to tolazoline.

PRECAUTIONS

For use only in a highly supervised setting such as an intensive care nursery. ■ Stimulates gastric secretion and may activate stress ulcers. Pretreat infants with antacids to prevent GI bleeding. ■ Use with caution in patients with known or suspected mitral stenosis. Priscoline may produce a rise or fall in pulmonary artery pressure and total pulmonary resistance.

Monitor: Vital signs, oxygenation, acid-base status, and fluid and electrolyte balance must be monitored and maintained. ▪ Observe for signs of systemic hypotension. Treat promptly. ▪ Effectiveness may be pH dependent. Acidosis may decrease effectiveness.

DRUG/LAB INTERACTIONS

Use caution with epinephrine; severe hypotension with exaggerated rebound will occur.

SIDE EFFECTS

Average dose: Cardiac arrhythmias, diarrhea, edema, flushing, GI hemorrhage, hematuria, hepatitis, hypertension, hypotension, increased pilomotor activity with tingling or chilliness, leukopenia, nausea, oliguria, pulmonary hemorrhage, rash, tachycardia, thrombocytopenia, tingling, vomiting.

Overdose: Hypotension and shock in addition to flushing, increased pilomotor activity, and peripheral vasodilation.

ANTIDOTE

Notify the physician of all side effects. If minor symptoms progress or major side effects appear, discontinue the drug immediately and notify the physician. Treat hypotension by placing patient in the Trendelenberg position. Administer IV fluids, and ephedrine or dopamine (Intropin) if necessary. Epinephrine and norepinephrine (Levophed) are contraindicated for hypotension. Further hypotension will occur. Treat all other side effects symptomatically and resuscitate as necessary.

TOLBUTAMIDE SODIUM

Diagnostic agent

Orinase Diagnostic

pH 8.0 to 9.8

USUAL DOSE

1 Gm. Specific procedure required (see Precautions and manufacturer's literature).

DILUTION

Diluent provided, 20 ml for 1 Gm. Prepare immediately before use and use within 1 hour. Must be completely dissolved and solution must be clear.

Storage: Store at 15° to 30° C.

INCOMPATIBLE WITH

Specific information not available. Consider specific use.

RATE OF ADMINISTRATION

A single dose equally distributed over 2 to 3 minutes.

ACTIONS

Lowers blood glucose concentration by stimulating the release of insulin from the beta cells of the pancreas. Will cause a rapid fall in blood sugar for 30 to 45 minutes followed by a return to normal limits in 90 to 180 minutes in normal individuals. Results in patients with pancreatic islet cell adenomas (insulinomas) are distinctively different.

INDICATIONS AND USES

Adjunct in the diagnosis of islet cell adenoma to prevent surgical intervention when it is not indicated. ▪ Has also been used to aid in the diagnosis of mild diabetes mellitus, pancreatic carcinoma, and acute pancreatitis.

CONTRAINDICATIONS

Children, hypersensitivity to tolbutamide or related sulfonylureas.

PRECAUTIONS

Results vary with laboratory methods. Use only a true glucose procedure (Somogyi-Nelson, Modified Folin-Wu, AutoAnalyzer, or glucose oxidase). ■ Physician will refer to manufacturer's literature for interpretation of results. ■ May cause severe and prolonged hypoglycemia with impaired renal or hepatic function. ■ Note Drug/lab interactions.

Monitor: A high-carbohydrate diet (150 to 300 Gm/day) must be eaten for 3 days before to the test. ■ To test for islet cell adenoma, draw a fasting blood glucose the morning of the test, administer tolbutamide, draw venous blood glucose samples 20, 30, 45, 60, 90, 120, 150, and 180 minutes after midpoint of tolbutamide administration. ■ Alternately, may draw venous blood samples for serum insulin levels before, and 10, 20, and 30 minutes after midpoint of tolbutamide administration. See manufacturer's literature for interpretation of test results. ■ Terminate the test with breakfast, oral glucose, or 50% glucose IV (followed by 10% dextrose in water as an infusion) depending on patient condition. Nondiabetics and individuals with atherosclerosis may develop a severe hypoglycemic reaction. If this occurs, terminate test after the 30-minute blood sample or sooner if indicated.

Maternal/child: Category C: not recommended for use during pregnancy; teratogenic in rats and prolonged severe hypoglycemia has occurred in newborns of mothers taking sulfonylureas. ■ Discontinue breast feeding.

DRUG/LAB INTERACTIONS

False-positive results can occur in patients with liver disease, alcohol hypoglycemia, idiopathic hypoglycemia of infancy, severe undernutrition, azotemia, sarcoma, or other extrapancreatic insulin-producing tumors. ■ Potentiated by beta-adrenergic blocking agents (e.g., propranolol [Inderal]), chloramphenicol, dicumarol, MAO inhibitors, phenylbutazone, probenecid, salicylates, and sulfonamides. Hypoglycemia may be severe and test results will not be accurate.

SIDE EFFECTS

Allergic reactions including anaphylaxis, burning sensation at injection site (too-rapid injection), thrombophlebitis. Hypoglycemia, mild (fatigue, hunger, nausea, nervousness, sweating, trembling, weakness) or severe (confusion, coma, lethargy, loss of consciousness, stupor), will occur.

ANTIDOTE

Notify physician and manage side effects as indicated by severity. Treat mild hypoglycemia with oral glucose. For severe hypoglycemia with loss of consciousness treat with 50% glucose IV and hospitalize. Follow with 10% dextrose in water as an IV infusion and maintain blood glucose above 100 mg/dl. Monitor for at least 48 hours; hypoglycemia may recur. Treat allergic reactions and resuscitate as necessary.

TOPOTECAN HYDROCHLORIDE

Antineoplastic
(Topoisomerase 1 inhibitor)

Hycamtin

pH 2.5 to 3.5

USUAL DOSE

Before giving the initial dose, the baseline neutrophil count must be at least 1,500/mm^3 and baseline platelet count must be at least 100,000/mm^3.

1.5 mg/M^2 as an infusion each day for 5 consecutive days (days 1 through 5 of a 21-day course). Begin the second course on day 22. A minimum of four courses is recommended; minimum time to response has been 9 to 12 weeks. Note Dose adjustments.

DOSE ADJUSTMENTS

Do not begin subsequent courses of topotecan until neutrophils recover to >1,000/mm^3, platelets recover to 100,000/mm^3, and hemoglobin recovers to 9mg/dl (with transfusion if necessary). ■ If severe neutropenia occurs (neutrophils ≤500/mm^3) during any course, either reduce dose for all subsequent courses by 0.25 mg/M^2 or, before resorting to dose reduction, give G-CSF (filgrastim) starting with day 6 (must be at least 24 hours after the final dose of that course). ■ Reduce dose to 0.75 mg/M^2 in patients with moderate impaired renal function (creatinine clearance 20 to 39 ml/min). There is inadequate data at this time to recommend a dose in severe renal impairment. ■ Dose adjustment may be required in the elderly because of age related renal impairment. ■ No dose adjustment required in patients with impaired hepatic function (bilirubin >1.5 to <10 mg/dl).

DILUTION

Specific techniques required; see Precautions: Reconstitute each 4 mg vial with 4 ml of SW (1 mg/ml). Withdraw the calculated dose and further dilute in 50 to 100 ml of NS or D5W.

Storage: Store unopened vials in cartons protected from light at controlled room temperature. Reconstituted solutions contain no preservative; use immediately. Solutions diluted for infusion are stable at room temperature in soft light for 24 hours.

INCOMPATIBLE WITH

Until specific information is available, should be considered incompatible in syringe or solution with any other drug because of toxicity and specific use.

RATE OF ADMINISTRATION

A single dose as an infusion evenly distributed over 30 minutes.

ACTIONS

A new class of antineoplastic agent that inhibits the enzyme topoisomerase 1 required for DNA replication. A topoisomerase 1 inhibitor, it is a semi-synthetic derivative of camptothecin. Metabolized through a specific process to its active lactone form. Causes cell death by damaging DNA produced during the S-phase of cell synthesis. Minor additional metabolism occurs in the liver. Terminal half-life is from 2 to 3 hours. Moderately bound to plasma protein (35%). Some excretion in urine.

INDICATIONS AND USES

Treatment of metastatic carcinoma of the ovary after failure of initial or subsequent chemotherapy

CONTRAINDICATIONS

Hypersensitivity to topotecan or any of its components. Not recommended for use during pregnancy, lactation, or in patients with severe bone marrow depression.

PRECAUTIONS

Follow guidelines for handling cytotoxic agents. See Appendix A, p. 893. ■ Administered by or under the direction of the physician specialist. ■ Adequate diagnostic and treatment facilities must be available. ■ Must have adequate bone marrow reserves. An 80% to 90% decrease in WBC count at nadir is typical after the first cycle of therapy. Neutropenia is not cumulative over time. ■ Use caution in patients with a history of allergies. ■ Use with caution in impaired renal function, clearance decreased.

Monitor: Baseline neutrophil count must be at least 1,500 cells/mm^3 and platelets at least 100,000 cell/mm^3 before the initial dose. ■ Obtain a baseline CBC with differential and platelets. ■ Monitor before each course and frequently during treatment. Platelet count must be 100,000/mm^3, neutrophils 1,000/mm^3, and hemoglobin 9 mg/dl before a course of therapy can be repeated. Anemia is frequent and transfusion is often indicated. ■ Baseline creatinine clearance and BUN suggested. ■ Monitor vital signs. ■ Maintain adequate hydration. ■ Nausea and vomiting are frequent and may be severe; use prophylactic administration of antiemetics to increase patient comfort. ■ Observe closely for S/S of infection. Prophylactic antibiotics may be indicated pending results of C/S in a febrile or non-febrile neutropenic patient. ■ Not a vesicant, but monitor injection site for inflammation and/or extravasation. ■ Expected nadir for neutrophils is 11 days, 15 days for platelets and hemoglobin.

Patient education: Nonhormonal birth control recommended. ■ Report any unusual or unexpected symptoms or side effects as soon as possible. ■ See Appendix D, p. 900.

Maternal/child: Category D: Avoid pregnancy, may cause fetal harm. ■ Discontinue breast feeding. ■ Safety and effectiveness for use in children not established.

Elderly: No dose adjustment necessary except in age-related renal impairment.

DRUG/LAB INTERACTIONS

Interaction of topotecan with other drugs has not been adequately studied. ■ May cause severe prolonged myelosuppression with cisplatin. ■ Concomitant administration of G-CSF (filgrastim) can prolong the duration of neutropenia. If used, do not administer before day 6, at least 24 hours after the final dose of topotecan.

SIDE EFFECTS

Bone marrow depression, primarily neutropenia, is the dose-limiting toxicity of topotecan. Abdominal pain, alopecia, anorexia, bone marrow toxicity (e.g., anemia {<10 mg/dl [96%], <8 mg/dl [40%]}, leukopenia {<3,000/mm^3 [98%], <1,000/mm^3 [32%]}, neutropenia {<1,500/mm^3 [98%], <500/mm^3 [81%]}, thrombocytopenia {<75,000/

mm^3 [63%], <25,000/mm^3 [26%]}), constipation, diarrhea, dyspnea, fatigue, fever, headache, infection with neutropenia <500/mm^3 (26%), nausea (77%), paresthesia, stomatitis, transient increases in AST (SGOT) and ALT (SGPT), vomiting (58%), weakness.

ANTIDOTE

Keep physician informed of all side effects. Withhold topotecan until myelosuppression has improved to minimum requirements. Neutropenia recovery may be aided by G-CSF (filgrastim) under specific conditions; see Dose adjustments or Drug/lab interactions. Anemia required RBC or whole blood tranfusions in 50% of patients. Thrombocytopenia may require platelet transfusion. Death can result from the progression of many side effects. No known antidote for overdose. Symptomatic and supportive treatment is indicated. Treat allergic reactions with oxygen, epinephrine, corticosteriods, and antihistamines.

TORSEMIDE INJECTION

Diuretic (loop)
Antihypertensive

Demadex

pH over 8.3

USUAL DOSE

IV and oral doses are therapeutically equivalent. Oral dose can replace an IV dose at any time. If diuretic response is not adequate titrate the recommended dose upward by doubling the dose until desired response achieved or maximum suggested dose reached.

Edema of congestive heart failure: 10 to 20 mg once daily. Note general instructions above; single doses over 200 mg have not been adequately studied to date.

Edema of chronic renal failure: 20 mg once daily. Note general instructions above; single doses over 200 mg have not been adequately studied to date.

Hepatic cirrhosis with ascites: 5 to 10 mg once daily. To prevent hypokalemia and metabolic alkalosis give in combination with an aldosterone antagonist (e.g., spironolactone [Aldactone]) or a potassium-sparing diuretic (e.g., dyazide). Note general instructions above; single doses over 40 mg have not been adequately studied to date.

Hypertension: 5 mg once daily. May be increased to 10 mg in 4 to 6 weeks if blood pressure reduction is inadequate. If response is still inadequate, the addition of other antihypertensive agents is recommended instead of larger doses of torsemide. Usually given orally.

Continuous infusion: Loading dose: As an IV injection 25 mg (2.5 ml) over 2 minutes. Follow with an infusion at 3.1 mg/hr (10 ml/hr).

DOSE ADJUSTMENTS

Higher doses may be required in renal failure. Note Drug/lab interactions.

DILUTION

Available as 10 mg/ml. May be given undiluted. Maybe given through Y-tube or three-way stopcock of infusion set. May be further diluted and given as a continuous infusion. Dilute 7.5 ml (75 mg) with NS to a total dose of 240 ml (10 ml/hr for 24 hours).

Storage: Store at controlled room temperature. Do not freeze.

INCOMPATIBLE WITH

Limited information available. Any drug with an acid pH]). Other loop diuretics (e.g., catecholamines [e.g., dopamine (Intropin), have many incompatibilities; consult pharmacist.

RATE OF ADMINISTRATION

Ototoxicity (usually reversible) has occurred with too rapid injection and doses over 200 mg. Flush IV line with NS before and after administration.

IV injection: Each 200 mg or fraction thereof over 2 minutes.

Continuous infusion: See Usual dose and Dilution.

ACTIONS

A sulfonamide type loop diuretic. Acts from within the ascending portion of the loop of Henle to excrete water, sodium, chlorides, and some potassium. Diuretic action correlates better with the rate of drug excretion in urine than with plasma concentration. Will produce diuresis in alkalosis or acidosis. Effects begin within 10 minutes and peak within 1 hour. Diuresis lasts 6 to 8 hours. Highly protein bound. Metabolized by the liver (80%). 20% eliminated via urinary excretion. Other loop diuretics cross the placental barrier and are secreted in breast milk; specific information not available for torsemide.

INDICATIONS AND USES

Treatment of edema associated with congestive heart failure, cirrhosis of the liver with ascites, and chronic renal failure. Used when a rapid onset of diuresis is desired or when oral administration is impractical.
- Treatment of hypertension.

CONTRAINDICATIONS

Known hypersensitivity to torsemide or to sulfonylureas and in anuric patients.

PRECAUTIONS

Tests to determine serum levels of torsemide not widely available
■ In patients with congestive heart failure and/or renal failure, a smaller dose is actually delivered to the ascending loop of Henle, resulting in less response at any given dose. ■ Use caution and improve basic condition first in hepatic coma, electrolyte depletion, and advanced cirrhosis of the liver. Initiation of therapy in the hospital is preferred. ■ Use extreme caution in patients sensitive to bumetanide (Bumex), furosemide (Lasix), or sulfonamides (including thiazide diuretics); may also be sensitive to torsemide. ■ In patients with hepatic disease with cirrhosis and ascites use a potassium-sparing diuretic (e.g., dyazide) or an aldosterone antagonist (e.g., spironalactone) concurrently to prevent hypokalemia and metabolic alkalosis.
■ Use caution in acute MI; excessive diuresis may precipitate shock.
■ In nonanuric renal failure, may cause marked increases in water and sodium excretion without impacting steady-state fluid retention. High doses (500 to 1,200 mg) have caused seizures. ■ May activate or exacerbate systemic lupus erythematosus. Chronic use in renal or hepatic disease has not been adequately studied. ■ Antihypertensive effects greater in black patients.

Monitor: Monitor blood pressure frequently, especially during initial

therapy. May precipitate excessive diuresis with water and electrolyte depletion. Dehydration, electrolyte imbalance, hypovolemia, prerenal axotemia, embolism, or thrombosis can occur. Routine checks on electrolyte panel, CO_2, and BUN are necessary during therapy. Potassium chloride and/or magnesium replacement may be required. ▪ Risk of hypokalemia greatest in patients with cirrhosis of the liver, during brisk diuresis, with inadequate oral electrolyte intake, or with concurrent administration of corticosteroids (e.g., prednisone). ▪ May increase blood glucose, serum cholesterol, and triglycerides. ▪ Slight increases in BUN, serum creatinine, and uric acid may occur, usually reverse when therapy discontinued. Sudden changes in fluid and electrolyte balance may precipitate hepatic coma in patients with hepatic disease and ascites. ▪ Rarely precipitates an attack of gout. ▪ Note Drug/lab interactions.
Patient education: Hypotension may cause dizziness; request assistance with ambulation. ▪ May cause a decrease in potassium levels and require a supplement. ▪ Possible skin photosensitivity. Avoid unprotected exposure to sunlight. ▪ Report cramps, dizziness, muscle weakness, or nausea promptly.
Maternal/child: Category B: use only if clearly needed during pregnancy, safety for use not established. ▪ Safety for use during lactation not established; other loop diuretics suggest discontinuing breast feeding. ▪ Safety and effectiveness in children under 18 not established. Administration of other loop diuretics to premature infants with edema due to patent ductus arteriosus and hyaline membrane disease may have caused renal calcifications; also other loop diuretics may have increased the risk of persistent patient ductus arteriosus in premature infants with hyaline membrane disease. Torsemide has not been studied in these situations.
Elderly: No specific age-related differences, dose adjustment not indicated. May be more susceptible to dehydration, observe carefully. ▪ Avoid rapid contraction of plasma volume and hemoconcentration. May cause thromboembolic episodes (e.g., CVA, pulmonary emboli).
DRUG/LAB INTERACTIONS
Concurrent administration with high-dose salicylates may cause salicylate toxicity. ▪ Probenicid decreases the diuretic activity of torsemide. ▪ May reduce renal clearance of spironolactone, but dose adjustment not required. ▪ Has been administered with beta-blockers (e.g., atenolol), ACE inhibitors (e.g., captopril), calcium-channel blockers (e.g., diltiazem), cimetidine (Tagamet), digoxin, and nitrates (e.g., nitroglycerin) without new or unexpected adverse events; however, torsemide has caused severe hypotension with ACE inhibitors in sodium- or volumedepleted patients. ▪ Does not affect protein binding of glyburide (Dia-Beta), or coumarin derivatives (e.g., warfarin). ▪ May cause excessive potassium depletion with amphotericin B (Fungizone, Abelcet), corticosteroids, thiazide diuretics (e.g., hydrochlorothiazide [HydroDiuril]). Monitor electrolytes closely. ▪ May cause cardiac arrhythmias with digitalis and other antiarrhythmic agents secondary to potassium and magnesium depletion. ▪ NSAIDs (e.g., indomethacin [Indocin] or salicylates [e.g., aspirin]) may cause retention of sodium and water and may decrease diuretic and antihypertensive effects. ▪ Antihypertensive effects may be increased by any hypotension-producing agent (e.g., lidocaine, nitroglycerin, nitroprusside, paclitaxel); reduced dose of the antihypertensive agent or

both drugs may be indicated. ■ May potentiate propranolol (Inderal), salicylates, muscle relaxants (e.g., mivacurium [Mivacron]), and hypotensive effect of other diuretics. ■ May increase ototoxicity in doses exceeding the usual or in conjunction with ototoxic drugs (e.g., cisplatin, aminoglycosides [e.g., amikacin, streptomycin, gentamicin], ethacrynic acid [Edecrin]). ■ May increase nephrotoxicity if given concurrently with any other nephrotoxic agent (e.g., amphotericin B, aminoglycosides [e.g., gentamicin], foscarnet [Foscavir], rifampin [Rifadin]). Concurrent use with amphotericin B is not recommended, especially in patients with some impaired renal function. ■ Anticoagulants (e.g., coumarin, heparin, streptokinase) may require dose adjustment; effects reduced by decreased plasma volumes and/or increased metabolism. ■ May be inhibited by phenytoin (Dilantin). ■ May reduce excretion of lithium and cause lithium toxicity. ■ May increase or decrease effectiveness of theophyllines.

SIDE EFFECTS

Arthralgia, constipation, cough, diarrhea, dizziness, dyspepsia, ECG abnormalities, edema, electrolyte imbalance, esophageal hemorrhage, excessive thirst, excessive urination, headache, hyperglycemia, hyperuricemia, hypokalemia, impotence, insomnia, myalgia, nervousness, ototoxicity (usually reversible), rhinitis, sore throat, and tinnitus have all been reported. Allergic reactions can occur. Hypocalcemia and hypomagnesemia have been minimal with usual doses.

Major: Anorexia, dizziness, drowsiness, dryness of the mouth, hypotension, increased BUN, lethargy; mental confusion, muscle cramps, fatigue, or pain; nausea and vomiting, oliguria, restlessness, tachycardia, thirst, or weakness may indicate severe electrolyte imbalance, hypovolemia, or prerenal azotemia.

Overdose: Circulatory collapse, dehydration, excessive diuresis, hemoconcentration, hypochloremic alkalosis, hyper- or hypochloremia, hyper-or hypokalemia, hypomagnesemia, hyper- or hyponatremia, hypotension, hypovolemia, vascular thrombosis, and embolism.

ANTIDOTE

Notify the physician of any side effect. Depending on severity the physician may treat the side effects symptomatically and either continue or discontinue torsemide. Fluid and electrolyte replacement may be indicated. If side effects are progressive or any major side effects or signs of overdose appear, discontinue the drug immediately and notify the physician. Treatment of overdose is symptomatic and aggressive. Hemodialysis is not effective in overdose. Resuscitate as necessary. Torsemide may be restarted at a lower dose after the patient is stable.

TRACE METALS
Nutritional supplement

chromium, ConTE-Pak-4, copper, iodine,manganese, molybdenum, M.T.E.-4, 5, 6, & 7, M.T.E.-4, 5, & 6 Concentrated, MulTE-Pak-4, MulTE-PAK-5, Multiple Trace Element, Multiple Trace Element Concentrated, Multiple Trace Element with Selenium, Multiple Trace Element with Selenium Concentrated, selenium, T.E.C., Trace Metals Additive in 0.9% NaCl, zinc

Multiple Trace Element Neonatal, Neotrace-4, Pediatric Multiple Trace Element, PedTE-PAK-4, Pedtrace-4, P.T.E.-4

USUAL DOSE
Available as single elements, selected combined elements in various strengths, and in combination with electrolytes. Selection of correct product based on minimum daily requirement and individual needs.

Zinc: 2.5 to 4 mg/day; add 2 mg in acute catabolic states. Increase to 12.2 mg/L of total parenteral nutrition (TPN) if there is fluid loss from the small bowel.

Copper: 0.5 to 1.5 mg/day.

Manganese: 0.15 to 0.8 mg/day.

Molybdenum: 20 to 120 mcg/day. Increase to 163 mcg/day for 21 days in deficiency states resulting from prolonged TPN.

Chromium: 10 to 15 mcg/day. Increase to 20 mcg/day with intestinal fluid loss.

Selenium: 20 to 40 mcg/day. Increase to 100 mcg/day for 31 days in deficiency states resulting from prolonged TPN.

Iodine: 1 to 2 mcg/kg of body weight/day. Increase to 2 to 3 mcg/kg/day in growing children, pregnant and lactating women.

PEDIATRIC DOSE
Zinc: 100 mcg/kg/day for full-term infants and children up to 5 years of age. 300 mcg/kg/day for premature infants with birth weights from 1,500 Gm to 3 kg.

Copper: 20 mcg/kg/day.

Manganese: 2 to 10 mcg/kg/day.

Molybdenum: Dosage must be calculated by extrapolation; consult pharmacist.

Chromium: 0.14 to 0.2 mcg/kg/day.

Selenium: 3 mcg/kg/day.

DOSE ADJUSTMENTS
Reduce or omit dose in impaired renal function.

DILUTION
Must be added to daily volume of IV infusion fluids including TPN.

INCOMPATIBLE WITH
None when used as directed.

RATE OF ADMINISTRATION
Administer properly diluted at rate prescribed for IV infusion fluids or TPN.

ACTIONS

All are basic elements present in the human body. Specific amounts required to initiate, facilitate, or maintain appropriate body systems.

INDICATIONS AND USES

Nutritional supplement to IV solutions given for total parenteral or central nutrition.

CONTRAINDICATIONS

Do not give direct IV; hypersensitivity to any component (especially iodides). Manganese contraindicated in presence of high manganese levels. Molybdenum without copper supplementation contraindicated in copper-deficient patients.

PRECAUTIONS

Selenium enhances vitamin E and decreases the toxicity of mercury, cadmium, and arsenic. ■ Patients with biliary tract obstruction may retain copper and manganese. ■ Avoid copper in patients with Wilson's disease (genetic disorder of copper metabolism). ■ Assess possibility of diabetes mellitus when giving chromium supplements to maintain normal glucose metabolism.

Monitor: Monitor serum trace metal concentration to avoid accumulation. Results will also determine use of a single element or a combined product.

Maternal/child: Category C: use in pregnancy only if clearly indicated. Use manganese with caution in the nursing mother. ■ May contain benzyl alcohol; may cause fatal "gasping" syndrome in premature infants.

DRUG/LAB INTERACTIONS

Therapeutic serum levels of copper and zinc will decrease if not given together.

SIDE EFFECTS

Toxicity is rare at recommended doses. Iodine may cause anaphylaxis.

ANTIDOTE

Dosage will be adjusted based on serum levels. Keep physician informed. Resuscitate as necessary.

TRANEXAMIC ACID

Antifibrinolytic
Antihemorrhagic

✣Cyclokapron, Cyklokapron

pH 6.5 to 7.5

USUAL DOSE

Dental extraction in patients with hemophilia: 10 mg/kg of body weight immediately before surgery. Follow with 25 mg/kg orally after surgery and for 2 to 8 days. 10 mg/kg IV may be given 3 to 4 times daily the day before surgery, followed by the above regimen. In patients unable to take oral medicine, use 10 mg/kg IV 3 to 4 times daily for 2 to 8 days. Normal renal function required.

DOSE ADJUSTMENTS

Reduce dose in impaired renal function; specific calculation required (see literature).

DILUTION

100 mg equals 1 ml of prepared solution. Further dilute a single dose with at least 50 ml compatible infusion solutions (e.g., NS, dextrose solutions in water or various concentrations of NS, Ringer's solution, amino acids, dextran). Heparin may be added to solution if indicated. Prepare solution immediately before use; discard any unused solution.

INCOMPATIBLE WITH

Blood, penicillins.

RATE OF ADMINISTRATION

100 mg or fraction thereof over at least 1 minute. Too-rapid infusion may cause hypotension.

ACTIONS

A synthetic amino acid with the specific action of inhibiting plasminogen activator substances; to a lesser degree inhibits plasmin activity. Increases fibrinogen activity in clot formation by inhibiting the enzyme required for destruction of formed fibrin. More potent than aminocaproic acid. Onset of action is prompt. Half-life approximately 2 hours. Readily excreted in the urine. Crosses the placental barrier. Secreted in breast milk.

INDICATIONS AND USES

Reduce or prevent hemorrhage and reduce the need for replacement therapy in hemophilia patients during and following tooth extraction.

CONTRAINDICATIONS

Acquired defective color vision, subarachnoid hemorrhage.

PRECAUTIONS

For short-term use only (2 to 8 days). ■ Use extreme caution; retinal changes, leukemia, hyperplasia of the biliary tract, cholangioma, and adenocarcinoma of the intrahepatic biliary system have been found in laboratory animal studies. ■ Rapid administration in any form may cause hypotension. ■ Whole blood transfusions may be given if necessary but must be given through a second infusion site.

Monitor: Use only in conjunction with general and specific tests to determine the amount of fibrinolysis present. ■ In repeated treatment or if treatment will last more than several (2 to 3) days, a complete ophthalmologic examination (visual acuity, color vision, eyeground, visual fields) should be done before and at regular intervals during treatment. Discontinue use if changes are found.

Maternal/child: Pregnancy Category B: use caution and only if clearly needed in pregnancy and lactation.

SIDE EFFECTS

Diarrhea, giddiness, hypotension, nausea and vomiting.

ANTIDOTE

All side effects may subside with reduced dosage or rate of administration. Discontinue use of drug if any changes are found during follow-up ophthalmologic examinations. Resuscitate as necessary.

TRIMETREXATE GLUCURONATE

Antiprotozoal
(Folate antagonist)

Neutrexin

USUAL DOSE

45 mg/M^2 once daily by IV infusion for 21 days. Must be given with concurrent leucovorin 20 mg/M^2 every 6 hours (total dose of 80 mg/M^2/day) to avoid potentially serious or life threatening toxicities. Leucovorin must be given every day of trimetrexate treatment and for 72 hours after the last trimetrexate dose. Leucovorin solution may be given prior to or following trimetrexate, but they can not be mixed together. Flushing of line before and after leucovorin with at least 10 ml of D5W is mandatory; See Incompatible with. See leucovorin monograph for appropriate IV administration information.

PEDIATRIC DOSE

(Investigational) Same as adult dose. See Maternal/child.

DOSE ADJUSTMENTS

Reduce dose based on the worst hematologic toxicity.

Dose modification for hematologic toxicity				
Toxicity grade	Neutrophils/mm^3	Platelets/mm^3	Trimetrexate dose (mg/M^2)	Leucovorin dose (mg/M^2)
1	> 1,000	>75,000	45 mg/M^2 once daily	20 mg/M^2 every 6 hr
2	750-1,000	50,000-75,000	45 mg/M^2 once daily	40 mg/M^2 every 6 hr
3	500-749	25,000-49,999	22 mg/M^2 once daily	40 mg/M^2 every 6 hr
4	< 500	<25,000	Day 1-9 any mg/M^2 discontinue Day 10-21 any mg/M^2 interrupt up to 96 hours	40 mg/M^2 every 6 hr

Prior to day 10, discontinue trimetrexate and give leucovorin 40 mg/M^2 every 6 hours for 72 hours. After day 10, trimetrexate dose may be withheld for up to 96 hours to allow counts to recover, continue leucovorin. If counts recover to grade 3 in 96 hours administer that specific dose as above. When counts recover to grade 2 administer that specific dose as above and maintain increased leucovorin dose for remainder of treatment. ▪ Leucovorin may be given orally if dose does not exceed 25 mg. Each dose should be rounded up to the next higher 25 mg increment. ▪ Interrupt trimetrexate if transaminase levels or alkaline phosphatase levels increase to more than 5 times the upper limit of normal range. Interrupt trimetrexate if serum creatinine levels increase to more than 2.5 mg/dl and the increase is thought to be secondary to trimetrexate. ▪ Interrupt trimetrexate if severe mucosal toxicity interferes with oral intake. ▪ Discontinue trimetrexate for an oral temperature over 40.5° C (105° F) not responsive to antipyretics. ▪ In all the above situations, continue leucovorin every 6 hours for 72 hours after trimetrexate is discontinued. ▪ Note Drug/lab interactions.

DILUTION

Specific techniques required; see Precautions. Reconstitute each 25 mg vial with 2 ml D5W or sterile water(12.5 mg/ml). A pale greenish yellow solution, must be clear and free from precipitation. Further dilute by using a 0.22 micron filter to add to D5W. Desired concentration range is 0.25 mg/ml to 2 mg/ml. A 100 mg dose in 50 ml diluent yields 2 mg/ml, in 400 ml diluent 0.25 mg/ml.

Storage: Store vials at controlled room temperature, protect from light. Reconstituted solution is stable at room temperature or refrigerated for 24 hours. Do not freeze. Discard after 24 hours.

INCOMPATIBLE WITH

Will cause immediate precipitation with leucovorin or any solution containing chloride ion.

RATE OF ADMINISTRATION

A single dose as an infusion over 60 to 90 minutes. Flush IV line before and after administration with 10 ml 5% dextrose in water.

ACTIONS

A nonclassic folate antagonist and synthetic inhibitor of the enzyme dihydrofolate reductase (DHFR). Results in the disruption of DNA, RNA, and protein synthesis, and causes cell death. Trimetrexate but not leucovorin is selectively transported into the *P. carinii* organism. The concurrent administration of leucovorin protects normal host cells from the cytotoxicity of trimetrexate without inhibiting trimetrexate's cytotoxicity to *P. carinii*. In one study distribution half-life ranged from 29 to 85 minutes and terminal half-life ranged from 13 to 19 hours. Metabolism in man is probably hepatic but has not been defined; does utilize the P_{450} enzyme system. 10% to 30% excreted unchanged in urine. Increased urine flow may increase clearance. Some excretion in feces. Crosses the placental barrier.

INDICATIONS AND USES

Alternative therapy with concurrent leucovorin to treat moderate-to-severe *Pneumocystis carinii* pneumonia (PCP) in immunocompromised patients, including those with AIDS, who are intolerant of or refractory to sulfamethoxazole-trimethoprim (SMZ/TMP) or pentamidine therapy or for whom either or both drugs are contraindicated.

Investigational uses: Treatment of *Pneumocystis carinii* pneumonia in children under 18 years. ▪ Treatment of non–small cell lung, prostate, and colorectal cancer.

CONTRAINDICATIONS

Clinically significant hypersensitivity to trimetrexate, leucovorin, or methotrexate.

PRECAUTIONS

Follow guidelines for handling cytotoxic agents. See Appendix A, p. 893. ▪ Administered by or under the direction of the physician specialist, with facilities for monitoring the patient and responding to any medical emergency. ▪ Must be used with concurrent leucovorin to avoid potentially serious or life-threatening complications including bone marrow suppression, oral and GI mucosal ulceration, and renal and hepatic dysfunction. ▪ Pharmacokinetics of trimetrexate have not been determined in patients with impaired renal or hepatic dysfunction. Use with caution; note Dose adjustments. ▪ Use with caution in patients with impaired hematologic function. ▪ Note Monitor and Drug/Lab interactions.

Monitor: Complete blood counts including an absolute neutrophil counts (ANC), and platelets, serum creatinine, BUN, AST, ALT and alkaline phosphatase should be monitored at least twice weekly throughout therapy. Carefully monitor patients who require concomitant therapy with nephrotoxic agents (e.g., aminoglycosides, antineoplastics, NSAIDs), myelosuppressive (e.g., antineoplastics, ganciclovir), or hepatotoxic (e.g., IV fat emulsion [prolonged use], NSAIDs, phenytoin [Dilantin]). ▪ Discontinue treatment with zidovudine during trimetrexate therapy, to allow for full therapeutic doses of trimetrexate. ▪ Monitor for symptoms of clinical deterioration, may have concurrent pulmonary conditions (e.g., bacterial, viral, or fungal pneumonia or mycobacterial diseases). ▪ Prophylactic antiemetics may be indicated. ▪ Note Dose adjustments, Precautions, and Drug/Lab interactions.

Patient education: Avoid pregnancy, nonhormonal birth control recommended. ▪ Leucovorin must be taken every 6 hours for a full 24 days, failure to do so can lead to fatal toxicity. ▪ Zidovudine will be discontinued during trimetrexate therapy. ▪ See Appendix D, p. 900.

Maternal/child: Category D: avoid pregnancy. Can cause significant maternal and fetotoxicity as well as skeletal, visceral, ocular, and cardiovascular abnormalities. ▪ Has caused degeneration of the testes and arrest of sperm formation in rats. ▪ Discontinue breast feeding. ▪ Safety and effectiveness in children under age 18 have not been established. Has been used under Compassionate Use Protocol in children with no serious or unexpected adverse effects.

Elderly: Consider age-related organ impairment (e.g., bone marrow reserve, renal, hepatic).

DRUG/LAB INTERACTIONS

Plasma concentrations may be altered by any other agent metabolized by a P_{450} enzyme system (e.g., cimetidine [Tagamet], erythromycin, fluconazole [Diflucan], ketoconazole [Nizoral], rifabutin [Mycobutin], rifampin [Rifadin]). ▪ Cimetidine may cause a significant reduction in trimetrexate metabolism and result in increased serum levels and toxicity. ▪ Acetaminophen may compete for metabolites and alter concentration of trimetrexate metabolites. ▪ Imidazole agents (e.g., clotrimazole, ketoconazole, miconazole [Monistat]) may alter trimetrexate metabolism, monitor carefully. ▪ Additive bone marrow depression may occur when used concurrently or consecutively with other bone marrow depressants (e.g., antineoplastics) or radiation. Reduced doses may be indicated.

SIDE EFFECTS

Myelosuppression from hematologic toxicity (e.g., anemia, neutropenia, thrombocytopenia) is the usual dose-limiting side effect. Anaphylaxis (one occurrence), confusion; elevated serum alkaline phosphatase, ALT, AST, bilirubin, and creatinine; fatigue, fever, GI and oral mucosal ulceration, hypocalcemia, hyponatremia, nausea/vomiting, rash pruritus, seizures (rare), and stomatitis can occur. May be difficult to distinguish from symptoms of underlying medical condition.

Overdose: Severe bone marrow suppression, oral and GI mucosal ulceration, renal and hepatic dysfunction.

ANTIDOTE

For accidental overdose, discontinue trimetrexate and give leucovorin 40 mg/M^2 every 6 hours for 3 days. Keep physician informed of all side effects. Myelosuppression, stomatitis, and GI toxicities can generally be managed by increasing the dose of leucovorin. Temporarily or permanently interrupt treatment for renal, hepatic, and mucosal toxicity and fever. Parameters described in Dose adjustments.

TROMETHAMINE

Tham, Tham-E

Alkalizing agent

pH 10.0 to 11.5

USUAL DOSE

Limit dose to amount needed to increase blood pH to normal limits (7.35 to 7.45) and to correct acid-base derangements. Tham-E contains electrolytes.

Acidosis: Required dose (ml of 0.3 molar solution) equal to body weight in kilograms × base deficit in mEq/L × 1.1.

Acidosis in cardiac bypass surgery: 9 ml/kg of body weight. 500 ml (18 Gm) is an average adult dose. Up to 1,000 ml has been used. Never exceed 500 mg/kg in any individual dose over less than 1 hour.

Correct acidity of ACD priming blood: Stored blood has a pH of 6.22 to 6.80. An average of 60 ml (15 to 77 ml) tromethamine to each 500 ml of stored blood is required to correct pH to 7.4.

Acidosis in cardic arrest: Use only if indicated. Never inject into cardiac muscle. Initial dose in an open chest is 62 to 185 ml (2 to 6 Gm). Additional doses should be based on evaluation of base deficit. If the chest is not open, give 111 to 333 ml (3.6 to 10.8 Gm); use a large peripheral vein. After arrest is reversed, additional amounts may be needed to control persistent acidosis.

DILUTION

May be given undiluted as an infusion or added to pump oxygenator blood, other priming fluid, or ACD blood.

INCOMPATIBLE WITH

Sufficient information not available. Should be administered alone because of specific use and potential side effects.

RATE OF ADMINISTRATION

Slow IV infusion recommended. 5 ml or less/min would deliver up to 300 ml in 1 hour. Rate dictated by patient's condition and intended use (see Usual dose and Precautions). Reduced rate may control venospasm.

ACTIONS

Acts as a proton acceptor and actively binds hydrogen ions in metabolic acids and carbonic acid. Releases bicarbonate anions. Rapidly excreted in the urine, it has an osmotic diuretic effect, increases urine output, urine pH, and excretion of fixed acids, CO_2 and electrolytes. Also capable of neutralizing acidic ions of the intracellular fluid.

INDICATIONS AND USES

Prevention and correction of systemic acidosis; particularly metabolic acidosis associated with cardiac bypass surgery, correction of acidity of ACD blood in cardiac bypass surgery, and cardiac arrest.

CONTRAINDICATIONS

Hypersensitivity to tromethamine, anuria, and uremia.

PRECAUTIONS

Intended for short-term use only (1 day). ■ Sodium bicarbonate or sodium lactate is effective in most acidotic situations and has fewer side effects. ■ Use extreme caution in impaired renal function or decreased urine output.

Monitor: Determine blood pH, P_{CO_2}, bicarbonate, glucose, and electrolytes before, during, and after administration. ■ Avoid overdose (total drug or too-rapid rate). Severe alkalosis and/or prolonged hypoglycemia may result. ■ Use a large peripheral vein. Determine absolute patency of vein; necrosis may result from extravasation. ■ May severely depress respiration; oxygen and controlled ventilation equipment must always be available. ■ ECG monitoring and frequent serum potassium measurements are required to rule out hyperkalemia in impaired renal function or decreased urine output. Decreased excretion of tromethamine may also occur resulting in toxicity.

Maternal/child: Pregnancy Category C: safety for use not established. Benefits must outweigh risks. ■ Severe hypoglycemia or severe hemorrhagic liver necrosis may occur in premature or full-term infants. ■ Discontinue breast feeding.

DRUG/LAB INTERACTIONS

Potentiates amphetamines, ephedrine, and quinidine. ■ Inhibits lithium, methotrexate, and salicylates.

SIDE EFFECTS

Hyperkalemia, hypoglycemia, phlebitis, respiratory depression, and thrombosis.

Overdose: Alkalosis, overhydration, severe prolonged hypoglycemia, soluted overload. May be due to total drug or too-rapid rate of administration.

ANTIDOTE

Notify physician of all side effects. Reduced rate of infusion may prevent hypoglycemia. Use glucose if indicated. Discontinue drug immediately for hyperkalemia or extravasation. Local infiltration with

1% procaine with hyaluronidase or phentolamine may reduce tissue necrosis. Use a no. 25 needle. Symptomatic treatment is indicated. Alternate drugs are indicated (sodium bicarbonate, sodium lactate).

TUBOCURARINE CHLORIDE

Neuromuscular blocking agent
(Nondepolarizing)
Anesthesia adjunct

Curare, ✹Tubarine

pH 2.5 to 5.0

USUAL DOSE

Aid to controlled ventilation: 16.5 mcg (0.0165 mg)/kg of body weight. Adjust as needed.

Muscle contraction or convulsions: 0.165 (1.1 units)/kg minus 3 mg (20 units). May repeat as necessary.

Adjunct to surgical anesthesia: 0.165 (1.1 units)/kg minus 3 mg (20 units). Average dose is 40 to 60 units (6 to 9 mg) at time of incision. May repeat 20 to 30 units if indicated. Maintain with 20 units as needed. Use of peripheral nerve stimulator recommended.

Diagnosis of myasthenia gravis: 4 to 33 mcg (0.004 to 0.033 mg)/kg.

PEDIATRIC DOSE

Adjunct to surgical anesthesia; neonates up to 4 weeks of age: 250 to 500 mcg (0.25 to 0.5 mg)/kg. Any subsequent dose required should be ⅕ to ⅙ of initial dose.

Infants over 4 weeks of age and children: 500 mcg (0.5 mg)/kg. See preceeding note for subsequent doses.

DOSE ADJUSTMENTS

Markedly reduced dose required with numerous drugs; see Drug/lab interactions. ■ Reduced dose required in prematurity (base on M^2 instead of mg/kg); acidosis and hypothermia if procedure required before they can be corrected. ■ Reduce dose by 20% to 33% with inhalant anesthetics (e.g., enflurane). ■ Reduced dose may be required in the elderly.

DILUTION

May be given undiluted in 3 mg/ml concentration, smaller doses may be diluted with NS to facilitate rate of administration.

Myasthenia testing: Dilute single dose to 4 ml with sterile NS. Use only clear solutions. Faint discoloration is acceptable.

INCOMPATIBLE WITH

Alkaline solutions such as barbiturates, trimethaphan (Artonad). Consider incompatible in syringe or solution with any other drug. Evaluation of predictable results imperative.

RATE OF ADMINISTRATION

A single dose over 60 to 90 seconds. Too-rapid injection will cause symptoms of overdose and histamine release resulting in severe bronchospasm and profound hypotension.

Myasthenia testing: 0.5 ml diluted medication over 2 minutes.

ACTIONS

A skeletal muscle relaxant. Causes paralysis by interfering with neural transmission at the myoneural junction. Onset of action is within 2 or 3 minutes and may last up to 60 minutes. Complete recovery from a single dose may take several hours. Most likely agent in this class to cause histamine release. Excreted primarily in urine. Crosses the placental barrier.

INDICATIONS AND USES

Muscle relaxation in severe muscle contraction or convulsion caused by disease, drugs, or electrical stimulation. ■ Diagnosis of myasthenia gravis if other tests inconclusive. ■ Adjunctive to general anesthesia to facilitate endotracheal intubation and to relax skeletal muscles during surgery or mechanical ventilation.

CONTRAINDICATIONS

Known sensitivity, patients in whom histamine release is definite hazard.

PRECAUTIONS

Administered by or under the direction of the anesthesiologist. ■ Repeated doses may produce cumulative effect. ■ Impaired pulmonary function or respiratory deficiencies can cause critical reactions. ■ Use caution in impaired liver or kidney function; recovery prolonged. ■ Myasthenia gravis increases sensitivity to drug. When using tubocurarine to aid in diagnosis of myasthenia gravis, terminate testing process within 2 to 3 minutes with 1.5 mg of neostigmine to avoid prolonged respiratory paralysis. ■ The action of this drug may be altered by electrolyte imbalances, acidosis, body temperature, some carcinomas, dehydration, and renal disease. ■ Hyperkalemia may cause cardiac arrhythmias and increased paralysis. ■ May contain bisulfites; use caution in patients with allergies.

Monitor: This drug produces apnea. Controlled artificial ventilation with oxygen must be continuous and under direct observation at all times. Maintain a patent airway. ■ Confirm adequate electrolyte levels (calcium, potassium, magnesium, sodium) before use. Consider withholding diuretics for at least 4 days before elective surgery. ■ Patient may be conscious and completely unable to communicate by any means. Tubocurarine has no analgesic properties. ■ Use of a peripheral nerve stimulator is recommended to monitor effectiveness of this drug. ■ Note Precautions and Drug/lab interactions.

Maternal/child: Pregnancy Category C: drug levels in fetus directly related to maternal dose. Use extreme caution in pregnancy; has caused fetal malformation. ■ Use caution in lactation; safety not established. ■ Premature infants and neonates may have increased sensitivity.

Elderly: Note Dose adjustments ■ Delay in onset time may be caused by slower circulation time in cardiovascular disease, old age, or edematous states; allow more time for drug to achieve maximum effect. ■ Recovery time may be extended.

DRUG/LAB INTERACTIONS

Potentiated by inhalant anesthetics (e.g., halothane, influrane), many antibiotics (e.g., gentamicin [Garamycin]), calcium and magnesium salts, CO_2, diuretics, muscle relaxants (e.g., diazepam [Valium]), lidocaine, propranolol (Inderal), quinidine, succinylcholine, verapamil (Isoptin), and others. Reduced dose of tubocurarine may be indicated.

Use with caution. ▪ Antagonized by acetylcholines, anticholinesterases, carbamazepine, and potassium.

SIDE EFFECTS

Airway closure caused by relaxation of epiglottis, pharynx, and
tongue muscles. Allergic reactions including anaphylaxis, histamine
release, profound hypotension, respiratory deficiency, respiratory
failure, severe bronchospasm, and shock may occur.

ANTIDOTE

All side effects are medical emergencies. Treat symptomatically. Controlled artificial ventilation must be continuous. Use a peripheral nerve
stimulator to determine degree of neuromuscular blockade. Edrophonium or neostigmine methylsulfate with atropine may help to reverse
muscle relaxation. Not effective in all situations; may aggravate
severe overdosage. Treat allergic reactions and resuscitate as
necessary.

UROKINASE

Thrombolytic agent

Abbokinase, Abbokinase Open-Cath

pH 6.0 to 7.5

USUAL DOSE

Pulmonary embolism: Abbokinase: 4,400 IU/kg of body weight is given as
an initial priming dose over 10 minutes. Follow with a continuous
infusion of 4,400 IU/kg/hr for 12 hours. Total volume of infusion must
not exceed 200 ml. To be sure entire dose is administered, follow entire
procedure with a flush of NS or D5W for infusion. Use a volume equal
to the volume of the catheter. Keep line open with this solution at 15
ml/hr. Follow with heparin therapy, see Monitor.

Coronary artery thrombi: Abbokinase: Intraarterial: Initially give a bolus dose
of heparin 2,500 to 10,000 units IV. Consider any heparin administered
in the previous 4 to 6 hours when calculating this dose. Follow with
prepared solution of urokinase directly into the coronary artery at 4
ml/min (6,000 IU/min) for up to 2 hours. Continue until artery is
maximally opened, usually 15 or 30 minutes after the initial breakthrough. Verify results with angiography. Average required total dosage
is 500,000 IU. Obtain coagulation parameters. Continue heparin therapy.

Intravenous: 2 to 3 million IU over 45 to 90 min, give total dose over 5
min, or ½ total dose over 5 min and balance as an infusion over 45 to 90
min.

IV catheter clearance: Abbokinase Open-Cath or Abbokinase: 5,000 IU (1 ml
specifically diluted solution). More or less can be used. Amount should
be equal to the volume of the catheter.

DILUTION

Abbokinase: Each vial (250,000 IU) must be diluted with 5.2 ml of sterile
water for injection without preservatives. Add diluent slowly, direct to
sides of vial, roll and tilt gently. Do not shake. Can terminally filter
through a 0.45 micron or smaller cellulose membrane filter. Reconstitute
immediately before use. Visually inspect; should be a clear, colorless
solution. Do not use highly colored solutions. Discard unused portions.

For IV infusion in pulmonary embolism: Each dose must be further diluted with sufficient NS to administer a total infusion of 195 ml.

For lysis of coronary artery thrombi: Intraarterial: Dilute three 250,000 IU vials as described. Add the contents of these three vials to 500 ml of D5W for infusion (1,500 IU/ml). *Intravenous:* Add contents of diluted vials to 500 ml D5W.

For IV catheter clearance: Use Abbokinase Open-Cath or add 1 ml of the initially reconstituted Abbokinase to 9 ml of sterile water for injection without preservatives (1 ml equals 5,000 IU). Prepare immediately before using and discard any solution remaining in vial after dose removed.

Storage: Refrigerate **Abbokinase**, do not freeze. Store **Abbokinase Open-Cath** at controlled room temperature.

INCOMPATIBLE WITH

Manufacturer recommends not mixing in syringe or solution with any other drug. Sometimes combined with small amounts of heparin to maintain patency of implant.

RATE OF ADMINISTRATION

Use of an infusion pump required in all situations.

Pulmonary embolism: Initial priming dose is delivered equally distributed over 10 minutes. Follow with continuous infusion of calculated total dose over 12 hours. Use of an infusion pump capable of administering the total volume (195 ml) over 12 hours is required. Keep vein open (see Usual dose).

Lysis of coronary artery thrombi: See Usual dose.

IV catheter clearance: Confirm occlusion by gently attempting to aspirate blood with a 10 ml syringe. Try to dissolve with heparin first; allow effects to diminish. If still present, slowly and gently inject specifically diluted and premeasured amount of urokinase into the catheter (usually 1 ml in a tuberculin syringe). Connect a 5 ml syringe to the catheter and wait 5 minutes. Gently aspirate to remove clot. Repeat aspiration every 5 minutes until clot clears or for 30 minutes. If unsuccessful, cap catheter for 30 to 60 minutes and attempt to aspirate again. If still unsuccessful, a second dose of urokinase may be required. Maintain absolute sterility of IV system in all situations. When successful, aspirate 5 ml of blood to ensure removal of clots and medication. Gently irrigate the catheter with 10 ml of NS. Reconnect to IV tubing.

Arterial catheter clearance: Use heparin initially as above. Inject urokinase as above and clamp end of occluded catheter(s) for 2 hours. Maintain sterility and aspirate as described above.

ACTIONS

An enzyme obtained from human kidney cells by tissue-culturing techniques. It converts plasminogen to plasmin, which degrades fibrin clots, fibrinogen, and other plasma proteins. This activation takes place both within a thrombus and on the surface. Onset of action is prompt. Half-life is 20 minutes. Some effects may last up to 12 to 24 hours. End products of this activity possess an anticoagulant effect. Bleeding may be very difficult to control.

INDICATIONS AND USES

Lysis of acute massive pulmonary emboli if one or more lobes are involved or if hemodynamics are unstable. ■ Lysis of coronary artery thrombi. JAMA standards identify thrombolytic agents as Class II therapy in patients younger than 70 years with chest pain consistent with acute MI and at least 0.1 mV of ST segment elevation in at least two ECG leads. Use in all other patients based on age, accurate diagnosis, and time from onset of chest pain. ■ Lysis of deep vein thrombosis. ■ Restore patency of IV catheters occluded by clotted blood or fibrin (includes central venous catheters).

Investigational uses: Lysis of clots in peripheral vascular disease (excluding thrombophlebitis in the calf). ■ Lysis of deep vein thrombosis (DVT). ■ Lysis of DVT through direct catheter placement, confirmed and observed with angiography. An extensive procedure; specialized equipment, techniques, and care required. Urokinase and heparin boluses and infusions given in specific sequences.

CONTRAINDICATIONS

Active internal bleeding, cerebrovascular accident within 2 months, intracranial or intraspinal surgery, intracranial neoplasm, hypersensitivity to urokinase, liver disease, visceral malignancy.

PRECAUTIONS

Administered only in the hospital under the direction of a physician knowledgeable in its use and with appropriate diagnostic and laboratory facilities available. ■ Diagnosis of pulmonary or other emboli should be confirmed. ■ Best results obtained if started within 5 to 7 days of onset of pulmonary emboli, 3 to 4 days of onset in DVT, and 3 days of onset of arterial thrombi. ■ For coronary catheter procedure, diagnosis of acute myocardial infarction must be confirmed and the site of the coronary thrombosis confirmed with selective angiography. Best results obtained within 4 to 6 hours of infarct. ■ Use caution in presence of atrial fibrillation. ■ Urokinase has less potential for allergic reaction than streptokinase and is indicated if repeated therapy necessary. ■ Will not dissolve drug precipitate or anything other than blood products. Use caution so as not to dislodge foreign bodies into the circulatory system. ■ Use extreme caution in the following situations: any surgical procedure, biopsy, lumbar puncture, thoracentesis, paracentesis, multiple cut-downs, or intraarterial diagnostic procedures within 10 days; ulcerative wounds; recent trauma with possible internal injury; visceral or intracranial malignancy; pregnancy and first 10 days postpartum; any lesion of GI or GU tract with a potential for bleeding (e.g., diverticulitis, ulcerative colitis); severe hypertension; acute or chronic hepatic or renal insufficiency; uncontrolled hypocoagulable state; chronic lung disease with cavitation; rheumatic valvular disease; recent cerebral embolism; subacute bacterial endocarditis; and any condition where bleeding might be hazardous or difficult to manage because of location.

Monitor: Establish a separate IV line for urokinase. ■ Observe patient continuously. Monitor hematocrit, platelet count, thrombin time (TT), and activated PTT (aPTT) or prothrombin time (PT) before therapy. TT or aPTT should be less than twice the normal control value before thrombolytic therapy is started. ■ In 4 hours and during therapy, TT or aPTT changes are monitored and will reflect effectiveness of treatment. Keep physician informed. Request specific parameters for notifying physician after initial supervised injection. ■ Maintain strict bed rest and apply pressure dressings to any recently invaded site. ■ A greater alteration of hemostatic status than with heparin; use care in handling

patient, avoid arterial puncture, venipuncture, and IM injection. Use extreme precautionary methods (use of radial artery, not femoral; extended pressure application of up to 30 minutes) if above procedures absolutely necessary. ■ Monitor for arrhythmias during therapy; atrial and ventricular arrhythmias can occur. ■ Intensive follow-up therapy with heparin is indicated. Do not use a loading dose with continuous heparin therapy. Thrombin time should be reduced to less than twice the normal control value before heparin therapy begins. Usually occurs in 3 to 4 hours. ■ Do not take blood pressure in lower extremities; thrombi may be dislodged. ■ Avoid force while attempting to clear catheters; may rupture catheter or dislodge clot into the circulation. Instruct the patient to exhale and hold his breath any time the catheter is not connected to the IV tubing or a syringe to prevent air from entering the open catheter and the circulatory system. ■ Note Drug/lab interactions. **Patient education:** Compliance with all measures to minimize bleeding (e.g., strict bed rest) is very important. ■ Avoid use of razors, toothbrushes, and other sharp items. ■ Use caution while moving to avoid excess bumping. ■ Report all episodes of bleeding and apply local pressure if indicated.
Maternal/child: Pregnancy Category B: use only when clearly needed and benefits outweigh risks. Note Precautions. ■ Safety for use in lactation and in children not established.
Elderly: Note Indications and Precautions. ■ May have poorer prognosis following MI and preexisting conditions that may increase risk of intracranial bleeding; select patients carefully to maximize benefits.

DRUG/LAB INTERACTIONS
Simultaneous use of anticoagulants not recommended except in lysis of coronary artery. Do not use either drug until the effects of the previous drug are diminished. ■ Avoid use of drugs that may alter platelet function (e.g., aspirin, indomethacin, phenylbutazone).

SIDE EFFECTS
Allergic reactions, arrhythmias, fever; bleeding can be life threatening.

ANTIDOTE
Notify physician of all side effects. Note even the minutest bleeding tendency. Therapy may have to be discontinued with blood loss and/or serious bleeding not controlled by local pressure. Whole blood, packed red blood cells, cryoprecipitate, fresh-frozen plasma, platelets, desmopressin, tranexamic acid and aminocaproic acid may all be indicated. Do not use dextran. Topical preparations of aminocaproic acid may stop minor bleeding. Consider protamine if heparin has been used. Treat bradycardia with atropine, reperfusion arrhythmias with lidocaine or procainamide, VT or VF may require cardioversion. Reduce rate promptly if hypotension occurs; if not resolved, vasopressors (e.g., dopamine [Intropin]), Trendelenburg position, and suitable plasma expanders (e.g., albumin, plasma protein fraction [Plasmanate], or hetastarch) may be indicated. Treat minor allergic reactions symptomatically. Discontinue drug and treat anaphylaxis as indicated; resuscitate as necessary.

VALPROATE SODIUM

Depacon

Anticonvulsant

pH 7.6

USUAL DOSE

Adults and children 10 years of age or older: For all indications optimal clinical response is usually achieved with doses <60 mg/kg/24 hr. Usual therapeutic range of plasma levels is 50 to 100 mcg/ml. A total daily dose exceeding 250 mg should be given in divided doses every 6 hours (studies used an every-6-hour regimen). Note Precautions, Monitor, and Drug/lab interactions. Transfer to oral dosing as soon as practical. Oral and IV doses are considered to be equivalent and should be given at previously established intervals (e.g., every 6 or 8 hours).

Complex partial seizures (monotherapy): Begin with an initial dose of 10 to 15 mg/kg/24 hr. May be increased by 5 to 10 mg/kg/week until desired clinical response achieved.

Complex partial seizures (conversion to monotherapy): Begin with an initial dose of 10 to 15 mg/kg/24 hr. May be increased by 5 to 10 mg/kg/week until desired clinical response achieved. Concomitant antiepilepsy drug (AED) dosage can usually be reduced by 25% every 2 weeks. Dose of AEDs may be decreased at the beginning of valproate therapy or delayed for 1 to 2 weeks to avoid unwanted seizures.

Complex partial seizures (adjunctive therapy): Begin with an initial dose of 10 to 15 mg/kg/24 hr. May be increased by 5 to 10 mg/kg/week until desired clinical response achieved.

Simple and complex absence seizures: Begin with an initial dose of 15 mg/kg/24 hr. May be increased by 5 to 10 mg/kg/week until seizures are controlled or side effects are dose limiting.

PEDIATRIC DOSE

No IV dose recommendations available for children under 10 years of age.

DOSE ADJUSTMENTS

Monitor plasma concentrations when transferring from oral to IV or IV to oral; dose increases or decreases may be indicated. ■ Reduce initial dose in the elderly; base subsequent doses on clinical response. ■ Reduced dose or discontinuation of therapy may be indicated if there is evidence of bruising, hemorrhage, or a disorder of hemostasis/coagulation. ■ Reduced doses and increased monitoring are indicated in hyperammonemia with or without lethargy or coma. Reduce dose further or discontinue if clinically significant symptoms occur (e.g., abnormal liver function tests, lethargy, coma). ■ No dose adjustments required for impaired renal function, gender, or race.

DILUTION

Each single dose should be diluted with at least 50 ml of D5W, NS, or LR.

Storage: Store vials at controlled room temperature (CRT). Diluted solutions stable at CRT for 24 hours. No preservative added; discard unused contents of vial.

INCOMPATIBLE WITH

Specific information not available.

RATE OF ADMINISTRATION

A single dose as an infusion over 60 minutes. Do not exceed a rate of 20 mg/min. Incidence of side effects is increased with too-rapid infusion.

ACTIONS

An anticonvulsant. A sodium salt of valproic acid. Therapeutic effect in epilepsy may result from increased brain concentrations of gamma-aminobutyric acid (GABA). Peak effect occurs at the end of a 60-minute infusion or 4 hours after an oral dose. Plasma protein binding is high and is concentration dependent. Concentration in CSF is similar to unbound concentrations in plasma (10%). When used as a single agent, terminal half-life ranges from 13 to 19 hours. Metabolized in the liver. 30% to 50% excreted in changed form in urine. Crosses placental barrier. Secreted in breast milk.

INDICATIONS AND USES

Use of IV product indicated in the following specific conditions when oral administration of valproate products (e.g., divalproex sodium [Depakote]) is temporarily not feasible. ■ Treatment of complex partial seizures occurring in isolation or with other seizures (monotherapy or adjunctive therapy). ■ Treatment of simple and complex absence seizures (monotherapy or adjunctive therapy). ■ Adjunctive treatment of multiple seizure types that include absence seizures.

CONTRAINDICATIONS

Known hypersensitivity to valproate products, patients with hepatic disease or significant hepatic dysfunction. ■ Not recommended for use in patients with acute head trauma or for the prophylaxis of post-traumatic seizures.

PRECAUTIONS

Use of IV valproate for more than 14 days has not been studied. ■ Has caused fatal hepatic failure. Risk further increased in patients who are on multiple anticonvulsants or have congenital metabolic disorders, severe seizure disorders with mental retardation, or organic brain disease. Children under 2 years of age are at greatest risk. Incidence of fatal hepatotoxicity decreases in progressively older patient groups. If valproate is used in patients with these increased risk factors or in children under 2 years of age with or without these increased risk factors, benefits must outweigh risks; use only as a sole agent with extreme caution. ■ Incidence of thrombocytopenia increases at total trough concentrations > 110 mcg/ml in females and > 135 mcg/ml in males. ■ Plasma protein binding is decreased and free fraction is increased in the elderly, in hyperlipidemic patients, in chronic hepatic disease, in impaired renal function, and in the presence of other drugs (note Drug/lab interactions). Total plasma concentrations may be normal, but free concentrations may be substantially elevated in these patients. ■ Reduce AED doses gradually to prevent status epilepticus in patients treated for major seizure activity.

Monitor: Obtain baseline platelet counts and coagulation tests and monitor during therapy. Repeat before planned surgery. ■ Obtain baseline liver function tests and monitor frequently during therapy, especially during the first 6 months. ■ Observe closely for S/S of hepatotoxicity (e.g., anorexia, facial edema, lethargy, loss of seizure control, malaise, weakness, vomiting). ■ Therapeutic serum levels for most patients will range from 50 to 100 mcg/ml, however, a good correlation has not been established between daily dose, serum levels, and therapeutic effect. ▪ Monitor antiepileptic concentrations more frequently whenever concomitant AEDs are being introduced or withdrawn and observe closely for seizure activity. ▪ Monitor serum concentrations more frequently if an asymptomatic elevation of ammonia occurs; may need to discontinue valproate sodium if hyperammonemia appears. ▪ Monitor serum concentrations more frequently if any of the risk factors listed in Dose adjustments or Precautions are present, and when any drugs that affect hepatic enzymes are introduced or discontinued (see Drug/lab interactions). ▪ Total serum valproic acid concentration is affected by variable free-fractions of drug; consider hepatic metabolism and protein binding when interpreting valproic acid concentrations. ▪ Note Dose adjustments, Precautions, and Drug/lab interactions for additional monitoring requirements.

Patient education: May cause drowsiness; determine effects before driving or operating any machinery. ▪ Consider birth control options.

Maternal/child: Category D; avoid pregnancy. Known to produce birth defects (e.g., spina bifida). Use during pregnancy only if essential for seizure management. Appropriate testing to detect birth defects is indicated. See package insert for additonal information. ▪ When used during pregnancy, valproate has caused clotting abnormalities, including afibrinogenemia in a newborn; monitor clotting parameters carefully. Has also caused hepatic failure in a newborn and an infant. ▪ Effects on testicular development and sperm production not known. ▪ Discontinue breast feeding. ▪ Neonates under 2 months have a markedly decreased ability to eliminate valproate compared to older children and adults. ▪ Children 3 months to 10 years have 50% higher clearance rates based on weight. ▪ IV product has not been studied in children under 2 years of age. ▪ Note Precautions and Monitor.

Elderly: Rate of clearance decreased, free fraction increased; (See Dose adjustments).

DRUG/LAB INTERACTIONS

Clearance increased and effectiveness reduced by drugs that induce hepatic enzymes (e.g., phenytoin [Dilantin], carbamazepine [Tegretol], phenobarbital [Luminal], primidone [Mysoline]); increased monitoring of valproate and concommitant drug concentrations indicated. ▪ Aspirin decreases protein binding, inhibits metabolism, and increases free concentration of valproate; use caution and monitor valproate concentrations if adminstered comcomittantly. ▪ Peak concentrations increased if coadministered with felbamate (Felbatol); reduced dose of valproate indicated. ▪ Rifampin (Rifadin) may increase clearance of valproate and require dose adjustment. ▪ Inhibits metabolism of barbiturates (e.g., phenobarbital) and primidone, increasing their effects. Monitor for neurological toxicity; obtain barbiturate serum levels and reduce barbiturate dose as indicated. ▪ May increase or decrease serum levels of carbamazepine. ▪ Concomittant use with clonazepam (Klonopin) may induce absence status in patients with a history of absence-type seizures. ▪ Displaces some protein-bound drugs, inhibits their metabolism, and increases their effects (e.g., carbamazepine, diazepam [Valium], phenytoin, tolbutamide [Orinase], warfarin [Coumadin]). Dose adjustments and serum concentrations may be indicated. Phenytoin with valproate has caused breakthrough seizures in patients with epilepsy; adjust dose of phenytoin as indicated by serum concentrations. ▪ Monitor coagulation tests if administered with anticoagulants (e.g., warfarin). ▪ Inhibits metabolism of ethosuximide (Zarontin); monitor serum concentrations of both drugs with concomitant administration. ▪ Markedly inhibits metabolism and increases effects of lamotrigine (Lamictal); reduce dose of lamotrigine when coadministered. ▪ Decreases clearance and may increase toxicity of zidovudine (AZT). ▪ See package insert for additional information about many drugs that do not present significant clinical interactions. ▪ May alter thyroid function tests. ▪ May cause false-positive urine ketone test.

SIDE EFFECTS

Abdominal pain, abnormal gait, chest pain, diarrhea, dizziness, elevated serum amylase, euphoria, hallucinations, headache, hyperesthesia, injection site reaction, insomnia, nausea, nervousness, pharyngitis, pneumonia, taste perversion, thrombocytopenia, tremor, vasodilation, vomiting. Frequency of elevated liver enzymes and thrombocytopenia may be dose related. Fatal hepatotoxicity (anorexia, facila edema, lethargy, loss of seizure control, malaise, sweating, weakness, vasodilation, vomiting) has occurred.

Overdose: Somnolence, deep coma, heart block. Some fatalities have been reported.

ANTIDOTE

Keep physician informed of all side effects. Some may respond to a decrease in the rate of administration. Discontinue immediately if signs of suspected or apparent significant hepatic dysfunction appear (e.g., hyperammonemia, elevated liver function tests). Hepatic dysfunction may progress after valproate is discontinued. Reduce dose or discontinue if bruising, hemorrhage, or abnormal coagulation parameters occur (e.g., thrombocytopenia). Maintain a patent airway and resuscitate as indicated. Support patient as required in treatment of overdose; monitor and maintain adequate urine output. Hemodialysis is effective in overdose. Naloxone (Narcan) may reverse CNS depressant effects in overdose but may also reverse antiepilepsy effects of valproate.

VANCOMYCIN HYDROCHLORIDE

Antibacterial
(Tricylic-glycopeptide)

Lyphocin, Vancocin, Vancoled, Vancor

pH 2.4 to 4.5

USUAL DOSE

500 mg every 6 hours or 1 Gm every 12 hours. Maximum dosage of 3 to 4 Gm/24 hr used only in extreme situations. Normal renal function required.

Prevention of bacterial endocarditis in penicillin-allergic patients having dental procedures or upper respiratory tract surgery or instrumentation: Adults and children over 27 kg (59½ lb); 1 Gm IV starting 1 hour before the procedure.

Children under 27 kg: 20 mg/kg of body weight starting 1 hour before the procedure. Dose may be repeated in 8 to 12 hours for high-risk patients. *Prevention of bacterial endocarditis in penicillin-allergic patients having GI or GU surgery or instrumentation: Adults and children over 27 kg (59 1/2 lb):* 1 Gm IV starting 1 hour before the procedure (gentamicin 1.5 mg/kg [not to exceed 80 mg] given concurrently). *Children under 27 kg:* 20 mg/kg starting 1 hour before the procedure (gentamicin 2 mg/kg [not to exceed 80 mg] given concurrently). Dose may be repeated in 8 to 12 hours for high-risk patients.

PEDIATRIC DOSE

10 mg/kg of body weight every 6 to 8 hours. Increase to 15 mg/kg if there is CNS involvement. Do not exceed 2 Gm in 24 hours. See Usual dose for specific uses.

NEONATAL DOSE

15 mg/kg as an initial dose. Follow with 10 mg/kg every 12 hours for *infants up to 1 week of age* and every 8 hours for *infants up to 1 month of age.* Interval extended to 24 hours in *neonates less than 7 days old and under 1 kg;* to 18 hours *in infants less than 7 days and between 1 kg and 2 kg or over 7 days and less than 1 kg.*

DOSE ADJUSTMENTS

Reduce total daily dose in the elderly and in impaired renal function.

DILUTION

Each 500 mg is initially diluted with 10 ml of sterile water for injection. Each 500 mg must be further diluted with 100 ml of NS or D5W and given as an intermittent infusion. If absolutely necessary, 1 to 2 Gm may be further diluted in sufficient amounts of the same infusion fluids and given over 24 hours. Not recommended. Also available pre-diluted and ready to use and in ADD-Vantage vials for use with ADD-Vantage diluent containers.

Storage: Store in refrigerator after initial dilution. Maintains potency for 2 weeks. Solutions prepared from ADD-vantage vials stable at room temperature for 24 hours.

INCOMPATIBLE WITH

Albumin, aminophylline, amobarbital (Amytal), aztreonam (Azactam), ceftazidime (Fortaz), chloramphenicol (Chloromycetin), chlorothiazide (Diuril), dexamethasone (Decadron), foscarnet (Foscavir), heparin, hydrocortisone sodium succinate (Solu-Cortef), idarubicin (Idamycin), methicillin (Staphcillin), penicillins, pentobarbital (Nembutal), phenobarbital (Luminal), phenytoin (Dilantin), piperacillin/tazobactam (Zosyn), prochlorperazine (Compazine), sargramostim (Leukine), secobarbital (Seconal), sodium bicarbonate, warfarin (Coumadin).

RATE OF ADMINISTRATION

A single dose properly diluted over 60 minutes. Preferred route of administration because of high incidence of thrombophlebitis. Severe hypotension, with or without red blotching of the face, neck, chest, and extremities, and cardiac arrest can occur with too-rapid injection.

ACTIONS

A very potent tricyclic glycopeptide antibiotic, it is bactericidal against gram-positive organisms. Well distributed in all body tissues and fluids including spinal fluid if the meninges are inflamed. Vancomycin is excreted in biologically active form in the urine.

INDICATIONS AND USES

Serious gram-positive infections (e.g, staphylococcal) infections including endocarditis, septicemia, bone, lower respiratory tract, and skin and skin structure infections that do not respond or are resistant to other less toxic antibiotics, such as penicillins or cephalosporins. ■ To substitute for contraindicated penicillin therapy if absolutely necessary. ■ Treatment of endocarditis caused by *Streptococcus viridans* or *S. bovis* concurrently with an aminoglycoside antibiotic; endocarditis caused by diphtheroids or *S. epidermidis* concurrently with rifampin and/or an aminoglycoside. ■ Prophylaxis against bacterial endocarditis in highrisk (rheumatic or congenital heart disease) patients undergoing dental, upper respiratory, GI, or GU surgery or instrumentation. ■ Parenteral form used orally for pseudomembranous colitis/staphylococcal enterocolitis caused by *C. difficile*.

CONTRAINDICATIONS

Known hypersensitivity to vancomycin.

PRECAUTIONS

Sensitivity studies necessary to determine susceptibility of the causative organism to vancomycin. ■ Prolonged use of drug may result in superinfection caused by overgrowth of nonsusceptible organisms. ■ Ototoxic and nephrotoxic. Use extreme caution in impaired hearing, impaired renal function, pregnancy, lactation, neonates, and the elderly. Oral vancomycin has a local effect only (e.g., in the bowel); not for systemic use.

Monitor: Blood levels of vancomycin and renal function tests are necessary when this drug is used. Auditory testing indicated with prolonged use. Draw vancomycin levels 1.5 to 2.5 hours after completion of an infusion. ■ Periodic monitoring of leukocyte count recommended in prolonged therapy. ■ Determine absolute patency of vein. Necrosis and sloughing will result from extravasation. Rotate injection sites every 2 to 3 days. ■ Observe for furry tongue, diarrhea, and foul-smelling stools. ■ Severe hypotension, with or without red blotching of the face, neck, chest, and extremities, and cardiac arrest can occur with too-rapid injection. Monitor blood pressure continuously during infusion to prevent a precipitous drop. ■ Note Drug/lab interactions.

Maternal/child: Pregnancy Category C: studies not conclusive. Use only if clearly needed. ■ Safety for use in lactation not established. ■ Neonates have immature renal function; blood levels may be excessive.

Elderly: Systemic and renal clearance may be reduced; dose reduction required.

DRUG/LAB INTERACTIONS

Use caution with dimenhydrinate (Dramamine), which can mask ototoxicity. ■ May potentiate nephrotoxicity of neuromuscular blocking antibiotics (e.g., gentamicin, tobramycin). ■ May be potentiated by other nephrotoxic, neurotoxic, or ototoxic drugs (e.g., cisplatin, ethacrynic acid [Edecrin], furosemide [Lasix]). ■ May enhance neuromuscular blockade with nondepolarizing muscle relaxants (e.g., pancuronium [Pavulon], mivacurium [Mivacron]). ■ May cause muscle paralysis and respiratory collapse with succinylcholine (Anectine). ■ May cause erythema and histamine-like flushing in children with anesthetics.

SIDE EFFECTS
Minor: Chills, dizziness, fever, macular rashes, nausea, pain at injection site, pruritus, tinnitus, urticaria.

Major: Anaphylaxis, cardiac arrest, dyspnea, eosinophilia, hearing loss, hypotension, interstitial nephritis, neutropenia, redneck or redman syndrome, renal failure, Stevens-Johnson syndrome (erythema multiforme [flu-like symptoms that can be fatal]), thrombophlebitis, wheezing.

ANTIDOTE
Notify the physician of all side effects. Hearing loss may progress even if drug is discontinued. If minor side effects are progressive or any major side effect occurs, discontinue the drug, treat allergic reaction, or resuscitate as necessary. Prevent severe hypotension by slowing infusion rate to 2 hours. Fluids, antihistamines, corticosteroids, and vasopressors (e.g., dopamine [Intropin]) may be required. Hemodialysis or CAPD will not decrease blood levels in toxicity.

VECURONIUM BROMIDE
**Neuromuscular blocking agent
(Nondepolarizing)
Anesthesia adjunct**

Norcuron   **pH 4.0**

USUAL DOSE
Must be individualized, depending on previous drugs administered and degree and length of muscle relaxation required. 0.08 to 0.1 mg/kg of body weight initially as an IV bolus. Patient should be unconscious before administration. Determine need for maintenance dose based on beginning symptoms of neuromuscular blockade reversal determined by a peripheral nerve stimulator. 0.01 to 0.015 mg/kg will be required in approximately 25 to 40 minutes and every 12 to 20 minutes thereafter to maintain muscle relaxation. Higher doses (0.15 to 0.28 mg/kg) at longer intervals have been given with proper ventilation without causing adverse cardiac effects.

PEDIATRIC DOSE
1 to 10 years of age: May require high end of initial adult dose and maintenance dose may be required on a more frequent basis.

DOSE ADJUSTMENTS
Reduce dose by 15% if administered more than 5 minutes after inhalation general anesthetics. ■ Reduce dose to 0.04 to 0.06 mg/kg if following succinylcholine administration. Succinylcholine must show signs of wearing off before vecuronium is given. Use caution. ■ Reduced dose required with numerous drugs, (See Drug/lab interactions). ■ Reduced dose may be required in renal or hepatic impairment. ■ Infants between 7 weeks and 1 year may require a slightly lower dose and recovery time will be extended.

DILUTION
Each 10 mg must be diluted with 5 ml sterile water for injection (supplied). May be given direct IV or 10 (20) mg may be further diluted in up to 100 ml NS, D5W, D5/NS, or LR and given as an infusion

0.1 (0.2) mg/ml concentration. Titrated to symptoms of neuromuscular blockade reversal.

Storage: Stable at room temperature before reconstitution. Store under refrigeration. Discard after 24 hours except if reconstituted with bacteriostatic water; stable refrigerated up to 5 days.

INCOMPATIBLE WITH
Alkaline solutions (e.g., barbiturates), diazepam (Valium).

RATE OF ADMINISTRATION
A single dose as an IV bolus over 30 to 60 seconds. If maintenance dose is given as an infusion, adjust rate to specific dose desired.

ACTIONS
A nondepolarizing skeletal muscle relaxant about one-third more potent than pancuronium with a shorter duration of neuromuscular blockade. Causes paralysis by interfering with neural transmission at the myoneural junction. Onset of action is dose dependent. Onset of action is within 30 seconds, produces maximum neuromuscular blockade within 3 to 5 minutes, and lasts about 25 minutes. It may take up to 60 minutes or more before complete recovery occurs. Up to three times the therapeutic dose has been given without significant changes of hemodynamic parameters in good risk surgical patients. Excreted as metabolites in bile and urine. Crosses the placental barrier.

INDICATIONS AND USES
Adjunctive to general anesthesia, to facilitate endotracheal intubation and to relax skeletal muscles during surgery or mechanical ventilation.

CONTRAINDICATIONS
Known hypersensitivity to vecuronium.

PRECAUTIONS
For IV use only. ■ Administered by or under the direct observation of the anesthesiologist. ■ Repeated doses have no cumulative effect if recovery is allowed to begin before administration. ■ Use extreme caution in patients with cirrhosis, cholestasis, obesity, or circulatory insufficiency. ■ Myasthenia gravis and other neuromuscular diseases increase sensitivity to drug. Can cause critical reactions.

Monitor: This drug produces apnea. Controlled artificial ventilation with oxygen must be continuous and under direct observation at all times. Maintain a patent airway. ■ Use a peripheral nerve stimulator to monitor response to vecuronium and avoid overdose. ■ Patient may be conscious and completely unable to communicate by any means. Has no analgesic properties. Respiratory depression with morphine may be preferred in some patients requiring mechanical ventilation. ■ Action is altered by dehydration, electrolyte imbalance, body temperatures, and acid-base imbalance. ■ Recovery time extended in infants 7 weeks to 1 year. ■ Note Drug/lab interactions.

Maternal/child: Category C: use in pregnancy only if use justifies potential risk to fetus. Has been used during cesarean section; monitor infant carefully. ■ Use caution during lactation. ■ Safety for use in infants under 7 weeks of age not established. ■ Some preparations contain benzyl alcohol; do not use in premature infants. ■ Note Dose adjustments.

DRUG/LAB INTERACTIONS
Potentiated by hypokalemia, some carcinomas, general anesthetics (e.g., enflurane, isoflurane, halothane), many antibiotics (e.g., clinda-

mycin [Cleocin], kanamycin [Kantrex], gentamicin [Garamycin]), polypeptide antibiotics (e.g., bacitracin, colistimethate), tetracyclines, diuretics, diazepam (Valium) and other muscle relaxants, magnesium sulfate, quinidine, morphine, meperidine, succinylcholine, verapamil, and others. May need to reduce dose of vecuronium. Use with caution. ■ Antagonized by acetylcholine, anticholinesterases, azathioprine, carbamazepine, phenytoin, and theophylline. ■ Succinylcholine must show signs of wearing off before vecuronium is given. Use caution.

SIDE EFFECTS

No side effects have occurred except with overdose: prolonged action resulting in respiratory insufficiency or apnea, airway closure caused by relaxation of epiglottis, pharynx, and tongue muscles. Hypersensitivity reactions including anaphylaxis are possible.

ANTIDOTE

All side effects are medical emergencies. Treat symptomatically. Controlled artificial ventilation must be continuous until full muscle control returns. Pyridostigmine (Mestinon) or neostigmine (Prostigmin) given with atropine will probably reverse the muscle relaxation but should not be required because of short time of effectiveness. Not effective in all situations, may aggravate severe overdose. Resuscitate as necessary.

VERAPAMIL HYDROCHLORIDE

Calcium channel blocker
Antiarrhythmic

Isoptin

pH 4.1 to 6.0

USUAL DOSE

5 to 10 mg initially (0.075 to 0.15 mg/kg of body weight). May cause transient bradycardia or hypotension. 10 mg (0.15 mg/kg) may be repeated in 30 minutes if needed to achieve appropriate response. Maximum total dose is 20 mg. JAMA recommendation is 2.5 to 5 mg every 15 min; repeat 5 to 10 mg every 15 to 30 min to total dose of 20 mg. Sometimes given as an infusion after initial bolus dose (*Investigational*).

PEDIATRIC DOSE

Infants up to 1 year of age: 0.1 to 0.2 mg/kg of body weight (usually 0.75 to 2 mg). Repeat in 30 minutes if indicated.

1 to 15 years of age: 0.1 to 0.3 mg/kg (usually 2 to 5 mg). Do not exceed 5 mg. Repeat in 30 minutes if response not adequate. Repeat dose should not exceed 10 mg as a single dose.

DOSE ADJUSTMENTS

Reduced dose may be required in hepatic or renal disease especially with repeat dosing. ■ Note Drug/lab interactions.

DILUTION

Direct IV: May be given undiluted through Y-tube or three-way stopcock of tubing containing dextrose 5%, sodium chloride 0.9%, or Ringer's solution for infusion or further diluted for infusion (1 mg/ml).

Infusion: (*Investigational*): Verapamil 100 mg (40 ml) diluted in 60 ml D5W equals 1 mg/ml. More diluent may be used (100 mg in 360 ml diluent equals 0.25 mg/ml). Use with extreme caution.

Storage: Protect from light. Do not use if discolored or particulate matter present. Discard unused solution.

INCOMPATIBLE WITH

Albumin, aminophylline, amphotericin B (Fungizone), ampicillin (Polycillin-N), dobutamine (Dobutrex), hydralazine (Apresoline), mezlocillin (Mezlin), nafcillin sodium, oxacillin (Prostaphlin), sodium bicarbonate, sodium lactate in PVC bags, sulfamethoxazole-trimethoprim. Will precipitate in any solution with a pH over 6.

RATE OF ADMINISTRATION

Direct IV: A single dose over 2 minutes for adults and children. Extend to 3 minutes in the elderly.

Infusion: Infusion pump required; separate IV line preferred to ensure accuracy and prevent accidental bolusing during addition of other fluids. Rate may be constant (e.g., 5 to 10 mg/hr) or titrated to heart rate.

ACTIONS

A calcium (and possibly sodium) ion inhibitor through slow channels. Slows conduction through SA and AV nodes, prolongs effective refractory period in the AV node, and reduces ventricular rates. Prevents reentry phenomena through the AV node. Reduces myocardial contractility, afterload, arterial pressure, vascular tone, and oxygen demand. Effective within 1 to 5 minutes. Hemodynamic effects last about 20 minutes, but antiarrhythmic effects may last up to 6 hours. Does not alter total serum calcium levels. Metabolized in the liver. Crosses the placental barrier. Excreted in urine and feces. Secreted in breast milk.

INDICATIONS AND USES

Treatment of supraventricular tachyarrhythmias including conversion to normal sinus rhythm of paroxysmal supraventricular tachycardia (includes Wolff-Parkinson-White and Lown-Ganong-Levine syndromes) ▪ Temporary control of rapid ventricular rate in atrial flutter or atrial fibrillation. ▪ Narrow complex PSVT not responsive to adenosine.

CONTRAINDICATIONS

Atrial fibrillation or flutter when associated with an accessory bypass tract (e.g., Wolff-Parkinson-White or Lown-Ganong-Levine syndromes), cardiogenic shock, congestive heart failure (severe) unless secondary to supraventricular tachyarrhythmia treatable with verapamil, known sensitivity to verapamil, second- or third-degree AV block, severe hypotension, sick sinus syndrome (unless functioning artificial pacemaker in place), patients receiving IV beta-adrenergic blocking drugs (e.g., propranolol [Inderal]) within 2 to 4 hours, and ventricular tachycardia.

PRECAUTIONS

Valsalva maneuver recommended before use of verapamil in all paroxysmal supraventricular tachycardias if clinically appropriate. ▪ Caution required in hepatic and renal disease, especially if repeated dosing is required. ▪ Use extreme caution in patients with hypertrophic cardiomyopathy. ▪ May cause ventricular fibrillation in patients with wide-complex ventricular tachycardia. ▪ May precipitate respiratory muscle failure in patients with muscular dystrophy or increase intracranial pressure during anesthesia induction in patients with supratentorial tumors. Use caution. ▪ Reduction of myocardial contractility may worsen CHF in patients with severe left ventricular dysfunction. ▪ Continue regular dosing on day of surgery and thereafter unless otherwise specified by physician. May cause severe angina or MI if discontinued. ▪ Recent studies indicate that verapamil inhibits thrombus formation and platelet aggregation.

Monitor: ECG monitoring during administration mandatory for infants and children, and during an infusion; recommended for all others. ▪ Document cardiac rhythm before therapy, with any significant change in type or rate, and at least every 4 hours. Note PR interval. ▪ Monitor blood pressure very closely, every 5 minutes times 3 or until reasonably stabilized, every 15 minutes times 4 and hourly thereafter. May need more frequent checks with increased drip rate. ▪ Emergency resuscitation drugs and equipment must always be available. ▪ Treat heart failure with digitalis and diuretics before using verapamil. ▪ Pulmonary wedge pressure above 20 mm Hg and/or ejection fraction below 20% to 30% indicates acute heart failure. ▪ Maintain bed rest until effects on heart rate, blood pressure and potential dizziness evaluated. ▪ Monitor for side effects (AV block) and digoxin levels when used concurrently with digitalis. ▪ Monitor for any unusual bleeding or bruising. ▪ Note Drug/lab interactions.

Maternal/child: Category C: safety for use in pregnancy not yet established; use only when clearly indicated. ▪ Discontinue breast feeding. ▪ Children under 6 months of age may not respond to treatment with verapamil. ▪ Severe hemodynamic side effects (e.g., bradycardia, hypotension, or a rapid ventricular rate in atrial flutter/fibrillation) can occur in infants and neonates. Use caution and monitor closely.

Elderly: May have an increased hypotensive effect; note Rate of administration. ▪ Consider reduced renal function; half-life may be prolonged. ▪ May cause drug induced tinnitus.

DRUG/LAB INTERACTIONS

Potentiates digoxin; lower dose may be appropriate. ▪ Do not give comcomitantly (within a few hours) with oral or IV beta-adrenergic blocking drugs (e.g., propranolol [Inderal]) (see Contraindications). Both drugs depress myocardial contractility and AV node conduction. ▪ Do not administer disopyramide (Norpace) within 48 hours before or 24 hours after verapamil. ▪ Potentiates cyclosporine and carbamazepine. ▪ Potentiates nondepolarizing muscle relaxants (e.g., tubocurarine); use lower doses of muscle relaxant and extreme caution. ▪ May cause excessive hypotension with other antihypertensive drugs (vasodilators and diuretics) and quinidine. ▪ May inhibit other highly protein-bound drugs (e.g., oral hypoglycemics, warfarin). Use caution. ▪ In two case reports AV block and severe hypotension occurred with clonidine.

SIDE EFFECTS

Abdominal discomfort, allergic reactions including anaphylaxis, asystole, bradycardia, dizziness, headache, second and third degree heart block, heart failure, hypotension (symptomatic), increased ventricular response in atrial flutter, fibrillation (Wolff-Parkinson-White and Lown-Ganong-Levine syndromes), nausea, PVCs, tachycardia.

ANTIDOTE

Discontinue verapamil and notify physician promptly if hypotension, bradycardia, or 2nd or 3rd degree heart block occurs. Keep physician informed of all side effects. Treatment will depend on clinical situation. Calcium chloride may reverse effects of verapamil and can be used in toxicity. Glucagon may also be used in toxicity (see glucagon monograph). Rapid ventricular response in atrial flutter/fibrillation should respond to cardioversion, procainamide, and/or lidocaine. Treat bradycardia, AV block, and asystole with standard AHA protocol (atropine, pacing). Levarterenol or dopamine will reverse hypotension. Treat allergic reactions or resuscitate as necessary.

VINBLASTINE SULFATE

Antineoplastic
(Mitotic inhibitor-vinca alkaloid)

Velban, ✽Velbe, Velsar, VLB   pH 3.5 to 5.0

USUAL DOSE

3.7 mg/M^2 initially. Administered once every 7 days, increasing the dose to specific amounts (5.5, 7.4, 9.25, 11.1 mg/M^2) a single step each week until the white blood cell count is decreased to 3,000 cells/ml, remission is achieved, or a maximum dose of 18.5 mg/M^2 is reached. Maintenance dose is one step below any dose that causes leukopenia (3,000 cells/ml or less), once every 7 to 14 days. Usually 5.5 to 7.4 mg/M^2. Continue treatment for 4 to 6 weeks. Up to 12 weeks often necessary.

PEDIATRIC DOSE

2.5 mg/M^2 initially. Use same procedure as for adult dose using steps to 3.75, 5.0, 6.25, and 7.5 mg/M^2. Maximum dose is 12.5 mg/M^2. Maintenance dose is calculated by same parameters as adult dose. Usually differs with each individual.

DOSE ADJUSTMENTS

Reduce dose by 50% if serum bilirubin above 3 mg/dl. ■ Often used with other antineoplastic drugs and corticosteroids in reduced doses to achieve tumor remission.

DILUTION

Specific techniques required; see Precautions. Each 10 mg is diluted with 10 ml of NS for injection. 1 mg equals 1 ml. Also available in liquid form (1 mg/ml). May be given direct IV or through Y-tube or three-way stopcock of a free-flowing IV infusion. Occasionally further diluted in 50 ml or more of D5W and given as an infusion.

Storage: Store in refrigerator before and after dilution. Potency maintained for 30 days after dilution if reconstituted with bacteriostatic NS.

INCOMPATIBLE WITH

Furosemide (Lasix), heparin. Consider toxicity and specific use.

RATE OF ADMINISTRATION

IV injection: Total desired dose, properly diluted, over 1 minute.

Infusion: A single dose over 20 to 30 minutes or as a continuous infusion prolonged over up to 96 hours. Extended infusion may increase vein irritation.

ACTIONS

An alkaloid of the periwinkle plant with antitumor activity. Cell cycle specific for M phase. Thought to interfere with the metabolic pathways of amino acids. Sometimes pharmacologically effective without any noticeable improvement in symptoms of malignancy. Cell energy production and synthesis of nucleic acid may also be inhibited. Some excretion through bile and urine.

INDICATIONS AND USES

To suppress or retard neoplastic growth. Remission and probable cure has been achieved with bleomycin and cisplatin in testicular malignancies. Response has been noted in Hodgkin's disease, non-Hodgkin's lymphomas, choriocarcinoma, Kaposi's sarcoma, mycosis fungoids, breast and renal cell malignancies. ■ Used to treat many other malignancies.

CONTRAINDICATIONS

Bacterial infection or leukopenia below 3,000 cells/ml.

PRECAUTIONS

Follow guidelines for handling cytotoxic agents. See Appendix A, p. 893. ■ Usually administered by or under the direction of the physician specialist. ■ For IV use only; fatal if given intrathecally. ■ May cause corneal ulceration with accidental contact to the eye. ■ Use caution in presence of ulcerated skin areas or impaired liver function.

Monitor: Determine absolute patency, quality of vein, and adequate circulation of extremity. Severe cellulitis may result from extravasation. Rinse syringe and needle with venous blood before withdrawal from the vein. ■ White blood cell count must be checked before each dose. Must be above 4,000 cells/ml. ■ Be alert for signs of bone marrow depression or infection. ■ Prophylactic antibiotics may be indicated pending results of C/S in a febrile neutropenic patient. ■ Observe for increased uric acid levels; may require increased doses of antigout agents; allopurinol (Zyloprim) preferred. ■ Maintain adequate hydration. ■ Prophylactic antiemetics may increase patient comfort. ■ Note Drug/lab interactions.

Patient education: Avoid pregnancy; nonhormonal birth control recommended ■ Report IV site burning or stinging promptly. ■ Report chills, fever, sore mouth or throat promptly. ■ Maintain adequate hydration; avoid constipation. ■ See Appendix D, p. 900.

Maternal/child: Category D: avoid pregnancy. May produce teratogenic effects on the fetus. Has a mutagenic potential. ■ Discontinue breast feeding. ■ Do not use diluents containing benzyl alcohol in premature infants.

Elderly: Leukopenic response may be increased in malnutrition or with skin ulcers.

DRUG/LAB INTERACTIONS

Inhibited by some amino acids, glutamic acid, and tryptophan. ■ Potentiated by other bone marrow depressants (e.g., antineoplastics, radiation therapy). ■ Do not administer live virus vaccines to patients receiving antineoplastic drugs. ■ Acute pulmonary reactions can occur with Mitomycin-C. ■ May inhibit effects of phenytoin (Dilantin), increased doses of phenytoin may be needed. ■ Erythomycin decreases metabolism and increases toxicity of vinblastine. ■ Use caution with any drug that inhibits P_{450} enzymes (e.g., calcium channel blockers [e.g., diltiazem (Cardizem), nicardipine (Cardene), verapamil (Isoptin)], antifungal agents [e.g., fluconazole (Diflucan), ketoconazole (Nizoral)], bromocriptine [Parlodel], cimetidine [Tagamet], clarithromycin [Biaxin], cyclosporine [Sandimmune], danazol [Medrol], metoclopramide [Reglan]); may increase vinblastine blood levels and increase toxicity.

SIDE EFFECTS

Usually dose related and not always reversible: abdominal pain, alopecia, anorexia, cellulitis, constipation, convulsions, diarrhea, dizziness, extravasation, gonadal suppression, headache, hemorrhage, ileus, leukopenia (severe), malaise, mental depression, myelosuppression, nausea, numbness, oral lesions, paresthesias, peripheral neuritis, pharyngitis, Raynaud's syndrome, reflex depression (deep tendon), skin lesions, thrombophlebitis, tumor site pain, vomiting, weakness.

ANTIDOTE

For extravasation, discontinue the drug immediately and administer into another vein. Hyaluronidase should be injected locally into extravasated area. Use a fine hypodermic needle. Elevate extremity. Moist heat may be helpful. Notify the physician of all side effects; symptomatic treatment is often indicated. Glutamic acid blocks toxicity of vinblastine, but also blocks its antineoplastic activity.

VINCRISTINE SULFATE

Antineoplastic
(Mitotic inhibitor-vinca alkaloid)

LCR, Oncovin, VCR, Vincasar PFS   pH 3.5 to 5.5

USUAL DOSE

1.4 mg/M^2 administered once every 7 days. Various dosage schedules have been used with caution.

PEDIATRIC DOSE

2 mg/M^2. For children weighing less than 10 kg (22 lb) or with a body surface area less than 1 M^2, give 0.05 mg/kg of body weight once a week.

DOSE ADJUSTMENTS

In impaired hepatic function, reduce initial doses to 0.05 to 1 mg/M^2 or by 50% if direct bilirubin above 3 mg/dl. May be increased gradually based on individual response. ▪ Usually given with other antineoplastic drugs and corticosteroids in reduced doses to achieve tumor remission. ▪ Note Drug/lab interactions.

DILUTION

Specific techniques required; see Precautions. Diluent provided, or each 1 mg is diluted with 10 ml of sterile water or NS. 0.1 mg equals 1 ml (may use as little as 2 ml diluent for each 1 mg). May be given direct IV or through Y-tube or three-way stopcock of a free-flowing IV infusion. Available in preservative-free solutions. Occasionally further diluted in 50 ml or more NS or D5W and given as an infusion.

Storage: Store in refrigerator before and after dilution. Potency maintained for 14 days after dilution. Label vial pertaining to mg/ml.

INCOMPATIBLE WITH

All solutions except NS or dextrose in water. pH must not be less than 3.5 or more than 5.5. Furosemide (Lasix), idarubicin (Idamycin). Consider toxicity and specific use.

RATE OF ADMINISTRATION

Direct IV: Total desired dose, properly diluted, over 1 minute.

Infusion: A single dose over 20 to 30 minutes or as a continuous infusion prolonged over up to 96 hours.

ACTIONS

An alkaloid of the periwinkle plant with antitumor activity. Cell cycle specific for the M phase. Well distributed except in spinal fluid, it is primarily excreted through bile and feces.

INDICATIONS AND USES

To suppress or retard neoplastic growth; good response experienced in leukemia, Hodgkin's disease, lymphosarcoma, oat cell, Wilm's tumor and others.

Investigational uses: Treatment of idiopathic thrombocytopenic purpura; treatment of Kaposi's sarcoma, breast and bladder cancer.

CONTRAINDICATIONS

Demyelinating form of Charcot-Marie-Tooth syndrome.

PRECAUTIONS

Follow guidelines for handling cytotoxic agents. See Appendix A, p. 893.
■ Administered by or under the direction of the physician specialist.
■ For IV use only. Fatal if given intrathecally. ■ Use extreme caution in combination with radiation therapy. ■ May cause corneal ulceration with accidental contact to the eye; flush eyes with water immediately.
■ Use caution in preexisting neuromuscular disease or impaired liver function.

Monitor: Determine absolute patency and quality of vein and adequate circulation of extremity. Severe cellulitis may result from extravasation.
■ Monitor CBC, platelets and evaluate neuro status before therapy and at frequent intervals. ■ Be alert for signs of bone marrow depression or infection. ■ Prophylactic antibiotics may be indicated pending results of C/S in a febrile neutropenic patient. ■ Observe for increased uric acid levels; may require increased doses of antigout agents; allopurniol (Zyloprim) preferred. ■ Maintain adequate hydration. ■ Prophylactic antiemetics may increase patient comfort. ■ Monitor for hyponatremia and inappropriate secretion of antidiuretic hormone (ADH); may require fluid limitation. ■ Use a laxative to prevent constipation. ■ Note Drug/lab interactions.

Patient education: Avoid pregnancy, nonhormonal birth control recommended. ■ Report IV site burning or stinging promptly. ■ See Appendix D, p. 900. ■ Use laxatives to avoid constipation.

Maternal/child: Category D: avoid pregnancy. May produce teratogenic effects on the fetus. Has a mutagenic potential. ■ Discontinue breast feeding.

Elderly: Neurotoxicity may be more severe (observe closely for constipation, ileus, and urinary retention).

DRUG/LAB INTERACTIONS

May cause severe bone marrow depression with other antineoplastic drugs or radiation therapy. ■ Use with asparaginase, or doxorubicin not recommended. Asparaginase inhibits the elimination of vincristine and increases its toxicity. One source suggests giving vincristine 12 to 24 hours before asparaginase; use caution. ■ Acute pulmonary reactions can occur with mitomycin-C. ■ Inhibited by glutamic acid. ■ Do not administer live virus vaccines to patients receiving antineoplastic drugs. ■ Inhibits digoxin and phenytoin, increased doses of these drugs may be required. ■ Use with filgrastim may induce a severe atypical neuropathy (foot pain, severe motor weakness).

SIDE EFFECTS

Frequently dose related and not always reversible: abdominal pain, alopecia, anaphylaxis, ataxia, bronchospasm, cellulitis, constipation, convulsions, cranial nerve damage, diarrhea, dysuria, extravasation, fever, foot-drop, gonadal suppression, headache, hypertension, hypotension, leukopenia (rare), muscle wasting, nausea, neuritic pain, oral lacerations, paralytic ileus, paresthesias, polyuria, reflex changes, sensory impairment, shortness of breath, SIADH, tingling and numbness of extremities, thrombocytopenia (rare), thrombophlebitis, upper colon impaction, uric acid nephropathy, vomiting, weakness, weight loss.

ANTIDOTE

For extravasation, discontinue the drug immediately and administer into another vein. Hyaluronidase or hydrocortisone sodium succinate (Solu-Cortef) may be injected locally into extravasated area. Use a fine hypodermic needle. Elevate extremity; moist heat may be helpful. Notify the physician of all side effects; symptomatic treatment is often indicated. Will probably reduce dose at earliest signs of neurological toxicity (tingling and numbness of extremities). Discontinue for inappropriate ADH secretion or hyponatremia. Treat with fluid restriction and diuretics. Phenobarbital may be needed for convulsions. Use enemas or cathartics to treat constipation or prevent ileus. Glutamic acid blocks toxicity of vincristine, but also blocks its antineoplastic activity. Folinic acid, 100 mg IV every 3 hours for 24 hours and then every 6 hours for at least 48 hours, may be helpful in overdose. Supportive measures still required.

✖VINDESINE SULPHATE

Antineoplastic
(Mitotic inhibitor-vinca alkaloid)

✖Eldisine   pH 4.2 to 4.5

USUAL DOSE

3 mg/M^2 administered once every 7 to 10 days. Repeat for 8 cycles. May be adjusted upward if necessary. Do not exceed 4 mg/M^2. Calculate carefully in presence of edema or ascites, overdose may be fatal. Decreased bone marrow function induced by disease will require full doses to restore marrow function. Will require constant monitoring.

PEDIATRIC DOSE

4 mg/M^2 administered once every 7 to 10 days. Repeat for 8 cycles. 2 mg/M^2/day for 2 consecutive days may be given as an alternate

regimen. Follow by 5 to 7 days without the drug and repeat for 8 cycles.

DOSE ADJUSTMENTS

Decrease dose in significant hepatic disease and in patients with bone marrow depression from previous treatment. May be increased gradually based on clinical response. ▪ Reduced dose may be required in the elderly (over 60). ▪ Note Precautions/Monitor.

DILUTION

Specific techniques required; see Precautions. Each 5 mg vial must be diluted with 5 ml of bacteriostatic NS. 1 mg equals 1 ml. Do not add to IV solutions. Must be given direct IV or through Y-tube or three-way stopcock of a free-flowing IV infusion.

Storage: Stable after dilution at room temperature for 24 hours and up to 14 days if refrigerated. Label vial pertaining to mg/ml.

INCOMPATIBLE WITH

May precipitate in any solution with a pH above 6. Manufacturer suggests not mixing with any other drug in syringe or solution.

RATE OF ADMINISTRATION

Total desired dose, properly diluted, over 1 to 3 minutes.

ACTIONS

An antineoplastic agent; a vinca alkaloid with properties similar to but more potent than vincristine and vinblastine. Cell cycle specific for the M phase. Can prevent invasion of normal tissue by malignant cells. Has been effective in patients who have relapsed on multiple-agent treatment that included vincristine. Well distributed through plasma and body tissues, it is primarily excreted through bile and feces.

INDICATIONS AND USES

Treatment of acute lymphocytic leukemia of childhood resistant to vincristine and non-oat cell lung cancer.

CONTRAINDICATIONS

Drug-induced severe granulocytopenia or thrombocytopenia; serious bacterial infections.

PRECAUTIONS

Follow guidelines for handling cytotoxic agents. See Appendix A, p. 893. ▪ Administered by or under the direction of the physician specialist. ▪ For IV use only; intrathecal administration of other vinca alkaloids has resulted in death. ▪ Use extreme caution in patients with impaired liver function, preexisting neuromuscular disease, or those taking other neurotoxic drugs (e.g., antineoplastics [cisplatin], phenothiazines [prochlorperazine]). Neurotoxicity may require dose reduction or discontinuation of vindesine. ▪ Prior radiation therapy or treatment with other antineoplastic agents may cause thrombocytopenia (platelets below 200,000/mm^3). Not common in patients with normal bone marrow function receiving once-a-week dosage. ▪ May cause corneal ulceration with accidental contact to the eye; flush eyes with water immediately.

Monitor: Monitor blood count 1 or 2 times weekly. Temporary leukopenia is an expected effect and is directly related to the dose. Discontinue or reduce dosage if abnormal depression of the bone marrow occurs (sustained white blood cell count below 2,500/mm^3). Maximum depression usually occurs in 3 to 5 days, and recovery of bone marrow should

occur 7 to 10 days after each dose. ▪ Strict adherence to recommended dose schedule is very important. Changes may result in increased side effects. ▪ Determine absolute patency and quality of vein and adequate circulation of extremity. Severe cellulitis and phlebitis with sloughing can result from extravasation. ▪ Be alert for any sign of infection. Infections must be brought under control before beginning therapy with vindesine. ▪ Prophylactic antibiotics may be indicated pending results of C/S in a febrile neutropenic patient. ▪ Maintain adequate hydration. ▪ Observe for increased uric acid levels; may require increased doses of antigout agents; allopurinol (Zyloprim) preferred. ▪ Prophylactic antiemetics may increase patient comfort. ▪ Use a stool softener to prevent impaction. Monitor bowel sounds to prevent obstipation. ▪ Inappropriate secretion of antidiuretic hormone (ADH) may require fluid limitation and diuretics (e.g., furosemide [Lasix]). ▪ Note Drug/lab interactions. *Patient education:* Report IV site burning or stinging promptly. ▪ Emphasize adherence to dose schedule. ▪ Avoid pregnancy, non-hormonal birth control recommended. ▪ See Appendix D, p. 900.
Maternal/child: Embryotoxic and may be teratogenic. Must be given with caution in men and women capable of conception. ▪ Discontinue breast feeding.

DRUG/LAB INTERACTIONS

Neurotoxicity increased by other neurotoxic drugs (e.g., antineoplastics [cisplatin], phenothiazines [prochlorperazine]); may require dose reduction or discontinuation of vindesine. ▪ Do not administer vaccine or chloroquine to patients receiving antineoplastic drugs.

SIDE EFFECTS

Frequently dose related and not always reversible: abdominal pain; alopecia; anorexia; cellulitis; constipation; convulsions; depression; diarrhea; epilation, chills, and fever; extravasation; generalized musculoskeletal pain; granulocytopenia; headache; jaw pain; leukopenia (rare); loss of deep tendon reflexes; macular skin rash;, malaise; nausea; neuritic pain; oral lacerations; pain in tumor site; paralytic ileus; peripheral neuritis; thrombocytopenia (rare); thrombophlebitis; tingling and numbness of extremities (paresthesias); upper colon impaction; vomiting.
Overdose: Cardiovascular collapse, ileus, inappropriate secretion of ADH, seizures, serious bone marrow depression, death.

ANTIDOTE

For extravasation, discontinue the drug immediately and administer into another vein. Hyaluronidase should be injected locally into extravasated area. Use a fine hypodermic needle. Moist heat may be helpful. Notify the physician of all side effects; symptomatic and supportive treatment is often indicated. Will probably reduce dose at earliest signs of neurologic toxicity (tingling and numbness of extremities). Discontinue or reduce dose with abnormal depression of bone marrow, blood transfusion may be required. Discontinue for inappropriate ADH secretion or hyponatremia. Glutamic acid blocks toxicity of vindesine but also blocks its antineoplastic activity. Diuretics and fluid restriction may be required for inappropriate secretion of ADH hormone. Diazepam (Valium) or phenobarbital may be required for seizures.

VINORELBINE TARTRATE

Antineoplastic
(Mitotic inhibitor-vinca alkaloid)

Navelbine, NVB

pH 3.5

USUAL DOSE

30 mg/M^2 administered once every 7 days until disease progression or dose-limiting toxicity. Calculate carefully in presence of edema or ascites. This same dose has been used in combination with cisplatin (120 mg/M^2 on day 1 and 21 followed by once every 6 weeks). Premedication with dexamethasone (Decadron) may be beneficial in patients who experience acute or subacute pulmonary reactions.

DOSE ADJUSTMENTS

Reduce or withhold dose based on hematologic toxicity or hepatic insufficiency (e.g., hyperbilirubinemia) on the day of treatment. See charts.

Granulocytes (cells/mm^3) on day of treatment	Dose of Navelbine
≥ 1,500	30 mg/M^2
1,000 to 1,499	15 mg/M^2
< 1,000	Do not administer. Repeat count in 1 week. If 3 consecutive weekly doses are held because granulocyte count is < 1,000 cells/mm^3, discontinue Navelbine

Note: For patients who, during treatment with Navelbine have experienced fever and/or sepsis while granulocytopenic or had 2 consecutive weekly doses held due to granulocytopenia, subsequent doses of Navelbine should be:

22.5 mg/M^2 for granulocytes ≥ 1,500 cells/mm^3 and
11.25 mg/M^2 for granulocytes 1,000 to 1,499 cells/mm^3

Total Bilirubin (mg/dL)	Dose of Navelbine
≤ 2	30 mg/M^2
2.1 to 3	15 mg/M^2
> 3	7.5 mg/M^2

Note: For patients with both hematologic toxicity and hepatic insufficiency administer the lower of the doses determined appropriate from the above tables.

DILUTION

Specific techniques required; see Precautions.

Direct IV: Each 10 mg (1 ml) must be further diluted with a minimum of 2 to 5 ml NS or D5W (2 ml diluent yields 3 mg/ml concentration, 5 ml yields 1.5 mg/ml concentration). Must be given into the side arm port of a free-flowing IV infusion.

Intermittent infusion: Each 10 mg (1 ml) must be further diluted with 4 to

19 ml NS or D5W, ½NS, D5/½NS, R, or LR (4 ml diluent yields 2 mg/ml concentration, 19 ml yields 0.5 mg/ml concentration). Other references recommend diluting a single dose to a minimum total volume of 100 ml. Must be given into the side arm port of a free-flowing IV infusion or may be given directly into a large central vein.

Storage: Refrigerate vials and protect from light; are stable at room temperature for up to 72 hours. Diluted solution stable for 24 hours.

INCOMPATIBLE WITH

All solutions except those specified in Dilution. Acyclovir, allopurinol (Zyloprim), aminophylline, amphotericin B (Fungizone), ampicillin, cefazolin (Kefzol), cefoperazone (Cefobid), cefotetan (Cefotan), ceftriaxone (Rocephin), cefuroxime (Zinacef), fluorouracil, furosemide (Lasix), ganciclovir (Cytovene), methylprednisolone (Solu-Medrol), mitomycin, piperacillin (Pipracil), sodium bicarbonate, thiotepa, sulfamethoxazole-trimethoprim (Bactrim).

COMPATIBLE WITH

Additive: Small amounts of potassium chloride.

Y-site: Chlorpromazine (Compazine), dexamethasone (Decadron), diphenhydramine (Benadryl), hydrocortisone sodium phosphate, hydrocortisone sodium succinate (Solu-Cortef), hydroxyzine (Vistaril), lorazepam (Ativan), meperidine (Demerol), metoclopramide (Reglan), morphine, ondansetron (Zofran), promethazine (Phenergan), and numerous others. Consult pharmacist.

RATE OF ADMINISTRATION

Inadequate flushing of the vein after administration may increase the risk of phlebitis.

Direct IV: Total desired dose, properly diluted over 6 to 10 minutes through the side arm port of a free-flowing IV. After administration, flush with at least 75 to 125 ml of diluent solution over 10 minutes or more. Up to 300 ml has been used as a flush.

Intermittent infusion: Total desired dose, properly diluted over 6 to 10 minutes. Other references recommend over 20 minutes. Must be given into the side arm port of a free-flowing IV infusion or may be given directly into a large central vein. Flush according to directions in Direct IV.

ACTIONS

An antineoplastic agent. A semisynthetic vinca alkaloid with chemical differences from other vinca alkaloids that may provide unique clinical benefits with a lower incidence of clinical neurotoxicity. Causes depolymerization of microtubules and inhibits microtubule assembly. May be more specific to mitotic microtubules. Cell-cycle specific and produces a blockade in the cell-cycle progression in G_2 and M phase. Elimination half-life is 27 to 43 hours. Metabolized in the liver. Excreted in bile, feces, and urine.

INDICATIONS AND USES

Treatment of unresectable advanced non-small cell lung cancer (ANSCLC), in ambulatory patients. Used as a single agent or in combination with cisplatin.

Investigational uses: Advanced breast cancer, ovarian and head and neck cancers, and lymphomas.

CONTRAINDICATIONS

Patients with an absolute neutrophil count less than 1,000 cells/mm^3.

PRECAUTIONS

Follow guidelines for handling cytotoxic agents. See Appendix A, p. 893. ■ Administered by or under the direction of the physician specialist. ■ For IV use only; intrathecal administration of other vinca alkaloids has resulted in death. ■ Adequate diagnostic and treatment facilities must be readily available. ■ Use extreme caution in patients with hepatic impairment, preexisting neuromuscular disease, or those taking other neurotoxic drugs (e.g., antineoplastics [cisplatin], phenothiazines [prochlorperazine]). ■ Prior radiation therapy or treatment with other antineoplastic agents may cause an increase in myelotoxicity; use with extreme caution.

Monitor: Monitor complete blood count, differential, platelets, and bilirubin on each day of treatment to determine correct dose and 1 or 2 times weekly. Temporary leukopenia is an expected effect. Maximum depression usually occurs in 7 to 10 days after the dose and recovery should occur within the following 7 to 14 days. ■ Monitor AST (SGOT) frequently. ■ Evaluate neurologic status frequently (e.g., constipation, decreased deep tendon reflexes, parasthesia). ■ Determine absolute patency and quality of vein and adequate circulation of extremity. Cellulitis and phlebitis with sloughing can result from extravasation. ■ Be alert for any sign of infection. Infections must be brought under control before beginning therapy with vinorelbine. ■ Use of prophylactic antibiotics may be indicated pending results of C/S in a febrile neutropenic patient. ■ Maintain adequate hydration. ■ Prophylactic antiemetics may increase patient comfort; haloperidol and oral dexamethasone have benefited some patients. ■ Use a laxative to prevent constipation. Monitor bowel sounds to prevent obstipation. ■ Monitor for hyponatremia and syndrome of inappropriate secretion of antidiuretic hormone (SIADH). ■ Note Drug/lab interactions.

Patient education: Report burning or stinging at IV site promptly. ■ Report chills, fever, difficulty breathing or shortness of breath promptly. ■ Avoid pregnancy; nonhormonal birth control recommended. ■ Take laxatives consistently to avoid constipation. ■ See Appendix D, p. 900.

Maternal/child: Category D: avoid pregnancy; may cause fetal harm. ■ Discontinue breast feeding. ■ Safety for use in children has not been investigated.

Elderly: Consider age-related organ impairment (kidney, liver, bone marrow reserve).

DRUG/LAB INTERACTIONS

Neurotoxicity may be increased by other neurotoxic drugs (e.g., antineoplastics [cisplatin], phenothiazines [prochlorperazine]); may require dose reduction or discontinuation of vinorelbine. ■ Do not administer live vaccines to patients receiving antineoplastic drugs. ■ Mitomycin-C may cause or aggravate acute pulmonary reactions (e.g., acute shortness of breath, bronchospasm). May require oxygen, bronchodilators, and/or corticosteroids. ■ Granulocytopenia significantly higher when used in combination with cisplatin. ■ Additive bone marrow depression may occur with radiation therapy and/or other bone marrow depressing agents (e.g., azathioprine [Imuran], chloramphenicol, melphalan [Alkeran]), dose reductions may be required. ■ Leukopenic effects may be increased by agents that cause similar blood dyscrasias (e.g., anticonvulsants, antidepressants, phenothiazines). ***Other vinca alkaloids cause interactions with the following drugs; vinorelbine has not been studied.*** ■ Use with asparaginase or doxorubicin may not be recommended or require specific scheduling. ■ May be potentiated by calcium channel blockers (e.g., verapamil). ■ May inhibit digoxin and phenytoin, increased doses of these drugs may be required. ■ Note Precautions.

SIDE EFFECTS

Alopecia (12%, mild); anemia (87%, mild to moderate); chest pain (7%); constipation (35%); diarrhea; dyspnea [2%] (acute and reversible shortness of breath may occur within a few hours); elevated total bilirubin and AST (SGOT); fatigue; hematologic toxicity [99%] (leukopenia and neutropenia are the most frequent and are dose-limiting); hemorrhagic cystitis (rare); jaw pain; loss of deep tendon reflexes (5%); nausea and vomiting (50% [23%]); pain and redness at injection site (38%); paralytic ileus (< 2%); peripheral neuropathy (31%, mild to moderate parasthesia and hypesthesia), phlebitis (10%); SIADH (few); subacute pulmonary reactions (4%, e.g., cough, dyspnea, hypoxemia, and interstitial infiltrates on chest x-ray); thrombocytopenia (rare), thrombocytosis (asymptomatic), tumor pain.

ANTIDOTE

For extravasation, discontinue the drug immediately and administer into another vein. Injection of hyaluronidase locally into the extravasated area may be helpful. Use a fine hypodermic needle. Elevate the extremity. Moist heat may be helpful. Notify the physician of all side effects; symptomatic treatment is often indicated. Discontinue for hyponatremia or SIADH, may require fluid limitation and diuretics (e.g., furosemide [Lasix]). Bone marrow toxicity is reversible after discontinuing vinorelbine. Blood transfusions may be indicated. Filgrastim (Neupogen), sargramostim (Leukine), or epoetin-alfa (Epogen) may be used to promote bone marrow recovery but may not be given until 24 hours after last dose of vinorelbine. Acute or chronic pulmonary reactions may be an allergic phenomena, corticosteroids (e.g., dexamethasone [Decadron]) may be helpful. Neurologic toxicity may be reversible.

WARFARIN SODIUM

Coumadin

Anticoagulant

pH 8.1 to 8.3

USUAL DOSE

Used primarily for patients on Coumadin when oral dosing is not feasible. IV and oral doses are the same. Dose must be individualized and adjusted based on Prothrombin Time (PT)/International Normalized Ratio (INR). An INR of greater than 4 appears to provide no additional benefit in most patients and is associated with a higher risk of bleeding. Loading doses may increase the incidence of complications and do not offer greater prompt anticoagulation protection. Heparin is preferred in situations requiring prompt anticoagulation.

Maintenance dose: 2 to 10 mg/day. Adjust dose to maintain desired INR.

Atrial fibrillation, prophylaxis and treatment of venous thromboembolism, prophylaxis and treatment of pulmonary embolism: Adjust dose to maintain an INR of 2 to 3.

Post-myocardial infarction: Usually initiated 2 to 4 weeks post-infarction and maintained long term. Adjust dose to maintain an INR of 2.5 to 3.5.

Mechanical heart valves: Adjust dose to maintain an INR of 2.5 to 3.5. Maintained long term.

Bioprosthetic heart valves: Adjust dose to maintain an INR of 2 to 3 for 12 weeks after valve insertion. Longer-term therapy may be required in patients with additional risk factors (e.g., atrial fibrillation, prior thromboembolism).

PEDIATRIC DOSE

Safety for use in children under age 18 not established, but is used. Usually given orally.

Prophylaxis and treatment of thromboembolic events: 0.1 mg/kg/24 hr. Adjust to desired PT/INR.

Maintenance dose: 0.05 to 0.34 mg/kg/24 hr.

DOSE ADJUSTMENTS

Use low initiation doses in the elderly, debilitated, and those with expected increased PT/INR responses. ■ Use lower end of dose range in patients at increased risk of bleeding or those on aspirin therapy. ■ Reduced dose is required in impaired hepatic function. ■ No dose adjustment is required in impared renal function. ■ Higher doses may be required in selected situations (e.g., patients with recurrent systemic embolism or mechanical prosthetic valves). The American College of Chest Physicians (ACCP) and the National Heart, Lung, and Blood Institute (NHLBI) suggest maintaining an INR of 3 to 4.5.

DILUTION

Reconstitute the 5-mg vial with 2.7 ml of SW (2 mg/ml).

Storage: Protect from light by storing in carton at controlled room temperature. Store reconstituted solution at room temperature and use within 4 hours. Do not refrigerate; discard any unused solution.

INCOMPATIBLE WITH

Amikacin, ascorbic acid, epinephrine, metaraminol (Aramine), oxytocin, promazine (Sparine), vancomycin.

RATE OF ADMINISTRATION

A single dose as an injection over 1 to 2 minutes.

ACTIONS

An anticoagulant that acts by inhibiting vitamin K—dependent coagulation factors (e.g., Factor II, VII, IX, and X) and the anticoagulant proteins C and S in the liver, resulting in a depression of their activities. An anticoagulant effect occurs within 24 hours; however, peak anticoagulant effect may be delayed for 72 to 96 hours. Effective half-life ranges from 20 to 60 hours. Effects may be more pronounced as daily maintenance doses overlap. Well-established clots are not dissolved, but growth is prevented. Metabolized by the liver to inactive metabolites and reduced metabolites. Excreted primarily in urine with small amounts excreted in bile. Crosses the placental barrier. Secreted in breast milk in an inactive form.

INDICATIONS AND USES

Prophylaxis and/or treatment of venous thrombosis and pulmonary embolism. ▪ Prophylaxis and or treatment of the thromboembolic complications of atrial fibrillation and/or cardiac valve replacement. ▪ Reduce the risk of death, recurrent myocardial infarction, and thromboembolic events such as stroke or systemic embolization after myocardial infarction. ▪ Treatment of patients receiving oral warfarin who are unable to take oral medication.

CONTRAINDICATIONS

Localized or general physical condition or circumstance in which the hazard of hemorrhage might be greater than the potential clinical benefits of anticoagulation (e.g., bleeding tendencies associated with active ulceration or overt bleeding of GI, GU, or respiratory tracts, CVA, aneurysms [cerebral or aortic], pericarditis, pericardial effusions, bacterial endocarditis; hemorrhagic tendencies or blood dyscrasias, inadequate laboratory facilities; major regional or lumbar block anesthesia; malignant hypertension; pregnancy; spinal puncture or other procedures with potential for uncontrollable bleeding; threatened abortion, eclampsia, preeclampsia; unsupervised patients who would find it difficult to cooperate [e.g., senility, alcoholism, or psychosis], and recent or contemplated surgery of the CNS, eye, or traumatic surgery resulting in large open surfaces).

PRECAUTIONS

For IV use only; do not administer IM. ▪ Determinations of whole blood clotting and bleeding times are not an accurate measurement to adjust dose. ▪ A severe aPTT elevation (>50 seconds) with a PT/INR in the normal range is an indicator of increased risk of postoperative hemorrhage. ▪ Use caution in the elderly or debilitated, severe to moderate impaired hepatic or renal function, severe to moderate hypertension, severe diabetes, with indwelling catheters, infectious diseases or disturbances of intestinal flora (e.g., sprue, antibiotic therapy), surgery or trauma involving large raw surfaces or that may result in internal bleeding, patients with a history of allergic problems, polycythemia vera, vasculitis, and known or suspected deficiency in protein C anticoagulant response. ▪ Increased PT/INR response may occur in patients with blood dyscrasias (See Contraindications) , cancer, collagen vascular disease, congestive heart failure, diarrhea, elevated temperature, hyperthyroidism, infectious hepatitis, jaundice, poor nutritional state, steatorrhea, or vitamin K deficiency. ▪ Decreased PT/INR response may occur in patients with edema, hereditary coumarin resistance, hyperlipidemia, hypothyroidism, or nephrotic syndrome. ▪ If dental procedures or surgery or other minor surgical procedures are necessary, the PT/INR should be adjusted to the lower end of the therapeutic range. Monitor PT/INR just prior to treatment. Operative site should be limited so local procedures for hemostasis can be used. Warfarin therapy may have to be interrupted; consider risks versus benefits.

Monitor: PT/INR must be done before initial injection. Frequent monitoring of PT/INR required (bedside monitoring units are now available that are very accurate). Usually repeated daily during initiation of therapy, every 1 to 4 weeks after PT/INR has stabilized in the therapeutic range. Monitor with any change in patient regimen that may affect treatment (e.g., diet, illness, change in drug regimen). Draw blood for prothrombin just before any heparin dose being given concomitantly. If heparin is given as a continuous infusion, PT/INR may be drawn at any time. ■ Note Precautions. ■ Has a narrow therapeutic range that can be affected by other drugs and dietary vitamin K. Note Drug/lab interactions. ■ Decrease dose gradually over 3 to 4 weeks.

Patient education: Nonhormonal birth control recommended. ■ Adhere to dose schedule; do not take or discontinue any prescription or over-the-counter medication without physician's approval. ■ Confirm procedure for missed dose. ■ Avoid alcohol. ■ Avoid any activity or sport that may result in traumatic injury. ■ Regular PT/INR testing and physician visits are imperative. ■ Notify physician of any illness (e.g., diarrhea, infection, fever) or unusual bleeding (e.g., increased menstrual flow, nosebleeds, tarry stools), headache, dizziness, or weakness. ■ Carry an ID stating that warfarin is being taken.

Maternal/child: Category X: avoid pregnancy. May cause fatal hemorrhage to the fetus, has caused birth deformities, and may cause abortion and/or still-birth. ■ PTs remained unchanged in infants nursing from mothers receiving warfarin. Premature infants have not been evaluated; use caution.

Elderly: Less warfarin is required to produce a therapeutic level of anti-coagulation in patients over 60 years of age; may have a greater than expected PT/INR response.

DRUG/LAB INTERACTIONS

Monitor PT/INR carefully when drugs are added or discontinued. ■ Numerous drug interactions can occur. Listed are some of the most significant. ■ Not recommended for concurrent use with streptokinase or urokinase; may be hazardous. ■ Risk of bleeding increased with amiodarone (Cordarone), aspirin, cimetidine (Tagamet), clofibrate (Atromid-S), cyclophosphamide (Cytoxan), erythromycin, fluconazole (Diflucan), heparin, isoniazid (Nydrazid), metronidazole (Flagyl), miconazole (Monistat IV), NSAIDs (e.g., ibuprofen [Motrin]), omeprazole (Prilosec), phenylbutazone (Butazolidin), propafenone (Rhythmol), propranolol (Inderal), sulfinpyrazone (Anturane), sulfonamides (e.g., SMX-TMP [Bactrim]), ticlopidine (Ticlid). Anticoagulant effects decreased and risk of blood clots increased by barbiturates (e.g., phenobarbital), carbamazepine (Tegretol), cholestyramine (Questran), griseofulvin (Fulvicin), penicillins (e.g., nafcillin [Unipen]), rifampin (Rifadin), sucralfate (Carafate), and increased oral vitamin K intake (e.g., leafy greens, supplements). ■ May inhibit metabolism and increase effects of nifedipine (Adalat), oral antidiabetic agents (e.g., tolbutamide [Orinase]), phenytoin (Dilantin); may cause toxicity.

SIDE EFFECTS

Bleeding when the PT/INR is within the therapeutic range (may unmask an unsuspected lesion [e.g., tumor, ulcer]), hemorrhage in any tissue or organ, necrosis and/or gangrene of skin and other tissues. Complications from systemic cholesterol microembolization (e.g., "purple toes syndrome") from release of atheromatous plaque emboli. Allergic reactions do occur.

ANTIDOTE

Keep physician informed of all side effects; some may be life-threatening. Discontinue if warfarin is suspected to be the cause of developing necrosis (e.g., "purple toes syndrome"); consider heparin therapy if anti-coagulation required. Phytonadione (Aquamephyton) is a specific antagonist and indicated in overdose or desired warfarin reversal (e.g., severe bleeding). Will impede subsequent anticoagulant therapy. Fresh whole blood, fresh frozen plasma, Factor IX complex (not purified Factor IX preparations, they increase PT levels) may be indicated.

ZIDOVUDINE
Antiviral

Azidothymidine, AZT, Compound S, Retrovir
pH 5.5

USUAL DOSE

Symptomatic HIV: 1 to 2 mg/kg every 4 hours. Initiate oral therapy as soon as possible (100 mg orally approximately equal to 1 mg/kg IV). Impaired renal or hepatic function may increase toxicity.

Prevention of maternal-fetal HIV transmission: 2 mg/kg of total body weight over 1 hour when labor begins. Follow with an infusion of 1 mg/kg/hr (of total body weight) until umbilical cord is clamped.

PEDIATRIC DOSE

Children 3 months to 12 years of age with symptomatic HIV: 0.5 to 1.8 mg/kg/hr as a continuous infusion. An alternate regimen is 100 mg/M^2 infused over 1 hour every 6 hours (4 doses daily) for 2 weeks. Follow with oral therapy. Do not exceed 200 mg in 6 hours.

NEONATAL DOSE

Prevention of maternal-fetal HIV transmission: 1.5 mg/kg infused over 30 minutes every 6 hours. Oral dosing preferred.

DOSE ADJUSTMENTS

May be required in anemia and/or with other drugs. Note Monitor and Drug/lab interactions.

DILUTION

Each 1 mg of the calculated dose must be diluted in at least 0.25 ml of D5W (4 mg/ml). For a 70 kg patient at 1 mg/kg, a 70 mg dose would be diluted in 17.5 ml (equals 4 mg/ml [70 mg in 35 ml equals 2 mg/ml]). More dilute solutions are preferred (e.g., 1 mg/ml).

Infusion: Dilute 1 Gm in 1,000 ml D5W (1 mg/ml), 500 mg in 500 ml (1 mg/ml), 1 Gm in 500 ml (2 mg/ml), or 1 Gm in 250 ml (4 mg/ml).

Storage: Store undiluted vials at 15° to 25° C (59° to 77° F). Protect from light. Stable after dilution for 8 hours at room temperature, 24 hours if refrigerated.

INCOMPATIBLE WITH

Blood products and protein solutions.

RATE OF ADMINISTRATION

Intermittent infusion: Each single dose properly diluted must be delivered at a constant rate over 1 hour. Avoid rapid infusion or IV bolus.

Continuous infusion: Prevention of maternal-fetal HIV transmission: 1 mg/kg/hr until umbilical cord clamped.

Pediatric continuous infusion: 0.5 to 1.8 mg/kg/hr.

Neonatal in prevention of maternal-fetal HIV transmission: A single dose infused over 30 min.

ACTIONS

An antiviral agent. Through a specific process this thymidine analog inhibits the in vitro replication and terminates the DNA chain of some retroviruses including HIV (HTLV III, LAV, or ARV). May also have antiviral activity against the Epstein-Barr virus. Metabolized by gluc-uronidation in the liver and excreted through the kidneys.

INDICATIONS AND USES

Decrease the severity of symptoms in symptomatic HIV (AIDS and advanced ARC) when the patient has a history of *Pneumocystis carinii* pneumonia (PCP) or an absolute CD4 (T4 helper/inducer) lymphocyte count of less than 200/mm^3. ■ Prevention of maternal-fetal HIV transmission. Protocol includes oral zidovudine beginning with week 14 to week 34 of gestation, IV dosing during labor, and zidovudine syrup or IV dosing to the newborn. ■ Oral form used in combination with many other agents.

CONTRAINDICATIONS

Life-threatening allergic reactions to any of the components.

PRECAUTIONS

Confirm history of *Pneumocystis carinii* and/or CD4 lymphocyte count of less than 200/mm^3 before beginning therapy. ■ Do not give IM. ■ Zidovudine has not been shown to reduce the risk of transmission to others. ■ Use with extreme caution in patients with bone marrow compromise as indicated by a granulocyte count of less than 1,000/mm^3 or hemoglobin below 9.5/dl. ■ Zidovudine resistance seems to develop more quickly in patients with advanced disease. ■ Decrease in CD4 count or clinical deterioration may be reversed with a switch to didanosine.

Monitor: Observe closely; not a cure for HIV infections. Patients may acquire illnesses associated with AIDS or ARC, including opportunistic infections. ■ Frequent blood counts are required. Hematologic toxicity, including granulocytopenia, severe anemia, and occasionally reversible pancytopenia are common. Anemia occurs most commonly after 4 to 6 weeks of therapy; dosage adjustments and/or transfusions may be required. ■ Monitor liver function. ■ Note Drug/lab interactions.

Patient education: Report abdominal pain, jaundice, muscle weakness, shortness of breath or rapid breathing promptly. ■ Requires close follow-up with physician, keep all appointments. ■ Check with physician before taking any other meds.

Maternal/child: Category C: safety for use during pregnancy has been evaluated. Considered reasonably safe for HIV-infected mothers only. Congenital deformities not increased in studies. ■ Discontinue breast feeding to reduce incidence of further transmission. ■ Safety for use in children under 12 years of age not established but has been used.

DRUG/LAB INTERACTIONS

Toxicity may be increased by nephrotoxic and/or cytotoxic drugs and/or drugs that interfere with red or white blood cell number and function (e.g., amphotericin B [Fungizone], dapsone, doxorubicin [Adriamycin], flucytosine, interferons, pentamidine [Pentam 300], vinblastine [Velban], vincristine [Oncovin], vindesine [Eldesine]). ■ Use caution with any drug metabolized by glucuronidation (e.g., acetaminophen, diazepam [Valium], morphine); toxicity of both drugs may be increased. ■ Probenicid may inhibit glucuronidation or reduce renal excretion of zidovudine increasing zidovudine toxicity. ■ Use with atovaquone (Mepron), fluconazole (Diflucan), or sulfamethoxazole-trimethoprim (Bactrim) may increase zidovudine serum levels. Acetaminophen (Anacin-3, Tylenol), aspirin, or indomethacin (Indocin), and rifamycins (e.g., rifampin [Rifadin], rifabutin [Mycobutin]) may reduce zidovudine serum levels, increase clearance, and reduce effectiveness. ■ Acetaminophen has increased the incidence of granulocytopenia. ■ Hematologic toxicity may be increased by nucleoside analogs being evaluated in AIDS and ARC patients (e.g., didanosine [DDI]) because of their effect on red or white blood cell numbers or function. The same analogs can affect DNA replication and may antagonize effects of zidovudine. Avoid concomitant administration. ■ Hematologic toxicity increased with ganciclovir (Cytovene) and interferons. ■ Phenytoin levels may increase or decrease; monitor carefully to assure proper dosing. ■ Phenytoin may also increase zidovudine levels by decreasing clearance. ■ Use with acyclovir may cause neurotoxicity (drowsiness, lethargy).

SIDE EFFECTS

Directly related to dose and duration and inversely related to T4 lymphocyte numbers. Anaphylaxis, anemia (severe), anorexia, asthenia, diaphoresis, diarrhea, dizziness, dyspepsia, dyspnea, fever, GI pain, granulocytopenia, headache, hepatomegaly (severe), insomnia, malaise, myalgia, myopathy and myositis, nausea, neutropenia, pancytopenia (reversible), paresthesia, rash, somnolence, taste perversion, vomiting. Suspect lactic acidosis if dyspnea, a fall in serum bicarbonate level, or tachypnea occurs.

ANTIDOTE

Notify physician of all side effects; most will be treated symptomatically. Moderate anemia or granulocytopenia may respond to a reduction in dose. Discontinue zidovudine for severe anemia (less than 7.5 g/dl or a 25% reduction from baseline) or severe granulocytopenia (less than 750/mm^3 or 50% reduction from baseline). Transfusions may be required. Rash may be the first sign of anaphylaxis; notify physician and treat with diphenhydramine (Benadryl), epinephrine (Adrenalin), and corticosteriods as indicated. Sulfamethoxazole-trimethoprim (Bactrim), pyrimethamine (Daraprim), and acyclovir (Zovirax) may be indicated to treat opportunistic infections.

APPENDIX A

Recommendations for the Safe Handling of Cytotoxic Drugs

INTRODUCTION

Cytotoxic drugs are toxic compounds and are known to have carcinogenic, mutagenic, and/or teratogenic potential. With direct contact they may cause irritation to the skin, eyes, and mucous membranes, and ulceration and necrosis of tissue. The toxicity of cytotoxic drugs dictates that the exposure of health-care personnel to these drugs should be minimized. At the same time, the requirement for maintenance of aseptic conditions must be satisfied.

POTENTIAL ROUTES OF EXPOSURE

This brochure reviews the routes through which exposure may occur and presents recommendations for the safe handling of parenteral cytotoxic drugs by pharmacists, nurses, physicians and other personnel who participate in the preparation and administration of these drugs to patients. These guidelines apply in any setting where cytotoxic drugs are prepared—including pharmacies, nursing units, clinics, physicians' offices and the home health care environment. The primary routes of exposure during the preparation and administration phases are through the inhalation of aerosolized drug or by direct skin contact.

During drug preparation, a variety of manipulations are used which may result in aerosol generation, spraying, and splattering. Examples of these manipulations include: the withdrawal of needles from drug vials; the use of syringes and needles or filter straws for drug transfer; the opening of ampules; and the expulsion of air from the syringe when measuring the precise volume of a drug. Pharmaceutical practice calls for the use of aseptic techniques and a sterile environment. Many pharmacies provide this sterile environment by using a horizontal laminar flow work bench. However, while this type of unit provides product protection, it may expose the operator and other room occupants to aerosols generated during drug preparation procedures. Therefore, a Class II laminar flow (vertical) biological safety cabinet that provides both product and operator protection is needed for the preparation of cytotoxic drugs. This is accomplished by filtering incoming and exhaust air through a high-efficiency particulate air (HEPA) filter. It should be noted that these filters are not effective for volatile materials because they do not capture vapors and gases. Personnel should be familiar with the capabilities, limitations and proper utilization of the biological safety cabinet selected.

During administration, clearing air from a syringe or infusion line and leakage at tubing, syringe, or stopcock connections should be avoided to prevent opportunities for accidental skin contact and aerosol generation. Dispose of syringes and unclipped needles into a leakproof and puncture-resistant container.

From U.S. Department of Health and Human Services, Public Health Service, National Institutes of Health: NIH Publication No. 92-2621. Prepared by the NIH Division of Safety and the NIH Clinical Center Pharmacy Department and Cancer Nursing Service.

The disposal of cytotoxic drugs and trace contaminated materials (e.g., gloves, gowns, needles, syringes, vials) presents a possible source of exposure to pharmacists, nurses and physicians as well as to ancillary personnel, especially the housekeeping staff. Excreta from patients receiving cytotoxic drug therapy may contain high concentrations of the drug. All personnel should be aware of this source of potential exposure and should take appropriate precautions to avoid accidental contact.

The potential risks to pharmacists, nurses and physicians from repeated contact with parenteral cytotoxic drugs can be effectively controlled by using a combination of specific containment equipment and certain work techniques which are described in the recommendations sections. For the most part, the techniques are merely an extension of good work practices by health-care and ancillary personnel, and similar in principle and practice to *Universal Precautions.*[1] These may be supplemented as deemed appropriate for the work being performed. By using these precautions, personnel are better able to minimize possible exposure to cytotoxic drugs.

RECOMMENDED PRACTICES FOR PERSONNEL PREPARING CYTOTOXIC DRUGS

Professionally accepted standards concerning the aseptic preparation of parenteral products should be followed. Only properly trained personnel should handle cytotoxic drugs.

Training sessions should be offered to new professionals as well as to technical and housekeeping personnel who may come in contact with these drugs. Safe handling should be the focus of such training.

A. Part 1—All procedures involved in the preparation of cytotoxic drugs should be performed in a Class II, Type A or Type B laminar flow biological safety cabinet. The cabinet exhaust should be discharged to the outdoors in order to eliminate the exposure of personnel to drugs that may volatilize after retention on filters of the cabinet. The cabinet of choice is a Class II, Type B which discharges exhaust to the outdoors and can be obtained with a bag-in/bag-out filter to protect the personnel servicing the cabinet and to facilitate disposal.

Part 2—Alternatively, a Class II, Type A cabinet can be equipped with a canopy or thimble unit which exhausts to the outdoors. For detailed information about the design, capabilities and limitations of various types of biological safety cabinets, refer to the National Sanitation Foundation Standard 49.[2]

B. The work surface of the safety cabinet should be covered with plastic-backed absorbent paper. This will reduce the potential for dispersion of droplets and spills and facilitate cleanup. This paper should be changed after any overt spill and at the end of each work shift.

C. Personnel preparing the drugs should wear unpowdered latex surgical gloves and a disposal gown with knit cuffs. Gloves should be changed

---

1. Centers for Disease Control. 1988. Update: Universal precautions for prevention of transmission of human immunodeficiency virus, hepatitis B virus, and other blood-borne pathogens in health-care settings. Morbidity and Mortality Weekly Report, 37(24): 377-382, 387-388.

2. National Science Foundation. Standard 49 for Class II (Laminar Flow) Biohazard Cabinetry.

regularly and immediately if torn or punctured. Protective clothing should not be worn outside of the drug preparation area. Overtly contaminated gowns require immediate removal and replacement. In case of skin contact with any cytotoxic drug, thoroughly wash the affected area with soap and water. However, do not abrade the skin by using a scrub brush. Flush the affected eye(s), while holding back the eyelid(s), with copious amounts of water for at least 15 minutes. Then seek medical evaluation by a physician.

D. Vials containing drugs requiring reconstitution should be vented to reduce the internal pressure with a venting device using a 0.22 micron hydrophobic filter or other appropriate means such as a chemotherapy dispensing pin. This reduces the probability of spraying and spillage.

E. If a chemotherapy dispensing pin is not used, a sterile alcohol pad should be carefully placed around the needle and vial top during withdrawal from the septum.

F. The external surfaces contaminated with a drug should be wiped clean with an alcohol pad prior to transfer or transport.

G. When opening the glass ampule, wrap it and then snap it at the break point using an alcohol pad to reduce the possibility of injury and to contain the aerosol produced. Use a 5 micron filter needle or straw when removing the drug solution.

H. Syringes and I.V. bottles containing cytotoxic drugs should be labeled and dated. Before these items leave the preparation area, an additional label reading, "Caution—Chemotherapy, Dispose of Properly" is recommended.

I. After completing the drug preparation process, wipe down the interior of the safety cabinet with water (for injection or irrigation) followed by 70% alcohol using disposable towels. All wastes are considered contaminated and should be disposed of properly.

J. Contaminated needles and syringes, I.V. tubing, butterfly clips, etc., should be disposed of intact to prevent aerosol generation and injury. Do not recap needles. Place these items in a puncture-resistant container along with any contaminated bottles, vials, gloves, absorbent paper, disposable gowns, gauze and other waste. The container should then be placed in a box labeled, "Cytotoxic waste only," sealed and disposed of according to Federal, state and local requirements. Linen contaminated with drugs, patient excreta or body fluids should be handled separately.

K. Hands should be washed between glove changes and after glove removal.

L. Cytotoxic drugs are categorized as regulated wastes and therefore, should be disposed of according to Federal, state and local requirements.

RECOMMENDED PRACTICES FOR PERSONNEL ADMINISTERING PARENTERAL CYTOTOXIC DRUGS

Some cytotoxic drugs are excreted from patients in high concentrations. Personnel should be knowledgeable regarding which drugs fit this description and take care to avoid skin contact and to minimize aerosol generation.

When disposing of excreta from patients, all personnel should wear gowns and latex surgical gloves.

A. A protective outer garment such as a closed-front surgical-type gown with knit cuffs should be worn. Gowns may be of the disposable or washable variety.

B. Disposable latex surgical gloves should be worn during those procedures where exposure to the drugs may result and when handling patient body fluids or excreta. When bubbles are removed from syringes or I.V. tubing, an alcohol pad should be placed carefully over the tip of such items in order to collect any of the cytotoxic drugs which may be inadvertently discharged. Discard gloves after each use and wash hands.

C. Contaminated needles and syringes and I.V. apparatus should be disposed of intact into a labeled, puncture-resistant container in order to minimize aerosol generation and risk of injury. Do not recap needles. The container, as well as contaminated materials should be placed in a box labeled, "Cytotoxic waste only." Linen overtly contaminated with any cytotoxic agent or excreta from a patient within 48 hours following drug administration, may be safely handled by using the procedures prescribed for isolation cases. For example, place the contaminated articles in a "yellow" cloth bag lined with a water-soluble plastic bag and then place into the washing machine. Linen without overt contamination can be handled by routine laundering procedures.

D. In case of skin contact with an cytotoxic drug, thoroughly wash the affected area with soap and water. However, do not abrade the skin by using a scrub brush. Flush affected eye(s), while holding back the eyelid(s), with copious amounts of water for at least 15 minutes. Then seek evaluation by a physician. Always wash hands after removing gloves.

Alternate Choices for Infrequently Used Drugs

An average of 15 new drugs has been included each year in *Intravenous Medications*. Although the goal has always been to make this reference as complete as possible, this rapid increase in new drugs requires some deletions to prevent *Intravenous Medications* from becoming too cumbersome to be useful. After extensive consultation, 33 drugs have been deleted. They were generally selected because they were rarely used and newer, sometimes more effective, drugs are now preferred for intravenous use for the same indications. The following list includes the deleted drugs and suggested alternates.

Deleted drug	Category	Suggested alternate(s)
*4 azlocillin (Azlin)	antibacterial	ticarcillin (Ticar), p. 833
*12 betamethasone	corticosteroid	dexamethasone (Decadron), p. 260
*8 biperiden lactate (Akineton)	antiparkinson agent	benztropine mesylate (Cogentin), p. 128
*8 brompheniramine maleate (Histaject)	antihistamine	diphenhydramine HCL (Benadryl), p. 294
*13 cephalothin sodium (Keflin)	D/C no longer available	
*8 cephradine sodium (Velosef)	antibacterial	cefazolin (Kefzol), p. 157
*13 chlorothiazide (Diuril)	diuretic	loop diuretics (e.g., furosemide [Lasix]), p.417
*13 chlorpheniramine maleate (Chlor-Trimeton)	antihistamine	diphenhydramine (Benadryl), p. 294
*13 colchicine	antigout agent	oral NSAIDs, intrasynovial steroids
*8 colistimethate sodium (Coly-Mycin M)	antibacterial organism-specific	aminoglycosides (e.g., gentamicin [Garamycin]), p. 429
*13 dexpanthenol (Ilopan)	GI stimulant	no equivalent; see 13th edition, p. 282
*13 dimenhydrinate	antihistamine/ antiemetic	diphenhydramine (Benadryl), p. 294, prochlorperazine (Compazine), p. 714, ondansetron (Zofran), p. 634

Deleted drug	Category	Suggested alternate(s)
*13 eflornithine (Ornidyl)	antiprotozoal Tx of sleeping sickness	no equivalent; see 13th edition, p. 364
*13 ethacrynic acid (Edecrin)	diuretic	loop diuretics (e.g., furosemide [Lasix]), p. 417
*13 fentanyl citrate with droperiodol (Innovar)	narcotic analgesic	fentanyl (Sublimaze), p. 385
*8 gallamine triethiodide (Flaxedil)	skeletal muscle relaxant	atracurium (Tracium), p. 116 pancuronium (Pavulon), p. 651
*8 lincomycin HC1 (Lincocin)	antimicrobial agent	clindamycin (Cleocin), p. 222
*13 mephentermine	vasopressor	phenylephrine (Neo-Synephrine), p. 676
*13 methicillin sodium	antibacterial	other penicillins
*13 methoxamine	vasopressor	other vasopressors
*13 mezlocillin sodium	antibacterial	ticarcillin (Ticar), p. 833
*14 miconazole	D/C no longer available	
*8 minocycline HC1 (Minocin)	tetracycline antibacterial	ampicillin, p. 76 erythromycin, p. 359 doxycycline (Vibramycin), p. 323
*8 nicotinic acid (Niacin) and nicotinamide (Niacinamide)	water-soluble B vitamin	well absorbed via other routes
*13 paraldehyde	parenteral no longer available in U.S.	
*13 phenolsullfonphtalein	replaced by newer renal function tests	
*8 polymyxin B sulfate	antibacilli organism-specific	aminoglycosides (e.g., gentamicin [Garamycin]), p. 429
*8 propiomazine HCL (Largon)	sedative and hypnotic	lorazepam (Ativan), p. 526 midazolam (Versed), p. 574

Deleted drug	Category	Suggested alternate(s)
*8 sodium lactate	alkalinizing agent	sodium bicarbonate, p. 791
*13 theophylline & 5% dextrose	bronchodilator	aminophylline, p. 58
*13 trimethaphan camsylate	D/C no longer available	
*8 urea-sterile USP (Ureaphil)	osmotic diuretic	mannitol, p. 535
*13 vidarabine	D/C no longer available	

*Information can be found in this previous edition of *Intravenous Medications*.

APPENDIX C

FDA Pregnancy Categories

No drug should be used during pregnancy unless clearly needed and the risks to the fetus are outweighed by the benefits to the mother.

Category A   Adequate studies have not demonstrated a risk to the fetus in any trimester.

Category B   May have caused adverse effects in animals, but no adverse effects have been demonstrated in humans in any trimester or no demonstrated risk in animals but there are no adequate studies in pregnant women.

Category C   Animal studies have shown an adverse effect but there are no adequate studies in pregnant women or no animal studies and no studies in pregnant women.

Category D   Definite fetal risks. May be given in spite of risks if needed in life-threatening conditions.

Category X   Will cause fetal abnormalities. Risk of use outweighs benefits. Not recommended for use at any time during pregnancy. Consider alternatives before treating a pregnant woman.

Consider all men and women capable of conception when any drug in Category D or Category X is to be administered. Discuss birth control options to avoid pregnancy if a specific drug in these categories must be administered. Some drugs require birth control for months after all dosing is complete. Research complete information and keep patient informed.

Information for Patients Receiving Immunosuppressive Agents

- Report any allergic or sensitivity reaction you may have had to drugs or food.
- Report any other medical problem you may have (especially exposure to chickenpox, herpes zoster, infections, bone marrow, heart, kidney, or liver problems).
- Provide a complete list of all medications you take, prescription and over the counter.
- In most situations birth control is essential and may be required for both patient and partner; consider options. Nonhormonal birth control reduces the possibility of drug interactions, but compliance is imperative. If there is any possibility you or your partner may be pregnant, inform your physician promptly.
- Discontinue breast feeding.
- Take only prescribed medication(s) in the exact amounts prescribed and at the times prescribed. This will help to maintain correct blood levels and avoid drug interactions.
- Confirm procedure if you should miss a dose. If any questions, notify physician.
- Confirm procedure for correct storage of your medication(s).
- Close monitoring by your physician is very important; keep all appointments and have all required lab work done on schedule. Your medications may interfere with some test results. Discuss with your physician.
- Do not take any immunizations without your physician's approval. Polio vaccine is especially virulent in your condition; request family members to defer immunization and either avoid friends who have been immunized or wear a protective mask covering your nose and mouth while visiting.
- Dental procedures may need to be completed before starting therapy or deferred until therapy is completed. Use caution with your toothbrush, toothpicks, or dental floss. Alternate methods of dental hygiene may be necessary should your gums become tender, inflamed, or bleed.
- Avoid anyone with an infection or fever. Report promptly any symptoms such as: chills, fever, cough, hoarseness, lower back or side pain, painful or difficult urination.
- Wash hands before touching your eyes or the inside of your nose.
- Report promptly any unusual bleeding, bruising, black tarry stools, blood in urine, or pinpoint red spots on your skin (petechiae).
- Avoid accidental cuts whenever possible (e.g., razors, fingernail and toenail clippers).
- Avoid contact sports where you might be bruised or injured.
- Drink adequate amounts of fluids to prevent increases in serum uric acid concentrations. Allopurinol (Zyloprim) and/or alkalinazation of urine may be required.
- Review all side effects with your physician. Confirm those that may be a special problem for you and discuss solutions and expectations.
- Anesthesia during dental, surgical, or emergency treatment may be a problem. Best to consult with your physician, but inform all health professionals of the medications you are taking before they treat you in any way.

General Dilution Chart (Grams to mg)

Amount of drug required in Grams	Amount of Diluent						
	1,000 ml	500 ml	250 ml	125 ml	100 ml	50 ml	25 ml
	mg/ml	mg/ml	mg/ml	mg/ml	mg/ml	mg/ml	mg/ml
20 Gm	20	40	80	160	200	400	800
19 Gm	19	38	76	152	190	380	760
18 Gm	18	36	72	144	180	360	720
17 Gm	17	34	68	136	170	340	680
16 Gm	16	32	64	128	160	320	640
15 Gm	15	30	60	120	150	300	600
14 Gm	14	28	56	112	140	280	560
13 Gm	13	26	52	104	130	260	520
12 Gm	12	24	48	96	120	240	480
11 Gm	11	22	44	88	110	220	440
10 Gm	10	20	40	80	100	200	400
9 Gm	9	18	36	72	90	180	360
8 Gm	8	16	32	64	80	160	320
7 Gm	7	14	28	56	70	140	280
6 Gm	6	12	24	48	60	120	240
5 Gm	5	10	20	40	50	100	200
4.5 Gm	4.5	9	18	36	45	90	180
4 Gm	4	8	16	32	40	80	160
3.5 Gm	3.5	7	14	28	35	70	140
3 Gm	3	6	12	24	30	60	120
2.5 Gm	2.5	5	10	20	25	50	100
2 Gm	2	4	8	16	20	40	80
1.5 Gm	1.5	3	6	12	15	30	60
1 Gm	1	2	4	8	10	20	40
0.5 Gm	0.5	1	2	4	5	10	20
0.25 Gm	0.25	0.5	1	2	2.5	5	10

To use chart:
1. Find mg/ml desired, track to amount of diluent desired and amount of drug in Grams required.
2. Find amount of drug in Grams required, track to diluent desired and/or mg/ml desired.
3. Find amount of diluent required, track to amount of drug in Grams and/or mg/ml desired.

Formula: Substitute any number for X

X Grams diluted in 1,000 ml = X mg/ml (1 Gram in 1,000 ml = 1 mg/ml)
X Grams diluted in 500 ml = 2 X mg/ml (1 Gram in 500 ml = 2 mg/ml)
X Grams diluted in 250 ml = 4 X mg/ml (1 Gram in 250 ml = 4 mg/ml)
X Grams diluted in 125 ml = 8 X mg/ml (1 Gram in 125 ml = 8 mg/ml)
X Grams diluted in 100 ml = 10 X mg/ml (1 Gram in 100 ml = 10 mg/ml)
X Grams diluted in 50 ml = 20 X mg/ml (1 Gram in 50 ml = 20 mg/ml)
X Grams diluted in 25 ml = 40 X mg/ml (1 Gram in 25 ml = 40 mg/ml)

Some variation occurs from manufacturer's overfill or if the drug is in liquid form. If absolute accuracy is required, these variations can be avoided by withdrawing an amount in ml from the diluent equal to manufacturer's overfill and/or an amount equal to the amount in ml of the drug. Consult the pharmacist for specific information on manufacturer's overfill of infusion fluids used in your facility.

General Dilution Chart (mg to mcg)

Amount of drug required in mg	Amount of Diluent						
	1,000 ml	500 ml	250 ml	125 ml	100 ml	50 ml	25 ml
	mcg/ml	mcg/ml	mcg/ml	mcg/ml	mcg/ml	mcg/ml	mcg/ml
20 mg	20	40	80	160	200	400	800
19 mg	19	38	76	152	190	380	760
18 mg	18	36	72	144	180	360	720
17 mg	17	34	68	136	170	340	680
16 mg	16	32	64	128	160	320	640
15 mg	15	30	60	120	150	300	600
14 mg	14	28	56	112	140	280	560
13 mg	13	26	52	104	130	260	520
12 mg	12	24	48	96	120	240	480
11 mg	11	22	44	88	110	220	440
10 mg	10	20	40	80	100	200	400
9 mg	9	18	36	72	90	180	360
8 mg	8	16	32	64	80	160	320
7 mg	7	14	28	56	70	140	280
6 mg	6	12	24	48	60	120	240
5 mg	5	10	20	40	50	100	200
4.5 mg	4.5	9	18	36	45	90	180
4 mg	4	8	16	32	40	80	160
3.5 mg	3.5	7	14	28	35	70	140
3 mg	3	6	12	24	30	60	120
2.5 mg	2.5	5	10	20	25	50	100
2 mg	2	4	8	16	20	40	80
1.5 mg	1.5	3	6	12	15	30	60
1 mg	1	2	4	8	10	20	40
0.5 mg	0.5	1	2	4	5	10	20
0.25 mg	0.25	0.5	1	2	2.5	5	10

To use chart:
1. Find mg/ml desired, track to amount of diluent desired and amount of drug in Grams required.
2. Find amount of drug in Grams required, track to diluent desired and/or mg/ml desired.
3. Find amount of diluent required, track to amount of drug in Grams and/or mg/ml desired.

Formula: Substitute any number for X

   X Grams diluted in 1,000 ml = X mg/ml (1 Gram in 1,000 ml = 1 mg/ml)
   X Grams diluted in 500 ml = 2 X mg/ml (1 Gram in 500 ml = 2 mg/ml)
   X Grams diluted in 250 ml = 4 X mg/ml (1 Gram in 250 ml = 4 mg/ml)
   X Grams diluted in 125 ml = 8 X mg/ml (1 Gram in 125 ml = 8 mg/ml)
   X Grams diluted in 100 ml = 10 X mg/ml (1 Gram in 100 ml = 10 mg/ml)
   X Grams diluted in 50 ml = 20 X mg/ml (1 Gram in 50 ml = 20 mg/ml)
   X Grams diluted in 25 ml = 40 X mg/ml (1 Gram in 25 ml = 40 mg/ml)

Some variation occurs from manufacturer's overfill or if the drug is in liquid form. If absolute accuracy is required, these variations can be avoided by withdrawing an amount in ml from the diluent equal to manufacturer's overfill and/or an amount equal to the amount in ml of the drug. Consult the pharmacist for specific information on manufacturer's overfill of infusion fluids used in your facility.

APPENDIX F

National Cancer Institute Common Toxicity Grading Criteria

Toxicity	0	1	2	3	4
			GRADE		
WBC	≥4	3 to 3.9	2 to 2.9	1 to 1.9	<1
Plt	WNL	75 to normal	50 to 74.9	25 to 49.9	<25
HgB	WNL	10 to normal	8 to 10	6.5 to 7.9	<6.5
Granulocytes/Bands	≥2	1.5 to 1.9	1 to 1.4	0.5 to 0.9	<0.5
Lymphocytes	≥2	1.5 to 1.9	1 to 1.4	0.5 to 0.9	<0.5
Hemorrhage (clinical)	none	mild, no transfusion	gross, 1 to 2 units transfusion per episode	gross, 3 to 4 units transfusion per episode	massive, ≥4 units transfusion per episode
Infection	none	mild	moderate	severe	life-threatening
Nausea	none	able to eat reasonable intake	intake significantly decreased but can eat	no significant intake	—
Vomiting	none	1 episode in 24 hrs	2 to 5 episodes in 24 hrs	6 to 10 episodes in 24 hrs	≥10 episodes in 24 hrs, or requiring parenteral support
Diarrhea	none	increase of 2 to 3 stools/day over pre-Rx	Increase of 4 to 6 stools/days, or nocturnal stools, or moderate cramping	Increase of 7 to 9 stools/day, or incontinence, or severe cramping	Increase of ≥10 stools/day, or grossly bloody diarrhea or need for parenteral support
Stomatitis	none	painless ulcers, erythema, or mild soreness	painful erythema, edema, or ulcers, but can eat	painful erythema, edema, or ulcers, and cannot eat	requires parenteral or enteral support
Bilirubin	WNL	—	<1.5 × N	1.5 to 3 × N	>3 × N

Continued

National Cancer Institute Common Toxicity Grading Criteria—cont'd

Toxicity	0	1	2	3	4
			GRADE		
Transaminase (SGOT, SGPT)	WNL	$\leq 2.5 \times N$	2.6 to $5 \times N$	5.1 to $20 \times N$	$>20 \times N$
Alk Phos or 5'nucleotidase	WNL	$\leq 2.5 \times N$	2.6 to $5 \times N$	5.1 to $20 \times N$	$>20 \times N$
Liver (clinical)	no change from baseline	—	—	pre-coma	hepatic coma
Creatinine	WNL	$<1.5 \times N$	1.5 to $3.0 \times N$	3.1 to $6 \times N$	$>6 \times N$
Proteinuria	no change	1+ or <0.3 to 1 g% or <3 g/L	2 to 3+ or 0.3 to 1 g% or 3 to 10 g/L	4+ or >1 g% or >10 g/L	nephrotic syndrome
Hematuria	neg	micro only	gross, no clots	gross + clots	requires transfusion
Alopecia	no loss	mild hair loss	pronounced or total hair loss	—	—
Pulmonary	none or no change	asymptomatic, with abnormality in PFT's	dyspnea or significant exertion	dyspnea at normal level of activity	dyspnea at rest
Cardiac dysrhythmias	none	asymptomatic, transient, requiring no therapy	recurrent or persistent, no therapy required	requires treatment	requires monitoring, or hypotension, or ventricular tachycardia, or fibrillation
Cardiac function	none	asymptomatic, decline of resting ejection fraction by more than 20% of baseline value	asymptomatic, decline of resting ejection fraction by more than 20% of baseline value	mild CHF, responsive to therapy	severe or refractory CHF

Cardiac ischemia	none	non-specific T-wave flattening	asymptomatic, ST and T-wave changes suggesting ischemia	angina without evidence of infarction	acute myocardial
Cardiac-pericardial	none	asymptomatic effusion, no intervention required	pericarditis (rub, chest pain, ECG changes)	symptomatic effusion; drainage required	tamponade; drainage urgently required
Hypertension	none or no change	asymptomatic, transient increase by greater than 20 mm Hg (D) or to >150/100 if previously WNL. No treatment required	recurrent or persistent increase by greater than 20 mm Hg (D) or to >150/100 if previously WNL. No treatment required	requires therapy	hypertensive crisis
Hypotension	none or no change	changes requiring no therapy (including transient orthostatic hypotension)	requires fluid replacement or other therapy but not hospitalization	requires therapy and hospitalization; resolves within 48 hrs of stopping the agent	requires therapy and hospitalization for >48 hrs after stopping the agent
Neuro–Sensory	none or no change	mild paresthesias, loss of deep tendon reflexes	mild or moderate objective sensory loss; moderate paresthesias	severe objective sensory loss or paresthesias that interfere with function	—
Neuro–Motor	none or no change	subjective weakness; no objective findings	mild objective weakness without significant impairment of function	objective weakness with impairment of function	paralysis
Neuro–Cortical	none	mild somnolence or agitation	moderate somnolence or agitation	severe somnolence, agitation, confusion, disorientation, or hallucinations	coma, seizures, toxic psychosis
Neuro–Cerebellar	none	slight incoordination, dysdiadochokinesis	intense tremor, dysmetria, slurred speech, nystagmus	locomotor ataxia	cerebellar necrosis
Neuro–Mood	no change	mild anxiety or depression	moderate anxiety or depression	severe anxiety or depression	suicidal ideation

Continued

National Cancer Institute Common Toxicity Grading Criteria—cont'd

Toxicity	0	1	2	GRADE 3	4
Neuro–Headache	none	mild	moderate or severe but transient	unrelenting and severe	—
Neuro–Constipation	none or no change	mild	moderate	severe	ileus >96 hrs
Neuro–Hearing	none or no change	asymptomatic, hearing loss on audiometry only	tinnitus	hearing loss interfering with function but correctable with hearing aid	deafness, not correctable
Neuro–Vision	none or no change	—	—	symptomatic subtotal loss of vision	blindness
Skin	none or no change	scattered macular or papular eruption or erythema that is asymptomatic	scattered macular or papular eruption or erythema with pruritus or other associated symptoms	generalized symptomatic macular, papular, or vesicular eruption	exfolliative dermatitis or ulcerating dermatitis
Allergy	none	transient rash, drug fever <38°C, 100.4°F	urticaria, drug fever = 38°C, 100.4°F mild broncho-spasm	serum sickness, broncho-spasm, requires parenteral meds	anaphylaxis
Fever in absence of infection	none	37.1 to 38°C 98.7 to 100.4°F	38.1 to 40°C 100.5 to 104°F	>40°C, >104°F for less than 24 hrs	>40°C (104°F) for more than 24 hrs or fever accompanied by hypotension

Local	none	pain	pain and swelling, with inflammation or phlebitis	ulceration	plastic surgery indicated
Weight gain/loss	<5%	5 to 9.9%	10 to 19.9%	≥20%	—
Hyperglycemia	<116	116 to 160	161 to 250	251 to 500	>500 or ketoacidosis
Hypoglycemia	>64	55 to 64	40 to 54	30 to 39	<30
Amylase	WNL	<1.5 × N	1.5 to 2.0 × N	2.1 to 5 × N	>5.1 × N
Hypercalcemia	<10.6	10.6 to 11.5	11.6 to 12.5	12.6 to 13.5	≥13.5
Hypocalcemia	>8.4	8.4 to 7.8	7.7 to 7	6.9 to 6.1	≤6
Hypomagnesemia	>1.4	1.4 to 1.2	1.1 to 0.9	0.8 to 0.6	≤0.5
Fibrinogen	WNL	0.99 to 0.75 × N	0.74 to 0.5 × N	0.49 to 0.25 × N	≤0.24 × N
Prothrombin time	WNL	1.01 to 1.25 × N	1.26 to 1.5 × N	1.51 to 2 × N	>2 × N
Partial thromboplastin time	WNL	1.01 to 1.66 × N	1.67 to 2.33 × N	2.34 to 3 × N	>3 × N
Headache	none	mild	moderate or severe but transient	unrelenting and severe	—
Aching pain (muscle or bone)	none	mild, transient; does not interfere with casual daily activity	moderate; interferes with usual daily activity	severe; interrupts usual daily activity	intractable
Chills	none	mild, transient	moderate	severe	intractable
Malaise	none	25% of time	50% of time	75% of time	100% of time
Fatigue/Asthenia	none	25% of time	50% of time	75% of time	100% of time
Anorexia	none	able to eat normal meals, loss of hunger	able to eat 2 meals/day with loss of hunger	able to eat 1 meal/day with loss of hunger	unable to eat a meal, some nutritional fluids tolerated

N = Normal, WNL = within normal limits.

Recently Approved Drugs

ALDESLEUKIN

Antineoplastic
Immunomodulator
Biological response modifier
Recombinant interleukin-2

interleukin-2 recombinant, Proleukin, rIL-2

pH 7.2 to 7.8

USUAL DOSE

Patient selection restricted. Prescreening and baseline studies required; note Precautions/Monitor.

Standard high-dose regimen: Intermittent IV: 600,000 IU/kg (0.037 mg/kg) every 8 hours for 14 doses. After 9 days of rest repeat for up to 14 more doses; this constitutes one course (two 5-day [14 or fewer doses] treatment cycles separated by a rest period of 9 days). Treat with 28 doses or until dose-limiting toxicity requiring ICU level support occurs.

Low-dose regimen (investigational): Intermittent IV: 72,000 IU/kg every 8 hours. Cycles same as standard high-dose regimen. Low-dose regimens are especially useful in patients at greater risk with a higher dose.

In all situations, evaluate for response 4 weeks after course completion and again before scheduling start of the next course. Additional courses are considered if there is some tumor shrinkage following the previous course, a CT scan rules out disease progression, and retreatment is not contraindicated. At least 7 weeks from hospital discharge should elapse before a second course is administered.

Sometimes given in combination with other agents (see Indications).

Investigational protocols: Other investigational protocols have been used (see below). These various protocols expressed doses of aldesleukin in Cetus, Roche, or International units. Aldesleukin is available only in International units, 1 Cetus unit = 6IU, 1 Roche unit = 3 IU. Results from studies include stable disease or disease regression with some decreased toxicity, but efficacy not established.

Continuous IV (Investigational): 18,000,000 IU/M^2/day as a continuous infusion. Each daily dose is given over 24 hours (interrupted as indicated by patient symptoms) for two 5-day cycles with 5 to 8 days of rest before the second cycle. Another investigational study administers the daily dose for 4 days followed by 3 days off. This cycle is repeated for 4 weeks followed by 2 weeks off. Based on patient tolerance, the entire sequence is usually repeated until some response occurs. Another investigational low-dose regimen given on an outpatient basis uses 18,000,000 IU given over 6 to 8 hours, Monday through Friday, 4 weeks on and 2 weeks off. Beginning with the second cycle, doses on day 1 and 2 are reduced to 9,000,000 IU. Other investigational studies are using SC injection.

DOSE ADJUSTMENTS

Doses are frequently withheld for toxicity. Doses are actually withheld, not reduced in amount. Median number of doses actually administered in a first course is 20. Continuous infusions can be interrupted as indicated by patient symptoms.

Hold doses and restart based on the following chart:

Hold dose for	May give next dose if
Cardiovascular:	
Atrial fibrillation, supraventricular tachycardia, bradycardia that requires treatment or is recurrent or persistent.	Patient is asymptomatic with full recovery to normal sinus rhythm.
Systolic BP < 90 mm Hg with increasing requirements for pressors.	Systolic BP ≥ 90 mm Hg and stable or improving requirements for pressors.
Any ECG change consistent with MI or ischemia with or without chest pain; suspicion of cardiac ischemia or CHF.	Patient is asymptomatic, MI has been ruled out, clinical suspicion of angina is low; there is no incidence of ventricular hypokinesia.
Pulmonary:	
O_2 saturation < 94% on room air or < 90% with 2 L O_2 by nasal prongs.	O_2 saturation > 94% on room air or > 90% with 2 L O_2 by nasal prongs.
Central Nervous System:	
Mental status changes (e.g., agitation, confusion, lethargy, somnolence). May result in coma.	Mental status changes completely resolved.
Body as a whole:	
Sepsis syndrome; patient is clinically unstable.	Sepsis syndrome has resolved, patient is clinically stable, infection is under treatment.
Urogenital:	
Serum creatinine > 4.5 mg/dl or a serum creatinine of ≥ 4 mg/dl in presence of severe volume overload, acidosis, or hyperkalemia.	Serum creatinine < 4 mg/dl, and fluid and electrolyte status is stable.
Persistent oliguria, urine output of < 10 ml/hr for 16 to 24 hr with rising serum creatinine.	Urine output > 10 ml/hr with a decrease of serum creatinine > 1.5 mg/dl or normalization of serum creatinine.
Digestive:	
Signs of hepatic failure including encephalopathy, increasing ascites, liver pain, hypoglycemia.	Discontinue for remainder of current course. If all signs of hepatic failure have resolved, may consider a new course of treatment in 7 weeks
Stool guaiac repeatedly > 3 to 4+.	Stool guaiac negative.
Skin:	
Bullous dermatitis or marked worsening of preexisting skin condition (avoid topical steroid therapy).	Resolution of all signs of bullous dermatitis.

▪ After withholding a dose, no dose should be given until patient is globally assessed and specific criteria for restarting aldesleukin are met.

DILUTION

Each 22,000,000 IU vial (1.3 mg) must be reconstituted with 1.2 ml of preservative-free SW (18,000,000 IU/ml [1.1 mg(1100mcg)/ml]). Sterile technique imperative. Direct diluent to side of vial and gently swirl to avoid excess foaming. Do not shake. Plastic infusion containers are preferred over glass. Do not use any filters for dilution or administration. Do not use any other diluent or infusion solution; may cause increased aggregation. Bring to room temperature before administration. Must be further diluted in D5W and given as an intermittent or continuous (investigational) IV. Desired concentration is 30 to 70 mcg/ml. The following chart provides an overview of upper and lower limits of Proleukin content within the IV diluent to remain within the 30 to 70 mcg/mL concentration:

Volume of IV Diluent (D5W)	Minimum Amount of Proleukin to Maintain ≥ 30 mcg/mL	Maximum Amount of Proleukin to Maintain ≤ 70 mcg/mL
*50 mL	1.5 mg (24.3 MIU)	3.5 mg (57 MIU)
100 mL	3 mg (49 MIU)	7 mg (114 MIU)
150 mL	4.5 mg (73 MIU)	10.5 mg (172 MIU)
200 mL	6 mg (97 MIU)	14 mg (229 MIU)
250 mL	7.5 mg (122 MIU)	17.5 mg (286 MIU)

*Recommended volume of IV diluent per package insert.

In specific concentrations albumin must be added to improve stability and maintain aldesleukin in an "aggregated state." To achieve a concentration of 0.1% add 1 ml of 5% (0.2 ml of 25%) albumin to each 50 ml of diluent (D5W). Albumin must be added before adding the reconstituted dose of aldesleukin. See chart below for concentrations requiring albumin at room temperature and body temperature administration.

Final concentration of Proleukin				
Route of Proleukin administration	1 to 30 mcg/mL	30 to 70 mcg/mL	70 to 100 mcg/mL	> 100 mcg/mL
Intermittent Short IV Infusion and Continuous Infusion at *room temperature* [15-30° C; 59-89° F]	Add albumin to a final concentration of 0.1%	Not necessary to add albumin	**Do not use Proleukin at this concentration due to poor stability**	Not necessary to add albumin
Continuous Infusion at *body temperature* [≥ 32° C (89° F)] (e.g., CADD Pump)	Add albumin to a final concentration of 0.1%	Add albumin to a final concentration of 0.1%	**Do not use Proleukin at this concentration due to poor stability**	Not necessary to add albumin

Manufacturer provides a worksheet to guide dilution for continuous IV infusion with a programmed infusion pump. Note Storage.

Storage: Store in refrigerator before and after reconstitution and dilution. Do not freeze. No stability problems will occur at controlled room temperature for 48 hours after dilution but has no preservatives. Do not use beyond expiration date on vial. Stable for up to 6 days in a programmed infusion pump in a concentration of 100 to 500 mcg/ml without the addition of albumin or in a concentration from 1 to 70 mcg/ml with the addition of albumin. Infusion pump has body temperature conditions.

INCOMPATIBLE WITH

Manufacturer states "do not mix with any other drug." Bacteriostatic water for injection or normal saline will increase aggregation.

Y-site: Ganciclovir (Cytovene), lorazepam (Ativan), pentamidine (Pentam 300), prochlorperazine (Compazine), promethazine (Phenergan).

RATE OF ADMINISTRATION

Intermittent IV: A single dose as an intermittent infusion over 15 minutes. Flush main line IV with D5W before and after each use. Manufacturer recommends that any keep-open IV in place for intermittent administration be D5W.

Continuous IV (investigational): A single dose equally distributed over 24 hours. Only compatible with D5W. May be administered through a programmed infusion pump. The Pharmacia Deltec CADD system has been used in clinical studies. Use of a central venous catheter is appropriate. All recommendations under Dilution (e.g., concentration and addition of albumin) are indicated.

ACTIONS

A genetically engineered recombinant protein that possesses the biologic activity of naturally occurring interleukin-2. It boosts immune system function by increasing production of immune system cells (e.g., T lymphocytes), inducing interferon-gamma activity, and enhancing the activity of other lymphokines. Lymphocytes exposed to interleukin-2 become capable of killing cancer cells and are called lymphokine activitated killer (LAK) cells. Clinically significant numbers of lymphokines become available as contrasted to a smaller quantity generated naturally. It can result in an immune response—related destruction of cancer cells and the reduction or elimination of tumor mass. 30% of a dose initally distributes to plasma and then to extravascular, extracellular spaces; 70% of a dose distributes rapidly into the liver, kidney, and lung. Half-life is from 13 to 85 minutes (distribution to elimination). Metabolized to amino acids in proximal convoluted tubules of the kidney. No active drug is found in urine. May cross blood-brain barrier. Not known if it crosses placental barrier or is secreted in breast milk.

INDICATIONS AND USES

Prescreening mandatory. Eligibility requirements for treatment are specific and directly impact response rate and toxicity (asymptomatic preferred; symptomatic and fully ambulatory may be considered). ■ Treatment of metastatic renal cell carcinoma in adults. May be used as a single agent, in combination with interferon-alfa, or in combination with interferon-alfa and 5-fluorouracil. Response rate is about 15% but may last 2 years; may be complete or partial. ■ Treatment of adults with metastatic melanoma. May be used as a single agent, in combination with interferon-alfa, in combination with chemotherapy, or in combination with interferon-alfa and chemotherapy. Several chemotherapy combinations have been used (Dartmouth regimen [carmustine, dacarbazine, cisplatin, and tamoxifen]; CVD regimen [cisplatin, vinblastine, and dacarbazine]). Response rate is about 16%; median duration of complete or partial response was 9 months.

Investigational uses: Kaposi's sarcoma in combination with zidovudine. ▪ Colorectal cancer. ▪ Non-Hodgkin's lymphoma. ▪ Lung cancer. ▪ Ovarian cancer.

CONTRAINDICATIONS

Abnormal thallium stress test or pulmonary function tests. ▪ Known hypersensitivity to interleukin-2 or any component of aldesleukin. ▪ Patients with organ allografts. ▪ Exclude from treatment any patient with significant cardiac, pulmonary, renal, hepatic or CNS impairment, any patient requiring treatment with steroidal agents, and any patient at higher risk for cardiovascular adverse events during periods of hypotension and fluid shifts.

Retreatment is permanently contraindicated in patients who experienced specific toxicities in a previous course of therapy, i.e.,

Organ system	Symptom
Cardiovascular	Sustained ventricular tachycardia ≥5 beats. Cardiac rhythm disturbances not controlled or unresponsive to management. Chest pain with ECG changes consistent with angina or myocardial infarction. Pericardial tamponade.
Pulmonary	Intubation required more than 72 hours.
Renal	Renal dysfunction requiring dialysis over 72 hours.
Central Nervous System	Coma or toxic psychosis lasting more than 48 hours. Repetitive or difficult to control seizures.
Gastrointestinal	Bowel ischemia or perforation. Bleeding requiring surgery.

PRECAUTIONS

Administered in the hospital under the supervision of a qualified physician (usually a medical oncologist and/or immunologist). Intensive care facilities and specialists in cardiopulmonary and/or intensive care medicine must be available. ▪ Capillary leak syndrome (CLS [extravasation of plasma proteins and fluid into the extravascular space and loss of vascular tone]) can begin immediately after aldesleukin treatment starts and results in hypotension and reduced organ perfusion that can be severe enough to result in death. ▪ Therapy should be restricted to patients with normal cardiac, pulmonary, renal (serum creatinine ≤ 1.5 mg/dl), hepatic, and CNS functions as defined by appropriate tests. Patients who have had a nephrectomy are eligible for treatment if serum creatinine is below 1.5 mg/dl (85% of patients in one study). ■ Use extreme caution in patients with normal thallium stress tests and pulmonary function tests who have a history of prior cardiac or pulmonary disease. ■ May exacerbate disease symptoms in clinically unrecognized or untreated CNS metastases. Thoroughly evaluate and treat CNS metastases prior to aldesleukin therapy. Should be neurologically stable and have a negative CT scan. ■ Use extreme caution in patients with a history of seizures (may cause seizures), patients with fixed requirements for large volumes of fluid (e.g., hypercalcemia), those with autoimmune disorders (e.g., Crohn's disease, ulcerative colitis, or psoriasis), previous cytotoxic drug therapy or radiation therapy, and patients sensitive to *Escherichia coli*-derived proteins. ■ May cause auto-immune disease and inflammatory disorders or exacerbate pre-existing conditions (e.g., Crohn's disease, scleroderma, inflammatory arthritis, oculobulbar myasthenia gravis, glomerulonephritis, cholecystitis, cerebral vasculitis, Steven's-Johnson syndrome, bullous pemphigoid). ■ Associated with impaired neutrophil function and an increased risk of disseminated infection, including sepsis and bacterial endocarditis. Preexisting bacterial infections should be adequately treated before beginning therapy. ■ Induces significant hypotension; discontinue antihypertensives during treatment. ■ May impair thyroid function, changes may suggest auto-immunity; thyroid replacement therapy has been required in a few patients. ■ May cause hyperglycemia and/or diabetes mellitus. ■ Note Drug/lab interactions.

Monitor: A central venous catheter (double or triple lumen) is frequently ordered on admission (required for continuous infusion). A minimum of two IV lines is usually required (one for the aldesleukin and its keep-open IV and one for other needed fluids and medications). One line could suffice if absolutely necessary since aldesleukin would be discontinued when colloids are administered. Flushing of line with D5W before and after aldesleukin is imperative. Ability to record CVP and draw blood samples should be available. ■ Admission chest x-ray, ECG, SMA-20, CBC with differential and platelet-count, T_3, T_4, PT, PTT, urinalysis and body weight should be obtained. Adequate pulmonary function, normal arterial blood gases, and normal ejection fraction and unimpaired wall motion (confirmed by thallium stress test and/or a stress echocardiogram) should be documented. ■ Continuous cardiac monitoring is indicated (required with blood pressure below 90 mm Hg or any cardiac irregularity). ■ Monitoring and flexibility in management of fluid and organ perfusion status is imperative. Requires constant management and balancing of effects of fluid shifts to prevent the consequences of hypovolemia (e.g., impaired organ function [such as breakdown of blood-brain barrier]) or fluid accumulation (e.g., edema, pulmonary edema, ascites, pulmonary effusion), which may exceed the patient's tolerance. ■ Assess hypovolemia by central venous catheterization and frequent central venous pressure monitoring. Administer colloids (albumin, plasmanate) or crystalloids (IV fluids) as indicated for a blood pressure drop of 20 mm Hg or greater or a CVP reading lower than 3 to 4 mm H_2O. ■ Neuro checks (note agitation, blurred vision, confusion, depression, irritability, and persistent somnolence). ■ Vital signs, and strict I and O are required every 2 to 4 hours (much more frequently as side effects develop). ▪ Weigh daily. ▪ Blood is drawn twice daily (AM: CBC with differential and platelet count, SMA-20, PT, PTT; PM: SMA-6, electrolytes and creatinine [to check if evening dose can be given; significant changes in creatinine usually do not occur in less than 12 hr]). ▪ Assess thyroid function periodically. ▪ An ECG and cardiac enzymes are indicated for any S/S of chest pain, murmurs, gallops, irregular rhythm or palpitations. A repeat thallium study is indicated for evidence of cardiac ischemia or CHF; may indicate ventricular hypokinesia due to myocarditis. ▪ Obtain a urinalysis as indicated, and draw a magnesium level for any respiratory problems, arrhythmias, or other electrolyte disturbances. ▪ Assess pulmonary function through examination, vital signs, and pulse oximetry. Arterial blood gases are indicated for any dyspnea or respiratory impairment. ▪ Some routine medications are indicated prophylactically to reduce incidence of side effects and to promote patient comfort. The morning of the first treatment begin acetaminophen 650 mg p.o. q 4 hr and indomethacin 25 mg q 6 hr (may increase nephrotoxicity) or naprosyn 500 mg q 12 hr p.o. for fever and arthralgia. Use ranitidine 150 mg p.o. q 12 hr or cimetidine 300 mg q 6 hr to prevent GI bleeding. Continue administration of these drugs until 12 hours after last dose of aldesleukin. Low-dose dopamine 1 to 5 mcg/kg can help maintain organ perfusion and urine output if given at initial onset of CLS before hypotension occurs. Give prophylactic ciprofloxacin 250 mg p.o. q 12 hr for patients with central venous lines (may be given IV [200 mg] or can substitute cefazolin, oxacillin, nafcillin, or vancomycin [must be active against *S. aureus*]; begin when line is placed and continue for 5 days after removal. Antiemetics, antidiarrheals, antichill/rigors (meperidine), antihistamines, and moisturizing skin lotions will also be used throughout treatment (note Antidote for specifics). ▪ If fever occurs several days into treatment or recurs after subsiding, assume infection first, then drug. Confusion, depression, or irritability may also suggest infection. Draw cultures; administer appropriate antibiotics. ▪ Patients who have had nephrectomies may be more at risk for increases in serum BUN or creatinine, electrolyteshifts, and reduced urine output. Evaluate fluid, electrolyte and acid base status promptly if any of the above occur. Gradual increases without other complications (marked fluid overload, hyperkalemia, acidosis) are frequently tolerated (serum creatinine must not exceed 4.5 mg/dl). ▪ Maintain pulmonary status as needed with O_2, diuretics (furosemide) and maintain serum bicarbonate above 15 mEq/L. Assess pulmonary status with chest x-rays. ▪ Monitor central and peripheral IV sites to reduce potential for infection. Change peripheral sites every 3 days. ▪ No restrictions on activity; use caution ambulating (orthostatic hypotension). ▪ No restrictions on diet. Encouragement may be required (anorexia and/or mouth sores). ▪ Specific preparation required for discharge; refer to literature. ▪ Manufacturer supplies excellent brochures with detailed guidelines in chart form on all aspects of monitoring, toxicity, and treatment for nurses and physicians. ▪ Complete review and adequate preparation of all aspects of this therapy with the patient and family are imperative. Can reduce psychological stress of toxicity. ▪ Tumor regression has continued for up to 12 months after one or more courses of therapy. ▪ Note Dose adjustments, Contraindications, and Antidote.

Patient education: Many side effects will occur; report any changes you perceive so they can be evaluated and treated if needed (e.g., changes in breathing, chest or other pain, temperature, mood, lightheadedness, fatigue). ▪ Request assistance for ambulation and always sit on the side of the bed first. ▪ Take only prescribed medications. ▪ Avoid alcohol. ▪ Use of effective contraceptive measures recommended for fertile men and women. ▪ Use 15 SPF sunscreen in sunlight to protect against photosensitivity. ▪ See Appendix D, p. 900, for additional information. ▪ Manufacturer supplies a patient education booklet; review thoroughly and discuss with your physicain and nurse.

Maternal/child: Pregnancy Category C: animal studies not conducted; effects unknown. Benefits must outweight risks. Contraceptive measures required before initial administration and throughout treatment. ▪ Discontinue breast feeding. ▪ Safety for use in children under 18 years of age not established; studies show responsiveness and toxicity similar.

Elderly: May not tolerate toxicity; use caution, consider age-related organ impairment.

DRUG/LAB INTERACTIONS

May cause interactions with psychotropic drugs (e.g, analgesics, antiemetics, narcotics, sedatives, tranquilizers) because aldesleukin also affects central nervous function. ▪ Concomitant use with cardiotoxic agents (e.g., doxorubicin [Adriamycin]), hepatotoxic agents (e.g., methotrexate, asparaginase), myelotoxic agents (e.g., cytotoxic chemotherapy, radiation therapy), and nephrotoxic agents (e.g., aminoglycosides, indomethacin) may increase toxicity in these organ systems and/or delay excretion of these agents increasing their toxicity. ▪ Effects may be potentiated by drugs that also cause blood dyscrasias (e.g., penicillins, phenothiazines). ▪ May cause severe allergic reactions with iodinated contrast media. ▪ Glucocorticoids (e.g., dexamethasone [Decadron]) reduce aldesleukin-induced side effects but also reduce its antitumor effectiveness. ▪ Aldesleukin-induced hypotension may be potentiated by beta-blockers (e.g., metoprolol, atenolol) and antihypertensive agents (e.g., nitroglycerin IV, nitroprusside). ▪ Concurrent use with interferon alfa may increase incidence of MI, myocarditis, ventricular hypokinesia, and severe rhabdomyolysis. ▪ May cause hypersensitivity reactions in patients receiving combination regimens (high-dose aldesleukin and antineoplastics [e.g., dacarbazine, cisplatin, tamoxifen, interferon-alfa]). ▪ Capable of altering numerous lab values, see literature.

SIDE EFFECTS

Frequent, predictable, often severe; are usually clinically manageable and frequently require intensive care management. Begin to occur shortly after therapy begins (chills, fatigue, fever, hypotension, nausea, vomiting). Frequency and severity are dose-related and schedule-dependent. Most are reversible within 2 or 3 days of discontinuation of therapy. Even with intensive management, side effects can progress to death.

Initially anorexia, arthralgia, chills, fatigue, fever, nausea, and vomiting occur. Initial symptoms of capillary leak syndrome are edema, electrolyte abnormalities, hypotension, oliguria, respiratory distress, significant weight gain, tachycardia. Effects of CLS **successively** result in *hypovolemia* which in turn leads to→ hypotension→ hypoperfusion→ sinus tachycardia→ angina → myocardial ischemia and infarction→ arrhythmias (supraventricular and ventricular)→ decreased renal perfusion→ prerenal azotemia→ oliguria→ anuria; *fluid retention/weight gain* which in turn leads to→ rales→ dyspnea→ cough→ tachypnea→ hypoxia→ pleural effusion→ respiratory insufficiency requiring intubation→ diarrhea→ edema of the bowel→ refractory acidosis→ edema→ ascites; *and breakdown of blood-brain barrier* (neuropsychiatric toxicity [e.g., agitation, combativeness, confusion, hallucinations, lethargy, psychosis, somolence]). Abdominal pain and GI bleeding may be related to diarrhea, vomiting, stomatitis, duodenal ulcer formation, bowel ischemia, infarction, or perforation. Cerebral edema and concomitant medications may impact many side effects. Lethargy and/or somnolence may lead to coma. Anemia and thrombocytopenia may occur; coagulation abnormalities (PT, PTT) reflect liver dysfunction. Hemodynamic effects similar to septic shock may be caused by tumor necrosis factor. Erythematous rash and pruritus (can progress to dry desquamation) can occur in almost all patients and are extremely uncomfortable. Note Precautions and Drug/lab interactions.

ANTIDOTE

Temporarily discontinue aldesleukin and notify physician immediately of arrhythmias or rhythm changes, chest pain, marked changes in heart rate, positive neuropsychiatric check (agitation, blurred vision, persistent extreme somnolence), systolic blood pressure below 90 mm Hg, apical heart rate over 120, temperature over 38° C (100.4° F), respirations over 25/min, complaints of dyspnea, decreased breath sounds, or increased sputum production, urinary output less than 200 ml/4 hr, CVP reading below 3 to 4 mm H_2O, weight increase over 4 kg or 10% of baseline over 5 days, abnormal blood or urine tests (e.g., serum bicarbonate < 15 mEq/L, serum creatinine > 4 to 4.5 mg/dl [based on gradual or sudden rise and if accompanied by other complications]), severe diarrhea associated with refractory acidosis, vomiting refractory to treatment, acute changes in GI status. May be restarted based on patient response. Hold any subsequent dose for failure to maintain organ perfusion (see Dose adjustments). Fever is routinely treated with acetaminophen and indomethacin or naprosyn; increased doses may be needed; administer rectally if nausea and vomiting are present. Suggested treatments include slow IV meperidine (Demerol) 25 to 50 mg for chills and rigidity; diphenoxylate (Lomotil) or loperamide (Imodium) p.o. for diarrhea (these meds may not help and diarrhea may be dose limiting); diphenhydramine (Benadryl) 25 mg p.o. q 6 hr, a soothing skin cream (Eucerin), and oatmeal baths for urticaria and pruritus; temazepam (Restoril) for insomnia; ondansetron (Zofran) or prochlorperazine (Compazine) for nausea. Treat edema with furosemide (Lasix). IV fluids, albumin or plasmanate, and Trendelenburg positioning are used to maintain fluid balance and blood pressure. If organ perfusion and blood pressure are not sustained by dopamine 2 to 5 mcg/kg as a continuous infusion, increase to 6 to 10 mcg/kg or add phenylephrine (1 to 5 mcg/kg/

min). Prolonged use of pressors at relatively high doses may cause cardiac arrhythmias. Treat arrhythmias as indicated (usually sinus or supraventricular tachycardia [adenosine, verapamil]). Use O_2 for decreased PaO_2. Use packed red blood cells for anemia and to ensure maximum oxygen carrying capacity. Platelet transfusions are indicated for thrombocytopenia or to reduce risk of GI bleeding. Special precautions may be required (e.g., avoid IM injections; test urine, emesis, stool, secretions for occult blood). All treatment is supportive; recovery should begin within a few hours of cessation of aldesleukin. With normalized blood pressure, diuretics (furosemide [Lasix]) can hasten recovery. Low-dose haloperidol (Haldol) may help severe mental status changes.

More rapid onset of dose-limiting toxicities will occur with overdose. **Dexamethasone (Decadron)** is indicated to counteract life-threatening toxicities. May result in loss of therapeutic effect.

LEPIRUDIN
Refludan

Anticoagulant

pH 7.0

USUAL DOSE

A baseline aPTT should be determined before initiation of therapy with lepirudin. To avoid a potential overdose, therapy should not be started in patients with a baseline aPTT ratio (patient aPTT at a given time over an aPTT reference value, usually median of the laboratory normal range for aPTT) of 2.5 or more.

Anticoagulation in adult patients with heparin-induced thrombocytopenia (HIT) and associated thromboembolic disease. Bolus dose: 0.4 mg/kg body weight (up to 110 kg).

Standard bolus injection volumes according to body weight for a 5 mg/mL concentration

Body Weight [kg]	Injection Volume	
	Dosage 0.4 mg/kg	Dosage 0.2 mg/kg*
50	4 mL	2 mL
60	4.8 mL	2.4 mL
70	5.6 mL	2.8 mL
80	6.4 mL	3.2 mL
90	7.2 mL	3.6 mL
100	8 mL	4 mL
≥110	8.8 mL	4.4 mL

*Dosage recommended for all patients with renal insufficiency.

Maintenance infusion: 0.15 mg/kg body weight (up to 110 kg)/hr for 2 to 10 days or longer as clinically indicated. Adjust rate to maintain an aPTT ratio of 1.5 to 2.5. See Dose adjustments and Precautions/ Monitor.

DOSE ADJUSTMENTS

Normally the initial dose depends on body weight. This is valid up to a body weight of 110 kg. In patients weighing more than 110 kg, the initial dose should not be increased beyond the 110 kg body weight dose (i.e., the initial bolus dose should not exceed 44 mg and the initial infusion rate should not exceed 16.5 mg/hr). ■ Any aPTT ratio outside of the target range (aPTT 1.5 to 2.5) should be confirmed before any dose adjustment if possible. If the confirmed aPTT ratio is above the target range, the infusion should be stopped for 2 hours and then restarted at half the previous infusion rate. If the confirmed aPTT ratio is below the target range, the infusion rate should be increased in 20% increments. ■ Dose reduction is required in patients with renal impairment as measured by a CrCl of < 60 ml/min or a serum creatinine >1.5 mg/dl. Reduce bolus dose to 0.2 mg/kg body weight. Adjust infusion rate as indicated in chart.

Reduction of infusion ratio in patients with renal impairment

Creatinine clearance [mL/min]	Serum creatinine [mg/DL]	Adjusted infusion rate	
		[% of standard initial infusion rate]	[mg/kg/h]
45–60	1.6–2	50%	0.075
30–44	2.1–3	30%	0.045
15–29	3.1–6	15%	0.0225
below 15*	above 6*	avoid or STOP infusion*	

*In hemodialysis patients or in case of acute renal failure (creatinine clearance below 15 mL/min or serum creatinine above 6 mg/dL). Infusion of lepirudin is to be avoided or stopped. Additional intravenous bolus doses of 0.1 mg/kg body weight should be considered every other day only if the aPTT ratio falls below the lower therapeutic limit of 1.5

■ There is limited data regarding concomitant use of lepirudin with thrombolytic therapy (e.g., alteplase [tPA, Activase], streptokinase [Streptase], urokinase [Abbokinase]). A dose reduction of 0.2 mg/kg body weight for the bolus dose and 0.1 mg/kg body weight/hr for the continuous infusion has been recommended. ■ In patients scheduled to receive a coumarin derivative for oral anticoagulation after lepirudin therapy, the rate should be decreased gradually until an aPTT ratio just above 1.5 is reached. Initiate oral anticoagulant therapy at this point. Discontinue lepirudin when an INR of 2 is reached. ■ Clearance of lepirudin is lower in women and in the elderly. Dose adjustments may be necessary.

DILUTION

Warm preparation to room temperature before administration.

Bolus: Reconstitute 50 mg vial with 1 ml of SW or NS and shake gently. Transfer the contents of the vial to a sterile syringe and further dilute with NS, SW, or D5W to a total volume of 10 ml. This provides a final concentration of 5 mg/ml which is suitable for bolus injection. Calculate volume of dilution to be administered. See Usual dose. Discard any unused solution.

Infusion: Reconstitute 2 vials with 1 ml each of SW or NS. Add the contents of both vials (100 mg) to 250 ml or 500 ml of NS or D5W to obtain a final concentration of 0.4 mg/ml or 0.2 mg/ml, respectively.

Storage: Store unopened vials at 2° to 25° C (36° to 77° F). Once reconstituted, lepirudin should be used immediately. Stable for 24 hours at room temperature (e.g., during infusion).

INCOMPATIBLE WITH

Data not available. Manufacturer states should not be mixed with other drugs except for SW, NS, or D5W.

RATE OF ADMINISTRATION

Bolus: A single dose over 15 to 20 seconds.

Infusion: Administer at the determined rate according to body weight. See Usual dose and Dose adjustments. An infusion rate of 0.21 mg/kg/hr should not be exceeded without checking for coagulation abnormalities, which might prevent an appropriate aPTT response.

Standard infusion rates according to body weight

Body Weight [kg]	Infusion rate at 0.15 mg/kg/h	
	500-mL infusion bag 0.2 mg/mL	250-mL infusion bag 0.4 mg/mL
50	38 mL/h	19 mL/h
60	45 mL/h	23 mL/h
70	53 mL/h	26 mL/h
80	60 mL/h	30 mL/h
90	68 mL/h	34 mL/h
100	75 mL/h	38 mL/h
≥110	83 mL/h	41 mL/h

ACTIONS

An anticoagulant that is a highly specific direct inhibitor of thrombin. A recombinant hirudin that is derived from yeast cells. One molecule of lepirudin binds to one molecule of thrombin, thereby blocking the thrombogenic activity of thrombin. Inhibits both free and clot-bound thrombin without requiring endogenous cofactors (i.e., mode of action is independent of antithrombin III and heparin cofactor II and is not inhibited by platelet factor 4.) Distribution is restricted primarily to the extracellular space. Excreted almost exclusively by the kidneys. Terminal half-life approximately 1.3 hours.

INDICATIONS AND USES

Anticoagulation in patients with heparin-induced thrombocytopenia (HIT) and associated thromboembolic disease to prevent further thromboembolic complications.

CONTRAINDICATIONS

Known hypersensitivity to hirudins.

PRECAUTIONS

Concomitant therapy with thrombolytic agents (e.g., alteplase [tPA, Activase], streptokinase [Streptase], urokinase [Abbokinase]) may increase the risk of bleeding, including life-threatening intracranial bleeding. Note Dose adjustments and Drug/lab interactions. ▪ Use with extreme caution and weigh risk versus benefit in all patients with an increased risk of bleeding. Conditions of conern include: recent significant surgery, anomaly of vessels or organs, bacterial endocarditis, severe uncontrolled hypertension, advanced renal impairment, hemorrhagic diathesis, recent puncture of large vessels, recent CVA, stroke, intracerebral surgery or other neuraxial procedures, recent organ biopsy, and recent major bleeding (e.g., intracranial, gastrointestinal, intraocular, or pulmonary bleeding). ▪ Hepatic impairment may enhance the antiocoagulant effect of lepirudin due to coagulation defects secondary to reduced generation of vitamin k-dependent coagulation factors. ▪ There is limited data regarding reexposure to lepirudin. A case of mild allergic skin reaction upon reexposure has been reported. ▪ Antihirudin antibody formation has been reported in about 40% of patients receiving lepirudin. This may increase the drug's anticoagulant effect. To date, there is no evidence that antibody formation may lead to an allergic reaction or to neutralization of lepirudin.

Monitor: Monitor renal function. CrCl is preferred method of monitoring. May use serum creatinine if CrCl is not available. Note Dose adjustments. ▪ Determine a baseline aPTT ratio. Infusion rate should be adjusted according to the aPTT ratio. Note Dose adjustments. An aPTT ratio should be determined 4 hours after the start of the infusion and 4 hours after any change in infusion rate. Follow-up aPTT ratios should be determined at least once daily. More frequent monitoring is recommended in patients with renal or hepatic impairment. ▪ Obtain baseline and monitor platelet count, hemoglobin, hematocrit, and occult blood in stool. ▪ Strict monitoring of aPTT indicated in prolonged therapy to monitor for antihirudin antibodies.

Patient education: Report all episodes of bleeding. ▪ Report tarry stools. ▪ Compliance with all measures to minimize bleeding is very important (e.g., avoid use of razors, toothbrushes, other sharp items). ▪ Use caution while moving to avoid excess bumping.

Maternal/child: Pregnancy category B: safety for use in pregnancy not established. Benefits must overweigh risks. ▪ In lactating women, the decision should be made to discontinue breast feeding or to discontinue the drug, taking into account the importance of the drug to the mother. ▪ Safety and efficacy have not been established for children. Was used during trials in two older children without adverse events.

Elderly: Clearance is reduced in the elderly, possibly due to age-related renal impairment. Note Dose adjustments.

DRUG/LAB INTERACTIONS

Concomitant treatment with thrombolytics (e.g., alteplase [tPA, Activase], reteplase [Retavase], streptokinase [Streptase], uronkinase [Abbokinase]) may increase the risk of bleeding complications and enhance the effect of lepirudin on aPTT prolongation. Note Dose adjustments. ▪ Concomitant treatment with coumarin derivatives (warfarin [Coumadin]) and drugs that affect platelet function (e.g., dipyridamole [Persantine], NSAIDs (e.g., ibuprofen [Motrin], naproxen [Naprosyn]) may also increase the risk of bleeding. ▪ Other thrombin-dependent coagulation assays will be changed by lepirudin.

SIDE EFFECTS
Bleeding is the most frequent adverse event.

Abnormal kidney or liver function, allergic reactions, fever, heart failure, infection, multiorgan failure, pericardial effusion, pneumonia, ventricular fibrillation.

ANTIDOTE
No specific antidote is available. If life-threatening bleeding develops and excessive plasma levels of lepirudin are suspected, immediately stop lepirudin infusion. Determine aPTT and hemoglobin and prepare for blood transfusion as appropriate. Follow current guidelines for treatment of shock as indicated [fluid, vasopressors (e.g., dopamine), Trendelenberg position, plasma expanders (e.g., albumin, hetastarch)]. Hemodialysis or hemofiltration may be useful in an overdose situation; see product insert for specifics.

TIROFIBAN HYDROCHLORIDE   Platelet aggregation inhibitor
Aggrastat   pH 5.5 to 6.5

USUAL DOSE
A *loading infusion* of 0.4 mcg/kg/min for 30 minutes followed by a *maintenance infusion* of 0.1 mcg/kg/min. Unless contraindicated, give in conjunction with aspirin (325 mg/day) and heparin. Administer a heparin bolus of 5,000 units followed by an infusion titrated to maintain an aPTT of 2 times control. Heparin and tirofiban may be administered through the same intravenous catheter. Duration of therapy will vary, depending on patient condition and procedures performed. In one major study, infusion was continued for 48 to 108 hours. The infusion should be continued through angiography and for 12 to 24 hours after angioplasty or artherectomy.

DOSE ADJUSTMENTS
Patients with severe renal insufficiency (CrCl < 30 ml/min) should receive half the usual rate of infusion. Note Rate of administration.
- Differences in plasma clearance based on age, race, gender, or mild to moderate hepatic insufficiency do not require dose adjustment.

DILUTION
Available premixed in a plastic container as an iso-osmotic solution containing 50 mcg/ml. Remove overwrap. Plastic may be somewhat opaque due to sterilization process. Opacity should diminish. Squeeze inner container to check for leak. Discard if leakage noted; sterility is impaired. Also available in vials containing 12.5 mg/50 ml. Vials must be diluted to same concentration as premixed solution before administration. Withdraw 100 ml from a 500 ml bag of NS or D5W and replace this volume with 100 ml of tirofiban (two 50 ml vials) or withdraw 50 ml from a 250 ml bag of NS or D5W and replace this volume with 50 ml tirofiban (one 50 ml vial). Mix well. Concentration of either solution is 50 mcg/ml. Do not use plastic connectors in a series connection.

Storage: Store unopened vials or premixed containers at 25° C (77° F).

Variations from 15° to 30° C (59° to 86° F) are acceptable for short periods. Protect from light during storage. Do not freeze. Discard unused solution 24 hours following the start of the infusion.

INCOMPATIBLE WITH

Data not available. Manufacturer states should not be mixed with other drugs except for NS or D5W. May be given through the same intravenous catheter as heparin.

RATE OF ADMINISTRATION

Loading infusion: 0.4 mcg/kg/min for 30 minutes.

Maintenance infusion: 0.1 mcg/kg/min.

Patient Weight [kg]	Most Patients		Severe Renal Impairment	
	30 Min Loading Infusion Rate (mL/hr)	Maintenance Infusion Rate (mL/hr)	30 Min Loading Infusion Rate (mL/hr)	Maintenance Infusion Rate (mL/hr)
30-37	16	4	8	2
38-45	20	5	10	3
46-54	24	6	12	3
55-62	28	7	14	4
63-70	32	8	16	4
71-79	36	9	18	5
80-87	40	10	20	5
88-95	44	11	22	6
96-104	48	12	24	6
105-112	52	13	26	7
113-120	56	14	28	7
121-128	60	15	30	8
129-137	64	16	32	8
138-145	68	17	34	9
146-153	72	18	36	9

ACTIONS

A non-peptide antagonist of the platelet glycoprotein (GP) IIb/IIIa receptor. It inhibits platelet aggregation by preventing the binding of fibrinogen to the receptor site on activated platelets. Inhibits platelet aggregation in a dose- and concentration-dependent manner. When given according to the recommended regimen, greater than 90% inhibition is attained by the end of the 30-minute infusion. Bleeding time is prolonged. Inhibition is reversible, with aggregation returning to baseline in > 90% of patients within 4 to 8 hours following cessation of the infusion. Has been shown to decrease the rate of a combined endpoint of death, new myocardial infarction, or refractory ischemia/repeat cardiac procedure (see literature). Half-life is approximately 2 hours. Cleared from the plasma primarily by renal excretion, with about 65% of the unchanged drug appearing in the urine and about 25% appearing in feces. Metabolism is limited.

INDICATIONS AND USES

Used in combination with heparin and aspirin for treatment of acute coronary syndrome (characterized by prolonged [> 10 minutes] or repetitive symptoms of cardiac ischemia occurring at rest or with minimal exertion, associated with either ischemic ST-T wave changes on electrocardiogram [ECG] or elevated cardiac enzymes. Includes "unstable angina" and "non-Q-wave myocardial infarction" but excludes myocardial infarction that is associated with Q-waves or non-transient ST-segment elevation). May be used in patients who are being medically managed and in those undergoing percutaneous transluminal coronary angioplasty (PTCA) or artherectomy.

CONTRAINDICATIONS

Known hypersensitivity to any component of the product, active internal bleeding or history of bleeding diathesis within the previous 30 days, a history of intracranial hemorrhage, intracranial neoplasm, arteriovenous malformation, or aneurysm, a history of thrombocytopenia following prior exposure to tirofiban, a history of stroke within 30 days or any history of hemorrhagic stroke, major surgical procedure or severe physical trauma within the previous month, history, symptoms or findings suggestive of aortic dissection, severe hypertension (systolic blood perssure > 180 mm Hg and/or diastolic blood pressure > 110 mm Hg), concomitant use of another parenteral GP IIb/IIIa inhibitor (e.g., abciximab [ReoPro]), acute pericarditis.

PRECAUTIONS

Use with caution in patients with platelet count < $150,000/mm^3$ and in patients with hemorrhagic retinopathy. ■ Use caution when given with drugs that affect hemostasis (e.g., warfarin [Coumadin]). Safety when used in combination with thrombolytic agents (e.g., alteplase [tPA, Activase], reteplase [Retavase], urokinase [Abbokinase], streptokinase [Streptase]) has not been established. Note Drug/lab interactions. ■ Use with caution in patients with renal insufficiency. Note Dose adjustments. ■ Bleeding is the most common complication encountered during therapy. Incidence may be slightly higher in females and the elderly. ■ Most major bleeding occurs at the arterial access site for cardiac catheterization. Care should be taken when attempting vascular access that only the anterior wall of the femoral artery is punctured.

Monitor: Obtain platelet count, hemoglobin, and hematocrit before therapy, within 6 hours following the loading infusion, and at least daily thereafter. More frequent monitoring may be indicated. ■ If platelet count drops to < $90,000/mm^3$, additional platelet counts should be performed to exclude pseudothrombocytopenia. If thrombocytopenia is confirmed, heparin and tirofiban should be discontinued and appropriate therapy initiated. ■ Obtain an aPTT 6 hours after the start of the heparin infusion. Adjust heparin infusion rate to maintain an aPTT 2 times control. ■ Patients receiving percutaneous coronary intervention who have a sheath in place should be maintained on complete bed rest with the head of the bed elevated 30 degrees and the affected limb restrained in a straight position. Monitor sheath insertion site(s) and distal pulses of affected leg(s) frequently while sheath is in place and for 6 hours after removal. Measure any hematoma and monitor for enlargement. ▪ Monitor the patient for signs of bleeding; take vital signs (avoiding automatic BP cuffs), observe any invaded sites at least every 15 minutes (e.g., sheaths, IV sites, cutdowns, punctures, foleys, NGs); watch for hematuria, hematemesis, bloody stool, pete-chiae, hematoma, flank pain, muscle weakness. Perform neuro checks frequently. If during thereapy bleeding cannot be controlled with pressure, tirofiban and heparin infusions should be discontinued. ▪ Use care in handling patient; minimize use of urinary catheters, nasotracheal intubation, and nasogastric tubes. Avoid arterial puncture, venipuncture, and IM injection. Use extreme precautionary methods and only compressible sites if these procedures are absolutely necessary (i.e., avoid subclavian or jugular veins). Apply pressure for 30 minutes to any invaded site and then apply pressure dressings. Saline or heparin locks suggested to facilitate blood draws. ▪ In patients receiving percutaneous coronary intervention, heparin should be discontinued 3 to 4 hours before pulling the sheath and an activated clotting time (ACT) < 180 seconds or an aPTT < 45 seconds should be documented. ▪ Care should be taken to obtain proper hemostatsis after removal of the sheath using standard compressive techniques followed by close observation. Sheath hemostatsis should be achieved at least 4 hours before hospital discharge.

Patient education: Compliance with all measures to minimize bleeding (e.g., strict bed rest, positioning) is imperative. ▪ Avoid use of razors, toothbrushes, and other sharp items. ▪ Use caution while moving to avoid excessive bumping. ▪ Report all episodes of bleeding and apply local pressure if indicated. ▪ Expect oozing from IV sites.

Maternal/child: Pregnancy category B: safety for use in pregnancy not established. Benefits must outweigh risks. ▪ In lactating women, the decision should be made to discontinue breast feeding or to discontinue the drug, taking into account the importance of the drug to the mother. ▪ Safety and efficacy have not been established for children.

Elderly: Clearance is reduced in the elderly, possibly due to age-related renal impairment. Dose adjustment is not necessary. Incidence of bleeding complications and other side effects increase somethwat but are similar to use of heparin as a single agent.

DRUG/LAB INTERACTIONS

All studies with tirofiban included the use of aspirin and heparin. Concomitant use, although indicated, increases the risk of bleeding. ▪ Use caution when given with drugs that affect hemostasis (e.g., thrombolytics [e.g., alteplase (tPA, Activase), reteplase (Retavase), urokinase (Abbokinase), streptokinase (Streptase)], oral anticoagulants [e.g., warfarin (Coumadin)], NSAIDs [e.g., ibuprofen (Motrin)], dipyr-idamole [Persantine], ticlopidine [Ticlid], selected antibiotics [e.g., cefamandole (Mandol), cefoperazone (Cefobid)]). ▪ Patients receiving omeprazole (Prilosec) or levothyroxine (Synthroid) concurrently with tirofiban had a higher clearance of tirofiban. Clinical significance of this observation is not known. ▪ The following drugs were co-administered with tirofiban in clinical trials: acebutolol (Monitan), acetaminophen (Tylenol), alprazolam (Xanax), amlodipine, aspirin, atenolol (Tenormin), bromazepam, captopril (Capoten), diazepam (Valium), digoxin, diltiazem (Cardizem), docusate sodium, enalapril (Vasotec), furosemide (Lasix), glyburide, heparin, insulin, isosorbide, lorazepam (Ativan), lovastatin (Mevacor), metoclopramide (Reglan), metoprolol (Lopressor), morphine, nifedipine (Procardia), nitrate preparations (e.g., nitroglycerin), oxazepam (Serax), potassium chloride, propranolol (Inderal), ranitidine (Zantac), simvastatin (Zocor), sucralfate (Sulcrate), and temazepam (Restoril). Plasma clearance of tirofiban was not affected by co-administration.

SIDE EFFECTS

Bleeding is the most frequent adverse event and is usually reported as mild or oozing. Laboratory findings related to bleeding include decrease in hemoglobin, hematocrit and platelet count and occult blood in urine and feces. Other side effects that occur at an incidence of > 1%, regardless of drug relationship, are bradycardia, dissection of the coronary artery, dizziness, edema, fever, headache, leg pain, nausea, pelvic pain, and sweating.

ANTIDOTE

Keep physician informed of laboratory values and side effects. Discontinue the infusion of tirofiban and heparin if any serious bleeding not controllable with pressure occurs. If platelet count drops to below 90,000 mm^3, obtain additional platelet counts to exclude pseudo-thrombocytopenia. If thrombocytopenia is confirmed, discontinue tirofiban and heparin. Platelet transfusion may be required. If a hypersensitivity reaction should occur, discontinue the infusion and treat as indicated by severity (e.g., epinephrine, dopamine (Inotropin), theophylline, antihistamines (e.g., diphenhydramine [Benedryl]), and/or corticosteroids as necessary).

No specific antidote is available. Overdosage should be treated by assessment of the patient's clinical condition and cessation or adjutment of the drug infusion as appropriate. Hemodialysis may be useful in an overdose situation.

Index

Bold type indicates generic drug name.
Italic type indicates drug categories and
listings.

927

NOTES

NOTES

NOTES

NOTES

NOTES

NOTES

NOTES

NOTES

Solution Compatibility Chart

Intravenous medication	D2½	D5	D10	D5 0.2 S	D5 0.45 S	D5 NS	NS	½NS	R	LR	D5R	D5LR
Acetazolamide	C	C	C	C	C	C	C	C	C	C	C	C
Acyclovir		C		C	C	C	C			C		C
Amikacin sulfate		C	C	C	C	C	C	C		C	C	C
Ascorbic acid	C	C	C	C	C	C	C	C	C	C	C	C
Aztreonam		C	C	C	C	C	C		C	C	C	C
Bethamethasone Na phosphate		C					C			C	C	C
Cefamandole nafate		C		C	C	C	C					C
Cefazolin Na		C	C	C	C	C	C		C	C		C
Cefonicid		C	C	C	C	C	C		C	C		C
Cefoperazone Na		C	C	C		C	C			C		C
Cefotaxime Na		C	C	C	C	C	C			C		
Cefoxitin Na		C	C	C	C	C	C		C	C		C
Ceftazidime		C	C	C	C	C	C		C	C		
Ceftizoxime Na		C	C				C		C	C		
Ceftriaxone Na		C	C	C	C	C	C			C		
Cefuroxime Na		C	C	C	C	C	C		C	C		
Cephalothin Na		C	C			C	C		C	C		C
Cephapirin Na		C	C	C	C	C	C		C	C	C	C
Chlorothiazide Na	C	C	C	C	C	C	C	C	C	C	C	C
Cimetidine		C	C	C	C	C	C		C	C		C
Cisplatin				C	C	C	C	C				
Clindamycin phosphate		C	C		C	C	C			C	C	
Cyclophosphamide		C				C	C	C		C	C	
Deferoxamine mesylate		C					C			C		
Dexmethasone Na phosphate		C	C	C	C	C	C			C	C	C
Dobutamine Hcl		C	C		C	C	C	C		C		C
Dopamine Hcl		C	C		C	C	C			C		C
Doxycycline hyclate		C					C		C	C		C
Edrophonium Cl		C					C			C	C	C
Enalaprilat		C				C	C					C
Famotidine		C	C				C			C		
Fentanyl citrate		C				C	C			C	C	C
Furosemide		C	C			C	C			C		C
Heparin Na	C	C		C	C	C		C	C		C	C
Hydrocortisone Na succinate		C				C	C	C				
Hydromorphone Hcl		C			C	C	C	C	C	C	C	C
Ifosfamide	C	C				C	C	C		C	C	
Imipenen-cilastin		C[4]	C[4]	C[4]	C[4]	C[4]	C[10]					
Insulin injection (regular)		C[P]	C		C		C[P]	C[P]	C	C	C	C
Kanamycin sulfate		C	C			C	C			C		
Leucovorin calcium		C	C				C		C	C		
Lidocaine Hcl		C[P]			C	C	C	C		C	C	
Meperidine Hcl	C	C	C	C	C	C	C	C	C	C	C	C
Metaraminol bitartrate		C	C			C	C		C[C]	C		C
Methicillin Na		C	C			C	C			C		C